ANTIBIOTIC ESSENTIALS

Ninth Edition

Edited by

Burke A. Cunha, MD, MACP

Chief, Infectious Disease Division
Winthrop-University Hospital
Mineola, New York
Professor of Medicine
State University of New York
School of Medicine
Stony Brook, New York

2010

PHYSICIANS' PRESS
A DIVISION OF JONES AND BARTLETT PUBLISHERS
Sudbury, Massachusetts
BOSTON TORONTO LONDON SINGAPORE

World Headquarters
Jones and Bartlett Publishers
40 Tall Pine Drive
Sudbury, MA 01776
978-443-5000
info@jbpub.com
www.jbpub.com

Jones and Bartlett Publishers Canada
6339 Ormindale Way
Mississauga, ON L5V 1J2
Canada

Jones and Bartlett Publishers International
Barb House, Barb Mews
London W6 7PA
United Kingdom

Jones and Bartlett's books and products are available through most bookstores and online booksellers. To contact Jones and Bartlett Publishers directly, call 800-832-0034, fax 978-443-8000, or visit our website at www.jbpub.com.

Substantial discounts on bulk quantities of Jones and Bartlett's publications are available to corporations, professional associations, and other qualified organizations. For details and specific discount information, contact the special sales department at Jones and Bartlett via the above contact information or send an email to specialsales@jbpub.com.

Production Credit
Senior Acquisitions Editor: Alison Hankey
Editorial Assistant: Sara Cameron
Production Editor: Daniel Stone
Composition: diacriTech, Chennai, India
Cover Design: Kristin E. Parker
Printing and Binding: Cenveo
Cover Printing: Cenveo

ISBN-13: 978-0-7637-9214-5

6048

Printed in the United States of America
14 13 12 11 10   10 9 8 7 6 5 4 3 2 1

ABOUT THE EDITOR

Burke A. Cunha, MD, is Chief, Infectious Disease Division at Winthrop-University Hospital, Mineola, New York; Professor of Medicine, State University of New York School of Medicine, Stony Brook, New York; and one of the world's leading authorities on the treatment of infectious diseases. During his 30-year career, he has written/edited more than 1150 articles, 185 book chapters, and 25 books on infectious diseases. He has received numerous teaching awards, including the prestigious Aesculapius Award for outstanding teaching. He also serves on the editorial boards of more than two dozen infectious disease journals, and is Infectious Disease Editor-in-Chief for eMedicine online. Dr. Cunha is a Fellow of the Infectious Disease Society of America, American Academy of Microbiology, American College of Clinical Pharmacology, Surgical Infection Society, and American College of Chest Physicians. He has had a lifelong interest in antimicrobial therapy, antibiotic resistance, pneumonias, surgical infections, infections in compromised hosts, zoonoses, FUOs, meningitis, endocarditis, nosocomial infections, and tropical medicine. Dr. Cunha is a Master of the American College of Physicians, awarded for achievement as a master clinician and teacher.

DEDICATION

for
Marie

"Grace in her steps,
Heaven in her eye,
In every gesture, dignity and love"

Milton

TABLE OF CONTENTS

CONTRIBUTORS

Burke A. Cunha, MD, MACP
Chief, Infectious Disease Division
Winthrop-University Hospital
Mineola, New York
Professor of Medicine
State University of New York
School of Medicine
Stony Brook, New York
All chapters except HIV Infection & Pediatric ID

Edward J. Bottone, PhD
Professor of Medicine
Professor of Microbiology
Professor of Pathology
Mount Sinai
School of Medicine
New York, New York
Medical Microbiology; Parasites, Fungi, Unusual Organisms

John L. Brusch, MD
Associate Chief of Medicine, Cambridge Health Alliance
Infectious Disease Service, Cambridge Health Alliance
Medical Director, Somerville Hospital
Assistant Professor of Medicine
Harvard Medical School
Boston, Massachusetts
Endocarditis: Therapy & Prophylaxis

Daniel Caplivski, MD
Assistant Professor of Medicine
Infectious Disease Division
Mt. Sinai School of Medicine
New York, New York
Fungal Stain Atlas

Dennis J. Cleri, MD
St. Francis Medical Center
Professor of Medicine
Seton Hall University
School of Graduate Medical Education
Trenton, New Jersey
Bioterrorism

Cheston B. Cunha, MD
Department of Medicine
Brown University School of Medicine
Rhode Island Hospital and The Miriam Hospital
Providence, Rhode Island
Infectious Disease Differential Diagnosis

Pierce Gardner, MD
John E. Fogarty International Center for Advanced Study in the Health Sciences
Senior Advisor, Clinical Research and Training
National Institutes of Health
Bethesda, Maryland
Prophylaxis and Immunization

Mark H. Kaplan, MD
Professor of Medicine
Infectious Diseases
University of Michigan School of Medicine
Ann Arbor, Michigan
HIV Drug Summaries

Douglas S. Katz, MD
Vice Chair for Clinical Research and Education
Director, Body CT
Winthrop-University Hospital
Mineola, New York
Professor of Clinical Radiology
State University of New York School of Medicine
Stony Brook, New York
Chest X-ray Atlas

Raymond Koff, MD
Clinical Professor of Medicine
University of Connecticut School of Medicine
Farmington, Connecticut
Viral Hepatitis: Therapy & Prophylaxis

Leonard R. Krilov, MD
Chief, Pediatric Infectious Disease Division
Winthrop-University Hospital
Mineola, New York
Professor of Pediatrics
State University of New York
School of Medicine
Stony Brook, New York
Pediatric Infectious Diseases

David W. Kubiak, PharmD
Infectious Disease Clinical Pharmacist
Brigham and Women's Hospital
Boston, Massachusetts
Antiretroviral Drug Summaries

George H. McCracken, Jr., MD
Distinguished Professor of Pediatric Infectious Disease and the Sarah M. and Charles E. Seay Chair in Pediatric Infectious Disease
University of Texas Southwestern Medical Center
Dallas, Texas
Pediatric Infectious Diseases

James H. McGuire, MD
Master Clinician,
Division of Infectious Diseases
Brigham and Women's Hospital
Professor of Medicine
Harvard Medical School
Boston, Massachusetts
Parasites, Fungi, Unusual Organisms

Nardeen Mickail, MD
Infectious Disease Division
Winthrop-University Hospital
Mineola, New York
and State University of New York
School of Medicine
Stony Brook, New York
Antimicrobial Drug Summaries

Robert Moore, MD
Chairman, Department of Radiology
Stony Brook University Hospital
Professor of Radiology
State University of New York School of Medicine
Stony Brook, New York
Chest X-ray Atlas

Ronald L. Nichols, MD
William Henderson Professor of Surgery
Professor of Microbiology and Immunology
Tulane University School of Medicine
New Orleans, Louisiana
Surgical Antimicrobial Prophylaxis and Therapy

Genovefa Papanicolaou, MD
Attending Physician
Memorial Sloan Kettering
Cancer Center
Infectious Disease Service
Associate Professor of Medicine
Weill Cornell Medical College
New York, New York
Transplant Infections

Michael F. Rein, MD
Professor Emeritus of Medicine
University of Virginia Health System
Charlottesville, Virginia
Sexually Transmitted Diseases

John H. Rex, MD
Adjunct Professor of Medicine, University of Texas Medical School, Houston, Texas
Vice-President and Medical Director for Infection
AstraZeneca Pharmaceuticals, Macclesfield, UK
Antifungal Therapy

Paul E. Sax, MD
Clinical Director, Division of Infectious Diseases and HIV Program
Division of Infectious Diseases
Brigham and Women's Hospital
Associate Professor of Medicine
Harvard Medical School
Boston, Massachusetts
HIV Infection

David Schlossberg, MD
Tuberculosis Control Program
Philadelphia Department of Health
Professor of Medicine
Temple University School of Medicine
Philadelphia, Pennsylvania
Tuberculosis

Paul E. Schoch, PhD
Director, Clinical Microbiology Laboratory
Winthrop-University Hospital
Mineola, New York
Medical Microbiology and Gram Stains Atlas

Daniel S. Siegal, MD
Department of Radiology
Mount Auburn Hospital
Harvard Medical School
Boston, Massachusetts
Chest X-ray Atlas

Stephanie Strollo, MD
Infectious Disease Division
Winthrop-University Hospital
Mineola, New York
and State University of New York School of Medicine

Stony Brook, New York
Initial Therapy of Isolates Pending Susceptibility Testing

Uzma Syed, MD
Infectious Disease Division
Winthrop-University Hospital
Mineola, New York
and State University of New York School of Medicine
Stony Brook, New York
Initial Therapy of Isolates Pending Susceptibility Testing

Damary C. Torres, PharmD
Clinical Pharmacy Specialist
Winthrop-University Hospital
Mineola, New York
Associate Clinical Professor of Pharmacy
College of Pharmacy, St. John's University
Queens, New York
Antimicrobial Drug Summaries

Kenneth F. Wagner, DO
Attending Physician, Infectious Disease
Consultant, National Naval Medical Center
Associate Professor of Medicine, Uniformed Services, University of the Health Sciences
F. Edward Hebert School of Medicine
Bethesda, Maryland
Parasites, Fungi, Unusual Organisms

ACKNOWLEDGMENTS

To accomplish the task of presenting the data compiled in this reference, a small, dedicated team of professionals was assembled. This team focused their energy and discipline for many months into typing, revising, designing, illustrating, and formatting the many chapters that make up this text. I wish to acknowledge Monica Crowder Kaufman, Lisa Lusardi, and Rebecca Smith for their important contribution. I would also like to thank the many contributors who graciously contributed their time and energy; and Mark Freed, MD, past President and Editor-in-Chief of Physicians' Press, for his vision, commitment, and guidance.

Burke A. Cunha, MD

NOTICE

Antibiotics Essentials has been developed as a concise, practical, and authoritative guide for the treatment of infectious diseases. Aside from Chapter 7, Pediatric Infectious Diseases, the book pertains to the treatment of infectious diseases and use of antimicrobial agents in adults. The clinical recommendations set forth in this book are those of the authors and are offered as general guidelines, not specific instructions for individual patients. Clinical judgement should always guide the physician in the selection, dosing, and duration of antimicrobial therapy for individual patients. Not all medications cited in this book have been accepted by the U.S. Food and Drug Administration for indications, and antimicrobial recommendations are not limited to indications in the package insert. The use of any drug should be preceded by careful review of the package insert, which provides indications and dosing approved by the U.S. Food and Drug Administration. The information provided in this book is not exhaustive, and the reader is referred to other medical references and the manufacturer's product literature for further information. Clinical use of the information provided and any consequences that may arise from its use is the responsibility of the prescribing physician. The authors, editors, and publisher do not warrant or guarantee the information herein contained and do not assume and expressly disclaim any liability for errors or omissions or any consequences that may occur from use of this information.

ABBREVIATIONS

ABE	acute bacterial endocarditis
ABM	acute bacterial meningitis
AFB	acid fast bacilli
AIHA	autoimmune hemolytic anemia
ANA	antinuclear antibody
ARDS	adult respiratory distress syndrome
A-V	atrio-ventricular
β-lactams	penicillins, cephalosporins, cephamycins (not monobactams or carbapenems)
BAL	bronchoalveolar lavage
BMT	bone marrow transplant
CAB	catheter associated bacteriuria
CABG	coronary artery bypass grafting
CAC	catheter associated candiduria
CAH	chronic active hepatitis
CA-MRSA	community-acquired MRSA (see p. 14)
CAP	community-acquired pneumonia
CD_4	CD_4 T-cell lymphocyte
CE	California encephalitis virus
CFS	chronic fatigue syndrome
CGD	chronic granulomatous disease
CIE	counter-immunoelectrophoresis
CLL	chronic lymphocytic leukemia
CMV	Cytomegalovirus
CNS	central nervous system
CO-MRSA	community-onset MRSA (see p. 16)
CoNS	coagulase-negative staphylococci
CPH	chronic persistent hepatitis
CPK	creatine phosphokinase
CrCl	creatinine clearance
CSD	cat scratch disease
CSF	cerebrospinal fluid
CT	computerized tomography
CVA	costovertebral angle
CVVH	continuous veno venous hemo filtration
CXR	chest x-ray
DFA	direct fluorescent antibody
DI	diabetes insipidus
DIC	disseminated intravascular coagulation
DM	diabetes mellitus
DOT	directly observed therapy
e.g.	for example
EBV	Ebstein-Barr virus
EEE	Eastern equine encephalitis
EEG	electroencephalogram
EIA	enzyme immunoassay
ELISA	enzyme-linked immunosorbent assay
EM	erythema migrans
EMB	ethambutol

Enterobacteriaceae:	Citrobacter, Edwardsiella, Enterobacter, E. coli, Klebsiella, Proteus, Providencia, Shigella, Salmonella, Serratia, Hafnia, Morganella, Yersinia
ESBLs	extended spectrum β-lactamases
esp	especially
ESR	erythrocyte sedimentation rate
ESRD	end-stage renal disease
ET	endotracheal
FTA-ABS	fluorescent treponemal antibody absorption test
FUO	fever of unknown origin
G6PD	glucose-6-phosphate dehydrogenase
GC	gonococcus/gonorrhea
GI	gastrointestinal
gm	gram
GU	genitourinary
HA-MRSA	hospital-acquired MRSA (see p. 16)
HAV	hepatitis A virus
HBcAb	hepatitis B core antibody
HBsAg	hepatitis B surface antigen
HBV	Hepatitis B virus
HCV	Hepatitis C virus
HDV	Hepatitis D virus
HEV	Hepatitis E virus
HFV	hepatitis F virus
HFHD	high flux hemodialysis
HFM	hand foot mouth disease
HD	hemodialysis
HGA	human granulocytic anaplasmosis
HGE	human granulocytic ehrlichiosis
HHV-6	human Herpes virus 6
HME	human monocytic ehrlichiosis
HMPV	Human metapneumovirus
HPS	Hanta virus pulmonary syndrome
HPV	human papilloma virus
HRIG	human rabies immune globulin
HSV	Herpes simplex virus
I & D	incision and drainage
IFA	immunofluorescent antibody
IgA	immunoglobulin A
IgG	immunoglobulin G
IgM	immunoglobulin M
INH	isoniazid
IP	intraperitoneal
IT	intrathecal
ITP	idiopathic thrombocytopenic purpura
IV	intravenous
IV/PO	IV or PO
IVDA	intravenous drug abuser

JE	Japanese encephalitis
kg	kilogram
L	liter
LCM	lymphocytic choriomeningitis
LDH	lactate dehydrogenase
LFTs	liver function tests
LGV	lymphogranuloma venereum
MAI	Mycobacterium avium-intracellulare
mcg	microgram
mcL	microliter
MDR	multidrug resistant
MDRSP	multidrug-resistant S. pneumoniae
mg	milligram
mL	milliliter
MIC	minimum inhibitory concentration
min	minute
MMR	measles, mumps, rubella
MRI	magnetic resonance imaging
MRSA	methicillin-resistant S. aureus
MRSE	methicillin-resistant S. epidermidis
MS	multiple sclerosis
MSSA	methicillin-sensitive S. aureus
MSSE	methicillin-sensitive S. epidermidis
MTT	methlytetrathiazole
MU	million units
MVP	mitral valve prolapse
NHAP	nursing home acquired pneumonia
NNRTI	non-nucleoside reverse transcriptase inhibitor
NP	nosocomial pneumonia
NRTI	nucleoside reverse transcriptase inhibitor
NSAIDS	nonsteroidal anti-inflammatory drugs
OI	opportunistic infection
PAN	polyarteritis nodosa
PBC	primary biliary cirrhosis
PBS	protected brush specimen
PCEC	purified chick embryo cells
PCN	penicillin
PCP	Pneumocystis (carinii) jiroveci pneumonia
PCR	polymerase chain reaction
PD	peritoneal dialysis
PDA	patent ductus arteriosus
PEP	post-exposure prophylaxis
PI	protease inhibitor
PML	progressive multifocal leukoencephalopathy
PMN	polymorphonuclear leucocytes
PO	oral
PPD	tuberculin skin test
PPIs	proton pump inhibitors
PPNG	penicillinase-producing N. gonorrhoeae
PVE	prosthetic valve endocarditis
PVL	Panton-Valentine leukocidin
PZA	pyrazinamide
q__d	every __ days
q__h	every __ hours
q month	once a month
q week	once a week
RA	rheumatoid arthritis
RBC	red blood cells
RE	regional ileitis (Crohn's disease)
RMSF	rocky mountain spotted fever
RUQ	right upper quadrant
RVA	rabies vaccine absorbed
SARS	severe acute respiratory syndrome
SBE	subacute bacterial endocarditis
SGOT/SGPT	serum transaminases
SLE	systemic lupus erythematosus
SOT	solid organ transplant
sp.	species
SPB	spontaneous bacterial peritonitis
SPEP	serum protein electrophoresis
SQ	subcutaneous
STD	sexually transmitted diseases
St. LE	Saint Louis encephalititis
TA	temporal arteritis
TAH/BSO	total abdominal hysterectomy/bilateral salpingoopherectomy
TB	M. tuberculosis
TEE	transesophageal echocardiogram
TEN	toxic epidermal necrolysis
TID	three times per day
TMP	trimethoprim
TMP–SMX	trimethoprim-sulfamethoxazole
TRNG	tetracycline-resistant N. gonorrhoeae
TSS	toxic shock syndrome
TTE	transthoracic echocardiogram
TTP	thrombotic thrombocytopenic purpura
TURP	transurethral resection of prostate
UC	ulcerative colitis
UTI	urinary tract infection
VA	ventriculoatrial
VAP	ventilator-associated pneumonia
VCA	viral capsid antigen
VEE	Venezuelan equine encephalitis virus
VISA	vancomycin-intermediate S. aureus
VLM	visceral larval migrans
VP	ventriculoperitoneal
VRE	vancomycin-resistant enterococci
VRSA	vancomycin-resistant S. aureus
VSE	vancomycin-sensitive enterococci
VZV	Varicella zoster virus
WBC	white blood cells
WNE	west nile encephalitis
XMRV	xenotropic murine leukemia related virus
yrs	years

Chapter 1

Overview of Antimicrobial Therapy

Burke A. Cunha, MD
Paul E. Schoch, PhD
Edward J. Bottone, PhD

Overview of Antimicrobial Therapy

Despite the ability of antimicrobial therapy to prevent/control infection, prescribing errors are common, including treatment of colonization, suboptimal empiric therapy, inappropriate combination therapy, dosing and duration errors, and mismanagement of apparent antibiotic failure. Inadequate consideration of antibiotic resistance potential, tissue penetration, drug interactions, and side effects, limit the effectiveness of antimicrobial therapy. *Antibiotic Essentials* is a concise, practical, and authoritative guide to the treatment and prevention of infectious diseases commonly encountered.

FACTORS IN ANTIBIOTIC SELECTION

A. Spectrum. Antibiotic spectrum refers to the range of microorganisms an antibiotic is usually effective against, and is the basis for empiric antibiotic therapy (Chapter 2). Antibiotics with "concentration-dependent" kinetics (e.g., quinolones, aminoglycosides) display increasing killing with increasing concentrations above MIC of organism; antibiotics with "time-dependent" kinetics (e.g., beta-lactams) do not.

B. Tissue Penetration. Antibiotics that are effective against a microorganism in vitro but unable to reach the site of infection are of little or no benefit to the host. Antibiotic tissue penetration depends on properties of the antibiotic (e.g., lipid solubility, molecular size) and tissue (e.g., adequacy of blood supply, presence of inflammation). Antibiotic tissue penetration is rarely problematic in acute infections due to increased microvascular permeability from local release of chemical inflammatory mediators. In contrast, chronic infections (e.g., chronic pyelonephritis, chronic prostatitis, chronic osteomyelitis) and infections caused by intracellular pathogens often rely on chemical properties of an antibiotic (e.g., high lipid solubility, small molecular size) for adequate tissue penetration. Antibiotics cannot be expected to eradicate organisms from areas that are difficult to penetrate or have impaired blood supply, such as abscesses, which usually require surgical drainage for cure. In addition, implanted foreign materials associated with infection usually need to be removed for cure, since microbes causing infections associated with prosthetic joints, shunts, and intravenous lines produce a slime/biofilm on plastic/metal surfaces that permits organisms to survive despite antimicrobial therapy.

C. Antibiotic Resistance. Bacterial resistance to antimicrobial therapy may be classified as natural/intrinsic or acquired, and as relative or absolute. Pathogens not covered by the usual spectrum of an antibiotic are termed *naturally/intrinsically* resistant (e.g., 25% of S. pneumoniae are naturally resistant to macrolides); *acquired* resistance refers to a previously susceptible pathogen that is no longer susceptible to an antibiotic (e.g., ampicillin-resistant H. influenzae). Organisms with *intermediate level (relative)* resistance manifests as an increase in minimum inhibitory concentrations (MICs), but are susceptible at achievable serum/tissue concentrations (e.g., penicillin-resistant S. pneumoniae). In contrast, organisms with *high level (absolute)* resistance manifests as a sudden increase in MICs during therapy, and cannot be overcome by higher-than-usual antibiotic doses (e.g., gentamicin-resistant P. aeruginosa). Most acquired antibiotic resistance is *agent-specific*, not a class specific, and is usually limited to one or two species. Resistance is *not* related, per se, to volume or duration of use. Some antibiotics have little resistance potential i.e., "low resistance" potential even when used in high volume; other antibiotics can induce resistance i.e., "high resistance" potential with little use.

Successful antibiotic resistance control strategies include eliminating antibiotics from animal feeds, microbial surveillance to detect resistance problems early, infection control precautions to limit/contain spread of clonal resistant species, restricted hospital formulary (i.e., controlled use of high resistance potential antibiotics), and preferential use of "low resistance" potential antibiotics by clinicians. Unsuccessful strategies include rotating formularies, restricted use of certain antibiotic classes (e.g., 3rd generation cephalosporins, fluoroquinolones), and use of combination therapy. In choosing between similar antibiotics, try to select an antibiotic with "low resistance" potential. Some antibiotics (e.g., ceftazidime) are also associated with increased prevalence of methicillin-resistant S. aureus (MRSA); other antibiotics (e.g., vancomycin) are associated with increased prevalence of vancomycin-resistant enterococci (VRE).

D. Safety Profile. Whenever possible, avoid antibiotics with serious/frequent side effects.

E. Cost. Switching early from IV to PO antibiotics is the single most important cost saving strategy in hospitalized patients, as the institutional cost of IV administration (~$10/dose) may exceed the cost of the antibiotic itself. Antibiotic costs can also be minimized by using antibiotics with long half-lives, and by choosing monotherapy over combination therapy. Other factors adding to the cost of antimicrobial therapy include the need for an obligatory second antimicrobial agent, antibiotic side effects (e.g., diarrhea, cutaneous reactions, seizures, phlebitis), and outbreaks of resistant organisms, which require cohorting and prolonged hospitalization.

FACTORS IN ANTIBIOTIC DOSING

Usual antibiotic dosing assumes normal renal and hepatic function. Patients with significant renal insufficiency and/or hepatic dysfunction may require dosage reduction in antibiotics metabolized/eliminated by these organs (Table 1.1). Specific dosing recommendations based on the degree of renal and hepatic insufficiency are detailed in Chapter 9.

A. Renal Insufficiency. Since most antibiotics eliminated by the kidneys have a wide "toxic-to-therapeutic ratio," dosing strategies are frequently based on formula-derived estimates of creatinine clearance (Table 1.1), rather than precise quantitation of glomerular filtration rates. Dosage adjustments are especially important for antibiotics with narrow toxic-to-therapeutic ratios, and for patients who are receiving other nephrotoxic medications or have preexisting renal disease.

Table 1.1. Dosing Strategies in Hepatic/Renal Insufficiency*

Hepatic Insufficiency

- Decrease total daily dose of hepatically-eliminated antibiotic by 50% in presence of clinically severe liver disease.
- **Alternative: Use antibiotic eliminated/inactivated by the renal route in usual dose.**

Renal Insufficiency

- If creatinine clearance ~ 40–60 mL/min, decrease dose of renally-eliminated antibiotic by 50% and maintain the usual dosing interval.
- If creatinine clearance ~10–40 mL/min, decrease dose of renally-eliminated antibiotic by 50% and double the dosing interval.
- **Alternative: Use antibiotic eliminated/inactivated by the hepatic route in usual dose.**

Major Route of Elimination			
Hepatobiliary		**Renal**	
Chloramphenicol	Nafcillin	Most β-lactams	Nitrofurantoin
Cefoperazone	Linezolid	Aminoglycosides	Fosfomycin
Doxycycline	INH/EMB/RIF	TMP–SMX	Amantadine
Minocycline	Pyrazinamide	Monobactams	Rimantadine
Telithromycin	Itraconazole	Carbapenems	Acyclovir
Moxifloxacin	Caspofungin	Polymyxin B	Valacyclovir
Macrolides	Micafungin	Colistin	Famciclovir
Clindamycin	Anidulafungin	Ciprofloxacin	Valganciclovir
Metronidazole	Ketoconazole	Levofloxacin	Oseltamavir
Tigecycline	Voriconazole	Gatifloxacin	Peramavir
Quinupristin/dalfopristin	Posaconazole	Gemifloxacin	Tetracycline
		Flucytosine	Daptomycin
		Fluconazole	Telavancin
		Vancomycin	Ceftobiprole

* See individual drug summaries in Chapter 11 for specific dosing recommendations. Creatinine clearance (CrCl) is used to assess renal function and can be estimated by the following formula: CrCl (mL/min) = [(140 – age) × weight (kg)] / [72 × serum creatinine (mg/dL)]. Multiply by 0.85 if female. It is important to recognize that due to age-dependent declines in renal function, elderly patients with "normal" serum creatinines may have CrCls requiring dosage adjustment. For example, a 70-year-old, 50-kg female with a serum creatinine of 1.2 mg/dL has an estimated CrCl of 34 mL/min.

1. **Initial and Maintenance Dosing in Renal Insufficiency.** For drugs eliminated by the kidneys, ***the initial dose is unchanged***, and the ***maintenance dose/dosing interval are modified in proportion to the degree of renal insufficiency (CrCl)***. Dosing adjustment problems in renal insufficiency can be circumvented by selecting an antibiotic with a similar spectrum that is eliminated by the hepatic route.

2. **Aminoglycoside Dosing.** Single daily dosing—adjusted for the degree of renal insufficiency after the loading dose is administered–has virtually eliminated the nephrotoxic potential of aminoglycosides, and is recommended for all patients,

including the critically ill (a possible exception is enterococcal endocarditis, where gentamicin dosing every 8 hours may be preferable). Aminoglycoside-induced tubular dysfunction is best assessed by quantitative renal tubular cast counts in urine, which more accurately reflect aminoglycoside nephrotoxicity than serum creatinine.

B. **Hepatic Insufficiency.** Antibiotic dosing for patients with hepatic dysfunction is problematic, since there is no hepatic counterpart to the serum creatinine to accurately assess liver function. In practice, antibiotic dosing is based on clinical assessment of the severity of liver disease. For practical purposes, dosing adjustments are usually not required for mild or moderate hepatic insufficiency. For severe hepatic insufficiency, dosing adjustments are usually made for antibiotics with hepatotoxic potential (Chapter 9). Relatively few antibiotics depend solely on hepatic inactivation/elimination, and dosing adjustment problems in these cases can be circumvented by selecting an appropriate antibiotic eliminated by the renal route.

C. **Combined Renal and Hepatic Insufficiency.** There are no good dosing adjustment guidelines for patients with hepatorenal insufficiency. If renal insufficiency is worse than hepatic insufficiency, antibiotics eliminated by the liver are often administered at half the total daily dose. If hepatic insufficiency is more severe than renal insufficiency, renally eliminated antibiotics are usually administered and dosed in proportion to renal function.

D. **Mode of Antibiotic and Excretion/Excretory Organ Toxicity.** The mode of elimination/excretion does not predispose to excretory organ toxicity per se, e.g., nafcillin (hepatically eliminated) is not hepatotoxic.

MICROBIOLOGY AND SUSCEPTIBILITY TESTING

A. **Overview.** In vitro susceptibility testing provides information about microbial sensitivities of a pathogen to various antibiotics and is useful in guiding therapy. Proper application of microbiology and susceptibility data requires careful assessment of the in vitro results to determine if they are consistent with the clinical context; if not, the clinical impression usually should take precedence.

B. **Limitations of Microbiology Susceptibility Testing**

1. ***In vitro* data do not differentiate between colonizers and pathogens.** Before responding to a culture report from the microbiology laboratory, it is important to determine whether the organism is a pathogen or a colonizer in the clinical context. As a rule, colonization should not be treated.

2. ***In vitro* data do not necessarily translate into *in vivo* efficacy.** Reports which indicate an organism is "susceptible" or "resistant" to a given antibiotic in vitro do not necessarily reflect in vivo activity. Table 1.2 lists antibiotic-microorganism combinations for which susceptibility testing is usually unreliable.

Table 1.2. Antibiotic-Organism Combinations for Which *In Vitro* Susceptibility Testing Does Not Predict *In Vivo* Effectiveness[1]

Antibiotic	"Susceptible" Organism
Penicillin	H. influenzae, Yersinia pestis
TMP–SMX	Klebsiella, Enterococci, Bartonella
Polymyxin B	Proteus, Salmonella
Imipenem	Stenotrophomonas maltophilia[2]
Gentamicin	Mycobacterium tuberculosis
Vancomycin	Erysipelothrix rhusiopathiae
Aminoglycosides	Streptococci, Salmonella, Shigella
Clindamycin	Fusobacteria, Clostridia, enterococci, Listeria
Macrolides	P. multocida
1st, 2nd generation cephalosporins	Salmonella, Shigella, Bartonella
3rd, 4th generation cephalosporins[4]	Enterococci, Listeria, Bartonella
All antibiotics except vancomycin, minocycline, quinupristin/dalfopristin, tigecycline, linezolid, daptomycin, ceftobiprole, telavancin	MRSA[3]

1. In vitro susceptibility *does not* predict in vivo activity; susceptibility data cannot be relied upon to guide therapy for antibiotic-organism combinations in this table.
2. Formerly Pseudomonas.
3. In spite of apparent in vitro susceptibility of many antibiotics against MRSA, only vancomycin, minocycline, quinupristin/dalfopristin, linezolid, daptomycin, ceftobiprole, telavancin, and tigecycline are effective in vivo.
4. Cefoperazone is the only cephalosporin with clinically useful anti-enterococcal activity against E. faecalis (VSE), *not* E. faecium (VRE).

3. ***In vitro* susceptibility testing is dependent on the microbe, methodology, and antibiotic concentration.** *In vitro* susceptibility testing by the microbiology laboratory *assumes* the isolate was recovered from *blood*, and is being exposed to *serum* concentrations of an antibiotic given in the *usual* dose. Since some body sites (e.g., bladder, urine) contain higher antibiotic concentrations than found in serum, and other body sites (e.g., CSF) contain lower antibiotic concentrations than found in serum, *in vitro* data may be misleading for non-bloodstream infections. For example, a Klebsiella pneumoniae isolate obtained from the CSF may be reported as "sensitive" to cefazolin even though cefazolin does not penetrate the CSF. Likewise, E. coli and Klebsiella urinary isolates are often reported as "resistant" to ampicillin/sulbactam despite *in vivo* efficacy, due to high antibiotic concentrations in the urinary tract. Antibiotics should be prescribed at the usual recommended doses; attempts to lower cost by reducing dosage may decrease antibiotic efficacy (e.g., cefoxitin 2 gm IV inhibits ~ 85% of B. fragilis isolates, whereas 1 gm IV inhibits only ~ 20% of strains).

4. **Unusual susceptibility patterns.** Organisms have predictable susceptibility patterns to antibiotics. When an isolate has an unusual susceptibility pattern (i.e., isolate of a species is inconsistent with its usual susceptibility pattern) (Table 1.3), further testing should be performed by the microbiology laboratory. Expanded susceptibility testing may be warranted.

Table 1.3. Unusual Susceptibility Patterns Requiring Further Testing

Organism	Unusual Susceptibility Patterns	Usual Susceptibility Patterns
Neisseria meningitidis	Penicillin resistant	Penicillin susceptible
Staphylococci	Vancomycin/clindamycin resistant; erythromycin susceptible	Vancomycin susceptible
Viridans streptococci	Vancomycin intermediate/ resistant	Vancomycin susceptible
S. pneumoniae	Vancomycin intermediate/ resistant	Vancomycin susceptible
Beta-hemolytic streptococci	Penicillin intermediate/ resistant	Penicillin susceptible
Enterobacteriaceae	Imipenem resistant	Imipenem susceptible
E. coli, P. mirabilis, Klebsiella	Cefoxitin/cefotetan resistant	2nd generation cephalosporin susceptible
Enterobacter, Serratia	Ampicillin/cefazolin susceptible	Ampicillin/cefazolin resistant
Morganella, Providencia	Ampicillin/cefazolin susceptible	Ampicillin/cefazolin resistant
Klebsiella	Cefotetan susceptible; ceftazidime resistant	Cefotetan resistant; ceftazidime susceptible
P. aeruginosa	Amikacin resistant; gentamicin/ tobramycin susceptible	Amikacin susceptible; gentamicin/ tobramycin resistant
Stenotrophomonas maltophilia	TMP–SMX resistant; imipenem susceptible	TMP–SMX susceptible

Isolates with unusual susceptibility patterns require further testing by the microbiology laboratory to verify the identity of the isolate and characterize resistance mechanism. Expanded susceptibility testing is indicated.

C. **Susceptibility Breakpoints for Streptococcus pneumoniae.** Because antibiotic susceptibility is, in part, concentration related, the Clinical and Laboratory Standards Institute (CLSI), formerly the National Committee for Clinical Laboratory Standards (NCCLS), has revised its breakpoints for S. pneumoniae susceptibility testing, which differentiate between meningeal and non-meningeal sites of pneumococcal infection (Table 1.5).

Table 1.4. Susceptibility Patterns of Multi-Drug Resistant Organisms (MDROs) and Extended-Spectrum Beta-Lactamase (ESBL) Organisms*

MDROs & ESBL Resistance Profiles
Resistance Profiles • MDRO Acinetobacter sp. ***resistant to ciprofloxacin and amikacin and ceftazidime*** • MDRO *Pseudomonas aeruginosa* ***resistant to amikacin and meropenem*** • ESBL *Klebsiella oxytoca* ***resistant to ceftazidime*** • ESBL *Klebsiella pneumoniae* ***resistant to ceftazidime*** • ESBL *Enterobacter sp.* ***resistant to ceftazidime*** • ESBL *Escherichia coli* ***resistant to ceftazidime*** • ESBL *Proteus mirabilis* ***resistant to ceftazidime***

* Most common ESBL producing organisms *Klebsiella, Enterobacter, E. coli.*

Table 1.5. CLSI Susceptibility Breakpoints for Streptococcus pneumoniae*

Antibiotic	MIC (mcg/mL)		
	Sensitive	**Intermediate**	**Resistant**
Amoxicillin (non-meningitis)	≤ 2	4	≥ 8
Amoxicillin-clavulanic acid (non-meningitis)	≤ 2/1	4/2	≥ 8/4
Penicillin (meningitis)	≤ 0.06	–	≥ 0.12
Penicillin (non-meningitis)	≤ 2	4	≥ 8
Azithromycin	≤ 0.5	1	≥ 2
Clarithromycin/erythromycin	≤ 0.25	0.5	≥ 1
Doxycycline/tetracycline	≤ 2	4	≥ 8
Telithromycin	≤ 1	2	≥ 4
Cefaclor	≤ 1	2	≥ 4
Cefdinir/cefpodoxime	≤ 0.5	1	≥ 2
Cefprozil	≤ 2	4	≥ 8
Cefuroxime axetil (oral)	≤ 1	2	≥ 4
Loracarbef	≤ 2	4	≥ 8
Cefepime (non-meningitis)	≤ 1	2	≥ 4

Table 1.5. CLSI Susceptibility Breakpoints for Streptococcus pneumoniae* (cont'd)

Antibiotic	MIC (mcg/mL)		
	Sensitive	Intermediate	Resistant
Cefepime (meningitis)	≤ 0.5	1	≥ 2
Cefotaxime (non-meningitis)	≤ 1	2	≥ 4
Cefotaxime (meningitis)	≤ 0.5	1	≥ 2
Ceftriaxone (non-meningitis)	≤ 1	2	≥ 4
Ceftriaxone (meningitis)	≤ 0.5	1	≥ 2
Imipenem	≤ 0.12	0.25–0.5	≥ 1
Meropenem	≤ 0.25	0.5	≥ 1
Ertapenem	≤ 1	2	> 4
Vancomycin	≤ 1	–	–
Moxifloxacin	≤ 1	2	≥ 4
Levofloxacin	≤ 2	4	≥ 8
TMP–SMX	≤ 0.5/9.5	1/19–2/38	≥ 4/78
Chloramphenicol	≤ 4	–	≥ 8
Clindamycin	≤ 0.25	0.5	≥ 1
Linezolid	≤ 2	–	–
Rifampin	≤ 1	2	≥ 4

CLSI = Clinical and Laboratory Standards Institute (formerly NCCLS = National Committee for Clinical Laboratory Standards) M100–S20 (2010).

* *Testing Conditions:* Medium: Mueller-Hinton broth with 2.5% lysed horse blood (cation-adjusted). Inoculum: colony suspension. Incubation: 35°C (20–24 hours).

D. Summary. In vitro susceptibility testing is useful in most situations, but should not be followed blindly. Many factors need to be considered when interpreting in vitro microbiologic data, and infectious disease consultation is recommended for all but the most straightforward susceptibility interpretation problems. IV-to-PO switch changes using antibiotics of the same or other antibiotic class is best made when the oral antibiotic can achieve similar blood/tissue levels as the IV antibiotic. For example, IV-to-PO switch from cefazolin 1 gm (IV) to cephalexin 500 mg (PO) may not be effective against all pathogens at all sites, since cephalexin 500 mg (PO) achieves much lower serum concentrations compared to cefazolin 1 gm (IV) (16 mcg/mL vs. 200 mcg/mL).

OTHER CONSIDERATIONS IN ANTIMICROBIAL THERAPY

A. **Bactericidal vs. Bacteriostatic Therapy.** For most infections, bacteriostatic and bactericidal antibiotics inhibit/kill organisms at the same rate, and **should not be a factor in antibiotic selection**. Bactericidal antibiotics have an advantage in certain infections, such endocarditis, meningitis, and febrile leukopenia, but there are exceptions even in these cases.

B. **Monotherapy vs. Combination Therapy. Monotherapy is preferred to combination therapy for nearly all infections.** In addition to cost savings, monotherapy results in less chance of medication error and fewer missed doses/drug interactions. Combination therapy may be useful for drug synergy or for extending spectrum beyond what can be obtained with a single drug. However, since drug synergy is difficult to assess and the possibility of antagonism always exists, antibiotics should be combined for synergy if synergy is based on actual testing. Combination therapy is not effective in preventing antibiotic resistance, except in very few situations (Table 1.6).

C. **Intravenous vs. Oral Switch Therapy.** Patients admitted to the hospital are usually started on IV antibiotic therapy, then switched to equivalent oral therapy after clinical improvement/defervescence (usually within 72 hours). **Advantages of early IV-to-PO switch programs include reduced cost, early hospital discharge, less need for home IV therapy, and virtual elimination of IV line infections**. Drugs well-suited for IV-to-PO switch or for treatment entirely by the oral route include doxycycline, minocycline, clindamycin, metronidazole, chloramphenicol, amoxicillin, trimethoprim-sulfamethoxazole, quinolones, and linezolid.

Table 1.6. Combination Therapy and Antibiotic Resistance

Examples of Antibiotic Combinations That Prevent Resistance
Anti-pseudomonal penicillin (carbenicillin) + aminoglycoside (gentamicin, tobramycin, amikacin)
Rifampin + other TB drugs (INH, ethambutol, pyrazinamide)
5-flucytosine + amphotericin B
Examples of Antibiotic Combinations That Do Not Prevent Resistance*
TMP–SMX
Aztreonam + ceftazidime
Cefepime + ciprofloxacin
Aminoglycoside + imipenem
Most other antibiotic combinations

* These combinations are often prescribed to prevent resistance when, in actuality, they do not.

Most infectious diseases should be treated orally unless the patient is critically ill, cannot take antibiotics by mouth, or there is no equivalent oral antibiotic. If the patient is able to take/absorb oral antibiotics, there is no difference in clinical outcome using equivalent IV or PO antibiotics. It is more important to think in terms of antibiotic spectrum, bioavailability and tissue penetration, rather than route of administration. **Nearly all non-critically ill patients should be treated in part or entirely with oral antibiotics.** When switching from IV to PO therapy, **the oral antibiotic chosen should have the same spectrum/degree of activity against the presumed/known pathogen and achieve the same blood and tissue levels as the equivalent IV antibiotic** (Table 1.7).

D. Duration of Therapy. Most bacterial infections in normal hosts are treated with antibiotics for 1–2 weeks. The duration of therapy may need to be extended in patients with impaired immunity (e.g., diabetes, SLE, alcoholic liver disease, neutropenia, diminished splenic function, etc.), chronic bacterial infections (e.g., endocarditis, osteomyelitis), chronic viral and fungal infections, or certain bacterial intracellular pathogens (Table 1.8). Infections such as HIV may require life-long therapy. Antibiotic therapy should ordinarily not be continued for more than 2 weeks, even if low-grade fevers persist (Table 1.8). Prolonged therapy offers no benefit, and increases the risk of adverse side effects, drug interactions, and superinfections.

Table 1.7. Bioavailability of Oral Antimicrobials

Bioavailability	Antimicrobials		
Excellent[1] (> 90%)	Amoxicillin Cephalexin Cefprozil Cefadroxil Clindamycin Quinolones	TMP TMP–SMX Doxycycline Minocycline Chloramphenicol Metronidazole	Linezolid Fluconazole Voriconazole Rifampin INH Pyrazinamide Cycloserine
Good[2] (60–90%)	Most beta-lactams Cefixime Cefpodoxime Ceftibuten Cefuroxime	Valacyclovir Famciclovir Valganciclovir Macrolides Cefaclor	EMB 5-Flucytosine Posaconazole Itraconazole (solution) Nitazoxanide (with food)
Poor[3] (< 60%)	Vancomycin	Cefdinir Cefditoren	Nitazoxanide (without food)

1. Oral administration results in ***equivalent blood/tissue levels*** as the same dose given IV (PO = IV).
2. Oral administration results in ***lower but effective blood/tissue levels*** than the same dose given IV (PO < IV).
3. Oral administration results in ***suboptimal blood/tissue levels***.

Table 1.8. Infectious Diseases Usually Requiring Prolonged Antimicrobial Therapy

Therapy	Infectious Diseases
3 weeks	Lymphogranuloma venereum (LGV), syphilis (late latent), H. pylori, chronic prostatitis
4 weeks	Chronic otitis media, chronic sinusitis, acute osteomyelitis, chronic pyelonephritis, brain abscess, SBE
6 weeks	Acute bacterial endocarditis (S. aureus, enterococcal), chronic osteomyelitis[4]
3 months	Lung abscess[1]
6 months	Pulmonary TB, extrapulmonary TB, Actinomycosis[2], Nocardia[3], prosthetic-related infections[5]
12 months	Whipple's disease
> 12 months	Lepromatous leprosy, HIV

1. Treat until resolved or until chest x-ray is normal/nearly normal and remains unchanged.
2. May require longer treatment; treat until resolved.
3. May require longer treatment in compromised hosts.
4. Adequate surgical debridement is required for cure.
5. Implanted foreign materials associated with infection (prosthetic valves, vascular grafts, joint replacements, hemodialysis shunts) should be removed as soon as possible after diagnosis. If removal is not feasible, then chronic suppressive therapy may be attempted, although clinical failure is the rule.

EMPIRIC ANTIBIOTIC THERAPY

Microbiology susceptibility data are not ordinarily available prior to initial treatment with antibiotics. Empiric therapy is based on directing coverage against the most likely pathogens, and takes into consideration drug allergy history, hepatic/renal function, possible antibiotic side effects, resistance potential, and cost. If a patient is moderately or severely ill, empiric therapy is usually initiated intravenously. Patients who are mildly ill, whether hospitalized or ambulatory, may be started on oral antibiotics with high bioavailability. Cultures of appropriate clinical specimens (e.g., blood, sputum, urine) should be obtained prior to starting empiric therapy to provide bacterial isolates for in vitro susceptibility testing. Empiric therapy for common infectious diseases is described in Chapter 2.

ANTIBIOTIC FAILURE

There are many possible causes of *apparent* antibiotic failure, including drug fever, antibiotic-unresponsive infections, and febrile non-infectious diseases. The most common error in the management of apparent antibiotic failure is changing/adding additional antibiotics instead of determining the cause (Tables 1.9, 1.10).

Table 1.9. Causes of Apparent/Actual Antibiotic Failure

Microbiologic Factors

- *In vitro* susceptibility but ineffective *in vivo*
- Antibiotic tolerance with gram-positive cocci
- Treating colonization (not infection)

Antibiotic Factors

- Inadequate coverage/spectrum
- Inadequate antibiotic blood levels
- Inadequate antibiotic tissue levels
- Decreased antibiotic activity in tissue
- Drug-drug interactions
  - Antibiotic inactivation
  - Antibiotic antagonism

Antibiotic Penetration Problems

- Undrained abscess
- Foreign body-related infection
- Protected focus (e.g., cerebrospinal fluid)
- Organ hypoperfusion/diminished blood supply
  - Chronic osteomyelitis
  - Chronic pyelonephritis

Non-infectious Diseases

- Medical disorders mimicking infection (e.g., SLE)
- Drug fever

Antibiotic-unresponsive Infectious Diseases

- Viral infections
- Fungal infections

Table 1.10. Clinical Features of Drug Fever

History

Many but not all individuals are atopic

Patients have been on a sensitizing medication for days or years "without a problem"

Physical exam

Relative bradycardia*

Fevers may be low- or high-grade, but usually range between 102°–104°F and may exceed 106°F

Patient appears "inappropriately well" for degree of fever

Laboratory tests

Elevated WBC count (usually with left shift)

Eosinophils almost always present, but eosinophilia is uncommon

Elevated erythrocyte sedimentation rate in majority of cases

Early, transient, mild elevations of serum transaminases (common)

Negative blood cultures (excluding contaminants)

* Relative bradycardia refers to heart rates that are inappropriately slow relative to body temperature (pulse must be taken simultaneously with temperature elevation). Applies to adult patients with temperature ≥ 102°F; does not apply to patients with second/third-degree heart block, pacemaker-induced rhythms, or those taking beta-blockers, diltiazem, or verapamil.

Relative Bradycardia

Temperature-Pulse Relationships

Temperature	Appropriate Pulse Response (beats/min)	Relative Bradycardia Pulse (beats/min)
106°F (41.1°C)	150	< 140
105°F (40.6°C)	140	< 130
104°F (40.7°C)	130	< 120
103°F (39.4°C)	120	< 110
102°F (38.9°C)	110	< 100

METHICILLIN-RESISTANT STAPHYLOCOCCUS AUREUS (MRSA)

MRSA infections occur most commonly in hospitals and healthcare settings (e.g., nursing homes, dialysis centers) but can occur in the community setting as well. MRSA infections are classified as hospital-acquired (HA-MRSA), community-onset (CO-MRSA), or community-acquired (CA-MRSA), which has implications for therapy (Table 1.11).

Table 1.11. Classification of MRSA Infections

MRSA Strain	Epidemiology & Microbiology	Therapy
Hospital *acquired* MRSA (HA-MRSA)*	Strains *originate within the hospital*, have SCC *mec* I,II,III genes, PVL+ (rare), and elaborate several *S. aureus* toxins.	Resistant to most antibiotics. Only vancomycin, quinupristin/dalfopristin, minocycline, linezolid, tigecycline, or daptomycin are *reliably* effective.
Community *onset* MRSA (CO-MRSA)*	Strains *originate in the hospital and later present from community*, have SCC *mec* I,II,III genes, PVL+ (rare) and elaborate several *S. aureus* toxins.	CO-MRSA strains are have the *same antibiotic susceptibility* as HA-MRSA strains and *should be treated as HA-MRSA*.

PVL = Panton-Valentine Leukocidin.

*CO-MRSA = HA-MRSA.

Adapted from: Cunha BA. Clinical Manifestations and Antimicrobial Therapy of Methicillin Resistant Staphylococcus aureus (MRSA). Clin Microbiol Infect 11:33–42, 2005 and Cunha BA: Simplified Clinical Approach to Community acquired MRSA (CA-MRSA) Infections. Journal of Hospital Infection 68:271–273, 2008.

Table 1.11. Classification of MRSA Infections (cont'd)

MRSA Strain	Epidemiology & Microbiology	Therapy
Community *acquired* MRSA (CA-MRSA)	*Only* MRSA infections "from the community" presenting as *severe pyomyositis or severe/ necrotizing community acquired MRSA pneumonia (with influenza)* should be considered as potentially due to CA-MRSA. *All other MRSA infections from the community should be clinically considered as CO-MRSA.* SCC *mec* IV, V genes. PVL+, (common). CA-MRSA PVL - Strains are *clinically indistinguishable* from MSSA or CO-MRSA. Elaborate the usual *S.aureus* toxins plus 18 other toxins.	CA-MRSA strains are susceptible to clindamycin, TMP–SMX, and doxycycline. Antibiotics used to treat CO-MRSA/HA-MRSA are also effective against CA-MRSA, but *not* vice versa.

PVL = Panton-Valentine Leukocidin.

*CO-MRSA = HA-MRSA.

Adapted from: Cunha BA. Clinical Manifestations and Antimicrobial Therapy of Methicillin Resistant Staphylococcus aureus (MRSA). Clin Microbiol Infect 11:33–42, 2005 and Cunha BA: Simplified Clinical Approach to Community acquired MRSA (CA-MRSA) Infections. Journal of Hospital Infection 68:271–273, 2008.

PITFALLS IN ANTIBIOTIC PRESCRIBING

- Use of antibiotics to treat non-infectious or antibiotic-unresponsive infectious diseases (e.g., viral infections) or colonization.
- Overuse of combination therapy. Monotherapy is preferred over combination therapy unless compelling reasons prevail, such as drug synergy or extended spectrum beyond what can be obtained with a single drug. Monotherapy reduces the risk of drug interactions and side effects, and is usually less expensive.
- Use of antibiotics for persistent fevers. For patients with persistent fevers on an antimicrobial regimens that appears to be failing, it is important to reassess the patient rather than add additional antibiotics. Causes of prolonged fevers include undrained septic foci, non-infectious medical disorders, and drug fevers. Undiagnosed causes of leukocytosis/low-grade fevers should not be treated with prolonged courses of antibiotics.
- Inadequate surgical therapy. Infections involving infected prosthetic materials or fluid collections (e.g., abscesses) often require surgical therapy for cure. For infections such as chronic osteomyelitis, surgery is the only way to cure the infection; antibiotics are useful only for suppression or to prevent local infectious complications.
- Home IV therapy. There is less need to use home IV therapy given the vast array of excellent oral antibiotics (e.g., doxycycline, minocycline, quinolones, TMP–SMX, linezolid).

REFERENCES AND SUGGESTED READINGS

CLSI (NCCLS). Performance standards for antimicrobial susceptibility testing: twelfth informational supplement M100-S16. NCCLS, Wayne, PA, 2006.

Cunha BA. Oral Antibiotic Therapy of Serious Systemic Infections. Med Clin N Am 90:1197–1222, 2006.

Cunha BA. Pseudomonas aeruginosa: Resistance and therapy. Semin Respir Infect 17:231–9, 2002.

Cunha BA. Clinical relevance of penicillin-resistant Streptococcus pneumoniae. Semin Respir Infect 17:204–14, 2002.

Cunha BA. Antimicrobial side effects. Medical Clinics of North America 85:149–185, 2001.

Cunha BA. Intravenous to oral antibiotic switch therapy. Drugs for Today 37:311–319, 2001.

Cunha BA. Effective antibiotic resistance and control strategies. Lancet 357:1307–1308, 2001.

Cunha BA. Factors in antibiotic selection for hospital formularies (part I). Hospital Formulary 33:558–572, 1998.

Cunha BA. Factors in antibiotic selection for hospital formularies (part II). Hospital Formulary 33:659–662, 1998.

Cunha BA. The significance of antibiotic false sensitivity testing with in vitro testing. J Chemother 9:25–33, 1997.

Cunha BA, Ortega A. Antibiotic failure. Medical Clinics of North America 79:663–672, 1995.

Daver NG, Shelburne SA, Atmar RL, et al. Oral step-down therapy is comparable to intravenous therapy for Staphylococcus aureus osteomyelitis. Journal of Infection 54:539–544, 2007.

Empey KM, Rapp RP, Evans ME. The effect of an antimicrobial formulary change on hospital resistance patterns. Pharmacotherapy 22:81–7, 2002.

Fenoll A, Gimenez MJ, Robledo O, et al. Influence of penicillin/amoxicillin non-susceptibility on the activity of third-generation cephalosporins against Streptococcus pneumoniae. Clin Microb & Infect Dis 27:75–80, 2008.

Johnson DH, Cunha BA. Drug fever. Infectious Disease Clinics of North America 10:85–91, 1996.

Jorgensen JH, Ferraro MJ. Antimicrobial Susceptibility Testing: A Review of General Principles and Contemporary Practices. Clin Infect Dis 49:1749–1755, 2009.

Leclercq R. Epidemiological and resistance issues in multi-drug resistant staphylococcal and enterococci. Clinical Microbiology and Infectious Diseases 15:224–231, 2009.

Lode HM. Clinical impact of antibiotic-resistant Gram-positive pathogens. Clin Microbiology Infect 15:212–217, 2009.

Patel SM, Saravolatz LD. Monotherapy Versus Combination Therapy. Med Clin N Am 90:1183–95, 2006.

Schlossberg D. Clinical Approach to Antibiotic Failure. Med Clin N Am 90:1265–77, 2006.

Tenover FC, Moellering RC. The rationale for revising the clinical and laboratory standards institute vancomycin minimal inhibitory concentration interpretive criteria for Staphylococcus aureus. Clinical Infect Dis 44:1208–1215, 2007.

Weinstein MP, Klugman KP, Jones RN. Rationale for Revised Penicillin Susceptibility Breakpoints versus *Streptococcus pneumoniae*: Coping with Antimicrobial Susceptibilityi in an Era of Resistance. Clin Infect Dis 48:1596–1600, 2009.

TEXTBOOKS

Amabile-Cuevas CF (ed). Antibiotic Resistance From Molecular Basics to Therapeutic Options. R.G. Landes Company, Austin, 1996.

Anaissie EJ, McGinnis MR, Pfaller MA (eds). Clinical Mycology. Churchill Livingstone, New York, 2003.

Baddour L,Gorbach SL (eds). Therapy of Infectious Diseases. Saunders, Philadelphia, Pennsylvania, 2003.

Bryskier A (ed). Antimicrobial Agents. ASM Press, Washington, D.C., 2005.

Chadwick DJ, Goode J (eds). Antibiotic Resistance: Origins, Evolution, Selection and Spread. John Wiley & Sons, New York, 1997.

Finch RG, Greenwood D, Norrby SR, Whitley RJ (eds). Antibiotic and Chemotherapy, 8th Edition. Churchill Livingstone, Edinburgh, Scotland, 2003.

Gorbach SL, Bartlett JG, Blacklow NR (eds). Infectious Diseases, 3rd Edition. Philadelphia, Lippincott, Williams & Wilkins, 2004.

Kucers A, Crowe S, Grayson ML, Hoy J (eds). The Use of Antibiotics, 5th Edition, Butterworth Heinemann, Oxford, England, 1997.

Mandell GL, Bennett JE, Dolin R (eds). Mandell, Douglas, and Bennett's Principles and Practice of infectious Diseases, 7th Edition. Philadelphia Elsevier Churchill Livingstone, 2010.

O'Grady F, Lambert HP, Finch RG, Greenwood D (eds). Antibiotic and Chemotherapy, 2nd Edition. Churchill, Livingston, New York, 1997.

Ristuccia AM, Cunha BA (eds). Antimicrobial Therapy. Raven Press, New York, 1984.

Scholar EM Pratt WB (eds). The Antimicrobial Drugs, 2nd Edition, Oxford University Press, New York, 2000.

Yoshikawa TT, Rajagopalan S (eds). Antibiotic Therapy for Geriatric Patients. Taylor & Francis Group, New York, 2006.

Yu V, Edwards G, McKinnon PS, Peloquin C, Morse G (eds). Antimicrobial Therapy and Vaccines, Volume II: Antimicrobial Agents, 2nd Edition. Esun, Technologies, Pittsburgh, Pennsylvania, 2005.

Chapter 2

Empiric Therapy Based on Clinical Syndrome

Burke A. Cunha, MD, Ronald L. Nichols, MD
John H. Rex, MD, Dennis J. Cleri, MD
David Schlossberg, MD

This chapter is organized by clinical syndrome, patient subset, and in some cases, specific organism. Clinical summaries immediately follow each treatment grid. Unless otherwise specified, **this chapter pertains to infectious diseases and antimicrobial agents in adults.** Therapeutic recommendations are based on antimicrobial effectiveness, reliability, cost, safety, and resistance potential. Switching to a more specific/narrow spectrum antimicrobial is not more effective than well-chosen empiric/initial therapy and usually results in increased cost and more side effects/drug interactions. The antimicrobial dosages in this section represent the usual dosages for normal renal and hepatic function. ***For any treatment category (i.e., preferred IV therapy, alternate IV therapy, PO therapy), recommended drugs are equally effective and not ranked by priority.*** Dosage adjustments, side effects, drug interactions, and other important prescribing information are described in the individual drug summaries in Chapter 11. Use of any drug should be preceded by careful review of the package insert, which provides indications and dosing approved by the U.S. Food and Drug Administration. *"IV-to-PO Switch"* in the last column of the shaded title bar in each treatment grid indicates the clinical syndrome should be treated either by IV therapy alone or IV followed by PO therapy, but *not* by PO therapy alone. *"PO Therapy or IV-to-PO Switch"* indicates the clinical syndrome can be treated by IV therapy alone, PO therapy alone, or IV followed by PO therapy (unless otherwise indicated in the footnotes under each treatment grid). Most patients on IV therapy should be switched to PO equivalent therapy after clinical improvement.

Empiric Therapy of CNS Infections

Acute Bacterial Meningitis (ABM) (see Color Atlas for CSF Gram stains)

Subset	Usual Pathogens	Preferred IV Therapy	Alternate IV Therapy	IV-to-PO Switch
Normal host	N. meningitidis H. influenzae S. pneumoniae	Ceftriaxone 2 gm (IV) q12h × 2 weeks	Meropenem 2 gm (IV) q8h × 2 weeks **or** Cefotaxime 3 gm (IV) q6h × 2 weeks **or** Ceftizoxime 3 gm (IV) q6h × 2 weeks	Chloramphenicol 500 mg (PO) q6h × 2 weeks
Elderly or malignancy	Listeria monocytogenes plus usual meningeal pathogens in normal hosts	Before culture results Ceftriaxone 2 gm (IV) q12h × 2 weeks **plus** Ampicillin 2 gm (IV) q4h × 2 weeks After culture results *Listeria present* Ampicillin 2 gm (IV) q4h × 2 weeks *Listeria not present* Treat as normal host	After culture results *Listeria present* TMP–SMX 5 mg/kg (IV) q6h × 2 weeks **or** Meropenem 2 gm (IV) q8h × 2 weeks **or** Chloramphenicol 500 mg (IV) q6h × 2 weeks *Listeria not present* Treat as for normal host, above	For Listeria meningitis only TMP–SMX 5 mg/kg (PO) q6h × 2 weeks **or** Chloramphenicol 500 mg (PO) q6h × 2 weeks For usual meningeal pathogens Chloramphenicol 500 mg (PO) q6h × 2 weeks

Acute Bacterial Meningitis (ABM) (see Color Atlas for CSF Gram stains) (cont'd)

Subset	Usual Pathogens	Preferred IV Therapy	Alternate IV Therapy	IV-to-PO Switch
CNS shunt infections (VA shunts) (Treat initially for MSSA; if later identified as MRSA, MSSE, or MRSE, treat accordingly)	S. aureus S. epidermidis (coagulase-negative staphylococci) CoNS	<u>MSSA/MSSE</u> Cefotaxime 3 gm (IV) q6h* **or** Ceftizoxime 3 gm (IV) q6h* <u>MRSA/MRSE</u> Linezolid 600 mg (IV) q12h*	<u>MSSA/MSSE</u> Cefepime 2 gm (IV) q8h* **or** Meropenem 2 gm (IV) q8h*<u>MRSA/ MRSE</u> Vancomycin 2 gm (IV) q12h* ± 20 mg (IT) q24h until shunt removal	<u>MSSE/MRSE</u> Linezolid 600 mg (PO) q12h* <u>MSSA/MRSA</u> Minocycline 100 mg (PO) q12h* **or** Linezolid 600 mg (PO) q12h*
CNS shunt infections (VP shunts)	E. coli K. pneumoniae Enterobacter S. marcescens	Ceftriaxone 2 gm (IV) q12h × 2 weeks after shunt removal	TMP–SMX 5 mg/kg (IV) q6h × 2 weeks after shunt removal	TMP–SMX 5 mg/kg (PO) q6h × 2 weeks after shunt removal
	MDR P. aeruginosa	Colistin 1.7 mg/kg (IV) q8h **plus either** Amikacin 10–40 mg (IT) q24h **or** Colistin 10 mg (IT) q24h × 2 weeks after shunt removal	Polymyxin B 1.25 mg/kg (IV) q8h **plus either** Amikacin 10–40 mg (IT) q24h **or** Polymyxin B 5 mg (IT) q24h × 3 days, then q48h × 2 weeks after shunt removal	
	MDR Acinetobacter baumanii	Ampicillin/sulbactam 4.5 gm (IV) q6h **or** Colistin 1.7 mg/kg (IV) q8h **plus either** Amikacin 10–40 mg (IT) q24h **or** Colistin 10 mg (IT) q24h × 2 weeks after shunt removal	Polymyxin B 1.25 mg/kg (IV) q8h **plus either** Amikacin 10–40 mg (IT) q24h **or** Polymyxin B 5 mg (IT) q24h × 3 days, then q48h × 2 weeks after shunt removal	

MSSA/MRSA = methicillin-sensitive/resistant S. aureus; MSSE/MRSE = methicillin-sensitive/resistant S. epidermidis. Duration of therapy represents total time IV or IV + PO. Most patients on IV therapy able to take PO meds should be switched to PO therapy after clinical improvement.

MDR = multidrug-resistant. Duration of therapy represents total time IV or IV + PO. Most patients on IV therapy able to take PO meds should be switched to PO therapy after clinical improvement.

* Treat for 1 week after shunt removal.

Clinical Presentation: Abrupt onset of fever, headache, stiff neck.
Diagnosis: CSF gram stain/culture.

Acute Bacterial Meningitis (Normal Hosts)

Diagnostic Considerations: Gram stain of centrifugated CSF is still the best diagnostic test. CSF antigen/CIE are unhelpful in establishing the diagnosis (many false-negatives). Blood cultures are positive for ABM pathogen in 80–90%. Typical CSF findings include a WBC count of 100–5000 cells/mm^3, elevated opening pressure, elevated protein and lactic acid levels (> 4–6 mmol/L), and a positive CSF gram stain. If the WBC is extremely high (> 20,000 cells/mm^3), suspect brain abscess with rupture into the ventricular system, and obtain a CT/MRI to confirm. S. pneumoniae meningitis is associated with cranial nerve abnormalities, mental status changes, and neurologic sequelae. With H. influenzae or S. pneumoniae meningitis, obtain a head CT/MRI to rule out other CNS pathology.
Pitfalls: If ABM is suspected, always perform lumbar puncture (LP) *before* obtaining a CT scan, since early antibiotic therapy is critical to prognosis. A CT/MRI should be obtained before LP *only* if a mass lesion/suppurative intracranial process is of primary concern, after blood cultures have been drawn. A stiff neck on physical examination has limited diagnostic value in the elderly, since nuchal rigidity may occur without meningitis (e.g., cervical arthritis) and meningitis may occur without nuchal rigidity. Recurrence of fever during the first week of H. influenzae meningitis is commonly due to subdural effusion, which usually resolves spontaneously over several days. Meningococcal meningitis may occur with or without meningococcemia. On gram stain, S. pneumoniae may be mistaken for H. influenzae, and Listeria may be mistaken for S. pneumoniae. Meningococcal meningitis may occur in those who received the meningococcal vaccine especially serogroup B not in meningococcal vaccine.
Therapeutic Considerations: Do not reduce meningeal antibiotic dosing as the patient improves. Repeat LP only if the patient is not responding to antibiotics after 48 hours; lack of response may be due to therapeutic failure, relapse, or a non-infectious CNS disorder. For S. pneumoniae meningitis, obtain penicillin MICs on all CSF isolates; nearly all penicillin-resistant strains have relatively low MICs (2–5 mcg/mL) and are susceptible to meningeal doses of beta-lactam antibiotics (e.g., ceftriaxone). All but the most highly penicillin-resistant pneumococci are still effectively treated with meningeal doses of beta-lactams. Highly resistant pneumococcal strains (rare in the CSF) may be treated for 2 weeks with meropenem 2 gm (IV) q8h, cefepime 2 gm (IV) q8h, linezolid 600 mg (IV) q12h, or vancomycin (IV/IT). Dexamethasone 0.15 mg/kg (IV) q6h × 4 days may be given to children with ABM to reduce the incidence/severity of neurologic sequelae, although the value of steroids in adult ABM is unclear; if used, give dexamethasone 30 minutes *before* the initial antibiotic dose.
Prognosis: Uniformly fatal without treatment. Case-fatality rates in treated adults are 10–20%. Neurological deficits on presentation are associated with a poor prognosis. Permanent neurological deficits are more frequent with S. pneumoniae than H. influenzae, even with prompt therapy. In meningococcal meningitis with meningococcemia, prognosis is related to the number of petechiae, with few or no neurological deficits in survivors.

Acute Bacterial Meningitis (Elderly Patients/Malignancy)

Diagnostic Considerations: Diagnosis by CSF gram stain/culture. ABM pathogens include usual pathogens in normal hosts plus Listeria monocytogenes, a gram-positive, aerobic, bacillus. Listeria is the most common ABM pathogen in patients with malignancies, and is a common pathogen in the elderly. With Listeria meningitis, CSF cultures are positive in 100%, but CSF gram stain is negative in 50%. Meningeal carcinomatosis is suggested by multiple cranial nerve abnormalities.

Pitfalls: "Diphtheroids" isolated from CSF should be speciated to rule out Listeria. Listeria are motile and hemolytic on blood agar plate, diphtheroids are not.
Therapeutic Considerations: Elderly patients and cancer patients with ABM require empiric coverage of Listeria plus other common pathogens in normal hosts (N. meningitidis, H. influenzae, S. pneumoniae). Specific monotherapy can be administered once the organism is known. Third-generation cephalosporins are not active against Listeria.
Prognosis: Related to underlying health of host.

Acute Bacterial Meningitis (CNS Shunt Infections)

Diagnostic Considerations: Diagnosis by CSF gram stain/culture. S. epidermidis meningitis usually occurs only with infected prosthetic implant material (e.g., CNS shunt/plate).
Pitfalls: Blood cultures are usually negative for shunt pathogens. CSF P. acnes cultures usually represent skin contamination. P. acnes is rarely a CNS shunt pathogen.
Therapeutic Considerations: 15% of S. epidermidis strains are resistant to nafcillin/clindamycin. In addition to systemic antibiotics in meningeal doses, adjunctive intraventricular/intrathecal antibiotics are sometimes given to control shunt infections before shunt removal. If vancomycin is used to treat CNS S. aureus (MSSA/MRSA) infection, I.T. dosing may be needed in addition to IV therapy.
Prognosis: Good if prosthetic material is removed.

Acute Non-Bacterial Meningitis/Chronic Meningitis

Subset	Usual Pathogens	Preferred IV Therapy	Alternate IV Therapy	PO Therapy or IV-to-PO Switch
Viral (aseptic)	EBV, VZV, LCM, Parvo B19, mumps, Enteroviruses, WNE. No effective therapy for most. For, HIV, effective therapy (see Chapter 5 and HIV Therapy)			
	HSV-1 HSV-2	IV Therapy: Acyclovir 10 mg/kg (IV) q8h × 10 days **or** Ganciclovir 5 mg/kg (IV) q12h × 10 days IV-to-PO Switch or PO Therapy: Acyclovir 800 mg (PO) 5x/day × 10 days **or** Valacyclovir 2 gm (PO) q6h × 10 days		
	HHV-6	Ganciclovir 5 mg/kg (IV) q12h × 2 weeks ± cidofovir 5 mg/kg (IV) plus probenecid q week × 2		
Primary amebic meningo-encephalitis	Naegleria fowleri	Amphotericin B deoxycholate 1 mg/kg (IV) q24h until cured **plus** Amphotericin B deoxycholate 1 mg into ventricles via Ommaya reservoir q24h until cured		
Lyme neuro-borreliosis	Borrelia burgdorferi	Ceftriaxone 1 gm (IV) q12h × 2 weeks **or** Minocycline 100 mg (IV) q12h × 2 weeks **or** Doxycycline 200 mg (IV) q12h × 3 days, then 100 mg (IV) q12h × 11 days		Minocycline 100 mg (PO) q12h × 2 weeks **or** Doxycycline 200 mg (PO) q12h × 3 days, then 100 mg (PO) q12h × 11 days (loading dose not needed PO if given IV with same drug)

Acute Non-Bacterial Meningitis/Chronic Meningitis

Subset	Usual Pathogens	Preferred IV Therapy	Alternate IV Therapy	PO Therapy or IV-to-PO Switch
Granulomatous amebic meningoencephalitis	Acanthamoeba	No proven treatment (amphotericin B, fluconazole, ketoconazole, itraconazole, flucytosine, rifampin, isoniazid, aminoglycosides, sulfonamides, pentamidine mostly with little success. Success reported in transplant recipient with IV pentamidine followed by itraconazole, and in AIDS patient with ketoconazole plus flucytosine)		
TB	M. tuberculosis	IV Therapy Not applicable	PO Therapy Begin with 4 drugs, as for pulmonary TB, but extend treatment for 9–12 months. Corticosteroids tapered over 1–2 months is helpful. If resistance is demonstrated or suspected, ID consultation is advised	
Fungal *Non-HIV*	Cryptococcus neoformans	Amphotericin B deoxycholate 0.7–1 mg/kg (IV) q24h × 2–6 weeks* **plus** Flucytosine 25 mg/kg (PO) q6h × 6 weeks*, **followed by** Fluconazole 800 mg (IV or PO) × 1 dose, then 400 mg (PO) q24h × 10 weeks*	Liposomal amphotericin B (AmBisome) 6 mg/kg (IV) q24h × 6–10 weeks† **or** Fluconazole 800 mg (IV or PO) × 1 dose, then 400 mg (PO) q24h × 10 weeks*	PO therapy alone Fluconazole may be given PO*
HIV	Cryptococcus neoformans: see p. 325 Blastomyces dermatitidis: see p. 264			
Chronic meningitis	M. tuberculosis, Brucella, Leptospirosis, T. pallidum, Cryptococcus, Coccidioidomycosis, Histoplasmosis, Toxoplasmosis, Toxocariasis, CMV, Neurocysticercosis, Neuroborreliosis, Enteroviruses			Treat pathogen after confirming diagnosis. Do not treat empirically

Duration of therapy represents total time PO (for TB), IV, or IV + PO.

* The 6-week amphotericin B deoxycholate plus flucytosine regimen is the classical approach to achieving a durable cure. Anecdotal data suggest that a shorter course followed by Fluconazole × 10 weeks (or longer) may be successful. ID consultation is advised.

† Other lipid-associated amphotericin B formulations at 3–5 mg/kg (IV) q24h may also be used (p. 513).

‡ Levofloxacin 500 mg or Moxifloxacin 400 mg.

Viral (Aseptic) Meningitis

Clinical Presentation: Headache, low-grade fever, mild meningismus, photophobia.

Diagnostic Considerations: Diagnosis by specific serological tests/viral culture. HSV-2 genital infections are often accompanied by mild CNS symptoms, which usually do not require anti-viral therapy. HSV-1 causes a variety of CNS infections, including meningitis, meningoencephalitis, and encephalitis (most common; see p. 25). HSV HHV-6, and WNE meningitis is indistinguishable clinically from other causes of viral meningitis. EBV meningitis is usually associated with clinical/laboratory features of EBV infectious mononucleosis; suspect the diagnosis in a patient with a positive monospot and unexplained meningoencephalitis. VZV meningitis is typically associated with cutaneous vesicular lesions (H. zoster), and usually does not require additional therapy beyond that given for shingles. LCM meningitis begins as a "flu-like" illness usually in the fall after hamster contact, and may have low CSF glucose. Enterovirus meningitis is often associated with a maculopapular rash, non-exudative pharyngitis, diarrhea, and rarely low CSF glucose. Aseptic meningitis due to mumps may present without parotid swelling ± acute deafness. Drug induced aseptic meningitis may have eosinophils in the CSF and little/no fever.

Pitfalls: Consider NSAIDs, TMP–SMX, and IV immunoglobulin as causes of drug induced aseptic meningitis.

Therapeutic Considerations: Treat specific pathogen.

Prognosis: Without neurological deficits, full recovery is the rule.

Primary Amebic Meningoencephalitis (PAM) (Naegleria fowleri)

Clinical Presentation: Acquired by freshwater exposure containing the protozoa, often by jumping into a lake/pool. Affects healthy children/young adults. Organism penetrates cribriform plate and enters CSF. Symptoms occur within 7 days of exposure and may be indistinguishable from fulminant bacterial meningitis, including headache, fever, anorexia, vomiting, signs of meningeal inflammation, altered mental status, coma. May complain of unusual smell/taste sensations early in infection. CSF has RBCs and very low glucose.

Diagnostic Considerations: Diagnosis by demonstrating organism in CSF. Worldwide distribution. Free-living freshwater amoeba flourish in warmer climates. Key to diagnosis rests on clinical suspicion based on history of freshwater exposure in previous 1–2 weeks.

Pitfalls: CSF findings resemble bacterial meningitis, but RBCs present.

Therapeutic Considerations: Often fatal despite early treatment.

Prognosis: Frequently fatal.

Granulomatous Amebic Meningoencephalitis (Acanthamoeba)

Clinical Presentation: Insidious onset with focal neurologic deficits ± mental status changes, seizures, fever, headache, hemiparesis, meningismus, ataxia, visual disturbances. May be associated with Acanthamoeba keratoconjunctivitis, skin ulcers, or disseminated disease. Usually seen only in immunocompromised/debilitated patients.

Diagnostic Considerations: Diagnosis by demonstrating organism in brain biopsy specimen. CT/MRI shows mass lesions. "Stellate cysts" characteristic of Acanthamoeba. Worldwide distribution. Strong association with extended wear of contact lenses. Differentiate from N. fowleri by culture.

Pitfalls: Not associated with freshwater exposure, unlike primary amebic meningoencephalitis (Naegleria fowleri). Resembles subacute/chronic meningitis. No trophozoites in CSF. Skin lesions may be present for months before onset of CNS symptoms.

Therapeutic Considerations: No proven treatment. Often fatal despite early treatment.
Prognosis: Usually fatal.

TB Meningitis (Mycobacterium tuberculosis)

Clinical Presentation: Subacute onset of non-specific symptoms. Fever usually present ± headache, nausea, vomiting. Acute presentation and cranial nerve palsies uncommon.
Diagnostic Considerations: Diagnosis by CSF AFB smear/culture; PCR of CSF is sensitive/specific. CSF may be normal but usually shows a mild lymphocytic pleocytosis, ↓ glucose, ↑ protein, and few RBCs.
Pitfalls: CSF may have PMN predominance early, before developing typical lymphocytic predominance. Eosinophils in CSF is not a feature of TB, and should suggest another diagnosis. Chest x-ray, PPD, and CSF smear/culture may be negative.
Therapeutic Considerations: Dexamethasone 4 mg (IV or PO) q6h × 4–8 weeks is useful to reduce CSF inflammation if given early.
Prognosis: Poor prognostic factors include delay in treatment, neurologic deficits, or hydrocephalus. Proteinaceous TB exudates may obstruct ventricles and cause hydrocephalus, which is diagnosed by CT/MRI and may require shunt.

Fungal (Cryptococcal) Meningitis (Cryptococcus neoformans)

Clinical Presentation: Insidious onset of non-specific symptoms. Headache most common. Chronic cases may have CNS symptoms for weeks to months with intervening asymptomatic periods. Acute manifestations are more common in AIDS, chronic steroid therapy, lymphoreticular malignancies. 50–80% of patients are abnormal hosts.
Diagnostic Considerations: C. neoformans is the most common cause of fungal meningitis, and the only encapsulated yeast in the CSF to cause meningitis. Diagnosis by CSF India ink preparations showing encapsulated yeasts/cryptococcal latex antigen by latex agglutination/culture. Rule out HIV and other underlying immunosuppressive diseases.
Pitfalls: CSF latex antigen titer may not return to zero. Continue treatment until titers decline/do not decrease further, and until CSF culture is negative for cryptococci. India ink preparations showing encapsulated yeasts of CSF are useful for initial infection, but should not be relied on to diagnose recurrent episodes, since smears may be positive despite negative CSF cultures (dead cryptococci may remain in CSF for years). Diagnosis of recurrences rests on CSF culture.
Therapeutic Considerations: Treat until CSF is sterile or CSF latex antigen titer is zero or remains near zero on serial lumbar punctures. After patient defervesces on deoxycholate/5FC, switch to oral fluconazole × 10 weeks. Lipid-associated formulations of amphotericin B may be used if amphotericin B deoxycholate cannot be tolerated (p. 513). HIV patients require life-long suppressive therapy with fluconazole 200 mg (PO) q24h. Expert consultation is strongly advised.
Prognosis: Good. Poor prognostic factors include no CSF pleocytosis, many organisms in CSF, and altered consciousness on admission.

Chronic Meningitis

Clinical Presentation: Same as acute meningitis, but signs/symptoms less prominent and clinical presentation is subacute (> 1 month). Chronic neuroborreliosis is extremely rare.
Diagnostic Considerations: Differential diagnosis is too broad for empiric treatment. Subacute/chronic clinical presentation allows time for complete diagnostic work-up. Culture CSF and obtain

CSF/serum tests to identify a specific pathogen, then treat. CNS Lyme is diagnosed by demonstrating B. burgdorferi antibody production in the CNS. A CSF-to-serum IgM Lyme titer ratio > 1:1 is diagnostic.

Pitfalls: If infectious etiology is not found, consider NSAIDs, SLE, meningeal carcinomatosis, sarcoidosis, etc. Chronic CMV or enterococcal meningitis should prompt search for underlying host defense defects/immunosuppression. Neuroborreliosis cannot be reliably diagnosed using CSF-to-serum IgM if antibiotics given before the LP (antibiotics change the ratio and render it useless).

Therapeutic Considerations: If suspicion of TB meningitis is high, empiric anti-TB treatment is warranted. Otherwise, treat only after diagnosing specific infection.

Prognosis: Related to underlying health of host. Prognosis with neuroborreliosis is good even with delayed treatment.

Encephalitis

Subset	Usual Pathogens	IV-to-PO Switch		
Herpes	HSV-1 HSV-2	IV Therapy: Acyclovir 10 mg/kg (IV) q8h × 10 days **or** ganciclovir 5 mg/kg (IV) q12h × 10 days IV-to-PO Switch or PO Therapy: Acyclovir 800 mg (PO) 5x/day × 10 days **or** Valacyclovir 2 gm (PO) q6h × 10 days		
	HHV-6	Ganciclovir 5 mg/kg (IV) q12h × 2 weeks ± cidofovir 5 mg/kg (IV) plus probenecid q week × 2		
Arbovirus	Usual Pathogens: California encephalitis (CE), Western equine encephalitis (WEE), Venezuelan equine encephalitis (VEE), Eastern equine encephalitis (EEE), St. Louis encephalitis (SLE), Japanese encephalitis (JE), West Nile encephalitis (WNE) IV/PO Therapy: Not applicable			
Mycoplasma	M. pneumoniae	Doxycycline 200 mg (IV) q12h × 3 days, then 100 mg (IV) q12h × 2 weeks	Minocycline 100 mg (IV) q12h × 2 weeks	Doxycycline 200 mg (PO) q12h × 3 days, then 100 mg (PO) q12h × 2 weeks* **or** Minocycline 100 mg (PO) q12h × 2 weeks
Listeria	L. monocytogenes	Treat the same as for Listeria meningitis (p. 18)		
HIV	see Chapter 5 p. 300			
Solid organ transplants, HIV/AIDS	CMV Toxoplasma gondii	For organ transplants, see p. 157. For HIV/AIDS, see p. 300		

Duration of therapy represents total time IV or IV + PO. Most patients on IV therapy able to take PO meds should be switched to PO therapy after clinical improvement.

* Loading dose is not needed PO if given IV with the same drug.

Herpes Encephalitis (HSV-1)

Clinical Presentation: Acute onset of fever and change in mental status without nuchal rigidity.

Diagnostic Considerations: EEG is best early (< 72 hours) presumptive test, showing unilateral temporal lobe abnormalities. Brain MRI is abnormal before CT scan, which may require several days before a temporal lobe focus is seen. Definitive diagnosis is by CSF PCR for HSV-1 DNA. Usually presents as encephalitis or meningoencephalitis; presentation as meningitis alone is uncommon. Profound decrease in sensorium is characteristic of HSV meningoencephalitis. CSF may have PMN predominance and low glucose levels, unlike other viral causes of meningitis.

Pitfalls: In normal hosts, HHV-6 may mimic HSV-1 encephalitis with a frontal/temporal focus on EEG.

Therapeutic Considerations: HSV is the only treatable common cause of viral encephalitis in normal hosts. Treat as soon as possible, since neurological deficits may be mild and reversible early on, but severe and irreversible later.

Prognosis: Related to extent of brain injury and early anti-HSV therapy.

Arboviral Encephalitis

Clinical Presentation: Acute onset of fever, headache, change in mental status days to weeks after inoculation of virus through the bite of an infected insect (e.g., mosquito/tick). May progress over several days to stupor/coma.

Diagnostic Considerations: Diagnosis by specific arboviral serology.

Pitfalls: Usually occurs in summer/fall. Diagnosis suggested by arboviral contact/travel history. Electrolyte abnormalities due to syndrome of inappropriate antidiuretic hormone (SIADH) may occur.

Therapeutic Considerations: Only supportive therapy is available at present.

Prognosis: Permanent neurological deficits are common, but not predictable. May be fatal.

Mycoplasma Encephalitis

Clinical Presentation: Acute onset of fever and change in mental status without nuchal rigidity.

Diagnostic Considerations: Diagnosis suggested by CNS and extra-pulmonary manifestations–sore throat, otitis, E. multiforme, soft stools/diarrhea–in a patient with community-acquired pneumonia, elevated IgM mycoplasma titers, and very high (≥ 1:1024) cold agglutinin titers. CSF shows mild mononucleosis/pleocytosis and normal/low glucose.

Pitfalls: CNS findings may overshadow pulmonary findings.

Therapeutic Considerations: Macrolides will treat pulmonary infection, but not CNS infection (due to poor CNS penetration).

Prognosis: With early treatment, prognosis is good without neurologic sequelae.

Listeria Encephalitis

Clinical Presentation: Fever/mental confusion (encephalitis/cerebritis) ± nuchal rigidity (meningoencephalitis).

Diagnostic Considerations: Diagnosis by LP. Suspect Listeria if CSF with "purulent profile" plus RBCs. Listeria seen on Gram stain of CSF in 50%; but culture positive in 100%.

Pitfalls: Not to be confused with other gram-positive bacilli (skin contaminants) isolated from CSF (diphtheroids). Listeria are motile and hemolytic on blood agar.

Therapeutic Considerations: 3rd generation cephalosporins not active against Listeria. In penicillin-tolerant patients, use meningeal dose ampicillin (not penicillin).

Prognosis: Good with early/adequate treatment. Related to degree of T lymphocyte dysfunction.

CMV Encephalitis (see p. 159)

Toxoplasma Encephalitis (see p. 326)

Brain Abscess/Subdural Empyema/Cavernous Vein Thrombosis/Intracranial Suppurative Thrombophlebitis

<table>
<thead>
<tr><th>Subset</th><th>Usual Pathogens</th><th>Preferred IV Therapy</th><th>Alternate IV Therapy</th><th>IV-to-PO Switch</th></tr>
</thead>
<tbody>
<tr><td colspan="5">Brain Abscess (Single Mass Lesion)</td></tr>
<tr><td>Open trauma</td><td>S. aureus (MSSA) Enterobacteriaceae P. aeruginosa</td><td>Meropenem 2 gm (IV) q8h × 2 weeks</td><td>Cefepime 2 gm (IV) q8h × 2 weeks</td><td>Not applicable</td></tr>
<tr><td>Neurosurgical procedure
(Treat initially for MSSA; if later identified as MRSA, MSSE or MRSE, treat accordingly)</td><td>S. aureus
S. epidermidis (CoNS)</td><td colspan="2"><u>MSSA</u>
Nafcillin 2 gm (IV) q4h × 2 weeks
or
<u>MRSA/MSSE/MRSE</u>
Linezolid 600 mg (IV) q12h × 2 weeks
or
Minocycline 100 mg (IV) q12h × 2 weeks</td><td><u>MSSA/MRSA/MSSE/MRSE</u>
Linezolid 600 mg (PO) q12h × 2 weeks
or
Minocycline 100 mg (PO) q12h × 2 weeks</td></tr>
<tr><td>Mastoid/otitic source</td><td>Enterobacter
Proteus</td><td colspan="3">Treat the same as for open trauma, above</td></tr>
<tr><td>Dental source</td><td>Oral anaerobes
Actinomyces</td><td colspan="2">Ceftriaxone 2 gm (IV) q12h × 2 weeks
plus
Metronidazole 500 mg (IV) q12h × 2 weeks</td><td>Ceftizoxime 3 gm (IV) q6h × 2 weeks</td></tr>
<tr><td>Subdural empyema/sinus source</td><td>Oral anaerobes
H. influenzae</td><td colspan="3">Treat the same as for dental source, above</td></tr>
<tr><td rowspan="2">Cardiac source (ABE; right-to-left shunt)</td><td>S. aureus (MSSA)
S. pneumoniae
H. influenzae</td><td>Ceftriaxone 2 gm (IV) q12h × 2 weeks</td><td colspan="2">Meropenem 2 gm (IV) q8h × 2 weeks</td></tr>
<tr><td>S. aureus (MRSA)</td><td colspan="2">Linezolid 600 mg (IV) q12h × 2 weeks
or
Vancomycin 2 gm (IV) q12h × 2 weeks
or
Minocycline 100 mg (IV) q12h × 2 weeks</td><td>Linezolid 600 mg (PO) q12h × 2 weeks
or
Minocycline 100 mg (PO) q12h × 2 weeks</td></tr>
</tbody>
</table>

Brain Abscess/Subdural Empyema/Cavernous Vein Thrombosis/Intracranial Suppurative Thrombophlebitis (cont'd)

Subset	Usual Pathogens	Preferred IV Therapy	Alternate IV Therapy	IV-to-PO Switch
Brain Abscess (Single Mass Lesion)				
Pulmonary source	Oral anaerobes Actinomyces	Ceftriaxone 2 gm (IV) q12h × 2 weeks **plus** Metronidazole 500 mg (IV) q12h × 2 weeks		Ceftizoxime 3 gm (IV) q6h × 2 weeks

MSSA/MRSA = methicillin-sensitive/resistant S. aureus; MSSE/MRSE = methicillin-sensitive/resistant S. epidermidis. Duration of therapy represents total time IV or IV + PO. Most patients on IV therapy able to take PO meds should be switched to PO therapy after clinical improvement.

Clinical Presentation: Variable presentation, with fever, change in mental status, cranial nerve abnormalities ± headache.

Diagnostic Considerations: Diagnosis by CSF gram stain/culture. If brain abscess is suspected, obtain head CT/MRI. Lumbar puncture may induce herniation.

Pitfalls: CSF analysis is negative for bacterial meningitis unless abscess ruptures into ventricular system.

Therapeutic Considerations: Treatment with meningeal doses of antibiotics is required. Large single abscesses may be surgically drained; multiple small abscesses are best treated medically.

Prognosis: Related to underlying source and health of host.

Brain Abscess (Mastoid/Otitic Source)

Diagnostic Considerations: Diagnosis by head CT/MRI demonstrating focus of infection in mastoid.

Pitfalls: Rule out associated subdural empyema.

Therapeutic Considerations: ENT consult for possible surgical debridement of mastoid.

Prognosis: Good. May require mastoid debridement for cure.

Brain Abscess (Dental Source)

Diagnostic Considerations: Diagnosis by panorex x-rays/gallium scan of jaw demonstrating focus in mandible/erosion into sinuses.

Pitfalls: Apical root abscess may not be apparent clinically.

Therapeutic Considerations: Large single abscess may be surgically drained. Multiple small abscesses are best treated medically. Treat until lesions on CT/MRI resolve or do not become smaller on therapy.

Prognosis: Good if dental focus is removed.

Brain Abscess (Subdural Empyema/Sinus Source)

Diagnostic Considerations: Diagnosis by sinus films/CT/MRI to confirm presence of sinusitis/bone erosion (cranial osteomyelitis/epidural abscess). Usually from paranasal sinusitis.

Pitfalls: Do not overlook underlying sinus infection, which may need surgical drainage.
Therapeutic Considerations: Obtain ENT consult for possible surgical debridement of sinuses.
Prognosis: Good prognosis if sinus is drained.

Brain Abscess (Cardiac Source; Acute Bacterial Endocarditis)

Diagnostic Considerations: Blood cultures often positive if brain abscess due to acute bacterial endocarditis (ABE) pathogen. Head CT/MRI shows multiple mass lesions.
Pitfalls: Do not overlook right-to-left cardiac shunt (e.g., patent foramen ovale, atrial septal defect) as source of brain abscess. Cerebral embolization results in aseptic meningitis in SBE, but septic meningitis/brain abscess in ABE (due to high virulence of pathogens).
Therapeutic Considerations: Multiple lesions suggest hematogenous spread. Use susceptibility of blood culture isolates to determine coverage. Meningeal doses are the same as endocarditis doses.
Prognosis: Related to location/size of CNS lesions and extent of cardiac valvular involvement.

Brain Abscess (Pulmonary Source)

Diagnostic Considerations: Diagnosis suggested by underlying bronchiectasis, empyema, cystic fibrosis, or lung abscess in a patient with a brain abscess.
Pitfalls: Brain abscesses are most often due to chronic suppurative lung disease (e.g., bronchiectasis, lung abscess/empyema), not chronic bronchitis/AECB.
Therapeutic Considerations: Lung abscess may need surgical drainage.
Prognosis: Related to extent/location of CNS lesions, drainage of lung abscess/empyema, and control of lung infection.

Empiric Therapy of HEENT Infections

Facial/Periorbital Cellulitis

Subset	Usual Pathogens	Preferred IV Therapy	Alternate IV Therapy	PO Therapy or IV-to-PO Switch
Facial cellulitis	Group A streptococci H. influenzae	Ceftriaxone 1 gm (IV) q24h × 2 weeks **or** Cefotaxime 2 gm (IV) q6h × 2 weeks **or** Ceftizoxime 2 gm (IV) q8h × 2 weeks	Quinolone* (IV) q24h × 2 weeks	Any oral 2nd or 3rd gen. cephalosporin × 2 weeks **or** Quinolone* (PO) q24h × 2 weeks

Duration of therapy represents total time IV, PO, or IV + PO. Most patients on IV therapy able to take PO meds should be switched to PO therapy soon after clinical improvement (usually < 72 hours).

* Levofloxacin 500 mg or Moxifloxacin 400 mg.

Clinical Presentation: Acute onset of warm, painful, facial rash without discharge, swelling, pruritus.
Diagnostic Considerations: Diagnosis by clinical appearance. May spread rapidly across face. Purplish hue suggests H. influenzae.
Pitfalls: If periorbital cellulitis, obtain head CT/MRI to rule out underlying sinusitis/CNS involvement. If secondary to an abrasion after contact with a saliva-contaminated surface, consider Herpes gladiatorum; lesions are painful/edematous and do not respond to antibiotic therapy for cellulitis.
Therapeutic Considerations: May need to treat × 3 weeks in compromised hosts (chronic steroids, diabetics, SLE, etc.).
Prognosis: Good with early treatment; worse if underlying sinusitis/CNS involvement.

Bacterial Sinusitis

Subset	Usual Pathogens	IV Therapy (Hospitalized)	PO Therapy or IV-to-PO Switch (Ambulatory)
Acute	S. pneumoniae H. influenzae M. catarrhalis	Quinolone† (IV) q24h × 1–2 weeks **or** Ceftriaxone 1 gm (IV) q24h × 1– 2 weeks **or** Doxycycline 200 mg (IV) q12h × 3 days, then 100 mg (IV) q12h × 11 days	Quinolone† (PO) q24h × 1–2 weeks **or** Amoxicillin/clavulanic acid XR 2 tablets (PO) q12h × 10 days **or** Doxycycline 200 mg (PO) q12h × 3 days, then 100 mg (PO) q12h × 11 days* **or** Cephalosporin‡ (PO) × 2 weeks **or** Clarithromycin XL 1 gm (PO) q24h × 2 weeks
Chronic	Same as acute + oral anaerobes	Requires prolonged antimicrobial therapy (2–4 weeks)	

Duration of therapy represents total time IV, PO, or IV + PO in adults. Most patients on IV therapy able to take PO meds should be switched to PO therapy soon after clinical improvement (usually < 72 hours). See Chapter 7 for pediatric therapy.
* Loading dose is not needed PO if given IV with the same drug.
† Moxifloxacin 400 mg × 7 days or Levofloxacin 750 mg × 5 days.
‡ Cefdinir 300 mg q12h or Cefditoren 400 mg q12h or Cefixime 400 mg q12h or Cefpodoxime 200 mg q12h.

Acute Bacterial Sinusitis (adults)

Clinical Presentation: Nasal discharge and cough frequently with headache, facial pain, and low-grade fever lasting > 10–14 days. Can also present acutely with high fever (≥ 104°F) and purulent nasal discharge ± intense headache lasting for ≥ 3 days. Other manifestations depend on the affected sinus: maxillary sinus: percussion tenderness of molars; maxillary toothache; local extension may cause osteomyelitis of facial bones with proptosis, retroorbital cellulitis, ophthalmoplegia; direct intracranial extension is rare; frontal sinus: prominent headache; intracranial extension may cause epidural/brain abscess, meningitis, cavernous sinus/superior sagittal sinus thrombosis; orbital extension may cause periorbital cellulitis; ethmoid sinus: eyelid edema and prominent tearing; extension may cause retroorbital pain/periorbital cellulitis and/or cavernous sinus/superior sagittal sinus thrombosis; sphenoid sinus: severe headache; extension into cavernous sinus may cause meningitis, cranial nerve paralysis [III, IV, VI], temporal lobe abscess, cavernous sinus thrombosis). Cough and nasal discharge are prominent in children.

Diagnostic Considerations: Diagnosis by sinus x-rays or CT/MRI showing complete sinus opacification, air-fluid levels, mucosal thickening. Consider sinus aspiration in immunocompromised hosts or treatment failures. In children, acute sinusitis is a clinical diagnosis; imaging studies are not routine.

Pitfalls: May present as periorbital cellulitis (obtain head CT/MRI to rule out underlying sinusitis). If CT/MRI demonstrates "post-septal" involvement, treat as acute bacterial meningitis. In children, transillumination, sinus tenderness to percussion, and color of nasal mucus are not reliable indicators of sinusitis.

Therapeutic Considerations: Treat for full course to prevent relapses/complications. Macrolides and TMP–SMX may predispose to drug-resistant S. pneumoniae (DRSP), and ≥ 30% of S. pneumoniae are naturally resistant to macrolides. Consider local resistance rates before making empiric antibiotic selections.

Prognosis: Good if treated for full course. Relapses may occur with suboptimal treatment. For frequent recurrences, consider radiologic studies and ENT consultation.

Chronic Bacterial Sinusitis (adults)

Clinical Presentation: Generalized headache, fatigue, nasal congestion, post-nasal drip lasting > 3 months with little/no sinus tenderness by percussion. Local symptoms often subtle. Fever is uncommon.

Diagnostic Considerations: Sinus films and head CT/MRI are less useful than for acute sinusitis (chronic mucosal abnormalities may persist after infection is treated). Many cases of chronic maxillary sinusitis are due to a dental cause; obtain odontogenic x-rays if suspected.

Pitfalls: Clinical presentation is variable/non-specific. Malaise and irritability may be more prominent than local symptoms. May be mistaken for allergic rhinitis. Head CT/MRI can rule out sinus tumor.

Therapeutic Considerations: Therapeutic failure/relapse is usually due to inadequate antibiotic duration, dose, or tissue penetration. Treat for full course. If symptoms persist after 4 weeks of therapy, refer to ENT for surgical drainage procedure.

Prognosis: Good if treated for full course. Relapses may occur with suboptimal treatment. For frequent recurrences, consider radiologic studies and ENT consultation.

Keratitis

Subset	Pathogens	Topical Therapy
Bacterial	S. aureus S. pneumoniae Bacillus cereus M. catarrhalis P. aeruginosa	Antibacterial eyedrops (ciprofloxacin, ofloxacin, or tobramycin/bacitracin/polymyxin B) hourly while awake × 2 weeks
Viral	HSV-1	Trifluridine 1% solution 1 drop hourly while awake × 2 days, then 1 drop q6h × 14–21 days ***or*** viral ophthalmic topical ointment (e.g., vidarabine) at bedtime × 14–21 days

Keratitis (cont'd)

Subset	Pathogens	Topical Therapy
Amebic	Acanthamoeba	Propamidine (0.1%), neomycin, gramicidin, or polymyxin B eyedrops hourly while awake × 1–2 weeks **or** polyhexamethylene biguanide (0.02%) eyedrops hourly while awake × 1–2 weeks **or** chlorhexidine (0.02%) eyedrops hourly while awake × 1–2 weeks

Clinical Presentation: Corneal haziness, infiltrates, or ulcers.
Diagnosis: Appearance of corneal lesions/culture.

Bacterial Keratitis

Diagnostic Considerations: Usually secondary to eye trauma. Always obtain ophthalmology consult.
Pitfalls: Be sure to culture ulcer. Unusual organisms are common in eye trauma.
Therapeutic Considerations: Treat until lesions resolve. Ointment easier/lasts longer than solutions. Avoid topical steroids.
Prognosis: Related to extent of trauma/organism. S. aureus, B. cereus, P. aeruginosa have worst prognosis.

Viral Keratitis (HSV-1)

Diagnostic Considerations: "Dendritic" corneal ulcers characteristic. Obtain ophthalmology consult.
Pitfalls: Small corneal ulcers may be missed without fluorescein staining.
Therapeutic Considerations: Treat until lesions resolve. Oral acyclovir is not needed. Avoid ophthalmic steroid ointment.
Prognosis: Good if treated early (before eye damage is extensive).

Amebic Keratitis (Acanthamoeba)

Diagnostic Considerations: Usually associated with extended use of soft contact lenses. Corneal scrapings are positive with calcofluor staining. Acanthamoeba keratitis is painful with typical circular, hazy, corneal infiltrate. Always obtain ophthalmology consult.
Pitfalls: Do not confuse with HSV-1 dendritic ulcers. Avoid topical steroids.
Therapeutic Considerations: If secondary bacterial infection, treat as bacterial keratitis.
Prognosis: No good treatment. Poor prognosis.

Conjunctivitis

Subset	Usual Pathogens	PO/Topical Therapy
Bacterial	M. catarrhalis H. influenzae S. pneumoniae N. meninsititis N. gonorrhea	Antibacterial eyedrops (ciprofloxacin, ofloxacin, moxifloxacin, or tobramycin/bacitracin/polymyxin B) q12h × 1 week plus antibacterial ointment (same antibiotic) at bedtime × 1 week

Conjunctivitis (cont'd)

Subset	Usual Pathogens	PO/Topical Therapy
Viral	Adenovirus	Not applicable
	VZV	Famciclovir 500 mg (PO) q8h × 10–14 days **or** Valacyclovir 1 gm (PO) q8h × 10–14 days
Chlamydial	C. trachomatis (trachoma)	Doxycycline 100 mg (PO) q12h × 1–2 weeks **or** Azithromycin 1 gm (PO) × 1 dose

Bacterial Conjunctivitis

Clinical Presentation: Profuse, purulent exudate from conjunctiva.

Diagnostic Considerations: Reddened conjunctiva; culture for specific pathogen.

Pitfalls: Do not confuse with allergic conjunctivitis, which itches and has a clear discharge.

Therapeutic Considerations: Obtain ophthalmology consult. Ointment lasts longer in eye than solution. Do not use topical steroids without an antibacterial.

Prognosis: Excellent when treated early, with no residual visual impairment.

Viral Conjunctivitis

Adenovirus

Clinical Presentation: Reddened conjunctiva, watery discharge, negative bacterial culture.

Diagnostic Considerations: Diagnosis by cloudy/steamy cornea with negative bacterial cultures. Clue is punctate infiltrates with a cloudy cornea. Extremely contagious; careful handwashing is essential. Obtain viral culture of conjunctiva for diagnosis.

Pitfalls: Pharyngitis a clue to adenoviral etiology (pharyngoconjunctival fever).

Therapeutic Considerations: No treatment available. Usually resolves in 1–2 weeks.

Prognosis: Related to degree of corneal haziness. Severe cases may take weeks to clear.

VZV Ophthalmicus

Diagnostic Considerations: Vesicles on tip of nose predict eye involvement.

Pitfalls: Do not miss vesicular lesions in external auditory canal in patients with facial palsy (Ramsey-Hunt Syndrome).

Therapeutic Considerations: Obtain ophthalmology consult. Topical steroids may be used if given with anti-VZV therapy.

Prognosis: Good if treated early with systemic antivirals.

Trachoma (C. trachomatis) Conjunctivitis

Diagnostic Considerations: Diagnosis by direct fluorescent antibody (DFA)/culture of conjunctiva.

Pitfalls: Do not confuse bilateral, upper lid, granular conjunctivitis of Chlamydia with viral/bacterial conjunctivitis, which involves both upper and lower eyelids.

Therapeutic Considerations: Ophthalmic erythromycin treatment is useful for neonates. Single-dose azithromycin may be associated with recurrence.

Prognosis: Excellent with early treatment.

Chorioretinitis

Subset	Usual Pathogens	Preferred IV Therapy	Alternate IV Therapy	PO Therapy or IV-to-PO Switch
Viral	CMV	See p. 334		
Fungal†	Candida albicans	Fluconazole 800 mg (IV) × 1 dose, then 400 mg (IV) q24h × 2 weeks‡ **or** Caspofungin 70 mg (IV) × 1 dose, then 50 mg (IV) q24h × 2 weeks‡	Amphotericin B deoxycholate 0.6 mg/kg (IV) q24h for total of 1 gm **or** Lipid-associated formulation of amphotericin B (p. 513) (IV) q24h × 3 weeks‡	Fluconazole 800 mg (PO) × 1 dose, then 400 mg (PO) q24h × 2 weeks*‡
Protozoal	Toxoplasma gondii	IV Therapy Not applicable	PO Therapy Pyrimethamine 75 mg (PO) × 1 dose, then 25 mg (PO) q24h × 6 weeks **plus either** Sulfadiazine 1 gm (PO) q6h × 6 weeks **or** Clindamycin 300 mg (PO) q8h × 6 weeks	

Duration of therapy represents total time IV, PO, or IV + PO. Most patients on IV therapy able to take PO meds should be switched to PO therapy after clinical improvement.

† Treat only IV or IV-to-PO switch.

* Loading dose is not needed PO if given IV with the same drug.

‡ Duration of therapy is approximate and should be continued until resolution of disease. Close follow-up with an ophthalmologist is required.

CMV Chorioretinitis (see p. 334)

Candida Chorioretinitis

Clinical Presentation: Small, raised, white, circular lesions on retina.

Diagnostic Considerations: Fundus findings similar to white, raised colonies on blood agar plates.

Pitfalls: Candida endophthalmitis signifies invasive/disseminated candidiasis.

Therapeutic Considerations: Treat as disseminated candidiasis.

Prognosis: Good with early treatment.

Toxoplasma Chorioretinitis

Clinical Presentation: Grey/black pigmentation of macula.

Diagnostic Considerations: Diagnosis by IgM IFA toxoplasmosis titers.

Pitfalls: Unilateral endophthalmitis usually indicates acquired toxoplasmosis; congenital toxoplasmosis is usually bilateral.

Therapeutic Considerations: Obtain ophthalmology consult. Treat only acute/active toxoplasmosis with visual symptoms; do not treat chronic chorioretinitis. Add folinic acid 10 mg (PO) q24h to prevent folic acid deficiency.

Prognosis: Related to degree of immunosuppression.

Endophthalmitis

Subset	Usual Pathogens	Preferred IV Therapy	Alternate IV Therapy	PO Therapy or IV-to-PO Switch
Bacterial (Treat initially for MSSA; if later identified as MRSA or S. epidermidis, treat accordingly)	Streptococci H. influenzae S. aureus (MSSA)	Intravitreal injection: Cefepime 2.25 mg/0.1 mL sterile saline × 1 dose; repeat × 1 if needed in 2–3 days **plus** Subconjunctival injection: Cefepime 100 mg/0.5 mL sterile saline q24h × 1–2 weeks **plus** Levofloxacin 500 mg (IV/PO) q12h × 1–2 weeks		
	S. aureus (MRSA) S. epidermidis (CoNS)	Intravitreal injection: Vancomycin 1 mg/0.1 mL sterile saline × 1 dose; repeat × 1 if needed in 2–3 days **plus** Subconjunctival injection: Vancomycin 2.5 mg/0.5 mL sterile saline q24h × 1–2 weeks **plus** Linezolid 600 mg (IV/PO) q12h × 1–2 weeks		
Fungal‡	C. albicans	Fluconazole 800 mg (IV) × 1 dose, then 400 mg (IV) q24h × 2 months	Voriconazole (see "usual dose," p. 695) × 2 months	Fluconazole (same as IV dose) **or** Voriconazole (see p. 695) × 2 months
	A. fumigatus A. flavus	Amphotericin B (intravitreal) 10 mcg (in 0.1 mL of saline) q2–3 days	Voriconazole (see "usual dose," p. 695) × 2 months	Voriconazole (see "usual dose," p. 695) × 2 months
TB	M. tuberculosis	Treat the same as for TB pneumonia (p. 52)		
Infected lens implant* (Treat initially for MSSA; if later identified as MRSA, treat accordingly)	Enterobacteriaceae S. aureus (MSSA)	Meropenem 1 gm (IV) q8h × 2 weeks **or** Cefepime 2 gm (IV) q8h × 2 weeks	Chloramphenicol 500 mg (IV) q6h × 2 weeks	Chloramphenicol 500 mg (PO) q6h × 2 weeks
	S. aureus (MRSA)	Linezolid 600 mg (IV) q12h × 2 weeks	Minocycline 100 mg (IV) q12h × 2 weeks	Linezolid 600 mg (PO) q12h × 2 weeks **or** Minocycline 100 mg (PO) q12h × 2 weeks

EMB = ethambutol; INH = isoniazid; MSSA/MRSA = methicillin-sensitive/resistant S. aureus; PZA = pyrazinamide. Duration of therapy represents total time IV, PO, or IV + PO. Most patients on IV therapy able to take PO meds should be switched to PO therapy after clinical improvement (usually < 72 hours).

* Treat only IV or IV-to-PO switch.

‡ Duration of therapy is approximate and should be continued until resolution of disease. Close follow-up with an ophthalmologist is required.

Bacterial Endophthalmitis

Clinical Presentation: Ocular pain/sudden vision loss.

Diagnosis: Post-op endophthalmitis occurs 1–7 days after surgery. Hypopyon seen in anterior chamber.

Pitfalls: Delayed-onset endophthalmitis may occur up to 6 weeks post-op. White intracapsular plaque is characteristic.

Therapeutic Considerations: Use steroids (dexamethasone 0.4 mg/0.1 mL intravitreal and 10 mg/1 mL subconjunctival) with antibiotics in post-op endophthalmitis. Also use systemic antibiotics for severe cases. Vitrectomy is usually necessary.

Prognosis: Related to pathogen virulence.

Fungal Endophthalmitis

Clinical Presentation: Slow deterioration in visual acuity ± eye pain. N fever. Antecedent/concomitant TPN, central IV line, prolonged antibiotic/immunosuppressive therapy, steroids, IVDA, or post-cataract surgery.

Diagnostic Considerations: Blood cultures frequently positive in Candida endophthalmitis. Small/round white lesions near retinal vessels. Cultures of aqueous/vitreous humors diagnostic.

Pitfalls: Symptoms develop insidiously with little/no eye pain or fever. Blood cultures negative with Aspergillus endophthalmitis.

Therapeutic Considerations: Penetration of antibiotic into vitreous humor requires high lipid solubility and inflammation. IV/intravitreous/subconjunctival antimicrobial choice depends on physiochemical properties of drug selected. Vitrectomy preferred by some.

If using intravitreal amphotericin B, there is no benefit in adding systemic IV therapy. Voriconazole penetrates CSF/eye, but clinical experience is limited. Based on limited data, caspofungin appears to have poor penetration into the vitreous and should not be relied upon to treat fungal endophthalmitis.

Prognosis: Best results with vitrectomy plus intravitreal antifungal therapy.

Tuberculous (TB) Endophthalmitis

Clinical Presentation: Raised retinal punctate lesions ± visual impairment.

Diagnostic Considerations: Signs of extraocular TB are usually present. Confirm diagnosis of miliary TB by liver/bone biopsy.

Pitfalls: TB endophthalmitis is a sign of disseminated TB.

Therapeutic Considerations: Treat as disseminated TB. Systemic steroids may be used if given with anti-TB therapy.

Prognosis: Related to degree of immunosuppression.

Infected Lens Implant

Diagnostic Considerations: Diagnosis by clinical appearance and culture of anterior chamber. Obtain ophthalmology consult.

Pitfalls: Superficial cultures are inadequate. Anterior chamber aspirate may be needed for culture.

Therapeutic Considerations: Infected lens must be removed for cure.
Prognosis: Good with early lens removal and recommended antibiotics.

External Otitis

Subset	Usual Pathogens	Preferred IV Therapy	Alternate IV Therapy	Topical Therapy or IV-to-PO Switch
Benign	P. aeruginosa	Use otic solutions only (ofloxacin 0.3%, tobramycin, polymyxin B); apply ear drops q6h × 1 week		
Malignant	P. aeruginosa	**One "A" drug ± one "B" drug:** **"A" drugs:** Meropenem 1 gm (IV) q8h **or** Cefepime 2 gm (IV) q8h **or** Piperacillin 4 gm (IV) q8h × 4–6 weeks **"B" drugs:** Ciprofloxacin 400 mg (IV) q12h **or** Levofloxacin 750 mg (IV) q24h × 4–6 weeks **or** Amikacin 1 gm (IV) q24h × 4–6 weeks		Ciprofloxacin 750 mg (PO) q12h **or** Levofloxacin 750 mg (PO) q24h × 4–6 weeks

Duration of therapy represents total time topically (benign), or IV + PO (malignant). Most patients on IV therapy able to take PO meds should be switched to PO therapy soon after clinical improvement (usually < 72 hours).

Benign External Otitis (Pseudomonas aeruginosa)

Clinical Presentation: Acute external ear canal drainage without perforation of tympanic membrane or bone involvement.
Diagnostic Considerations: Diagnosis suggested by external ear drainage after water exposure. Usually acquired from swimming pools ("swimmers ear"). Not an invasive infection.
Pitfalls: Be sure external otitis is not associated with perforated tympanic membrane, which requires ENT consultation and systemic antibiotics.
Therapeutic Considerations: Treat topically until symptoms/infection resolve.
Prognosis: Excellent with topical therapy.

Malignant External Otitis (Pseudomonas aeruginosa)

Clinical Presentation: External ear canal drainage with bone involvement.
Diagnostic Considerations: Diagnosis by demonstrating P. aeruginosa in soft tissue culture from ear canal plus bone/cartilage involvement on x-ray. Usually affects diabetics. CT/MRI of head shows bony involvement of external auditory canal.
Pitfalls: Rare in non-diabetics.
Therapeutic Considerations: Requires surgical debridement plus antibiotic therapy for cure.
Prognosis: Related to control of diabetes mellitus.

Acute Otitis Media

Subset	Usual Pathogens	IM Therapy	PO Therapy
Initial uncomplicated bacterial infection	S. pneumoniae H. influenzae M. catarrhalis	Ceftriaxone 50 mg/kg (IM) × 1 dose	Amoxicillin 1 gm or 10 mg/kg (PO) q8h × 10 days **or** Clarithromycin 7.5 mg/kg (PO) q12h × 10 days **or** Azithromycin 10 mg/kg (PO) × 1 dose, then 5 mg/kg (PO) q24h × 4 days
Treatment failure or resistant organism*	MDRSP Beta-lactamase positive H. influenzae	Ceftriaxone 50 mg/kg (IM) q24h × 3 doses	Amoxicillin/clavulanic acid ES-600 90 mg/kg/day (PO) in 2 divided doses × 10 days† **or** Cephalosporin† (PO) × 10 days

MDRSP = multidrug-resistant S. pneumoniae. Pediatric doses are provided; acute otitis media is uncommon in adults. For chronic otitis media, prolonged antimicrobial therapy is required.

* Treatment failure = persistent symptoms and otoscopy abnormalities 48–72 hours after starting initial antimicrobial therapy. For risk factors for MDRSP, see Therapeutic Considerations.

† ES-600 = 600 mg amoxicillin/5 mL. Cephalosporins: Cefuroxime axetil 15 mg/kg (PO) q12h or Cefdinir 7 mg/kg (PO) q12h or 14 mg/kg (PO) q24h or Cefpodoxime 5 mg/kg (PO) q12h may be used.

Acute Otitis Media

Clinical Presentation: Fever, otalgia, hearing loss. Nonspecific presentation is more common in younger children (irritability, fever). Key to diagnosis is examination of the tympanic membrane. Uncommon in adults.

Diagnostic Considerations: Diagnosis is made by finding an opaque, hyperemic, bulging tympanic membrane with loss of landmarks and decreased mobility on pneumatic otoscopy.

Pitfalls: Failure to remove cerumen (inadequate visualization of tympanic membrane) and reliance on history of ear tugging/pain are the main factors associated with overdiagnosis of otitis media. Otitis media with effusion (i.e., tympanic membrane retracted or in normal position with decreased mobility or mobility with negative pressure; fluid present behind the drum but normal in color) usually resolves spontaneously and should not be treated with antibiotics.

Therapeutic Considerations: Risk factors for infection with MDRSP S. pneumoniae include antibiotic therapy in past 30 days, failure to respond within 48–72 hours of therapy, day care attendance, and antimicrobial prophylaxis. Macrolides and TMP–SMX may predispose to DRSP, and 25% of S. pneumoniae are naturally resistant to macrolides.

Prognosis: Excellent, but tends to recur. Chronic otitis, cholesteatomas, mastoiditis are rare complications. Tympanostomy tubes/adenoidectomy for frequent recurrences of otitis media are the leading surgical procedures in children.

Mastoiditis

Subset	Usual Pathogens	Preferred IV Therapy	Alternate IV Therapy	PO Therapy or IV-to-PO Switch
Acute	S. pneumoniae H. influenzae S. aureus (MSSA)	Ceftriaxone 1–2 gm (IV) q24h × 2 weeks **or** Cefotaxime 2 gm (IV) q6h × 2 weeks **or** Cefepime 2 gm (IV) q12h × 2 weeks	Moxifloxacin 400 mg (IV) q24h × 2 weeks **or** Levofloxacin 500 mg (IV) q24h × 2 weeks	Moxifloxacin 400 mg (PO) q24h × 2 weeks **or** Levofloxacin 500 mg (PO) q24h × 2 weeks
Chronic	S. pneumoniae H. influenzae P. aeruginosa S. aureus (MSSA) Oral anaerobes	Meropenem 1 gm (IV) q8h × 4 weeks **or** Cefepime 2 gm (IV) q8h × 4 weeks	Quinolone* (IV) × 4–6 weeks	Quinolone* (PO) × 4–6 weeks

Duration of therapy represents total time IV, PO, or IV + PO. Most patients on IV therapy able to take PO meds should be switched to PO therapy soon after clinical improvement (usually < 72 hours).

* Levofloxacin 750 mg (IV or PO) q24h or Moxifloxacin 400 mg (IV or PO) q24h.

Acute Mastoiditis

Clinical Presentation: Pain/tenderness over mastoid with fever.

Diagnostic Considerations: Diagnosis by CT/MRI showing mastoid involvement.

Pitfalls: Obtain head CT/MRI to rule out extension into CNS presenting as acute bacterial meningitis.

Prognosis: Good if treated early.

Chronic Mastoiditis

Clinical Presentation: Subacute pain/tenderness over mastoid with low-grade fever.

Diagnostic Considerations: Diagnosis by CT/MRI showing mastoid involvement. Rarely secondary to TB (diagnose by AFB smear/culture of bone biopsy or debrided bone).

Pitfalls: Obtain head CT/MRI to rule out CNS extension.

Therapeutic Considerations: Usually requires surgical debridement for cure. Should be viewed as chronic osteomyelitis. If secondary to TB, treat as skeletal TB.

Prognosis: Progressive without surgery. Poor prognosis with associated meningitis/brain abscess.

Suppurative Parotitis

Subset	Usual Pathogens	Preferred IV Therapy	Alternate IV Therapy	PO Therapy or IV-to-PO Switch
Parotitis	S. aureus (MSSA) Entero-bacteriaceae Oral anaerobes	Meropenem 500 mg (IV) q8h × 2 weeks **or** Quinolone* (IV) q24h × 2 weeks	Ceftriaxone 1 gm (IV) q24h × 2 weeks **or** Ceftizoxime 2 gm (IV) q8h × 2 weeks	Quinolone* (PO) q24h × 2 weeks

Duration of therapy represents total time IV, PO, or IV + PO. Most patients on IV therapy able to take PO meds should be switched to PO therapy soon after clinical improvement (usually < 72 hours).

* Levofloxacin 500 mg or Moxifloxacin 400 mg.

Clinical Presentation: Unilateral parotid pain/swelling with discharge from Stensen's duct ± fever.
Diagnostic Considerations: Diagnosis by clinical presentation, ↑ amylase, CT/MRI demonstrating stone in parotid duct/gland involvement.
Pitfalls: Differentiate from unilateral mumps by purulent discharge from Stensen's duct.
Therapeutic Considerations: If duct is obstructed, remove stone.
Prognosis: Good with early therapy/hydration.

Pharyngitis/Chronic Fatigue Syndrome (CFS)

Subset	Usual Pathogens	PO Therapy
Bacterial	Group A streptococci	Amoxicillin 1 gm (PO) q8h × 7–10 days **or** Cefprozil 500 mg (PO) q12h × 7–10 days **or** Clindamycin 300 mg (PO) q8h × 7–10 days **or** Clarithromycin XL 1 gm (PO) q24h × 7–10 days **or** Azithromycin 500 mg (PO) × 1 dose, then 250 mg (PO) q24h × 4 days
Membranous	Arcanobacterium (Corynebacterium) hemolyticum	Doxycycline 100 mg (IV or PO) q12h × 1–2 weeks **or** Clarithromycin XL 1 gm (PO) q24h × 1–2 weeks **or** Azithromycin 500 mg (IV or PO) × 1 dose then 250 mg (IV or PO) q24h × 1–2 weeks **or** Cephalosporin (IV or PO) × 1–2 wks
	C. diphtheriae	Diphtheria antitoxin (p. 166) ± penicillin or macrolide
Viral	Respiratory viruses, EBV, CMV, HHV-6	Not applicable. EBV/CMV do not cause primary pharyngitis, but pharyngitis part of infectious mononucleosis syndrome, along with hepatitis and lymph node involvement. See viral hepatitis (pp. 95–96)

Pharyngitis/Chronic Fatigue Syndrome (CFS) (cont'd)

Subset	Usual Pathogens	PO Therapy
Other	M. pneumoniae C. pneumoniae	Quinolone* (PO) q24h × 1 week **or** Doxycycline 100 mg (PO) q12h × 1 week **or** Clarithromycin XL 1 gm (PO) q24h × 1 week **or** Azithromycin 500 mg (PO) × 1 dose, then 250 mg (PO) q24h × 4 days
Chronic fatigue syndrome.[†]		

* Levofloxacin 500 mg or Moxifloxacin 400 mg.

† Not a cause of pharyngitis, pathogen unknown (not EBV) but may be caused by xenotropic murine leukemia related virus (XMRV). See therapeutic considerations (p. 43).

Bacterial Pharyngitis

Clinical Presentation: Acute sore throat with fever, bilateral anterior cervical adenopathy, and elevated ASO titer. No hoarseness.

Diagnostic Considerations: Diagnosis of Group A streptococcal pharyngitis by elevated ASO titer after initial sore throat and positive throat culture. Rapid strep tests unnecessary, since delay in culture results (~1 week) still allows adequate time to initiate therapy and prevent acute rheumatic fever. Group A streptococcal pharyngitis is rare in adults > 30 years.

Pitfalls: Gram stain of throat exudate differentiates Group A streptococcal colonization (few or no PMNs) from infection (many PMNs) in patients with a positive throat culture or rapid strep test. Neither throat culture nor rapid strep test alone differentiates colonization from infection.

Therapeutic Considerations: Benzathine penicillin 1.2 mu (IM) × 1 dose can be used as an alternative to oral therapy. Penicillin, erythromycin, and ampicillin fail in 15% of cases due to poor penetration into oral secretions or beta-lactamase producing oral organisms.

Prognosis: Excellent. Treat within 10 days to prevent acute rheumatic fever.

Membranous Pharyngitis

Clinical Presentation: A. hemolyticum presents with a scarlet fever-like rash and membranous pharyngitis. C. diphtheriae pharyngitis has no fever/rash.

Diagnostic Considerations: Diagnosis by throat culture/recovery of organism in patients with scarlatiniform rash.

Pitfalls: A. hemolyticum must be differentiated from C. diphtheriae on culture.

Therapeutic Considerations: For A. hemolyticum, doxycycline or erythromycin are more active than beta-lactams. Penicillin or macrolides are preferred for C. diphtheriae. C. diphtheriae should be treated with antitoxin ASAP since antibiotic therapy is adjunctive.

Prognosis: Related to degree of airway obstruction. Good with early treatment of A. hemolyticum. Diphtheria prognosis related to early antitoxin treatment and to presence/severity of toxic myocarditis.

Viral Pharyngitis

Clinical Presentation: Acute sore throat. Other features depend on specific pathogen.

Diagnostic Considerations: Most cases of viral pharyngitis are caused by respiratory viruses, and are frequently accompanied by hoarseness, but not high fever, pharyngeal exudates, palatal petechiae, or posterior cervical adenopathy. Other causes of viral pharyngitis (EBV, CMV, HHV-6) are usually associated with posterior cervical adenopathy and ↑ SGOT/SGPT. EBV mono may present with exudative or non-exudative pharyngitis, and is diagnosed by negative ASO titer with a positive mono spot test or elevated EBV IgM viral capsid antigen (VCA) titer. Before mono spot test turns positive (may take up to 8 weeks), a presumptive diagnosis of EBV mono can be made by ESR and SGOT, which are elevated in EBV and normal in Group A streptococcal pharyngitis. If EBV mono spot is negative, retest weekly × 8 weeks; if still negative, obtain IgM CMV/toxoplasmosis titers to diagnose the cause of "mono spot negative" pharyngitis.

Pitfalls: 30% of patients with viral pharyngitis have Group A streptococcal colonization. Look for viral features to suggest the correct diagnosis (leukopenia, lymphocytosis, atypical lymphocytes).

Therapeutic Considerations: Symptomatic care only. Short-term steroids should only be used in EBV infection if airway obstruction is present/imminent. Since 30% of patients with viral pharyngitis are colonized with Group A streptococci, do not treat throat cultures positive for Group A streptococci if non-streptococcal pharyngitis features are present (e.g., bilateral posterior cervical adenopathy).

Prognosis: Related to extent of systemic infection. Post-viral fatigue is common. CMV may remain active in liver for 6–12 months with mildly elevated serum transaminases.

Mycoplasma/Chlamydophilia (Chlamydia) Pharyngitis

Clinical Presentation: Acute sore throat ± laryngitis. Usually non-exudative.

Diagnostic Considerations: Diagnosis by elevated IgM M. pneumoniae or C. pneumoniae titers. Consider diagnosis in patients with non-exudative pharyngitis without viral or streptococcal pharyngitis. Mycoplasma pharyngitis is often accompanied by otitis/bullous myringitis.

Pitfalls: Patients with C. pneumoniae frequently have laryngitis, which is not a feature of EBV, CMV, Group A streptococcal, or M. pneumoniae pharyngitis.

Therapeutic Considerations: Treatment of C. pneumoniae laryngitis results in rapid (~ 3 days) return of normal voice, which does not occur with viral pharyngitis.

Prognosis: Excellent.

Chronic Fatigue Syndrome (CFS)

Clinical Presentation: Fatigue > 1 year with cognitive impairment ± mild pharyngitis.

Diagnostic Considerations: Rule out other causes of chronic fatigue (cancer, adrenal/thyroid disease, etc.) before diagnosing CFS. HHV-6/Coxsackie B titers are usually elevated. Some have ↓ natural kill (NK) cells/activity. ESR ~ 0. Crimson crescents in the posterior pharynx are common.

Pitfalls: ↑ VCA IgG EBV titers is common in CFS, but EBV does not cause CFS. Do not confuse CFS with fibromyalgia, which has muscular "trigger points" and no cognitive impairment. CFS and fibromyalgia may coexist.

Therapeutic Considerations: No specific therapy is available. Patients with ↓ NK cells may benefit from beta-carotene 50,000 U (PO) q24h × 3 weeks. Patients with ↑ C. pneumoniae titers may benefit from doxycycline 100 mg (PO) q24h × 3 weeks or azithromycin 250 mg (PO) q24h × 2 weeks.
Prognosis: Cyclical illness with remissions and flares (precipitated by exertion). Avoid exercise.

Thrush (Oropharyngeal Candidiasis)

Subset	Pathogens	PO Therapy
Fungal	C. albicans	Fluconazole 200 mg (PO) × 1 dose, then 100 mg (PO) q24h ×† weeks **or** Posaconazole 100 mg (PO) q12h × 1 day, then 100 mg (PO) q24h × 13 days **or** Clotrimazole 10 mg troches (PO) 5x/day ×† weeks **or** Itraconazole 200 mg (PO) q24h ×† weeks
	Fluconazole-resistant Candida species	Posaconazole 400 mg (PO) q12h ×† weeks* **or** Voriconazole 200 mg (PO) q12h ×† weeks* **or** Caspofungin 70 mg (IV) × 1, then 50 mg (IV) q24h ×† weeks* **or** Itraconazole 200 mg (PO) q12h ×† weeks*

* Duration of therapy depends on underlying disease and clinical response.
† See fluconazole unresponsive esophagitis (p. 595).

Thrush (Oropharyngeal Candidiasis)

Clinical Presentation: White coated tongue or oropharynx. White adherent plaques may be on any part of the oropharynx.
Diagnostic Considerations: Gram stain/culture of white plaques demonstrates yeasts (Candida). Culture and susceptibility testing of causative fungus is useful in analyzing failure to respond to therapy.
Pitfalls: Lateral, linear, white, striated tongue lesions may resemble thrush but really represent hairy leukoplakia. Hairy leukoplakia should suggest HIV. Thrush may occur in children, alcoholics, diabetics, those receiving steroids/antibiotic therapy, or HIV.
Therapeutic Considerations: Almost all infections are caused by C. albicans, a species that is usually susceptible to fluconazole. Fluconazole-unresponsive infections may be caused by infection with fluconazole-resistant C. albicans (most common explanation), infection with a fluconazole-resistant non-albicans species (rare), noncompliance with therapy (common), or drug interactions (e.g., concomitant usage of rifampin, which markedly reduced azole blood levels). For suspected fluconazole-resistance, a trial with another azole is appropriate as cross-resistance is not universal.
Prognosis: Non-HIV/AIDS patients respond well to therapy, particularly when the predisposing factor is eliminated/decreased (i.e., antibiotics discontinued, steroids reduced, etc.). HIV/AIDS patients may require longer courses of therapy and should be treated until cured. Relapse is frequent in HIV/AIDS patients, and institution of effective antiretroviral therapy is the most effective general strategy.

Mouth Ulcers/Vesicles

Subset	Usual Pathogens	Preferred IV Therapy	Alternate IV Therapy	PO Therapy or IV-to-PO Switch
Vincent's angina	Borrelia Fusobacterium	Clindamycin 600 mg (IV) q8h × 2 weeks	Ceftizoxime 2 gm (IV) q8h × 2 weeks **or** Any beta-lactam (IV) × 2 weeks	Clindamycin 300 mg (PO) q8h × 2 weeks **or** Amoxicillin/clavulanic acid 500/125 mg (PO) q8h × 2 weeks
Ludwig's angina	Group A streptococci	Clindamycin 600 mg (IV) q8h × 2 weeks	Ceftizoxime 2 gm (IV) q8h × 2 weeks **or** Any beta-lactam (IV) × 2 weeks	Clindamycin 300 mg (PO) q8h × 2 weeks **or** Amoxicillin/clavulanic acid 500/125 mg (PO) q8h × 2 weeks
Stomatitis	Normal mouth flora	Not applicable		
Herpangina	Coxsackie A virus	Not applicable		
Herpes gingivo-stomatitis	HSV-1	PO Therapy Valacyclovir 500 mg (PO) q12h × 1 week **or** Famciclovir 500 mg (PO) q12h × 1 week **or** Acyclovir 400 mg (PO) 5x/day × 1 week		
Herpes labialis (cold sores/ fever blisters)	HSV-1 (recurrent)	PO Therapy Valacyclovir 2 gm (PO) q12h × 1 day (2 doses) started at onset of symptoms (tingling/burning) **or** Acyclovir 400 mg (PO) 5x/day × 1 week **or** Famciclovir 500 mg (PO) q12h × 1 week Topical Therapy Penciclovir 1% cream q2h while awake × 4 days **or** Acyclovir 5% cream 5x/d × 4 days		
Aphthous ulcers	Normal mouth flora	Not applicable		

Duration of therapy represents total time IV, PO, or IV + PO. Most patients on IV therapy able to take PO meds should be switched to PO therapy soon after clinical improvement (usually < 72 hours).

Clinical Presentation: Painful mouth ulcers/vesicles without fever.

Vincent's Angina (Borrelia/Fusobacterium)

Diagnostic Considerations: Foul breath, poor dental hygiene/pyorrhea. Painful/bleeding gums.

Pitfalls: Do not attribute foul breath to poor dental hygiene without considering other serious causes (e.g., lung abscess, renal failure).

Therapeutic Considerations: After control of acute infection, refer to dentist.

Prognosis: Excellent with early treatment.

Ludwig's Angina (Group A streptococci)

Diagnostic Considerations: Fever with elevated floor of mouth is diagnostic. Massive neck swelling may be evident.

Pitfalls: C_{1q} deficiency has perioral/tongue swelling, but n fever or floor of mouth elevation. Rarely, Ludwig's, angina may be due to F. necrophorum.

Therapeutic Considerations: Surgical drainage is not necessary. May need airway emergently; have tracheotomy set at bedside.

Prognosis: Early airway obstruction has adverse impact on prognosis.

Stomatitis (normal mouth flora)

Diagnostic Considerations: Diagnosis based on clinical appearance.

Pitfalls: Do not miss a systemic cause (e.g., acute leukemia).

Therapeutic Considerations: Painful; treat symptomatically.

Prognosis: Related to severity of underlying systemic disease.

Herpangina (Coxsackie A virus)

Diagnostic Considerations: Ulcers located posteriorly in pharynx. No gum involvement or halitosis.

Pitfalls: Do not confuse with anterior vesicular lesions of HSV.

Therapeutic Considerations: No good treatment available. Usually resolves spontaneously in 2 weeks.

Prognosis: Good, but may be recurrent.

Herpes Gingivostomatitis (HSV-1)

Diagnostic Considerations: Anterior ulcers in pharynx. Associated with bleeding gums, not halitosis.

Pitfalls: Do not miss a systemic disease associated with bleeding gums (e.g., acute myelogenous leukemia). Periodontal disease is not usually associated with oral ulcers.

Therapeutic Considerations: Oral analgesic solutions may help in swallowing.

Prognosis: Excellent with early treatment.

Herpes Labialis (Cold Sores/Fever Blisters) (HSV-1)

Diagnostic Considerations: Caused by recurrent HSV-1 infection, which appears as painful vesicular lesions on/near the vermillion border of lips. Attacks may be triggered by stress, sun exposure, menstruation, and often begin with pain or tingling before vesicles appear. Vesicles crust over and attacks usually resolve by 1 week. "Fever blisters" are not triggered by temperature elevations per se, but may accompany malaria, pneumococcal/meningococcal meningitis. Diagnosis is clinical.

Pitfalls: Do not confuse with perioral impetigo; impetigo has crusts (not vesicles), is itchy (not painful), and does not involve the vermillion border of the lips.

Therapeutic Considerations: Treatment is not always needed. If valacyclovir if used, it should be started when pain/tingling appear to decrease symptoms/vesicles/duration of attack. Valacyclovir is of no proven value once vesicles have appeared. Non-prescription topical products (docosanol 10%,

tetracaine cream) may decrease pain/itching. Once-daily suppressive therapy may be considered for frequent recurrences or during times of increased risk (e.g., sun exposure). Sun screen may be helpful.
Prognosis: Tends to be recurrent in normal hosts. May be severe in compromised hosts.

Aphthous Ulcers (normal mouth flora)

Diagnostic Considerations: Usually an isolated finding. Ulcers are painful.
Pitfalls: May be a clue to systemic disorder (e.g., Behcet's syndrome). Mouth ulcers in SLE are painless.
Therapeutic Considerations: Usually refractory to all treatment and often recurrent. Steroid ointment (Kenalog in orabase) may be helpful.
Prognosis: Good, but tends to recur.

Deep Neck Infections, Lemierre's Syndrome, Severe Dental Infections

Subset	Usual Pathogens	Preferred IV Therapy	Alternate IV Therapy	IV-to-PO Switch
Deep neck infections (lateral pharyngeal, retro-pharyngeal, prevertebral space)	Oral anaerobes Oral streptococci	Meropenem 500 mg (IV) q8h × 2 weeks **or** Tigacycline 100 mg (IV) × 1 dose, then 100 mg (IV) q24h or 50 mg (IV) q12h × 2 weeks **or** Piperacillin 4 gm (IV) q8h × 2 weeks	Clindamycin 600 mg (IV) q8h × 2 weeks **or** Ceftizoxime 2 gm (IV) q8h × 2 weeks **or** Ertapenem 1 gm (IV) q24h × 2 weeks	Clindamycin 300 mg (PO) q8h × 2 weeks **or** Doxycycline 200 mg (PO) q12h × 3 days, then 100 mg (PO) q12h × 11 days*
Lemierre's Syndrome	Fusobacterium necrophorum	Treat as deep neck infection, above		
Severe dental infections	Oral anaerobes Oral streptococci	Clindamycin 600 mg (IV) q8h × 2 weeks **or** Piperacillin 4 gm (IV) q8h × 2 weeks	Ertapenem 1 gm (IV) q24h × 2 weeks **or** Meropenem 1 gm (IV) q8h × 2 weeks	Clindamycin 300 mg (PO) q8h × 2 weeks **or** Doxycycline 200 mg (PO) q12h × 3 days, then 100 mg (PO) q12h × 11 days*

Duration of therapy represents total time IV or IV + PO. Most patients on IV therapy able to take PO meds should be switched to PO therapy after clinical improvement.
* Loading dose is not needed PO if given IV with the same drug.

Clinical Presentation: Neck pain and fever.
Diagnosis: Clinical presentation plus confirmatory CT/MRI scan.

Deep Neck Infections (lateral pharyngeal, retropharyngeal, prevertebral space)

Diagnostic Considerations: Patients are usually toxemic with unilateral posterior pharyngeal soft tissue mass on oral exam. Neck stiffness may be present with retropharyngeal space infection/abscess.

Pitfalls: Retropharyngeal "danger space" infection may extend to mediastinum and present as mediastinitis.

Therapeutic Considerations: Obtain ENT consult for surgical drainage.

Prognosis: Poor without surgical drainage.

Lemierre's Syndrome

Clinical Presentation: Jugular vein septic thrombophlebitis with fever, toxemic appearance, and tenderness over angle of jaw/jugular vein.

Diagnostic Considerations: May present as multiple septic pulmonary emboli. Usually follows recent dental infection.

Pitfalls: Suspect Lemierre's syndrome in patients with sore throat and shock.

Therapeutic Considerations: If unresponsive to antibiotic therapy, may need venotomy.

Prognosis: Poor with septic pulmonary emboli/shock.

Severe Dental Infections

Diagnostic Considerations: Obtain CT/MRI of jaws to rule out osteomyelitis or abscess.

Pitfalls: Chronic drainage in a patient with an implant is diagnostic of chronic osteomyelitis/abscess until proven otherwise.

Therapeutic Considerations: Abscesses must be drained for cure.

Prognosis: Poor prognosis and recurrent without adequate surgical drainage.

Epiglottitis

Subset	Usual Pathogens	Preferred IV Therapy	Alternate IV Therapy	IV-to-PO Switch
Epiglottitis	S. pneumoniae H. influenzae Respiratory viruses	Ceftriaxone 1 gm (IV) q24h × 2 weeks **or** Ceftizoxime 2 gm (IV) q8h × 2 weeks	Ertapenem 1 gm (IV) q24h × 2 weeks **or** Meropenem 500 mg (IV) q8h × 2 weeks **or** Imipenem 500 mg (IV) q6h × 2 weeks **or** Moxifloxacin 400 mg (IV) q24h × 2 weeks **or** Levofloxacin 500 mg (IV) q24h × 2 weeks	Moxifloxacin 400 mg (PO) q24h × 2 weeks **or** Levofloxacin 500 mg (PO) q24h × 2 weeks **or** Cefprozil 500 mg (PO) q12h × 2 weeks

Duration of therapy represents total time IV or IV + PO. Most patients on IV therapy able to take PO meds should be switched to PO therapy after clinical improvement.

Clinical Presentation: Stridor with upper respiratory infection.
Diagnostic Considerations: Lateral film of neck shows epiglottic edema. Neck CT/MRI may help if neck films are non-diagnostic.
Pitfalls: Do not attempt to culture the epiglottis (may precipitate acute upper airway obstruction).
Therapeutic Considerations: Treat empirically as soon as possible. Obtain ENT consult.
Prognosis: Early airway obstruction is associated with an adverse prognosis.

Empiric Therapy of Lower Respiratory Tract Infections

Acute Bacterial Exacerbation of Chronic Bronchitis (AECB)

Subset	Pathogens	PO Therapy
AECB	S. pneumoniae H. influenzae M. catarrhalis	Quinolone* (PO) q24h × 5 days **or** Amoxicillin/clavulanic acid 500/125 mg (PO) q12h × 5 days **or** Clarithromycin XL 1 gm (PO) q24h × 5 days **or** Doxycycline 100 mg (PO) q12h × 5 days **or** Azithromycin 500 mg (PO) × 3 days

* Moxifloxacin 400 mg or Levofloxacin 500 mg.

Clinical Presentation: Productive cough and negative chest x-ray in a patient with chronic bronchitis.
Diagnostic Considerations: Diagnosis by productive cough, purulent sputum, and chest x-ray negative for pneumonia. H. influenzae is relatively more common than other pathogens.
Pitfalls: Do not obtain sputum cultures in chronic bronchitis; cultures usually reported as normal/mixed flora and should not be used to guide therapy.
Therapeutic Considerations: Treated with same antibiotics as for community-acquired pneumonia, since pathogens are the same (even though H. influenzae is relatively more frequent). Respiratory viruses/C. pneumoniae may initiate AECB, but is usually followed by bacterial infection, which is responsible for symptoms and is the aim of therapy. Bronchodilators are helpful for bronchospasm. Macrolide-resistant S. pneumoniae is an important clinical problem (prevalence ≥ 30%).
Prognosis: Related to underlying cardiopulmonary status.

Mediastinitis

Subset	Usual Pathogens	IV Therapy	IV-to-PO Switch
Following esophageal perforation or thoracic surgery	Oral anaerobes	Preferred: Piperacillin 4 gm (IV) q8h × 2 wks **or** Ampicillin/sulbactam 3 gm (IV) q6h × 2 wks Alternate: Meropenem 1 gm (IV) q8h × 2 weeks or Ertapenem 1 gm (IV) q24h × 2 weeks	Amoxicillin/ clavulanic acid 500/125 mg (PO) q8h × 2 weeks **or** Quinolone* (PO) q24h × 2 weeks

Duration of therapy represents total time IV or IV + PO. Most patients on IV therapy able to take PO meds should be switched to PO therapy after clinical improvement.

* Moxifloxacin 400 mg or Levofloxacin 500 mg.

Diagnostic Considerations: Chest x-ray usually shows perihilar infiltrate in mediastinitis. Pleural effusions from esophageal tears have elevated amylase levels.

Pitfalls: Do not overlook esophageal tear in mediastinitis with pleural effusions.

Therapeutic Considerations: Obtain surgical consult if esophageal perforation is suspected.

Prognosis: Related to extent, location, and duration of esophageal tear/mediastinal infection.

Community-Acquired Pneumonia (CAP) (see Color Atlas for Sputum Gram stains and Chapter 8 for differential diagnosis of CXR patterns)

Subset	Usual Pathogens*	Alternate IV Therapy	PO Therapy or IV-to-PO Switch
Pathogen unknown	S. pneumoniae¶ H. influenzae M. catarrhalis B. pertussis Legionella sp. Mycoplasma pneumoniae Chlamydophilia (Chlamydia) pneumoniae	Quinolone† (IV) q24h **or combination therapy with** Ceftriaxone 1 gm (IV) q24h × 1–2 weeks **plus either** Doxycycline‡ (IV) × 1–2 weeks **or** Azithromycin 500 mg (IV) q24h × 1–2 weeks (minimum 2 doses before switching to PO therapy)	Quinolone† (PO) q24h **or** Doxycycline‡ (PO) × 1–2 weeks **or** Macrolide†† (PO) q24h × 1–2 weeks

Duration of therapy represents total time IV or IV, PO, or IV + PO. Most patients on IV therapy able to take PO meds should be switched to PO therapy after clinical improvement.

* Compromised hosts may require longer courses of therapy.

† Moxifloxacin 400 mg × 1–2 weeks or Levofloxacin 750 mg × 5 days (or 500 mg × 1–2 weeks).

†† Azithromycin 500 mg or Clarithromycin XL 1 gm.

¶ Macrolides should not be used in areas where *macrolide-resistant S. pneumoniae (MRSP) or multidrug-resistant S. pneumoniae (MDRSP)* strains are prevalent.

‡ Doxycycline 200 mg (IV or PO) q12h × 3 days, then 100 mg (IV or PO) q12h × 4–11 days.

Community-Acquired Pneumonia (CAP) (cont'd)

Subset	Usual Pathogens*	Preferred IV Therapy	Alternate IV Therapy	PO Therapy or IV-to-PO Switch
Typical bacterial pathogens	S. pneumoniae¶ H. influenzae M. catarrhalis B. pertussis	Quinolone† (IV) q24h × 1–2 weeks **or** Ertapenem 1 gm (IV) q24h × 1–2 weeks **or** Ceftriaxone 1 gm (IV) q24h × 1–2 wks **or** Tigecycline 100 mg (IV) × 1 dose, 50 mg (IV) q12h × 1–2 weeks**	Doxycycline‡ (IV) × 1–2 weeks **or** Azithromycin 500 mg (IV) q24h × 1–2 weeks (minimum 2 doses before switching to PO therapy)	(see unknown pathogen) **or** Amoxicillin/ clavulanic acid XR 2 tablets (PO) q12h × 7–10 days **or** Cefprozil 500 mg (PO) q12h × 1–2 weeks
	K. pneumoniae*	Meropenem 1 gm (IV) q8h × 2 weeks **or** Ertapenem 1 gm (IV) q24h × 2 weeks	Quinolone§ (IV) q24h × 2 weeks **or** Ceftriaxone 1 gm (IV) q24 × 2 weeks	Quinolone§ (PO) q24h × 2 weeks
Atypical pathogens *Zoonotic*	C. psittaci (psittacosis) Coxiella burnetii (Q fever) Francisella tularensis (tularemia)	Doxycycline 200 mg (IV) q12h × 3 days, then 100 mg (IV) q12h × 2 weeks	Quinolone†† (IV) q24h × 2 weeks	Doxycycline 200 mg (PO) q12h × 3 days, then 100 mg (PO) q12h × 11 days **or** Quinolone†† (PO) q24h × 2 weeks

* Compromised hosts may require longer courses of therapy.

† Moxifloxacin 400 mg × 1–2 weeks or Levofloxacin 750 mg × 5 days (or 500 mg × 1–2 weeks).

§ Moxifloxacin 400 mg or Levofloxacin 500 mg.

¶ Macrolides should not be used in areas where *macrolide-resistant S. pneumoniae (MRSP) or multidrug-resistant S. pneumoniae (MDRSP)* strains are prevalent.

‡ Doxycycline 200 mg (IV or PO) q12h × 3 days, then 100 mg (IV or PO) q12h × 4–11 days.

†† Moxifloxacin 400 mg or Levofloxacin 500 mg.

** Tigecycline indicated for S. pneumoniae (PCN sensitive), H. influenzae (β-lactamase –), and Legionella CAP.

Community-Acquired Pneumonia (CAP) (cont'd)

Subset	Usual Pathogens*	Preferred IV Therapy	Alternate IV Therapy	PO Therapy or IV-to-PO Switch
Non-zoonotic	Legionella sp.‡ Mycoplasma pneumoniae‡ C. pneumoniae‡	Moxifloxacin 400 mg (IV) q24h × 1–2 weeks **or** Levofloxacin 500 mg (IV) q24h × 1–2 weeks **or** Tigecycline 100 mg (IV) × 1 dose, then 50 mg (IV) q12h × 1–2 weeks**	Azithromycin 500 mg (IV) q24h × 1–2 weeks (minimum of 2 doses before switching to PO therapy) **or** Doxycycline 200 mg (IV) q12h × 3 days, then 100 mg (IV) q12h × 4–11 days	Quinolone† (PO) q24h × 1–2 weeks **or** Doxycycline 200 mg (PO) q12h × 3 days, then 100 mg (PO) q12h × 4–11 days **or** Azithromycin 500 mg (PO) q24h × 1–2 weeks **or** Clarithromycin XL 1 gm (PO) q24h × 1–2 weeks
Influenza *Severe*§	Influenza A Avian influenza (H_5N_1) Swine influenza (H_1N_1)	Oseltamivir (Tamiflu) 75 mg (PO) q12h × 5 days¶ **plus either** Rimantadine 100 mg (PO) q12h × 7–10 days¶¶ **or** Amantadine 200 mg (PO) q24h × 7–10 days¶¶		Start treatment as soon as possible after onset of symptoms, preferably within 2 days. Rimantadine/amantadine miss Influenza B. Oseltamivir may be ineffective against human seasonal influenza/avian influenza (H_5N_1), but appears effective against swine influenza (H_1N_1)
Influenza *Mild or moderate*	Influenza A/B Swine influenza (H_1N_1)	Oseltamivir (Tamiflu) 75 mg (PO) q24h × 5 days	Zanamivir (Relenza) 10 mg (2 puffs via oral inhaler) q12h × 5 days	

* Compromised hosts may require longer courses of therapy.

§ If CXR shows multiple rapidly cavitating infiltrates, begin empiric anti-MSSA/CA-MRSA therapy with vancomycin, linezolid or tigacycline, together with anti-influenza therapy.

† Moxifloxacin 400 mg or Levofloxacin 500 mg.

‡ May require prolonged therapy: Legionella (2–3 weeks); Mycoplasma (2 weeks); Chlamydia (2 weeks).

** Tigecycline indicated for Legionella CAP.

¶ Serious neuropsychiatric symptoms (delirium/behavioral abnormalities, panic attacks, convulsions) may occur in some children and adults. See drug summary for details.

¶¶ Although resistance common, these drugs may improve oxygenation in severe cases of influenza A, on ventilatory support.

Community-Acquired Pneumonia (CAP) (cont'd)

Subset	Usual Pathogens*	Preferred IV Therapy	Alternate IV Therapy	PO Therapy or IV-to-PO Switch
Influenza *(Post-influenza bacterial CAP)*	S. pneumoniae H. influenzae	Quinolone‡ (IV) q24h × 2 weeks **plus either** Nafcillin 2 gm (IV) q4h × 2 weeks **or** Clindamycin 600 mg (IV) q8h × 2 weeks	Ceftriaxone 1 gm (IV) q24h × 2 wks **plus either** Vancomycin 1 gm (IV) q12h × 2 weeks **or** Linezolid 600 mg (IV) q12h × 2 weeks	Quinolone‡ (PO) q24h × 2 weeks
Chickenpox pneumonia	VZV	Acyclovir 5–10 mg/kg (IV) q8h × 10 days		Valacyclovir 1–2 gm (PO) q8h × 10 days
Aspiration	Oral anaerobes S. pneumoniae H. influenzae M. catarrhalis	Ceftriaxone 1 gm (IV) q24h × 2 weeks **or** Quinolone† (IV) q24h × 2 weeks	Doxycycline 200 mg (IV) q12h × 3 days, then 100 mg (IV) q12h × 11 days	Quinolone† (PO) q24h × 2 weeks **or** Doxycycline 200 mg (PO) q12h × 3 days, then 100 mg (PO) q12h × 4–11 days** **or** Amoxicillin/ clavulanic acid XR 2 tablets (PO) q12h × 2 weeks **or** Clarithromycin XL 1 gm (PO) q24h × 2 weeks
Tuberculosis (TB)	M. tuberculosis	INH 300 mg (PO) q24h × 6 months **plus** Rifampin 600 mg (PO) q24h × 6 months **plus** PZA 25 mg/kg (PO) q24h × 2 months **plus** EMB 15 mg/kg (PO) q24h (until susceptibilities known)††		
Non-tuberculous (atypical tuberculosis) Mycobacteria	Mycobacterium avium-intracellulare (MAI)	Treat for 6 months after sputum negative for MAI: Ethambutol 15 mg/kg (PO) q24h **plus either** (Clarithromycin 500 mg (PO) q12h **or** Azithromycin 500 mg (PO) q24h) **plus either** (rifampin or rifabutin). May substitute a quinolone (PO)† q24h for one rifamycin		

Duration of therapy represents total time IV or IV, PO, or IV + PO.

* Compromised hosts predisposed to organisms listed, but may be infected by usual pathogens in normal hosts.

† Moxifloxacin 400 mg or Levofloxacin 500 mg.

†† If isolate is sensitive, discontinue EMB and continue as above to complete 6 months. If INH-resistant, continue EMB, rifampin and PZA to complete 6 months. If any other resistance is present, obtain infectious disease or pulmonary consult.

‡ May require prolonged therapy: Legionella (2–3 weeks); Mycoplasma (2 weeks); Chlamydia (2 weeks).

** Loading dose is not needed PO if given IV with the same drug.

Community-Acquired Pneumonia (CAP) (cont'd)

Subset	Usual Pathogens*	Preferred IV Therapy	Alternate IV Therapy	PO Therapy or IV-to-PO Switch
	M. kansasii	Preferred therapy Rifampin 600 mg (PO) q24h **plus** INH 300 mg (PO) q24h **plus** pyridoxine 50 mg (PO) q24h **plus** EMB 15 mg/kg (PO) q24h. Treat × 18 months with 12 months of negative sputum Alternate therapy Clarithromycin 500 mg (PO) q12h **plus** INH 900 mg (PO) q24h **plus** pyridoxine 50 mg (PO) q24h **plus** EMB 25 mg kg (PO) q24h **plus** sulfamethoxazole 1 gm (PO) q8h. Treat × 18 months with 12 months of negative sputum For severe cases, add streptomycin 0.5–1 gm (IM) 3x/week during first 3 months of preferred/alternate therapy		
Chronic alcoholics	K. pneumoniae S. pneumoniae H. influenzae M. catarrhalis	Ceftriaxone 1 gm (IV) q24h × 2 weeks **or** Ertapenem 1 gm (IV) q24h × 2 weeks **or** Meropenem 1 gm (IV) q24h × 2 weeks	Ceftriaxone 1 gm (IV) q24h × 2 weeks **or** Quinolone† (IV) q24h × 2 weeks	Quinolone (PO) q24h × 2 weeks
Bronchiectasis, cystic fibrosis	S. maltophilia B. cepacia Alcaligenes xyloxidans	Preferred: Meropenem 2 gm (IV) q8h¶ **or** Cefepime 2 gm (IV) q8h¶ **or** Minocycline 100 mg (IV) q12h¶ **or** TMP–SMX 2.5 mg/kg (IV) q6h¶ Alternate: Quinolone (IV) q24h¶		TMP–SMX 1 SS tablet (PO) q6h¶ **or** Quinolone‡ (PO) q24h **or** Minocycline 100 mg (PO) q12h¶
	P. aeruginosa	Meropenem 2 gm (IV) q8h¶	Quinolone** **or** Cefepime 2 gm (IV) q8h¶ ± Amikacin 1 gm (IV) q24h¶	Levofloxacin 750 mg (PO) q24h¶ **or** Ciprofloxacin 750 mg (PO) q12h
	MDR P. aeruginosa	Colistin 80 mg or 1.7 mg/kg (IV) q8h¶ ± Rifampin 600 mg (PO) q24h¶	Polymyxin B 1–1.25 mg/kg (IV) q12h¶¥ **or** Doripenem 1g (IV) q8h¶	Colistin or Polymyxin B 80 mg q8h (via nebulizer aerosol)¶¥§

* Compromised hosts predisposed to organisms listed, but may be infected by any of the usual pathogens in normal hosts.
¶ Treat until cured.
† Treat only IV or IV-to-PO Switch.
‡ Moxifloxacin 400 mg or Levofloxacin 500 mg.
¥ 1 mg colistin = 12,500 IU; 1 mg Polymyxin B = 10,000 IU.
§ for recurrent infections use 160 mg q8h.
** Loading dose is not needed PO if given IV with the same drug.

Community-Acquired Pneumonia (CAP) (cont'd)

Subset	Usual Pathogens*	Preferred IV Therapy	Alternate IV Therapy	PO Therapy or IV-to-PO Switch
Nursing home-acquired pneumonia (NHAP)	H. influenzae S. pneumoniae M. catarrhalis	Ceftriaxone 1 gm (IV) q24h × 2 weeks **or** Quinolone‡ (IV) q24h × 2 weeks **or** Doxycycline 200 mg (IV) q12h × 3 days; then 100 mg (IV) q12h × 2 weeks	Ertapenem 1 gm (IV) q24h × 2 weeks **or** Cefepime 2 gm (IV) q12h × 2 weeks	Quinolone‡ (PO) q24h × 2 weeks **or** Doxycycline 200 mg (PO) q12h × 3 days, then 100 mg (PO) q12h × 11 days
Organ transplants†	CMV	Ganciclovir 5 mg/kg (IV) q12h until clinical improvement followed by valganciclovir 900 mg (PO) q12h until cured **plus** CMV immunoglobulin (CMV-IG) 500 mg/kg (IV) q48h × 2 weeks		
	PCP	Treat same as for chronic steroid therapy† (next page)		
Chronic steroid therapy† (next page)	Aspergillus	Voriconazole (see "usual dose," p. 695)¶	Lipid-associated formulation of amphotericin B (p. 513)¶ **or** Caspofungin 70 mg (IV) × 1 then 50 mg (IV) q24h¶ **or** (high risk nephrotoxicity) amphotericin B deoxycholate 1–1.5 mg/kg (IV) q24h¶	Voriconazole (see "usual dose," p. 695)¶ **or** Posaconazole 200 mg q6h initially, then 400 mg q12h when disease stabilized¶ **or** Itraconazole 200 mg (IV) q12h × 2 days then 200 mg (PO) q12h**¶

CO/CA-MRSA = community-onset/community-acquired methicillin-resistant S. aureus (see p. 53). Duration of therapy represents total time IV or IV, PO, or IV + PO.

* Compromised hosts predisposed to organisms listed but may be infected by usual pathogens in normal hosts.

¶ Treat until cured.

‡ Moxifloxacin 400 mg or Levofloxacin 500 mg.

** Levofloxacin 750 mg (IV) q24h or Ciprofloxacin 750 mg (IV) q12h.

Community-Acquired Pneumonia (CAP) (cont'd)

Subset	Usual Pathogens*	Preferred IV Therapy	Alternate IV Therapy	PO Therapy or IV-to-PO Switch
	P. (carinii) jiroveci (PCP)	TMP–SMX 5 mg/kg (IV) q6h × 3 weeks‡	Pentamidine 4 mg/kg (IV) q24h × 3 weeks‡	TMP–SMX 5 mg/kg (PO) q6h × 3 weeks **or** Atovaquone 750 mg (PO) of q12h **or** Dapsone 100 mg (PO) of q24h
Other pathogens	For Blastomyces, Histoplasma, Coccidioides, Paracoccidioides, Actinomyces, Nocardia, Pseudallescheria boydii, Sporothrix, Mucor, see pp. 264–266			

¶ Treat until cured.
† Treat only IV or IV-to-PO Switch.
* Compromised hosts predisposed to organisms listed, but may be infected by usual pathogens of normal hosts.
** Loading dose is not needed PO if given IV with the same drug.
‡ Steroid dosage: Prednisone 40 mg (PO) q12h on days 1–5, then 40 mg (PO) q24h on days 6–10, then 20 mg (PO) q24h on days 11–21. Methylprednisolone (IV) can be substituted at 75% of prednisone dose.

Clinical Presentation: Fever, cough, respiratory symptoms, chest x-ray consistent with pneumonia. Typical CAPs present only with pneumonia without extrapulmonary findings.
Diagnosis: Identification of organism on sputum gram stain/culture. Same organism is found in blood if blood cultures are positive. Also see Chapter 8 for typical chest x-ray patterns.

Community-Acquired Pneumonia (Typical Bacterial Pathogens)

Diagnostic Considerations: Sputum is useful if a single organism predominates and is not contaminated by saliva. Purulent sputum, pleuritic chest pain, pleural effusion favor typical pathogens.
Pitfalls: Obtain chest x-ray to verify the diagnosis and rule out non-infectious mimics (e.g., heart failure).
Therapeutic Considerations: Do not switch to narrow-spectrum antibiotic after organism is identified on gram stain/blood culture. Pathogen identification is important for prognostic and public health reasons, not for therapy. Severity of CAP is related to the degree of cardiopulmonary/immune dysfunction and impacts the length of hospital stay, not the therapeutic approach or antibiotic choice.
Prognosis: Related to cardiopulmonary status and splenic function.

Community-Acquired Pneumonia (Pertussis)

Clinical Presentation: Rhinorrhea over 1–2 weeks (catarrhal stage) progressing to paroxysms of cough (paroxysmal stage) lasting 2–4 weeks, often with a characteristic inspiratory whoop, followed by a convalescent stage lasting 1–2 weeks during which cough paroxysms decrease in frequency/ severity. Fever is low grade or absent. In children < 6 months, whoop is frequently absent and apnea may occur. Older children/adults may present with persistent cough (without whoop) lasting 2–6 weeks.

Diagnostic Considerations: A positive DFA for Bordetella pertussis from a nasopharyngeal swab (NP). May be cultured by beside inoculation from NP swab of Bordet-gengou media. "Shaggy heart" on chest x-ray is characteristic. The only CAP with > 60% lymphocytosis.

Pitfalls: Be sure to consider pertussis in older children and adults with prolonged coughing illness.

Therapeutic Considerations: By the paroxysmal stage, antibiotics have minimal effect on the course of the illness but are indicated to decrease transmission.

Prognosis: Good, despite the prolonged course.

Community-Acquired Pneumonia (Atypical Pathogens)

Clinical Presentation: CAP with extra-pulmonary symptoms, signs, or laboratory abnormalities.

Diagnosis: Confirm by specific serological tests.

Non-Zoonotic Infections (Legionella sp., M. pneumoniae, C. pneumoniae)

Diagnostic Considerations: Each atypical pathogen has a different and characteristic pattern of extra-pulmonary organ involvement. Legionaire's disease is suggested by relative bradycardia, ⇉ PO_4^-, ↑ SGOT, microscopic hematuria, abdominal pain, diarrhea.

Zoonotic Infections (Psittacosis, Q fever, Tularemia)

Diagnostic Considerations: Zoonotic contact history is key to presumptive diagnosis: psittacosis (parrots and relatives); Q fever (sheep, parturient cats); tularemia (rabbit, deer, deer fly bite).

Pitfalls: Organisms are difficult/dangerous to grow. Do not culture. Use serological tests for diagnosis.

Therapeutic Considerations: Q fever endocarditis requires prolonged therapy.

Prognosis: Good except for Q fever with complications (e.g., myocarditis, SBE).

Zoonotic Infections (Severe Acute Respiratory Syndrome; SARS)

Presentation: Fever, dry cough, myalgias, diarrhea in some. Auscultation of the lungs resembles viral influenza (i.e., quiet, no rales). Biphasic infection: fever decreases after few days, patient improves, then fever recurs in a few days and patients become short of breath/hypoxic. Chest x-ray shows bilateral interstitial (diffuse) infiltrates. WBC and platelet counts are usually normal or slightly decreased. Relative lymphopenia present early. Mild increases in SGOT/SGPT, LDH, CPK are common.

Diagnostic Considerations: Diagnosis by viral isolation or specific SARS serology. Important to exclude influenza A, Legionnaires' disease and tularemic pneumonia.

Pitfalls: Should not be confused with viral influenza (a 3-day illness). Patients with SARS deteriorate during week 2 when influenza patients are recovering. Early, chest x-ray in SARS has discrete infiltrates (unlike influenza unless superimposed CAP) that may be ovoid. Late, ARDS on chest x-ray.

Therapeutic Considerations: Most patients are severely hypoxemic and require oxygen/ventilatory support. In a preliminary study, some patients benefitted from corticosteroids (pulse-dosed

methylprednisolone 500 mg [IV] q24h × 3 days followed by taper/step down with prednisone [PO] to complete 20 days) plus Interferon alfacon-1 (9 mcg [SQ] q24h × at least 2 days, increased to 15 mcg/d if no response) × 8–13 days. Ribavirin of no benefit.
Prognosis: Related to underlying cardiopulmonary/immune status/ARDS. Frequently fatal.
Pitfalls: Failure to respond to beta-lactams should suggest diagnosis of atypical CAP.
Therapeutic Considerations: Treat Legionella × 4 weeks. Treat Mycoplasma or Chlamydia × 2 weeks.
Prognosis: Related to severity of underlying cardiopulmonary disease.

Avian Influenza (Influenza virus, type A (H_5N_1)

Clinical Presentation: Influenza following close contact with infected poultry. Recent outbreaks in humans in Asia. Human-to-human transmission reported. Often fulminant respiratory illness rapidly followed by ARDS/death.
Diagnostic Considerations: Often acute onset of severe influenza illness ± diarrhea/conjunctival suffusion with leukopenia, lymphopenia, mildly ↑ serum transaminases and ↑ LDH. Diagnosis by hemagglutin-specific RT-PCR for avian influenza or culture of respiratory secretions.
Pitfalls: Although avian influenza is caused by influenza A virus, the hemagglutinin inhibition serological test used to diagnose influenza A is insensitive to avian hemagglutinin, resulting in negative testing.
Therapeutic Considerations: Antivirals must be given early to be effective. Avian influenza strains may be resistant to oseltamivir and amantadine/rimantadine. Oseltamivir 150 mg dose may be more effective than 75 mg dose. Even if resistant, amantadine/rimantadine should be given to increase peripheral airway dilatation/oxygenation.
Prognosis: Often fulminant infection with ARDS/death.

Influenza (Seasonal human) types A/B

Clinical Presentation: Acute onset of fever, headache, myalgias/arthralgias, sore throat, prostration, dry cough. Myalgias most pronounced in lower back/legs. Eye pain is common. Rapid high fever initially, which decreases in 2–3 days. Severity ranges from mild flu to life-threatening pneumonia.
Diagnostic Considerations: Mild cases with headache, sore throat, and rhinorrhea resemble the common cold/respiratory viruses (influenza-like illnesses) and can be caused by type A or B. Severe flu is usually due to type A. Rapid diagnosis by DFA of respiratory secretions (nasopharyngeal swabs). Influenza virus may be cultured in viral media from respiratory secretions and typed. Swine flu may be presumptively identified in patients with a "flu-like" illness with prominent N/V that test positive for influenza A.
Pitfalls: Influenza pneumonia has no auscultatory finding in the chest, and the chest x-ray is normal/near normal. Severe influenza pneumonia is accompanied by an oxygen diffusion defect (↑ A-a gradient), and patients are hypoxemic/cyanotic. Pleuritic chest pain indicates pleural irritation ± pleural effusion, which is characteristic of bacterial CAPs. Viral pneumonias are not associated with pleuritic chest pain, but Influenza virus can invade the intercostal muscles to mimic pleuritic chest pain. Chest x-ray in early influenza is normal/near normal without focal/segmental

infiltrates or pleural effusion. Infiltrates on chest x-ray with viral pneumonia indicate concurrent/ subsequent bacterial pneumonia. Ask about antecedent "flu/flu-like illness" if CAP presents with fulminant/severe necrotizing pneumonia in a normal host. Not all cases of swine flu test positive for influenza A.

Therapeutic Considerations: Mild/moderate influenza can be treated with neuraminidase inhibitors (Tamiflu/Relenza), which reduce symptoms by 1–2 days. Start treatment within 2 days of symptom onset. Reduce the dose of Tamiflu to 75 mg (PO) q48h for CrCl 10–30 cc/min. Relenza is generally not recommended for patients with underlying COPD/asthma (increased risk of bronchospasm) and should be discontinued if bronchospasm or a decline in respiratory function occurs. For severe influenza/pneumonia, treat with rimantadine or amantadine, which may increase peripheral airway dilatation/oxygenation. Reduce the dose of rimantadine to 100 mg (PO) q24h in the elderly, severe liver dysfunction, or CrCl < 10 cc/min. Flu with bacterial CAP is often due to S. aureus with post influenza CAP usually due to S. pneumoniae or H. influenzae (p. 52).

Prognosis: Good for mild/moderate flu. Severe flu may be fatal due to influenza pneumonia with profound hypoxemia. Prognosis is worse if presents with bacterial pneumonia, particularly if due to S. aureus. Influenza with necrotizing community-acquired (CA) MSSA/MRSA CAP is frequently fatal. Prognosis is worst for CA-MRSA Panton-Valentine Leukocidin (PVL)-positive strains. Dry cough/ fatigue may persist for weeks after influenza.

Table 2.1. Winthrop-University Hospital Infectious Disease Division's Point System for Diagnosing Severe Influenza A in Adults

Presentation	Clinical Features	Point Score
Symptoms		
Onset	Acute	+5
Prostration	Acute/severe	+5
Generalized muscle soreness	Severe	+5
Pain behind eyes neck/back	Severe	+5
Signs		
Fever (>102°F)	Present	+2
Dry cough	Present	–4
Coryza	Present	+1
Conjuctival suffusion	Otherwise unexplained	+5
Hemoptysis	Otherwise unexplained	+5
Blood-tinged/	Present	+3
purulent sputum	Present	–3
Localized rales	Otherwise unexplained	+5
Cyanosis	Shock	+5
Vascular collapse		

Table 2.1. Winthrop-University Hospital Infectious Disease Division's Point System for Diagnosing Severe Influenza A in Adults (cont'd)

Presentation	Clinical Features	Point Score
Laboratory Tests		
Leukocytosis	Present	–4
Leukopenia	Otherwise unexplained	+3
Lymphopenia	Otherwise unexplained Otherwise	+3
Thrombocytopenia	unexplained	+3
Chest x-ray	Minimal or no infiltrates (very early)	+3
	Focal segmental infiltrate*	–5
	Bilateral diffuse interstitial infiltrates (≤ 1 day)	+5
	Severe hypoxemia/(A-a gradient > 30)	+5
	Mild/no hypoxemia	–5
	Pleural effusion	–5
	Likelihood of Influenza A	
Total Points	> 20 Influenza A very ***likely***	
	10–20 Mild/moderate influenza A ***likely***	
	< 10 Influenza A ***unlikely*** (influenza B or influenza-like illness likely)	

* If or onset with present, suggests S. aureus (MSSA/CA-MCSA)

Table 2.2. The 3 Clinical Presentations of Influenza A Pneumonia in Adults

Clinical features at time of onset	Severity	Usual Pathogens
• Influenza pneumonia (***no focal/lobar CXR infiltrates***)	Mild → often fatal	Influenza (human, avian, swine)
• Influenza pneumonia (***with multiple rapidly cavitating infiltrates***)	Severe → rapidly fatal	Influenza (human, avian, swine) plus MSSA/CA-MRSA
• Influenza pneumonia (***followed by non-cavitating focal/ lobar infiltrates*** (*after ~1 week of improvement*))	Mild/moderate → rarely fatal (unless underlying cardiopulmonary disease/ Immunodeficiency)	S. pneumoniae, H. influenzae

Swine Influenza (H_1N_1) Pneumonia

A. Clinical Presentation: Swine influenza (H_1N_1) may present as a mild illness with fever, cough, and loose stool/diarrhea to severe viral pneumonia requiring ventilation that may rapidly progress to ARDS/death. Because the clinical presentation resembles that of human seasonal influenza, patients with swine influenza (H_1N_1) pneumonia as well as other viral pneumonias typically present as influenza-like illnesses (ILIs). Unlike human seasonal influenza, swine influenza (H_1N_1) pneumonia affects primarily young healthy adults. As with human seasonal influenza, swine influenza (H_1N_1) may affect children, pregnant females, and the elderly with co-morbid conditions. In adults, swine influenza (H_1N_1) pneumonia typically presents with high fevers > 102° F (not uncommonly initial fevers are 103° F - 104° F) usually with shaking chills and severe myalgias but some patients have low grade fevers. Swine influenza (H_1N_1) pneumonia patients with fevers > 102° F do not have a pulse temperature deficit, i.e., relative bradycardia. Patients may complain of headache or sore throat. Dry cough is characteristic but a productive cough with thin mucoid sputum is also common. Depending upon on the severity of swine influenza (H_1N_1) pneumonia, patients are variably short of breath. Conjunctival suffusion is rare. Lungs are clear to auscultation. Patients often have loose stools/diarrhea but abdominal pain is not part of the clinical presentation. Swine influenza (H_1N_1) pneumonia clinically resembles human seasonal influenza, avian influenza CMV or adenoviral CAP. CXR early (< 48 hours) typically is clear or may show accentuated bibasilar lung markings resembling basilar atelectasis. CXR later (> 48 hours) typically shows bilateral patchy interstitial infiltrates. Consolidation may occur later, but cavitations or pleural effusions are not features of swine influenza (H_1N_1) pneumonia. Degree of hypoxemia is related to the severity of swine influenza (H_1N_1) pneumonia. In adults, non-specific laboratory clues to swine influenza (H_1N_1) pneumonia include otherwise unexplained relative lymphopenia (< 21%) +/– thrombocytopenia. Atypical lymphocytes are not a feature of swine influenza (H_1N_1) pneumonia. Unlike in human seasonal and avian influenza (H_5N_1), leukopenia is rare in swine influenza (H_1N_1) pneumonia in adults and when present is not an isolated feature and usually accompanies or follows relative lymphopenia/thrombocytopenia. Most patients with swine influenza (H_1N_1) pneumonia have highly elevated CPKs and mildly elevated serum transaminases (SGOT/SGPT). Serum LDH is variably elevated. Elevated cold agglutinin titers are not a feature of swine influenza (H_1N_1) pneumonia. Nosocomial transmission occurs. In children with swine influenza (H_1N_1) pneumonia, leukocytosis is the rule and relative lymphopenia is not universal as it is with adults.

B. Diagnostic Considerations: Definitive diagnosis is by RT-PCR of oropharyngeal/respiratory secretions/lung tissue. Rapid screening tests for influenza A, if positive, correlate fairly well with RT-PCR positivity. However, rapid influenza A tests are associated with up to 30% false negatives. Therefore, a negative rapid influenza A test does not rule out swine influenza (H_1N_1). Respiratory fluorescent antibody (FA) viral testing may or may not be associated with a positive rapid influenza A/positive RT-PCR tests. Discordant testing results with rapid influenza A, respiratory FA viral panel, and RT-PCR may be due to variability of specimens rather than differences in test sensitivity/specificity. All tests may be negative in autopsy proven cases of swine influenza (H_1N_1) pneumonia whose lungs are RT-PCR positive.

C. Pitfalls: Since swine influenza (H_1N_1) pneumonia presents as an ILI, care must be taken to rule out other viral pneumonias as well as mimics of viral pneumonia. During the swine influenza (H_1N_1) pandemic, the most frequent diagnostic error was to assume a negative rapid influenza A test was predictive of a negative RT-PCR test. In adults with ILIs and negative rapid influenza A tests, clinical criteria are helpful in identifying swine influenza (H_1N_1) pneumonia and differentiating them from other viral pneumonias and typical/atypical bacterial CAP (Table 2.2). The CXR is important in identifying possible causes of atypical/typical bacterial CAP. Legionnaires' disease in particular, has some clinical features in common with swine influenza (H_1N_1) pneumonia. Importantly, any focal/lobar infiltrate on CXR should suggest typical/atypical CAP; *not* swine influenza (H_1N_1) pneumonia. While human seasonal influenza may present together with *S. aureus* (MSSA/MRSA) CAP or subsequently after an interval of improvement (5-7 days) with *S. pneumoniae* or *H. influenzae* CAP, this does not appear to be the case with swine influenza (H_1N_1) pneumonia (or avian influenza (H_5N_1) pneumonia). Swine influenza (H_1N_1) pneumonia on CXR appears initially with clear lung fields and with subsequent bilateral patchy infiltrates, but *not* with focal/lobar infiltrates. In patients with severe swine influenza (H_1N_1) pneumonia on ventilatory support over time, may develop consolidation overtime on CXR/chest CT and may develop ARDS. Late occurring consolidation should not be confused with lobar consolidation seen early with typical/atypical bacterial CAP. In adults, although relative lymphopenia is a consistent laboratory marker for swine influenza (H_1N_1) pneumonia, clinicians must be careful to be sure that relative lymphopenia is not due to a pre-existing disorder. (Table 2.3) On CXR, cavitations or pleural effusions are not a feature of swine influenza (H_1N_1) pneumonia and their presence argues against the diagusosis. In terms of non-specific laboratory tests, a highly elevated serum ferritin level ($\geq 2 \times$ normal) or otherwise unexplained hypophosphatemia strongly argue against the diagnosis of swine influenza (H_1N_1) pneumonia and instead points to Legionnaires' disease. Such patients will have focal/lobar infiltrates and other features of Legionnaires' disease, i.e., relative bradycardia which will readily differentiate Legionnaires' disease from swine influenza (H_1N_1) pneumonia. Also, patients with Legionnaires disease do not present with the severe myalgias characteristic of swine influenza (H_1N_1) penumonia. Loose stools/diarrhea may occur with both Legionnaires' disease and swine influenza (H_1N_1) pneumonia but abdominal pain in a patient with CAP suggests Legionnaires' disease until proven otherwise. Headache and mental confusion may occur in both swine influenza (H_1N_1) and Legionnaires' disease. Otherwise, unexplained microscopic hematuria points to Legionnaires' disease rather than swine influenza (H_1N_1) pneumonia. Cold agglutinins and atypical lymphocytes may occur in pediatric cases but in adults the presence of elevated cold agglutinins titers or atypical lymphocytes in the peripheral smear should suggest an alternate diagnosis, e.g., adenoviral or CMV pneumonia. Diagnostic tests for swine influenza (H_1N_1) pneumonia may all be negative. In autopsy proven cases of swine influenza (H_1N_1) pneumonia with negative rapid influenza A, negative respiratory FA viral, negative respiratory viral culture, and a negative RT-PCR tests have had positive RT-PCR in lung tissue.

D. Therapeutic Considerations: Swine influenza (H_1N_1) appears to respond to oseltamivir. There are no benefits to steroids. Although amantadine or rimantadine are ineffective against swine influenza (H_1N_1), patients who are severely hypoxemic may benefit from amantadine or rimantadine by increasing peripheral airway dilatation/oxygenation. If the CXR in swine influenza (H_1N_1) pneumonia has no lobar/focal infiltrates, there is no need to treat with empiric antimicrobial therapy. Patients (without swine influenza (H_1N_1) pneumonia) presenting with ILIs and lobar/focal infiltrates should be worked up and treated for typical/atypical bacterial CAPs. With swine influenza (H_1N_1) pneumonia with multiple lobar/focal infiltrates that rapidly cavitate (< 72 hours) empiric anti-MSSA/CA-MRSA therapy should be given with oseltamivir.

In patients unable to take oval oseltamivir, IV peramivir may be given. (See p. 650 for dosing recommendations.) For patients with swine influenza (H_1N_1) pneumonia that improves and after 5–7 days re-present with focal segmental/lobar (non-cavitating) infiltrates, treat as for typical CAP to cover S. pneumoniae or H. influenzae.

E. Prognosis: In immuncompetent adults, prognosis is related to severity of swine influenza (H_1N_1) pneumonia. The severity of the myalgias appears to correlate with the degree of CPK elevation. The degree and duration of relative lymphopenia has important diagnostic and prognostic implications. The longer a patient with swine influenza (H_1N_1) pneumonia has profound relative lymphopenia the worse the prognosis. Clinical improvement is preceded by an increase in the percentage of relative lymphocytes followed by an increase in the platelet count. With swine influenza (H_1N_1), prognosis is directly related to the severity of pneumonia and its associated oxygen diffusion defect, i.e., degree/duration of severe hypoxemia.

Table 2.3. Swine Influenza (H_1N_1) Pneumonia: Winthrop-University Infectious Disease Division's Weighted Diagnostic Point Score System for Hospitalized Adults with Negative Rapid Influenza Diagnostic Tests (RIDTs)

ILI with dry cough, fever > 102°F and a CXR *without* focal/segmental lobar infiltrates with negative RIDTs:

• Myalgias†	+5
• Relative lymphopenia*†	+5
• Elevated CPKs†	+3
• Elevated serum transaminases (SGOT/SGPT)†	+2
• Thrombocytopenia†	+5

Argues *against* the diagnosis of Swine influenza (H_1N_1) Pneumonia:

• Relative bradycardia†	−5
• No thrombocytopenia	−5
• Leukopenia (alone)†	−2
• Atypical lymphocytes†	−1
• Highly elevated serum ferritin levels (> 2 x n)†	−5
• Hypophosphatemia†	−3

Table 2.3. Swine Influenza (H_1N_1) Pneumonia: Winthrop-University Infectious Disease Division's Weighted Diagnostic Point Score System for Hospitalized Adults with Negative Rapid Influenza Diagnostic Tests (RIDTs) (cont'd)

Swine influenza Diagnostic Point Score Totals:	
• ***Probable*** swine influenza (H_1N_1) =	> 15
• ***Possible*** swine influenza (H_1N_1) =	10–15
• ***Unlikely*** swine influenza (H_1N_1) =	< 10

† Otherwise unexplained.
* Other causes of relative lymphopenia: Infectious causes: CMV, HHV-6, HHV-8, HIV, miliary TB, Legionella, typhoid fever, Q fever, bracellosis, SARS, malaria, babesiosis, influenza, (human, avian), RMSF, histoplasmosis, dengue fever, chickungunya fever, ehrlichiosis, prevovirus B19, HPS, WNE, viral hepatitis (early); Noninfectious causes: cytoxic drugs, steroids, sarcoidosis, SLE, lymphoma, RA, radiation therapy, Wiskott-Aldrich syndrome, Whipple's disease, severe combine immunodeficiency disease (SCID), common variable immune deficiency (CVID), Di George's syndrome, Nezelof's syndrome, intestinal lymphgiectasia, constrictive pericarditis, tricuspid regurgitation, Kawasaki's disease, idiopathic CD_4 cytopenia, Wegener's granulomatosis, acute/chromic renal failure, hemodialysis, myasthenia gravis, celiac disease, alcoholic circhosis, coronary byepass, CHF, acute pancreatitis, carcinomas (terminal).

Table 2.4. Swine Influenza (H_1N_1) Pneumonia: Case Definitions in Hospitalized Adults

Definite Swine Influenza (H_1N_1) Pneumonia (Laboratory Criteria) Diagnosis
ILI with dry cough, temperature > 102°F and *without* focal/segmental lobar infiltrates ***plus one or more of these positive tests:*** • Rapid influenza A test • Respiratory fluorescent antibody (FA) viral panel • RT-PCR for swine influenza (H_1N_1)
Probable Swine Influenza (H_1N_1) Pneumonia (Clinical Criteria) Diagnosis*
ILI with dry cough, temperature > 102°F with myalgias and a CXR without focal segmental/lobar infiltrates and negative RIDTs ***plus*** • Relative lymphopenia† • Thrombocytopenia† • Elevated CPKs†

† Otherwise unexplained.
* Diagnostic tests negative for other viral CAP pathogens (CMV, SARS, HPS, RSV, metapneumoviruses, parainfluenza viruses, adenoviruses).

Table 2.5. Rapid Clinical Diagnosis of Swine Influenza (H_1N_1) Pneumonia in Hospitalized Adults with Negative Rapid Influenza Diagnostic Tests (RIDTs): Diagnostic Swine Influenza Triad

Probable Swine Influenza (H_1N_1) Pneumonia (Clinical Criteria) Diagnosis
ILI with dry cough, temperature > 102°F and myalgias with a CXR *without* focal/segmental lobar infiltrates *with negative RIDTs* (see Table 2.4)* ***plus any 3 of the following***§: • Relative lymphopenia† • Thrombocytopenia† • Elevated SGOTs/SGPTs† • Elevated CPKs†

† Otherwise unexplained.
* Diagnostic tests negative for other viral CAP pathogens (CMV, SARS, HPS, RSV, metapneumoviruses, parainfluenza viruses, adenoviruses).
§ Present during first 3 days of hospitalization.

Aspiration Pneumonia

Diagnostic Considerations: Sputum not diagnostic. No need for transtracheal aspirate culture.
Pitfalls: Lobar location varies with patient position during aspiration.
Therapeutic Considerations: Oral anaerobes are sensitive to all beta-lactams and most antibiotics used to treat CAP. Additional anaerobic (B. fragilis) coverage is not needed.
Prognosis: Related to severity of CNS/esophageal disease.

CAP in HIV (*Sputum Negative for AFB*) *(for PCP, see p. 317)*

Clinical Presentation: CAP in HIV patient with focal infiltrate(s) and normal/slightly depressed CD_4.
Diagnostic Considerations: Diagnosis by sputum gram stain/culture ± positive blood cultures (bacterial pathogens) or Legionella/Chlamydia serology (atypical pathogens). Blood cultures most often positive for S. pneumoniae/H. influenzae. Cover S. aureus in IV drug users with preterminal disease.
Pitfalls: Atypical chest x-ray appearance is not uncommon. Treat syndrome of CAP, not chest x-ray. CAP in HIV does not resemble PCP, which presents with profound hypoxemia without focal infiltrates.
Therapeutic Considerations: Treat the same as CAP in normal hosts.
Prognosis: Clinically resolves the same as CAP in normal hosts.

Tuberculous (TB) Pneumonia

Clinical Presentation: Community-acquired pneumonia with single/multiple infiltrates.
Diagnostic Considerations: Diagnosis by sputum AFB smear/culture. Respiratory isolation important. Lower lobe effusion common in lower lobe primary TB. Reactivation TB is usually bilateral/apical ± old, healed Ghon complex; cavitation/fibrosis are common, but pleural effusion and adenopathy are absent.
Pitfalls: Primary TB may present as CAP and improve transiently with quinolone therapy. Reactivation TB presents as chronic pneumonia.

Therapeutic Considerations: 1–2 weeks of therapy is usually required to eliminate AFBs from sputum.
Prognosis: Related to underlying health status.

Mycobacterium avium-intracellulare (MAI) Pneumonia

Clinical Presentation: Community-acquired pneumonia in normal hosts or immunosuppressed/HIV patient with focal single/multiple infiltrates indistinguishable from TB.
Diagnostic Considerations: Diagnosis by AFB culture. In HIV, MAI may disseminate, resembling miliary TB. MAI typically lingular with "tree in bud" appearance on chest CT. BHA more frequent than with TB. No cavitation with MAI (vs. TB). Diagnosis by culture of blood, liver, or bone marrow.
Pitfalls: Must differentiate TB from MAI by AFB culture, since therapy for MAI differs from TB.
Therapeutic Considerations: MAI in normal hosts is readily treatable, but MAI in HIV patients requires life-long suppressive therapy after initial treatment.
Prognosis: Good in normal hosts. In HIV related to degree of immunosuppression/CD_4 count.

Mycobacterium kansasii Pneumonia

Clinical Presentation: Subacute CAP resembling TB/MAI infection that can occur in clusters/outbreaks.
Diagnostic Considerations: Chest x-ray infiltrates/lung disease plus M. kansasii in a single sputum specimen. M. kansasii can cause disseminated infection, like TB, and is diagnosed by culturing M. kansasii from sputum, blood, liver, or bone marrow.
Pitfalls: M. kansasii in sputum with a normal chest x-ray does not indicate infection.
Therapeutic Considerations: M. kansasii is more readily treatable than TB. Use the alternate regimen for rifampin-resistant strains.
Prognosis: Good in normal hosts. May be rapidly progressive/fatal without treatment in HIV patients.

Pneumonia in Chronic Alcoholics

Diagnostic Considerations: Klebsiella pneumoniae usually occurs only in chronic alcoholics, and is characterized by blood-flecked "currant jelly" sputum and cavitation (typically in 3–5 days).
Pitfalls: Suspect Klebsiella in "pneumococcal" pneumonia that cavitates. Empyema is more common than pleural effusion.
Therapeutic Considerations: Monotherapy with newer anti-Klebsiella agents is as effective or superior to "double-drug" therapy with older agents.
Prognosis: Related to degree of hepatic/splenic dysfunction.

Post-Viral Influenza Pneumonia

Diagnostic Considerations: S. aureus pneumonia usually only affects patients *concurrently* with viral influenza pneumonia, and is characterized by cyanosis and rapid cavitation on chest x-ray. Do not diagnose staphylococcal pneumonia without these signs (see pp. 51–52).
Pitfalls: Bacterial pneumonia may be superimposed or follow viral influenza pneumonia.
Therapeutic Considerations: Usually no need to cover MRSA for post-viral influenza CAP.
Prognosis: Related to severity of influenza pneumonia.

Bronchiectasis/Cystic Fibrosis

Diagnostic Considerations: Cystic fibrosis/bronchiectasis is characterized by viscous secretions ± low grade fevers; less commonly may present as lung abscess. Onset of pneumonia/lung abscess heralded by cough/decrease in pulmonary function.

Pitfalls: Sputum colonization is common (e.g., S. maltophilia, B. cepacia, P. aeruginosa); may not reflect pathogens.

Therapeutic Considerations: Important to select antibiotics with low resistance potential and good penetration into respiratory secretions (e.g., quinolones, meropenem).

Prognosis: Related to extent of underlying lung disease/severity of infection.

Nursing Home-Acquired Pneumonia (NHAP)

Diagnostic Considerations: Difficult to obtain sputum in elderly/debilitated patients. H. influenzae is common; K. pneumoniae is uncommon in non-alcoholics, even in this population.

Pitfalls: Resembles community-acquired pneumonia in terms of pathogens and length of hospital stay, not nosocomial pneumonia.

Therapeutic Considerations: Treat as community-acquired pneumonia, not nosocomial pneumonia. No need to cover P. aeruginosa or GNBs.

Prognosis: Related to underlying cardiopulmonary status.

Pneumonia in Organ Transplants

Clinical Presentation: CAP with perihilar infiltrates and hypoxemia.

Diagnostic Considerations: CMV is diagnosed by stain/culture of lung biopsy.

Therapeutic Considerations: Treat as CMV pneumonia if CMV is predominant pathogen on lung biopsy. CMV may progress despite ganciclovir therapy.

Prognosis: Related to degree of immunosuppression.

Pneumonia in Chronic Steroid Therapy

If fungal infection is suspected, obtain lung biopsy to confirm diagnosis/identify causative organism. Non-responsiveness to appropriate antibiotics should suggest fungal infection. Avoid empirically treating fungi; due to the required duration of therapy, it is advantageous to confirm the diagnosis by lung biopsy first. Prognosis related to degree of immunosuppression.

Acute Aspergillus Pneumonia

Clinical Presentation: Chest x-ray shows progressive necrotizing pneumonia (bilateral in half) unresponsive to antibiotics. Characteristic of early Aspergillus pneumonia is the "halo sign". A few days later the halo decreases in size. After a week after the appearance of the halo sign, the "air crescent sign" is typically present. Usually seen only in compromised hosts.

Diagnostic Considerations: Diagnosis by lung biopsy (not broncho-alveolar lavage) demonstrating hyphae invading lung parenchyma/blood vessels. Usually occurs only in patients receiving chronic steroids or cancer chemotherapy, organ transplants, leukopenic compromised hosts, or patients with chronic granulomatous disease.

Pitfalls: Invasive Aspergillus pneumonia does not occur in normal hosts.

Prognosis: Cavitation is a good prognostic sign. Prognosis related to degree of immunosuppression.

Lung Abscess/Empyema

Subset	Usual Pathogens	Preferred IV Therapy	Alternate IV Therapy	PO Therapy or IV-to-PO Switch
Lung abscess/ empyema	Oral anaerobes S. aureus K. pneumoniae S. pneumoniae	Clindamycin 600 mg (IV) q8h* **or** Piperacillin/ tazobactam 3.375 gm (IV) q8h*	Meropenem 1 gm (IV) q8h* **or** Ertapenem 1 gm (IV) q24h*	Clindamycin 300 mg (PO) q8h* **or** Quinolone† (PO) q24h*
Bronchiectasis, cystic fibrosis (P. aeruginosa): see p. 53				

* Treat until resolved. Duration of therapy represents total time IV, PO, or IV + PO. Most patients on IV therapy able to take PO meds should be switched to PO therapy soon after clinical improvement (usually < 72 hours).

† Moxifloxacin 400 mg or levofloxacin 500 mg.

Clinical Presentation: Lung abscess presents as single/multiple cavitary lung lesion(s) with fever. Empyema presents as persistent fever/pleural effusion without layering on lateral decubitus chest x-ray.

Diagnostic Considerations: In lung abscess, plain film/CT scan demonstrates cavitary lung lesions appearing > 1 week after pneumonia. Most CAPs are not associated with pleural effusion, and few develop empyema. In empyema, pleural fluid pH is ≤ 7.2; culture purulent exudate for pathogen.

Pitfalls: Pleural effusions secondary to CAP usually resolve rapidly with treatment. Suspect empyema in patients with persistent pleural effusions with fever.

Therapeutic Considerations: Chest tube/surgical drainage needed for empyema. Treat lung abscess until it resolves (usually 3–12 months).

Prognosis: Good if adequately drained.

Nosocomial Pneumonia (NP) / Hospital-Acquired Pneumonia (HAP) / Ventilator-Associated Pneumonia (VAP)

Subset	Usual Pathogens	Preferred IV Therapy	Alternate IV Therapy	IV-to-PO Switch
Empiric therapy	P. aeruginosa* E. coli K. pneumoniae S. marcescens (S. aureus)†	Meropenem 1 gm (IV) q8h × 1–2 weeks **or** Doripenem 1 gm (IV) q8h × 2 weeks **or** Levofloxacin 750 mg (IV) q24h × 1–2 weeks **or** Piperacillin/tazobactam 4.5 gm (IV) q6h ***plus*** amikacin 1 gm (IV) q24h × 1–2 wks		Levofloxacin 750 mg (PO) q24h × 1–2 weeks **or** Ciprofloxacin 750 mg (PO) q12h × 1–2 weeks

Duration of therapy represents total time IV or IV + PO. Most patients on IV therapy able to take PO meds should be switched to PO therapy after clinical improvement.

* For confirmed P. aeruginosa NP/VAP, combination therapy preferred.

† MSSA/HA-MRSA are common colonizers of respiratory secretions in ventilated patients, but *rarely* cause NP/HAP/VAP.

Nosocomial Pneumonia (NP) / Hospital-Acquired Pneumonia (HAP) / Ventilator-Associated Pneumonia (VAP) (cont'd)

Subset	Usual Pathogens	Preferred IV Therapy	Alternate IV Therapy	IV-to-PO Switch
Specific therapy	P. aeruginosa*‡	Meropenem 1 gm (IV) q8h × 2 weeks **or** Doripenem 1 gm (IV) q8h × 2 weeks† **plus either** Levofloxacin 750 mg (IV) q24h × 2 wks **or** Ciprofloxacin 400 mg (IV) q8h × 2 wks **or** Amikacin 1 gm (IV) q24h × 2 weeks		Levofloxacin 750 mg (PO) q24h × 2 weeks **or** Ciprofloxacin 750 mg (PO) q12h × 2 weeks
	MDR Klebsiella or MDR Acinetobacter	Meropenem 1 gm (IV) q8h × 2 weeks **or** Doripenem 1 gm (IV) q8h × 2 weeks†		
	MDR P. aeruginosa	Meropenem 1 gm (IV) q8h × 2 weeks **or** Colistin 1.7 mg/kg (IV) q8h × 2 weeks **or** Polymyxin B 1–1.25 mg/kg (IV) q12h × 2 weeks **or** Doripenem 1 gm (IV) q8h × 2 weeks†		
	HSV-1**	Acyclovir 5 mg/kg (IV) q8h × 10 days		Valacyclovir 1 gm (PO) q8h × 10 days

Duration of therapy represents total time IV or IV + PO.

* For proven P. aeruginosa NP/VAP, combination therapy preferred.

‡ P. aeruginosa NP/VAP shows multiple infiltrates with rapid cavitation in <72 h on CXR ± otherwise unexplained blood cultures for P. aeruginosa (BCs - in inhalation acquired P. aeruginosa VAP and BCs + in hematogenously acquired P. aeruginosa NP/VAP).

† Give as a 4 hour infusion.

** Presents late in course of VAP as "failure to wean", does *not* present initially as VAP.

Clinical Presentation: Pulmonary infiltrate compatible with a bacterial pneumonia occurring ≥ 1 week in-hospital ± fever/leukocytosis.

Diagnostic Considerations: CXR infiltrates with leukocytosis and fever are nonspecific/nondiagnostic of NP/VAP. Definitive diagnosis by lung biopsy. P. aeruginosa is a common colonizer in ventilated patients. P. aeruginosa VAP manifests as a necrotizing pneumonia with rapid cavitation (< 72 hours), microabscesses, and blood vessel invasion. S. aureus (MSSA/MRSA) is a very rare cause of NP/VAP despite being cultured from 25% of ET tube respiratory secretions. Acinetobacter/Legionella NP/VAP occur usually in outbreak situations.

Pitfalls: No rationale for covering non-pulmonary pathogens colonizing respiratory secretions in ventilated patients (Enterobacter, B. cepacia, S. maltophilia, Citrobacter, Flavobacterium, Enterococci); these organisms rarely if ever cause NP/VAP. Semi-quantitative BAL/protected brush specimens may reflect airway colonization. Even tissue biopsy is needed for definitive diagnosis of P. aeruginosa NP/VAP. MSSA/MRSA are common colonizers of respiratory secretions and are not uncommon pathogens causing tracheobronchitis in ventilated patients. MSSA/MRSA necrotizing/rapidly cavitating NP/VAP is rare.

Therapeutic Considerations: NP (HAP/VAP) is defined as pneumonia acquired > 5 hospital days. So called "early" NP occurring < 5 days of hospitalization, which may be due to S. pneumoniae (including DRSP strains) or H. influenzae, actually represents CAP that manifests early after hospital admission. Empiric therapy recommendations (p. 67) cover "early" and "late" NP/VAP pathogens. Monotherapy is as effective as combination therapy for non-P. aeruginosa NP/VAP, but 2-drug therapy is recommended for confirmed P. aeruginosa NP/VAP. If MSSA/MRSA nectorizing/rapidly cavitating NP/VAP present, may be treated with vancomycin, quinupristin/dalfopristin or linezolid (see drug summaries in Chapter 11). After 2 weeks of appropriate antibiotic therapy, non-progressive/stable pulmonary infiltrates with fever and leukocytosis are usually due to a non-infectious cause, rather than persistent infection. Anaerobes are not pathogens in NP/VAP.

Prognosis: Related to underlying cardiopulmonary status.

Empiric Therapy of Cardiovascular Infections

Subacute Bacterial Endocarditis (SBE)

Subset	Usual Pathogens	Preferred IV Therapy	Alternate IV Therapy	PO Therapy or IV-to-PO Switch
No obvious source or oral	Veridans streptococci*† Group B, C, G streptococci, S. bovis (PCN MIC < 0.12 mcg/ml)	Ceftriaxone 2 gm (IV) q24h × 2 weeks*‡ **plus** Gentamicin 120 mg (IV) q24h × 2 weeks* **or monotherapy with** Ceftriaxone 2 gm (IV) q24h × 4 weeks	Penicillin G 3 mu (IV) q4h × 2 weeks*‡ **plus** Gentamicin 120 mg (IV) q24h × 2 weeks* **or** Vancomycin 1 gm (IV) q12h × 2 weeks **or** Linezolid 600 mg (IV) q12h × 4 weeks	Amoxicillin 1 gm (PO) q8h × 4 weeks **or** Linezolid 600 mg (PO) q12h × 4 weeks

* If relatively PCN resistant (MIC 0.12–0.5 mcg/ml) or if no intra/extra cardiac complications treat × 4 weeks.

† S. mitis (S. mitior), S. oralis, S. gordonii, S. parasanguis, S. sanguis, S. mutans, S. sobrinus, S. thermophilus, S. angiosus, S. milleri, S. intermedius, S. constellatus.

‡ In PCN allergic patients, Vancomycin 1 gm (IV) q12h × 2 weeks.

Subacute Bacterial Endocarditis (SBE) (cont'd)

Subset	Usual Pathogens	Preferred IV Therapy	Alternate IV Therapy	PO Therapy or IV-to-PO Switch
	Nutritionally-variant streptococci (NVS) pyridoxal B_6 dependent streptocci[‡]	As above, but treat × 6 weeks	As above, but treat × 6 weeks	As above, but treat × 6 weeks
GI/GU source likely (Treat initially for E. faecalis (VSE); if later identified as E. faecium (VRE), treat accordingly)	E. faecalis (VSE)[†]	Ampicillin 2 gm (IV) q4h × 4–6 weeks or Vancomycin 1 gm (IV) q12h × 4–6 weeks **plus** Gentamicin 80 mg (IV) q8h or 120 mg (IV) q12h × 4–6 weeks	Meropenem 1 gm (IV) q8h × 4–6 weeks **or** Linezolid 600 mg (IV) q12h × 4–6 weeks	Linezolid 600 mg (PO) q12h × 4–6 weeks
	E. faecium (VRE)[†]	Linezolid 600 mg (IV) q12h × 4–6 weeks **or** Quinupristin/dalfopristin 7.5 mg/kg (IV) q8h × 4–6 weeks		Linezolid 600 mg (PO) q12h × 4–6 weeks
GI source	S. (bovis) gallolyticus (Non-enterococcal group D streptococci)	Treat the same as "no obvious source" subset (p. 69)		

VRE = vancomycin-resistant enterococci. Duration of therapy represents total time IV, PO, or IV + PO. Most patients on IV therapy able to take PO meds should be switched to PO therapy soon after clinical improvement.

† Symptoms < 3 months → treat × 4 weeks.
Symptoms > 3 months → treat × 6 weeks.

‡ *NVS (nutritionally variant streptococci)* include: Abiotrophia defectivus, Granulicata adjacens/elegans.

Subacute Bacterial Endocarditis (SBE) (cont'd)

Subset	Usual Pathogens	Preferred IV Therapy	Alternate IV Therapy	PO Therapy or IV-to-PO Switch
Apparent "culture negative" SBE*	Hemophilus sp. Actinobacillus actinomycetem-comitans Cardiobacterium hominis Eikenella corrodens Kingella kingae	Ceftriaxone 2 gm (IV)/(IM) q24h × 4 weeks **or** Any 3rd generation cephalosporin (IV) × 4 weeks **or** Cefepime 2 gm (IV) q12h × 4 weeks	Ampicillin 2 gm (IV) q4h × 4 weeks **plus** Gentamicin 120 mg (IV) q24h × 4 weeks **or monotherapy with** Quinolone† (IV) q24h × 4–6 weeks	Quinolone† (PO) q24h × 4–6 weeks
True "culture negative" SBE*	Legionella Coxiella burnetii (Q fever) Chlamydophilia (Chlamydia) psittaci	Quinolone† (IV) q24h × 4–6 weeks	Doxycycline 200 mg (IV) q12h × 3 days, then 100 mg (IV) q12h × 4–6 weeks	Quinolone† (PO) q24h × 4–6 weeks **or** Doxycycline 200 mg (PO) q12h × 3 days, then 100 mg (PO) q12h × 4–6 weeks**
Brucella SBE†	Brucella melitensis, abortus, canis, suis	Doxycycline 200 mg (IV) q12h × 3 days, then 100 mg (IV) q12h × 4–6 weeks **plus** Gentamicin 120 mg (IV) q24h × 4–6 weeks	Quinolone (IV) q24h† × 4–6 weeks **plus** Rifampin 300 mg (PO) q12h × 4–6 weeks	Quinolone† (PO) q24h × 4–6 weeks **or** Doxycycline 200 mg (PO) q12h × 3 days, then 100 mg (PO) q12h × 4–6 weeks**

* Slow growing/fastidious organisms may require ↑ CO_2 and prolonged incubation 2–4 weeks.
† Levofloxacin 500 mg (IV or PO) or Moxifloxacin 400 mg (IV or PO).
** Loading dose is not needed PO if given IV with the same drug.

Clinical Presentation: Subacute febrile illness ± localizing symptoms/signs in a patient with a heart murmur. Peripheral manifestations are commonly absent with early diagnosis/treatment.
Diagnosis: Positive blood cultures plus vegetation on transthoracic/transesophageal echo.

SBE (No Obvious Source)

Diagnostic Considerations: Most common pathogen is veridans streptococcal. Source is usually from the mouth, although oral/dental infection is usually inapparent clinically.
Pitfalls: Vegetations without positive blood cultures or peripheral manifestations of SBE are not diagnostic of endocarditis. SBE vegetations may persist after antibiotic therapy, but are sterile.
Therapeutic Considerations: In penicillin-allergic (anaphylactic) patients, vancomycin may be used alone or in combination with gentamicin. Follow ESR weekly to monitor antibiotic response. No need to repeat blood cultures unless patient has persistent fever or is not responding clinically. Two-week treatment is acceptable for uncomplicated veridans streptococcal SBE. Treat nutritionally-variant streptococci (NVS) (B_6/pyridoxal dependent streptococci) same as veridans streptococcal SBE.
Prognosis: Related to extent of embolization/severity of heart failure.

SBE (GI/GU Source Likely)

Diagnostic Considerations: Commonest pathogens from GI/GU source are Enterococci (especially) E. faecalis). If S. bovis, look for GI polyp, tumor. Enterococcal SBE commonly follows GI/GU instrumentation.
Therapeutic Considerations: E. faecalis SBE may be treated with ampicillin alone; gentamicin may be added if synergy testing is positive (e.g., isolate sensitive to < 500 mcg/mL of gentamicin). Do not add gentamicin if MIC > 500 mcg/mL. For penicillin-allergic patients, use vancomycin plus gentamicin; vancomycin alone is inadequate for enterococcal (E. faecalis) SBE. Treat enterococcal PVE the same as for native valve enterococcal SBE. Treat S. bovis SBE the same as S. viridans SBE. Non-enterococcal Group D streptococci (S. bovis) is penicillin sensitive, unlike Group D enterococci (E. faecalis).
Prognosis: Related to extent of embolization/severity of heart failure.

Apparent "Culture Negative" SBE

Diagnostic Considerations: Culture of HACEK organisms may require enhanced CO_2/special media (Castaneda vented bottles) and prolonged incubation (2–4 weeks). True "culture negative" SBE is rare, and is characterized by peripheral signs of SBE, a murmur, vegetation (by TTE/TEE), and negative blood cultures.
Pitfalls: Most cases of "culture negative" SBE are not in fact culture negative SBE, but are due to fastidious organisms eg (HACEK group) that are not reported growing as rapidly in blood cultures (5 days with automated blood culture techniques) as non-fastidious SBE pathogens.
Therapeutic Considerations: Follow clinical improvement with serial ESRs, which should return to pretreatment levels with therapy. Verification of cure by negative blood culture is not needed if patient is afebrile and clinically well. Serial TTEs/TEEs show decreasing vegetation size during effective therapy. Sterile vegetations may persist after antibiotic therapy.
Prognosis: Related to extent of embolization/severity of heart failure.

True "Culture Negative" SBE

Diagnostic Considerations: Diagnosis by specific serology. Large vessel emboli suggests culture negative SBE in patients with negative blood cultures but signs of SBE.
Pitfalls: Do not diagnose culture negative SBE in patients with a heart murmur and negative blood cultures if peripheral SBE manifestations are absent.
Therapeutic Considerations: Treatment is based on specific organism identified by diagnostic tests.
Prognosis: Related to extent of embolization/severity of heart failure.

Acute Bacterial Endocarditis (ABE)

Subset	Usual Pathogens	Preferred IV Therapy	Alternate IV Therapy	PO Therapy or IV-to-PO Switch
Normal hosts* (Treat initially for MRSA; if later identified as MSSA, treat accordingly)	S. aureus (MRSA)	***Treat (IV)*** × ***4–6 weeks*** **with either** Daptomycin 6 mg/kg (IV) q24h × 4–6 weeks **or** Linezolid 600 mg (IV) q24h × 4–6 weeks **or** Quinupristin/dalfopristin 7.5 mg/kg (IV) q8h × 4–6 weeks **or** Vancomycin 1 gm (IV) q12h × 4–6 weeks **or** Minocycline 100 mg (IV) q12h × 4–6 weeks		Linezolid 600 mg (PO) q12h × 4–6 wks **or** Minocycline 100 mg (PO) q12h × 4–6 wks
	S. aureus (MSSA)	Nafcillin 2 gm (IV) q4h × 4–6 weeks **or** Cefazolin 1 gm (IV) q8h × 4–6 weeks **or** any carbapenem (IV) × 4–6 weeks **or** any MRSA agent (above) × 4–6 weeks		Linezolid 600 mg (PO) q12h × 4–6 wks **or** Minocycline 100 mg (PO) q12h × 4–6 wks **or** Cephalexin 1 gm (PO) q6h × 4–6 weeks
IV drug abusers (IVDAs)† (Treat as MRSA before culture results; treat according to pathogen after culture results)	S. aureus (MRSA)	Before culture results Vancomycin 1 gm (IV) q12h × 4 weeks **plus either** Gentamicin 120 mg (IV) q12h × 4 weeks **or** Amikacin 500 mg (IV) q24h × 4 weeks	After culture results Daptomycin 6 mg/kg (IV) q24h × 4 weeks **or** Linezolid 600 mg (IV) q12h × 4 weeks **or** Minocycline 100 mg (IV) q12h × 4 weeks **or** Vancomycin 1 gm (IV) q12h × 4 weeks	After culture results Linezolid 600 mg (PO) q12h × 4 weeks **or** Minocycline 100 mg (PO) q12h × 4 weeks

MRSA/MSSA = methicillin-resistant/sensitive S. aureus. Duration of therapy represents total time IV, PO, or IV + PO. Most patients on IV therapy able to take PO meds should be switched to PO therapy after clinical improvement.

* Treat IV or with IV-to-PO switch therapy.

† *MSSA/MRSA TV ABE may be treated IV/PO × 2 weeks if no intra cardiac or CNS complications.* Pulmonary septic emboli are a feature of TV ABE and are not, per se, an extracardiac complication.

Acute Bacterial Endocarditis (ABE) (cont'd)

Subset	Usual Pathogens	Preferred IV Therapy	Alternate IV Therapy	PO Therapy or IV-to-PO Switch
IV drug abusers (cont'd)	S. aureus (MSSA)	Before culture results Treat the same as MRSA	After culture results Nafcillin 2 gm (IV) q4h × 4 weeks **or** Cefazolin 1 gm (IV) q8h × 4 weeks **or** Daptomycin 6 mg/kg (IV) q24h × 4 weeks **or** Linezolid 600 mg (IV) q12h × 4 weeks **or** Minocycline (IV) 100 mg (IV) q12h × 4 weeks **or** Any carbapenem (IV) × 4 weeks	After culture results Linezolid 600 mg (PO) q12h × 4 weeks **or** Minocycline 100 mg (PO) q12h × 4 weeks **or** Cephalexin 1 gm (PO) q6h × 4 weeks
	P. aeruginosa* S. marcesens Aerobic GNBs	Before culture results Meropenem 1 gm (IV) q8h **or** Piperacillin 4 gm (IV) q6h	After culture results **One "A" drug ± one "B" drug** **"A" Drugs** Meropenem 1 gm (IV) q8h × 4–6 weeks **or** Doripenem 1 gm (IV) q8h × 4–6 weeks **"B" Drugs** Amikacin 500 mg (IV) q24h × 4–6 weeks **or** Aztreonam 2 gm (IV) q8h × 4–6 weeks	After culture results Ciprofloxacin 750 mg (PO) q12h × 4–6 weeks **or** Levofloxacin 750 mg (PO) q24h × 4–6 weeks

MRSA/MSSA = methicillin-resistant/sensitive S. aureus. Duration of therapy represents total time IV, PO, or IV + PO. Most patients on IV therapy able to take PO meds should be switched to PO therapy after clinical improvement.

* Treat IV or with IV-to-PO switch therapy.

Acute Bacterial Endocarditis (ABE)

Diagnostic Considerations: Clinical criteria for MRSA/MSSA ABE: continuous/high-grade bacteremia (repeatedly 3/4 or 4/4 positive blood cultures), fever (temperature usually ≥ 102°F), no, new or changing murmur, and vegetation by transesophageal/transthoracic echocardiogram.

Pitfalls: Obtain a baseline TTE for comparative purposes should ABE be complicated by valve destruction, heart failure or ring/perivalvular abscess. Obtain infectious disease and cardiology consultations. In MSSA/MRSA ABE patients initially treated with vancomycin, resistance to deptomycin may occur during therapy.

Therapeutic Considerations: Treat for 4–6 weeks. Follow teichoic acid antibody titers weekly in S. aureus ABE, which fall (along with the ESR) with effective therapy. If MSSA/MRSA ABE unresponsive (persistent high grade bacteremia) to appropriate antibiotic therapy or if a myocardial/paravalvular abscess present that cannot be surgically drained, "high dose" daptomycin 12 mg/kg (IV) q24h may be effective. With daptomycin resistant MSSA/MRSA strains, Quinupristin dalfopristin 7.5 mg/kg (IV) q8h may be effective.
Prognosis: Related to extent of embolization/severity of valve destruction/heart failure.

Acute Bacterial Endocarditis (IV Drug Abusers)

Diagnostic Considerations: Clinically IVDAs with S. aureus usually have relatively mild ABE, permitting oral treatment.
Pitfalls: IVDAs with new aortic or tricuspid regurgitation should be treated IV ± valve replacement.
Therapeutic Considerations: After pathogen is isolated, may switch from IV to PO regimen to complete treatment course.
Prognosis: Prognosis is better than ABE in normal hosts if not complicated by abscess, valve regurgitation, or heart failure.

Prosthetic Valve Endocarditis (PVE)

Subset	Usual Pathogens	Before Culture Results	After Culture Results
Early PVE (< 60 days post-PVR)	S. aureus (MSSA/MRSA) Enterobacteriaceae	Vancomycin 1 gm (IV) q12h **plus** Gentamicin 120 mg (IV) q24h	<u>MSSA/Enterobacteriaceae</u> Cefotaxime 3 gm (IV) q6h × 6 weeks **or** Ceftizoxime 4 gm (IV) q8h × 6 weeks **or** Cefepime 2 gm (IV) q8–12h × 6 weeks **or** Meropenem 1 gm (IV) q8h × 6 weeks <u>MSSA/MRSA†</u> Daptomycin 6 mg/kg (IV) q24h × 6 weeks **or** Linezolid 600 mg (IV or PO) q12h × 6 weeks **or** Vancomycin 1 gm (IV) q12h × 6 weeks* **or** Minocycline 100 mg (IV or PO) q12h × 6 weeks

MSSA/MRSA = methicillin-sensitive/resistant S. aureus. Duration of therapy represents total time IV or IV + PO. Most patients on IV therapy able to take PO meds should be switched to PO therapy after clinical improvement.
† MRSA drugs also effective against MSSA.
* ± Rifampin 300 mg (PO) q12h × 6 weeks.

Prosthetic Valve Endocarditis (PVE) (cont'd)

Subset	Usual Pathogens	Before Culture Results	After Culture Results
Late PVE (> 60 days post-PVR)	Veridans streptococci S. epidermidis (CoNS)	Meropenem 1 gm (IV) q8h **or combination therapy with** Vancomycin 1 gm (IV) q12h **plus** Gentamicin 120 mg (IV) q24h	<u>Veridans streptococci</u> Ceftriaxone 2 gm (IV) q24h × 6 weeks **or** Meropenem 1 gm (IV) q8h × 6 weeks **or** Ertapenem 1 gm (IV) q24h × 6 weeks <u>CoNS</u> Linezolid 600 mg (IV or PO) q12h × 6 weeks **or** Vancomycin 1 gm (IV) q12h × 6 weeks*

MSSA/MRSA = methicillin-sensitive/resistant S. aureus; MSSE/MRSE = methicillin-sensitive/resistant S. epidermidis. Duration of therapy represents total time IV or IV + PO. Most patients on IV therapy able to take PO meds should be switched to PO therapy after clinical improvement.

* ± Rifampin 300 mg (PO) q12h × 6 weeks.

Clinical Presentation: Prolonged fevers and chills following prosthetic valve replacement (PVR).

Diagnosis: High-grade blood culture positivity (3/4 or 4/4) with endocarditis pathogen and no other source of infection.

<u>Early PVE (< 60 days post-PVR)</u>

Diagnostic Considerations: Blood cultures persistently positive. Temperature usually ≤ 102°F.

Pitfalls: Obtain baseline TTE/TEE. Premature closure of mitral leaflet is early sign of impending aortic valve regurgitation.

Therapeutic Considerations: Patients improve clinically on treatment, but are not cured without valve replacement. Replace valve as soon as possible (no advantage in waiting).

Prognosis: Related to extent of embolization/severity of heart failure.

<u>Late PVE (> 60 days post-PVR)</u>

Pitfalls: Culture of removed valve may be negative, but valve gram stain will be positive.

Therapeutic Considerations: Late PVE resembles veridans streptococcal SBE clinically. Valve removal for S. epidermidis PVE may be necessary for cure.

Prognosis: Related to extent of embolization/severity of heart failure.

Pericarditis/Myocarditis

Subset	Usual Pathogens	Preferred Therapy
Diptheritic myocarditis	C. diphtheriae	Treat same as diphtheriae (p. 166)
Viral	Coxsackie, influenza	No treatment for Coxsackie, for influenza therapy (p. 166)
Lyme myocarditis	B. burgdorferi	Ceftriaxone 1 gm (IV) q24h × 2 weeks **or** Doxycycline 100 mg (IV) q12h × 2 weeks
TB pericarditis	M. tuberculosis	Treat same as pulmonary TB (p. 52). Add a tapering dose of corticosteroids × 4–8 weeks
Suppurative pericarditis	S. pneumoniae S. aureus	Treat same as lung abscess/ empyema (p. 67)

Clinical Presentation: Viral pericarditis presents with acute onset of fever/chest pain (made worse by sitting up) following a viral illness. Viral myocarditis presents with heart failure, arrhythmias ± emboli. TB pericarditis is indolent in presentation, with ↑ jugular venous distension (JVD), pericardial friction rub (40%), paradoxical pulse (25%), and chest x-ray with cardiomegaly ± left-sided pleural effusion. Suppurative pericarditis presents as acute pericarditis (patients are critically ill). Develops from contiguous (e.g., pneumonia) or hematogenous spread (e.g., S. aureus bacteremia). Lyme often presents with varying degrees of heart block (including complete heart block) ± signs of myocarditis.

Diagnostic Considerations: Pericarditis/effusion manifests cardiomegaly with decreased heart sounds ± tamponade. Diagnosis by culture/biopsy of pericardial fluid or pericardium for viruses, bacteria, or acid-fast bacilli (AFB). Diagnosis of myocarditis is clinical ± myocardial biopsy.

Pitfalls: Consider other causes of pericardial effusion (malignancy, esp. if bloody effusion, uremia, etc). Rule out treatable non-viral causes of myocarditis (e.g., RMSF, Lyme, diphtheria). Suspect Lyme disease in any person without heart disease with exposure to endemic area who presents with otherwise unexplained heart block. Lyme IgM titers may be negative early when patients present with heart block.

Therapeutic Considerations: No specific treatment for viral myocarditis/pericarditis. TB pericarditis is treated the same as pulmonary TB ± pericardiectomy. Suppurative pericarditis is treated the same as lung abscess plus surgical drainage (pericardial window). Heart block in Lyme disease rapidly reverses with therapy, but a temporary pacemaker may be needed until heart block is reversed.

Prognosis: For viral pericarditis, the prognosis is good, but viral myocarditis may be fatal. For TB pericarditis, the prognosis is good if treated before constrictive pericarditis/adhesions develop. Suppurative pericarditis is often fatal without early pericardial window/antibiotic therapy. With Lyme myocarditis/heart block, prognosis is good if treatment is started early when diagnosis is suspected.

Central IV Line (CVC) and Pacemaker Infections

Subset	Usual Pathogens	Preferred IV Therapy	Alternate IV Therapy	IV-to-PO Switch
CVC (temporary) *Bacterial* (Treat initially for MSSA; if later identified as MRSA, treat accordingly)	S. aureus (MSSA) Aerobic GNBs	Meropenem 1 gm (IV) q8h* **or** Cefepime 2 gm (IV) q12h*	Ceftizoxime 2 gm (IV) q8h* **or** Cefotaxime 2 gm (IV) q6h*	Quinolone‡ (PO) q24h*
	S. aureus (MRSA/MSSA§)	Daptomycin 6 mg/kg (IV) q24h* **or** Linezolid 600 mg (IV) q12h* **or** Quinupristin/dalfopristin 7.5 mg/kg (IV) q8h* **or** Vancomycin 1 gm (IV) q12h*		Linezolid 600 mg (PO) q12h* **or** Minocycline 100 mg (PO) q12h*
Candida¶	C. albicans	Treat the same as for Candidemia (p. 150)		
(Treat initially for C. albicans; if later identified as non-albicans Candida, treat accordingly).	Non-albicans Candida	Treat the same as for Candidemia (p. 150)		
CVC (semi-permanent Hickman/Broviac) *Bacterial*	S. aureus (MSSA/MRSA)	Daptomycin 6 mg/kg (IV) q24h* **or** Linezolid 600 mg (IV) q12h* **or** Quinupristin/dalfopristin 7.5 mg/kg (IV) q8h* **or** Vancomycin 1 gm (IV) q12h*		Linezolid 600 mg (PO) q12h* **or** Minocycline 100 mg (PO) q12h*

MSSA/MRSA = methicillin-sensitive/resistant S. aureus.

‡ Levofloxacin 500 mg or Moxifloxacin 400 mg.

* Treat × 2 weeks after line removal.

¶ For candidemia not associated with IV lines, see pp. 148–149.

§ MRSA drugs also effective against MSSA.

Central IV Line (CVC) and Pacemaker Infections (cont'd)

Subset	Usual Pathogens	Preferred IV Therapy	Alternate IV Therapy	IV-to-PO Switch
	S. epidermidis (CoNS)	Daptomycin 6 mg/kg (IV) q24h* **or** Linezolid 600 mg (IV) q12h* **or** Quinupristin/dalfopristin 7.5 mg/kg (IV) q8h* **or** Vancomycin 1 gm (IV) q12h*		Linezolid 600 mg (PO) q12h*
Pacemaker wire/generator infection (Treat initially for S. aureus; if later identified as S. epidermidis, treat accordingly)	S. aureus (MSSA/MRSA)	Daptomycin 6 mg/kg (IV) q24h**† **or** Linezolid 600 mg (IV) q12h**† **or** Quinupristin/dalfopristin 7.5 mg/kg (IV) q8h**† **or** Vancomycin 1 gm (IV) q12h**†		Linezolid 600 mg (PO) q12h**† **or** Minocycline 100 mg (PO) q12h**†
	S. epidermidis (CoNS)	Daptomycin 6 mg/kg (IV) q24h**† **or** Linezolid 600 mg (IV) q12h† **or** Quinupristin/dalfopristin 7.5 mg/kg (IV) q8h† **or** Vancomycin 1 gm (IV) q12h†		Linezolid 600 mg (PO) q12h†

MSSA/MRSA = methicillin-sensitive/resistant S. aureus; MSSE/MRSE = methicillin-sensitive/resistant S. epidermidis.

* Treat × 2 weeks after line removal.

† Treat × 2 weeks after wire/generator removal.

** Obtain teichoic acid antibody titers after 2 weeks. If titers are 1:4 or less, 2 weeks of therapy is sufficient. If titers are > 1:4, rule out endocarditis and complete 4–6 weeks of therapy.

Central IV Line (CVC) and Pacemaker Infections (cont'd)

Subset	Usual Pathogens	Preferred IV Therapy	Alternate IV Therapy	IV-to-PO Switch
Septic thrombophlebitis (Treat initially for MSSA; if later identified as MRSA, treat accordingly)	S. aureus (MSSA)	Nafcillin 2 gm (IV) q4h × 2 weeks* **or** Linezolid 600 mg (IV) q12h × 2 weeks* **or** Meropenem 1 gm (IV) q8h × 2 weeks*	Ceftizoxime 2 gm (IV) q8h × 2 weeks* **or** Cefotaxime 2 gm (IV) q6h × 2 weeks*	Linezolid 600 mg (PO) q12h × 2 weeks* **or** Clindamycin 300 mg (PO) q8h × 2 weeks* **or** Cephalexin 1 gm (PO) q6h × 2 weeks*
	S. aureus (MRSA)	Linezolid 600 mg (IV) q12h × 2 weeks* **or** Vancomycin 1 gm (IV) q12h × 2 weeks* **or** Quinupristin/dalfopristin 7.5 mg/kg (IV) q8h × 2 weeks*		Linezolid 600 mg (PO) q12h × 2 weeks* **or** Minocycline 100 mg (PO) q12h × 2 weeks*

MSSA/MRSA = methicillin-sensitive/resistant S. aureus. Duration of therapy represents total time IV or IV + PO. Most patients on IV therapy able to take PO meds should be switched to PO therapy after clinical improvement.

* Obtain teichoic acid antibody titers after 2 weeks. If titers are < 1:4, 2 weeks of therapy is sufficient. If titers are ≥ 1:4, rule out ABE and complete 4–6 weeks of therapy.

† Treat × 2 weeks after wire/generator removal.

CVC (Temporary) Infections

Clinical Presentation: Temperature ≥ 102°F ± IV site erythema.

Diagnostic Considerations: Diagnosis by semi-quantitative catheter tip culture with ≥ 15 colonies plus blood cultures with same pathogen. If no other explanation for fever and line has been in place ≥ 7 days, remove line and obtain semi-quantitative catheter tip culture. Suppurative thrombophlebitis presents with hectic/septic fevers and pus at IV site ± palpable venous cord.

Pitfalls: Temperature ≥ 102°F with IV line infection, in contrast to phlebitis.

Therapeutic Considerations: Line removal is usually curative, but antibiotic therapy is usually given for 1 week after IV line removal for gram-negative bacilli or 2 weeks after IV line removal for S. aureus (MSSA/MRSA). Antifungal therapy is usually given for 2 weeks after IV line removal for Candidemia.

Prognosis: Good if line is removed before endocarditis/metastatic spread.

CVC (Semi-Permanent) Hickman/Broviac Infection

Clinical Presentation: Fever ± IV site erythema.

Diagnostic Considerations: Positive blood cultures plus gallium scan pickup on catheter is diagnostic.

Pitfalls: Antibiotics will lower temperature, but patient will usually not be afebrile without line removal.

Therapeutic Considerations: Lines usually need to be removed for cure. Rifampin 600 mg (PO) q24h may be added to IV/PO regimen if pathogen is S. aureus.

Prognosis: Good with organisms of low virulence.

Pacemaker Wire/Generator Infection

Clinical Presentation: Persistently positive blood cultures without endocarditis in a pacemaker patient.

Diagnostic Considerations: Positive blood cultures with gallium scan pickup on wire/pacemaker generator is diagnostic. Differentiate wire from pacemaker pocket infection by chest CT/MRI.

Pitfalls: Positive blood cultures are more common in wire infections than pocket infections. Blood cultures may be negative in both, but more so with pocket infections.

Therapeutic Considerations: Wire alone may be replaced if infection does not involve pacemaker generator. Replace pacemaker generator if involved; wire if uninvolved can usually be left in place.

Prognosis: Good if pacemaker wire/generator replaced before septic complications develop.

Septic Thrombophlebitis

Clinical Presentation: Temperature ≥ 102°F with local erythema and signs of sepsis.

Diagnostic Considerations: Palpable venous cord and pus at IV site when IV line is removed.

Pitfalls: Suspect diagnosis if persistent bacteremia and no other source of infection in a patient with a peripheral IV.

Therapeutic Considerations: Remove IV catheter. Surgical venotomy is usually needed for cure.

Prognosis: Good if removed early before septic complications develop.

Vascular Graft Infections

Subset	Usual Pathogens	Preferred IV Therapy	Alternate IV Therapy	IV-to-PO Switch
AV graft/shunt infection (Treat initially for MRSA, etc.; if later identified as MSSA, treat accordingly)	S. aureus (MRSA)	Daptomycin 6 mg/kg (IV) q24h*† **or** Linezolid 600 mg (IV) q12h dose*†	Vancomycin 1 gm (IV) q12h*† **or** Minocycline 100 mg (IV) q12h†	Linezolid 600 mg (PO) q12h† **or** Minocycline 100 mg (PO) q12h†

MRSA/MSSA = methicillin-resistant/sensitive S. aureus. Duration of therapy represents total time IV or IV + PO. Most patients on IV therapy able to take PO meds should be switched to PO therapy after clinical improvement.

* Follow with maintenance dosing for renal failure (CrCl < 10 mL/min) and type of dialysis (see Chapter 9).

† If ABE not present, treat for 2 weeks after graft is removed/replaced.

Vascular Graft Infections (cont'd)

Subset	Usual Pathogens	Preferred IV Therapy	Alternate IV Therapy	IV-to-PO Switch
	S. aureus (MSSA) E. faecalis (VSE) aerobic GNBs	Meropenem 1 gm (IV) q8h*† **or** Piperacillin 4 gm (IV)*† **or** Moxifloxacin 400 mg (IV) q24h†	Vancomycin 1 gm (IV) q12h*† **plus** Gentamicin 120 mg (IV) q24h*†	Moxifloxacin 400 mg (IV or PO) q24h*†
Aortic graft infection	S. aureus (MSSA) Aerobic GNBs P. aeruginosa	Meropenem 1 gm (IV) q8h† **or** Cefepime 2 gm (IV) q12h†	Piperacillin 4 gm (IV) q8h† **or** Moxifloxacin 400 mg (IV) q24h†	Moxifloxacin 400 mg (PO) q24h† **or** Levofloxacin 750 mg (PO) q24h†

MRSA/MSSA = methicillin-resistant/sensitive S. aureus. Duration of therapy represents total time IV or IV + PO. Most patients on IV therapy able to take PO meds should be switched to PO therapy after clinical improvement.

* Follow with maintenance dosing for renal failure (CrCl < 10 mL/min) and type of dialysis (see Chapter 9).

† If ABE not present, treat for 2 weeks after graft is removed/replaced.

AV Graft Infection

Clinical Presentation: Persistent fever/bacteremia without endocarditis in a patient with an AV graft on hemodialysis.

Diagnostic Considerations: Diagnosis by persistently positive blood cultures and gallium scan pickup over infected AV graft. Gallium scan will detect deep AV graft infection not apparent on exam.

Pitfalls: Antibiotics will lower temperature, but patient will usually not become afebrile without AV graft replacement.

Therapeutic Considerations: Graft usually must be removed for cure. MRSA is a rare cause of AV graft infection; if present, treat with linezolid 600 mg (IV or PO) q12h until graft is removed/replaced.

Prognosis: Good if new graft does not become infected at same site.

Aortic Graft Infection

Clinical Presentation: Persistently positive blood cultures without endocarditis in a patient with an aortic graft.

Diagnostic Considerations: Diagnosis by positive blood cultures plus gallium scan pickup over infected aortic graft or abdominal CT/MRI scan.

Pitfalls: Infection typically occurs at anastomotic sites.

Therapeutic Considerations: Graft must be removed for cure. Operate as soon as diagnosis is confirmed (no value in waiting for surgery). MRSA is a rare cause of AV graft infection; if present, treat with linezolid 600 mg (IV or PO) q12h until graft is replaced.

Prognosis: Good if infected graft is removed before septic complications develop.

Empiric Therapy of GI Tract Infections

Esophagitis

Subset	Usual Pathogens	Preferred IV Therapy	Alternate IV Therapy	PO Therapy or IV-to-PO Switch
Fungal	Candida albicans	Fluconazole 200 mg (IV or PO) × 1 dose, then 100 mg (IV or PO) q24h × 2–3 weeks	Anidulafungin 100 mg (IV or PO) × 1 dose then 50 mg (IV) q24h × 2–3 weeks **or** Caspofungin 50 mg (IV) q24h × 2–3 weeks **or** Micafungin 150 mg (IV) q24h × 2–3 weeks **or** Amphotericin B deoxycholate 0.5 mg/kg (IV) q24h × 2–3 weeks **or** Itraconazole 200 mg (IV) q12h × 2 days, then 200 mg (IV) q24 h × 2–3 weeks	Fluconazole 200 mg (PO) × 1 dose, then 100 mg (PO) q24h × 2–3 weeks* **or** Posaconazole 100 mg (PO)q12h × 1 day, then 100 mg (PO) q24h × 2 weeks **or** Itraconazole 200 mg (PO) solution q24h × 2–3 weeks
Viral	HSV-1	Acyclovir 5 mg/kg (IV) q8h × 3 weeks	Valacyclovir 500 mg (PO) q12h × 3 weeks **or** Famciclovir 500 mg (PO) q12h × 3 weeks	
	CMV	Ganciclovir 5 mg/kg (IV) q12h × 3 weeks	Valganciclovir 900 mg (PO) q12h × 3 weeks	

Duration of therapy represents total time IV, PO, or IV + PO. Most patients on IV therapy able to take PO meds should be switched to PO therapy soon after clinical improvement (usually < 72 hours).

* Loading dose is not needed PO if given IV with the same drug.

Clinical Presentation: Pain on swallowing.
Diagnosis: Stain/culture for fungi/HSV/CMV on biopsy specimen.

Fungal (Candida) Esophagitis

Diagnostic Considerations: Rarely if ever in normal hosts. Often (but not always) associated with Candida in mouth. If patient is not alcoholic or diabetic and is not receiving antibiotics, test for HIV.
Pitfalls: Therapy as a diagnostic trial is appropriate. Suspect CMV-related disease and proceed to endoscopy if a patient with a typical symptom complex fails to respond to antifungal therapy.
Therapeutic Considerations: In normal hosts, treat for 1 week after clinical resolution. HIV patients respond more slowly than normal hosts and may need higher doses/treatment for 2–3 weeks after clinical resolution (p. 329).
Prognosis: Related to degree of immunosuppression.

Viral Esophagitis

Diagnostic Considerations: Rarely in normal hosts. May occur in the immunosuppressed.
Pitfalls: Viral and non-viral esophageal ulcers look similar; need biopsy for specific viral diagnosis.
Therapeutic Considerations: In normal hosts, treat for 2–3 weeks after clinical resolution. HIV patients respond more slowly and may need treatment for weeks after clinical resolution.
Prognosis: Related to degree of immunosuppression.

Peptic Ulcer Disease (H. pylori)

Triple Therapy	Quadruple Therapy	Sequential Therapy
PPI + amoxicillin 1 gm (PO) q12h ***plus either*** clarithromycin 500 mg (PO) q12h ***or*** tinidazole (or metronidazole) 500 mg (PO) q12h all × 2 weeks	PPI + metronidazole 500 mg (PO) q12h + doxycycline 100 mg (PO) q12h + bismuth subsalicylate 525 mg tabs (PO) q6h all × 2 weeks	***5 days:*** PPI + amoxicillin 1 gm (PO) q12h; ***next 5 days:*** PPI ***plus*** either clarithromycin 500 (PO) q12h ***or*** levofloxacin 500 mg (PO) q24h

Diagnostic Considerations: Invasive: rapid urease test, histology, culture. **Non-invasive:** serum ELISA test, urea breath test, stool (monoclonal antibody) antigen test.
Pitfalls: False negative tests with antibiotics, bismuth, PPIs.
Therapeutic Considerations: See grid. For therapeutic failure: ***substitute*** bismuth (for amoxicillin) or ***substitute*** nitazoxanide 1 gm (PO) q12h (for clarithromycin, metronidazole or tinidazole) all × 2 weeks. *1 week of therapy often fails.*
Test of Cure: Urea breath test → 4–6 weeks post-therapy. Stool antigen test → 6–8 weeks post-therapy. *Stop PPIs 2 weeks before re-testing for cure.*

Gastric Perforation

Subset	Usual Pathogens	Preferred IV Therapy	Alternate IV Therapy	IV-to-PO Switch
Gastric perforation	Oral anaerobes	Cefazolin 1 gm (IV) q8h × 1–3 days	Any beta-lactam (IV) × 1–3 days	Amoxicillin 1 gm (PO) q8h × 1–3 days **or** Cephalexin 500 mg (PO) q6h × 1–3 days **or** Quinolone* (PO) q24h × 1–3 days

* Levofloxacin 500 mg or Moxifloxacin 400 mg.

Clinical Presentation: Presents acutely with fever and peritonitis.
Diagnostic Considerations: Obtain CT/MRI of abdomen for perforation/fluid collection.
Pitfalls: No need to cover B. fragilis with perforation of stomach/small intestine.
Therapeutic Considerations: Obtain surgical consult for possible repair.
Prognosis: Good if repaired.

Infectious Diarrhea/Typhoid (Enteric) Fever

Subset	Usual Pathogens	Preferred Therapy	Alternate Therapy
Acute watery diarrhea	E. coli (ETEC, EHEC) Campylobacter Yersinia Salmonella Vibrio sp.	Quinolone† (IV or PO) × 5 days	Doxycycline 100 mg (IV or PO) q12h × 5 days **or** TMP–SMX 1 DS tablet (PO) q12h × 5 days
C. difficile diarrhea colitis	Clostridium difficile	Diarrhea: Vancomycin 250 mg (PO) q6h × 7–10 days‡ **or** Nitazoxanide 500 mg (PO) q12h × 7–10 days Colitis: Metronidazole 1 gm (IV) q24h (moderate) or 500 mg (IV/PO) q6-8h (severe) until cured. For colitis with microscopic/ clinical peritonitis, consider adding Ertapenem 1 gm (IV) q24h until peritonitis component resolved **or** Nitazoxanide 500 mg (PO) q12h until cured (moderate/ severe). For colitis with microscopic/clinical peritonitis, consider adding Ertapenem 1 gm (IV) q24h until peritonitis component resolved **or** Tigacycline 200 mg (IV) × 1 dose, then 100 mg (IV) q24h or 50 mg (IV) q12h until *colitis resolved	Diarrhea: Metronidazole 250 mg (PO) q6h × 7–10 days Colitis: If unresponsive to Metronidazole (IV/PO), use Nitazoxanide 500 mg (PO) q12h until cured

Duration of therapy represents total time IV, PO, or IV + PO. Most patients on IV therapy able to take PO meds should be switched to PO therapy soon after clinical improvement (usually < 72 hours).

* May also present as acute watery diarrhea.

† Ciprofloxacin 400 mg (IV) or 500 mg (PO) q12h or Levofloxacin 500 mg (IV or PO) q24h or Moxifloxacin 400 mg (IV or PO) q24h.

‡ If C. difficile diarrhea on oral Vancomycin 125/250 mg (PO) q6h not improving after 72 hours, increase Vancomycin dose to 500 mg (PO) q6h.

Infectious Diarrhea/Typhoid (Enteric) Fever (cont'd)

Subset	Usual Pathogens	Preferred Therapy	Alternate Therapy
Cytomegalovirus colitis	CMV	Normal hosts: Valganciclovir 900 mg (PO) q12h × 21 days HIV/ARDS: see p. 324	
Typhoid (enteric) fever	Salmonella typhi/ paratyphi	Quinolone† (IV or PO) × 10–14 days **or** TMP–SMX 5 mg/kg (IV or PO) q6h × 10–14 days	Chloramphenicol 500 mg (IV or PO) q6h × 10–14 days **or** any 3rd gen cephalosporin (IV or PO) × 10–14 days **or** Azithromycin 1 gm (PO) q24h × 5 days
Chronic watery diarrhea	Giardia lamblia*	Nitazoxanide 500 mg (PO) q12h × 5 days	Albendazole 400 mg (PO) q24h × 5 days **or** Quinacrine 100 mg (PO) q8h × 5 days
	Cryptosporidia*	Nitazoxanide 500 mg (PO) q12h × 5 days	Paromomycin 500–750 mg (PO) q8h until response **or** Azithromycin 600 mg (PO) q24h × 4 weeks
	Isospora Cyclospora*	TMP–SMX 1 DS tablet (PO) q12h × 2–4 weeks	
Acute dysentery	Entamoeba histolytica	Preferred therapy: Metronidazole 750 mg (PO) q8h × 10 days **followed by either** Iodoquinol 650 mg (PO) q8h × 20 days **or** Paromomycin 500 mg (PO) q8h × 7 days Alternate therapy: Tinidazole 1 gm (PO) q12h × 3 days	
	Shigella	Quinolone† (IV or PO) × 3 days	TMP–SMX 1 DS tablet (PO) q12h × 3 days **or** Azithromycin 500 mg (IV or PO) q24h × 3 days

Duration of therapy represents total time IV, PO, or IV + PO. Most patients on IV therapy able to take PO meds should be switched to PO therapy soon after clinical improvement (usually < 72 hours).

* May also present as acute watery diarrhea.

† Ciprofloxacin 400 mg (IV) or 500 mg (PO) q12h or Levofloxacin 500 mg (IV or PO) q24h or Moxifloxacin 400 mg (IV or PO) q24h.

Acute Watery Diarrhea

Clinical Presentation: Acute onset of watery diarrhea without blood/mucus.

Diagnostic Considerations: Diagnosis by culture of organism from stool specimens.

Pitfalls: Recommended antibiotics are active against most susceptible enterotoxigenic bacterial pathogens causing diarrhea, but not viruses/parasites. Concomitant transient lactase deficiency may prolong diarrhea if dairy products are taken during an infectious diarrhea.

Therapeutic Considerations: Avoid norfloxacin and ciprofloxacin due to resistance potential. V. cholerae may be treated with a single dose of any oral respiratory quinolone or doxycycline.
Prognosis: Excellent. Most recover with supportive treatment.

Clostridium difficile Diarrhea/Colitis

Clinical Presentation: Voluminous watery diarrhea following exposure to C. difficile contaminated fomites, exposure to patients with C. difficle, recent cancer chemotherapy or antibiotic therapy with some, but not most, antibiotics. May be associated with quinolones and proton pump inhibitors (PPIs). Among antibiotics, clindamycin and β-lactams are most frequent inducers of toxin production. Rarely due to aminoglycosides, azthreonam, linezolid, doxycycline, minocycline, TMP–SMX, carbapenems, daptomycin, TMP–SMX, vancomycin, ceftriaxone, or tigacycline.
Diagnostic Considerations: Watery diarrhea with positive C. difficile stool toxin. A single positive C. difficle stool toxin test is sufficiently sensitive/specific for diagnosis (endpoint is end of diarrhea, not stool toxin negativity); If negative, no need to repeatedly retest. If C. difficle colitis suspected in C. difficile positive patients with fever/prominent leukocytosis/abdominal pain confirm diagnosis of C. difficile colitis by abdominal CT scan.
Pitfalls: C. difficile colitis is suggested by the presence of otherwise unexplained leukocytosis, ↑ ESR, abdominal pain and often temperature > 102°F; confirm diagnosis with CT/MRI of abdomen. Virulent strains of C. difficile may present with colitis with temperature ≤ 102°F, leukocytosis (often very high, i.e., 25–50 K/mm^3), and little/no abdominal pain; confirm diagnosis with CT/MRI of abdomen. Radiographically C. difficile colitis is a pancolitis. Segmental colitis suggests a non-C. difficile etiology, i.e., ischemic colitis. C. difficile toxin test may remain positive in stools for weeks following resolution of diarrhea; do not treat positive stool toxin test. In patients receiving enteral feeds, diarrhea is likely due to enteral feeds (high infusion rates/high osmotic loads) rather than C. difficile. Norovirus diarrhea may mimic C. difficile diarrhea or concurrent outbreaks may occur. Vancomycin (IV/PO) is *not* useful for C. difficile colitis.
Therapeutic Considerations: For C. difficile diarrhea oral vancomycin or nitazoxanide are preferred; metronidazole frequently fails. Rifaxamin often ineffective. C. difficile diarrhea begins to improve (≤ 3 days) and usually resolves by 5–7 days, although some patients require 10 days of therapy. If no improvement with vancomycin ↑ dose to 500 mg (PO) q6h or use nitazoxanide. Do not treat C. difficile toxin-negative diarrhea with vancomycin or metronidazole. For relapses/recurrences, treat with vancomycin 500 mg (PO) q6h × 1 month. For repeat relapses oral vancomycin (full dose; do *not* taper) × 2 or 3 months until resolved. For C. difficle colitis, treat until colitis resolves and follow with serial ESRS/abdominal CT scans. Add aerobic GNB coverage for microscopic/gross peritonitis with meropenem or ertapenem. Tigacycline highly effective monotherapy in C. difficle colitis; and also provides anti-B fragilis coverage for microscopic clinical peritonitis C. difficile virulent epidemic strain is type B1 (toxinotype III), produces 20 × the amount of toxin A/B compared to less virulent strains due to deletion of TcdC gene. ***Avoid*** anti-motility agents, e.g., loperamide with C. difficile diarrhea which may result in C. difficile colitis/toxic megacolon.
Prognosis: Prognosis with C. difficile diarrhea is excellent. With C. difficile colitis prognosis is related to strain virulence/severity of the colitis.

Typhoid (Enteric) Fever (Salmonella typhi/Paratyphi)

Clinical Presentation: High fevers (> 102°F) increasing in a stepwise fashion accompanied by relative bradycardia in a patient with watery diarrhea/constipation, headache, abdominal pain, cough/sore throat ± Rose spots.

Diagnostic Considerations: Most community-acquired watery diarrheas are not accompanied by temperatures > 102°F and relative bradycardia. Diagnosis is confirmed by demonstrating Salmonella in blood, bone marrow, Rose spots, or stool cultures. Culture of bone marrow is the quickest/most reliable method of diagnosis. WBC count is usually low/low normal. Leukocytosis should suggest another diagnosis or bowel perforation, which may occur during 2nd week of typhoid fever.

Pitfalls: Rose spots are few/difficult to see and not present in all cases. Typhoid fever usually presents with constipation, not diarrhea. Suspect another diagnosis in the absence of headache.

Therapeutic Considerations: 2nd generation cephalosporins, aztreonam, and aminoglycosides are ineffective. Since Salmonella strains causing enteric fever are intracellular pathogens, treat for a full 2 weeks to maximize cure rates/minimize relapses. Treat relapses with the suggested antibiotics × 2–3 weeks. Salmonella excretion into feces usually persists < 3 months. Persistent excretion > 3 months suggests a carrier state—rule out hepatobiliary/urinary calculi.

Prognosis: Good if treated early. Poor with late treatment/bowel perforation.

Chronic Watery Diarrhea

Clinical Presentation: Watery diarrhea without blood/mucus lasting > 1 month.

Diagnostic Considerations: Diagnosis by demonstrating organisms/cysts in stool specimens. Multiple fresh daily stool samples often needed for diagnosis especially for protozoan parasites.

Pitfalls: Concomitant transient lactase deficiency may prolong diarrhea if dairy products are consumed during an infectious diarrhea.

Therapeutic Considerations: Cryptosporidia and Isospora are being recognized increasingly in acute/chronic diarrhea in normal hosts.

Prognosis: Excellent in well-nourished patients. Untreated patients may develop malabsorption.

Giardia lamblia

Clinical Presentation: Acute/subacute onset of diarrhea, abdominal cramps, bloating, flatulence. Incubation period 1–2 weeks. Malabsorption may occur in chronic cases. No eosinophilia.

Diagnostic Considerations: Diagnosis by demonstrating trophozoites or cysts in stool/antigen detection assay. If stool exam and antigen test are negative and Giardiasis is suspected, perform "string test"/duodenal aspirate and biopsy.

Pitfalls: Cysts intermittently excreted into stool. Usually need multiple stool samples for diagnosis. Often accompanied by transient lactose intolerance.

Therapeutic Considerations: Nitazoxanide effective therapy. Diarrhea may be prolonged if milk (lactose-containing) products are ingested after treatment/cure. May need repeat courses of therapy.

Prognosis: Related to severity of malabsorption and health of host.

Cryptosporidia

Clinical Presentation: Acute/subacute onset of diarrhea. Usually occurs in HIV/AIDS patients with CD_4 counts < 200. Biliary cryptosporidiosis is seen only in HIV; may present as acalculous cholecystitis or sclerosing cholangitis with RUQ pain, fever, ↑ alkaline phosphatase, but bilirubin is normal.

Diagnostic Considerations: Diagnosis by demonstrating organism in stool/intestinal biopsy specimen. Cholera-like illness in normal hosts. Chronic watery diarrhea in compromised hosts.

Pitfalls: Smaller than Cyclospora. Oocyst walls are smooth (not wrinkled) on acid fast staining.
Therapeutic Considerations: Nitazoxanide effective therapy.
Prognosis: Related to adequacy of fluid replacement/underlying health of host.

Cyclospora

Clinical Presentation: Acute/subacute onset of diarrhea. Incubation period 1–14 days.
Diagnostic Considerations: Diagnosis by demonstrating organism in stool/intestinal biopsy specimen. Clinically indistinguishable from cryptosporidial diarrhea (intermittent watery diarrhea without blood or mucus). Fatigue/weight loss common.
Pitfalls: Oocysts only form seen in stool and are best identified with modified Kinyoun acid fast staining. Acid fast fat globules stain pink with acid fast staining. "Wrinkled wall" oocysts are characteristic of Cyclospora, not Cryptosporidia. Oocysts are twice the size of similar appearing Cryptosporidia (~ 10 μm vs. 5 μm).
Therapeutic Considerations: Nitazoxanide effective therapy.
Prognosis: Related to adequacy of fluid replacement/underlying health of host.

Acute Dysentery

Entamoeba histolytica

Clinical Presentation: Acute/subacute onset of bloody diarrhea/mucus. Fecal WBC/RBCs due to mucosal invasion. E. histolytica may also cause chronic diarrhea. Colonic ulcers secondary to E. histolytica are round and may form "collar stud" abscesses.
Diagnostic Considerations: Diagnosis by demonstrating organism/trophozoites in stool/intestinal biopsy specimen. Serology is negative with amebic dysentery, but positive with extra-intestinal forms. Test to separate E. histolytica from non-pathogenic E. dispar cyst passers. On sigmoidoscopy, ulcers due to E. histolytica are round with normal mucosa in between, and may form "collar stud" abscesses. In contrast, ulcers due to Shigella are linear and serpiginous without normal intervening mucosa. Bloody dysentery is more subacute with E. histolytica compared to Shigella.
Pitfalls: Intestinal perforation/abscess may complicate amebic colitis. Rule out infectious causes of bloody diarrhea with mucus before diagnosing/treating inflammatory bowel disease (IBD). Obtain multiple stool cultures for bacterial pathogens/parasites. Do not confuse E. histolytica in stool specimens with E. hartmanni, a non-pathogen protozoa similar in appearance but smaller in size.
Therapeutic Considerations: E. histolytica cyst passers should be treated, but metronidazole is ineffective against cysts. Recommended antibiotics treat both luminal and hepatic E. histolytica. Use paromomycin 500 mg (PO) q8h × 7 days for asymptomatic cysts.
Prognosis: Good if treated early. Related to severity of dysentery/ulcers/extra-intestinal amebiasis.

Shigella

Clinical Presentation: Acute onset of bloody diarrhea/mucus.
Diagnostic Considerations: Diagnosis by demonstrating organism in stool specimens. Shigella ulcers in colon are linear, serpiginous, and rarely lead to perforation.
Therapeutic Considerations: Shigella dysentery is more acute/fulminating than amebic dysentery. Shigella has no carrier state, unlike Entamoeba.
Prognosis: Good if treated early. Severity of illness related to Shigella species: S. dysenteriae (most severe) > S. flexneri > S. boydii/S. sonnei (mildest).

Cholecystitis

Subset	Usual Pathogens	Preferred IV Therapy	Alternate IV Therapy	PO Therapy or IV-to-PO Switch
Normal host	E. coli Klebsiella E. faecalis (VSE)	Meropenem 500 mg (IV) q8h* **or** Piperacillin/tazobactam 3.375 gm (IV) q6h* **or** Tigacyline 100 mg (IV) × 1 dose, then 50 mg (IV) q12h	Cefazolin 1 gm (IV) q8h* ± Ampicillin 1 gm (IV) q6h* **or** Quinolone‡ (IV)*	Quinolone‡ (PO)*
Emphysematous cholecystitis†	Clostridium perfringens E. coli	Meropenem 500 mg (IV) q8h¶ **or** Piperacillin/tazobactam 3.375 gm (IV) q6h¶	Ertapenem 1 gm (IV) q24h¶ **or** Ticarcillin/clavulanate 3.1 gm (IV) q6h¶	Clindamycin 300 mg (PO) q8h¶

Duration of therapy represents total time IV, PO, or IV + PO. Most patients on IV therapy able to take PO meds should be switched to PO therapy after clinical improvement.

† Treat only IV or IV-to-PO switch.

‡ Ciprofloxacin 400 mg (IV) or Levofloxacin 500 mg (IV or PO) q24h or Moxifloxacin 400 mg (IV or PO) q24h.

* If no cholecystectomy, treat × 5–7 days. If cholecystectomy is performed, treat × 3–4 days post-operatively.

¶ Treat × 4–7 days after cholecystectomy.

Cholecystitis

Clinical Presentation: RUQ pain, fever usually ≤ 102°F, positive Murphy's sign, no percussion tenderness over right lower ribs.

Diagnostic Considerations: Diagnosis by RUQ ultrasound/positive HIDA scan.

Pitfalls: No need to cover B. fragilis.

Therapeutic Considerations: Obtain surgical consult for possible cholecystectomy.

Prognosis: Related to cardiopulmonary status.

Emphysematous Cholecystitis

Clinical Presentation: Clinically presents as cholecystitis. Usually in diabetics.

Diagnostic Considerations: RUQ/gallbladder gas on flat plate of abdomen.

Pitfalls: Requires immediate cholecystectomy.

Therapeutic Considerations: Usually a difficult/prolonged post-op course.

Prognosis: Related to speed of gallbladder removal.

Cholangitis

Subset	Usual Pathogens	Preferred IV Therapy	Alternate IV Therapy	IV-to-PO Switch
Normal host	E. coli Klebsiella E. faecalis (VSE)	Meropenem 500 mg (IV) q8h* **or** Tigecycline 100 mg (IV) × 1 dose, then 100 mg (IV) q24h **or** 50 mg (IV) q12h* **or** Piperacillin/tazobactam 3.375 gm (IV) q6h* **or** Doripenem 500 mg (IV) q8h	Ampicillin/ sulbactam 3 gm (IV) q6h* **or** Imipenem 500 mg (IV) q6h* **or** Cefoperazone 2 gm (IV) q12h*	Ciprofloxacin 500 mg (PO) q12h* **or** Levofloxacin 500 mg (PO) q24h* **or** Moxifloxacin 400 mg (PO) q24h*

Duration of therapy represents total time IV or IV + PO. Most patients on IV therapy able to take PO meds should be switched to PO therapy after clinical improvement.

* Treat until resolved (usually 5–7 days).

Clinical Presentation: RUQ pain, fever > 102°F, positive Murphy's sign, percussion tenderness over right lower ribs.

Diagnostic Considerations: Obstructed common bile duct on ultrasound/CT/MRI of abdomen.

Pitfalls: Charcot's triad (fever, RUQ pain, jaundice) is present in only 50%.

Therapeutic Considerations: Obtain surgical consult to relieve obstruction. Continue antibiotics for 4–7 days after obstruction is relieved.

Prognosis: Related to speed of surgical relief of obstruction.

Gallbladder Wall Abscess/Perforation

Subset	Usual Pathogens	Preferred IV Therapy	Alternate IV Therapy	IV-to-PO Switch
Gallbladder wall abscess/ perforation	E. coli Klebsiella E. faecalis (VSE)	Piperacillin/ tazobactam 3.375 gm (IV) q6h* **or** Tigecycline 100 mg (IV) × 1 dose, then 50 mg (IV) q12h* **or** Meropenem 500 mg (IV) q8h*	Ampicillin/ sulbactam 3 gm (IV) q6h* **or** Cefoperazone 2 gm (IV) q12h* **or** Doripenem 1 gm (IV) q8h	Ciprofloxacin 500 mg (PO) q12h* **or** Levofloxacin 500 mg (PO) q24h* **or** Moxifloxacin 400 mg (PO) q24h*

Duration of therapy represents total time IV or IV + PO.

* Treat until resolved (usually 1–2 weeks).

Clinical Presentation: RUQ pain, fever ≤ 102°F, positive Murphy's sign, no percussion tenderness over right lower ribs.
Diagnostic Considerations: Diagnosis by CT/MRI of abdomen. Bile peritonitis is common.
Pitfalls: Bacterial peritonitis may be present.
Therapeutic Considerations: Obtain surgical consult for possible gallbladder removal. Usually a difficult and prolonged post-op course.
Prognosis: Related to removal of gallbladder/repair of perforation.

Acute Pancreatitis

Subset	Usual Pathogens	Preferred IV Therapy	Alternate IV Therapy	IV-to-PO Switch
Edematous pancreatitis	None	Not applicable	Not applicable	Not applicable
Hemorrhagic/ necrotizing pancreatitis	Aerobic GNBs B. fragilis	Meropenem 500 mg (IV) q8h* **or** Ertapenem 1 gm (IV) q24h* **or** Imipenem 500 mg (IV) q6h*	Piperacillin 4 gm (IV) q8h* **or** Ampicillin/sulbactam 1.5 gm (IV) q6h* **or** Ticarcillin/ clavulanate 3.1 gm (IV) q6h*	Clindamycin 300 mg (PO) q8h* **plus** Levofloxacin 500 mg (PO) q24h* **or monotherapy with** Moxifloxacin 400 mg (PO) q24h*

Duration of therapy represents total time IV or IV + PO and varies depending on the clinical response. Most patients on IV therapy able to take PO meds should be switched to PO therapy after clinical improvement.
* Treat until resolved (usually 1–2 weeks).

Edematous Pancreatitis
Clinical Presentation: Sharp abdominal pain with fever ≤ 102°F ± hypotension.
Diagnostic Considerations: Diagnosis by elevated serum amylase and lipase levels with normal methemalbumin levels. May be drug-induced (e.g., steroids).
Pitfalls: Amylase elevation alone is not diagnostic of acute pancreatitis.
Therapeutic Considerations: NG tube is not needed. Aggressively replace fluids.
Prognosis: Good with adequate fluid replacement.

Hemorrhagic/Necrotizing Pancreatitis
Clinical Presentation: Sharp abdominal pain with fever ≤ 102°F ± hypotension. Grey-Turner/Cullen's sign present in some.
Diagnostic Considerations: Mildly elevated serum amylase and lipase levels with high methemalbumin levels.
Pitfalls: With elevated lipase, amylase level is inversely related to severity of disease.
Therapeutic Considerations: Obtain surgical consult for possible peritoneal lavage as adjunct to antibiotics. Serum albumin/dextran are preferred volume expanders.
Prognosis: Poor with hypocalcemia or shock.

Pancreatic Abscess/Infected Pancreatic Pseudocyst

Subset	Usual Pathogens	Preferred IV Therapy	Alternate IV Therapy	IV-to-PO Switch
Infected pancreatic pseudocyst/ pancreatic abscess	Aerobic GNBs B. fragilis	Meropenem 500 mg (IV) q8h* **or** Piperacillin/ tazobactam 3.375 gm (IV) q6h* **or** Ertapenem 1 gm (IV) q24h*	Ampicillin/sulbactam 1.5 gm (IV) q6h* **or** Ticarcillin/ clavulanate 3.1 gm (IV) q6h* **or** Imipenem 500 mg (IV) q6h* **or** Doripenem 500 mg (IV) q8h	Moxifloxacin 400 mg (PO) q24h* **or combination therapy with** Clindamycin 300 mg (PO) q8h* **plus** Quinolone† (PO)*

Duration of therapy represents total time IV or IV + PO.
† Ciprofloxacin 500 mg q12h or Levofloxacin 500 mg q24h.
* Treat until resolved.

Clinical Presentation: Follows acute pancreatitis or develops in a pancreatic pseudocyst. An infected pancreatic pseudocyst is an abscess equivalent. Fevers usually ≥ 102°F.
Diagnostic Considerations: CT/MRI of abdomen demonstrates pancreatic abscess.
Pitfalls: Peritoneal signs are typically absent.
Prognosis: Related to size/extent of abscess and adequacy of drainage.

Liver Abscess

Subset	Usual Pathogens	Preferred IV Therapy	Alternate IV Therapy	PO Therapy or IV-to-PO Switch
Liver abscess	Aerobic GNBs Enterococci (VSE) B. fragilis	Piperacillin/ tazobactam 3.375 gm (IV) q6h* **or** Tigecycline 100 mg (IV) × 1 dose, then 50 mg (IV) q12h* **or** Meropenem 500 mg (IV) q8h* **or**	Quinolone† (IV)* **plus either** Metronidazole 1 gm (IV) q24h* **or** Clindamycin 600 mg (IV) q8h*	Amoxicillin/clavulanic acid 875/125 mg (PO) q12h* **or** Moxifloxacin 400 mg (PO) q24h* **or combination therapy with** Quinolone† (PO)* **plus either**

Duration of therapy represents total time IV, PO, or IV + PO.
* Treat until abscess(es) are no longer present or stop decreasing in size on CT scan.
† Ciprofloxacin 400 mg (IV) or 500 mg (PO) q12h or Levofloxacin 500 mg (IV or PO) q24h.

Liver Abscess (cont'd)

Subset	Usual Pathogens	Preferred IV Therapy	Alternate IV Therapy	PO Therapy or IV-to-PO Switch
		Moxifloxacin 400 mg (IV) q24h* **or** Sulbactam/ampicillin 3 gm (IV) q6h		Metronidazole 500 mg (PO) q12h* **or** Clindamycin 300 mg (PO) q8h*
	E. histolytica	See p. 271		

Duration of therapy represents total time IV, PO, or IV + PO.

* Treat until abscess(es) are no longer present or stop decreasing in size on CT scan.

† Ciprofloxacin 400 mg (IV) or 500 mg (PO) q12h or Levofloxacin 500 mg (IV or PO) q24h.

Clinical Presentation: Fever, RUQ tenderness, negative Murphy's sign, and negative right lower rib percussion tenderness.
Diagnostic Considerations: Diagnosis by CT/MRI scan of liver and aspiration of abscess. CT shows multiple lesions in liver. Source is usually either the colon (diverticulitis or diverticular abscess with portal pyemia) or retrograde infection from the gallbladder (cholecystitis or gallbladder wall abscess).
Pitfalls: Bacterial abscesses are usually multiple and involve multiple lobes of liver; amebic abscesses are usually solitary and involve the right lobe of liver.
Therapeutic Considerations: Liver laceration/trauma usually requires ~ 2 weeks of antibiotics.
Prognosis: Good if treated early.

Hepatosplenic Candidiasis

Subset	Usual Pathogens	Preferred IV Therapy	Alternate IV Therapy	IV-to-PO Switch
Hepato-splenic candidiasis	Candida albicans	Fluconazole 800 mg (IV) × 1 dose, then 400 mg (IV) q24h × 2–4 weeks **or** Micafungin 100 mg (IV) q24h × 2–4 weeks **or** Caspofungin 70 mg (IV) × 1 dose, then 50 mg (IV) q24h × 2–4 weeks	Ambisome (L-Amb) (p. 525) (IV) q24h × 2–4 weeks **or** Amphotericin B deoxycholate 0.7 mg/kg (IV) q24h × 2–4 weeks	Fluconazole 800 mg (PO) × 1 dose, then 400 mg (PO) q24h × 2–4 weeks* **or** Itraconazole 200 mg (PO) solution q12h × 2–4 weeks

Duration of therapy represents total time IV or IV + PO. Most patients on IV therapy able to take PO meds should be switched to PO therapy after clinical improvement.

* Loading dose is not needed PO if given IV with the same drug.

Clinical Presentation: New high spiking fevers with RUQ/LUQ pain after 2 weeks in a patient with afebrile leukopenia.
Diagnostic Considerations: Diagnosis by abdominal CT/MRI showing mass lesions in liver/spleen.
Pitfalls: Do not overlook RUQ tenderness and elevated alkaline phosphatase in leukopenic cancer patients as a clue to the diagnosis.
Therapeutic Considerations: Treat until liver/spleen lesions resolve. Should be viewed as a form of disseminated disease.
Prognosis: Related to degree/duration of leukopenia.

Granulomatous Hepatitis (BCG)

Subset	Pathogen	Preferred Therapy
BCG hepatitis	Bacille Calmette-Guérin (BCG)	INH 300 mg (PO) q24h × 6 months + rifampin 600 mg (PO) q24h × 6 months

Clinical Presentation: Fever, chills, anorexia, weight loss, hepatomegaly ± RUQ pain days to weeks after intravesicular BCG for bladder cancer.
Diagnostic Considerations: ↑ alkaline phosphatase > ↑ SGOT/SGPT. Liver biopsy is negative for AFB/positive for granulomas.
Pitfalls: Exclude other causes of hepatomegaly.
Therapeutic Considerations: INH plus rifampin × 6 months is curative.
Prognosis: Excellent with early treatment.

Viral Hepatitis

Subset	Pathogens	PO/SQ Therapy
Acute	HAV, HBV, HCV, HDV, HEV, EBV, CMV (see below): no acute therapy	
Chronic	HBV	Treat × 1 year with either adefovir (Hepsera) 10 mg (PO) q24h **or** Entecavir (Baraclude) 0.5 mg (PO) q24h (1 mg PO q24h if lamivudine-refractory) **or** adefovir (Hepsera) 10 mg (PO) q24h. Pegasys in a dose of 180 mcg/week (SQ) for 1 year without ribavirin is an option
	HCV	Pegylated interferon (Pegasys) alfa-2a (40 KD) 180 mcg/week (SQ) × 48 weeks *plus* ribavirin 500–600 mg (PO) q12h × 48 weeks (for Genotype 1) **or** 24 weeks (for Genotype 2 or 3) (see pp. 646–647 for dosage adjustments), **or** Pegylated interferon (Peg-Intron) alfa-2b (12 KD) 1 mcg/kg/week (SQ) × 1 year (see Table 2.6 and pp. 646–647 for dosing adjustments), **or** Pegylated interferon (Peg-Intron) alfa-2b (12 KD) 1.5 mcg/kg/week (SQ) × 1 year (see Table 2.7 and pp. 646–647 for dosing adjustments) *plus* ribavirin 400 mg (PO) q12h × 1 year
	HDV	Prolonged treatment with pegylated interferon in the same or larger doses as used in chronic hepatitis B has been successful in a small number of patients

Viral Hepatitis (cont'd)

Subset	Pathogens	PO/SQ Therapy

Table 2.6. Recommended PEG-Intron Monotherapy Dosing

Weight (kg)	PEG Interferon alfa-2b		
	Vial Strength (mcg/0.5 mL)	Amount to Administer (mcg)	Volume to Administer (mL)
≤ 45	50	40	0.4
46–56		50	0.5
57–72	80	64	0.4
73–88		80	0.5
89–106	120	96	0.4
107–136		120	0.5
137–160	150	150	0.5

Table 2.7. Recommended PEG-Intron Combination Therapy Dosing

Weight (kg)	PEG Interferon alfa-2b		
	Vial Strength (mcg/0.5 mL)	Amount to Administer (mcg)	Volume to Administer (mL)
< 40	50	50	0.5
40–50	80	64	0.4
51–60		80	0.5
61–75	120	96	0.4
76–85		120	0.5
> 85	150	150	0.5

Acute Viral Hepatitis

Clinical Presentation: Anorexia, malaise, RUQ tenderness, temperature ≤ 102°F ± jaundice.

Diagnostic Considerations: Diagnosis by elevated IgM anti-HAV, HBsAg or IgM anti-HBc, or anti-HCV with HCV RNA with markedly elevated serum transaminases (SGOT ≥ 1000). Serum alkaline phosphatase is normal/mildly elevated. Percussion tenderness over right lower ribs distinguishes liver from gallbladder problem.

Pitfalls: In patients without jaundice (anicteric hepatitis), rule out other hepatitic viruses (EBV, CMV).

Therapeutic Considerations: Patients feel better after temperature falls/jaundice appears.

Prognosis: Excellent for hepatitis A (does not progress to chronic hepatitis). Hepatitis B and C may progress to chronic hepatitis/cirrhosis. Serum transaminases are not a good predictor/indicator of liver injury in hepatitis C.

EBV/CMV Hepatitis

Clinical Presentation: Same as acute viral hepatitis plus bilateral posterior cervical adenopathy and fatigue.

Diagnostic Considerations: EBV hepatitis occurs as part of infectious mononucleosis and may be the presenting sign in older adults. CMV hepatitis presents as a "mono-like" infection in normal hosts. Like EBV, CMV hepatitis in normal hosts is part of a systemic infection. In compromised hosts, particularly bone marrow/solid organ transplants (BMT/SOT), CMV hepatitis may be the primary manifestation of CMV infection. In the normal host, EBV and CMV infectious mono/hepatitis can be diagnosed by serology (positive mono spot test, ↑ EBV VCA IgM titer, ↑ CMV IgM titer). In BMT/SOT, CMV infection/hepatitis is diagnosed by liver biopsy, PCR, or semi-quantitative CMV antigenic assay.

Pitfalls: In normal hosts and BMT/SOT patients with unexplained ↑ SGOT/SGPT, consider CMV hepatitis in the differential diagnosis and order appropriate diagnostic tests.

Therapeutic Considerations: CMV hepatitis may be treated in normal hosts with valganciclovir 900 mg (PO) q12h × 21 days.

Prognosis: EBV/CMV hepatitis is usually self-limiting in normal hosts. The prognosis of CMV hepatitis in BMT/SOT is related to the degree of immunosuppression and rapidity of treatment.

Chronic Viral Hepatitis

Clinical Presentation: Persistently or intermittently elevated serum transaminases but in some cases transaminases are persistently in the normal range. In the latter, serologic and virologic markers are necessary for diagnosis.

Diagnostic Considerations: Chronic hepatitis B is diagnosed by HBsAg and HBV DNA. Chronic hepatitis C is diagnosed by anti-HCV and HCV RNA. Liver biopsy may be used to grade and stage the degree of liver injury.

Pitfalls: Do not confuse viral hepatitis with lupoid/autoimmune hepatitis, which may present in similar fashion but with elevated ANAs. With both HCV and HBV, rule out co-infection with HIV.

Therapeutic Considerations: For chronic hepatitis B, use entecavir (Baraclude) or adefovir (Hepsera) until HBV DNA levels become undetectable, ALT normalizes, and HBeAg seroconversion occurs (then continue for additional 6 months). Tenofovir is also effective in HBV/HIV co-infection and is likely to be approved for use in HBV. For chronic hepatitis C, continue treatment for 48 weeks (in Genotype 1) or for a full 24 weeks (in Genotype 2 or 3); if no EVR, discontinue treatment. Pegasys monotherapy results in a sustained viral response in 30%. Pegasys plus ribavirin results in a 56% response.

Prognosis: Sustained viral clearance results in a good prognosis.

Intraabdominal or Pelvic Peritonitis/Abscess

Subset	Usual Pathogens	Preferred IV Therapy	Alternate IV Therapy	PO Therapy or IV-to-PO Switch
Mild/ moderate peritonitis	Entero- bacteriaceae B. fragilis	Moxifloxacin 400 mg (IV) q24h¥ **or** Cefoxitin 2 gm (IV) q6h¥	Ampicillin/ sulbactam 1.5 gm (IV) q6h¥ **or combination therapy with** Clindamycin 600 mg (IV) q8h¥ *plus* Aztreonam 2 gm (IV) q8h¥	Moxifloxacin 400 mg (PO) q24h¥ **or** Amoxicillin/clavulanic acid 875/125 mg (PO) q12h¥ **or combination therapy with** Clindamycin 300 mg (PO) q8h¥ *plus* Quinolone¶ (PO) q24h¥
Severe peritonitis‡ (e.g, appendicitis, diverticulitis)	Entero- bacteriaceae B. fragilis	Meropenem 500 mg (IV) q8h¥ **or** Tigecycline 100 mg (IV) × 1 dose, then 50 mg (IV) q12h¥ **or** Piperacillin/ tazobactam 3.375 gm (IV) q6h¥ **or** Ertapenem 1 gm (IV) q24h¥	Ampicillin/ sulbactam 3 gm (IV) q6h¥ **or** Doripenem 500 mg (IV) q8h **or combination therapy with** Metronidazole 1 gm (IV) q24h¥ **plus either** Ceftriaxone 1 gm (IV) q24h¥ **or** Quinolone¶ (IV)¥	Moxifloxacin 400 mg (PO) q24h¥ **or** Amoxicillin/clavulanic acid 875/125 mg (PO) q12h¥
Fungal peritonitis/ abscess	C. albicans Non-albicans Candida	Treat as for Candidemia (p. 150)		
Spontaneous bacterial peritonitis (SBP)‡	Entero- bacteriaceae S. pneumoniae (children)	Ceftriaxone 1 gm (IV) q24h × 1–2 wks **or** Quinolone¶ (IV) × 1–2 weeks	Aztreonam 2 gm (IV) q8h × 1–2 weeks **or** Any aminoglycoside (IV) q24h × 1–2 wks	Quinolone¶ (PO) × 1–2 weeks **or** Amoxicillin/clavulanic acid 875/125 mg (PO) q12h × 1–2 weeks

Duration of therapy represents total time IV, PO, or IV + PO.

‡ Treat only IV or IV-to-PO switch.

¶ Moxifloxacin 400 mg (IV or PO) q24h or Levofloxacin 500 mg (IV or PO) q24h.

¥ Duration of therapy as clinically indicated or for 5–7 days following corrective surgery.

Intraabdominal or Pelvic Peritonitis/Abscess (cont'd)

Subset	Usual Pathogens	Preferred IV Therapy	Alternate IV Therapy	PO Therapy or IV-to-PO Switch
Chronic TB peritonitis	M. tuberculosis	Not applicable		Treat the same as pulmonary TB (p. 52)
CAPD-associated peritonitis‡	S. epidermidis (CoNS) S. aureus (MSSA) Entero-bacteriaceae Non-ferment-ative GNBs	*Before culture results* Vancomycin 1 gm (IV) loading dose* **plus** Gentamicin 5 mg/kg or 240 mg (IV) loading dose*	*After culture results* *MSSA/Enterobacteriaceae* Meropenem 1 gm (IV) loading dose* *MRSA* Vancomycin 1 gm (IV) loading dose* **or** Linezolid 600 mg (IV or PO)	

MSSA/MRSA = methicillin-sensitive/resistant S. aureus. Duration of therapy represents total time IV, PO, or IV + PO.

‡ Treat only IV or IV-to-PO switch.

* Follow with maintenance dosing × 2 weeks after culture results are available. For maintenance dosing, use renal failure (CrCl < 10 mL/min) and post-peritoneal dialysis dosing (Chapter 9).

Intraabdominal or Pelvic Peritonitis/Abscess (Appendicitis/Diverticulitis/Septic Pelvic Thrombophlebitis)

Clinical Presentation: Spiking fevers with acute abdominal pain and peritoneal signs. In diverticulitis, the pain is localized over the involved segment of colon. Appendicitis ± perforation presents as RLQ pain/rebound tenderness or mass. Peri-diverticular abscess presents the same as intraabdominal/pelvic abscess, most commonly in the LLQ. Septic pelvic thrombophlebitis (SPT) presents as high spiking fevers unresponsive to antibiotic therapy following delivery/pelvic surgery.

Diagnostic Considerations: Diagnosis by CT/MRI scan of abdomen/pelvis.

Pitfalls: Tympany over liver suggests abdominal/visceral perforation. Pelvic peritonitis/abscess presents the same as intraabdominal abscess/peritonitis, but peritoneal signs are often absent.

Therapeutic Considerations: Patients with ischemic/inflammatory colitis should be treated the same as peritonitis, depending on severity. Obtain surgical consult for repair/lavage or abscess drainage. In SPT, fever rapidly falls when heparin is added to antibiotics.

Prognosis: Related to degree/duration of peritoneal spillage and rapidity/completeness of lavage. Prognosis for SPT is good if treated early and clots remain limited to pelvic veins.

Spontaneous Bacterial Peritonitis (SBP)

Clinical Presentation: Acute or subacute onset of fever ± abdominal pain.

Diagnostic Considerations: Diagnosis by positive blood cultures of SBP pathogens. For patients with abdominal pain, ascites, and a negative CT/MRI, paracentesis ascitic fluid with > 500 WBCs and > 100 PMNs predicts a positive ascitic fluid culture and is diagnostic of SBP. Some degree of splenic dysfunction usually exists, predisposing to infection with encapsulated organisms.

Pitfalls: Do not overlook GI source of peritonitis (e.g, appendicitis, diverticulitis); obtain CT/MRI.

Therapeutic Considerations: B. fragilis/anaerobes are not common pathogens in SBP, and B. fragilis coverage is unnecessary.
Prognosis: Related to degree of hepatitic/splenic dysfunction.

Chronic Tuberculous Peritonitis (Mycobacterium tuberculosis)

Clinical Presentation: Abdominal pain with fevers, weight loss, ascites over 1–3 months.
Diagnostic Considerations: "Doughy consistency" on abdominal palpation. Diagnosis by AFB on peritoneal biopsy/culture.
Pitfalls: Chest x-ray is normal in ~ 70%. Increased incidence in alcoholic cirrhosis.
Therapeutic Considerations: Treated the same as pulmonary TB.
Prognosis: Good if treated early.

CAPD-Associated Peritonitis

Clinical Presentation: Abdominal pain ± fever in a CAPD patient.
Diagnostic Considerations: Diagnosis by gram stain/culture and ↑ WBC count in peritoneal fluid.
Pitfalls: Fever is often absent.
Therapeutic Considerations: Treat with systemic antibiotics ± antibiotics in dialysate.
Prognosis: Good with early therapy and removal of peritoneal catheter.

Empiric Therapy of Genitourinary Tract Infections

Dysuria-Pyuria Syndrome (Acute Urethral Syndrome)

Subset	Usual Pathogens	IV Therapy	PO Therapy
Acute urethral syndrome	S. saprophyticus C. trachomatis E. coli < 10^5 cfu/mL	Not applicable	Doxycycline 100 mg (PO) q12h × 10 days **or** Quinolone (PO)* × 7 days

* Ciprofloxacin 500 mg q12h or Levofloxacin 500 mg q24h.

Clinical Presentation: Dysuria, frequency, urgency, lower abdominal discomfort, fevers < 102°F.
Diagnostic Considerations: Diagnosis by symptoms of cystitis with pyuria and no growth or low concentration of E. coli (≤ 10^3 colonies/mL) by urine culture. Clue to S. saprophyticus is alkaline urinary pH and RBCs in urine.
Pitfalls: Resembles "culture negative" cystitis.
Therapeutic Considerations: S. saprophyticus is susceptible to most antibiotics used to treat UTIs.
Prognosis: Excellent.

Cystitis (see Color Atlas for Urine Gram stains)

Subset	Usual Pathogens	Therapy
Bacterial	Enterobacteriaceae E. faecalis (VSE) S. agalactiae (group B streptococci) S. saprophyticus	Amoxicillin 500 mg (PO) × q12h × 3 days **or** TMP–SMX 1 SS tablet (PO) × q12h × 3 days **or** Quinolone (PO)* q24h × 3 days **or** Nitrofurantoin 100 mg (PO) q12h × 3 days
Fungal	C. albicans	Fluconazole 200 mg (PO) × 1 dose, then 100 mg (PO) q24h × 4 days
	Fluconazole-resistant Candida isolates or fluconazole-refractory disease	Amphotericin B deoxycholate 0.3 mg/kg (IV) × 1 dose

* Ciprofloxacin XR 500 mg or Levofloxacin 500 mg.
† C. albicans cystitis: See page 102, Catheter-associated candiduria.
‡ Fluconazole-resistant: See page 102.

Bacterial Cystitis

Clinical Presentation: Dysuria, frequency, urgency, lower abdominal discomfort, fevers < 102°F.
Diagnostic Considerations: Pyuria plus bacteriuria.
Pitfalls: Compromised hosts (chronic steroids, diabetes, SLE, cirrhosis, multiple myeloma) may require 3–5 days of therapy. A single dose of amoxicillin or TMP–SMX may be sufficient in acute uncomplicated cystitis in normal hosts.
Therapeutic Considerations: Pyridium 200 mg (PO) q8h after meals × 24–48h is useful to decrease dysuria (inform patients urine will turn orange).
Prognosis: Excellent in normal hosts.

Candidal Cystitis

Diagnostic Considerations: Marked pyuria, urine nitrate negative ± RBCs. Speciate if not C. albicans.
Pitfalls: Lack of response suggests renal candidiasis or a "fungus ball" in the renal collecting system.
Therapeutic Considerations: If fluconazole fails, use amphotericin. For chronic renal failure/dialysis patients with candiduria, use amphotericin B deoxycholate bladder irrigation (as for catheter-associated candiduria, below). Removal of devices and correction of anatomic abnormalities are critical to success.
Prognosis: Patients with impaired host defenses, abnormal collecting systems, cysts, renal disease or stones are prone to recurrent UTIs/urosepsis.

Catheter-Associated Bacteriuria/Candiduria*

Subset	Usual Pathogens	Therapy
Catheter-associated bacteriuria (CAB)†	E. coli E. faecalis (VSE)	Nitrofurantoin 100 mg (PO) q12h × 3–5 days **or** Amoxicillin 500 mg (PO) q12h × 3–5 days
	E. faecium (VRE)	Nitrofurantoin 100 mg (PO) q12h × 3–5 days
	MDR Klebsiella MDR Acinetobacter MDR P. aeruginosa	Colistin 1.7 mg/kg (IV) q8h × 3–5 days Polymyxin B 1 mg/kg (IV) of q12h × 3–5 days Doripenem 500 mg (IV) q8h × 3–5 days Fosomycin 3 gm (PO) q24h × 3–5 days
Catheter-associated candiduria (CAC)†	C. albicans	Fluconazole 200 mg (PO) × 1 dose, then 100 mg (PO) q24h × 2 weeks
	Fluconazole-resistant C. albicans/non-albicans Candida	Amphotericin B deoxycholate 0.3–0.6 mg/kg q24h × 1–7 days **or** Flucytosine 25 mg/kg QID (PO) × 7–10 days **or** Amphotericin B deoxycholate bladder irrigation (continuous: 50 mg in 1 liter sterile water over 24h × 1–2 days; intermittent: 50 mg in 200–300 ml sterile water q6-8h × 1–2 days)§

VSE/VRE = vancomycin-sensitive/resistant enterococci.

* Remove/replace Foley catheter before initiating antibiotic therapy.

† Treat CAB/CAC in compromised hosts, e.g., cirrhosis, SLE, DM, myeloma, steroids, immunosuppressives, and those with renal disease.

§ Limited efficacy.

Clinical Presentation: Indwelling urinary (Foley) catheter with bacteriuria and pyuria; no symptoms.

Diagnostic Considerations: Pyuria plus bacteriuria/candiduria. Usually afebrile or temperature < 101°F.

Pitfalls: Bacteriuria/candiduria often represent colonization, not infection. Persistent candiduria after amphotericin B deoxycholate bladder irrigation suggests renal candidiasis.

Therapeutic Considerations: Compromised hosts (diabetes, SLE, chronic steroids, multiple myeloma, cirrhosis) may require therapy for duration of catheterization. If bacteriuria/candiduria does not clear with appropriate therapy, change the catheter. For chronic renal failure/dialysis patients with candiduria, use amphotericin B deoxycholate bladder irrigation. Efficacy of therapy of catheter-associated candiduria is limited and relapse is frequent unless the catheter can be replaced or (preferably) removed. Avoid treating catheter-associated bacteriuria in normal hosts without GU tract abnormalities/disease.

Prognosis: Excellent in normal hosts. Untreated bacteriuria/candiduria in compromised hosts may result in ascending infection (e.g., pyelonephritis) or bacteremia/candidemia.

Epididymitis

Subset	Usual Pathogens	Preferred IV Therapy	Alternate IV Therapy	PO Therapy or IV-to-PO Switch
Acute *Young males*	C. trachomatis	Doxycycline 200 mg (IV) q12h × 3 days, then 100 mg (IV) q12h × 4 days	Levofloxacin 500 mg (IV) q24h × 7 days	Doxycycline 200 mg (PO) q12h × 3 days, then 100 mg (PO) q12h × 7 days* **or** Levofloxacin 500 mg (PO) q24h × 10 days **or** Ofloxacin 300 mg (PO) q12h × 10 days
Elderly males	P. aeruginosa	Cefepime 2 gm (IV) q8h × 10 days **or** Meropenem 1 gm (IV) q8h × 10 days	Ciprofloxacin 400 mg (IV) q12h × 10 days **or** Levofloxacin 750 mg (IV) q24h × 10 days	Ciprofloxacin 750 mg (PO) q12h × 10 days
Chronic	M. tuberculosis Blastomyces dermatiditis	Treat the same as pulmonary TB (p. 52) or pulmonary blastomycosis (p. 264)		

Duration of therapy represents total time IV, PO, or IV + PO. Most patients on IV therapy able to take PO meds should be switched to PO therapy soon after clinical improvement (usually < 72 hours).

* Loading dose is not needed PO if given IV with the same drug.

Acute Epididymitis (Chlamydia trachomatis/Pseudomonas aeruginosa)

Clinical Presentation: Acute unilateral testicular pain ± fever.

Diagnostic Considerations: Ultrasound to rule out torsion or tumor.

Pitfalls: Rule out torsion by absence of fever and ultrasound.

Therapeutic Considerations: Young males respond to treatment slowly over 1 week. Elderly males respond to anti-Pseudomonal therapy within 72 hours.

Prognosis: Excellent in young males. Related to health of host in elderly.

Chronic Epididymitis (Mycobacterium tuberculosis/ Blastomyces dermatiditis)

Clinical Presentation: Chronic epididymoorchitis with epididymal nodules.

Diagnostic Considerations: Diagnosis by AFB on biopsy/culture of epididymis. TB epididymitis is always associated with renal TB. Blastomyces epididymitis is a manifestation of systemic infection.

Pitfalls: Vasculitis (e.g., polyarteritis nodosum) and lymphomas may present the same way.

Therapeutic Considerations: Treated the same as pulmonary TB/blastomycosis.

Prognosis: Good.

Acute Pyelonephritis (see Color Atlas for Urine Gram stains)

Subset	Usual Pathogens	Preferred IV Therapy	Alternate IV Therapy	PO Therapy or IV-to-PO Switch
Acute pyelonephritis (Treat initially based on urine gram stain; see therapeutic considerations, below)	Entero-bacteriaceae	Ceftriaxone 1 gm (IV) q24h × 2 weeks **or** Quinolone† (IV) × 2 weeks	Meropenem 500 mg (IV) q8h × 2 weeks **or** Aztreonam 2 gm (IV) q8h × 2 weeks **or** Gentamicin 240 mg (IV) q24h × 2 weeks	Quinolone† (PO) × 2 weeks **or** Amoxicillin 1 gm (PO) q8h × 2 weeks
	Enterococcus faecalis (VSE)§	Ampicillin 1 gm (IV) q4h × 2 weeks **or** Linezolid 600 mg (IV) q12h × 2 weeks **or** Meropenem 500 mg (IV) q8h × 2 weeks	Quinolone† (IV) × 2 weeks	Amoxicillin 1 gm (PO) q8h × 2 weeks **or** Linezolid 600 mg (PO) q12h × 2 weeks **or** Quinolone† (PO) × 2 weeks
	Enterococcus faecium (VRE)	Linezolid 600 mg (IV) q12h × 2 weeks	Quinupristin/ dalfopristin 7.5 mg/kg (IV) q8h × 2 weeks **or** Doxycycline 200 mg (IV) q12h × 3 days, then 100 mg q12h × 2 weeks	Linezolid 600 mg (PO) q12h × 2 weeks **or** Doxycycline 200 mg (PO) q12h × 3 days, then 100 mg (PO) q12h × 2 weeks*

VSE/VRE = vancomycin-sensitive/resistant enterococci. Duration of therapy represents total time IV, PO, or IV + PO. Most patients on IV therapy able to take PO meds should be switched to PO therapy after clinical improvement (usually < 72 hours).

* Loading dose is not needed PO if given IV with the same drug.

† Ciprofloxacin XR 1000 mg (PO) q24h or Ciprofloxacin 400 mg (IV) q12h or Levofloxacin 500 mg (IV or PO) q24h.

§ Treat vancomycin resistant E. faecalis as VRE.

Chronic Pyelonephritis/Renal TB

Subset	Usual Pathogens	Preferred IV Therapy	Alternate IV Therapy	PO Therapy or IV-to-PO Switch
Chronic pyelonephritis	Entero-bacteriaceae	IV Therapy Not applicable		Quinolone† (PO) × 4–6 weeks **or** TMP–SMX 1 DS tab (PO) q12h × 4–6 weeks **or** Doxycycline 200 mg (PO) q12h × 3 days, then 100 mg (PO) q12h × 4–6 weeks total
Renal TB	M. tuberculosis	IV Therapy Not applicable		Treated the same as pulmonary TB (p. 52)

Duration of therapy represents total time IV, PO, or IV + PO. Most patients on IV therapy able to take PO meds should be switched to PO therapy after clinical improvement (usually < 72 hours).

† Ciprofloxacin XR 1000 mg (PO) q24h or Ciprofloxacin 400 mg (IV) q12h or Levofloxacin 500 mg (IV or PO) q24h.

Acute Bacterial Pyelonephritis (Enterobacteriaceae, E. faecalis/faecium)

Clinical Presentation: Unilateral CVA tenderness with fevers ≥ 102°F.

Diagnostic Considerations: Bacteriuria plus pyuria with unilateral CVA tenderness and temperature ≥ 102°F. Bacteremia usually accompanies acute pyelonephritis; obtain blood and urine cultures.

Pitfalls: Temperature decreases in 72 hours with or without antibiotic treatment. If temperature does not fall after 72 hours of antibiotic therapy, suspect renal/perinephric abscess.

Therapeutic Considerations: Initial treatment is based on the urinary gram stain: If gram-negative bacilli, treat as Enterobacteriaceae. If gram-positive cocci in chains (enterococcus), treat as E. faecalis; if enterococcus is subsequently identified as E. faecium, treat accordingly. Acute pyelonephritis is usually treated initially for 1–3 days IV, then switched to PO to complete 4 weeks of antibiotics to minimize progression to chronic pyelonephritis. Obtain a CT/MRI in persistently febrile patients after 72 hours of antibiotics to rule out renal calculi, obstruction, abscess, or xanthomatous pyelonephritis.

Prognosis: Excellent if first episode is adequately treated with antibiotics for 4 weeks.

Chronic Bacterial Pyelonephritis (Enterobacteriaceae)

Clinical Presentation: Previous history of acute pyelonephritis with same symptoms as acute pyelonephritis but less CVA tenderness/fever.

Diagnostic Considerations: Diagnosis by CT/MRI showing changes of chronic pyelonephritis plus bacteriuria/pyuria. Urine cultures may be intermittently negative before treatment. Chronic pyelonephritis is bilateral pathologically, but unilateral clinically.

Pitfalls: Urine culture may be intermittently positive after treatment; repeat weekly × 4 to confirm urine remains culture-negative.

Therapeutic Considerations: Treat × 4–6 weeks. Impaired medullary vascular blood supply/renal anatomical distortion makes eradication of pathogen difficult.
Prognosis: Related to extent of renal damage.

Renal TB (Mycobacterium tuberculosis)

Clinical Presentation: Renal mass lesion with ureteral abnormalities (pipestem, corkscrew, or spiral ureters) and sterile pyuria. Painless unless complicated by ureteral obstruction.
Diagnostic Considerations: Combined upper/lower urinary tract abnormalities ± microscopic hematuria/urinary pH ≤ 5.5. Diagnosis by culture of TB from urine.
Pitfalls: Chest x-ray is normal in 30%, but patients are PPD–positive. Rule out other infectious/inflammatory causes of sterile pyuria (e.g., Trichomonas, interstitial nephritis).
Therapeutic Considerations: Treat the same as pulmonary TB.
Prognosis: Good if treated before renal parenchymal destruction/ureteral obstruction occur.

Renal Abscess (Intrarenal/Perinephric)

Subset	Usual Pathogens	Preferred IV Therapy	Alternate IV Therapy	PO Therapy or IV-to-PO Switch
Cortical (Treat initially for MSSA; if later identified as MRSA, treat accordingly)	S. aureus	MSSA: Nafcillin 2 gm (IV) q4h* **or** Ceftriaxone 1 gm (IV) q24h* **or** Clindamycin 600 mg (IV) q8h* MRSA: Linezolid 600 mg (IV) q12h* **or** Minocycline 100 mg (IV) q12h*	MSSA Meropenem 500 mg (IV) q8h* **or** Ertapenem 1 gm (IV) q24h* MRSA Vancomycin 1 gm (IV) q12h*	MSSA/MRSA Linezolid 600 mg (PO) q12h* **or** Minocycline 100 mg (PO) q12h*
Medullary	Entero-bacteriaceae	Quinolone (IV)†*	TMP–SMX 2.5 mg/kg (IV) q6h*	Quinolone (PO)†*

MSSA/MRSA = methicillin-sensitive/resistant S. aureus. Duration of therapy represents total time IV, PO, or IV + PO. Most patients on IV therapy able to take PO meds should be switched to PO therapy soon after clinical improvement.
* Treat until renal abscess resolves completely or is no longer decreasing in size on CT/MRI.
† Ciprofloxacin XR 1000 mg (PO) q24h or Ciprofloxacin 400 mg (IV) q12h or Levofloxacin 500 mg (IV or PO) q24h.

Clinical Presentation: Similar to pyelonephritis but fever remains elevated after 72 hours of antibiotics.
Diagnostic Considerations: Obtain CT/MRI to diagnose perinephric/intra-renal abscess and rule out mass lesion. Cortical abscesses are usually secondary to hematogenous/contiguous spread. Medullary abscesses are usually due to extension of intrarenal infection.

Pitfalls: Urine cultures may be negative with cortical abscesses.
Therapeutic Considerations: Most large abscesses need to be drained. Multiple small abscesses are managed medically. Obtain urology consult.
Prognosis: Related to degree of baseline renal dysfunction.

Prostatitis/Prostatic Abscess

Subset	Usual Pathogens	Preferred IV Therapy	Alternate IV Therapy	PO Therapy or IV-to-PO Switch
Acute prostatitis/ acute prostatic abscess	Entero-bacteriaceae	Quinolone* (IV) × 2 weeks **or** Ceftriaxone 1 gm (IV) q24h × 2 weeks	TMP–SMX 2.5 mg/kg (IV) q6h × 2 weeks **or** Aztreonam 2 gm (IV) q8h × 2 weeks	Quinolone* (PO) × 2 weeks **or** Doxycycline 200 mg (PO) q12h × 3 days, then 100 mg (PO) q24h × 11 days **or** TMP–SMX 1 SS tablet (PO) q12h × 2 weeks
Chronic prostatitis	Entero-bacteriaceae	IV therapy not applicable	Quinolone* (PO) × 1–3 months **or** Doxycycline 100 mg (PO) q24h × 1–3 months **or** TMP–SMX 1 DS tablet (PO) q12h × 1–3 months	

Duration of therapy represents total time IV, PO, or IV + PO. Most patients on IV therapy able to take PO meds should be switched to PO therapy soon after clinical improvement (usually < 72 hours).

* Ciprofloxacin XR 1000 mg (PO) q24h or Ciprofloxacin 400 mg (IV) q12h or Levofloxacin 500 mg (IV or PO) q24h.

Acute Prostatitis/Acute Prostatic Abscess (Enterobacteriaceae)

Clinical Presentation: Acute prostatitis presents as an acute febrile illness in males with dysuria and no CVA tenderness. Prostatic abscess presents with hectic/septic fevers without localizing signs.
Diagnostic Considerations: Acute prostatitis is diagnosed by bacteriuria plus pyuria with exquisite prostate tenderness, and is seen primarily in young males. Positive urine culture is due to contamination of urine as it passes through infected prostate. Prostatic abscess is diagnosed by transrectal ultrasound or CT/MRI of prostate.
Pitfalls: Do not overlook acute prostatitis in males with bacteriuria without localizing signs, or prostatic abscess in patients with a history of prostatitis.

Therapeutic Considerations: Treat acute prostatitis for 2 full weeks to decrease progression to chronic prostatitis. Prostatic abscess is treated the same as acute prostatitis plus surgical drainage.
Prognosis: Excellent if treated early with full course of antibiotics (plus drainage for prostatic abscess).

Chronic Prostatitis (Enterobacteriaceae)

Clinical Presentation: Vague urinary symptoms (mild dysuria ± low back pain), history of acute prostatitis, and little or no fever.
Diagnostic Considerations: Diagnosis by bacteriuria plus pyuria with "boggy prostate" ± mild tenderness. Urine/prostate expressate is culture positive. Chronic prostatitis with prostatic calcifications (rectal ultrasound) will not clear with antibiotics; treat with transurethral resection of prostate (TURP).
Pitfalls: Commonest cause of treatment failure is inadequate duration of therapy.
Therapeutic Considerations: In sulfa-allergic patients, TMP alone may be used in place of TMP–SMX.
Prognosis: Excellent if treated × 1–3 months. Prostatic abscess is a rare but serious complication (may cause urosepsis).

Urosepsis (see Color Atlas for Urine Gram stains)

Subset	Usual Pathogens	Preferred IV Therapy	Alternate IV Therapy	IV-to-PO Switch
Community-acquired (Treat initially based on urine gram stain)	Entero-bacteriaceae	Ceftriaxone 1 gm (IV) q24h × 7 days **or** Quinolone† (IV) × 7 days	Amikacin 1g (IV) q24h × 7 days **or** Aztreonam 2 gm (IV) q8h × 7 days	Quinolone† (PO) × 7 days **or** TMP–SMX 1 SS tablet (PO) q12h × 7 days
	E. faecalis (VSE) Group B streptococci	Ampicillin 2 gm (IV) q4h × 7 days	Meropenem 500 mg (IV) q8h × 7 days	Amoxicillin 1 gm (PO) q8h × 7 days **or** Quinolone† (PO) × 7 days
(No urine gram stain)	Entero-bacteriaceae E. faecalis (VSE) Group B streptococci	Piperacillin/tazobactam 3.375 mg (IV) q6h × 7 days **or** Meropenem 500 mg (IV) q8h × 7 days	Meropenem 500 mg (IV) q8h × 7 days **or** Doripenem 500 mg (IV) q8h × 7 days	Quinolone† (PO) × 7 days

Duration of therapy represents total time IV or IV + PO. Most patients on IV therapy able to take PO meds should be switched to PO therapy after clinical improvement.

† Ciprofloxacin XR 1000 mg (PO) q24h or Ciprofloxacin 400 mg (IV) q12h or Levofloxacin 500 mg (IV or PO) q24h.

Urosepsis (see Color Atlas of Urine Gram stains) (cont'd)

Subset	Usual Pathogens	Preferred IV Therapy	Alternate IV Therapy	IV-to-PO Switch
Related to urological procedure (Treat intially for P. aeruginosa, etc; if later identified as non-aeruginosa Pseudomonas, treat accordingly)	P. aeruginosa Enterobacter Klebsiella Serratia	Quinolone† (IV) × 7 days **or** Cefepime 2 gm (IV) q8h × 7 days **or** Meropenem 500 mg (IV) q8h × 7 days **or** Doripenem 500 mg (IV) q8h × 7 days	Piperacillin 4 gm (IV) q8h × 7 days **or** Aztreonam 2 gm (IV) q8h × 7 days **or** Amikacin 1g (IV) q24h × 7 days	Quinolone† (PO) × 7 days
	Non-aeruginosa Pseudomonas (B. cepacia, S. maltophilia)	Meropenem 500 mg (IV) q8h × 7 days	TMP–SMX 2.5 mg/kg (IV) q6h × 7 days **or** Cefepime 2 gm (IV) q8h × 7 days	TMP–SMX 1 SS tablet (PO) q12h × 7 days **or** Quinolone† (PO) × 7 days

Duration of therapy represents total time IV or IV + PO. Most patients on IV therapy able to take PO meds should be switched to PO therapy after clinical improvement.

† Ciprofloxacin XR 1000 mg (PO) q24h or Ciprofloxacin 400 mg (IV) q12h or Levofloxacin 750 mg (IV or PO) q24h.

Community-Acquired Urosepsis

Clinical Presentation: Sepsis from urinary tract source.

Diagnostic Considerations: Blood and urine cultures positive for same uropathogen. If patient does not have diabetes, SLE, cirrhosis, myeloma, steroids, pre-existing renal disease or obstruction, obtain CT/MRI of GU tract to rule out abscess/obstruction. Prostatic abscess is rarely a cause of urosepsis.

Pitfalls: Mixed gram-positive/negative urine cultures suggest specimen contamination or enterovesicular fistula.

Therapeutic Considerations: Empiric treatment is based on urine gram stain. If urine gram stain shows pyuria and gram-positive cocci, treat as group D enterococci (E. faecalis-VSE). If gram-negative bacilli, treat as Enterobacteriaceae. S. aureus/S. pneumoniae are not uropathogens.

Prognosis: Related to severity of underlying condition causing urosepsis and health of host.

Urosepsis Following Urological Procedures

Clinical Presentation: Sepsis within 24 hours after GU procedure.

Diagnostic Considerations: Blood and urine cultures positive for same uropathogen. Use pre-procedural urine culture to identify uropathogen and guide therapy.

Pitfalls: If non-aeruginosa Pseudomonas in urine/blood, switch to TMP–SMX pending susceptibilities.

Therapeutic Considerations: Empiric P. aeruginosa monotherapy will cover most other uropathogens.

Prognosis: Related to severity of underlying condition causing urosepsis and health of host.

Pelvic Inflammatory Disease (PID), Salpingitis, Tuboovarian Abscess, Endometritis/Endomyometritis, Septic Abortion

Subset	Usual Pathogens	IV Therapy	PO Therapy or IV-to-PO Switch
Hospitalized patients†	B. fragilis Entero-bacteriaceae N. gonorrhoeae C. trachomatis C. sordelli§ (septic abortion)	**Monotherapy with** Moxifloxacin 400 mg (IV) q24h × 2 weeks **or combination therapy with** Doxycycline 200 mg (IV) q12h × 3 days, then 100 mg (IV) q12h × 11 days **plus either** Piperacillin 4 gm (IV) q6h × 2 weeks **or** Meropenem 500 mg (IV) q8h × 2 weeks **or** Ertapenem 1 gm (IV) q24h × 3–10 days **or** Cefoxitin 2 gm (IV) q6h × 2 weeks **or** Cefotetan 2 gm (IV) q12h × 2 weeks **Alternate combination therapy** Doxycycline 200 mg (IV) q12h × 3 days, then 100 mg (IV) q12h × 11 days **plus** Ampicillin/sulbactam 3 gm (IV) q6h × 2 weeks **or** Quinolone‡ (IV) q24h × 2 weeks **plus** Metronidazole 1 gm (IV) q24h × 2 weeks	**Monotherapy with** Moxifloxacin 400 mg (PO) q24h × 2 weeks
Outpatients (mild PID only)	N. gonorrhoeae C. trachomatis B. fragilis Entero-bacteriaceae	Moxifloxacin 400 mg (PO) q24h × 2 weeks** **or** Doxycycline 100 mg (PO) q12h × 2 weeks	

Duration of therapy represents total time IV, PO, or IV + PO. Most patients on IV therapy able to take PO meds should be switched to PO therapy after clinical improvement.

† Treat only IV or IV-to-PO switch for salpingitis, tuboovarian abscess, endometritis, endomyometritis, septic abortion, or severe PID.

‡ 500 mg (PO) q12h or levofloxacin 500 mg (IV or PO) q24h or ofloxacin 400 mg (IV or PO) q12h.

** Recent increases in gonococcal resistance to quinolones suggest need for careful follow-up during/after therapy.

§ Antibiotic therapy of septic abortion same as salpingitis/endometritis plus evacuation of uterine contents.

Clinical Presentation: PID/salpingitis presents with cervical motion/adnexal tenderness, lower quadrant abdominal pain, and fever. Endometritis/endomyometritis presents with uterine tenderness ± cervical discharge/fever. Endomyometritis is the most common post-partum infection.
Diagnostic Considerations: Unilateral lower abdominal pain in a female without a non-pelvic cause suggests PID/salpingitis.
Pitfalls: Obtain CT/MRI of abdomen/pelvis to confirm diagnosis and rule out other pathology or tuboovarian abscess.
Therapeutic Considerations: Tuboovarian abscess usually requires drainage/removal ± TAH/BSO, plus antibiotics (p. 110) × 1–2 weeks after drainage/removal. Septic abortion is treated the same as endometritis/endomyometritis plus uterine evacuation.
Prognosis: Related to promptness of treatment/adequacy of drainage if tuboovarian abscess. Late complications of PID/salpingitis include tubal scarring/infertility.

Empiric Therapy of Sexually Transmitted Diseases

Urethritis/Cervicitis

Subset	Usual Pathogens	IM Therapy	PO Therapy
Gonococcal (GC)	N. gonorrhoeae	Ceftriaxone 125 mg (IM) × 1 dose Alternate 3rd gen. cephalosporin 250–500 mg (IM) × 1 dose	Cefixime 400 mg (PO) × 1 dose **or** Cefpodoxime 400 mg (PO) × 1 dose **or** Azithromycin 2 gm (PO) × 1 dose**
Non-gonococcal (NGU)	C. trachomatis U. urealyticum M. genitalium	Not applicable	Azithromycin 1 gm (PO) × 1 dose **or** Doxycycline 100 mg (PO) q12h × 7 days **or** Quinolone* (PO) × 7 days **or** Erythromycin 500 mg (PO) q6h × 7 days
	Trichomonas vaginalis	Not applicable	Tinidazole 2 gm (PO) × 1 dose **or** Metronidazole 2 gm (PO) × 1 dose

* Levofloxacin 500 mg q24h or Moxifloxacin 400 mg q24h or Ofloxacin 300 mg q12h.
** Increased resistance, test of cure essential.

Gonococcal Urethritis/Cervicitis (Neisseria gonorrhoeae)

Clinical Presentation: Purulent penile/cervical discharge with burning/dysuria 3–5 days after contact.

Diagnostic Considerations: Rapid diagnosis in males by Gram stain of urethral discharge showing gram-negative diplococci; urethral cultures also positive. In females, diagnosis requires identification of organism by culture or DNA probe, not Gram stain. Rapid diagnosis in males/females by DNA probe. Obtain throat/rectal culture for N. gonorrhoeae. Co-infections are common; obtain VDRL and HIV serologies.

Pitfalls: Gram stain of cervical discharge showing gram-negative diplococci is not diagnostic of N. gonorrhoeae; must confirm by culture. N. gonorrhoeae infections are asymptomatic in 10% of men and 70% of women.

Therapeutic Considerations: Failure to respond suggests re-infection or infection with another agent (e.g., Trichomonas, Ureaplasma). Treat pharyngeal/rectal with ceftriaxone or cefixime. Spectinomycin is ineffective in pharyngeal GC, but spectinomycin 2 gm (IM) × 1 dose may be used to treat rectal/disseminated disease (not currently available in US).

Prognosis: Good even with disseminated infection.

Non-Gonococcal Urethritis/Cervicitis (Chlamydia/Ureaplasma/Mycoplasma)

Clinical Presentation: Mucopurulent penile/cervical discharge ± dysuria ~ 1 week after contact.

Diagnostic Considerations: Diagnosis by positive chlamydial PCR/Ureaplasma or Mycoplasma culture of urethral/cervical discharge. Evaluate urethral/cervical discharge to rule out N. gonorrhoeae. Co-infections are common; obtain syphilis and HIV serologies.

Pitfalls: C. trachomatis infections are asymptomatic in 25%.

Therapeutic Considerations: Failure to respond to doxycycline therapy suggests re-infection or Trichomonas/Ureaplasma/Mycoplasma infection. Failure to respond to azithromycin or a quinolone suggests trichomoniasis.

Prognosis: Tubal scarring/infertility in chronic infection.

Trichomonas Urethritis/Cervicitis (Trichomonas vaginalis)

Clinical Presentation: Frothy, pruritic vaginal discharge.

Diagnostic Considerations: Trichomonas by wet mount/culture on special media.

Pitfalls: Classic "strawberry cervix" is infrequently seen.

Therapeutic Considerations: Use week-long regimen if single dose fails. Resistance now recognized as a cause of treatment failure.

Prognosis: Excellent if partner is also treated.

Vaginitis/Balanitis

Subset	Usual Pathogens	PO Therapy
Bacterial vaginosis/ vaginitis	Polymicrobial (Gardnerella vaginalis, Mobiluncus, Prevotella, M. hominis, etc)	Tinidazole 1 gm (PO) × 5 days **or** 2 gm (PO) × 2 days **or** Clindamycin 300 mg (PO) q12h × 7 days
Candida vaginitis/balanitis	Candida	Fluconazole 150 mg (PO) × 1 dose†

† Those failing to respond should be treated with Fluconazole 200 mg (PO) × 1 dose then 100 mg (PO) q24h × 1 week.

Bacterial Vaginosis/Vaginitis

Clinical Presentation: Non-pruritic vaginal discharge with "fishy" odor.
Diagnostic Considerations: Diagnosis by "clue cells" in vaginal fluid wet mount. Vaginal pH ≥ 4.5.
Pitfalls: "Fishy" odor from smear of vaginal secretions intensified when 10% KOH solution is added (positive "whiff test").
Therapeutic Considerations: As an alternative to oral therapy, clindamycin cream 2% intravaginally qHS × 7 days (avoid in pregnancy) or metronidazole gel 0.075% 1 application intravaginally q12h × 5 days can be used.
Prognosis: Complications include premature rupture of membranes, premature delivery, increased risk of PID. Recurrences very common.

Candida Vaginitis/Balanitis

Clinical Presentation: Pruritic white plaques in vagina/erythema of glans penis.
Diagnostic Considerations: Diagnosis by gram stain/culture of whitish plaques.
Pitfalls: Rule out Trichomonas, which also presents with pruritus in females.
Therapeutic Considerations: Uncomplicated vaginitis (mild sporadic infections in healthy individuals) responds readily to single-dose therapy. Complicated vaginitis (severe, recurrent, or in difficult-to-control diabetes) often requires ≥ 7 days of therapy (daily topical therapy or 2 doses of fluconazole 150 mg given 72h apart). Non-albicans infections respond poorly to azoles. Topical boric acid (600 mg/d in a gelatin capsule × 14 days) is often effective in this setting.
Prognosis: Good with systemic therapy. Diabetics/uncircumcised males may need prolonged therapy.

Genital Vesicles (Genital Herpes) (HSV-2/HSV-1)

Subset	PO Therapy
Initial therapy	Acyclovir 200 mg (PO) 5×/day × 10 days **or** Famciclovir 500 mg (PO) q12h × 7–10 days **or** Valacyclovir 1 gm (PO) q12h × 3 days
Recurrent/ intermittent therapy (< 6 episodes/year)	Acyclovir 200 mg (PO) 5×/day × 5 days **or** Famciclovir (normal host: 125 mg [PO] q12h × 5 days **or** 1 gm [PO] q12h × 1 day*; HIV-positive: 500 mg [PO] q12h × 7 days) **or** Valacyclovir (normal host: 500 mg [PO] q24h × 5 days; HIV-positive: 1 gm [PO] q12h × 7–10 days)**
Chronic suppressive therapy (> 6 episodes/year)	Acyclovir 400 mg (PO) q12h × 1 year **or** Famciclovir 250 mg (PO) q12h × 1 year **or** Valacyclovir (normal host: 1 gm [PO] q24h × 1 year; HIV-positive: 500 mg [PO] q12h × 1 year)

* Patient initiated therapy to be started immediately when recurrence begins.
** Short-course therapy with valaciclovir 500 mg (PO) q12h × 3 days or acyclovir 800 mg (PO) q8h × 2 days also effective.

Clinical Presentation: Painful vesicles/ulcers on genitals with painful bilateral regional adenopathy ± low-grade fever.
Diagnostic Considerations: Diagnosis by clinical presentation may be misleading.
Pitfalls: 70% of newly acquinal gential herpes is due to HSV-1. Elevated IgG HSV-2 titer indicates past exposure, not acute infection. HSV-2 IgM titers may be negative.

Therapeutic Considerations: If concomitant rectal herpes, increase acyclovir to 800 mg (PO) q8h × 7 days. For recurrent genital herpes, use acyclovir or valacyclovir (dose same as primary infection) for 7 days after each relapse. Recurrent episodes of HSV-2 are less painful than primary infection, and inguinal adenopathy is less prominent/painful.
Prognosis: HSV-2 tends to recur, especially during the first year. HSV-1 recurrences less frequent.

Genital Ulcers

Subset	Usual Pathogens	IM Therapy	PO Therapy
Primary syphilis	Treponema pallidum	Benzathine penicillin 2.4 mu (IM) × 1 dose	Doxycycline 100 mg (PO) q12h × 2 weeks
Chancroid	Hemophilus ducreyi	Ceftriaxone 250 mg (IM) × 1 dose <u>Alternate</u>: Any 3rd generation cephalosporin 250–500 mg (IM) × 1 dose	Azithromycin 1 gm (PO) × 1 dose **or** Quinolone* (PO) × 3 days **or** Erythromycin base 500 mg (PO) q6h × 7 days

* Ciprofloxacin 500 mg q12h or levofloxacin 500 mg or moxifloxacin 400 mg q24h.

Primary Syphilis (Treponema pallidum)

Clinical Presentation: Painless, indurated ulcers (chancres) with bilateral painless inguinal adenopathy. Syphilitic chancres are elevated, clean and raised, but not undermined.
Diagnostic Considerations: Diagnosis by spirochetes on darkfield examination of ulcer exudate. Elevated non-treponemal (VDRL/RPR) titers after 1 week.
Pitfalls: Non-treponemal (VDRL/RPR) titers fall slowly within 1 year; failure to decline suggests treatment failure/HIV. Even after effective treatment some patients remain VDRL/RPR positive for life (serofast).
Therapeutic Considerations: Parenteral penicillin is the preferred antibiotic for all stages of syphilis. If treatment fails and VDRL/RPR titers do not decline, obtain HIV serology.
Prognosis: Good with early treatment.

Chancroid (Hemophilus ducreyi)

Clinical Presentation: Ragged, undermined, painful ulcer(s) + painful unilateral inguinal adenopathy.
Diagnostic Considerations: Diagnosis by streptobacilli in "school of fish" configuration on gram-stained smear of ulcer exudate/culture of H. ducreyi/PCR.
Pitfalls: Co-infection is common; obtain Syphilus and HIV serologies.
Therapeutic Considerations: In HIV, multiple dose regimens or azithromycin is preferred. Resistance to erythromycin/ciprofloxacin has been reported.
Prognosis: Good with early treatment.

Suppurating Inguinal Adenopathy

Subset	Pathogens	IV Therapy	PO Therapy
Lympho-granuloma venereum (LGV)	Chlamydia trachomatis (L_{1-3} serotypes)	Not applicable	Doxycycline 100 mg (PO) q12h × 3 wks **or** Erythromycin 500 mg (PO) q6h × 3 weeks
Granuloma inguinale (Donovanosis)	Klebsiella (Calymmato-bacterium) granulomatis	Not applicable	Azithromycin 1 gm (PO) q week until cured. Doxycycline 100 mg (PO) q12h × until cured **or** Erythromycin 500 mg (PO) q6h × until cured **or** TMP–SMX 1 DS (PO) q12h × until cured **or** Ciprofloxacin 500 mg (PO) q12h × until cured

Lymphogranuloma Venereum (Chlamydia trachomatis) LGV

Clinical Presentation: Unilateral inguinal adenopathy ± discharge/sinus tract.

Diagnostic Consideration: Diagnosis by very high Chlamydia trachomatis L_{1-3} titers. Do not biopsy site (often does not heal and may form a fistula). May present as FUO.

Pitfalls: Initial papule not visible at clinical presentation. Biopsy shows granulomas; may be confused with perianal Crohn's disease.

Therapeutic Considerations: Rectal LGV may require additional courses of treatment.

Prognosis: Fibrotic perirectal/pelvic damage does not reverse with therapy.

Granuloma Inguinale (Klebsiella [Calymmatobacterium] granulomatis) Donovanosis

Clinical Presentation: Pseudolymphadenopathy ("groove sign") with painless inguinal ulcers.

Diagnostic Considerations: Donovan bodies ("puffed-wheat" appearance) in tissue biopsy.

Pitfalls: No true inguinal adenopathy, as opposed to LGV infection.

Therapeutic Considerations: Doxycycline or erythromycin preferred. Continue therapy until lesions are healed.

Prognosis: Good if treated early.

Genital/Perianal Warts (Condylomata Acuminata)

Subset	Pathogens	Therapy
Genital/ perianal warts	Human papilloma virus (HPV)	Podophyllin 10–25% in tincture of benzoin or podofilox or imiquimod (patient applies) **or** surgical/laser removal/ cryotherapy with liquid nitrogen **or** cidofovir gel (1%) QHS × 5 days every other week for 6 cycles **or** trichloracetic acid (TCA)/bichloracetic acid (BCA) **or** intralesional interferon. Sinecatechins (15% ointment) q8h × 4 months

Clinical Presentation: Single/multiple verrucous genital lesions ± pigmentation, without inguinal adenopathy.

Diagnostic Considerations: Diagnosis by clinical appearance. Genital warts are usually caused by HPV types 6, 11. Anogenital warts caused by HPV types 16,18,31,33,35 and others are associated with cervical neoplasia. Females with anogenital warts need serial cervical PAP smears to detect cervical dysplasia/neoplasia.

Pitfalls: Most HPV infections are asymptomatic.

Therapeutic Considerations: Cidofovir cures/halts HPV progression in 50% of cases.

Prognosis: Related to HPV serotypes with malignant potential (HPV types 16,18,31,33,35). Preventative (not therapeutic) vaccines now available.

Syphilis

Subset	Pathogen	IV/IM Therapy	PO Therapy
Primary, secondary, or early latent (duration < 1 year) syphilis	Treponema pallidum	Benzathine penicillin 2.4 mu (IM) × 1 dose	Doxycycline 100 mg (PO) q12h × 2 weeks
Late latent (duration > 1 year) or tertiary syphilis	Treponema pallidum	Benzathine penicillin 2.4 mu (IM) weekly × 3 weeks	Doxycycline 100 mg (PO) q12h × 4 weeks
Neurosyphilis	Treponema pallidum	Penicillin G 3–4 mu (IV) q4h or continuous infusion × 10–14 days Alternate: Procaine penicillin 2.4 mu (IM) q24h × 10–14 days plus probenecid 500 mg (PO) q6h × 10–14 days **or monotherapy with** Ceftriaxone 2 gm (IV) q24h × 10–14 days	Doxycycline 100 mg (PO) q12h × 4 weeks **or** Minocycline 100 mg (PO) q12h × 4 weeks

Duration of therapy represents total time IV, IM, or PO. All stages of syphilis in HIV/AIDS patients usually respond to therapeutic regimens recommended for normal hosts. Syphilis in pregnancy should be treated according to the stage of syphilis; penicillin-allergic pregnant patients should be desensitized and treated with penicillin.

Primary Syphilis (Treponema pallidum)

Clinical Presentation: Painless, indurated ulcer(s) (chancre) with bilateral painless inguinal adenopathy.

Diagnostic Considerations: Diagnosis by spirochetes on darkfield examination of ulcer exudate. Elevated Non-treponemal (VDRL/RPR) or treponemal (TPPA) titers after 1 week.

Pitfalls: VDRL/RPR titers fall slowly within 1 year; failure to decline suggests treatment failure.

Therapeutic Considerations: Parenteral penicillin is the preferred antibiotic for all stages of syphilis; if treatment fails and VDRL/RPR titers do not decline, obtain HIV serology.

Prognosis: Good with early treatment.

Secondary Syphilis (Treponema pallidum)

Clinical Presentation: Facial/truncal macular, papular, papulosquamous, non-pruritic, non-tender, symmetrical rash which may involve the palms/soles. Usually accompanied by generalized adenopathy. Typically appears 4–10 weeks after primary chancre, although stages may overlap. Alopecia, condyloma lata, mucous patches, iritis/uveitis may be present. Renal involvement ranges from mild proteinuria to nephrotic syndrome. Without treatment, spontaneous resolution occurs after 3–12 weeks.

Diagnostic Considerations: Diagnosis by clinical findings and VDRL/RPR in high titers (≥ 1:256). After treatment, VDRL titers usually return to non-reactive within 2 years. Syphilitic hepatitis is characterized by elevated alkaline phosphatase > elevated SGOT.

Pitfalls: If only undiluted serum is tested, prozone phenomenon may render VDRL/RPR falsely negative.

Therapeutic Considerations: Parenteral penicillin is the preferred antibiotic for all stages of syphilis.

Prognosis: Excellent with early treatment.

Latent Syphilis (Treponema pallidum)

Clinical Presentation: Patients are asymptomatic with elevated non-treponemal titers and reactive treponemal tests.

Diagnostic Considerations: Diagnosis by positive serology ± prior history, but no signs/symptoms of syphilis. Asymptomatic syphilis < 1 year in duration is termed "early" latent syphilis; asymptomatic syphilis > 1 year/unknown duration is termed "late" latent syphilis. Secondary syphilis may relapse in up to 25% of patients with early latent syphilis, but relapse is rare in late latent syphilis. Evaluate patients for neurosyphilis.

Pitfalls: Treponemal tests (FTA-ABS, MHA-TP, TPPA) usually remain positive for life, even after adequate treatment.

Therapeutic Considerations: Parenteral penicillin is the preferred antibiotic for all stages of syphilis. Repeat VDRL/RPR titers at 6, 12, and 24 months; therapeutic response is defined as a 4-fold reduction in VDRL titers (2 tube dilutions).

Prognosis: Excellent even if treated late.

Tertiary Syphilis (Treponema pallidum)

Clinical Presentation: May present with aortitis, neurosyphilis, iritis, or gummata 5–30 years after initial infection.

Diagnostic Considerations: Diagnosis by history of syphilis plus positive serological tests with signs/symptoms of late syphilis.

Pitfalls: Treat for signs of neurosyphilis on clinical exam or LP, even if VDRL/RPR are non-reactive.

Therapeutic Considerations: Parenteral penicillin is the preferred antibiotic for all stages of syphilis.

Prognosis: Related to extent of end-organ damage.

Neurosyphilis (Treponema pallidum)

Clinical Presentation: Patients are often asymptomatic, but may have ophthalmic/auditory symptoms, cranial nerve abnormalities, tabes dorsalis, paresis, psychosis, or signs of meningitis/dementia.

Diagnostic Considerations: Diagnosis by elevated CSF VDRL titers; no need to obtain CSF FTA-ABS titers. Diagnosis confirmed if CSF has pleocytosis (> 5 WBCs/hpf) or increased protein (> 50 mg/dL), and positive VDRL.

Pitfalls: Persistent CSF abnormalities suggest treatment failure. CSF VDRL (60% sensitive) may be negative in neurosyphilis.

Therapeutic Considerations: Parenteral penicillin is the preferred antibiotic for all stages of syphilis. CSF abnormalities should decrease in 6 months and return to normal after 2 years; repeat lumbar puncture 6 months after treatment. Failure rate with ceftriaxone is 20%.

Prognosis: Related to extent of end-organ damage.

Empiric Therapy of Bone and Joint Infections

Septic Arthritis/Bursitis

Subset	Usual Pathogens	Preferred IV Therapy	Alternate IV Therapy	PO Therapy or IV-to-PO Switch
Acute (Treat initially based on gram stain of synovial fluid. If gram-positive cocci in clusters, treat initially for MRSA; if later identified as MSSA, treat accordingly)	S. aureus (MSSA)	Ceftriaxone 1 gm (IV) q24h × 3 weeks **or** Cefazolin 1 gm (IV) q8h × 3 weeks **or** Clindamycin 600 mg (IV) q8h × 3 weeks	Nafcillin 2 gm (IV) q4h × 3 weeks **or** Meropenem 500 mg (IV) q8h × 3 weeks **or** Ertapenem 1 gm (IV) q24h × 3 weeks	Cephalexin 1 gm (PO) q6h × 3 weeks **or** Clindamycin 300 mg (PO) q8h× 3 weeks **or** Quinolone* (PO) q24h × 3 weeks
	S. aureus (MRSA)	Linezolid 600 mg (IV) q12h × 3 weeks **or** Quinupristin/dalfopristin 7.5 mg/kg (IV) q8h × 3 weeks **or** Minocycline 100 mg (IV) q12h × 3 weeks		Linezolid 600 mg (PO) q12h × 3 weeks **or** Minocycline 100 mg (PO) q12h × 3 weeks
	Group A,B,C,G streptococci	Ceftriaxone 1 gm (IV) q24h × 3 weeks **or** Clindamycin 600 mg (IV) q8h × 3 weeks	Cefazolin 1 gm (IV) q8h × 3 weeks **or** Quinolone* (IV) q24h × 3 weeks	Clindamycin 300 mg (PO) q8h × 3 weeks **or** Cephalexin 500 mg (PO) q6h × 3 weeks **or** Quinolone* (PO) q24h × 3 weeks

* Moxifloxacin 400 mg or levofloxacin 500 mg.

Septic Arthritis/Bursitis (cont'd)

Subset	Usual Pathogens	Preferred IV Therapy	Alternate IV Therapy	PO Therapy or IV-to-PO Switch
Acute (cont'd)	Entero-bacteriaceae	Ceftriaxone 1 gm (IV) q24h × 3 weeks **or** Cefepime 2 gm (IV) q12h × 3 weeks **or** Cefotaxime 2 gm (IV) q6h × 3 weeks **or** Ceftizoxime 2 gm (IV) q8h × 3 weeks	Aztreonam 2 gm (IV) q8h × 3 weeks **or** Quinolone‡ (IV) × 3 weeks	Quinolone‡ (PO) × 3 weeks
	P. aeruginosa	Meropenem 1 gm (IV) q8h × 3 weeks **or** Cefepime 2 gm (IV) q8h × 3 weeks	Aztreonam 2 gm (IV) q8h × 3 weeks **or** Piperacillin 4 gm (IV) q8h × 3 weeks	Ciprofloxacin 750 mg (PO) q12h × 3 weeks
	N. gonorrhoeae (PSNG/PPNG)	Ceftriaxone 1 gm (IV) q24h × 2 weeks **or** Ceftizoxime 2 gm (IV) q8h × 2 weeks	Ciprofloxacin 400 mg (IV) q24h × 2 weeks **or** Moxifloxacin 400 mg (IV) q24h × 2 weeks **or** Levofloxacin 500 mg (IV) q24h × 2 weeks	Ciprofloxacin 500 mg (PO) q24h × 2 weeks **or** Moxifloxacin 400 mg (PO) q24h × 2 weeks **or** Levofloxacin 500 mg (PO) q24h × 2 weeks

‡ Ciprofloxacin 400 mg (IV) q12h or 750 mg (PO) 12h or Moxifloxacin 400 mg (IV or PO) q24h or Levofloxacin 750 mg (IV or PO) q24h.

Septic Arthritis/Bursitis (cont'd)

Subset	Usual Pathogens	Preferred IV Therapy	Alternate IV Therapy	PO Therapy or IV-to-PO Switch
Acute (cont'd)	Brucella	Streptomycin 1 gm (IM) q24h × 3 weeks **plus** Doxycycline 200 mg (IV) q12h × 3 days, then 100 mg (IV) q12h for 3-week total course	Gentamicin 5 mg/kg (IV) q24h × 3 weeks **plus** Doxycycline 200 mg (IV) q12h × 3 days, then 100 mg (IV) q12h for 3-week total course	Doxycycline 200 mg (PO) q12h × 3 days, then 100 mg (PO) q12h for 3-week total course† **plus** Rifampin 600 mg (PO) q24h × 3 weeks
	Salmonella	Ceftriaxone 2 gm (IV) q24h × 2–3 weeks **or** Quinolone* (IV) × 2–3 weeks	Aztreonam 2 gm (IV) q8h × 2–3 weeks **or** TMP–SMX 2.5 mg/kg (IV) q6h × 2–3 weeks	Quinolone* (PO) × 2–3 weeks **or** TMP–SMX 1 DS tablet (PO) q12h × 2–3 weeks
Secondary to animal bite wound	Pasteurella multocida Streptobacillus moniliformis Eikinella corrodens	Piperacillin/ tazobactam 3.375 gm (IV) q6h × 2 weeks **or** Ampicillin/ sulbactam 3 gm (IV) q6h × 2 weeks **or** Ticarcillin/ clavulanate 3.1 gm (IV) q6h × 2 weeks	Meropenem 1 gm (IV) q8h × 2 weeks **or** Ertapenem 1 gm (IV) q24h × 2 weeks **or** Doxycycline 200 mg (IV) q12h × 3 days, then 100 mg (IV) q12h × 11 days	Amoxicillin/ clavulanic acid 875/125 mg (PO) q12h × 2 weeks **or** Doxycycline 200 mg (PO) q12h × 3 days, then 100 mg (PO) q12h × 11 days† **or** Moxifloxacin 400 mg (PO) q24h × 2 weeks

† Loading dose is not needed PO if given IV with the same drug.

* Ciprofloxacin 400 mg (IV) or 500 mg (PO) q12h or Levofloxacin 500 mg (IV or PO) q24h or Moxifloxacin 400 mg (IV or PO) q24h.

Septic Arthritis/Bursitis (cont'd)

Subset	Usual Pathogens	Preferred IV Therapy	Alternate IV Therapy	PO Therapy or IV-to-PO Switch
Fungal arthritis	Coccidioides immitis	Not applicable	Itraconazole 200 mg (PO) solution q12h × 12 months or until cured* **or** Fluconazole 800 mg (PO) q24h until cured*	
	Sporothrix schenckii	Not applicable	Itraconazole 200 mg (PO) q12h until cured*	
TB arthritis	M. tuberculosis	Not applicable	Treat the same as for pulmonary TB (p. 52) except treat for 6–9 months	

MSSA/MRSA = methicillin-sensitive/resistant S. aureus. Duration of therapy represents total time IV, PO, or IV + PO. Most patients on IV therapy able to take PO meds should be switched to PO therapy after clinical improvement.

* Itraconazole solution provides more reliable absorption than capsules.

Acute Septic Arthritis/Bursitis

Clinical Presentation: Acute joint pain with fever. Septic joint unable to bear weight. Septic bursitis presents with pain on joint motion, but patient is able to bear weight.

Diagnostic Considerations: Diagnosis by demonstrating organisms in synovial fluid by stain/culture. In septic bursitis (knee most common), there is pain on joint flexion (although the joint can bear weight), and synovial fluid findings are negative for septic arthritis. Except for N. gonorrhoeae, polyarthritis is not usually due to bacterial pathogens. Post-infectious polyarthritis is usually viral in origin, most commonly due to parvovirus B19, rubella, or HBV.

Pitfalls: Reactive arthritis may follow C. jejuni, Salmonella, Shigella, Yersinia, N. gonorrheae C. trachomatis, or C. difficile infections. Synovial fluid cultures are negative. Reactive arthritis is usually asymmetrical and is monoarticular/oligoarticular.

Therapeutic Considerations: See specific pathogen, below. Treat septic bursitis as septic arthritis.

Staphylococcus aureus (MSSA/MRSA)

Diagnostic Considerations: Painful hot joint; unable to bear weight. Diagnosis by synovial fluid pleocytosis and positive culture for joint pathogen. Examine synovial fluid to rule out gout (doubly birefringent crystals) and pseudogout (calcium pyrophosphate crystals). May occur in setting of endocarditis with septic emboli to joints; other manifestations of endocarditis are usually evident.

Pitfalls: Rule out causes of non-infectious arthritis (sarcoidosis, Whipple's disease, Ehlers-Danlos, etc.), which are less severe, but may mimic septic arthritis. In reactive arthritis following urethritis (C. trachomatis, Ureaplasma urealyticum, N. gonorrhoeae) or diarrhea (Shigella, Campylobacter, Yersinia, Salmonella), synovial fluid culture is negative, and synovial fluid WBCs counts are usually < 10,000/mm^3 with normal synovial fluid lactic acid and glucose. Do not overlook infective endocarditis in mono/polyarticular MSSA/MRSA septic arthritis without apparent source.

Therapeutic Considerations: For MRSA septic arthritis, vancomycin penetration into synovial fluid is poor; use linezolid instead. Immobilization of infected joint during therapy is helpful. Local installation of antibiotics into synovial fluid has no advantage over IV/PO antibiotics.

Prognosis: Treat as early as possible to minimize joint damage. Repeated aspiration/open drainage may be needed to preserve joint function.

Group A, B, C, G Streptococci

Diagnostic Considerations: Usually monoarticular. Not usually due to septic emboli from endocarditis.

Prognosis: Related to extent of joint damage and rapidity of antibiotic treatment.

Enterobacteriaceae

Diagnostic Considerations: Diagnosis by isolation of gram-negative bacilli from synovial fluid.

Pitfalls: Septic arthritis involving an unusual joint (e.g., sternoclavicular, sacral) should suggest IV drug abuse until proven otherwise.

Therapeutic Considerations: Joint aspiration is essential in suspected septic arthritis of the hip and may be needed for other joints; obtain orthopedic surgery consult. Local installation of antibiotics into joint fluid is of no proven value.

Prognosis: Related to extent of joint damage and rapidity of antibiotic treatment.

Pseudomonas aeruginosa

Diagnostic Considerations P. aeruginosa septic arthritis/osteomyelitis may occur after water contaminated puncture wound (e.g., nail puncture of heel through shoes). Sternoclavicular/sacroiliac joint involvement is common in IV drug abusers (IVDAs).

Pitfalls: Suspect IVDA in P. aeruginosa septic arthritis without a history of trauma.

Therapeutic Considerations: If ciprofloxacin is used, treat with 750 mg (not 500 mg) dose for P. aeruginosa septic arthritis/osteomyelitis.

Prognosis: Related to extent of joint damage and rapidity of antibiotic treatment.

Neisseria gonorrhoeae

Diagnostic Considerations: Gonococcal arthritis may present as a monoarticular arthritis, or multiple joints may be affected as part of gonococcal arthritis-dermatitis syndrome (disseminated gonococcal infection). Bacteremia with positive blood cultures occurs early during rash stage while synovial fluid cultures are negative. Joint involvement follows with typical findings of septic arthritis and synovial fluid cultures positive for N. gonorrhoeae; blood cultures are negative at this stage. Acute tenosynovitis is often a clue to gonococcal septic arthritis.

Pitfalls: Spectinomycin is ineffective against pharyngeal gonorrhea.

Therapeutic Considerations: Gonococcal arthritis-dermatitis syndrome is caused by very susceptible strains of N. gonorrhoeae. Cephalosporins also eliminate incubating syphilis.

Prognosis: Excellent with arthritis-dermatitis syndrome; worse with only monoarticular arthritis.

Brucella sp.

Diagnostic Considerations: Usually evidence of brucellosis elsewhere (meningitis, SBE, epididymoorchitis). Diagnosis by blood/joint cultures.

Pitfalls: Brucella has predilection for bones/joints e.g., vertebra, sacroiliac joints. Suspect in patients with an unusual affect with back abdominal pain. May present as an FUO.

Therapeutic Considerations: Some patients may require 6 weeks of antibiotic therapy.
Prognosis: Related to severity of infection and underlying health of host.

Salmonella sp.

Diagnostic Considerations: Occurs in sickle cell disease and hemoglobinopathies. Diagnosis by blood/joint cultures.
Pitfalls: S. aureus, not Salmonella, is the most common cause of septic arthritis in sickle cell disease.
Prognosis: Related to severity of infection and underlying health of host.

Septic Arthritis Secondary to Animal Bite Wound

Clinical Presentation: Penetrating bite wound into joint space.
Diagnostic Considerations: Diagnosis by smear/culture of synovial fluid/blood cultures.
Pitfalls: May develop metastatic infection from bacteremia.
Therapeutic Considerations: Treat for at least 2 weeks of combined IV/PO therapy.
Prognosis: Related to severity of infection and underlying health of host.

Chronic Septic Arthritis

Clinical Presentation: Subacute/chronic joint pain with decreased range of motion and little or no fever. Able to bear weight on joint.
Diagnostic Considerations: Diagnosis by smear/culture of synovial fluid/synovial biopsy.

Coccidioides immitis

Diagnostic Considerations: Must grow organisms from synovium/synovial fluid for diagnosis.
Pitfalls: Synovial fluid the same as in TB (lymphocytic pleocytosis, low glucose, increased protein).
Therapeutic Considerations: Oral therapy is preferred; same cure rates as amphotericin regimens. HIV/AIDS patients need life-long suppressive therapy.
Prognosis: Related to severity of infection and underlying health of host.

Sporothrix schenckii

Diagnostic Considerations: Usually a monoarticular infection secondary to direct inoculation/trauma.
Pitfalls: Polyarticular arthritis suggests disseminated infection.
Therapeutic Considerations: SSKI is useful for lymphocutaneous sporotrichosis, not bone/joint involvement.
Prognosis: Excellent for localized disease (e.g., lymphocutaneous sporotrichosis). In disseminated disease, prognosis is related to host factors.

Mycobacterium tuberculosis (TB)

Diagnostic Considerations: Clue is subacute/chronic tenosynovitis over involved joint. Unlike other forms of septic arthritis, which are usually due to hematogenous spread, TB arthritis may complicate adjacent TB osteomyelitis. Synovial fluid findings include lymphocytic pleocytosis, low glucose, and increased protein.
Pitfalls: Send synovial fluid/biopsy for AFB smear/culture in unexplained chronic monoarticular arthritis.
Therapeutic Considerations: TB arthritis is usually treated for 9–12 months.
Prognosis: Related to severity of infection and underlying health of host.

Lyme Disease*/Lyme Arthritis

Subset	Usual Pathogens	Preferred IV Therapy	Alternate IV Therapy	PO Therapy or IV-to-PO Switch
Lyme disease	Borrelia burgdorferi	Ceftriaxone 1 gm (IV) q24h × 2 weeks	Ceftizoxime 2 gm (IV) q8h × 2 weeks	Amoxicillin 1 gm (PO) q8h × 2 weeks **or** Doxycycline 200 mg (PO) q12h × 3 days, then 100 mg (PO) q12h × 11 days†
Lyme arthritis		Ceftriaxone 1 gm (IV) q24h × 4 weeks	Ceftizoxime 2 gm (IV) q8h × 4 weeks	Amoxicillin 1 gm (PO) q8h × 4 weeks **or** Doxycycline 200 mg (PO) q12h × 3 days, then 100 mg (PO) q12h × 4 weeks

Duration of therapy represents total time IV, PO, or IV + PO. Most patients on IV therapy able to take PO meds should be switched to PO therapy after clinical improvement.

* See p. 21 for Lyme neuroborreliosis and p. 76 for Lyme myocarditis.

† Doxycycline therapy × 10 days as effective as 2 weeks.

‡ For adult patients intolerant of Amoxicillin, Doxycycline, and Cefuroxime axetil, Azithromycin (500 mg orally per day for 7–10 days), Clarithromycin (500 mg orally twice per day for 14–21 days, if the patient is not pregnant), or Erythromycin (500 mg orally 4 times per day for 14–21 days) may be given. The recommended dosages of these agents for children are as follows: Azithromycin, 10 mg/kg per day (maximum of 500 mg per day); Clarithromycin, 7.5 mg/kg twice per day (maximum of 500 mg per dose); and Erythromycin, 12.5 mg/kg 4 times per day (maximum of 500 mg per dose).

Lyme Disease

Clinical Presentation: Can manifest acutely or chronically with local or disseminated disease following bite of tick infected with Borrelia spirochete. Erythema migrans (expanding, erythematous, annular lesion with central clearing) occurs in ~ 75% within 2 weeks of tick bite and may be associated with fever, headache, arthralgias/myalgias, meningismus. Other possible acute manifestations include meningitis, encephalitis, Bell's palsy, peripheral neuropathy, mild hepatitis, myocarditis with heart block, or arthritis. Chronic disease may present with arthritis, peripheral neuropathy, meningoencephalitis, or acrodermatitis chronica atrophicans (usually > 10 years after infection).

Diagnostic Considerations: Diagnosis by clinical presentation plus elevated IgM Lyme titers (IFA/ELISA). If Lyme titer is borderline or suspected to be a false-positive, obtain an IgM Western blot to confirm the diagnosis. IgM titers may take 4–6 weeks to increase after tick bite. Ixodes ticks are the principal vector; small rodents are the primary reservoir. In the United States, most cases occur in the coastal Northeast, upper Midwest, California, and western Nevada.

Pitfalls: Rash is not always seen, and tick bite is often painless and goes unnoticed (tick often spontaneously falls off after 1–2 days of feeding). Do not overlook Lyme disease in patients with unexplained heart block in areas where Ixodes ticks are endemic. Highest failure rater with macrolide therapy.
Therapeutic Considerations: B. burgdorferi is highly susceptible to all beta-lactams. For Bell's palsy or neuroborreliosis, minocycline (100 mg PO q12h × 2 weeks) may be preferred to doxycycline. Symptoms may persist for 1 year or more after adequate therapy. No rationale to re-treat persistent symptoms.
Prognosis: Excellent in normal hosts.

Lyme Arthritis

Clinical Presentation: Acute Lyme arthritis presents with joint pain, decreased range of motion, ability to bear weight on joint, and little or no fever. Chronic Lyme arthritis resembles rheumatoid arthritis.
Diagnostic Considerations: Usually affects children and large weight-bearing joints (e.g., knee). Acute Lyme arthritis is diagnosed by clinical presentation plus elevated IgM Lyme titer. Chronic Lyme arthritis is suggested by rheumatoid arthritis-like presentation with negative ANA and rheumatoid factor, and positive IgG Lyme titer and synovial fluid PCR.
Pitfalls: Acute Lyme arthritis joint is red but not hot, in contrast to septic arthritis. In chronic Lyme arthritis, a negative IgG Lyme titer essentially rules out chronic Lyme arthritis, but an elevated IgG Lyme titer indicates only past exposure to B. burgdorferi and is not diagnostic of Lyme arthritis. Joint fluid in chronic Lyme disease is usually negative by culture, but positive by PCR; synovial fluid PCR, however, does not differentiate active from prior infection.
Therapeutic Considerations: IgG Lyme titers remain elevated for life, and do not decrease with treatment. Joint symptoms often persist for months/years after effective antibiotic therapy due to autoimmune joint inflammation; treat with anti-inflammatory drugs, not repeat antibiotic courses. Oral therapy as effective as IV therapy.
Prognosis: Good in normal hosts. Chronic/refractory arthritis may develop in genetically predisposed patients with DRW 2/4 HLA types.

Infected Joint Prosthesis

Subset	Usual Pathogens	Preferred IV Therapy	Alternate IV Therapy	IV-to-PO Switch
Staphylococcal (Treat initially for MSSA; if later identified as MRSA/CoNS, treat accordingly)	S. epidermidis (CoNS)	Linezolid 600 mg (IV) q12h* **or** Vancomycin 1 gm (IV) q12h*	Cefotaxime 2 gm (IV) q6h*† **or** Ceftizoxime 2 gm (IV) q8h*†	Linezolid 600 mg (PO) q12h*
	S. aureus (MSSA)	Nafcillin 2 gm (IV) q4h* **or** Ceftriaxone 1 gm (IV) q24h*† **or** Cefazolin 1 gm (IV) q8h*	Meropenem 1 gm (IV) q8h* **or** Clindamycin 600 mg (IV) q8h*	Clindamycin 300 mg (PO) q8h* **or** Linezolid 600 mg (PO) q12h* **or** Cephalexin 1 gm (PO) q6h*

Infected Joint Prosthesis (cont'd)

Subset	Usual Pathogens	Preferred IV Therapy	Alternate IV Therapy	IV-to-PO Switch
Staphylococcal (cont'd)	S. aureus (MRSA)	Linezolid 600 mg (IV) q12h* **or** Vancomycin 1 gm (IV) q12h* **or** Minocycline 100 mg (IV) q12h* **or** Quinupristin/dalfopristin 7.5 mg/kg (IV) q8h*		Linezolid 600 mg (PO) q12h* **or** Minocycline 100 mg (PO) q12h*

MRSA/MSSA = methicillin-resistant/sensitive S. aureus; MSSE/MRSE = methicillin-sensitive/resistant S. epidermidis. Duration of therapy represents total time IV or IV + PO. Most patients on IV therapy able to take PO meds should be switched to PO therapy after clinical improvement.

* Treat for 1 week after joint prosthesis is replaced.

† Only if MSSE strain susceptible.

Clinical Presentation: Pain in area of prosthesis with joint loosening/instability ± low-grade fevers.

Diagnostic Considerations: Infected prosthesis is suggested by prosthetic loosening/lucent areas adjacent to prosthesis on plain films ± positive blood cultures. Diagnosis confirmed by bone scan. Use joint aspiration to identify organism.

Pitfalls: An elevated ESR with prosthetic loosening suggests prosthetic joint infection. Mechanical loosening without infection is comon many years after joint replacement, but ESR is normal.

Therapeutic Considerations: Infected prosthetic joints usually must be removed for cure. Replacement prosthesis may be inserted anytime after infected prosthesis is removed. To prevent infection of new joint prosthesis, extensive debridement of old infected material is important. If replacement of infected joint prosthesis is not possible, chronic suppressive therapy may be used with oral antibiotics; adding rifampin 300 mg (PO) q12h may be helpful. TMP–SMX 5 mg/kg (PO) q6h may be successful in long-term suppression/cure in total hip replacement (treat × 6 months) or total knee replacement (treat × 9 months) due to susceptible strains of MSSA/MSSE.

Prognosis: Related to adequate debridement of infected material when prosthetic joint is removed.

Osteomyelitis

Subset	Usual Pathogens	Preferred IV Therapy	Alternate IV Therapy	PO Therapy or IV-to-PO Switch
Acute (Treat initially for MSSA; if later identified as MRSA or Enterobacteriaceae, treat accordingly)	S. aureus (MRSA)	Linezolid 600 mg (IV) q12h × 4–6 weeks **or** Quinupristin/dalfopristin 7.5 mg/kg (IV) q8h × 4–6 weeks **or** Minocycline 100 mg (IV) q12h × 4–6 weeks **or** Vancomycin 2 gm (IV) q12h × 4–6 weeks		Linezolid 600 mg (PO) q12h × 4–6 weeks **or** Minocycline 100 mg (PO) q12h × 4–6 weeks

Osteomyelitis (cont'd)

Subset	Usual Pathogens	Preferred IV Therapy	Alternate IV Therapy	PO Therapy or IV-to-PO Switch
Acute (cont'd)	S. aureus (MSSA)	Cefazolin 1 gm (IV) q8h × 4–6 weeks **or** Ceftriaxone 1 gm (IV) q24h × 4–6 weeks **or** Meropenem 500 mg (IV) q8h × 4–6 weeks	Cefotaxime 2 gm (IV) q6h × 4–6 weeks **or** Ceftizoxime 2 gm (IV) q8h × 4–6 weeks	Clindamycin 300 mg (PO) q8h × 4–6 weeks **or** Cephalexin 1 gm (PO) q6h × 4–6 weeks **or** Quinolone‡ (PO) q24h × 4–6 weeks
	Entero-bacteriaceae	Ceftriaxone 1 gm (IV) q24h × 4–6 wks **or** Quinolone† (IV) × 4–6 weeks **or monotherapy with** Tigacycline 100 mg (IV) × 1 dose, then 50 mg (IV) q12h¶	Cefotaxime 2 gm (IV) q6h × 4–6 wks **or** Ceftizoxime 2 gm (IV) q8h × 4–6 wks	Quinolone† (PO) × 4–6 weeks
Chronic *Diabetes mellitus*	Group A, B streptococci S. aureus (MSSA) E. coli P. mirabilis K. pneumoniae B. fragilis S. aureus (MRSA)¶	Meropenem 500 mg (IV) q8h* **or** Piperacillin/tazobactam 3.375 gm (IV) q6h* **or** Ertapenem 1 gm (IV) q24h*¶ **or combination therapy with** Ceftriaxone 1 gm (IV) q24h* **plus** Metronidazole 1 gm (IV) q24h*	Moxifloxacin 400 mg (IV) q24h* **or** Ceftizoxime 2 gm (IV) q8h* **or** Ampicillin/sulbactam 3 gm (IV) q6h* **or combination therapy with** Clindamycin 600 mg (IV) q8h* **plus** Quinolone¥ (IV)*	Clindamycin 300 mg (PO) q8h* **plus** Quinolone¥ (IV)* **or monotherapy with** Moxifloxacin 400 mg (PO) q24h*
Chronic *Peripheral vascular disease (non-diabetics)*	S. aureus Group A, B streptococci Entero-bacteriaceae	Ceftriaxone 1 gm (IV) q24h × 2–4 weeks **or** Ceftizoxime 2 gm (IV) q8h × 2–4 weeks	Clindamycin 600 mg (IV) q8h × 2–4 weeks **plus** Quinolone§ (IV) q24h × 2–4 weeks	Clindamycin 300 mg (PO) q8h × 2–4 weeks **plus** Quinolone§ (PO) q24h × 2–4 weeks

Osteomyelitis (cont'd)

Subset	Usual Pathogens	Preferred IV Therapy	Alternate IV Therapy	PO Therapy or IV-to-PO Switch
Chronic *Peripheral vascular disease (non-diabetics)* (cont'd)	Above pathogens/ MRSA	Tigacycline 100 mg (IV) × 1 dose, then 50 mg (IV) q12h × 2–4 weeks **or** Linezolid 600 mg (IV) q12h × 2–4 weeks	Minocycline 100 mg (IV) q12h × 2–4 weeks **plus either** Levofloxacin 500 mg (IV) q24h **or** Ceftriaxone 1 gm (IV) q24h × 2–4 weeks	Minocycline 100 mg (PO) q12h × 2–4 weeks **plus** Levofloxacin 500 mg (PO) q24h × 2–4 weeks
	Above pathogens/ B. fragilis (foul discharge)	Tigacycline 100 mg (IV) × 1 dose, then 50 mg (IV) q12h × 2–4 weeks	Moxifloxacin 400 mg (IV) q24h × 2–4 weeks **or** Ertapenem 1 gm (IV) q24h × 2–4 weeks	Moxifloxacin 400 mg (PO) q24h × 2–4 weeks
TB osteomyelitis	M. tuberculosis	Treat the same as pulmonary TB (p. 52), but extend treatment to 6–9 months		

MSSA/MRSA = methicillin-sensitive/resistant S. aureus. Duration of therapy represents total time IV, PO, or IV + PO. Most patients on IV therapy able to take PO meds should be switched to PO therapy soon after clinical improvement.

* Treat for 1 week after adequate debridement or amputation.
‡ Moxifloxacin 400 mg or Levofloxacin 500 mg.
† Ciprofloxacin 400 mg (IV) or 500 mg (PO) q12h or Levofloxacin 750 mg (IV or PO) q24h or Moxifloxacin 400 mg (IV or PO) q24h.
¥ Ciprofloxacin 400 mg (IV) or 500 mg (PO) q12h or Levofloxacin 750 mg (IV or PO) q24h.
¶ If pathogen unkown or MRSA likely (use tigacycline or Minocycline plus Levofloxacin, above) and treat for 4–6 weeks after adequate debridement or 1 week after amputation.
§ Moxifloxacin 400 mg or Levofloxacin 750 mg.

Acute Osteomyelitis

Clinical Presentation: Tenderness over infected bone. Fever and positive blood cultures common.
Diagnostic Considerations: Diagnosis by elevated ESR with positive bone scan. Bone biopsy is not needed for diagnosis. Bone scan is positive for acute osteomyelitis in first 24 hours.
Pitfalls: Earliest sign on plain films is soft tissue swelling; bony changes evident after 2 weeks.
Therapeutic Considerations: Treat 4–6 weeks with antibiotics. Debridement is not necessary for cure.
Prognosis: Related to adequacy/promptness of treatment.

Chronic Osteomyelitis

Diabetes Mellitus

Clinical Presentation: Afebrile or low-grade fever with normal WBC counts and deep penetrating ulcers ± draining sinus tracts.
Diagnostic Considerations: Diagnosis by elevated ESR and bone changes on plain films. Bone scan is not needed for diagnosis. Bone biopsy is preferred method of demonstrating organisms, since blood cultures are usually negative and cultures from ulcers/sinus tracts are unreliable.

Pitfalls: P. aeruginosa is a common colonizer and frequently cultured from deep ulcers/sinus tracts, but is not a pathogen in chronic osteomyelitis in diabetics.
Therapeutic Considerations: Surgical debridement is needed for cure; antibiotics alone are ineffective. Revascularization procedures usually do not help, since diabetes is a microvascular disease. Do not culture penetrating foot ulcers/draining sinus tracts; culture results reflect superficial flora. Bone biopsy during debridement is the best way to identify pathogen; if biopsy not possible, treat empirically.
Prognosis: Related to adequacy of blood supply/surgical debridement.

Non-Diabetics with Peripheral Vascular Disease (PVD)

Clinical Presentation: Absent or low-grade fever with normal WBC counts ± wet/dry digital gangrene.
Diagnostic Considerations: Diagnosis by clinical appearance of dusky/cold foot ± wet/dry gangrene. Chronic osteomyelitis secondary to PVD/open fracture is often polymicrobial.
Pitfalls: Wet gangrene usually requires surgical debridement/antibiotic therapy; dry gangrene may not.
Therapeutic Considerations: Surgical debridement needed for cure. Antibiotics alone are ineffective. Revascularization procedure may help treat infection by improving local blood supply.
Prognosis: Related to degree of vascular compromise.

TB Osteomyelitis (Mycobacterium tuberculosis)

Clinical Presentation: Presents similar to chronic bacterial osteomyelitis. Vertebral TB (Pott's disease) affects disk spaces early and presents with chronic back/neck pain ± inguinal/paraspinal mass.
Diagnostic Considerations: Diagnosis by AFB on biopsy/culture of infected bone. PPD–positive.
Pitfalls: Chest x-ray is normal in 50%. May be confused with cancer or chronic bacterial osteomyelitis.
Therapeutic Considerations: Treated the same as TB arthritis.
Prognosis: Good for non-vertebral TB/vertebral (if treated before paraparesis/paraplegia).

Empiric Therapy of Skin and Soft Tissue Infections

Cellulitis, Erysipelas, Impetigo, Lymphangitis (cSSSIs)

Subset	Usual Pathogens	Preferred IV Therapy	PO Therapy or IV-to-PO Switch
Above-the-waist (Treat initially for MSSA; if later identified as MRSA, treat accordingly)	S. aureus (MRSA)	Tigecycline 100 mg (IV) × 1 dose, then 50 mg (IV) q12h × 2 weeks **or** Linezolid 600 mg (IV) q12h × 2 weeks **or** Vancomycin 1 gm (IV) q12h × 2 weeks **or** Quinupristin/dalfopristin 7.5 mg/kg (IV) q12h × 2 weeks **or** Daptomycin 4 mg/kg (IV) q24h × 2 weeks **or** Minocycline 100 mg (IV) q12h × 2 weeks	Linezolid 600 mg (PO) q12h × 2 weeks **or** Minocycline 100 mg (PO) q12h × 2 weeks

Cellulitis, Erysipelas, Impetigo, Lymphangitis (cSSSIs) (cont'd)

Subset	Usual Pathogens	Preferred IV Therapy		PO Therapy or IV-to-PO Switch
Above-the-waist (cont'd)	Group A streptococci S. aureus (MSSA)	Ceftriaxone 1–2 gm (IV) q24h × 2 weeks **or** Cefazolin 1 gm (IV) q8h × 2 weeks	Nafcillin 2 gm (IV) q4h × 2 weeks **or** Clindamycin 600 mg (IV) q8h × 2 weeks	Cephalexin 500 mg (PO) q6h × 2 weeks **or** Clindamycin 300 mg (PO) q6h × 2 weeks
Below-the-waist	S. aureus (MRSA)	Treat the same as for above-the-waist cellulitis (MRSA); see above		
(Treat initially for MSSA; if later identified as MRSA, treat accordingly)	Group A, B streptococci P. mirabilis K. pneumoniae E. coli S. aureus (MSSA)	Quinolone* (IV) q24h × 2 weeks **or** Ceftriaxone 1–2 gm (IV) q24h × 2 weeks **or** Cefazolin 1 gm (IV) q8h × 2 weeks	Piperacillin/tazobactam 3.375 gm (IV) q6h × 2 weeks **or** Ampicillin/sulbactam 3 gm (IV) q6h × 2 weeks **or** Ticarcillin/clavulanate 3.1 gm (IV) q6h × 2 weeks	Cephalexin 500 mg (PO) q6h × 2 weeks **or combination therapy with** Clindamycin 300 mg (PO) q6h × 2 weeks **plus** Quinolone* (PO) q24h × 2 weeks

MRSA/MSSA = methicillin-resistant/sensitive S. aureus. Duration of therapy represents total time IV, PO, or IV + PO. Most patients on IV therapy able to take PO meds should be switched to PO therapy soon after clinical improvement.

* Moxifloxacin 400 mg or Levofloxacin 750 mg.

Clinical Presentation: Cellulitis presents as warm, painful, non-pruritic skin erythema without discharge. Impetigo is characterized by vesiculopustular lesions, most commonly on the face/extremities. Erysipelas resembles cellulitis but is raised and sharply demarcated. Mastitis presents as cellulitis/abscess of the breast and is treated the same as cellulitis above the waist.

Diagnostic Considerations: Diagnosis by clinical appearance ± culture of pathogen from aspirated skin lesion(s). Group B streptococci are important pathogens in diabetics. Lower extremity cellulitis tends to recur. Chronic edema of an extremity predisposes to recurrent/persistent cellulitis.

Pitfalls: Streptococcal and staphylococcal cellulitis may be indistinguishable clinically, but regional adenopathy/lymphangitis favors Streptococci, and bullae favors S. aureus.

Therapeutic Considerations: Lower extremity cellulitis requires ~ 1 week of antibiotics to improve. Patients with peripheral vascular disease, chronic venous stasis, alcoholic cirrhosis, and diabetes take 1–2 weeks longer to improve and often require 3–4 weeks of treatment. Treat mastitis as cellulitis above-the-waist, and drain surgically if an abscess is present.

Prognosis: Related to degree of micro/macrovascular insufficiency.

Complicated Skin/Skin Structure Tissue Infections (cSSSIs)

Subset	Usual Pathogens	Preferred IV Therapy		IV-to-PO Switch
Mixed aerobic-anaerobic deep soft tissue infection	Entero-bacteriaceae Group A streptococci S. aureus (MSSA) Anaerobic streptococci Fusobacterium	Tigecycline† 100 mg (IV) × 1 dose, then 50 mg (IV) q12h × 2 weeks **or** Piperacillin/tazobactam 3.375 gm (IV) q6h × 2 weeks **or** Meropenem 500 mg (IV) q8h × 2 weeks	Moxifloxacin 400 mg (IV) q24h × 2 weeks **or** Doripenem 500 mg (IV) q8h **or** Ertapenem 1 gm (IV) q24h × 2 weeks **or** Imipenem 500 mg (IV) q6h × 2 weeks	Moxifloxacin 400 mg (PO) q24h × 2 weeks **or combination therapy with** Clindamycin 300 mg (PO) q8h × 2 weeks **plus** Quinolone* (PO) × 2 weeks
Clostridial myonecrosis (gas gangrene)	Clostridium sp.	Preferred IV Penicillin G 10 mu (IV) q4h × 2 weeks **or** Clindamycin 600 mg (IV) q8h × 2 weeks **or** Piperacillin 4 gm (IV) q8h × 2 weeks	Alternate IV Meropenem 1 gm (IV) q8h × 2 weeks **or** Ertapenem 1 gm (IV) q24h × 2 weeks	Not applicable
Necrotizing fasciitis/ synergistic gangrene/ Fournier's gangrene	Group A strep Entero-bacteriaceae Anaerobic streptococci S. aureus (MSSA)	Piperacillin/tazobactam 3.375 gm (IV) q6h × 2 weeks **or** Meropenem 1 gm (IV) q8h × 2 weeks	Clindamycin 600 mg (IV) q8h × 2 weeks **plus** Quinolone* (IV) × 2 weeks	Clindamycin 300 mg (PO) q8h × 2 weeks **plus** Quinolone* (PO) × 2 weeks
Severe cellulitis, fascitis, phegmons, abscesses	MSSA/MRSA	Daptomycin 6 mg/kg (IV) q24h × 2 weeks **or** Linezolid 600 mg (IV) q12h × 2 weeks **or** Telavancin 10 mg/kg (IV) q24h × 2 weeks		Linezolid 600 mg (PO) q12h × 2 weeks **or** Minocycline 100 mg (PO) q12h × 2 weeks

CA-MRSA = community-acquired methicillin-resistant S. aureus (see p. 15), MSSA = methicillin-sensitive S. aureus. Duration of therapy represents total time IV or IV + PO. Most patients on IV therapy able to take PO meds should be switched to PO therapy after clinical improvement.

* Ciprofloxacin 400 mg (IV) or 500 mg (PO) q12h or Levofloxacin 750 mg (IV or PO) q24h.

† Tigecycline may be used if MRSA or VRE is suspected in addition to usual pathogens.

Complicated Skin/Skin Structure Tissue Infections (cSSSIs) (cont'd)

Subset	Usual Pathogens	Preferred IV Therapy	IV-to-PO Switch
Pyomyositis/ necrotizing abscesses	Community-acquired MRSA (CA-MRSA)§	Daptomycin 6 mg/kg (IV) q24h × 2 weeks **or** Linezolid 600 mg (IV) q12h × 2 weeks	Linezolid 600 mg (PO) q12h × 2 weeks **or** Minocycline 100 mg (PO) q12h × 2 weeks

CA-MRSA = community-acquired methicillin-resistant S. aureus (see p. 15), MSSA = methicillin-sensitive S. aureus.

§ CA-MRSA PVL-positive strains (see p. 15).

Mixed Aerobic/Anaerobic Deep Soft Tissue Infection

Clinical Presentation: Local pain/tenderness ± gross gas deep in soft tissues and usually high fevers. More common in diabetics.

Diagnostic Considerations: Diagnosed clinically. Bacteriologic diagnosis by gram stain/culture of aspirated fluid. Patients usually have high fevers. Wound discharge is foul when present.

Pitfalls: Gross crepitance/prominent gas in soft tissues on x-ray suggests a mixed aerobic/anaerobic necrotizing infection, not gas gangrene.

Therapeutic Considerations: Prompt empiric therapy and surgical debridement may be lifesaving.

Prognosis: Related to severity of infection, adequacy of debridement, and underlying health of host.

Gas Gangrene (Clostridial Myonecrosis)

Clinical Presentation: Fulminant infection of muscle with little or n fever. Infected area is extremely painful, indurated, and discolored with or without bullae.

Diagnostic Considerations: Diagnosis is clinical. Aspiration of infected muscle shows few PMNs and gram-positive bacilli without spores (C. perfringens only). Gas gangrene is not accompanied by high fever. Patients are often apprehensive with relative bradycardia ± diarrhea. Wound discharge, if present, is sweetish and not foul. Rapidly progressive hemolytic anemia is characteristic.

Pitfalls: Gas gangrene (clostridial myonecrosis) has little visible gas on plain film x-rays; abundant gas should suggest a mixed aerobic/anaerobic infection, not clostridial gas gangrene.

Therapeutic Considerations: Surgical debridement is life saving and the only way to control infection.

Prognosis: Related to speed/extent of surgical debridement. Progression/death may occur in hours.

Necrotizing Fasciitis/Synergistic Gangrene

Clinical Presentation: Acutely ill patient with high fevers and extreme local pain without gas in tissues. If scrotum involved (± abdominal wall involvement), the diagnosis is Fournier's gangrene.

Diagnostic Considerations: Diagnosis by CT/MRI of involved extremity showing infection confined to one or more muscle compartments/fascial planes. Patients are febrile and ill. Gas is not present on exam or x-rays. May be polymicrobial or due to a single organism. Foul smelling exudate from infected soft tissues indicates anaerobes are present.
Pitfalls: Extreme pain in patients with deep soft tissue infections should suggest a compartment syndrome/necrotizing fasciitis. No hemolytic anemia, diarrhea, or bullae as with gas gangrene.
Therapeutic Considerations: Control/cure of infection requires surgical decompression of infected compartment, debridement of dead tissue in necrotizing fasciitis, and antimicrobial therapy.
Prognosis: Related to rapidity/extent of surgical debridement.

Severe Cellulitis, Fascitis, Phegmons, Abscesses

Clinical Presentation: MSSA/MRSA cellulitis often accompanied by bullae. Fascitis presents with pain out of proportion to clinical findings in the distribution of fascial planes, a phegmon (pre-abscess before abscess wall forms) presents with pain ± overlying cellulitis. MSSA/MRSA abscesses are clinically indistinguishable from other abscesses, but remain the most common pathogens in cSSSI abscesses.
Diagnostic Considerations: Diagnosis of cellulitis and abscesses is clinical. Demonstration of fascitis, phegmons, of abscesses are by imaging studies by CT/MRI.
Pitfalls: Bullae with cellulitis should suggest MSSA/MRSA (not group A streptococci). Bullae in DM/ bullous diseases are not accompanied by fever/cellulitis.
Therapeutic Considerations: Cellulitis and phegmons may be treated with antibiotic therapy alone. Fasciitis and abscesses usually require debridement (fascitis) or drainage (abscesses).
Prognosis: Good if treated appropriately/early.

Pyomyositis/Necrotizing Abscesses (Community-Acquired MRSA)

Clinical Presentation: Abrupt onset of severe/deep muscle infection ± large abscesses should suggest community-acquired MRSA (CA-MRSA).
Diagnostic Considerations: The diagnosis of CA-MRSA is made on the basis of the distinctively fulminant/severe clinical presentation and by culturing MRSA from muscle/abscess. If available, test isolate for SCC *mec* IV ± Panton-Valentine leukocidin (PVL) gene.
Pitfalls: CA-MRSA susceptible to clindamycin, TMP–SMX, and doxycycline.
Therapeutic Considerations: Prompt/complete incision and drainage of abscesses and early use of anti-CA-MRSA drugs may be life-saving. Antibiotics effective against CA-MRSA (TMP–SMX, clindamycin, doxycycline) are ineffective against CO-MRSA/HA-MRSA; antibiotics effective against CO-MRSA/ HA-MRSA are also effective against CA-MRSA (see p. 15). Use minocycline instead of doxycline which is rapidly effective. Doxycycline resistances with CA-MRSA of concern Minocycline more effective than TMP-SMX or clindamycin for CA-MRSA.
Prognosis: Related to presence of CA-MRSA with PVL gene. CA-MRSA PVL negative infections are similar in severity to MSSA infections.

Skin Ulcers

Subset	Usual Pathogens	Preferred IV Therapy	Alternate IV Therapy	PO Therapy or IV-to-PO Switch
Decubitus ulcers *Above the waist*	Group A streptococci E. coli, P. mirabilis K. pneumoniae S. aureus (MSSA) S. aureus (MRSA)†	Cefazolin 1 gm (IV) q8h* **or** Ceftriaxone 1 gm (IV) q24h*	Cefotaxime 2 gm (IV) q6h* **or** Ceftizoxime 2 gm (IV) q8h*	Cephalexin 500 mg (PO) q6h*
Below the waist	Group A streptococci E. coli P. mirabilis K. pneumoniae B. fragilis S. aureus (MSSA) S. aureus (MRSA)‡	Meropenem 500 mg (IV) q8h* **or** Tigecycline 100 mg (IV) × 1 dose, then 50 mg (IV) q12h* **or** Piperacillin/ tazobactam 3.375 gm (IV) q6h* **or** Ertapenem 1 gm (IV) q24h*	Moxifloxacin 400 mg (IV) q24h* **or combination therapy with** Clindamycin 600 mg (IV) q6h* **plus either** Ciprofloxacin 400 mg (IV) q12h* **or** Levofloxacin 500 mg (IV) q24h*	Moxifloxacin 400 mg (PO) q24h* **or combination therapy with** Clindamycin 300 mg (PO) q8h* **plus either** Ciprofloxacin 500 mg (PO) q12h* **or** Levofloxacin 500 mg (PO) q24h*

Duration of therapy represents total time IV, PO, or IV + PO. Most patients on IV therapy able to take PO meds should be switched to PO therapy soon after clinical improvement.

* Treat Stages I/II (superficial) decubitus ulcers with local care. If no underlying chronic osteomyelitis, treat Stages III/IV (deep) decubitus ulcers with antibiotics for 1–2 weeks after adequate debridement.

† MRSA (above-the-waist): Preferred IV therapy: also add either Daptomycin 4 mg/kg (IV) q24h* or Linezolid 600 mg (IV) q12h*. Alternate IV therapy: also add either Vancomycin 1 gm (IV) q12h* or Minocycline 100 mg (IV) q12h*. PO therapy or IV-to-PO switch: Quinolone (PO) q24h* plus either Linezolid 600 mg (PO) q12h* or Minocycline 100 mg (PO) q12h*.

‡ MRSA (below-the-waist): Preferred IV therapy: Tigecycline 100 mg (IV) × 1 dose then 50 mg (IV) q12h*, or combination therapy with either [Meropenem 1 gm (IV) q8h* or Piperacillin/Tazobactam 3.375 gm (IV) q6h* or Ertapenem 1 gm (IV) q24h] plus either [Daptomycin 4 mg/kg (IV) q24h* or Linezolid 600 mg (IV) q12h*]. Alternate IV therapy: Moxifloxacin 400 mg (IV) q24h* plus either Vancomycin 1 gm (IV) q12h* or Minocycline 100 mg (IV) q12h*. PO therapy or IV-to-PO switch: Moxifloxacin 400 mg (PO) q24h* plus either Linezolid 600 mg (PO) q12h* or Minocycline 100 mg (PO) q12h*.

Skin Ulcers (cont'd)

Subset	Usual Pathogens	Preferred IV Therapy	Alternate IV Therapy	PO Therapy or IV-to-PO Switch
Diabetic foot ulcers (deep/ complicated) (Treat initially for MSSA; if later identified as Group A streptococci, MRSA, etc., treat accordingly)	S. aureus (MRSA)	Daptomycin 4 mg/kg (IV) q24h† **or** Linezolid 600 mg (IV) q12h† **or** Telavancin 10 mg/kg (IV) q24h† **or** Tigacycline 100 mg (IV) × 1 dose, then 50 mg (IV) q12h†	Vancomycin 1 gm (IV) q12h†	Linezolid 600 mg (PO) q12h† **or** Minocycline 100 mg (PO) q12h†
	Group A, B streptococci S. aureus (MSSA) E. coli P. mirabilis K. pneumoniae B. fragilis	Meropenem 500 mg (IV) q8h† **or** Moxifloxacin 400 mg (IV) q24h† **or** Ertapenem 1 gm (IV) q24h† **or** Piperacillin/ tazobactam 3.375 gm (IV) q6h† **or** Doripenem 500 mg (IV) q8h	Cefoperazone 2 gm (IV) q12h **or** Ceftizoxime 2 gm (IV) q8h† **or** Ampicillin/ sulbactam 3 gm (IV) q6h† **or combination therapy with** [Ceftriaxone 1 gm (IV) q24h† *plus* Metronidazole 1 gm (IV) q24h†] **or** [Clindamycin 600 mg (IV) q8h† *plus either* Ciprofloxacin 400 mg (IV) q12h† *or* Levofloxacin 750 mg (IV) q24h†]	Moxifloxacin 400 mg (PO) q24h† **or combination therapy with** Minocycline 100 mg (PO) q12h† **or** Clindamycin 300 mg (PO) q8h† **plus either** Ciprofloxacin 500 mg (PO) q12h† **or** Levofloxacin 500 mg (PO) q24h†
	Any pathogen(s) above ***plus*** S. aureus (MRSA)	IV Therapy: **Combination therapy with** a MRSA drug *plus* a non-MRSA drug (see above) PO Therapy or IV-to-PO Switch: MRSA drug (PO) *plus* a non-MRSA drug (PO) (see above)		

† Treat until adequate debridement/amputation and then for 1 week after adequate debridement or amputation.

Skin Ulcers (cont'd)

Subset	Usual Pathogens	Preferred IV Therapy	Alternate IV Therapy	PO Therapy or IV-to-PO Switch
Ischemic foot ulcers	S. aureus (MRSA)	Treat the same as for deep/complicated diabetic foot ulcers, above		
(Treat initially for MSSA; if later identified as Gp. A strep, MRSA, etc., treat accordingly)	Group A streptococci E. coli S. aureus (MSSA)	Cefazolin 1 gm (IV) q8h × 2 weeks **or** Ceftriaxone 1 gm (IV) q24h × 2 weeks	Clindamycin 600 mg (IV) q8h × 2 weeks ***plus*** Quinolone* (IV) q24h × 2 weeks	Quinolone* (PO) q24h × 2 weeks
	Any pathogen(s) above ***plus*** S. aureus (MRSA)	IV Therapy: **Combination therapy with** a MRSA drug ***plus*** a non-MRSA drug (see diabetic foot ulcers) PO Therapy or IV-to-PO Switch: MRSA drug ***plus*** a non-MRSA drug (see diabetic foot ulcers)		

MSSA = methicillin-sensitive S. aureus. Duration of therapy represents total time IV, PO, or IV + PO. Most patients on IV therapy able to take PO meds should be switched to PO therapy soon after clinical improvement.

* Levofloxacin 750 mg or Moxifloxacin 400 mg.

Decubitus Ulcers

Clinical Presentation: Painless ulcers with variable depth and infectious exudate $\pm$ fevers $\leq$ 102°F.

Diagnostic Considerations: Diagnosis by clinical appearance. Obtain ESR/bone scan to rule out underlying osteomyelitis with deep (Stage III/IV) decubitus ulcers.

Pitfalls: Superficial decubitus ulcers do not require systemic antibiotics.

Therapeutic Considerations: Deep decubitus ulcers require antibiotics and debridement, superficial ulcers do not. Coverage for B. fragilis is needed for deep perianal decubitus ulcers. Good nursing care is important in preventing/limiting extension of decubitus ulcers.

Prognosis: Related to fecal contamination of ulcer and bone involvement (e.g., osteomyelitis).

Diabetic Foot Ulcers/Chronic Osteomyelitis

Clinical Presentation: Ulcers/sinus tracts on bottom of foot/between toes; usually painless. Fevers $\leq$ 102°F and a foul smelling exudate are common.

Diagnostic Considerations: In diabetics, deep, penetrating, chronic foot ulcers/draining sinus tracts are diagnostic of chronic osteomyelitis. ESR $\geq$ 100 mm/hr in a diabetic with a foot ulcer/sinus tract is diagnostic of chronic osteomyelitis. Foot films confirm chronic osteomyelitis. Bone scan is needed only in acute osteomyelitis.

Pitfalls: Do not rely on culture results of deep ulcers/sinus tracts to choose antibiotic coverage, since cultures reflect skin colonization, not bone pathogens. Treat empirically.

Therapeutic Considerations: B. fragilis coverage is required in deep penetrating diabetic foot ulcers/fetid foot infection. P. aeruginosa is often cultured from diabetic foot ulcers/sinus tracts, but represents colonization, not infection. P. aeruginosa is a "water" organism that colonizes feet from moist socks/dressings, irrigant solutions, or whirlpool baths. Surgical debridement is essential for cure of chronic osteomyelitis in diabetics. Treat superficial diabetic foot ulcers the same as cellulitis in non-diabetics (p. 129).

Prognosis: Related to adequacy of debridement of infected bone.

Ischemic Foot Ulcers

Clinical Presentation: Ulcers often clean/dry ± digital gangrene. No fevers/exudate.

Diagnostic Considerations: Diagnosis by clinical appearance/location in a patient with peripheral vascular disease. Ischemic foot ulcers most commonly affect the toes, medial malleoli, dorsum of foot, or lower leg.

Pitfalls: In contrast to ulcers in diabetics, ischemic ulcers due to peripheral vascular disease usually do not involve the plantar surface of the foot.

Therapeutic Considerations: Dry gangrene should not be treated with antibiotics unless accompanied by signs of systemic infection. Wet gangrene should be treated as a mixed aerobic/anaerobic infection. Both dry/wet gangrene may require debridement for cure/control. Do not rely on ulcer cultures to guide treatment; treat empirically if necessary. Evaluate for revascularization.

Prognosis: Related to degree of vascular insufficiency.

Skin Abscesses/Infected Cysts (Skin Pustules, Skin Boils, Furunculosis) (uSSSIs/cSSSIs)

Subset	Usual Pathogens	Preferred IV Therapy	Alternate IV Therapy	PO Therapy or IV-to-PO Switch
cSSSIs Severe skin abscesses (Treat initially for MSSA; if later identified as MRSA, treat accordingly)	S. aureus (MRSA)	Tigecycline 100 mg (IV) × 1 dose, then 50 mg (IV) q12h × 2 weeks **or** Linezolid 600 mg (IV) q12h × 2 weeks **or** Daptomycin 4 mg/kg (IV) q24h × 2 weeks **or** Telavancin 10 mg/kg (IV) q24h × 2 weeks **or** Minocycline 100 mg (IV) q12h × 2 weeks **or** Vancomycin 1 mg (IV) q12h × 2 weeks		Linezolid 600 mg (PO) q12h × 2 weeks **or** Minocycline 100 mg (PO) q12h × 2 weeks
	S. aureus (MSSA)	Vancomycin 1 gm (IV) q12h × 2 weeks **or** Clindamycin 600 mg (IV) q8h × 2 wks **or** Ceftriaxone 1 gm (IV) q24h × 2 weeks	Cefazolin 1 gm (IV) q8h × 2 weeks **or** Nafcillin 2 gm (IV) q4h × 2 weeks	Cephalexin 500 mg (PO) q6h × 2 weeks **or** Clindamycin 300 mg (PO) q8h × 2 weeks

MRSA/MSSA = methicillin-resistant/sensitive S. aureus. Duration of therapy represents total time IV, PO, or IV + PO. Most patients on IV therapy able to take PO meds should be switched to PO therapy soon after clinical improvement

Skin Abscesses/Infected Cysts (Skin Pustules, Skin Boils, Furunculosis) (uSSSIs/cSSSIs) (cont'd)

Subset	Usual Pathogens	Preferred IV Therapy	Alternate IV Therapy	PO Therapy or IV-to-PO Switch
uSSSIs *Infected pilonidal cysts*	Group A streptococci E. coli P. mirabilis K. pneumoniae S. aureus (MSSA)	Ceftriaxone 1 gm (IV) q24h × 2 weeks **or** Ceftizoxime 2 gm (IV) q8h × 2 weeks **or** Cefoxitin 2 gm (IV) q6h × 2 weeks	Levofloxacin 500 mg (IV) q24h × 2 weeks **or** Moxifloxacin 400 mg (IV) q24h × 2 weeks	Levofloxacin 500 mg (PO) q24h × 2 weeks **or** Moxifloxacin 400 mg (PO) q24h × 2 weeks
Hydradenitis suppurativa	S. aureus (MSSA)	Not applicable	TMP–SMX 1 SS tablet (PO) q12h × 2–4 weeks **or** Clindamycin 300 mg (PO) q8h × 2–4 weeks **or** Minocycline 100 mg (PO) q12h × 2–4 weeks	
	S. aureus (MRSA)	Not applicable	Minocycline 100 mg (PO) q12h × 2–4 weeks	

MRSA/MSSA = methicillin-resistant/sensitive S. aureus. Duration of therapy represents total time IV, PO, or IV + PO. Most patients on IV therapy able to take PO meds should be switched to PO therapy soon after clinical improvement.
uSSSIs = uncomplicated SSSIs.
cSSSIs = complicated SSSIs.

Skin Abscesses

Clinical Presentation: Warm painful nodules ± bullae, low-grade fever ± systemic symptoms, no lymphangitis. Skin boils/furunculosis present as acute, chronic, or recurrent skin pustules, and remain localized without lymphangitis.

Diagnostic Considerations: Specific pathogen diagnosed by gram stain of abscess. Recurring S. aureus abscesses are not uncommon and should be drained. Blood cultures are rarely positive. Suspect Job's syndrome if recurring abscesses with peripheral eosinophilia. Skin boils/furunculosis are diagnosed by clinical appearance (skin pustules).

Pitfalls: Recurring S. aureus skin infections may occur on immune basis but immunologic studies are usually negative.

Therapeutic Considerations: Repeated aspiration of abscesses may be necessary. Surgical drainage is required if antibiotics fail. Treat boils/furunculosis as in hydradenitis suppurativa.

Prognosis: Excellent if treated early.

Infected Pilonidal Cysts

Clinical Presentation: Chronic drainage from pilonidal cysts.
Diagnostic Considerations: Diagnosis by clinical appearance. Deep/systemic infection is rare.
Pitfalls: Culture of exudate is usually unhelpful.
Therapeutic Considerations: Surgical debridement is often necessary.
Prognosis: Good with adequate excision.

Hydradenitis Suppurativa

Clinical Presentation: Chronic, indurated, painful, raised axillary/groin lesions ± drainage/sinus tracts.
Diagnostic Considerations: Diagnosis by clinical appearance/location of lesions. Infections are often bilateral and tend to recur.
Pitfalls: Surgical debridement is usually not necessary unless deep/extensive infection.
Therapeutic Considerations: Most anti-S. aureus antibiotics have poor penetration and usually fail.
Prognosis: Good with recommended antibiotics. Surgery, if necessary, is curative.

Skin Vesicles (Non-Genital)

Subset	Pathogen	Therapy
Herpes simplex	Herpes simplex virus (HSV)	Acyclovir 400 mg (PO) q8h × 10 days **or** Valacyclovir 1 gm (PO) q12h × 7–10 days **or** Famciclovir 250 mg (PO) q8h × 10 days
Chickenpox	Varicella zoster virus (VZV)	Acyclovir 800 mg (PO) q6h × 5 days **or** Famciclovir 500 mg (PO) q8h × 5 days **or** Valacyclovir 1 gm (PO) q8h × 5 days
Herpes zoster *Dermatomal (shingles)*	Varicella zoster virus (VZV)	Acyclovir 800 mg (PO) 5x/day × 7–10 days **or** Famciclovir 500 mg (PO) q8h × 7–10 days **or** Valacyclovir 1 gm (PO) q8h × 7–10 days
Disseminated		IV therapy: Acyclovir 10 mg/kg (IV) q8h × 7–10 days PO therapy: Famciclovir 500 mg (PO) q8h × 7–10 days or Valacyclovir 1 gm (PO) q8h × 7–10 days
Herpes whitlow	HSV-1	Acyclovir 400 mg (PO) q8h × 7–10 days **or** Valacyclovir 1 gm (PO) q12h × 7–10 days **or** Famciclovir 250 mg (PO) q8h × 7–10 days

Herpes Simplex (HSV)

Clinical Presentation: Painful, sometimes pruritic vesicles that form pustules or painful erythematous ulcers. Associated with fever, myalgias.
Diagnostic Considerations: Diagnosis by clinical appearance and demonstration of HSV by culture of vesicle fluid/vesicle base. May be severe in HIV/AIDS.

Pitfalls: Painful vesicular lesions surrounded by prominent induration distinguishes HSV from insect bites (pruritic) and cellulitis (no induration).
Therapeutic Considerations: Topical acyclovir ointment may be useful early when vesicles erupt, but is ineffective after vesicles stop erupting. For severe/refractory cases, use acyclovir 5 mg/kg (IV) q8h × 2–7 days, then if improvement, switch to acyclovir 400 mg (PO) q8h to complete 10-day course.
Prognosis: Related to extent of tissue involvement/degree of cellular immunity dysfunction.

Chickenpox (VZV)

Clinical Presentation: Abrupt appearance of discrete/diffuse pruritic vesicles. Appear in successive crops over 3 days, then no more new lesions. Patients do not appear toxic.
Diagnostic Considerations: Chickenpox lesions are central and typically concentrated on the trunk, although vesicles may also occur in the mouth, GI or GU tract. Vesicles are seen at different stages of development, and are superficial with the classic "dew drop on a rose petal" appearance. Tzanck test is positive in chickenpox (negative in smallpox).
Pitfalls: Vesicles are not deep/umbilicated like smallpox. Smallpox patients are sick/toxic, and vesicles are at the same stage of development in each anatomical area. Vesicles begin and are concentrated on the face with smallpox.
Therapeutic Considerations: Begin therapy as early as possible before appearance of successive crops of vesicles appear. Treat VZV pneumonia early with acyclovir.
Prognosis: Children do better than adults. Worst prognosis in smokers/pregnancy (may develop chickenpox/VZV pneumonia).

Herpes Zoster (VZV)

Clinical Presentation: Painful, vesicular eruption in dermatomal distribution. Pain may be difficult to diagnose.
Diagnostic Considerations: Diagnosis by appearance/positive Tzanck test of vesicle base scrapings.
Pitfalls: Begin therapy within 2 days of vesicle eruption.
Therapeutic Considerations: Higher doses of acyclovir are required for VZV than HSV. See p. 337 for disseminated VZV, ophthalmic nerve/visceral involvement, or acyclovir-resistant strains.
Prognosis: Good if treated early. Some develop painful post-herpetic neuralgia of involved dermatomes.

Herpes Whitlow

Clinical Presentation: Multiple vesicopustular lesions on fingers and hands. Lymphangitis, adenopathy, fever/chills are usually present, suggesting a bacterial infection.
Diagnostic Considerations: Common in healthcare workers giving patients oral care/suctioning.
Pitfalls: No need for antibiotics even though lesions appear infected with "pus."
Therapeutic Considerations: Never incise/drain herpes whitlow; surgical incision will flare/prolong the infection.
Prognosis: Excellent, unless incision/drainage has been performed.

Wound Infections (for rabies, see pp. 354, 364)

Subset	Usual Pathogens	Preferred IV Therapy	Alternate IV Therapy	PO Therapy or IV-to-PO Switch
Animal bite wounds	Group A strep P. multocida Capnocytophaga canimorsus (DF2) S. aureus (MSSA)	Piperacillin/ tazobactam 3.375 gm (IV) q6h × 2 weeks **or** Tigecycline 100 mg (IV) × 1 dose, then 50 mg (IV) q12h × 2 weeks **or** Ampicillin/ sulbactam 3 gm (IV) q6h × 2 weeks	Meropenem 500 mg (IV) q8h × 2 weeks **or** Imipenem 500 mg (IV) q6h × 2 weeks **or** Ertapenem 1 gm (IV) q24h × 2 weeks	Amoxicillin/ clavulanic acid 500/125 mg (PO) q8h or 875/125 mg (PO) q12h × 2 weeks **or** Doxycycline 200 mg (PO) q12h × 3 days, then 100 mg (PO) q12h × 11 days
Human bite wounds	Oral anaerobes Group A strep E. corrodens S. aureus (MSSA)	Same as for animal bite wounds, above	Same as for animal bite wounds, above	Same as for animal bite wounds, above
Cat scratch disease (CSD)	Bartonella henselae (invasive disease)	Doxycycline 200 mg (IV) q12h × 3 days, then 100 mg (IV) q12h × 4–8 weeks **or** Azithromycin 500 mg (IV) q24h × 4–8 weeks	Chloramphenicol 500 mg (IV) q6h × 4–8 weeks **or** Erythromycin 500 mg (IV) q6h × 4–8 weeks	Doxycycline 200 mg (PO) q12h × 3 days, then 100 mg (PO) q12h × 4–8 weeks* **or** Azithromycin 250 mg (PO) q24h × 4–8 weeks **or** Quinolone‡ (PO) × 4–8 weeks
	B. henselae (lymphaden-opathy only)	<u>PO therapy:</u> Azithromycin 500 mg (PO) × 1 dose, then 250 mg (PO) × 4 days		

MSSA = methicillin-sensitive S. aureus. Duration of therapy represents total time IV, PO, or IV + PO.

* Loading dose is not needed PO if given IV with the same drug.

‡ Ciprofloxacin 400 mg (IV) or 500 mg (PO) q12h or Levofloxacin 500 mg (IV or PO) q24h or Moxifloxacin 400 mg (IV or PO) q24h.

Wound Infections (cont'd) (for rabies, see pp. 354, 364)

Subset	Usual Pathogens	Preferred IV Therapy	Alternate IV Therapy	PO Therapy or IV-to-PO Switch
Burn wounds (severe)†	Group A streptococci S. aureus (MSSA) Enterobacter P. aeruginosa	Doripenem 1g (IV) q8h × 2 weeks **or** Meropenem 1 gm (IV) q8h × 2 weeks	Cefepime 2 gm (IV) q8h × 2 weeks **or** Cefoperazone 2 gm (IV) q12h × 2 weeks	Not applicable
Freshwater-exposed wounds	Aeromonas hydrophilia	Quinolone‡ (IV) × 2 weeks **or** TMP–SMX 2.5 mg/kg (IV) q6h × 2 weeks	Ceftriaxone 1 gm (IV) q24h × 2 weeks **or** Aztreonam 2 gm (IV) q8h × 2 weeks **or** Gentamicin 240 mg (IV) q24h × 2 weeks	Quinolone‡ (PO) × 2 weeks **or** TMP–SMX 1 SS tablet (PO) q12h × 2 weeks
Saltwater-exposed wounds	Vibrio vulnificus Vibrio sp.	Doxycycline 200 mg (IV) q12h × 3 days, then 100 mg (IV) q12h × 11 days **or** Quinolone‡ (IV) × 2 weeks	Ceftriaxone 2 gm (IV) q12h × 2 weeks **or** Chloramphenicol 500 mg (IV) q6h × 2 weeks	Doxycycline 200 mg (PO) q12h × 3 days, then 100 mg (PO) q12h × 11 days* **or** Quinolone‡ (PO) × 2 weeks

MSSA = methicillin-sensitive S. aureus. Duration of therapy represents total time IV, PO, or IV + PO. Most patients on IV therapy able to take PO meds should be switched to PO therapy soon after clinical improvement.

† Treat only IV or IV-to-PO switch.

* Loading dose is not needed PO if given IV with the same drug.

‡ Ciprofloxacin 400 mg (IV) or 500 mg (PO) q12h or Levofloxacin 500 mg (IV or PO) q24h or Moxifloxacin 400 mg (IV or PO) q24h.

Animal Bite Wounds (for rabies, see p. 354)

Clinical Presentation: Cellulitis surrounding bite wound.

Diagnostic Considerations: Diagnosis by culture of bite wound exudate. Deep bites may also cause tendinitis/osteomyelitis, and severe bites may result in systemic infection with bacteremia.

Pitfalls: Avoid erythromycin in penicillin-allergic patients (ineffective against P. multocida).

Therapeutic Considerations: For facial/hand bites, consult a plastic surgeon.

Prognosis: Related to adequacy of debridement and early antibiotic therapy.

Human Bite Wounds

Clinical Presentation: Cellulitis surrounding bite wound.

Diagnostic Considerations: Diagnosis by culture of bite wound exudate. Infection often extends to involve tendon/bone.

Pitfalls: Compared to animal bites, human bites are more likely to contain anaerobes, S. aureus, and Group A streptococci.

Therapeutic Considerations: Avoid primary closure of human bite wounds.

Prognosis: Related to adequacy of debridement and early antibiotic therapy.

Cat Scratch Disease (Bartonella henselae)

Clinical Presentation: Subacute presentation of obscure febrile illness associated with cat bite/contact. Usually accompanied by adenopathy.

Diagnostic Considerations: Diagnosis by wound culture/serology for Bartonella. Cat scratch fever/disease may follow a cat scratch, but a lick from a kitten contaminating an inapparent micro-laceration is more common. May present as an FUO. Culture of exudate/node is unlikely to be positive, but silver stain of biopsy material shows organisms.

Pitfalls: Rule out lymphoma, which may present in similar fashion.

Therapeutic Considerations: For invasive disease, treat until symptoms/signs resolve. For lymphadenopathy, oral azithromycin decreases the size of nodes but may not reduce fever/systemic symptoms. Bartonella are sensitive in vitro to cephalosporins and TMP–SMX, but these antibiotics are ineffective in vivo.

Prognosis: Related to health of host.

Burn Wounds

Clinical Presentation: Severe (3rd/4th degree) burns ± drainage.

Diagnostic Considerations: Semi-quantitative bacterial counts help differentiate colonization (low counts) from infection (high counts). Burn wounds quickly become colonized.

Pitfalls: Treat only infected 3rd/4th degree burn wounds with systemic antibiotics.

Therapeutic Considerations: Meticulous local care/eschar removal/surgical debridement is key in preventing and controlling infection.

Prognosis: Related to severity of burns and adequacy of eschar debridement.

Freshwater-Exposed Wounds (Aeromonas hydrophilia)

Clinical Presentation: Fulminant wound infection with fever and diarrhea.

Diagnostic Considerations: Diagnosis by stool/wound/blood culture.

Pitfalls: Suspect A. hydrophilia in wound infection with fresh water exposure followed by diarrhea.

Therapeutic Considerations: Surgical debridement of devitalized tissue may be necessary.

Prognosis: Related to severity of infection and health of host.

Saltwater-Exposed Wounds (Vibrio vulnificus/Vibrio sp.)

Clinical Presentation: Fulminant wound infection with fever, painful hemorrhagic bullae, diarrhea.

Diagnostic Considerations: Diagnosis by stool/wound/blood culture. Vibrio vulnificus is a fulminant, life-threatening infection that may be accompanied by hypotension.

Pitfalls: Suspect V. vulnificus in acutely ill patients with fever, diarrhea, and bullous lesions after salt-water exposure.

Therapeutic Considerations: Surgical debridement of devitalized tissue may be necessary.
Prognosis: Related to extent of infection and health of host.

Superficial Fungal Infections of Skin and Nails

Subset	Usual Pathogens	Topical Therapy	PO Therapy
Mucocutaneous (local/non-disseminated) candidiasis	C. albicans	Clotrimazole 1% cream twice daily × 2 weeks	Fluconazole 400 mg (PO) × 1 dose, then 200 mg (PO) q24h × 2 weeks
Tinea corporis (body ringworm)	Trichophyton rubrum Epidermophyton floccosum Microsporum canis Trichophyton mentagrophytes	Clotrimazole 1% cream twice daily × 4–8 weeks **or** Miconazole 2% cream twice daily × 2 weeks **or** Econazole 1% cream twice daily × 2 weeks	Terbinafine 250 mg (PO) q24h × 4 weeks **or** Ketoconazole 200 mg (PO) q24h × 4 weeks **or** Fluconazole 200 mg (PO) weekly × 4 weeks
Tinea capitis (scalp ringworm)	Same as Tinea corporis, above	Selenium sulfide shampoo daily × 2–4 weeks	Same as Tinea corporis, above
Tinea cruris (jock itch)	T. cruris	Same as Tinea corporis, above	Same as Tinea corporis, above
Tinea pedis (athlete's foot)	Same as Tinea corporis, above	Same as Tinea corporis, above	Terbinafine 250 mg (PO) q24h × 2 weeks **or** Ketoconazole 200 mg (PO) q24h × 4 weeks **or** Itraconazole 200 mg (PO)* q24h × 4 weeks

* Itraconazole solution provides more reliable absorption than itraconazole capsules.

Superficial Fungal Infections of Skin and Nails (cont'd)

Subset	Usual Pathogens	Topical Therapy	PO Therapy
Tinea versicolor (pityriasis)	Malasezzia furfur (Pityrosporum orbiculare)	Clotrimazole cream (1%) or miconazole cream (2%) or ketoconazole cream (2%) daily × 7 days	Ketoconazole 200 mg (PO) q24h × 7 days **or** Itraconazole 200 mg (PO)* q24h × 7 days **or** Fluconazole 400 mg (PO) × 1 dose
Onychomycosis (nail infection)	Epidermophyton floccosum Trichophyton mentagrophytes Trichophyton rubrum C. albicans	Not applicable	Terbinafine 250 mg (PO) q24h × 6 weeks (fingernail infection) or 12 weeks (toenail infection) **or** Itraconazole 200 mg (PO)* q24h 1 week per month × 2 months (fingernail infection) or 3 months (toenail infection) **or** Fluconazole 200 mg (PO) q24h 1 week per month × 3 months (fingernail infection) or 6 months (toenail infection)

* Itraconazole solution provides more reliable absorption than itraconazole capsules.

Mucocutaneous (Local/Non-disseminated) Candidiasis

Clinical Presentation: Primary cutaneous findings include an erythematous rash with satellite lesions, which may be papular, pustular, or ulcerated. Lesions can be limited or widespread over parts of body. Chronic mucocutaneous candidiasis manifests as recurrent candidal infections of skin, nails, or mucous membranes.

Diagnostic Considerations: Diagnosis by demonstrating organism by stain/culture in tissue specimen. In HIV/AIDS, Candida is very common on skin/mucous membranes.

Pitfalls: Do not confuse with the isolated, multinodular lesions of disseminated disease, which may resemble ecthyma gangrenosa or purpura fulminans.

Therapeutic Considerations: Diabetics and other compromised hosts may require prolonged therapy. In contrast to local disease, nodular cutaneous candidiasis represents disseminated disease (p. 287).

Prognosis: Related to extent of disease/host defense status.

Tinea Corporis (Body Ringworm)

Clinical Presentation: Annular pruritic lesions on trunk/face with central clearing.

Diagnostic Considerations: Diagnosis by clinical appearance/skin scraping.

Pitfalls: Do not confuse with erythema migrans, which is not pruritic.

Therapeutic Considerations: If topical therapy fails, treat with oral antifungals.

Prognosis: Excellent.

Tinea Capitis (Scalp Ringworm)

Clinical Presentation: Itchy, annular scalp lesions.

Diagnostic Considerations: Scalp lesions fluoresce with ultraviolet light. Culture hair shafts.

Pitfalls: T. capitis is associated with localized areas of alopecia.

Therapeutic Considerations: Selenium sulfide shampoo may be used first for 2–4 weeks. Treat shampoo Failures with oral ketoconazole, terbinafine, or fluconazole.

Prognosis: Excellent.

Tinea Cruris (Jock Itch)

Clinical Presentation: Groin, inguinal, perineal, or buttock lesions that are pruritic and serpiginous with scaling borders/central clearing.

Diagnostic Considerations: Diagnosis by clinical appearance/culture.

Pitfalls: Usually spares penis/scrotum, unlike Candida.

Therapeutic Considerations: In addition to therapy, it is important to keep area dry.

Prognosis: Excellent.

Tinea Pedis (Athlete's Foot)

Clinical Presentation: Painful cracks/fissures between toes.

Diagnostic Considerations: Diagnosis by clinical appearance/skin scraping.

Pitfalls: Must keep feet dry or relapse/reinfection may occur.

Therapeutic Considerations: In addition to therapy, it is important to keep area dry.

Prognosis: Excellent.

Tinea Versicolor (Pityriasis)

Clinical Presentation: Oval hypo- or hyperpigmented scaly lesions that coalesce into large confluent areas typically on upper trunk; chronic/relapsing.

Diagnostic Considerations: Diagnosis by clinical appearance and culture of affected skin lesions.

Pitfalls: M. furfur also causes seborrheic dermatitis, but seborrheic lesions are typically on the face/scalp.

Therapeutic Considerations: If topical therapy fails, treat with oral antifungals. Treat non-scalp seborrheic dermatitis with ketoconazole cream (2%) daily until cured.

Prognosis: Excellent.

Dermatophyte Nail Infections

Clinical Presentation: Chronically thickened, discolored nails.

Diagnostic Considerations: Diagnosis by culture of nail clippings.

Pitfalls: Nail clipping cultures often contaminated by bacterial/fungal colonizers. Green nail discoloration suggests P. aeruginosa, not a fungal nail infection; treat with ciprofloxacin 500 mg (PO) q12h × 2–3 weeks.

Therapeutic Considerations: Lengthy therapy is required. However, terbinafine and itraconazole remain bound to nail tissue for months following dosing and thus therapy with these compounds is not continued until clearance of the nail bed.

Prognosis: Excellent if infection is totally eradicated from nail bed. New nail growth takes months.

Skin Infestations

Subset	Usual Pathogens	Therapy
Scabies	Sarcoptes scabiei	Treat whole body with Permethrin cream 5% (Elimite); leave on for 8–10 hours **or** Ivermectin 18 mg (three 6-mg pills) (PO) × 1 dose
Head lice	Pediculus humanus var. capitis	Shampoo with Permethrin 5% (Elimite) or 1% (NIX) cream × 10 minutes
Body lice	Pediculus humanus var. corporis	Body lice removed by shower. Removed clothes should be washed in hot water or sealed in bags for 1 month, or treated with DDT powder 10% or malathion powder 1%
Pubic lice (crabs)	Phthirus pubis	Permethrin 5% (Elimite) or 1% (NIX) cream × 10 minutes to affected areas

Scabies (Sarcoptes scabiei)

Clinical Presentation: Punctate, serpiginous, intensely pruritic black spots in webbed spaces of hands/feet and creases of elbows/knees.

Diagnostic Considerations: Diagnosis by visualization of skin tracts/burrows. Incubation period up to 6 weeks after contact. Spread by scratching from one part of body to another.

Pitfalls: Mites are not visible, only their skin tracks, but mites may be scraped out of tracts for diagnosis.

Therapeutic Considerations: Permethrin cream is usually effective. If itching persists after treatment, do not retreat (itching is secondary to hypersensitivity reaction of eggs in skin burrows). Treat close contacts. Vacuum bedding/furniture.

Prognosis: Norwegian scabies is very difficult to eradicate.

Head Lice (Pediculus humanus var. capitis)

Clinical Presentation: White spots may be seen on hair shafts of head/neck, but not eyebrows.

Diagnostic Considerations: Nits on hair are unhatched lice eggs, seen as white dots attached to hair shaft. May survive away from body × 2 days.

Pitfalls: May need to retreat in 7 days to kill any lice that hatched from surviving nits.

Therapeutic Considerations: Shampoo with Permethrin 5% (Elimite) or 1% (NIX) cream kills lice/nits. Clothes and non-washables should be tied off in plastic bags × 2 weeks to kill lice. Alternately, wash and dry clothes/bed linens; heat from dryer/iron kills lice.

Prognosis: Related to thoroughness of therapy.

Body Lice (Pediculus humanus var. corporis)

Clinical Presentation: Intense generalized pruritus.

Diagnostic Considerations: Smaller than head lice and more difficult to see. May survive away from body × 1 week.

Pitfalls: Body lice live in clothes; leave only for a blood meal, then return to clothing.

Therapeutic Considerations: Can survive in seams of clothing × 1 week.

Prognosis: Good if clothes are also treated.

Pubic Lice (Phthirus pubis) Crabs

Clinical Presentation: Genital pruritus.

Diagnostic Considerations: Seen on groin, eyelashes, axilla. May survive away from body × 1 day.

Pitfalls: Smaller than head lice, but easily seen.

Therapeutic Considerations: Treat partners. Wash, dry, and iron clothes; heat from dryer/iron kills lice. Non-washables may be placed in a sealed bag × 7 days.

Prognosis: Good if clothes are also treated.

Ischiorectal/Perirectal Abscess

Subset	Pathogens	Preferred Therapy
Ischiorectal/ perirectal abscess	Enterobacteriaceae B. fragilis	Treat the same as mild/severe peritonitis (p. 98) ± surgical drainage depending on abscess size/severity

Clinical Presentation: Presents in normal hosts with perirectal pain, pain on defecation, leukocytosis, erythema/tenderness over abscess ± fever/chills. In febrile neutropenia, there is only tenderness.

Diagnostic Considerations: Diagnosis by erythema/tenderness over abscess or by CT/MRI.

Pitfalls: Do not confuse with perirectal regional enteritis (Crohn's disease) in normal hosts, or with ecthyma gangrenosum in febrile neutropenics.

Therapeutic Considerations: Antibiotic therapy may be adequate for mild cases. Large abscesses require drainage plus antibiotics × 1–2 weeks post-drainage. With febrile neutropenia, use an antibiotic that is active against both P. aeruginosa and B. fragilis (e.g., meropenem).

Prognosis: Good with early drainage/therapy.

Sepsis/Septic Shock

Sepsis/Septic Shock

Subset	Usual Pathogens	Preferred IV Therapy	Alternate IV Therapy	IV-to-PO Switch
Unknown source	Enterobacteriaceae B. fragilis E. faecalis (VSE)†	Meropenem 1 gm (IV) q8h × 2 weeks **or** Tigacycline 100 mg (IV) × 1 dose, then 50 mg (IV) q12h × 2 weeks **or** Piperacillin/ tazobactam 3.375 gm (IV) q6h × 2 weeks	Quinolone* (IV) × 2 weeks **plus either** Metronidazole 1 gm (IV) q24h × 2 weeks **or** Clindamycin 600 mg (IV) q8h × 2 weeks	Moxifloxacin 400 mg (PO) q24h × 2 weeks

VSE/VRE = vancomycin-sensitive/resistant enterococci. Duration of therapy represents total time IV or IV + PO.

* Ciprofloxacin 400 mg (IV) q12h or Levofloxacin 500 mg (IV or PO) q24h.

† Treat initially for E. faecalis (VSE); if later identified as E. faecium (VRE), treat accordingly (see urosepsis, pp. 151–152).

Sepsis/Septic Shock (cont'd)

Subset	Usual Pathogens	Preferred IV Therapy	Alternate IV Therapy	IV-to-PO Switch
Lung source *Community-acquired pneumonia*§	S. pneumoniae H. influenzae K. pneumoniae	Quinolone‡ (IV) q24h × 2 weeks **or** Ceftriaxone 1 gm (IV) q24h × 2 weeks	Any 2nd generation cephalosporin (IV) × 2 weeks **or** Cefepime 2 gm (IV) q12h × 2 weeks	Quinolone‡ (PO) q24h × 2 weeks **or** Doxycycline 200 mg (PO) q12h × 3 days, then 100 mg (PO) q12h × 11 days
Nosocomial pneumonia	P. aeruginosa K. pneumoniae E. coli S. marcescens	Same as ventilator-associated pneumonia (p. 67)		
Central IV line sepsis *Bacterial* (Treat initially for MRSA; if later identified as MSSA, etc., treat accordingly)	S. epidermidis (CoNS) S. aureus (MSSA) Klebsiella Enterobacter Serratia	Meropenem 1 gm (IV) q8h × 2 weeks **or** Cefepime 2 gm (IV) q12h × 2 wks	Ceftriaxone 1 gm (IV) q24h × 2 wks **or** Quinolone* (IV) q24h × 2 wks	Quinolone* (PO) q24h × 2 weeks **or** Cephalexin 500 mg (PO) q6h × 2 weeks
	S. aureus (MRSA)	Daptomycin 6 mg/kg (IV) q24h × 2 weeks **or** Linezolid 600 mg (IV) q12h × 2 weeks **or** Quinupristin/dalfopristin 7.5 mg/kg (IV) q8h × 2 weeks **or** Vancomycin 1 gm (IV) q12h × 2 weeks		Linezolid 600 mg (PO) q12h × 2 weeks **or** Minocycline 100 mg (PO) q12h × 2 weeks

MRSA/MSSA = methicillin resistant/sensitive S. aureus. Duration of therapy represents total time IV or IV + PO.

* Moxifloxacin 400 mg or Levofloxacin 500 mg.

‡ Levofloxacin 750 mg (IV) q24h or Moxifloxacin 400 mg (IV) q24h.

§ Uncomplicated by cardiopulmonary decompensation/failure, CAP does not present with hypotension/shock in normal hosts. Hyposplenia/asplenia should be suspected if CAP presents with hypotension/shock in patients with good cardiopulmonary function.

Sepsis/Septic Shock (cont'd)

Subset	Usual Pathogens	Preferred IV Therapy	Alternate IV Therapy	IV-to-PO Switch
Candidemia (Unless species is known, empiric therapy as for non-albicans/possibly fluconazole-resistant Candida is preferred if recent prior azole therapy, severe illness, neutropenia or high risk for infection with C. glabrata or C. krusei)	Candida albicans (or other fluconazole-susceptible species)¶	If less critically ill, not neutropenic, and no recent azole exposure: fluconazole is usual first choice alternates an echinocandin may be used. In critically ill, neutropenia or recent azole exposure: an echinocandin is preferred. Fluconazole 800 mg (IV) × 1, then 400 mg (IV) q24h × 2 weeks† **or** Anidulafungin 200 mg (IV) × 1 dose, then 100 mg (IV) q24h × 2 weeks† **or** Micafungin 100 mg (IV) q24h × 2 weeks† **or** Caspofungin 70 mg (IV) × 1 dose, then 50 mg (IV) q24h × 2 weeks† **or** Lipid-associated formulation of amphotericin B (p. 513) (IV) q24h × 2 weeks† **or** Amphotericin B deoxycholate 0.7 mg/kg (IV) q24h × 2 weeks† **or** Voriconazole (see "usual dose," p. 695)		Fluconazole 400 mg (PO) q24h × 2 weeks† **or** Voriconazole (see "usual dose," p. 695)
	Non-albicans Candida¶ (possibly fluconazole-resistant)	Choices are as for C. albicans (see above), but Fluconazole should *not* be used and an echinocandin is preferred. Use an Amphotericin or Voriconazole primarily if additional mould coverage is desired Anidulafungin 200 mg (IV) × 1 dose, then 100 mg (IV) q24h × 2 weeks† **or** Micafungin 100 mg (IV) q24h × 2 weeks† **or** Caspofungin (see C. albicans, above) **or** Lipid amphotericin B (p. 513) (IV) q24h† **or** Amphotericin B deoxycholate (see C. albicans, above) × 2 weeks† **or** Voriconazole (see "usual dose," p. 695) × 2 weeks¶† **or** Itraconazole (see C. albicans, above)		Voriconazole (see "usual dose," p. 695) × 2 weeks¶†

¶ Best agent depends on infecting species. Fluconazole-susceptibility varies predictably by species. C. glabrata (usually) and C. krusei (almost always) are resistant to Fluconazole. C. lusitaniae is often resistant to amphotericin B (deoxycholate and lipid-associated formulations). Others are generally susceptible to all agents.

† Treat candidemia for 2 weeks after negative blood cultures.

Sepsis/Septic Shock (cont'd)

Subset	Usual Pathogens	Preferred IV Therapy	Alternate IV Therapy	IV-to-PO Switch
Intra-abdominal/ pelvic source	Enterobacteriaceae B. fragilis	Meropenem 500 mg (IV) q8h × 2 weeks **or** Tigacycline 100 mg (IV) × 1 dose, then 50 mg (IV) q12h × 2 weeks **or** Ertapenem 1 gm (IV) q24h × 2 weeks **or** Doripenem 500 mg (IV) q8h × 2 weeks **or** Piperacillin/ tazobactam 3.375 gm (IV) q6h × 2 weeks	**Combination therapy with either** Ceftriaxone 1 gm (IV) q24h × 2 weeks **or** Levofloxacin 500 mg (IV) q24h × 2 weeks **plus** Metronidazole 1 gm (IV) q24h × 2 weeks	Moxifloxacin 400 mg (PO) q24h × 2 weeks **or combination therapy with** Clindamycin 300 mg (PO) q8h × 2 weeks **plus either** Ciprofloxacin 500 mg (PO) q12h × 2 weeks **or** Levofloxacin 500 mg (PO) q24h × 2 weeks
Urosepsis *Community-acquired*	Enterobacteriaceae E. faecalis (VSE)	Quinolone (IV)* × 1–2 weeks **or** Piperacillin/ tazobactam 3.375 gm (IV) q6h × 1–2 weeks	Meropenem 500 mg (IV) q8h × 1–2 weeks **or** Doripenem 500 mg (IV) q8h × 1–2 weeks	Quinolone (PO)* × 1–2 weeks
	E. faecium (VRE)	Linezolid 600 mg (IV) q12h × 1–2 weeks	Quinupristin/ dalfopristin 7.5 mg/kg (IV) q8h × 1–2 weeks	Linezolid 600 mg (PO) q12h × 1–2 weeks **or** Minocycline 100 mg (PO) q12h × 1–2 weeks

Sepsis/Septic Shock (cont'd)

Subset	Usual Pathogens	Preferred IV Therapy	Alternate IV Therapy	IV-to-PO Switch
Nosocomial	P. aeruginosa Entero-bacteriaceae	Meropenem 1 gm (IV) q8h × 1–2 weeks **or** Doripenem 1 gm (IV) q8h × 1–2 weeks	Piperacillin/tazobactam 3.375 gm (IV) q6h × 1–2 weeks *plus* Amikacin 1 gm (IV) q24h × 1–2 weeks **or** Aztreonam 2 gm (IV) q8h × 1–2 wks **or** Cefepime 2 gm (IV) q12h × 1–2 weeks **or** Colistin 1.7 mg/kg (IV) q8h × 1–2 weeks	Quinolone (PO)* × 1–2 weeks
Urosepsis *Group D enterococci*	E. faecalis (VSE)	Ampicillin 2 gm (IV) q4h × 1–2 weeks **or** Linezolid 600 mg (IV) q12h × 1–2 weeks **or combination therapy with** Vancomycin 1 gm (IV) q12h × 1–2 weeks **plus** Gentamicin 240 mg (IV) q24h × 1–2 weeks		Amoxicillin 1 gm (PO) q8h × 1–2 weeks **or** Quinolone* (PO) × 1–2 weeks
	E. faecium (VRE)	Linezolid 600 mg (IV) q12h × 1–2 weeks **or** Quinupristin/dalfopristin 7.5 mg/kg (IV) q8h × 1–2 weeks		Linezolid 600 mg (PO) q12h × 1–2 weeks **or** Minocycline 100 mg (PO) q12h × 3 days, then 100 mg (PO) q12h × 4–11 days
Overwhelming sepsis with purpura (asplenia or hyposplenia)	S. pneumoniae H. influenzae N. meningitidis	Ceftriaxone 2 gm (IV) q24h × 2 weeks **or** Levofloxacin 500 mg (IV) q24h × 2 weeks	Cefepime 2 gm (IV) q12h × 2 weeks **or** Cefotaxime 2 gm (IV) q6h × 2 weeks	Levofloxacin 500 mg (PO) q24h × 2 weeks **or** Amoxicillin 1 gm (PO) q8h × 2 weeks
Steroids (high chronic dose)	Aspergillus	Treat as Aspergillus pneumonia (p. 54)		

Sepsis/Septic Shock (cont'd)

Subset	Usual Pathogens	Preferred IV Therapy	Alternate IV Therapy	IV-to-PO Switch
Miliary TB	M. tuberculosis	Treat as pulmonary TB (p. 52) plus steroids × 1–2 wks		
Miliary BCG (disseminated)	Bacille Calmette-Guérin (BCG)	Treat with 4 anti-TB drugs (INH, rifampin, ethambutol, cycloserine) q24h × 6–12 months plus steroids (e.g., prednisolone 40 mg q24h) × 1–2 weeks		
Septic shock	Gram-negative or gram-positive bacteria	Empiric site appropriate antimicrobial therapy plus surgical decompression/drainage if needed		

Duration of therapy represents total time IV or IV + PO.

* Ciprofloxacin 400 mg (IV) or 500 mg (PO) q12h or Levofloxacin 750 mg (IV or PO) q24h.

Sepsis (Unknown Source)

Clinical Presentation: Abrupt onset of high spiking fevers, rigors ± hypotension.

Diagnostic Considerations: Diagnosis suggested by high-grade bacteremia (2/4–4/4 positive blood cultures) with unexplained hypotension. Rule out pseudosepsis (GI bleed, myocardial infarction, pulmonary embolism, acute pancreatitis, adrenal insufficiency, etc.). Sepsis usually occurs from a GI, GU, or IV source, so coverage is directed against GI and GU pathogens if IV line infection is unlikely.

Pitfalls: Most cases of fever/hypotension are *not* due to sepsis. Before the label of "sepsis" is applied to febrile/hypotensive patients, first consider treatable/reversible mimics (see p. 148).

Therapeutic Considerations: Resuscitate shock patients initially with rapid adequate volume replacement, followed by pressors, if needed. Do not give pressors before volume replacement or hypotension may continue/worsen. Use normal saline, plasma expanders, or blood for volume replacement, not D_5W. If patient is persistently hypotensive despite volume replacement, consider relative adrenal insufficiency: Obtain a serum cortisol level, then give cortisone 100 mg (IV) q6h × 24–72h; blood pressure will rise promptly if relative adrenal insufficiency is the cause of volume-unresponsive hypotension. Do not add/change antibiotics if patient is persistently hypotensive/febrile; look for GI bleed, myocardial infarction, pulmonary embolism, pancreatitis, undrained abscess, adrenal insufficiency, or IV line infection. Drain abscesses as soon as possible. Remove IV lines if the entry site is red or a central line has been in place for ≥ 7 days and there is no other explanation for fever/hypotension. In addition to antibiotic therapy/surgical drainage, selected patients with severe sepsis may benefit from activated protein C (Xigris); bleeding is the most serious side effect; avoid in patients with active bleeding, coagulopathy, or platelets < 60,000/mm^3.

Prognosis: Related to severity of septic process and underlying cardiopulmonary/immune status.

Sepsis (Lung Source)

Clinical Presentation: Normal hosts with community-acquired pneumonia (CAP) do not present with sepsis. CAP with sepsis suggests the presence of impaired immunity/hyposplenic function (see "sepsis in hyposplenia/asplenia," p. 155). Nosocomial pneumonia uncommonly presents as (or is complicated by) sepsis with otherwise unexplained hypotension.

Diagnostic Considerations: Impaired splenic function may be inferred by finding Howell-Jolly bodies (small, round, pinkish or bluish inclusion bodies in red blood cells) in the peripheral blood smear. The number of Howell-Jolly bodies is proportional to the degree of splenic dysfunction.

Pitfalls: CAP with hypotension/sepsis should suggest hyposplenic function, impaired immunity, or an alternate diagnosis that can mimic CAP/shock. Be sure to exclude acute MI, acute heart failure/COPD, PE/infarction, overzealous diuretic therapy, concomitant GI bleed, and acute pancreatitis.

Therapeutic Considerations: Patients with malignancies, myeloma, or SLE are predisposed to CAP, which is not usually severe or associated with shock. Be sure patients with CAP receiving steroids at less than "stress doses" do not have hypotension/shock from relative adrenal insufficiency. In patients with SLE, try to distinguish between lupus pneumonitis and CAP; lupus pneumonitis usually occurs as part of a lupus flare, CAP usually does not.

Prognosis: Related to underlying cardiopulmonary/immune status. Early treatment is important.

Sepsis (Central IV Line [CVC] Source)

Clinical Presentation: Temperature ≥ 102°F ± IV site erythema.

Diagnostic Considerations: Diagnosis by semi-quantitative catheter tip culture with ≥ 15 colonies plus blood cultures with same pathogen. If no other explanation for fever and line has been in place ≥ 7 days, remove CVC and obtain semi-quantitative catheter tip culture. Suppurative thrombophlebitis presents with hectic/septic fevers and pus at IV site ± palpable venous cord.

Pitfalls: Temperature ≥ 102°F with CVC infection, in contrast to phlebitis (temperature ≤ 102°F). Acute bacterial endocarditis (ABE) may complicate intracardiac or CVC (not peripheral) infection.

Therapeutic Considerations: Line removal is usually curative, but antibiotic therapy is usually given for 1 week after CVC removal for gram-negative bacilli or 2 weeks after CVC removal for S. aureus (MSSA/MRSA). Antifungal therapy is also usually given for 2 weeks after CVC removal for candidemia. Dilated ophthalmoscopy by an ophthalmologist is important to exclude candidal endophthalmitis following candidemia.

Prognosis: Good if CVC is removed before endocarditis/metastatic spread.

Sepsis (Intra-abdominal/Pelvic Source)

Clinical Presentation: Fever, peritonitis ± hypotension. Usually a history of an intra-abdominal disorder that predisposes to sepsis (e.g., diverticulosis, gallbladder disease, recent intra-abdominal/pelvic surgery). Signs and symptoms are referable to the abdomen/pelvis.

Diagnostic Considerations: Clinical presentation plus imaging studies (e.g., abdominal/pelvic CT or MRI to demonstrate pathology) are diagnostic.

Pitfalls: Elderly patients may have little/no fever and may not have rebound tenderness. Be sure to exclude intra-abdominal mimics of sepsis (e.g., GI bleed, pancreatitis).

Therapeutic Considerations: Empiric coverage should be directed against aerobic gram-negative bacilli plus B. fragilis. Anti-enterococcal coverage is not essential. Antibiotic therapy is ineffective unless ruptured viscus is repaired, obstruction is relieved, abscesses are drained.

Prognosis: Related to rapidity/adequacy of abscess drainage and repair/lavage of ruptured organs. The preoperative health of the host is also important.

Sepsis (Urinary Source)

Clinical Presentation: Fever/hypotension in a patient with diabetes mellitus, SLE, myeloma, pre-existing renal disease, stone disease, or partial/total urinary tract obstruction.

Diagnostic Considerations: Urine gram stain determines initial empiric coverage. Pyuria is also present. Diagnosis confirmed by culturing the same isolate from urine and blood.

Pitfalls: Pyuria without bacteriuria and bacteremia due to same pathogens is not diagnostic of urosepsis. Urosepsis does not occur in normal hosts; look for host defect (e.g., diabetes, renal disease).

Therapeutic Considerations: If stones/obstruction are not present, urosepsis resolves rapidly with appropriate therapy. Delayed/no response suggests infected/obstructed stent, stone, partial/total urinary tract obstruction, or renal abscess.

Prognosis: Good if stone/stent removed, obstruction relieved, abscess drained. Fatalities rare with urosepsis.

Sepsis (Hyposplenia/Asplenia)

Clinical Presentation: Presents as overwhelming septicemia/shock with petechiae.

Diagnostic Considerations: Diagnosis by gram stain of buffy coat of blood or by blood cultures. Organism may be stained/cultured from aspirated petechiae. Howell-Jolly bodies in the peripheral smear are a clue to decreased splenic function. Conditions associated with hyposplenism include sickle cell trait/disease, cirrhosis, rheumatoid arthritis, SLE, systemic necrotizing vasculitis, amyloidosis, celiac disease, chronic active hepatitis, Fanconi's syndrome, IgA deficiency, intestinal lymphangiectasia, intravenous gamma-globulin therapy, myeloproliferative disorders, non-Hodgkin's lymphoma, regional enteritis, ulcerative colitis, Sezary syndrome, splenic infarcts/malignancies, steroid therapy, systemic mastocytosis, thyroiditis, infiltrative diseases of spleen, mechanical compression of splenic artery/spleen, Waldenstrom's macroglobulinemia, hyposplenism of old age, congenital absence of spleen.

Pitfalls: Suspect hyposplenia/asplenia in unexplained overwhelming infection.

Therapeutic Considerations: In spite of early aggressive antibiotic therapy and supportive care, patients often die within hours from overwhelming infection, especially due to S. pneumoniae.

Prognosis: Related to degree of splenic dysfunction.

Sepsis (Chronic High-Dose Steroids)

Clinical Presentation: Subacute onset of fever with disseminated infection (Candida, Aspergillus) in multiple organs.

Diagnostic Considerations: Diagnosis by positive blood cultures for fungi or demonstration of invasive fungal infection from tissue biopsy specimens. Sepsis is most commonly due to fungemia.

Pitfalls: Obtain blood cultures to diagnose fungemias and rule out bacteremias (uncommon).

Therapeutic Considerations: Empirical approach is the same as for invasive candidiasis (page 150) or invasive *aspergillosis* (page 156 and page 160). Therapy focused solely on candidiasis (e.g., fluconazole alone) should be used only if *aspergillosis* seems unlikely following careful review of the epidemiologic and clinical presentation.

Prognosis: Related to degree of immunosuppression.

Miliary (Disseminated) TB (Mycobacterium tuberculosis)

Clinical Presentation: Unexplained, prolonged fevers without localizing signs.

Diagnostic Considerations: Diagnosis by AFB on biopsy/culture of liver or bone marrow.

Pitfalls: Chest x-ray is negative early in 1/3. Subtle miliary (2 mm) infiltrates on chest x-ray 1–4 weeks).

Therapeutic Considerations: Treated the same as pulmonary TB.

Prognosis: Death within weeks without treatment.

Miliary (Disseminated) BCG (Bacille Calmette-Guérin)

Clinical Presentation: Fever, circulatory collapse, DIC days to weeks after intravesicular BCG.

Diagnostic Considerations: Usually occurs in compromised hosts (e.g., transplants, active TB, congenital/acquired immunodeficiencies [e.g., HIV], leukemias/lymphomas). Rare in normal hosts.

Pitfalls: Avoid intravesicular BCG immediately after traumatic catheterization, bladder biopsy, TURP.

Therapeutic Considerations: Treat with 4 anti-TB drugs plus steroids. Do not repeat BCG therapy.

Prognosis: Good with early treatment.

Febrile Neutropenia

Febrile Neutropenia

Subset	Usual Pathogens	Preferred IV Therapy	Alternate IV Therapy	IV-to-PO Switch
Febrile leukopenia ***< 7 days***	P. aeruginosa Entero-bacteriaceae S. aureus (MSSA)	Meropenem 1 gm (IV) q8h* **or** Levofloxacin 750 mg (IV) q24h*	Cefepime 2 gm (IV) q8h* **or** Doripenem 1 gm (IV) q8h*	Ciprofloxacin 750 mg (PO) q12h* **or** Levofloxacin 750 mg (PO) q24h*
> 7 days	C. albicans Non-albicans Candida Aspergillus	Micafungin 100 mg (IV) q24h* **or** Voriconazole (see "usual dose," p. 695)* **or** Caspofungin 70 mg (IV) × 1 dose, then 50 mg (IV) q24h* **or** Lipid-associated formulation of amphotericin B (IV) (p. 513) q24h*	Amphotericin B deoxycholate 1.5 mg/kg (IV) q24h until 1–2 gm given	Itraconazole 200 mg (PO) q12h* **or** Voriconazole (see "usual dose," p. 695)*

MSSA = methicillin-sensitive S. aureus. Duration of therapy represents total time IV or IV + PO.

* Treat until neutropenia resolves.

Clinical Presentation: Incidence of infection rises as PMN counts fall below 1000/mm^3.
Diagnostic Considerations: Febrile neutropenia < 7 days ± positive blood cultures. After blood cultures are drawn, anti-P. aeruginosa coverage should be initiated. Do not overlook ischiorectal or perirectal abscess as sources of fever.
Pitfalls: Suspect fungemia if abrupt rise in temperature occurs after 7 days of appropriate anti-P. aeruginosa antibiotic therapy. Fungemias usually do not occur in first 7 days of neutropenia.
Therapeutic Considerations: If a patient is neutropenic for > 2 weeks and develops RUQ/LUQ pain/increased alkaline phosphatase, suspect hepatosplenic candidiasis; confirm diagnosis with abdominal CT/MRI showing mass lesions in liver/spleen and treat as systemic/invasive candidiasis (p. 78). S. aureus is not a common pathogen in neutropenic compromised hosts without central IV lines, and B. fragilis/anaerobes are not usual pathogens in febrile neutropenia. If IV line infection/perirectal abscess are ruled out, consider tumor fever or drug fever before changing antibiotic therapy. If febrile neutropenia persists after 1 week of antibiotic therapy, treat empirically for Aspergillus with amphotericin B deoxycholate, caspofungin, voriconazole, or itraconazole.
Prognosis: Related to degree and duration of neutropenia.

Infections in Organ Transplants

Infections in Organ Transplants

Subset	Usual Pathogens	Preferred IV Therapy	Alternate IV Therapy	PO Therapy or IV-to-PO Switch
BACTEREMIA OR CANDIDEMIA				
Bone marrow transplant ***(BMT)*** *(leukopenic pre-engraftment)* *< 7 days Bacteremia*	P. aeruginosa Entero-bacteriaceae S. aureus (MSSA) Veridans streptococci	Meropenem 1 gm (IV) q8h* **or** Piperacillin 4 gm (IV) q6h* **or** Cefepime 2 gm (IV) q8h*	Quinolone† (IV) q24h* **plus either** Aztreonam 2 gm (IV) q8h* **or** Amikacin 1 gm (IV) q24h*	Quinolone† (PO) q24h* **or** Ciprofloxacin 750 mg (PO) q12h*

BMT/SOT = bone marrow/solid organ transplant, CO/HA-MRSA = community-onset/hospital-acquired methicillin-resistant S. aureus (see p. 14), MSSA = Methicillin-sensitive S. aureus.

† Levofloxacin 750 mg or Moxifloxacin 400 mg.

* Treat until neutropenia resolves.

Infections in Organ Transplants (cont'd)

Subset	Usual Pathogens	Preferred IV Therapy	Alternate IV Therapy	PO Therapy or IV-to-PO Switch
> 7 days Candidemia	C. albicans Non-albicans Candida	Micafungin 100 mg (IV) q24h Ambisome (L-Amb) (p. 513) (IV) q24h* **or** Caspofungin 70 mg (IV) × 1 dose, then 50 mg (IV) q24h* **or** Anidulafungin 200 mg (IV) × 1 dose, then 100 mg (IV) q24h **or** Voriconazole (see "usual dose," p. 695)*¶	Itraconazole 200 mg (IV) q12h × 2 days, then 200 mg (IV) q24h*¶ **or** Amphotericin B deoxycholate 0.6–1.5 mg/kg (IV) q24h until 1–2 gm given (significant toxicity likely—alternate therapy preferred)	Itraconazole 200 mg (PO) q12h*¶ **or** Voriconazole (see "usual dose," p. 695)*¶ **or** Fluconazole 800 mg (PO) × 1, then 400 mg (PO) q24h*‡
Solid organ transplant ***(SOT)*** *Bacteremia* (Treat initially for MRSA; if later identified as MSSA, treat accordingly)	S. aureus (MSSA) Enterobacteriaceae	Meropenem 1 gm (IV) q8h × 2 wks **or** Ceftriaxone 1 gm (IV) q24h × 2 wks	Quinolone† (IV) q24h × 2 wks **or** Cefepime 2 gm (IV) q12h × 2 weeks	Quinolone† (PO) q24h × 2 wks **or** Cephalexin 500 mg (PO) q6h × 2 weeks
	S. aureus (CO-MRSA/ HA-MRSA)	Linezolid 600 mg (IV) q12h × 2 wks **or** Daptomycin 6 mg/kg (IV) q24h × 2 wks **or** Vancomycin 1 gm (IV) q12h × 2 weeks **or** Quinupristin/dalfopristin 7.5 mg/kg (IV) q8h × 2 wks		Linezolid 600 mg (PO) q12h **or** Minocycline 100 mg (PO) q12h × 2 wks
Candidemia	C. albicans	Same as for sepsis (p. 150) × 2 weeks¶	Same as for sepsis (p. 150) × 2 weeks¶	Same as for sepsis (p. 150), except use higher dose of fluconazole: 1600 mg (PO) × 1, then 800 mg (PO) q24h × 2 weeks‡

BMT/SOT = bone marrow/solid organ transplant, CO/HA-MRSA = community-onset/hospital-acquired methicillin-resistant S. aureus (see p. 14), MSSA = methicillin-sensitive S. aureus.

† Levofloxacin 750 mg or Moxifloxacin 400 mg.

* Treat until neutropenia resolves.

‡ Loading dose is not needed PO if given IV with the same drug.

¶ Significant drug interactions are possible with usual immunosuppressive agents (e.g., tacrolimus). Review all concomitant medications for potential interactions.

Infections in Organ Transplants (cont'd)

Subset	Usual Pathogens	Preferred IV Therapy	Alternate IV Therapy	PO Therapy or IV-to-PO Switch
	Non-albicans Candida*	Same as for IV line sepsis (p. 149)¶	Same as for IV line sepsis (p. 149), except use higher dose of fluconazole: 1600 mg (IV) × 1, then 800 mg (IV) q24h × 2 weeks¶	Same as for IV line sepsis (p. 149), except use higher dose of fluconazole: 1600 mg (PO) × 1, then 800 mg (PO) q24h × 2 weeks‡¶
CNS INFECTIONS				
Encephalitis/ meningitis	CMV HHV-6	Induction therapy Either Ganciclovir 5 mg/kg (IV) q12h × 2 weeks 900 mg (PO) q12h × 3 weeks **in conjunction with** CMV immunoglobulin (CMV-IG) 500 mg/kg (IV) q48h × 2 weeks For ganciclovir-induced neutropenia, Foscarnet 60 mg/kg (IV) q8h can be substituted for Ganciclovir until WBC ↑ to 2500–5000 WBC/mm^3. G-CSF 1–8 mcg/kg (IV) q24h can be given if neutropenia is prolonged/severe Maintenance therapy (following induction therapy) Valganciclovir 900 mg (PO) q24h × 3 months **plus** CMV-IG 100 mg/kg (IV) q48h × 3 months		
	CMV, ganciclovir-resistant CMV (MIC ≥ 3 mcg/mL)	Induction Therapy: Ganciclovir 5 mg/kg (IV) q24h × 2 weeks **plus** Foscarnet 90 mg/kg (IV) q12h × 2 weeks **plus** CMV immunoglobulin (CMV-IG) 500 mg/kg (IV) q48h × 2 weeks Maintenance Therapy (following induction therapy): Ganciclovir 5 mg/kg (IV) q24h × 2 weeks **plus** Foscarnet 90 mg/kg (IV) q24h × 2 weeks **with or without** CMV immunoglobulin (CMV-IG) 100 mg/kg (IV) q48h × 3 months		
	Listeria, HSV, C. neoformans, M. tuberculosis treated the same as in normal hosts (pp. 22–23)			

‡ Loading dose is not needed PO if given IV with the same drug.

* Fluconazole-susceptibility varies predictably by species. C. glabrata (usually) and C. krusei (almost always) are resistant to fluconazole. C. lusitaniae is often resistant to amphotericin B (deoxycholate and lipid-associated formulations). Others are generally susceptible to all agents.

¶ Significant drug interactions are possible when voriconazole or itraconazole is administered with usual immunosuppressive agents (e.g., tacrolimus). Review all concomitant medications for potential interactions.

Infections in Organ Transplants (cont'd)

Subset	Usual Pathogens	Preferred IV Therapy	Alternate IV Therapy	PO Therapy or IV-to-PO Switch
Brain abscess/ mass lesion	Aspergillus	Voriconazole (see "usual dose," p. 695) until cured¶	Ambisome (L-Amb) (p. 513) (IV) q24h until cured **or** Amphotericin B deoxycholate 1.5 mg/kg (IV) q24h until cured	Voriconazole (see "usual dose," p. 695) until cured¶
	Nocardia	TMP–SMX 5 mg/ kg (IV) q6h **or** Minocycline 200 mg (IV) q12h until clinical improvement, then (PO) therapy until cured	Linezolid 600 mg (IV) q12h until clinical improvement, then (PO) therapy until cured	TMP–SMX 2 DS (PO) q8h **or** Minocycline 200 mg (PO) q12h **or** Linezolid 600 mg (PO) q12h until cured
	T. gondii	<u>Preferred Therapy</u> Sulfadiazine 1–1.5 gm (PO) q6h + pyrimethamine 200 mg (PO) × 1 dose then 50 mg (PO) q6h + folinic acid 10 mg (PO) q24h × 6–8 weeks until CT/MRI clinical response. Follow with sulfadiazine 1 gm (PO) q12h + pyrimethamine 50 mg (PO) q24h + folinic acid 10 mg (PO) q24h until cured <u>Alternate Therapy</u> Clindamycin 600 mg (IV or PO) q6h + pyrimethamine 200 mg (PO) × 1 dose then 50 mg (PO) q6h + folinic acid 10 mg (PO) q24h × 6–8 weeks until CT/MRI clinical response. Follow with sulfadiazine 1 gm (PO) q12h + pyrimethamine 50 mg (PO) q24h + folinic acid 10 mg (PO) q24h until cured		
	C. neoformans	Treat the same as in chronic meningitis (p. 22)		
PNEUMONIAS				
Focal/segmental infiltrates *Acute*	S. pneumoniae Legionella	Treat the same as in normal hosts (pp. 49–55)		

¶ Significant drug interactions are possible when Voriconazole or Itraconazole is administered with usual immunosuppressive agents (e.g., tacrolimus). Review all concomitant medications for potential interactions.

Infections in Organ Transplants (cont'd)

Subset	Usual Pathogens	Preferred IV Therapy	Alternate IV Therapy	PO Therapy or IV-to-PO Switch
Subacute	Aspergillus	<u>Preferred Therapy</u> Voriconazole (see "usual dose," p. 695) until cured*¶ **or** Lipid-associated amphotericin B (p. 513) (IV) q24h until cured **or** Amphotericin B deoxycholate 1–1.5 mg/kg (IV) q24h until 2–3 grams given <u>Alternate Therapy</u> Itraconazole 200 mg (IV) q12h × 2 days, then 200 mg (IV) q24h × 1–2 weeks, then 200 mg (PO) solution q12h until cured¶		
	M. tuberculosis C. neoformans	For TB, see p. 52. For C. neoformans, see p. 266		
Diffuse infiltrates	S. stercoralis (hyperinfection syndrome)	<u>Preferred Therapy</u> Ivermectin 200 mcg/kg (PO) q24h until cured <u>Alternate Therapy</u> Thiabendazole 25–50 mg/kg (PO) q12h (max. 3 gm/day) until cured		
	PCP/RSV	Treat the same as in other compromised hosts (p. 322)		
	CMV	Treat the same as CMV pneumonia (p. 54)		
HEPATITIS				
Viral hepatitis	CMV	Treat the same as for CMV pneumonia (p. 54)		
	HBV, HCV	Treat the same as in normal hosts (p. 95)		

Duration of therapy represents total time PO, IV, or IV + PO. Most patients on IV therapy able to take PO meds should be switched to PO therapy after clinical improvement.

* If < 40 kg, use 100 mg (PO) maintenance dose.

¶ Significant drug interactions are possible when Voriconazole or Itraconazole is administered with usual immunosuppressive agents (e.g., tacrolimus). Review all concomitant medications for potential interactions.

Bacteremia/Candidemia (Bacteremia)

Clinical Presentation: Fever and shaking chills ± localizing signs. If localizing signs are present, the organ involved indicates the origin of the bacteremia (e.g., urinary tract findings suggest urosepsis).

Diagnostic Considerations: Diagnosis is clinical and is confirmed by positive blood cultures.

Pitfalls: 3/4 or 4/4 positive blood cultures indicates bacteremia. Even 1/4 positive blood cultures of an unusual pathogen may be clinically significant in BMT/SOT. The significance of 1/4 blood cultures with coagulase-negative staphylococci is less clear. S. epidermidis bacteremia is usually IV-line related, but in some compromised hosts, it may be pathogenic without an IV line focus.

Therapeutic Considerations: In SOT, coverage should be directed against S. aureus (MSSA) and Enterobacteriaceae. Anti-P. aeruginosa coverage is not needed since these patients are not neutropenic. If the source of infection is a central IV line, the line should be removed. In pre-engraftment BMT, coverage should be directed against P. aeruginosa until leukopenia resolves. Continued fever after 1 week of appropriate antibiotic therapy suggests the presence of fungemia.

Prognosis: Good with early antibiotic therapy and, if appropriate, IV line removal.

Bacteremia/Candidemia (Candidemia)

Clinical Presentation: Fever and shaking chills ± localizing signs. If localizing signs are present, the organ involved indicates the origin of the fungemia (e.g, reddened central IV line site suggests IV line-related fungemia).

Diagnostic Considerations: Candida and Aspergillus are the commonest fungi associated with fungemia in BMT/SOT. Non-albicans Candida are more commonly cultured from the blood than C. albicans.

Pitfalls: Do not assume that all Candida are C. albicans. Non-albicans Candida are more common in SOT patients. Empiric therapy should be directed against non-albicans Candida pending speciation, which will also cover C. albicans (including fluconazole-resistant strains). Because mortality/morbidity associated with fungemia exceeds that of bacteremia, empiric therapy should be started as soon as fungemia is suspected.

Prognosis: Related to underlying immune status and promptness of empiric antifungal therapy.

CNS Infections (Encephalitis/Meningitis)

Clinical Presentation: Typical encephalitis/meningitis presentation (fever, headache, stiff neck, change in mental status).

Diagnostic Considerations: CSF usually reveals a lymphocytic predominance with a normal or ↑ CSF lactic acid and low glucose. The diagnosis of HSV/CMV encephalitis can be made by CSF PCR.

Pitfalls: Patients with Listeria encephalitis often have a negative CSF Gram stain, but Listeria nearly always grow on CSF culture. HSV/Listeria encephalitis typically have RBCs in the CSF. Head CT/MRI rules out CNS mass lesions and is negative in encephalitis/meningitis.

Therapeutic Considerations: CMV encephalitis is rare but treatable, resulting in clinical/radiological improvement. However, neurological deficits usually remain. CMV retinitis, common in HIV (p. 300), is unusual in BMT/SOT.

Prognosis: Related to underlying immune status and promptness of therapy.

CNS Infections (Brain Abscess/Mass Lesions)

Clinical Presentation: BMT/SOT patients with brain abscesses/mass lesions present with seizures/cranial nerve abnormalities. Mental status is clear, in contrast to patients with encephalitis, and nuchal rigidity is absent, in contrast to patients with meningitis.

Diagnostic Considerations: Head CT/MRI is the preferred diagnostic modality, and brain biopsy is the definitive diagnostic method. CSF analysis is not usually helpful in mass lesions, with the exception of infection due to M. tuberculosis or C. neoformans. With C. neoformans, the CSF cryptococcal antigen test is positive, and the CSF India ink preparation may be positive. With M. tuberculosis, acid fast testing of the CSF is sometimes positive, but culture has a higher yield and PCR is the preferred diagnostic modality.

Pitfalls: Patients with brain abscesses/mass lesions should have a head CT/MRI before lumbar puncture. To avoid herniation during lumbar puncture when a mass lesion is present, lumbar puncture should be performed by an experienced operator, and a minimal amount of CSF should be withdrawn.

Therapeutic Considerations: M. tuberculosis and C. neoformans are readily treatable. Be sure to use antimicrobial therapy that penetrates into CSF/brain. If TMP, TMP–SMX, or minocycline cannot be used for CNS Nocardia, linezolid may be useful.

Prognosis: Related to underlying immune status and promptness of therapy.

Pneumonias (Focal or Segmental Pulmonary Infiltrates)

Clinical Presentation: Acute or subacute community-acquired pneumonia (CAP) with respiratory symptoms and fever.

Diagnostic Considerations: BMT/SOT patients with focal/segmental infiltrates are most commonly infected with the usual CAP pathogens affecting normal hosts (e.g., S. pneumoniae, H. influenzae, Legionella). The clinical presentation of CAP in organ transplants is indistinguishable from that in normal hosts. However, BMT/SOT patients presenting subacutely with focal/segmental infiltrates are usually infected with pulmonary pathogens with a slower clinical onset (e.g., Nocardia, Aspergillus). Empiric therapy will not cover all possible pathogens; tissue biopsy is necessary for definitive diagnosis and specific therapy. Preferred diagnostic modalities include transbronchial lung biopsy, percutaneous thin needle biopsy, or open lung biopsy, not BAL.

Pitfalls: Patients presenting with subacute onset of CAP have a different pathogen distribution than those presenting with acute CAP. PCP/CMV does not present with focal/segmental infiltrates.

Therapeutic Considerations: BMT/SOT patients with acute onset of CAP are treated with the same antibiotics used to treat CAP in normal hosts. Empiric coverage is directed against both typical and atypical bacterial pathogens. If no improvement in clinical status after 72 hours, proceed to lung biopsy to identify non-bacterial pathogens (e.g., Nocardia, Aspergillus).

Prognosis: Best with acute focal/segmental infiltrates. Not as good with subacute or chronic focal/segmental infiltrates.

Pneumonias (Diffuse Pulmonary Infiltrates)

Clinical Presentation: Insidious onset of interstitial pneumonia usually accompanied by low-grade fevers. Focal/segmental infiltrates are absent.

Diagnostic Considerations: Bilateral diffuse infiltrates, which can be minimal or extensive, fall into two clinical categories: those with and without hypoxemia/↑ A-a gradient. Diffuse pulmonary infiltrates without hypoxemia suggest a noninfectious etiology (e.g., CHF, pulmonary drug reaction, pulmonary hemorrhage). The differential diagnosis of diffuse pulmonary infiltrates with hypoxemia includes PCP, CMV, HSV, RSV, others. For interstitial infiltrates with hypoxemia, the chest x-ray may be only minimally abnormal, but gallium/indium scans reveal intense bilateral, diffuse lung uptake, explaining the apparent discrepancy between clinical status and chest x-ray findings. RSV/HSV may be detected by specific monoclonal antibody tests of respiratory secretions. CMV/PCP require tissue biopsy for definitive diagnosis. A highly elevated LDH suggests the possibility of PCP. Transbronchial biopsy is preferable, but BAL may be used. The incidence of CMV pneumonia is highest in lung transplants. CMV has a predilection for infecting the transplanted organ. (T. gondii myocarditis is the most common opportunistic infection in the transplanted heart.)

Pitfalls: Because infections in BMT/SOT are sequential, the majority of patients with PCP pneumonia may have underlying CMV as well. In BMT, CMV found alone on lung biopsy suggests it is the primary pathogen. Serological tests are unhelpful for CMV; a semiquantitative CMV antigenemic assay is preferred. Candida pneumonia does not exist as a separate entity but only as part of disseminated/invasive candidiasis.

Therapeutic Considerations: Nocardia and Aspergillus should be treated aggressively until lesions resolve. Among the subacute diffuse pneumonias, PCP is readily treatable. Initiate treatment for CMV pneumonia with ganciclovir IV; after clinical improvement, complete therapy with valganciclovir (PO) until cured. If after treatment, there is an ↑ in CMV antigen levels, treat pre-emptively to prevent CMV pneumonia with valganciclovir 900 mg (PO) q24h until CMV antigen levels return to previous levels. Specific therapy exists for HSV and RSV but not adenovirus or HHV-6/7.

Prognosis: Related to underlying immune status, promptness of therapy, and general health of host.

Hepatitis (Viral)

Clinical Presentation: Fever < 102°F with ↑ SGOT/SGPT ± RUQ pain.

Diagnostic Considerations: Because CMV is of such critical importance in BMT/SOT, CMV testing should always be done in organ transplants with ↑ SGOT/SGPT. The best test for CMV is semiquantitative CMV antigenemia assay (better than shell vial culture assay). Most patients undergoing organ transplant are immunized for HBV pre-transplant. HCV serology and EBV IgM VCA titers should be ordered. ↑ incidence of HCV in HIV patients. Viral hepatitis is usually accompanied by some degree of leukopenia. A few atypical lymphocytes may be present, and serum transaminases can be mildly or markedly elevated. CMV infectious mono is the commonest manifestation of CMV infection in BMT/SOT patients. CMV has a predilection for infecting the organ transplanted, and CMV hepatitis is particularly common in liver transplants. Anicteric hepatitis is more common than icteric hepatitis.

Pitfalls: The diagnosis of active CMV hepatitis in organ transplant patients is critical because it is an immunomodulating virus, adding to the net immunosuppressive effect of immunosuppressive therapy. Do not rely on CMV IgM/IgG titers for the diagnosis.

Therapeutic Considerations: CMV and HCV should be treated aggressively to minimize their potentiating immunoregulatory defects, which may predispose to nonviral opportunistic pathogens. CMV antigen levels increase before CMV infection; therefore, when CMV antigen levels increase, begin early pre-emptive therapy with valganciclovir 900 mg (PO) q24h until CMV antigen levels return to previous levels. There is no treatment for EBV or HDV.

Prognosis: Treated early, CMV responds well to therapy. HCV is more difficult to treat. Preserved functional capacity of the liver and early treatment are good prognostic factors. The incidence of hepatoma is increased with HCV (and markedly increased with HCV in HIV patients). Prognosis of HCV is worse with hepatoma.

Toxin-Mediated Infectious Diseases

Toxin-Mediated Infectious Diseases

Subset	Usual Pathogens	IV Therapy	PO Therapy or IV-to-PO Switch
Toxic shock syndrome (TSS)* (Treat initially for MRSA; if later identified as MSSA, treat accordingly)	S. aureus (MRSA)	Preferred IV Therapy Vancomycin 1 gm (IV) q12h × 2 weeks **or** Linezolid 600 mg (IV) q12h × 2 weeks Alternate IV Therapy Minocycline 100 mg (IV) q12h × 2 weeks **or** Quinupristin/dalfopristin 7.5 mg/kg (IV) q8h × 2 weeks	Linezolid 600 mg (PO) q12h × 2 weeks **or** Minocycline 100 mg (PO) q12h × 2 weeks
	S. aureus (MSSA)	Preferred IV Therapy Cefazolin 1 gm (IV) q8h × 2 weeks Alternate IV Therapy Nafcillin 2 gm (IV) q4h × 2 weeks **or** Clindamycin 600 mg (IV) q8h × 2 weeks	Cephalexin 500 mg (PO) q6h × 2 weeks **or** Clindamycin 300 mg (PO) q6h × 2 weeks
	Clostridium sordelli	Preferred IV Therapy Penicillin G 10 mu (IV) q4h × 2 weeks **or** Clindamycin 600 mg (IV) q8h × 2 weeks **or** Piperacillin 4 gm (IV) q8h × 2 weeks Alternate IV Therapy Meropenem 1 gm (IV) q8h × 2 weeks **or** Ertapenem 1 gm (IV) q24h × 2 weeks	Not applicable
Botulism (food, infant, wound)	Clostridium botulinum	Preferred Therapy 2 vials of type-specific trivalent (types A,B,E) or polyvalent (types A,B,C,D,E) antitoxin (IV)	Alternate Therapy Amoxicillin 1 gm (PO) q8h × 7 days (wound botulism only)

MRSA/MSSA = methicillin-resistant/sensitive S. aureus. Duration of therapy represents total time IV, PO, or IV + PO. Most patients on IV therapy able to take PO meds should be switched to PO therapy after clinical improvement.

* Treat only IV or IV-to-PO switch.

Toxin-Mediated Infectious Diseases (cont'd)

Subset	Usual Pathogens	IV Therapy	PO Therapy or IV-to-PO Switch
Tetanus	Clostridium tetani	Preferred Therapy Tetanus immune globulin (TIG) antitoxin 3000–10,000 units (IM) (50% into deltoid, 50% into wound site) **plus either** Penicillin G 4 mu (IV) q4h × 10 days **or** Doxycycline 200 mg (IV or PO) q12h × 3 days, then 100 mg (IV or PO) × 7 days	Alternate Therapy Tetanus immune globulin (TIG) antitoxin 3000–10,000 units (IM) (50% into deltoid, 50% into wound site) **plus** Metronidazole 1 gm (IV) q12h × 10 days
Diphtheria (pharyngeal, nasal, wound, myocarditis)	Coryne-bacterium diphtheriae	Diphtheria antitoxin (IV) over 1 hour (pharyngeal diphtheria = 40,000 units; nasopharyngeal diphtheria = 60,000 units; systemic diphtheria or diphtheria > 3 days duration = 100,000 units) **plus either** Penicillin G 1 mu (IV) q4h × 14 days **or** Erythromycin 500 mg (IV) q6h × 14 days	Diphtheria antitoxin (IV) over 1 hour (pharyngeal diphtheria = 40,000 units; nasopharyngeal diphtheria = 60,000 units; systemic diphtheria or diphtheria > 3 days duration = 100,000 units) **plus** Procaine penicillin 600,000 units (IM) q24h × 14 days

Duration of therapy represents total time IV, PO, or IV + PO. Most patients on IV therapy able to take PO meds should be switched to PO therapy after clinical improvement.

Toxic Shock Syndrome (S. aureus)

Clinical Presentation: Scarlatiniform rash ± hypotension. Spectrum ranges from minimal infection to multiorgan system failure/shock. ↑ CPK common.

Diagnostic Considerations: Diagnosis by clinical presentation with mucous membrane, renal, liver, and skin involvement/culture of TSS-1 toxin-producing strain of S. aureus from mouth, nares, vagina, or wound.

Pitfalls: Toxic shock syndrome wound discharge is clear, not purulent.

Therapeutic Considerations: Remove source of toxin production if possible (e.g., remove tampon, drain collections). Support organ dysfunction until recovery.

Prognosis: Good in early/mild form. Poor in late/multisystem disease form.

Toxic Shock Syndrome (C. sordelli)

Clinical Presentation: Resembles clostridial myonecrosis (gas gangrene) with soft tissue necrotizing infection are local edema. Hypotension with acute onset of nausea/vomiting and weakness characteristic. Associated with IVDA (black tar heroin), trauma, parturition, abortion, cadaver graft surgery. Hemoconcentration with leukocytosis typical; leukemoid reactions common with WBC counts > 50k/mm^3.

Diagnostic Considerations: Clinical diagnosis. Culture of C. sordelli from necrotic soft tissue.

Pitfalls: Gas gangrene like clinical presentation but with hemoconcentration not hemolytic anemia. Nausea/vomiting instead of diarrhea as with gas gangrene. Shock with no/low fever and ↑ WBC should suggest the diagnosis. Muscle involvement (clostridial myonecrosis) and bullae typical of gas gangrene not a feature of C. sordelli TSS.

Therapeutic Considerations: Early/adequate debridement critical. Anti-anerobic antibiotics and supportive measures important.

Prognosis: Like gas gangrene, prognosis related to early diagnosis and early/adequate surgical debridement.

Botulism (Clostridium botulinum)

Clinical Presentation: Descending symmetrical paralysis beginning with cranial nerve involvement, induced by botulinum toxin. Onset begins with blurry vision, followed rapidly by ocular muscle paralysis, difficulty speaking, and inability to swallow. Respiratory paralysis may occur in severe cases. Mental status is unaffected. Usual incubation period is 10–12 hours. Incubation is shortest for Type E strain (hours), longest for Type A strain (up to 10 days), and is inversely proportional to the quantity of toxin consumed (food botulism). Wound botulism (Types A or B) may follow C. botulinum entry into IV drug abuser injection site, surgical or traumatic wounds. Infant (< 1 year) botulism (most commonly Type A or B) is acquired from C. botulinum containing honey. Patients with botulism are afebrile, and have profuse vomiting without diarrhea.

Diagnostic Considerations: Detection of botulinum toxin from stool, serum, or food (especially home canned foods with neutral or near neutral pH [~ 7] or smoked fish [Type E]) is diagnostic of food botulism. Wound botulism is diagnosed by culturing C. botulinum from the wound or by detecting botulinum toxin in the serum.

Pitfalls: Clinical diagnosis based on descending paralysis with cranial nerve involvement in an afebrile patient must be differentiated from Guillain-Barre (fever, ascending paralysis, sensory component) and polio (fever, pure ascending motor paralysis). Do not diagnose botulism in the absence of ocular/pharyngeal paralysis.

Therapeutic Considerations: Antitoxin neutralizes only unbound toxin, and does not reverse toxin-induced paralysis. Botulism is a toxin-mediated infection and antibiotic therapy (wound botulism) is adjunctive. Guanidine has been used with variable effect. Ventilator support is needed for respiratory paralysis. Bioterrorist botulism presents clinically and is treated the same as naturally-acquired botulism.

Prognosis: Good if treated early, before respiratory paralysis.

Tetanus (Clostridium tetani)

Clinical Presentation: Begins with jaw stiffness/difficulty chewing induced by C. tetani toxin (tetanospasmin). Trismus rapidly follows with masseter muscle spasm, followed by spasm of the abdominal/back muscles. Rigidity and convulsions may occur. Patients are afebrile unless there is hypothalamic involvement (central fever), in which case fevers may exceed 106°F. Usual incubation period is 3–21 days.

Diagnostic Considerations: Diagnosis suggested by muscle spasms/rigidity in a patient with trismus.

Pitfalls: In rabies, muscle spasms are localized and usually involve the face/neck, rather than primary involvement of the extremities, as in tetanus.

Therapeutic Considerations: Tetanus is self-limited with intensive supportive care. Sedation is important, and avoidance of all stimuli is mandatory to reduce the risk of convulsions. Avoid unnecessary handling/movement of patient. Antitoxin is effective only in neutralizing unbound toxin. Tracheostomy/respiratory support can be lifesaving in severe cases.

Prognosis: Good if not complicated by spinal fractures, aspiration pneumonia, or CNS involvement (hyperpyrexia, hyper/hypotension).

Diphtheria (Corynebacterium diphtheriae)

Clinical Presentation: Within 1 week following insidious onset of sore throat without fever, pharyngeal patches coalesce to form a gray diphtheric membrane (surrounded by a red border), which is adherent/bleeds easily when removed. Membrane begins unilaterally; may extend to the soft palate, uvula and contralateral posterior pharynx; are accompanied by prominent bilateral anterior adenopathy; become necrotic (green/black); and have a foul odor (fetor oris). Submandibular edema ("bull neck") and hoarseness (laryngeal stridor) precede respiratory obstruction/death. Cutaneous diphtheria may follow C. diphtheriae contaminated wounds (traumatic, surgical) or insect/human bites, and is characterized by a leathery eschar (cutaneous membrane) covering a deep punched out ulcer. Serosanguineous discharge is typical of nasal diphtheria (membrane in nares). Diphtheric myocarditis may complicate any form of diphtheria (most commonly follows pharyngeal form), and usually occurs in the second week, but may occur up to 8 weeks after infection begins. Diphtheric polyneuritis is a common complication. Cardiac/neurologic complications are due to elaboration of a potent toxin.

Diagnostic Considerations: Diagnosis is suggested by unilateral membranous pharyngitis/palatal paralysis, absence of fever, and relative tachycardia. Diagnosis is confirmed by culture of C. diphtheriae from nares, membrane, or wound.

Pitfalls: Differentiated from Arcanobacterium (Corynebacterium) haemolyticum (which also Forms a pharyngeal membrane) by culture and absence of scarlatiniform rash with C. diphtheriae.

Therapeutic Considerations: Antibiotic therapy treats the infection and stops additional toxin production. Antitoxin is effective against unbound toxin, but will not reverse toxin-mediated myocarditis/neuropathy. Serum sickness is common 2 weeks after antitoxin. Respiratory/cardiac support may be lifesaving.

Prognosis: Poor with airway obstruction or myocarditis. Myocarditis may occur despite early treatment.

Bioterrorist Agents

Bioterrorist Agents in Adults¶

Subset	Pathogen	IV/IM Therapy	IV-to-PO Switch
Anthrax *Inhalation, oropharyngeal, gastrointestinal*	Bacillus anthracis	Quinolone* (IV) × 2 weeks **or** Doxycycline 200 mg (IV) q12h × 3 days, then 100 mg (IV) q12h × 11 days‡ **or** Penicillin G 4 MU (IV) q4h ± clindamycin 600 mg (IV) q8h × 2 weeks	Quinolone* (PO) × 2 weeks **or** Doxycycline 200 mg (PO) q12h × 3 days, then 100 mg (PO) q12h × 11 days (loading dose not needed PO if given IV). Duration of IV + PO therapy = 60 days
Cutaneous		Treat severe cases with same (PO) antibiotics as for inhalation anthrax	
Meningitis		If penicillin susceptible, treat with Penicillin G4 MU (IV) q24h **or** Meropenem 2 gm (IV) q8h for at least 2 weeks or markedly improved and complete 60–100 days of therapy as described in the inhalation, oropharyngeal or gastrointestinal forms, in addition to quinolones or doxycycline. Consider adjunctive steroid therapy. Penicillin should NOT be used as a single agent	
Tularemia pneumonia	Francisella tularensis	Streptomycin 1 gm (IM) q12h × 10 days **or** Gentamicin 5 mg/kg (IM or IV) q24h × 10 days **or** Doxycycline 200 mg (IV) q12h × 3 days, then 100 mg (IV) q12h × 11–18 days‡ **or** Chloramphenicol 500 mg (IV) q6h × 14 days **or** Quinolone* (IV) × 10 days If meningitis: add chloramphenicol	Doxycycline 200 mg (PO) q12h × 3 days, then 100 mg (PO) q12h × 11–18 days (loading dose not needed PO if given IV) **or** Quinolone* (PO) × 10 days If meningitis suspected: add chloramphenicol

Duration of therapy represents total treatment time.

‡ Patients who remain critically ill after Doxycycline 200 mg (IV) q12h × 3 days should continue receiving 200 mg (IV) q12h for the full course of therapy. For patients who have improved after 3 days, the dose may be decreased to 100 mg (IV or PO) q12h to complete the course of therapy. Total duration of IV + PO therapy = 60 days.

* Ciprofloxacin 400 mg (IV) q12h or 500 mg (PO) q12h or Levofloxacin 500 mg (IV or PO) q24h.

¶ Additional information can be obtained at www.bt.cdc.gov. For post-exposure prophylaxis, see p. 350.

Bioterrorist Agents in Adults¶ (cont'd)

Subset	Pathogen	IV/IM Therapy	IV-to-PO Switch
Pneumonic plague	Yersinia pestis	Treat the same as tularemic pneumonia	
Botulism	Clostridium botulinum	Contrary to the package insert, administer 50 mg/kg up to 1 vial of type-specific trivalent (types A,B,E) or polyvalent (types A,B,C,D,E) antitoxin (IV) after skin testing. Antitoxin administration is not repeated (circulating antitoxin's half-life = 5–8 days). Treatment with 1 vial resulted in adverse effects in < 1%; treatment with 2–4 times present dose resulted in hypersensitivity reactions in 9%. Antibiotics do not neutralize toxin	
Smallpox	Variola virus	Smallpox vaccine ≤ 4 days after exposure	
Ebola	Ebola virus	No specific therapy. Supportive therapy can be life saving	

Duration of therapy represents total treatment time.

* Ciprofloxacin 400 mg (IV) q12h or 500 mg (PO) q12h or Levofloxacin 500 mg (IV or PO) q24h.

¶ Additional information can be obtained at www.bt.cdc.gov. For post-exposure prophylaxis, see p. 350.

‡ Patients who remain critically ill after Doxycycline 200 mg (IV) q12h × 3 days should continue receiving 200 mg (IV) q12h for the full course of therapy. For patients who have improved after 3 days, the dose may be decreased to 100 mg (IV or PO) q12h to complete the course of therapy. Total duration of IV + PO therapy = 60 days.

Anthrax (B. anthracis)

Clinical Presentation: Bioterrorist anthrax usually presents as cutaneous or inhalational anthrax. Cutaneous anthrax has the same clinical presentation as naturally-acquired anthrax: Lesions begin as painless, sometimes mildly pruritic papules, usually on the upper extremities, neck, or face, and evolve into a vesicular lesion which may be surrounded by satellite lesions. A "gelatinous halo" surrounds the vesicle as it evolves into an ulcer, and a black eschar eventually develops over the ulcer. Inhalational anthrax is a biphasic illness. Initially, there is a viral illness-like prodrome with fever, chills, and myalgias with chest discomfort 3–5 days after inhaling anthrax spores. Bacteremia is common. Patients often improve somewhat over the next 1–2 days, only to rapidly deteriorate and become critically ill with high fevers, dyspnea, cyanosis, crushing substernal chest pain, and shock. Oropharyngeal anthrax presents with fever, soft tissue edema, painful cervical adenopathy. Lesions in oropharynx ulcerate in ~ 2 weeks. GI anthrax presents with fever, malaise ± syncope, followed in 24 hours by mild nausea/vomiting, severe abdominal pain, and then ascites, ↑ abdominal pain, flushed face, and shock.

Diagnostic Considerations: Cutaneous anthrax is a clinical diagnosis suggested by the lack of pain relative to the size of the lesion. A presumptive microbiologic diagnosis is made by finding gram-positive bacilli in the fluid from the gelatinous halo surrounding the ulcer or from under the eschar. Blood cultures may reveal B. anthracis. Definitive diagnosis depends on identifying B. anthracis from culture of the skin lesions or blood cultures. Inhalation anthrax is suspected in patients with fevers, chest pain, and mediastinal widening accompanied by bilateral pleural effusions on chest x-ray. If chest x-ray findings are equivocal, then a chest CT/MRI is recommended to demonstrate mediastinal lymph node enlargement. Inhalational anthrax presents as a hemorrhagic mediastinitis, not community-acquired pneumonia. The diagnosis is clinical but supported by Gram stain of hemorrhagic pleural fluid demonstrating gram-positive bacilli. Patients with inhalational anthrax often have positive blood cultures and may have associated anthrax meningitis. If meningitis is present, the CSF is hemorrhagic and CSF Gram stain shows gram-positive bacilli, which, when cultured, is B. anthracis.

Pitfalls: Cutaneous anthrax is most often initially confused with ringworm or a brown recluse spider bite. Subacute/chronic lesions may initially resemble ringworm, but the skin lesion in ringworm has an annular configuration, is painless, and is accompanied by prominent pruritus, particularly at the edges of the lesion. Patients with ringworm have no fever or systemic symptoms. Brown recluse spider bites produce extremely painful lesions with irregular edges, which eventually develop a necrotic center followed by eschar formation. The lesions of the brown recluse spider bite are irregular, not accompanied by fever, and intensely painful. In contrast, cutaneous anthrax lesions are painless, round, and are not primarily pruritic in nature. Be alert to the possibility of smallpox following outbreaks of other bioterrorist agents such as anthrax, as the genome of smallpox is easily modified and can be incorporated into bacteria.

Therapeutic Considerations: B. anthracis is highly susceptible to nearly all antibiotics; in the U.S. bioterrorist experience, no strains were resistant to antibiotics. Traditionally, penicillin has been used to treat natural anthrax, but because of concern for resistant bioterrorist strains, doxycycline or quinolones are preferred. Because meningitis is frequently associated with inhalational anthrax, penicillin in (IV) meningeal doses may be added as a second or third antibiotic to quinolones or doxycycline. For meningeal anthrax use penicillin G or meropenem in meningeal doses. Clindamycin is active against B. anthracis and has been used in combination therapy because of its potential anti-exotoxin activity. Some patients seemed to respond somewhat better when clindamycin 600 mg (IV) q8h or 300 mg (PO) q8h plus rifampin 300 mg (PO) q12h is added to either a quinolone or doxycycline. Corticosteroids should be considered for severe mediastinal edema or meningitis. Depending upon antimicrobial susceptibility testing, rifampin, vancomycin, penicillin, ampicillin, chloramphenicol, imipenem, clindamycin or clarithromycin may be added if the need arises. Prolonged therapy of 100 days with or without anthrax vaccine has been recommended by some authors. Three doses of anthrax vaccine (BioThraxT, formerly AVA - anthrax vaccine absorbed) have been recommended by the ACIP and the John Hopkins Working Group on Civilian Bio-Defense with antimicrobials for prophylaxis after aerosolized exposure, but as it is not licensed, it must be administered under an IND application. Some B. anthracis strains produce cephalosporinase and inducible beta-lactamase that make penicillins drugs less suitable for initial therapy. In general, the organism is resistant to trimethoprim-sulfamethoxazole.

Prognosis: Prognosis of cutaneous anthrax is uniformly good. With inhalational anthrax, prognosis is related to the inhaled dose of the organism, underlying host status, and rapidity of initiating antimicrobial therapy. Inhalational anthrax remains a highly lethal infectious disease, but with early intervention/supportive care, some patients survive. Patients with associated anthrax meningitis have a poor prognosis.

Tularemic Pneumonia (F. tularensis)

Clinical Presentation: Fever, chills, myalgias, headache, dyspnea and a nonproductive cough may occur, but encephalopathy is absent. Chest x-ray resembles other causes of community-acquired pneumonia, but tularemic pneumonia is usually accompanied by hilar adenopathy and pleural effusion, which is serosanguineous or frankly bloody. Cavitation sometimes occurs. Relative bradycardia is not present and serum transaminases are not elevated.

Diagnostic Considerations: Tularemic pneumonia can resemble other atypical pneumonias, but in a patient presenting with community-acquired pneumonia, the presence of hilar adenopathy with pleural effusions should suggest the diagnosis. F. tularensis may be seen in the Gram stain of the sputum or bloody pleural effusion fluid as a small, bipolar staining, gram-negative bacillus. Diagnosis is confirmed serologically or by culture of the organism from respiratory fluid/blood.

Pitfalls: Gram-negative bacilli in the sputum may resemble Y. pestis but are not bipolar staining. Chest x-ray may resemble inhalational anthrax (hilar adenopathy/mediastinal widening). Both tularemic pneumonia and inhalational anthrax may be accompanied by bloody pleural effusions. In contrast to inhalational anthrax (which may be accompanied by anthrax meningitis), CNS involvement is not a feature of tularemic pneumonia.

Therapeutic Considerations: Streptomycin is the antibiotic traditionally used to treat tularemia. Gentamicin may be substituted for streptomycin if it is not available. Doxycycline, chloramphenicol, or a quinolone are also effective.

Prognosis: Depends on inoculum size and health of host. Mortality rates for severe untreated infection can be as high as 30%, although early treatment is associated with mortality rates < 1%.

Pneumonic Plague (Y. pestis)

Clinical Presentation: Bioterrorist plague presents as pneumonic plague and has the potential for person-to-person spread. After an incubation period of 1–4 days, the patient presents with acute onset of fever, chills, headache, myalgias and dizziness, followed by pulmonary manifestations including cough, chest pain, dyspnea. Hemoptysis may occur, and increasing respiratory distress and circulatory collapse are common. Compared to community-acquired pneumonia, patients presenting with plague pneumonia are critically ill. Sputum is pink and frothy and contains abundant bipolar staining gram-negative bacilli. Chest x-ray is not diagnostic.

Diagnostic Considerations: Yersinia pestis may be demonstrated in sputum Gram stain (bipolar staining gram-negative bacilli) and may be recovered from blood cultures. Laboratory confirmation requires isolation of Y. pestis from body fluid or tissue culture. Consider the diagnosis in any critically ill patient with pneumonia and bipolar staining gram-negative bacilli in the sputum.

Pitfalls: Plague pneumonia can resemble tularemic pneumonia, but there are several distinguishing features. Unlike plague, tularemic pneumonia is usually associated with hilar enlargement and pleural effusion. Although gram-negative bacilli may be present in the sputum of patients with tularemia, the organisms are not bipolar staining.

Therapeutic Considerations: Streptomycin is the preferred drug for pneumonic plague. Doxycycline or a quinolone is also effective.

Prognosis: Depends on inoculum size, health of the host, and the rapidity of treatment. Left untreated, mortality rates exceed 50%. ARDS, DIC, and other manifestations of gram-negative sepsis are more common when treatment is delayed.

Botulism (C. botulinum) (see p. 170)

Smallpox

Clinical Presentation: After an incubation period of 1–12 days, typical smallpox is heralded by high fever, headache, and gastrointestinal complaints (vomiting, colicky pain). No rash is present at this time. After 1–2 days, the fever decreases to near normal level, and macules begin to appear on the head, usually at the hairline. Macules progress to papules, then vesicles, then finally pustules. The rash begins on the face/head and rapidly spreads to the extremities with relative sparing of the trunk. The mucous membranes of the oropharynx and upper/lower airways are also affected early. Lesions initially are umbilicated, then later lose their umbilication. The fully formed smallpox pustule is located deep in the dermis. The appearance of the pustules is accompanied by recrudescence of fever. Hemorrhagic smallpox is a fulminant form of smallpox that begins with petechial lesions in a "swimming trunk" distribution and results in widespread hemorrhage into the skin and mucous membranes. Patients look toxemic and have high fevers with no other signs of smallpox; death from toxemia often occurs before the typical rash appears.

Diagnostic Considerations: Smallpox is most likely to be confused with chickenpox or drug eruptions. Patients with chickenpox are less toxemic and the lesion distribution is different from smallpox. Chickenpox lesions occur in crops for the first 72 hours, then stop. The lesions of chickenpox are superficial, not deep in the dermis like smallpox, and chickenpox vesicles are predominantly centripetal rather than centrifugal. The chickenpox vesicle has been described as a "dewdrop on a rose petal" because of its fragility and superficial location on the skin. If there is any doubt, a Tzanck test should be performed by unroofing the vesicle, scraping cells from the base of the vesicle, and staining the cells. A positive Tzanck test indicates chickenpox, not smallpox. Alternatively, a monoclonal VZV test can be performed on vesicle base cells. Drug eruptions are not accompanied by toxemia and are usually accompanied by relative bradycardia if fever is present.

Pitfalls: Smallpox is easily missed before the rash and is difficult to diagnose. Look for the combination of high fever/headache with gastrointestinal symptoms (e.g., abdominal pain) that precedes the rash. GI complaints may be confused with appendicitis. A petechial rash in a swimming trunk distribution does not occur with any other infectious disease and should immediately suggest smallpox. Recently human monkeypox has occurred in the Western Hemisphere after transmission via imported African rodent pets. After an incubation period of 7–19 days, patients develop fever, headache, and malaise. Skin lesions appear on head, trunk, and extremities (including palms/soles). Rash begins like smallpox as macules, then papules, and finally umbilicated vesicles. Some exudative pharyngitis/tonsillitis with cervical adenopathy may be present. Encephalitis is very rare. Laboratory results are nonspecific. Unlike smallpox, human monkeypox patients are not toxic, have pharyngitis/tonsillitis with cervical adenopathy, and have focal hemorrhage into some lesions (in hemorrhagic smallpox, hemorrhages are extensive/widespread). Patients immunized against smallpox are unlikely to acquire human monkeypox.

Therapeutic Considerations: Smallpox vaccination should be initiated as soon as the diagnosis is suspected. Smallpox vaccine may be given at full strength or in a 1:5 dilution, which is also protective. Cidofovir may prove useful but dose for smallpox is not established.

Prognosis: Variable in typical smallpox, with deep, permanent scarring, especially on the face. Hemorrhagic smallpox is highly lethal.

Ebola/Lassa Fever

Clinical Presentation: After an incubation period of 3–9 days, abrupt onset of high fevers, severe headache/myalgias followed by diarrhea, extreme malaise. Hemorrhagic phenomenon–GI, renal, vaginal, conjunctival bleeding-occur at 5–7 days. Patients rapidly become critically ill. Fever is biphasic. Patients usually have leukopenia, thrombocytopenia, and hepatic/renal dysfunction. Conjunctival suffusion is also an early finding in half the cases. If a patient is not a traveler from an endemic area (e.g., Africa), suspect bioterrorist Ebola/Lassa fever. Lassa fever differs from Ebola in having prominent head/neck edema. CNS finding (oculogyric crisis, seizures, deafness) are characteristic of Lassa fever.

Diagnostic Considerations: Ebola is a hemorrhagic fever clinically indistinguishable from Yellow fever and other African hemorrhagic fevers (e.g., Lassa fever, Marburg virus disease). Presumptive diagnosis is clinical; definitive diagnosis is confirmed by specific virologic/serologic studies.

Pitfalls: Patients with Ebola may complain initially of a sore throat and dry cough, with or without chest pain. Diarrhea/abdominal pain is not uncommon. The rash is maculopapular before it becomes hemorrhagic. Failure to consider the diagnosis may occur early when sore throat/GI symptoms are prominent (i.e., before hemorrhagic manifestations appear).

Therapeutic Considerations: There is no specific therapy available for Ebola infection. Supportive therapy can be life saving.

Prognosis: Varies with severity of infection and health of the host.

REFERENCES AND SUGGESTED READINGS

Azad AF. Pathogenic rickettsiae as bioterrorism agents. Clin Infec Dis 45 Suppl 1:S52–S55, 2007.

Alvarez-Lerma F, Grau S, Alvarez-Beltran. Levofloxacin in the treatment of ventilator-associated pneumonia. Clin Microbiol Infect 12:81–92, 2006.

Artenstein AW, Opal SM, Cristofaro P, et al. Chloroquine enhances survival in Bacillus anthracis intoxication. J Infect Dis 190:1655–1660, 2004.

Baddour LM, Bettmann MA, Bolger AF, et al. Nonvascular cardiovascular device-related infections. Circulation 108:2015–2031, 2003.

Bartlett JG. Antibiotic-associated diarrhea. N Engl J Med 346:334–339, 2002.

Bartlett JG, Inglesby TV, JR, Bono L. Management of anthrax. Clin Infect Dis 35:851–858, 2002.

Bouza E, Burillo A, Munoz P. Antimicrobial Therapy of Clostridium difficile-Associated Diarrhea. Med Clin N Am 90:1141–63, 2006.

Boyce JM. Methicillin-resistant Staphylococcus aureus. Lancet Infect Dis 5:653–663, 2005.

Bradley SF. Infections in long-term-care residents. Infect Med 22:168–172, 2005.

Bratu S. Therapeutic Approach to Complicated Skin and Soft Tissue Infections: Methicillin-susceptible and Methicillin-resistant Staphylococcus aureus. Antibiotics for Clinicians 10:S35–28, 2006.

Breman JG, Henderson DA. Diagnosis and management of smallpox. N Engl J Med 346:1300–1308, 2002.

Carratala J, Martin-Herrero JE, Mykietiuk A, Garcia-Rey C. Clinical experience in the management of community-acquired pneumonia: lessons from the use of fluoroquinolones. Clin Microbiol Infect 12: 2–11, 2006.

Castro P, Soriano A, Escrich C, Villalba G, et al. Linezolid treatment of ventriculoperitoneal shunt infection without implant removal. Eur J Clin Microbiol Infect Dis 24:603–06, 2005.

Celebi G, Baruonu F, Ayoglu F, et al. Tularemia, a reemerging disease in northwest Turkey: epidemiological investigation and evaluation of treatment responses. Jpn J Infect Dis 59:229–234, 2006.

Centers for Disease Control. Anthrax Q & A: preventive therapy. Downloaded from http://www/bt.cdc.gov/ agent/anthrax/faq/preventive.asp. November 13, 2006, page last modified March 25, 2005.

Centers for Disease Control. Abstract: "Consensus statement: tularemia as a biological weapon: medical and public health management" http://www.bt.cec.gov/agent/tularemia/tularemia-biological-weapon-abstract.asp#4, November 14, 2006.

Centers for Disease Control. Botulism: treatment overview for clinicians. Downloaded from http://www.bt.cdc.gov/ agent/Botulism/clinicians/treatment.asp, November 14, 2006.

Chastre J, Wolff M, Fagon JY, et al. Comparison of 8 vs 15 days of antibiotic therapy for ventilator-associated pneumonia in adults. JAMA 290:2588–2598, 2003.

Chen XM, Leithly JS, Paya CV, et al. Cryptosporidiosis. N Engl J Med 346:1723–1731, 2002.

Chiou CC, Does Penicillin Remain the Drug of Choice for Pneumococcal Pneumonia in View of Emerging in Vitro Resistance? Clin Infect Dis 42:234–7, 2006.

Cieslak TJ, Christopher GW, Kortepeter MG, et al. Immunization against potential biological warfare agents. Clin Infect Dis 30:843–850, 2000.

Collins J, Ali-Ibrahim A, Smoot DT. Antibiotic Therapy for Helicobacter pylori. Med Clin N Am 90:1125–40, 2006.

Cono J, Craga JD, Jamieson DJ, et al. Prophylaxis and treatment of pregnant women for emerging infections and bioterrorism emergencies. Emerg Infect Dis 12:1631–1637, 2006.

Cunha BA. Antibiotic selection in the penicillin-allergic patient. Med Clin North Am 90:1257–64, 2006.

Cunha BA. Antimicrobial Therapy of Multidrug-Resistant Streptococcus pneumoniae, Vancomycin-Resistant Enterococci, and Methicillin-Resistant Staphylococcus aureus. Med Clin North Am 90:1165–82, 2006.

Cunha BA. The atypical pneumonias: clinical diagnosis and importance. Clin Microbiol Infect 12:12–4, 2006.

Cunha BA. Oral antibiotic therapy of serious systemic infections. Med Clin North Am 90:1197–222, 2006.

Cunha BA. Persistent S. aureus Bacteremia: Clinical Pathway for Diagnosis and Treatment. Antibiotics for Clinicians 10:S39–46, 2006.

Cunha BA. Staphylococcal aureus Acute Bacterial Endocarditis (ABE): Clinical Pathway for Diagnosis and Treatment. Antibiotics for Clinicians 10:S29–33, 2006.

Cunha BA. Ventilator-associated pneumonia: monotherapy is optimal if chosen wisely. Crit Care 10:141, 2006.

Cunha BA, Hamid N, Kessler H, Parchuri S. Daptomycin cure after cefazolin treatment failure of Methicillin-sensitive Staphylococcus aureus (MSSA) tricuspid valve acute bacterial endocarditis from a peripherally inserted central catheter (PICC) line. Heart and Lung 34:442–7, 2005.

Cunha BA. Herpes Simplex-1 (HSV-1) Pneumonia. Infect Dis Practice 29:375–78, 2005.

Cunha BA. Malaria vs. Typhoid Fever: A Diagnostic Dilemma? Am J of Med 118:1442–43, 2005.

Cunha BA. Methicillin-resistant Staphylococcus aureus: clinical manifestations and antimicrobial therapy. Clin Microbiol Infect 11:33–42, 2005.

Cunha BA. Pseudomonas aeruginosa: Resistance and therapy. Semin Respir Infect 17:231–9, 2002.

Cunha BA. Clinical relevance of penicillin-resistant Streptococcus pneumoniae. Semin Respir Infect 17: 204–14, 2002.

Cunha BA. Smallpox: An Oslerian primer. Infectious Disease Practice 26:141–148, 2002.

Cunha BA. Strategies to control the emergence of resistant organisms. Semin Respir Infect 17:250–258, 2002.

Cunha BA. Osteomyelitis in the elderly. Clin Infect Dis 35:287–273, 2002.

Cunha BA. Bioterrorism in the emergency room: Anthrax, tularemia, plague, ebola and smallpox. Clinical Microbiology & Infection 8:489–503, 2002.

Cunha BA. Central nervous system infections in the compromised host. A diagnostic approach. Infect Dis Clin 15:67–590, 2001.

Cunha BA. Effective antibiotic resistance and control strategies. Lancet 357:1307–1308, 2001.

Cunha BA. Nosocomial pneumonia: Diagnostic and therapeutic considerations. Medical Clinics of North America 85:79–114, 2001.

Cunha BA. Community acquired pneumonia: diagnostic and therapeutic considerations. Medical Clinics of North America 85:43–77, 2001.

Cunha BA. Antimicrobial selection in the penicillin allergic patient. Drugs for Today 37:337–383, 2001.

Cunha BA. Pneumonias in the compromised host. Infect Dis Clin 15:591–612, 2001.

Cunha BA. Community-acquired pneumonias re-revisited. Am J Med 108:436–437, 2000.

Daneman N, McGeer, Green K, Low DE. Macrolide Resistance in Bacteremic Pneumococcal Disease: Implications for Patient Management. Clin Infect Dis 43:432–8, 2006.

Demirturk N, Usluer G, Ozgunes I, et al. Comparison of different treatment combinations for chronic hepatitis B infection. J Chemother 14:285–9, 2002.

DiBisceglie AM. Combination therapy for hepatitis B. Gut 50:443–5, 2002.

Eckburg PB, Schneider JJ, Renault CA. Avian influenza in humans: A practical review for clinicians. Infect Med 22:535–542, 2005.

Falagas ME, Kasiakou SK. Colistin: The revival of polymyxins for the management of multidrug-resistant gram-negative bacterial infections. Clin Infect Dis 40:1333–1341, 2005.

Falagas ME, Matthaiou DK, Vardakas KZ. Fluoroquinolones vs B-Lactams for Empirical Treatment of Immunocompetent Patients with Skin and Soft Tissue Infections: A Meta-analysis of Randomized Controlled Trials. Mayo Clin Proc 81:1553–66, 2006.

Falagas ME, Siempos II,Bliziotis IA, Panos GZ. Impact of Initial Discordant Treatment with B-Lactam Antibiotics on Clinical Outcomes in Adults with Pneumococcal Pneumonia: A Systematic Review. Mayo Clin Proc 81:1567–74, 2006.

Fihn SD. Acute uncomplicated urinary tract infection in women. N Engl J Med 349:259–66, 2003.

File TM Jr. Community-acquired pneumonia. Lancet 362:1991–2001, 2003.

Fishman, JA. Infection in solid-organ transplant recipients. N Engl J Med 357:2601–2614, 2007.

Frieden TR, Sterling TR, Munsiff SS, et al. Tuberculosis. Lancet 362:887–99, 2003.

Fujitani S, Yu VL. Quantitative Cultures for Diagnosing Ventilator-Associated Pneumonia: A Critique. Clin Infect Dis 43:S104–5, 2006.

Furin J, Nardell EA. Multidrug-resistant tuberculosis: An update on the best regimens. J Respir Dis 27:172–82, 2006.

Gagliotti C, Nobilio L, Milandri M, et al. Macrolide Prescriptions and Erythyromycin Resistance or Streptococcus pyogenes. Clin Infect Dis 42:1153–6, 2006.

Garau J. Role of beta-lactam agents in the treatment of community-acquired pneumonia. Eur J Clin Micrbiol Infect Dis 24:83–99, 2005.

Giamarellou H, Treatment options for multidrug-resistant bacteria. Anti Infect Ther 4:601–18, 2006.

Gomes CC, Vormittag E, Santos CR, Levin AS. Nosocomial Infection with Cefalosporin-Resistant Klebsiella pneumoniae Is Not Associated With Increased Mortality. Infect Control and Hosp Epidemiol 27:907–12, 2006.

Gould IM. The clinical significance of methicillin-resistant *Staphylococcus aureus*. J Hosp Infect 61:277–282, 2005.

Grabenstein JD. Vaccines: Countering anthrax: vaccines and immunoglobulins. Clin Infect Dis 46:129–136, 2008.

Grover SS, Sharma M, Chattopadhya D, Kapoor H, et al. Phenotypic and genotypic detection of ESBL mediated cephalosporin resistance in Klebsiella pneumoniae: Emergence of high resistance against cefepime, the fourth generation cephalosporin. Journal of Infection 53:279–88, 2006.

Gupta R, Warren T, Wald A. Genital herpes. Lancet 370:2127–2137, 2007.

Hassoun A, Spera R, Dunkel J. Tularemia and Once-Daily Gentamycin. Antimicrob Agents and Chemotherapy 50:824, 2006.

Haque NZ, Zervos MJ. Vancomycin-Resistant Enterococcal Infections: Clinical Manifestations and Management. Infections in Medicine 23:14–19, 2006.

Hayakawa K, Nakagawa K. Treatment of Infected Total Knee Arthroplasty. Infect Diseases in Clin Practice 14:211–215, 2006.

Heldman AW, Hartert TV, Ray SC, et al. Oral antibiotic treatment of right-sided staphylococcal endocarditis in injection drug users: prospective randomized comparison with parenteral therapy. Am J Med 101: 68–76, 1996.

Hotchkiss RS, Karl IE. The pathophysiology and treatment of sepsis. N Engl J Med 348:138–50, 2003.

Huang H, Flynn NM, King JH, et al. Comparisons of Community-Associated Methicillin-Resistant Staphylococcus aureus (MRSA) and Hospital-Associated MSRA Infections in Sacramento, California. Journal of Clinical Microbiology. 44:2423–28, 2006.

Johnson DH, Cunha BA. Infections in alcoholic cirrhosis. Infectious Disease Clinics 16:363–372, 2001.

Johnson LB, Saravolatz LD. Community-Acquired MRSA: Current Epidemiology and Management Issues. Infections in Medicine 23:6–10, 2006.

Joseph SM, Peiris MD, D. Phil et al. The severe acute respiratory syndrome. N Engl J Med 349:2431–41, 2003.

Kanafani ZA, Khalife N, Kanj SS, Araj GF, Khalifeh M, Sharara AI. Antibiotic use in acute cholecystitis: practice patterns in the absence of evidence-based guidelines. J Infect 51:128–134, 2005.

Kauffman CA. Endemic mycoses in patients with hematologic malignancies. Semin Respir Infect 17:106–12, 2002.

Kauffman CA. Managing fungal pneumonias: a review of the new therapies. J Crit Illness 20:30–35, 2005.

Kawai N, Idematsu H, Iwaki N, et al. Comparisons of the Effectiveness of Zanamivir and Oseltamivir against Influenza A/H_1N_1, A/H3N2, and B. Clin Infect Dis 48:996–99, 2009.

Khardori N, Kanchanapoom T. Overview of biological terrorism: Potential agents and preparedness. Clin Microbiol News 27:1, 2005.

Kim AI, Saab S. Treatment of hepatitis C. Am J Med 118:808–815, 2005.

Kimberlin DW, Rouse DJ. Genital herpes. N Engl J Med 350:1970–7, 2004.

Kremery V, Barnes AJ. Non-albicans Candida spp. causing fungaemia: pathogenicity and antifungal resistance. J Hosp Infect 50:243–60, 2002.

Lai CL, Ratziu V, Yuen MF, et al. Viral hepatitis B. Lancet 362:2089–94, 2003.

Leather HL, Wingard JR. Infections following hematopoietic stem cell transplantation. Infect Dis Clin North Am 15:483–520, 2001.

Len O, Gavalda J, Aguado, JM, et al. Valganciclovir as treatment for cytomegalovirus disease in solid organ transplant recipients. Clin Infect Dis 46:20–27, 2008.

Linden PK. Treatment options for vancomycin-resistant enterococcal infections. Drugs 62: 425–41, 2002.

Lipsky BA, Berendt AR, Deery HG, et al. Diagnosis and Treatment of Diabetic Foot Infectionss. Clin Infect Dis 39:885–910, 2004.

Loddenkemper R, Sagebiel D, Brendel A. Strategies against multidrug-resistant tuberculosis. Eur Respir J Suppl 36:66s-77s, 2002.

Lok AS. Chronic hepatitis B. N Engl J Med 346:1682–3, 2002.

Lok AS, MacMahon BJ. Chronic hepatitis B. Hepatology 45:507–539, 2007.

Maartens G, Wilinson RJ. Tuberculosis. Lancet 370:2030–2043, 2007.

Mancino P, Ucciferri C, Falasca K, et al. Methicillin-resistant Staphylococcus epidermidis (MRSE) endocarditis treated with linezolid. Scand J Infect Dis 40:67–73, 2008.

McLaughlin SP, Carson CC. Urinary tract infections in women. Med Clin North Am 88:417–29, 2004.

Metlay JP, Fishman NO, Joffe MM, et al. Macrolide Resistance in Adults with Bacteremic Pneumococcal Pneumonia. Emerging Infect Dis 12:1223–30, 2006.

Minnaganti V, Cunha BA. Infections associated with uremia and dialysis. Infect Dis Clin 16:385–406, 2001.

Musher DM, Musher BJ. Contagious acute gastrointestinal infections. N Engl J Med 351:2417–27, 2004.

Musher DM, Aslam S, Logan N, Nallacheru S, Bhaila I, Borchert F, Hamill RJ. Relatively poor outcome after treatment of Clostridium difficile colitis with metronidazole. Clin Infect Dis 40:1586–1590, 2005.

Mylonakis E, Calderwood SB. Infective endocarditis in adults. N Engl J Med 345:1318, 2001.

Naas T, Fortineau N, SpicqC, Robert J, Jarlier V, Nordmann P. Three-year survey of community-acquired methicillin-resistant Staphylococcus aureus producing Panton-Valentine leukocidin in a French university hospital. J Hosp Infect 61:321–329, 2005.

Nicholson KG, Wood JM, Zambon M. Influenza. Lancet 362:1733–45, 2003.

Parry CM, Hien TT, Dougan G, et al. Typhoid fever. N Engl J Med 347:1770–82, 2002.

Paterson DL, Bonomo RA. Extended-spectrum ß-Lactamase: a clinical update. Clin Microbiol Rev 18:657–686, 2005.

Paya CV. Prevention of cytomegalovirus disease in recipients of solid-organ transplants. Clin Infect Dis 15:596–603, 2001.

Peipert JF. Genital Chlamydial Infections. N Engl J Med 349:2424–30, 2003.

Perea S, Patterson TF. Invasive Aspergillus infections in hematologic malignancy patients. Semin Respir Infect 17:99–105, 2002.

Peterson LR. Penicillin for Treatment of Pneumococcal Pneumonia: Does In Vitro Resistance Really Matter? Clin Infect Dis 42:224–33, 2006.

Pfaller MA, Segreti J. Overview of the Epidemiological Profile and Laboratory Detection of Extended-Spectrum B-Lactamases. Clin Infect Dis 42:S153–63, 2006.

Piccirillo JF. Acute bacterial sinusitis. N Engl J Med 351:902–10, 2004.

Rao N, White GJ. Successful treatment of Enterococcus faecalis prosthetic valve endocarditis with linezolid. Clin Infect Dis 35:902–4, 2002.

Razonable RR. Management of Cytomegalovirus Infection After Renal Transplantation. Infect Dis in Clinical Practice 17:220–230, 2009.

Relman DA. Bioterrorism preparedness: what practitioners need to know. Infect Med 18:497–515, 2001.

Rex JH. Approach to the treatment of systemic fungal infectious. In: Kelley WN (ed), Kelley's Textbook of Internal Medicine, 4th ed., 2279–2281, 2000.

Rex JH, Anaissie EF, Boutati E, et al. Systemic antifungal prophylaxis reduces invasive fungal infections in acute myelogenous leukemia: a retrospective review of 833 episodes of neutropenia in 322 adults. Leukemia 16:1197–1199, 2002.

Rivkina A, Rybalov S. Chronic hepatitis B: current and future treatment options. Pharmacotherapy 22:721–37, 2002.

Robinson DA, Sutcliffe JA, Tweodros W, et al. Evolution and Global Dissemination of Macrolide-Resistant Group A Streptococci. Antimicrobial Agents and Chemotherapy 50:2903–11, 2006.

Rodriguez-Bano J. Selection of empiric therapy in patients with catheter-related infections. Clin Microbiol Infect 8:275–81, 2002.

Ross AGP, Bartley PB, Sleigh AC, et al. Schistosomiasis. N Engl J Med 346:1212–1220, 2002.

Rovers MM, Schilder AGM, Zielhuis GA, et al. Otitis media. Lancet 363:465–73, 2004.

Ruhe JJ, Monson T, Bradsher RW, Menon A. Use of long-acting tetracyclines for methicillin-resistant Staphylococcus aureus infections: case series and review of the literature. Clin Infect Dis 40:1429–1434, 2005.

Sadaba B, Azanza JR, Campanero MA, Garcia-Quetglas E. Relationship between pharmacokinetics and pharmacodynamics of β-lactams and outcome. Clin Microbiol Infect 10:990–990, 2004.

Safdar A, Bryan CS, Stinfon S, et al. Prosthetic valve endocarditis due to vancomycin-resistant Enterococcus faecium: treatment with chloramphenicol plus minocycline. Clin Infect Dis 34:61–3, 2002.

Schlossberg D. Treatment of multi-drug resistant turberculosis. Antibiotics for Clinicians 9:317–321, 2005.

Slenczka W, Klenk HD. Fort years of Marburg virus. J Infect Dis 196:S131–S135, 2007.

Small PM, Fujiwara PI. Management of tuberculosis in the United States. N Engl J Med 345:189–200, 2001.

Sobel J. Botulism. Clin Infect Dis 41:1167–1173, 2005.

Sobel JD, Wiesenfeld HC, Martens M, et al. Maintenance fluconazole therapy for recurrent vulvovaginal candidiasis. N Engl J Med 351:876–83, 2004.

Spellberg BJ, Filler SG, Edwards JE. Current treatment strategies for disseminated candidiasis. Clin Infect Dis 42:244–251, 2006.

Stanek G, Strle F. Lyme borreliosis. Lancet 362:1639–47, 2003.

Strader DB, Wright T, Thomas DL, et al. Diagnosis, management, and treatment of hepatitis C. Hepatology 39:1147–1171, 2004.

Syndman DR. Use of valganciclovir for prevention and treatment of cytomegalovirus disease. Clin Infect Dis 46:28–29, 2008.

Tegnell A, Wahren B, Elgh G. Smallpox - eradicated, but a growing terror threat. Clin Microbiol Infect 8:504–509, 2002.

Thielman NM, Guerrant RL. Acute infectious diarrhea. N Engl J Med 350:38–47, 2004.

Tolkoff-Rubin NE, Rubin RH. Recent advances in the diagnosis and management of infection in the organ transplant recipient. Semin Nephrol 20:148–163, 2000.

Topic A, Skerk V, Puntaric A, et al. Azithromycin: 1.0 or 3.0 Gram Dose in the Treatment of Patients with Asymptomatic Urogenital Chlamydial Infections. Journal of Chemotherapy 18:115–16, 2006.

Tunkel AR, Hartman BJ, Kaplan SL, et al. Practical Guidelines for the Management of Bacterial Meningitis. Clin Infect Dis 39:1267–84, 2004.

van de Beek D, de Gans J, Spanjaard L, et al. Clinical features and prognostic factors in adults with bacterial meningitis. N Engl J Med 351:1849–59, 2004.

van de Beek D, de Gans J,Tunkel AR, Wijdicks EFM. Community-acquired bacterial meningitis in adults. N Engl J Med 354:44–53, 2006.

Viale P, STefani S. Vascular Catheter-Associated Infections: A Microbiological and Therapeutic Update. Journal of Chemotherapy 18:235–49, 2006.

Villegas MV, Quinn JP. An Update on Antibiotic-Resistant Gram-Negative Bacteria. Infections in Medicine 23:23–27, 2006.

Walsh TJ, Rex JH. All catheter-related candidemia is not the same: assessment of the balance between the risks and benefits of removal of vascular catheters. Clin Infect Dis 34:600–602, 2002.

Wareham DW, Bean DC. In Vitro Activities of Polymyxin B, Imipenem and Rifampin against Multidrug-Resistant Acinetobacter baumannii. Antimicrobial Agents and Chemotherapy 50:825–26, 2006.

Wormser, GP. Discovery of new infections diseases Bartonella species. N Engl J of Med 356:2346–2347, 2007.

Wormser, GP. Early Lyme Disease. N Engl J Med 354:2794–801, 2006.

GUIDELINES

Bisno AL, Gerber MA, Gwaltney JM Jr, Kaplan EL, Schwartz RH. Practice guidelines for the diagnosis and management of group A streptococcal pharyngitis. Infectious Diseases Society of America. Clin Infect Dis 35:113–25, 2002.

Chapman SW, Bradsher RW Jr, Cambell CD Jr, et al. Practice guidelines for the management of patients with blastomycosis. Infectious Diseases Society of America. Clin Infect Dis 30:679–83, 2000.

Cordonnier C, Pautas C, Maury S, Vekhoff A, et al. Empirical versus preemptive antifungal therapy for high-risk, febrile, neutropenic patients: A randomized, controlled trial. Clin Infect Dis 48:1042–1051, 2009.

Dworkin RH, Johnson RW, Breuer J. Recommendations for the Management of Herpes Zoster. Clin Infect Dis 44:S1–26, 2007.

Dykewicz CA. Summary of the guidelines for preventing opportunistic infectious among hematopoietic stem cell transplant recipients. Clin Infect Dis 33:139–44, 2001.

Galgiani JN, Ampel NM, Blair JE, et al. Coccidioidomycosis. Clin Infect Dis 41:1217–23, 2005.

Goodman EL. Practice guidelines for evaluating new fever in critically ill adult patients. Clin Infect Dis 30:234, 2000.

Guerrant RL, Van Gilder T, Sterner TS, Thielman NM, Slutsker L, et al. Practice guidelines for the management of infectious diarrhea. Clin Infect Dis 15:321–4, 2001.

Guidelines for the Management of Adults with Hospital-acquired, Ventilator-associated, and Healthcare-associated Pneumonia. Am J Respir Crit Care Med 171:388–416, 2005.

Horsburgh CR Jr, Feldman S, Ridzon R. Practice guidelines for the treatment of tuberculosis. Clin Infect Dis 31:633–9, 2000.

Hughes WT, Armstrong D, Bodey GP, Bow EJ, Brown AE, Calandra T. 2002 guidelines for the use of antimicrobial agents in neutropenic patients with cancer. Clin Infect Dis 34:730–51, 2002.

Kauffman CA, Hajjeh R, Chapman SW. Practice guidelines for the management of patients with sporotrichosis. For the mycoses study group, Infectious Diseases Society of America. Clin Infect Dis 30:684–7, 2000.

Lipsky BA, Berendt AR, Deery HG, et al. Diagnosis and treatment of diabetic foot infections. Infect Dis 39:885–910, 2004.

Mandell LA, Wunderink RG, Anzueto A, et al. Infectious Diseases Society of America/American Thoracic Society consensus guidelines on the management of community-acquired pneumonia in adults. Clin Infect Dis 44(S2):S27–S72, 2007.

Marr K, Boeckh M. Practice guidelines for fungal infections: a risk-guided approach. Clin Infect Dis 32:331–51, 2001.

Mermel LA, Farr BM, Sheretz RJ, Raad II, O'Grady N, Harris JS, Craven DE. Guidelines for the management of intravascular catheter-related infections. Clin Infect Dis 32:1249–82, 2001.

Mermel LA, Allon M, Bouza E, Craven DE, et al. Clinical practice guidelines for the diagnosis and management of intravascular catheter-related infection: 2009 update by the Infectious Diseases Society of America. Clin Infect Dis 49:1–45, 2009.

Nicolle LE, Bradley S, Colgan R, et al. Infectious Diseases Society of America guidelines for the diagnosis and treatment of asymptomatic bacteriuria in adults. Clin Infect Dis 40:643–54, 2005.

O'Grady NP, Barie PS, Bartlett JG, et al. Practice guidelines for evaluating new fever in critically ill adult patients. Clin Infect Dis 26:1042–1059, 1998.

Pappas PG, Rex JH, Sobel JD, et al. Guidelines for treatment of candidiasis. Clin Infect Dis 38:161–89, 2004.

Pappas PG, Kauffman CA, Andes D, et al. Clinical Practice Guidelines for the Management of Candidiasis: 2009 Update by the Infectious Diseases Society of America. Clin Infect Dis 48:503–535, 2009.

Rolston KV. The Infectious Diseases Society of America 2002 guidelines for the use of antimicrobial agents in patients with cancer and neutropenia: salient features and comments. Clin Infect Dis 39 Suppl 1:S44-8, 2004.

Saag MS, Graybill RJ, Larsen RA, Pappas PG, et al. Practice guidelines for the management of cryptococcal disease. Infectious Diseases Society of America. Clin Infect Dis 30:710-8, 2000.

Sobel JD. Practice guidelines for the treatment of fungal infections. For the Mycoses Study Group. Infectious Diseases Society of America. Clin Infect Dis 30:652, 2000.

Solomkin JS, Mazuski JE, Bradley JS, et al. Diagnosis and Management of Complicated Intra-abdominal Infection in Adults and Children: Guidelines by the Surgical Infection Society and the Infectious Diseases Society of America. Clin Infect. Dis 50:133–164, 2010.

Solomon JS, Mazuski JE, Baron EJ, et al. Guidelines for the Selection of Anti-infective Agents for Complicated Intra-abdominal Infections. Clin Infect Dis 37:997–1005, 2003.

Stevens DA, Dan VL, Judson MA, Morrison VA, et al. Practice guidelines for diseases caused by Aspergillus. Infectious Diseases Society of America. Clin Infect Dis 30:696–709, 2000.

Stevens DL, Bisno AL, Chambers HF, et al. Practice guidelines for the diagnosis and management of skin and soft-tissue infections. Clin Infect Dis 41:1373–1406, 2005.

Talmor M, Li P, Barie PS. Acute paranasal sinusitis in critically ill patients: guidelines for prevention, diagnosis, and treatment. Clin Infect Dis 25:1441–6, 1997.

Tice AD, Rehm SJ, Dalovisio JR, et al. Practice guidelines for outpatient parenteral antimicrobial therapy. IDSA guidelines. Clin Infect Dis 38:1651–72, 2004.

Tunkel AR, Hartman BJ, Kaplan SL, et al. Practice guidelines for the management of bacterial meningitis. Clin Infect Dis 39:1267–1284, 2004.

Update to CDC's Sexually Transmitted Diseases Treatment Guidelines, 2006: Fluoroquinolones no longer recommended for treatment of gonococcal infections. MMWR 56:332–336, 2007.

U.S. Preventive Services Task Force. Screening for Syphilis Infection in Pregnancy: U.S. Preventive Services Task Force Reaffirmation Recommendation Statement. Ann Intern Med 150:705–709, 2009.

Van Bambeke F, Michot J-M, Van Eldere J, Tulkens PM. Quinolones in 2005: an update. Clin Microbiol Infect 11:256–280, 2005.

Walker M, Kublin JG, Zunt JR. Parasitic central nervous system infections in immunocompromised hosts: Malaria, microsporidiosis, Leishmaniasis, and African trypanosomiasis. Clin Infect Dis 42:115–125, 2006.

Warren JW, Abrutyn E, Hebel JR, Johnson JR, et al. Guidelines for antimicrobial treatment of uncomplicated acute bacterial cystitis and acute pyelonephritis in women. Infectious Diseases Society of America. Clin Infect Dis 29:745–58, 1999.

Wheat LJ, Freifeld AG, Kleiman MB, et al. Clinical practice guidelines for the management of patients with histoplasmosis: 2007 update by the Infectious Diseases Society of America. Clin Infect Dis 45:807–25, 2007.

Wheat LJ, Musial CE, Jenny-Avital E. Diagnosis and management of central nervous system histoplasmosis. Clin Infect Dis 40:844–852, 2005.

Workowski KA. Sexually transmitted diseases treatment guidelines. Clin Infect Dis 44:S73–174, 2007.

Wormser GP, Nadelman RB, Battwyler RJ, et al. Practice guidelines for the treatment of Lyme disease. Infectious Disease Society of America. Clin infect Dis 31 (Suppl 1):1–14, 2000.

Yu VL, Ramirez J, Roig J, et al. Legionnaires disease and the updated IDSA guidelines for community-acquired pneumonia. Clin Infect Dis 39:1734–7, 2004.

TEXTBOOKS

Arikan S Rex JH (eds). Antifungal Drugs in Manual of Clinical Microbiology, 8th Edition, 2003.

Baddour L, Gorback SL (eds). Therapy of Infectious Diseases. Saunders, Philadelphia, Pennsylvania, 2003.

Bodey GP, Fainstein V (eds). Candidiasis. New York, Raven Press, 1985.

Bowden RA, Ljungman P, Paua CV (eds). Transplant Infections, 2nd Edition Lippincott Williams & Wilkins, Philadelphia, Pennsylvania, 2003.

Brandstetter R, Cunha BA, Karetsky M (eds). The Pneumonias. Mosby, Philadelphia, 1999.

Brook I (ed). Sinusitis. Taylor & Francis Group, New York, New York, 2006.

Brusch, JL. Infective Endocarditis: Management in the Era of Intravascular Devices. Informa Healthcare, New York 2007.

Bryskier A (ed). Antimicrobial Agents. ASM Press, Washington, D.C., 2005.

Calderone RA (ed). Candida and Candidiasis. ASM Press, Washington DC, 2002.

Cimolai N (ed). Laboratory Diagnosis of Bacterial Infections. New York, Marcel Dekker, 2001.

Cohen DM, Rex JH. Antifungal Therapy. In: Scholssberg DM (ed). Current therapy of infectious diseases, 1996.

Cook GC. (eds). Manson's Tropical Diseases, 21st Edition. W.B. Saunders Company Ltd., London, 2003.

Cunha BA (ed). Infectious Disease in Critical Care Medicine, 3rd Edition. Informa Healthcare, New York, 2010.

Cunha BA (ed). Tick-Borne Infectious Diseases. Marcel Dekker, New York, 2005.

Cunha BA (ed). Infectious Disease in the Elderly. John Wright & Co., London, 1988.

Despommier DD, Gwadz RW Hotez PJ, Knirsh CA (eds). Parasitic Diseases, 5th Edition Apple Tree Productions, LLC, New York, New York, 2005.

Faro S, Soper DE (eds). Infectious Diseases in Women. WB Saunders Company, Philadelphia, 2001.

Glauser MP, Pizzo PA (eds). Management of Infection in Immunocompromised Patients. W.B. Saunders, London, England, 2000.

Gorbach SL, Bartlett JG, Blacklow NR (eds). Infectious Diseases, ed 3. Philadelphia, Lippincott, Williams & Wilkins, 2004.

Guerrant RL, Walker DH, Weller PF (eds). Tropical Infectious Disease: Principles, Pathogens & Practice. Churchill Livingstone, Philadelphia, 1999.

Halperin JJ. Encephalitis: Diagnosis and Treatment. Informa Healthcare, New York, 2008.

Hauser AR, Rello J (eds). Severe Infections Caused by Pseudomonas Aeruginosa. Kluwer Academic Publishers, Boston, Massachusetts, 2003.

Lutwick L, Lutwick SM. Beyond Anthrax; The Weaponization of Infectious Diseases.

Madkour MM (ed). Tuberculosis. Springer-Verlag, Berlin Germany, 2004.

Maertens JA, Marr KA. Diagnosis of Fungal Infections. Informa Healthcare, New York, 2007.

Mandell GL, Bennett JE, Dolin R (eds). Mandell, Douglas, and Bennett's Principles and Practice of infectious Diseases, 7th Edition. Philadelphia, Elsevier Churchill Livingstone, 2010.

McMillan A, Young H, Ogilvie MM, Scott GR (eds). Clinical practice in Sexually Transmissible Infections, Saunders, London, England, 2002.

Pilch RF, Ziliinskas RA (eds). Encyclopedia of Bioterrorism Defense. Wiley-Liss, Hoboken, New Jersey, 2005.

Raoult D, Parola P. Rickettsial Diseases. Informa Healthcare, New York, 2007.

Rex JH, Sobel JD, Powderly WB. Candida Infections. In: Yu VL, Jr., Merigan TC, Jr., and Barriere SL (eds.). Antimicrobial Therapy & Vaccines. Williams Wilkins, Baltimore, MD, 1998.

Rex JH, Pappas PG. Hematogenously Disseminated Fungal Infections. In: Anaissie EJ, Pfaller MA, McGinnis M (eds.), Clinical Mycology, Churchill-Livingstone, Edinburgh, 2002.

Rom WN, Garay SM (eds). Tuberculosis. Lippincott Williams & Wilkins, Philadelphia, Pennsylvania, 2004.

Scheld W, Whitley R, Marra C (eds). Infections of the Central Nervous System, 3rd Edition. Lippincott Williams & Wilkins, Philadelphia, 2005.

Schlossberg D (ed). Medical Interventions for Bioterrorism and Emerging Infections. Handbooks in Healthcare Co., Newtown, Pennsylvania, 2004.

Schlossberg D (ed). Current Therapy of Infectious Disease 3rd Edition. Mosby-Yearbook, St. Louis, 2008.

Schlossberg D (ed). Tuberculosis & Nontuberculous Mycobacterial Infections, 5th Edition, New York, McGraw-Hill, 2006.

Singh N, Aguado JM (eds). Infectious Complications in Transplant Patients. Kluwer Academic Publishers, Boston, 2000.

Studahl M, Cinque P, Bergstrom T (eds). Herpes Simplex Viruses. Taylor & Francis Group, New York, New York, 2006.

Wingard JR, Anaissie EL (eds). Fungal Infections in the Immunocompromised Patient. Taylor & Francis Group, Boca Raton, Florida, 2005.

Woods JB (ed). USAMRIID's Medical management of biological casualties handbook, 6th Edition, US Army Medical Research Institute of Infections Disease, Fort Detrick, Frederick, Maryland, 2005.

Yoshikawa TT, Rajagopalan S (eds). Antibiotic Therapy for Geriatric Patients. Taylor & Francis Group, New York, New York, 2006.

Yu, V, Edwards G, McKinnon PS, Peloquin C, Morse G (eds). Antimicrobial Therapy and Vaccines, Volume II: Antimicrobial Agents, 2nd Edition ESun Technologies, Pittsburgh, Pennsylvania, 2005.

Chapter 3

Antibiotic Susceptibility Profiles and Initial Therapy of Isolates Pending Susceptibility Results

Burke A. Cunha, MD, Paul E. Schoch, PhD, Edward J. Bottone, PhD, John H. Rex, MD, Stephanie Strollo, MD, Uzma Syed, MD

***See Color Atlas for CSF, Sputum, and Urine Gram stains**

To determine if an isolate is likely to be susceptible to an antibiotic, see **Antibiotic Susceptibility Profiles (Tables 3.1–3.3).**

When bacteria are isolated from a body site and reported, the clinical significance of the organism should be determined before deciding on potential antibiotic treatment.

The tables in this chapter serve as a guide to the clinical significance of isolates recovered from various body sites. In general, isolates listed as pathogens (P) should be treated with antibiotics, while those listed as non-pathogens (NP), colonizers (C), or skin contaminants (C*) ordinarily should not. **To determine the clinical significance of an isolate in selecting appropriate initial antibiotic therapy pending susceptibility testing (see Tables 3.5–3.8).**

Table 3.1. Antibiotic Susceptibility Profiles (Penicillins, Macrolides, Tetracyclines, and Others)

	Penicillins							Anti-Pseudomonal Penicillins				Macrolides				Tetra-Cyclines			Miscellaneous				
ORGANISMS	Penicillin G (IV)	Penicillin V (PO)	Ampicillin (IV/PO)	Ampicillin/Sulbactam (IV)	Amoxicillin (PO)	Amoxicillin/ Clavulanate (PO)	Nafcillin (IV)	Ticarcillin (IV)	Ticarcillin/ Clavulanate (IV)	Piperacillin (IV)	Piperacillin/ Tazobactam (IV)	Erythromycin (IV/PO)	Clarithromycin (PO)	Azithromycin (IV/PO)	Telithromycin (PO)	Tetracycline (IV/PO)	Doxycycline (IV/PO)	Minocycline (IV/PO)	Clindamycin (IV/PO)	Metronidazole (IV/PO)	Rifampin (PO)	TMP-SMX (IV/PO)	Chloramphenicol (IV/PO)
Aerobic Gram Positive Cocci (Clusters)																							
Staphylococcus aureus (MSSA)	0	0	1	2	0	2	3	0	0	0	3	3	0	0	0	0	2	1	1	0	2	1	2
Staphylococcus aureus (HA/CO-MRSA)	0	0	0	0	0	0	0	0	0	0	0	0	0	0	0	0	2†	1	2†	0	2	3†	0
S. aureus (CA-MRSA)	0	0	0	0	0	0	0	0	0	0	0	0	0	0		0	2	1	2	0	0	2	0
S. *epidermidis* (CoNS)	0	0	0	0	0	0	0	0	0	0	0	0	0	0	0	0	2	2	2	0	2	2	0
Aerobic Gram Positive Cocci (Chains)																							
Enterococcus faecalis (VSE)	0	0	1	2	1	1	0	2	2	2	2	3	0	0	0	0	0	0	0	0	0	3	3

1 = Preferred antibiotic–High degree of activity against the isolate and likely to be clinically effective, most strains susceptible, has a favorable PK/PD characteristics, has a good safety profile, and has a "low resistance" potential (see Chapter 11 Drug Summaries for antibiotic dosing details). 2 = Alternate choice–With many attributes of a preferred antibiotic. 3 = Acceptable, but preferably select an alternate antibiotic. 0 = No activity or no data or limited experience. † = Preferably use another CA-MRSA antibiotic, e.g., minocycline.

Table 3.1. Antibiotic Susceptibility Profiles (Penicillins, Macrolides, Tetracyclines, and Others) (cont'd)

	Penicillins							Anti-Pseudomonal Penicillins				Macrolides				Tetra-Cyclines			Miscellaneous				
ORGANISMS	Penicillin G (IV)	Penicillin V (PO)	Ampicillin (IV/PO)	Ampicillin/Sulbactam (IV)	Amoxicillin (PO)	Amoxicillin/ Clavulanate (PO)	Nafcillin (IV)	Ticarcillin (IV)	Ticarcillin/ Clavulanate (IV)	Piperacillin (IV)	Piperacillin/ Tazobactam (IV)	Erythromycin (IV/PO)	Clarithromycin (PO)	Azithromycin (IV/PO)	Telithromycin (PO)	Tetracycline (IV/PO)	Doxycycline (IV/PO)	Minocycline (IV/PO)	Clindamycin (IV/PO)	Metronidazole (IV/PO)	Rifampin (PO)	TMP-SMX (IV/PO)	Chloramphenicol (IV/PO)
Enterococcus faecium (VRE)[††]	0	0	0	0	0	0	0	0	0	0	0	0	0	0	0	0	0	3	0	0	0	0	3
Group A, B, C, F, G	1	1	2	2	1	2	0	2	2	2	2	3	3	3	0	0	0	0	1	0	0	0	3
Streptococcus (bovis) galloyticus	1	1	2	2	1	2	0	2	2	2	2	3	0	0	0	0	0	0	0	0	0	0	0
Viridans streptococci (S. mitior, milleri, mitis, mutans, oralis, sanguis, parasanguis, salivarius)	1	1	2	2	1	2	0	2	2	2	3	3	3	3	0	0	0	0	2	0	0	0	3
Aerobic Gram Positive Cocci (Pairs)																							
Streptococcus pneumoniae (PSSP)	1	1	3*	2	1	2	0	2	2	2	2	3*	3*	3*	2	3*	1	2	1	0	3*	3*	3
Streptococcus pneumoniae (PRSP)	1	0	0*	2	1	2	0	3	3	3	3	0	0	0	2	0	1	1	2	0	2	0	3
Streptococcus pneumoniae (MDRSP)	0	0	0	0	0	0	0	0	0	0	0	0	0	0	2	0	2	3	3	0	3	0	3

Aerobic Gram Negative Cocci (Pairs)																							
Neisseria gonorrhoeae	0	0	0	2	0	2	0	0	2	0	2	3	0	2	0	3*	2	2	0	0	2	0	3
Neisseria meningitidis	1	2	2	2	2	2	0	2	0	2	0	0	0	0	0	0	3	3	0	0	2	0	2
Aerobic Gram Positive Bacilli																							
Bacillus anthracis	2	3	2	3	2	3	0	0	0	0	0	3	3	3	0	2	1	0	2	0	2	0	2
Corynebacterium diphtheriae	2	2	0	0	0	0	0	0	0	0	0	0	0	0	0	0	0	0	0	0	0	0	0
Corynebacterium jeikeium (JK)	0	0	0	0	0	0	0	0	0	0	0	0	0	0	0	0	0	0	0	0	2	0	0
Listeria monocytogenes	2	2	1	2	1	2	0	2	2	2	2	3	0	0	0	3	3	3	0	0	2	1	1
Nocardia	0	0	0	0	0	0	0	0	0	0	0	0	0	0	0	3	1	2	0	0	0	1	0
Aerobic Gram-Negative Bacilli																							
Acinetobacter sp.	0	0	0	1	0	0	0	0	3	0	3	0	0	0	0	0	3	2	0	0	3	3	0
Aeromonas hydrophila	0	0	0	3	0	3	0	3	3	3	3	0	0	0	0	0	2	3	0	0	0	2	2
Bordetella sp.	0	0	0	0	0	0	0	0	0	0	0	1	1	1	3	3	3	3	0	0	3	2	3
Brucella sp.	0	0	0	0	0	0	0	0	0	0	0	0	0	0	0	3	2	3	0	0	3	3	3

1 = Preferred antibiotic—High degree of activity against the isolate and likely to be clinically effective, most strains susceptible, has a favorable PK/PD characteristics, has a good safety profile, and has a "low resistance" potential (see Chapter 11 Drug Summaries for antibiotic dosing details). 2 = Alternate choice—With many attributes of a preferred antibiotic. 3 = Acceptable, but preferably select an alternate antibiotic. 0 = No activity or no data or limited experience. * = May be effective initially but as a "high resistance" antibiotic potential, resistance may develop during/after therapy.

†† = Same for vancomycin resistant E. faecalis. *PSSP = Penicillin sensitive S. pneumoniae; PRSP = Penicillin resistant S. pneumoniae; MDRSP = Multidrug resistant S. pneumoniae.*

Table 3.1. Antibiotic Susceptibility Profiles (Penicillins, Macrolides, Tetracyclines, and Others) (cont'd)

ORGANISMS	Penicillins							Anti-Pseudomonal Penicillins				Macrolides				Tetra-Cyclines			Miscellaneous				
	Penicillin G (IV)	Penicillin V (PO)	Ampicillin (IV/PO)	Ampicillin/Sulbactam (IV)	Amoxicillin (PO)	Amoxicillin/ Clavulanate (PO)	Nafcillin (IV)	Ticarcillin (IV)	Ticarcillin/ Clavulanate (IV)	Piperacillin (IV)	Piperacillin/ Tazobactam (IV)	Erythromycin (IV/PO)	Clarithromycin (PO)	Azithromycin (IV/PO)	Telithromycin (PO)	Tetracycline (IV/PO)	Doxycycline (IV/PO)	Minocycline (IV/PO)	Clindamycin (IV/PO)	Metronidazole (IV/PO)	Rifampin (PO)§	TMP-SMX (IV/PO)	Chloramphenicol (IV/PO)
Burkholderia (Pseudomonas) cepacia	0	0	0	0	0	0	0	0	0	0	0	0	0	0	0	0	3	2	0	0	0	3	3
Citrobacter sp.	0	0	0	0	0	0	0	3	3	3	3	0	0	0	0	0	0	0	0	0	0	3	3
Enterobacter sp.	0	0	0	0	0	0	0	3	3	3	3	0	0	0	0	0	0	0	0	0	0	3	0
Escherichia coli	0	0	3*	2	2	2	0	2	2	2	2	0	0	0	0	0	2	3	0	0	0	3	2
Francisella tularensis	0	0	0	0	0	0	0	0	0	0	0	0	0	0	0	0	2	0	0	0	3	3	3
Haemophilus sp.	0	0	3*	2	2	2	0	3	2	3	2	0	3	3	2	3*	1	3	0	0	3	3	2
Klebsiella sp.	0	0	0	2	0	3	0	0	3	3	3	0	0	0	0	0	0	0	0	0	0	0	3
Moraxella catarrhalis	0	0	0	3	0	3	0	3	2	3	2	0	0	3	2	3	1	3	0	0	0	3*	3
Morganella sp.	0	0	0	3	0	0	0	3	3	3	3	0	0	0	0	0	0	0	0	0	0	3*	3
P. aeruginosa	0	0	0	0	0	0	0	3	3	3	3	0	0	0	0	0	0	0	0	0	0	0	0
Proteus sp.	0	0	0	3	0	0	0	3	3	3	3	0	0	0	0	0	0	0	0	0	0	3*	3
Providencia sp.	0	0	0	3	0	0	0	3	3	3	3	0	0	0	0	0	0	0	0	0	0	3*	3
Salmonella sp.	0	0	0	3	3	3	0	3	3	3	3	0	0	3	0	3*	2	0	0	0	0	3	2

Serratia marcescens	0	0	0	0	0	0	0	0	3	0	3	0	0	0	0	0	0	0	0	0	0	3	0
Shigella sp.	0	0	0	3	3	3	0	3	3	3	3	0	0	3	0	0	3	3	0	0	0	3*	2
Stenotrophomonas (Pseudomonas) maltophilia	0	0	0	0	0	0	0	0	3	0	3	0	0	0	0	0	0	3	0	0	0	2	3
Vibrio vulnificus	0	0	0	0	0	0	0	0	0	0	0	0	0	0	0	3	1	3	0	0	0	0	3
Yersinia enterocolitica	0	0	0	2	0	3	0	3	2	2	2	0	0	0	0	0	0	0	0	0	0	1	2
Anaerobic Gram Positive Cocci (chains)																							
Peptostreptococcus	1	1	2	2	2	2	0	2	2	2	2	3	3	3	0	3	2	2	2	2	0	0	2
Anaerobic Gram Positive Bacilli																							
Actinomyces sp.	1	1	1	2	1	2	0	0	0	0	0	2	2	2	0	2	2	2	2	0	0	0	0
Anaerobic Gram Negative Bacilli																							
Bacteroides fragilis group (B. distasonis, ovatus, thetaiotaomicron, vulgatus)	0	0	0	2	0	2	0	2	2	2	2	3	3	3	0	3	2	2	1	1	0	0	2
Prevotella sp.	1	1	1	1	1	1	0	2	2	2	2	2	2	2	2	2	2	2	1	1	0	0	2

1 = Preferred antibiotic—High degree of activity against the isolate and likely to be clinically effective, most strains susceptible, has a favorable PK/PD characteristics, has a good safety profile, and has a "low resistance" potential (see Chapter 11 Drug Summaries for antibiotic dosing details).
2 = Alternate choice—With many attributes of a preferred antibiotic.
3 = Acceptable, but preferably select an alternate antibiotic.
0 = No activity or no data or limited experience.
* = May be effective initially but as a "high resistance" antibiotic potential, resistance may develop during/after therapy.
§ = Always use in combination with another antibiotic.
† = Preferably use another CA-MRSA antibiotic, e.g., minocycline.

Table 3.2. Antibiotic Susceptibility Profiles (Cephalosporins)

	CEPHALOSPORINS																					
	1st GC (IV)	2nd GCs (IV)			3rd/4th GCs (IV)				Anti-Pseudomonal 3rd GC (IV)		1st GCs (PO)		2nd GCs (PO)				3rd GCs (PO)					Anti-MRSA Cephalosporin
ORGANISMS	Cefazolin (IV)	Cefoxitin (IV)	Cefuroxime (IV)	Cefotetan (IV)	Cefotaxime (IV)	Ceftizoxime (IV)	Ceftriaxone (IV)	Cefepime (IV)	Cefoperazone (IV)	Ceftazidime (IV)	Cefadroxil (PO)	Cephalexin (PO)	Cefaclor (PO)	Loracarbef (PO)	Cefprozil (PO)	Cefuroxime axetil (PO)	Cefixime (PO)	Ceftibuten (PO)	Cefpodoxime (PO)	Cefdinir (PO)	Cefditoren (PO)	Ceftobiprole (IV)
Aerobic Gram Positive Cocci (Clusters)																						
Staphylococcus aureus (MSSA)	1	2	2	3	2	2	2	2	2	3	2	1	3	0	3	2	0	0	2	2	0	2
Staphylococcus aureus (HA/CO-MRSA)	0	0	0	0	0	0	0	0	0	0	0	0	0	0	0	0	0	0	0	0	0	2
S. aureus (CA-MRSA)	0	0	0	0	0	0	0	0	0	0	0	0	0	0	0	0	0	0	0	0	0	2
S. epidermidis (CoNS)	3	3	3	3	3	3	3	3	3	0	0	0	0	0	0	0	0	0	0	0	0	2
Aerobic Gram Positive Cocci (Chains)																						

Enterococcus faecalis (VSE)	0	0	0	0	0	0	0	0	3	0	0	0	0	0	0	0	0	0	0	0	0	0
Enterococcus faecium (VRE)	0	0	0	0	0	0	0	0	0	0	0	0	0	0	0	0	0	0	0	0	0	0
Group A, B, C, F, G	1	2	2	2	1	1	1	2	1	3		1	2		1	2	2	3	2	2	2	2
Streptococcus (bovis) galloyticus	1	2	2	2	1	1	1	2	1	3		1	2		2	2	2	3	2	2	2	2
Viridans streptococci (S. mitior, milleri, mitis, mutans, oralis, sanguis, par sanguis, salivarius)	1	2	2	2	1	1	1	2	1	2		1	2	3	2	2	2	3	2	2	2	2
Aerobic Gram Positive Cocci (Pairs)																						
Streptococcus pneumoniae (PSSP)	1	2	2	2	2	2	1	3	2	3	1	1	2	2	1	2	3	0	3	3	3	2
Streptococcus pneumoniae (PRSP)	1	2	2	2	2	2	1	3	2	3	1	1	2	2	1	2	2	0	2	2	3	2

1 = Preferred antibiotic—High degree of activity against the isolate and likely to be clinically effective, most strains susceptible, has a favorable PK/PD characteristics, has a good safety profile, and has a "low resistance potential" (see Chapter 11 Drug Summaries for antibiotic dosing details). 2 = Alternate choice—With many attributes of a preferred antibiotic. 3 = Acceptable, but preferably select an alternate antibiotic. 0 = No activity or no data or limited experience.

Table 3.2. Antibiotic Susceptibility Profiles (Cephalosporins) (cont'd)

	CEPHALOSPORINS																						
	1st GC (IV)	2nd GCs (IV)			3rd/4th GCs (IV)				Anti-Pseudomonal 3rd GC (IV)		1st GCs (PO)		2nd GCs (PO)				3rd GCs (PO)					Anti-MRSA Cephalosporin
ORGANISMS	Cefazolin (IV)	Cefoxitin (IV)	Cefuroxime (IV)	Cefotetan (IV)	Cefotaxime (IV)	Ceftizoxime (IV)	Ceftriaxone (IV)	Cefepime (IV)	Cefoperazone (IV)	Ceftazidime (IV)	Cefadroxil (PO)	Cephalexin (PO)	Cefaclor (PO)	Loracarbef (PO)	Cefprozil (PO)	Cefuroxime axetil (PO)	Cefixime (PO)	Ceftibuten (PO)	Cefpodoxime (PO)	Cefdinir (PO)	Cefditoren (PO)	Ceftobiprole (IV)
Streptococcus pneumoniae (MDRSP)	1	2	2	2	2	2	1	3	2	3	1	1	2	2	1	2	2	0	2	2	3	2
Aerobic Gram Negative Cocci (Pairs)																						
Neisseria gonorrhoeae	2	2	2	3	2	2	1	2	2	3	0	0	3	3	3	3	1	3	2	2	2	+
Neisseria meningitidis	3	3	2	3	2	3	1	2	2	3	0	0	3	3	3	3	3	3	0	0	0	3
Aerobic Gram Positive Bacilli																						
Bacillus anthracis	0	0	0	0	0	0	0	0	0	0	0	0	0	0	0	0	0	0	0	0	0	0
Corynebacterium diphtheriae	0	0	0	0	0	0	0	0	0	0	0	0	0	0	0	0	0	0	0	0	0	0

Corynebacterium jeikeium (JK)	0	0	0	0	0	0	0	0	0	0	0	0	0	0	0	0	0	0	0	0	0	0
Listeria monocytogenes	0	0	0	0	0	0	0	0	0	0	0	0	0	0	0	0	0	0	0	0	0	0
Nocardia sp.	0	0	3	0	3	0	3	0	0	0	0	0	0	0	0	0	0	0	0	0	0	0
Aerobic Gram-Negative Bacilli																						
Acinetobacter sp.	0	0	0	0	0	0	0	2	0	3	0	0	0	0	0	0	0	0	0	0	0	3
Aeromonas hydrophila	0	3	3	3	2	2	2	2	2	3	0	0	0	0	0	3	3	3	0	0	0	2
Bordetella pertussis	0	0	0	0	0	0	0	0	0	0	0	0	0	0	0	0	0	0	0	0	0	0
Brucella sp.	3	2	2	2	2	2	2	0	0	3	0	0	0	3	3	2	0	0	0	0	0	0
Burkholderia (Pseudomonas) cepacia	2	0	0	0	3	3	3	3	0	2	0	0	0	0	0	0	0	3	0	0	0	0
Campylobacter sp.	0	0	0	0	0	0	0	0	0	0	0	0	0	0	0	0	0	0	0	0	0	0
Citrobacter sp.	0	2	3	3	2	2	2	1	0	2	0	0	0	0	0	3	0	0	0	0	0	0
Enterobacter sp.	0	3	3	3	2	2	2	1	0	3	0	0	0	0	0	0	0	0	0	0	0	0
Escherichia coli	2	2	2	2	1	1	1	2	1	2	2	2	2	2	2	2	2	2	2	2	2	2
Francisella tularensis	0	0	0	0	0	0	0	0	0	0	0	0	0	0	0	0	0	0	0	0	0	0

1 = Preferred antibiotic—High degree of activity against the isolate and likely to be clinically effective, most strains susceptible, has a favorable PK/PD characteristics, has a good safety profile, and has a "low resistance potential" (see Chapter 11 Drug Summaries for antibiotic dosing details). 2 = Alternate choice—With many attributes of a preferred antibiotic. 3 = Acceptable, but preferably select an alternate antibiotic. 0 = No activity or no data or limited experience.

Table 3.2. Antibiotic Susceptibility Profiles (Cephalosporins) (cont'd)

	CEPHALOSPORINS																					
	1st GC (IV)	2nd GCs (IV)			3rd/4th GCs (IV)				Anti-Pseudomonal 3rd GC (IV)		1st GCs (PO)		2nd GCs (PO)				3rd GCs (PO)					Anti-MRSA Cephalosporin
ORGANISMS	Cefazolin (IV)	Cefoxitin (IV)	Cefuroxime (IV)	Cefotetan (IV)	Cefotaxime (IV)	Ceftizoxime (IV)	Ceftriaxone (IV)	Cefepime (IV)	Cefoperazone (IV)	Ceftazidime (IV)	Cefadroxil (PO)	Cephalexin (PO)	Cefaclor (PO)	Loracarbef (PO)	Cefprozil (PO)	Cefuroxime axetil (PO)	Cefixime (PO)	Ceftibuten (PO)	Cefpodoxime (PO)	Cefdinir (PO)	Cefditoren (PO)	Ceftobiprole (IV)
Haemophilus sp.	3	2	2	2	1	1	1	1	1	2	1	1	3	2	2	1	1	2	2	2	2	2
Klebsiella sp.	2	2	2	2	1	1	1	2	2	2	2	2	2	2	2	2	2	2	2	2	2	2
Moraxella catarrhalis	3	3	2	2	2	2	2	2	2	2	2	2	2	2	2	2	2	2	2	2	2	2
Morganella sp.	3	3	3	3	2	2	2	2	2	3	0	0	0	0	0	3	3	0	0	0	0	0
P. aeruginosa	0	0	0	0	0	0	0	0	2	3	0	0	0	0	0	0	0	0	0	0	0	0
Providencie sp.	3	3	3	3	2	2	2	2	2	3	0	0	0	0	0	3	3	0	0	0	0	0
Proteus sp.	3	3	3	3	2	2	2	2	2	3	0	0	0	0	0	3	3	0	0	0	0	0
Salmonella sp.	0	3	3	3	1	1	1	2	2	3	0	0	0	0	0	0	0	0	0	0	0	0
Serratia marcescens	0	3	0	2	1	1	1	1	1	2	0	0	0	0	0	0	0	0	3	0	3	0
Shigella sp.	0	3	0	3	2	2	2	2	2	3	0	0	0	0	0	0	0	0	0	0	0	0
Stenotrophomonas (Pseudomonas) maltophilia	0	0	0	0	0	0	0	0	0	0	0	0	0	0	0	0	0	0	3	0	0	0

Vibrio vulnificus	0	0	0	0	2	0	0	0	0	2	0	0	0	0	0	0	0	0	0	0	0	
Yersinia enterocolitica	0	3	3	3	2	2	2	2	2	3	0	0	0	0	0	0	2	2	0	2	0	0
Anaerobic Gram Positive Cocci (chains)																						
Peptostreptococcus	2	2	2	2	2	2	2	2	3	3	2	2	3	2	2	2	0	0	0	0	0	0
Anaerobic Gram Positive Bacilli																						
Actinomyces sp.	0	0	0	0	3	3	2	0	3	0	0	0	0	0	0	0	0	0	0	0	0	0
Anaerobic Gram Negative Bacilli																						
Bacteroides fragilis group (B distasonis, ovatus, thetaiotaomicron, vulgatus)	0	2	0	2	3	2	0	0	2	0	0	0	0	0	0	0	0	0	0	0	0	0
Prevotella sp.	2	2	2	2	2	2	2	2	2	0	2	2	2	2	2	2	2	2	2	2	2	2

1 = Preferred antibiotic—High degree of activity against the isolate and likely to be clinically effective, most strains susceptible, has a favorable PK/PD characteristics, has a good safety profile, and has a "low resistance potential" (see Chapter 11 Drug Summaries for antibiotic dosing details).

2 = Alternate choice—With many attributes of a preferred antibiotic.

3 = Acceptable, but preferably select an alternate antibiotic.

0 = No activity or no data or limited experience.

* = May be effective initially but as a "high resistance" antibiotic potential, resistance may develop during/after therapy.

§ = Always use in combination with another antibiotic.

Table 3.3. Antibiotic Susceptibility Profiles (Aminoglycosides, Fluoroquinolones, Carbapenems, and Others)

	Amino-Glycosides			Fluoro-Quinolones			Miscellaneous										Carbapenems			
ORGANISMS	Gentamicin (IV)	Tobramycin (IV)	Amikacin (IV)	Ciprofloxacin (IV/PO)	Levofloxacin (IV/PO)	Moxifloxacin (IV/PO)	Colistimethate/ Polymyxin B (IV)	Aztreonam (IV)	Tigecycline (IV)	Vancomycin (IV)	Quinupristin/ dalfopristin (IV)	Linezolid (IV/PO)	Daptomycin (IV)	Telavancin (IV)	Nitrofurantoin † (PO)	Fosfomycin † (PO)	Imipenem (IV)	Meropenem (IV)	Ertapenem (IV)	Doripenem (IV)
Aerobic Gram Positive Cocci (Clusters)																				
Staphylococcus aureus (MSSA)	2	3	3	3*	2	2	0	0	1	3	1	1	1	1	0	0	2	2	2	2
Staphylococcus aureus (HA/CO-MRSA)	0	0	0	0	0	0	0	0	1	2	1	1	1	1	0	3	0	0	0	0
S. aureus (CA-MRSA)	0	0	0	0	0	0	0	0	1	1	1	1	1	1	0	0	0	0	0	0
S. epidermidis (CoNS)	0	0	0	0	3	3	0	0	1	1	1	1	1	1	0	0	3	3	3	3
Aerobic Gram Positive Cocci (Chains)																				
Enterococcus faecalis (VSE)	0	0	0	0	3	2	0	0	1	2	0	1	2	0	1	3	2	2	0	3
Enterococcus faectium (VRE)	0	0	0	0	0	0	0	0	1	0	1	1	2	3	1	3	0	0	0	3

Group A, B, C, F, G	0	0	0	0	3	2	0	0	2	2	3	2	2	2	2	0	2	2	2	2
Streptococcus (bovis) galloyticus	0	0	0	0	3	2	0	0	2	2	2	2	2	2	0	0	2	2	0	2
Viridans streptococci (S. mitior, milleri, mitis, mutans, oralis, sanguis, parasanguis, salivarius)	0	0	0	0	3	2	0	0	2	2	2	2	2	2	0	0	2	2	0	2
Aerobic Gram Positive Cocci (Pairs)																				
Streptococcus pneumoniae (PSSP)	0	0	0	3*	1	1	0	0	1	2	2	2	3	2	0	0	2	2	2	2
Streptococcus pneumoniae (PRSP)	0	0	0	3*	1	1	0	0	1	2	2	2	3	2	0	0	2	2	2	2
Streptococcus pneumoniae (MDRSP)	0	0	0	3*	1	1	0	0	1	2	2	2	3	2	0	0	2	2	2	2
Aerobic Gram Negative Cocci (Pairs)																				
Neisseria gonorrhoeae	0	0	0	1	1	2	0	2	0	0	0	0	0	0	0	0	3	3	0	3
Neisseria meningitidis	0	0	0	2	2	2	0	2	0	0	0	0	0	0	0	0	2	2	0	2
Aerobic Gram Positive Bacilli																				

1 = Preferred antibiotic–High degree of activity against the isolate and likely to be clinically effective, most strains susceptible, has a favorable PK/PD characteristics, has a good safety profile, and has a "low resistance" potential (see Chapter 11 Drug Summaries for antibiotic dosing details). 2 = Alternate choice–With many attributes of a preferred antibiotic. 3 = Acceptable, but preferably select an alternate antibiotic. 0 = No activity or no data or limited experience. * = May be effective initially but as a "high resistance" antibiotic potential, resistance may develop during/after therapy.

Table 3.3. Antibiotic Susceptibility Profiles (Aminoglycosides, Fluoroquinolones, Carbapenems, and Others) (cont'd)

	Amino-Glycosides			Fluoro-Quinolones			Miscellaneous										Carbapenems			
ORGANISMS	Gentamicin (IV)	Tobramycin (IV)	Amikacin (IV)	Ciprofloxacin (IV/PO)	Levofloxacin (IV/PO)	Moxifloxacin (IV/PO)	Colistimethate/ Polymyxin B (IV)	Aztreonam (IV)	Tigecycline (IV)	Vancomycin (IV)	Quinupristin/ dalfopristin (IV)	Linezolid (IV/PO)	Daptomycin (IV)	Telavancin (IV)	Nitrofurantoin † (PO)	Fosfomycin † (PO)	Imipenem (IV)	Meropenem (IV)	Ertapenem (IV)	Doripenem (IV)
Bacillus anthracis	0	0	0	1	1	1	0	0	0	0	0	0	0	0	0	0	0	0	0	0
Corynebacterium diphtheriae	0	0	0	0	0	0	0	0	0	3	0	0	0	0	0	0	0	0	0	0
Corynebacterium jeikeium (JK)	0	0	0	0	0	0	0	0	2	1	3	2	0	0	0	0	0	0	0	0
Listeria monocytogenes	3	3	3	0	0	0	0	0	3	0	3	3	0	0	0	0	3	2	0	0
Nocardia	0	0	2	0	0	0	0	0	0	0	0	3	0	0	0	0	3	2	0	0
Aerobic Gram-Negative Bacilli																				
Acinetobacter sp.	1	2	2	3*	2	3	2	1	2*	0	0	0	0	0	0	0	2*	1	0	1
Aeromonas hydrophila	2	2	2	1	1	1	0	3	2	0	0	0	0	0	0	0	2	2	3	0
Bordetella sp.	0	0	0	3	3	3	0	0	0	0	0	0	0	0	0	0	3	3	3	0

Brucella sp.	2	0	0	3	3	0	0	0	0	0	0	0	0	0	0	0	0	0	0	0
Burkholderia (Pseudomonas) cepacia	0	0	0	3*	3	3	0	0	0	0	0	0	0	0	0	0	3	2	3	0
Campylobacter sp.	3	0	0	1	1	1	0	0	0	0	0	0	0	0	0	0	3	3	3	3
Citrobacter sp.	1	1	2	3	2	3	3	0	2	0	0	0	0	0	2	0	1	1	1	1
Enterobacter sp.	1	1	1	2*	2	2	3	2	2	0	0	0	0	0	3	3	1	1	1	1
Escherichia coli	2	2	1	2	2	2	3	2	1	0	0	0	0	0	2	2	2	2	2	2
Francisella tularensis	1	3	0	2	2	2	0	0	0	0	0	0	0	0	0	0	0	0	0	0
Haemophilus sp.	3	3	3	2	2	2	0	3	2	0	0	0	0	0	0	0	2	2	2	2
Moraxella catarrhalis	3	3	3	2	2	2	0	2	2	0	0	0	0	0	0	0	2	2	2	2
Morganella sp.	2	2	1	3	2	2	2	2	0	0	0	0	0	0	0	2	2	2	2	2
P. aeruginosa	3	3	1	1*	1	0	1	1*	0	0	0	0	0	0	0	1	2*	1	0	1
Proteus sp.	2	2	1	3	2	2	2	2	0	0	0	0	0	0	0	2	2	2	2	2
Providencia sp.	2	2	1	3	2	2	2	2	0	0	0	0	0	0	0	2	2	2	2	2
Salmonella sp.	0	0	0	1	1	1	3	2	2	0	0	0	0	0	0	0	2	2	2	2
Serratia marcescens	3	2	3	1*	1	2	0	2	2	0	0	0	0	0	3	3	2	2	2	2
Shigella sp.	3	3	3	1	1	1	3	2	2	0	0	0	0	0	0	0	2	2	2	2

1 = Preferred antibiotic—High degree of activity against the isolate and likely to be clinically effective, most strains susceptible, has a favorable PK/PD characteristics, has a good safety profile, and has a "low resistance" potential (see Chapter 11 Drug Summaries for antibiotic dosing details). 2 = Alternate choice—With many attributes of a preferred antibiotic. 3 = Acceptable, but preferably select an alternate antibiotic. 0 = No activity or no data or limited experience. * = May be effective initially but as a "high resistance" antibiotic potential, resistance may develop during/after therapy.

Table 3.3. Antibiotic Susceptibility Profiles (Aminoglycosides, Fluoroquinolones, Carbapenems, and Others) (cont'd)

	Amino-Glycosides			Fluoro-Quinolones			Miscellaneous										Carbapenems			
ORGANISMS	Gentamicin (IV)	Tobramycin (IV)	Amikacin (IV)	Ciprofloxacin (IV/PO)	Levofloxacin (IV/PO)	Moxifloxacin (IV/PO)	Colistimethate/ Polymyxin B (IV)	Aztreonam (IV)	Tigecycline (IV)	Vancomycin (IV)	Quinupristin/ dalfopristin (IV)	Linezolid (IV/PO)	Daptomycin (IV)	Telavancin (IV)	Nitrofurantoin † (PO)	Fosfomycin † (PO)	Imipenem (IV)	Meropenem (IV)	Ertapenem (IV)	Doripenem (IV)
Stenotrophomonas (Pseudomonas) maltophilia	0	0	0	3	2	2	2	0	3	0	0	0	0	0	0	0	0	0	0	0
Vibrio vulnificus	0	0	0	3	3	3	3	0	3	0	0	0	0	0	0	0	0	0	0	0
Yersinia enterocolitica	2	2	2	2	2	2	0	2	3	0	0	0	0	0	0	0	0	0	0	0
Anaerobic Gram Positive Cocci (chains)**																				
Peptostreptococcus	0	0	0	0	0	3	0	0	2	3	3	2	0	0	0	0	2	2	2	2
Anaerobic Gram Positive Bacilli																				
Actinomyces sp.	0	0	0	0	0	3	0	0	3		3	0	0	0	0	0	2	2	2	0

Anaerobic Gram Negative Bacilli																				
Bacteroides fragilis group (B distasonis, ovatus, thetaiotaomicron, vulgatus)	0	0	0	0	0	2	0	0	1	0	3	0	0	0	0	0	1	1	1	1
Prevotella sp.	0	0	0	2	2	2	0	0	2	0	0	0	0	0	0	0	2	2	2	2

1 = Preferred antibiotic—High degree of activity against the isolate and likely to be clinically effective, most strains susceptible, has a favorable PK/PD characteristics, has a good safety profile, and has a "low resistance" potential (see Chapter 11 Drug Summaries for antibiotic dosing details).

2 = Alternate choice—With many attributes of a preferred antibiotic.

3 = Acceptable, but preferably select an alternate antibiotic.

0 = No activity or no data or limited experience.

* = May be effective initially but as a "high resistance" antibiotic potential, resistance may develop during/after therapy.

† = For lower tract infections (UTIs)/catheter associated bacteriuria (CAB).

Isolates by Gram Stain Characteristics, Morphologic Arrangement, Oxygen Requirement

AEROBIC ISOLATES

*** Oxidase negative.**
† Catalase positive.

CAPNOPHILIC ISOLATES+

+ Capnophilic organisms grow best under increased CO^2 tension.

ANAEROBIC ISOLATES

++ Microaerophilic organisms. Grow best under decreased O_2 concentration.
*** Oxidase negative.**
† Catalase positive.

YEASTS/FUNGI

Alphabetical Index of Isolates

Table 3.4. Key Factors in Antibiotic Selection When Isolate Known

- **Select an antibiotic with a high degree of activity against the presumed pathogen** (*not colonizer*).
- **Dose appropriate for the target tissue to assure therapeutic/effective concentrations at site of infection**. If necessary, adjust dose ↑ for tissue targets that require higher doses, e.g., bacterial meningitis, endocarditis, etc., or ↓ dose for sites with antibiotic concentrations that are above serum concentrations, e.g., skin, urine, etc.
- **Select an empiric antibiotic with a "low resistance" potential** avoid, if possible, antibiotics with a "high resistance" potential (also with a high degree of activity against the presumed pathogen). Select a "low resistance" potential antibiotic for the same/different class with a high degree of activity.
- **Select antibiotic with a good safety profile** and minimal potential for drug-drug interactions.
- **Select antibiotic that is relatively cost effective** (that first takes into account the above principles).
- **Preferentially use PO antibiotics** unless patient critically ill, unable to take oral medications, or if no oral equivalent antibiotic available.

Table 3.5. Clinical Significance of AEROBIC Isolates Pending Susceptibility Testing

GRAM-POSITIVE COCCI (CLUSTERS)			
Isolate	**Isolate Significance**	**Therapy**	**Comments**
Staphylococcus aureus (MSSA/MRSA) (also see p. 14)	• CSF = C*, P (CNS shunts) • Blood = C*, P (from soft tissue/bone infection, abscess, IV line infection, ABE, PVE) • Sputum = C, P (S. aureus pneumonia is rare; usually only after viral influenza) • Urine = C, P (S. aureus in urine is usually due to skin contamination or rarely overwhelming S. aureus bacteremia) • Stool = C, P (enterocolitis) • Wound = C, P (cellulitis, abscess)	MSSA: Nafcillin (IV), Cefazolin (IV), Clindamycin (IV/PO), a "respiratory quinolone" (IV/PO), Minocycline (IV/PO), Daptomycin (IV), any carbapenem (IV), Linezolid (IV/PO), Tigecycline (IV), Telavancin (IV) Hospital-acquired MRSA (HA-MRSA)/ Community-onset MRSA (CO-MRSA): Daptomycin (IV), Linezolid (IV/PO), Tigecycline (IV), Vancomycin (IV), Minocycline (IV/PO), Quinupristin/ dalfopristin (IV), Telavancin (IV) Community acquired MRSA (CA-MRSA): Doxycycline*, TMP–SMX, Clindamycin VISA/VRSA: Linezolid (IV/PO), Daptomycin (IV), Telavancin (IV)	MSSA: For oral treatment, 1st generation cephalosporins are better than oral anti-staphylococcal penicillins (e.g., dicloxacillin) MRSA: *in-vitro susceptibility testing is unreliable*; treat MRSA infections empirically. Do not treat MRSA colonization. *Do not substitute doxycycline for minocycline for MRSA*. Most effective drugs for MRSA are vancomycin, linezolid, quinupristin/ dalfopristin, minocycline, daptomycin, tigecycline Community-acquired MRSA (CA-MRSA) SCC *mec* IV, V CA-MRSA has different susceptibilities than HA-MRSA/CO-MRSA (see p. 14). CA-MRSA strains with Panton-Valentin Leukocidin PVL+ gene cause two distinct clinical syndromes: severe necrotizing pneumonia (with viral influenza) and severe necrotizing fasciitis/pyomyositis. CA-MRSA is usually susceptible to doxycycline (but minocycline (IV/PO) preferred), TMP–SMX, clindamycin. *Drugs effective against HA-MRSA/CO-MRSA are also effective against CA-MRSA. However, drugs effective against CA-MRSA are may not be effective against HA-MRSA/CO-MRSA* MSSA/MRSA: Noncontinuous low-grade blood culture positivity indicates skin contamination during venipuncture. Continuous high-grade

C = colonizer; C = skin contaminant; NP = non-pathogen at site; P = pathogen at site; (IV/PO) = IV or PO. See p. ix for all other abbreviations.*

* Minocycline (IV/PO) preferred.

Table 3.5. Usual Clinical Significance of AEROBIC Isolates Pending Susceptibility Testing (cont'd)

GRAM-POSITIVE COCCI (CLUSTERS)				
Isolate	**Isolate Significance**	**Preferred Therapy**	**Alternate Therapy**	**Comments**
				blood culture positivity (3/4 or 4/4) indicates intravascular infection or abscess <u>VISA/VRSA:</u> MICs for vancomycin sensitive (VSSA), heteroresistant vancomycin intermediate (hVISA), intermediate (VISA), and resistant (VRSA) S. aureus are < 4 mcg/mL, < 4 mcg/mL (with subpopulations > 4 mcg/mL), 8–16 mcg/mL, and ≥ 32 mcg/mL, respectively.
Staphylococcus epidermidis (MSSE/MRSE) or coagulase-negative staphylococci (CoNS) Staphylococcus lugdunensis	• CSF = C*, P (CNS shunts) • Blood = C*, P (from IV lines, infected implants, prosthetic valve endocarditis [PVE], rarely from native valve subacute bacterial endocarditis [SBE]) • Sputum = C • Urine = C (may be reported as S. saprophyticus; request novobiocin sensitivity to differentiate S. epidermidis from other coagulase-negative staphylococci)	<u>MSSE:</u> Linezolid (IV/PO), Daptomycin (IV), Vancomycin (IV), Telavancin (IV), any carbapenem (IV), a "respiratory quinolone" (IV/PO), Minocycline (IV/PO) <u>MRSE:</u> Linezolid (IV/PO), Daptomycin (IV), Vancomycin (IV), Quinupristin/dalfopristin (IV), Minocycline (IV/PO)		Usually non-pathogenic in absence of prosthetic/implant materials. Common cause of PVE; rare cause of native valve SBE. Treat foreign body-related infection until foreign body is removed. S. lugdunensis is a CoNS but is often misidentified as S. aureus since it produces "clumping factor" which gives a + rapid short tube coagulase test (long tube test –) although a CoNS resembles S. aureus in terms of invasiveness/virulence. Unlike S. aureus, S. lugdensis is pan-sensitive to antibiotics which is another clue the isolate is not S. aureus. S. lugdensis bacteremia associated with community acquired (not nosocomial) SBE.

	• Stool = NP • Wound = C, P (infected foreign body drainage)			
Staphylococcus saprophyticus (coagulase-negative staphylococci)	• CSF = NP • Blood = NP • Sputum = NP • Urine = P (cystitis, pyelo) • Stool = NP • Wound = NP	<u>Preferred therapy</u> Amoxicillin (PO) TMP–SMX (PO) Nitrofurantoin (PO) <u>Alternate therapy</u> Any quinolone (PO) Any 1st generation cephalosporin (PO)		S. saprophyticus UTI is associated with a urinary "fishy odor," alkaline urine pH, and microscopic hematuria. Novobiocin sensitivity differentiates coagulase-negative staphylococci (sensitive) from S. saprophyticus (resistant).
GRAM-POSITIVE COCCI (CHAINS)				
Enterococcus faecalis (VSE)	• CSF = NP (except from S. stercoralis hyperinfection or V-P shunt infection) • Blood = C*, P (from GI/GU source, SBE) • Sputum = NP • Urine = C, P (cystitis, pyelonephritis) • Stool = NP • Wound = C, P (cellulitis)	<u>Non-SBE</u> Ampicillin (IV) Amoxicillin (PO) Meropenem (IV) Piperacillin (IV) Linezolid (IV/PO) Tigecycline (IV) Daptomycin (IV) <u>SBE</u> Gentamicin + ampicillin (IV) or vancomycin (IV) Meropenem (IV) Piperacillin (IV) Linezolid (IV/PO)	<u>Non-SBE</u> Cefoperazone (IV) Chloramphenicol (IV) Levofloxacin (IV/PO) Moxifloxacin (IV/PO) Nitrofurantoin (PO) (UTIs only) <u>SBE</u> Any quinolone (IV/PO) Cefoperazone (IV)	Sensitive to ampicillin, not penicillin. Cause of intermediate (Severity between ABE and SBE) endocarditis, hepatobiliary infections, and UTIs. Enterococci (E. faecalis, E. faecium) are the only cause of SBE (below the waist) from GI/GU sources. Permissive pathogen (i.e., usually does not cause infection alone) in the abdomen/ pelvis. Cefoperazone is the only cephalosporin with anti-E. faecalis (VSE) activity (MIC ~ 32 mcg/mL). Quinupristin/dalfopristin is not active against E. faecalis (VSE). Treat vancomycin resistant E. faecalis as VRE (see E. faecium VRE p. 208).

C = colonizer; C = skin contaminant; NP = non-pathogen at site; P = pathogen at site; (IV/PO) = IV or PO. See p. xi for all other abbreviations.*

Table 3.5. Usual Clinical Significance of AEROBIC Isolates Pending Susceptibility Testing (cont'd)

GRAM-POSITIVE COCCI (CHAINS)				
Isolate	**Isolate Significance**	**Preferred Therapy**	**Alternate Therapy**	**Comments**
Enterococcus faecium (VRE)	• CSF = NP (except from S. stercoralis hyperinfection or V-P shunt infection) • Blood = C*, P (from GI/GU source, SBE) • Sputum = C • Urine = C, P (cystitis, pyelo) • Stool = NP • Wound = C, P (cellulitis)	<u>Non-SBE</u> Linezolid (IV/PO), quinupristin/dalfopristin (IV), doxycycline (IV/PO), tigecycline (IV), chloramphenicol (IV/PO), nitrofurantoin (PO) (UTIs only) <u>SBE</u> Linezolid (IV/PO) Quinupristin/dalfopristin (IV)		Same spectrum of infection as E. faecalis. Colonization common; infection uncommon. Fecal carriage is intermittent but prolonged. In vitro sensitivity = in vivo efficacy. Increased prevalence of E. faecalis (VRE) related to vancomycin IV (not PO) use. Nitrofurantoin preferred for VRE lower UTIs/catheter-associated bacteriuria.
Group A streptococci	• CSF = C*, P (rare cause of ABM) • Blood = P (from skin/soft tissue infection) • Sputum = P (rare cause of CAP) • Urine = NP • Stool = NP • Wound = C, P (cellulitis) • Throat = C, P (pharynx is colonized with Group A streptococci in ~ 30% of patients with EBV mono)	Amoxicillin (PO) Any β-lactam (IV/PO)	Penicillin (PO) Clindamycin (IV/PO)	For Group A streptococcal pharyngitis, amoxicillin is preferred over penicillin. Clindamycin is best for elimination of carrier states, and for penicillin-allergic patients with streptococcal pharyngitis. Any β-lactam is equally effective against Group A streptococci. Nafcillin is the most active anti-staphylococcal penicillin against Group A streptococci. Erythromycin is no longer reliable against Group A streptococci due to increasing resistance. Doxycycline has little/no activity against Group A streptococci.

Group B streptococci (S. agalactiae)	• CSF = P • Blood = P (from IV line/urine source, SBE) • Sputum = NP • Urine = P (CAB, UTIs, especially in diabetics, elderly) • Stool = NP • Wound = C, P (diabetic foot infections)	<u>Non-SBE, non-CNS</u> Clindamycin (IV/PO) Any 1st, 2nd, 3rd generation cephalosporin (IV/PO) <u>SBE</u> Ceftriaxone (IV) Penicillin (IV) Vancomycin (IV) <u>CNS</u> Ceftriaxone (IV) Penicillin (IV)	<u>Non-SBE, non-CNS</u> Vancomycin (IV) Amoxicillin (PO) <u>SBE</u> Meropenem (IV) Ertapenem (IV) Linezolid (IV/PO) <u>CNS</u> Chloramphenicol (IV) Linezolid (IV/PO)	Cause of UTIs and IV line infections in diabetics and the elderly. Cause of neonatal meningitis. Infection is uncommon in the general population. Rarely a cause of SBE in non-pregnant adults. Aminoglycosides and tetracyclines are ineffective of Doxy.
Group C, F, G streptococci	• CSF = P (meningitis) • Blood = P (from skin/soft tissue infection, SBE) • Sputum = P (rare cause of CAP) • Throat = C (especially with viral pharyngitis), P (pharyngitis in medical personnel) • Urine = NP • Stool = NP • Wound = P (cellulitis)	Ceftriaxone (IV) Penicillin (IV) Ampicillin (IV) Clindamycin (IV/PO)	Vancomycin (IV) Amoxicillin (PO) Any 1st, 2nd, 3rd generation cephalosporin (IV) Meropenem (IV) Ertapenem (IV)	Group C, G streptococci may cause pharyngitis, wound infections, and rarely SBE. Group G streptococci associated with malignancies. Common pharyngeal colonizers in medical personnel.

C = colonizer; C = skin contaminant; NP = non-pathogen at site; P = pathogen at site; (IV/PO) = IV or PO. See p. xi for all other abbreviations.*

Table 3.5. Usual Clinical Significance of AEROBIC Isolates Pending Susceptibility Testing (cont'd)

Isolate	Isolate Significance	Preferred Therapy	Alternate Therapy	Comments
GRAM-NEGATIVE COCCI (CHAINS)				
Streptococcus (bovis) gallolyticus	• CSF = NP • Blood = P (SBE from GI source) • Sputum = NP • Urine = NP • Stool = NP • Wound = NP	Ceftriaxone (IV) Ampicillin (IV) Clindamycin (IV/PO)	Vancomycin (IV) Amoxicillin (PO) Any 1st, 2nd, 3rd generation cephalosporin (IV)	Associated with GI malignancies. Non-enterococcal Group D streptococci (e.g., S. bovis) are sensitive to penicillin.
Viridans streptococci (S. mitior, milleri, mitis, mutans, oralis, sanguis, parasanguis, salivarius)	• CSF = NP (aseptic meningitis with SBE) • Blood = C*, P (1° bacteremia, SBE) • Sputum = NP • Urine = NP • Stool = NP • Wound = NP	Ceftriaxone (IV) Penicillin (IV)	Amoxicillin (PO) Any 1st, 2nd, 3rd generation cephalosporin (IV/PO) Meropenem (IV) Ertapenem (IV) Vancomycin (IV)	Viridans streptococci are commonly isolated from blood cultures. Low-grade blood culture positivity (1/4) indicates contamination during venipuncture. Continuous/high-grade blood culture positivity (3/4 or 4/4) indicates SBE until proven otherwise. S. milleri is associated with metastatic abscesses.
GRAM-POSITIVE COCCI (PAIRS)				
Leuconostoc	• CSF = NP • Blood = P (PVE) • Sputum = NP • Urine = P (UTIs) • Stool = NP • Wound = NP	Penicillin (IV) Ampicillin (IV) Clindamycin (IV/PO)	Amoxicillin (PO) Erythromycin (IV) Minocycline (IV/PO) Clarithromycin XL (PO)	Coccobacillary forms resemble streptococci/enterococci. Cause of infection in compromised hosts. Rare cause of IV line infection. Usually vancomycin-resistant.
Streptococcus pneumoniae	• CSF = P (ABM) • Blood = P (from respiratory tract source)	<u>Multidrug Resistant S. pneumoniae (MDRSP)</u> A "respiratory quinolone" (IV/PO); telithromycin (PO); ertapenem (IV);		Penicillin-resistant S. pneumoniae (PRSP) are still sensitive to full-dose/high-dose β-lactams. If possible, avoid macrolides, as > 30% of S. pneumoniae are macrolide resistant (MRSP).

	• Sputum = C, P • Urine = NP • Stool = NP • Wound = P (cellulitis only in SLE)	meropenem (IV); cefepime (IV); linezolid (IV/PO); vancomycin (IV) Sensitive or relatively PCN-resistant Doxycycline (IV/PO); any cephalosporin (IV/PO); clindamycin (IV/PO); amoxicillin/clavulanic acid (PO)		(~ 20–25% are naturally resistant and 10–15% acquire macrolide resistance).
GRAM-NEGATIVE COCCI (PARIS)				
Neisseria gonorrhoeae (GC)	• CSF = NP • Blood = P (from pharyngitis, proctitis, ABE) • Sputum = NP • Urine = P (urethritis) • Stool = NP • Wound = NP • Rectal discharge = P (GC proctitis)	Penicillin-sensitive N. gonorrhoeae (PSNG) Ceftriaxone (IV/IM) Any quinolone (IV/PO) PRNG Ceftriaxone (IV/IM)	Penicillin-sensitive N. gonorrhoeae (PSNG) Penicillin (IV/IM) Amoxicillin (PO) Doxycycline (IV/PO) PPNG Spectinomycin (IM) Any quinolone (PO) Any 1st, 2nd, 3rd gen. cephalosporin (IV/IM)	Cause of "culture negative" right-sided ABE. May be cultured from synovial fluid/blood in disseminated GC infection (arthritis-dermatitis syndrome). Spectinomycin is ineffective against pharyngeal GC/incubating syphilis. PRNG are tetracycline-resistant (TRNG). GC strains from Hawaii/California have increased quinolone resistance; use cefixime or ceftriaxone for such strains. Treat possible Chlamydia trachomatis co-infection and sexual partners.
Neisseria meningitidis	• CSF = P (ABM) • Blood = P (acute/chronic meningococcemia) • Sputum = C, P (only in closed populations, e.g., military recruits)	Penicillin (IV) Ampicillin (IV) Any 3rd generation cephalosporin (IV)	Chloramphenicol (IV) Cefepime (IV) Meropenem (IV)	In ABM, do not decrease meningeal dose of β-lactam antibiotics as patient improves, since CSF penetration/concentration decreases as meningeal inflammation decreases. Chloramphenicol is an excellent choice for penicillin-allergic patients. Preferred meningococcal prophylaxis is an oral quinolone (single dose).

C = colonizer; C = skin contaminant; NP = non-pathogen at site; P = pathogen at site; (IV/PO) = IV or PO.* *See p. xi for all other abbreviations.*

Table 3.5. Usual Clinical Significance of AEROBIC Isolates Pending Susceptibility Testing (cont'd)

Isolate	Isolate Significance	Preferred Therapy	Alternate Therapy	Comments
GRAM-NEGATIVE COCCI (PARIS)				
	• Urine C, P (urethritis rarely) • Stool = NP • Wound = NP			
GRAM-POSITIVE BACILLI				
Arcanobacterium (Corynebacterium) haemolyticum	• CSF = NP • Blood = NP • Sputum = P (oropharyngeal secretions) • Urine = NP • Stool/Wound = NP	Doxycycline (PO)	Erythromycin (PO) Azithromycin (PO) Any 1st, 2nd, 3rd generation cephalosporin (PO) Clarithromycin XL (PO)	Causes membranous pharyngitis with scarlet fever-like rash. Differentiate from C. diphtheriae by culture. Penicillin and ampicillin are less effective than erythromycin or doxycycline.
Bacillus anthracis (naturally acquired) (For potential bioterrorist anthrax, see p. 169)	• CSF = P (ABM) • Blood = P (septicemia; isolation required; dangerous) • Sputum = P (mediastinitis; anthrax pneumonia rare) • Urine = NP • Stool = NP • Wound = P (ulcer; isolation required; dangerous)	Penicillin (IV) Doxycycline (IV/PO) Any quinolone (IV/PO)	Amoxicillin (PO) Ampicillin (IV)	Doxycycline may be used for therapy/outbreak prophylaxis. Streptobacillary configuration in blood. Causes hemorrhagic meningitis, wound infections, and bacteremia. Quinolones are effective. Alert microbiology laboratory of potentially biohazardous specimens.

Bacillus cereus, subtilis, megaterium	• CSF = NP • Blood = C*, P (leukopenic compromised hosts) • Sputum = NP • Urine = NP • Stool = NP • Wound = NP	Vancomycin (IV) Clindamycin (IV/PO)	Meropenem (IV) Any quinolone (IV/PO)	Soil organisms not commonly pathogenic for humans. Suspect pseudoinfection if isolated from clinical specimens. Look for soil/dust contamination of blood culture tube top/apparatus. Rare pathogen in leukopenic compromised hosts.
Corynebacterium diphtheriae	• CSF = NP • Blood = NP • Sputum = P (oropharyngeal secretions) • Urine = NP • Stool = NP • Wound = P (wound diphtheria)	Penicillin (IV) Erythromycin (IV) Clindamycin (IV/PO)	Doxycycline (IV/PO) Clarithromycin XL (PO) Rifampin (PO)	Administer diphtheria antitoxin as soon as possible (p. 166). Antibiotic therapy is adjunctive, since diphtheria is a toxin-mediated disease. Patients may die unexpectedly from toxin-induced myocarditis during recovery.
Corynebacterium jeikeium (JK)	• CSF = C*, P (CSF shunts) • Blood = C*, P (from IV lines) • Sputum = NP • Urine/Stool = NP • Wound = C	Vancomycin (IV) Linezolid (IV/PO)	Quinupristin/ dalfopristin (IV)	Cause of IV line/foreign body infections. In-vitro testing is not always reliable. Highly resistant to most anti-gram positive antibiotics.
Erysipelothrix rhusiopathiae	• CSF = NP • Blood = P (from SBE) • Sputum = NP • Urine = NP • Stool = NP • Wound = P (chronic erysipelas-like skin lesions)	Penicillin (IV) Ampicillin (IV)	Any 3rd generation cephalosporin (IV) Any quinolone (IV/PO)	Cause of "culture-negative" SBE. Susceptible to clindamycin but resistant to vancomycin.

C = colonizer; C = skin contaminant; NP = non-pathogen at site; P = pathogen at site; (IV/PO) = IV or PO. See p. xi for all other abbreviations.*

Table 3.5. Usual Clinical Significance of AEROBIC Isolates Pending Susceptibility Testing (cont'd)

GRAM-POSITIVE BACILLI				
Isolate	**Isolate Significance**	**Preferred Therapy**	**Alternate Therapy**	**Comments**
Listeria monocytogenes	• CSF = P (ABM) • Blood = P (1° bacteremia, SBE) • Sputum = NP • Urine = NP • Stool = NP • Wound = NP	Ampicillin (IV) Amoxicillin (PO) Chloramphenicol (IV) <u>CNS</u> Ampicillin (IV) TMP–SMX (IV/PO) Chloramphenicol (IV/PO) <u>SBE</u> Ampicillin (IV)	Doxycycline (IV/PO) Erythromycin (IV) Meropenem (IV) <u>CNS</u> Meropenem (IV) (Meningeal dosed) Linezolied (IV/PO) <u>SBE</u> Meropenem (IV) Linezolied (IV/PO)	Listeria ABM is common in T-cell deficiencies (e.g., lymphoma, steroids, HIV). Causes SBE in normal hosts, and is the commonest cause of bacteremia in non-neutropenic cancer patients. 3rd generation cephalosporins are ineffective against Listeria.
Nocardia asteroides, brasiliensis	• CSF = P (brain abscess) • Blood = P (from lung/soft tissue source) • Sputum = P (pneumonia, lung abscess) • Urine/Stool = NP • Wound = P (skin lesions from direct inoculation or dissemination)	TMP–SMX (IV/PO) Minocycline (IV/PO)	Imipenem (IV) plus either amikacin (IV) or any 3rd generation cephalosporin (IV)	Branched, filamentous, beady hyphae are typical, but coccobacillary and bacillary forms are also common. Nocardia are gram-positive, aerobic, and acid fast. Linezolid is active against Nocardia and may be effective if other agents cannot be used. Quinolones and macrolides are usually ineffective.
Rhodococcus equi	• CSF = NP • Blood = P (from pneumonia, lung abscess)	Any quinolone (IV/PO) Vancomycin (IV)	Erythromycin (IV) Imipenem (IV) Meropenem (IV)	Causes TB-like community-acquired pneumonia in AIDS patients. Filamentous bacteria break into bacilli/cocci. Aminoglycosides and β-lactams are relatively ineffective.

	• Sputum = P (pneumonia with abscess/cavitation) • Urine = NP • Stool = NP • Wound = NP		Doxycycline (IV/PO) TMP–SMX (IV/PO)	
GRAM-NEGATIVE BACILLI				
Acinetobacter baumannii, lwoffi, calcoaceticus, haemolyticus	• CSF = C*, P (ABM) • Blood = P (from IV line, lung, or urine source) • Sputum = C, P (VAP) • Urine = C, P (CAB) • Stool = NP • Wound = C (common), P (rare)	Any carbapenem (IV) Ampicillin/ sulbactam (IV)	Colistin Polymyxin B Any 3rd generation cephalosporin (IV) (except ceftazidime) Cefepime (IV)	Colonization common; infection uncommon. Occurs in outbreaks of ventilator-associated pneumonia. Usually associated with respiratory support equipment. Test susceptibility to each carbapenem (may be susceptible to one but not others). Use meropenem for MDR susceptible isolates. For meropenem resistant MDR isolates, use colistin, polymyxin B, tigacycline or doripenem.
Actinobacillus actinomycetem-comitans	• CSF = NP • Blood = P (from abscess, SBE) • Sputum = NP • Urine/Stool = NP • Wound = P (from abscess, draining fistulous tract)	Any quinolone (IV/PO) Any 3rd generation cephalosporin (IV/PO)	Penicillin (IV) + gentamicin (IV) TMP–SMX (IV/PO)	Cause of "culture-negative" SBE. One of the HACEK organisms. Found with Actinomyces in abscesses. Resistant to erythromycin and clindamycin.
Aeromonas hydrophila	• CSF = NP • Blood = P (from wound, urine, or GI source) • Sputum = NP • Urine = C, P (CAB) • Stool = P (diarrhea) • Wound = P (cellulitis)	Gentamicin (IV) TMP–SMX (IV/PO) Any quinolone (IV/PO)	Doxycycline (IV/PO) Any 3rd generation cephalosporin (IV/PO) Any carbapenem (IV) Aztreonam (IV)	Cause of wound infection, septic arthritis, diarrhea, and necrotizing soft tissue infection resembling gas gangrene.

C = colonizer; C = skin contaminant; NP = non-pathogen at site; P = pathogen at site; (IV/PO) = IV or PO. See p. xi for all other abbreviations.*

Table 3.5. Usual Clinical Significance of AEROBIC Isolates Pending Susceptibility Testing (cont'd)

GRAM-NEGATIVE BACILLI				
Isolate	**Isolate Significance**	**Preferred Therapy**	**Alternate Therapy**	**Comments**
Alcaligenes (Achromobacter) xylosoxidans	• CSF = P (rarely ABM) • Blood = P (from urine) • Sputum = NP • Urine = P (CAB) • Stool = NP • Wound = P (cellulitis rare)	Imipenem (IV) Meropenem (IV) Any 3rd generation cephalosporin (IV/PO)	Any quinolone (IV/PO) Cefepime (IV) Aztreonam (IV)	Water-borne pathogen resembling Acinetobacter microbiologically. Resistant to aminoglycosides and 1st, 2nd generation cephalosporins.
Bartonella henselae, quintana, bacilliformis	• CSF = NP • Blood = P (from skin source, SBE) • Sputum = NP • Urine = NP • Stool = NP • Wound = P (skin lesions)	Doxycycline (IV/PO) Azithromycin (PO)	Clarithromycin XL (PO) Any quinolone (IV/PO) Any aminoglycoside (IV)	B. henselae (bacteremia, endocarditis, peliosis hepatis, bacillary angiomatosis); B. quintana (relapsing, trench fever, bacillary angiomatosis); B. bacilliformis (Oroyo fever, Carrion's disease). May present as FUO. TMP–SMX and cephalosporins are ineffective.
Bordetella pertussis, parapertussis	• CSF = NP • Blood = P (from respiratory tract source) • Sputum = C, P (pertussis) • Urine = NP • Stool = NP • Wound = NP	Erythromycin (IV) Clarithromycin XL (PO) Azithromycin (IV/PO)	Any quinolone (IV/PO) TMP–SMX (IV/PO) Doxycycline (IV/PO)	Causes pertussis in children and incompletely/non-immunized adults. Macrolides remain the preferred therapy. Resistant to penicillins, cephalosporins, and aminoglycosides.

Brucella abortus, canis, suis, melitensis	• CSF = P (meningitis) • Blood = P (from abscess, SBE) • Sputum = NP • Urine = P (pyelonephritis) • Stool/Wound = NP	Doxycycline (IV/PO) + gentamicin (IV) Doxycycline + streptomycin (IM)	TMP–SMX (IV/PO) + gentamicin (IV) Doxycycline (IV/PO) + rifampin (PO) Any quinolone (IV/PO) + rifampin (PO)	Causes prolonged relapsing infection. Zoonotic cause of brucellosis/Malta fever. Resistant to penicillins.
Burkholderia (Pseudomonas) cepacia	• CSF = NP • Blood = P (usually from IV line/urinary tract infection) • Sputum = C (not a cause of VAP) • Urine = C • Stool = NP • Wound = NP	TMP–SMX (IV/PO)	A "respiratory quinolone" (IV/PO) Minocycline (IV/PO) Chloramphenicol (IV/PO)	Rare cause of urosepsis following urologic instrumentation. Common water-borne colonizer in intensive care units. Opportunistic pathogen in cystic fibrosis/bronchiectasis. Resistant to aminoglycosides, colistin, and polymyxin B.
Burkholderia (Pseudomonas) pseudomallei	• CSF = NP • Blood = P (from septicemic melioidosis) • Sputum = P (chronic cavitary pneumonia) • Urine = NP • Stool = NP • Wound = NP	TMP–SMX (IV/PO) Ceftazidime (IV)	Imipenem (IV) Meropenem (IV) Chloramphenicol (IV)	Causes melioidosis (acute/chronic). Chronic melioidosis resembles reactivation TB, but in lower lobe distribution. Resistant to aminoglycosides.
Campylobacter fetus	• CSF = P (ABM) • Blood = P (from vascular source)	Gentamicin (IV) Imipenem (IV)	Chloramphenicol (IV) Ampicillin (IV)	Causes invasive infection with spread to CNS. CNS infection may be treated with meningeal doses of chloramphenicol, ampicillin, or a

C = colonizer; C = skin contaminant; NP = non-pathogen at site; P = pathogen at site; (IV/PO) = IV or PO. See p. xi for all other abbreviations.*

Table 3.5. Usual Clinical Significance of AEROBIC Isolates Pending Susceptibility Testing (cont'd)

GRAM-NEGATIVE BACILLI				
Isolate	**Isolate Significance**	**Preferred Therapy**	**Alternate Therapy**	**Comments**
	• Sputum = NP • Urine = NP • Stool = NP • Wound = NP	Meropenem (IV)	Any 3rd generation cephalosporin (IV)	3rd generation cephalosporin. Resistant to erythromycin.
Campylobacter jejuni	• CSF = NP • Blood = P (from GI source) • Sputum = NP • Urine = NP • Stool = P (diarrhea) • Wound = NP	Any quinolone (IV/PO) Erythromycin (PO) Doxycycline (IV/PO)	Azithromycin (PO) Clarithromycin XL (PO)	Commonest cause of acute bacterial diarrhea. Resistant to TMP–SMX.
Cardiobacterium hominis	• CSF = NP • Blood = P (from SBE) • Sputum = NP • Urine = NP • Stool = NP • Wound = NP	Penicillin (IV) + gentamicin (IV) Ampicillin (IV) + gentamicin (IV)	Any 3rd generation cephalosporin (IV) + gentamicin (IV)	Pleomorphic bacillus with bulbous ends. Often appears in clusters resembling rosettes. Cause of "culture-negative" SBE (one of the HACEK organisms). Rare cause of abdominal abscess. Grows best with CO_2 enhancement. Resistant to macrolides and clindamycin.
Chromobacterium violaceum	• CSF = NP • Blood = P (from wound infection) • Sputum = NP • Urine = NP • Stool = NP • Wound = P (drainage from deep soft tissue infection)	Gentamicin (IV) Doxycycline (IV/PO)	Chloramphenicol (IV)	Cause of cutaneous lesions primarily in tropical/subtropical climates. Often mistaken for Vibrio or Alcaligenes. Resistant to β-lactams.

Chryseobacterium (Flavobacterium) meningosepticum	• CSF = P (ABM) • Blood = P (from IV line infection, PVE) • Sputum = NP • Urine = C, P (from urologic instrumentation) • Stool = NP • Wound = C, P (cellulitis)	CNS TMP–SMX (IV/PO) Non-CNS Vancomycin (IV) + rifampin (PO) Any quinolone (IV/PO)	CNS Chloramphenicol (IV) Non-CNS Clarithromycin XL (PO) + rifampin (PO) Clindamycin (IV/PO)	Rare cause of ABM in newborns and PVE in adults. Only unencapsulated Flavobacterium species. Clindamycin, clarithromycin, and vancomycin are useful only in non-CNS infections. Resistant to aztreonam and carbapenems.
Citrobacter diversus, freundii, koseri	• CSF = C*, P (from NS procedure) • Blood = C*, P (from IV line/urinary tract infection) • Sputum = C (not pneumonia) • Urine = C, P (from urologic instrumentation) • Stool = NP • Wound = C, P (rarely in compromised hosts)	Any carbapenem (IV) Cefepime (IV) Any quinolone (IV/PO)	Aztreonam (IV) Piperacillin (IV) Any 3rd generation cephalosporin (IV)	Common wound/urine colonizer. Rare pathogen in normal hosts. Often aminoglycoside resistant. (C. freundii is usually more resistant than C. koseri).
Edwardsiella tarda	• CSF = NP • Blood = P (from liver abscess) • Sputum/Urine = NP • Stool = P • Wound C, P (wound infection)	Ampicillin (IV) Amoxicillin (PO) Any quinolone (IV/PO)	Doxycycline (IV/PO) Any 3rd generation cephalosporin (IV/PO)	Cause of bacteremia, usually from liver abscess or wound source.

C = colonizer; C = skin contaminant; NP = non-pathogen at site; P = pathogen at site; (IV/PO) = IV or PO. See p. xi for all other abbreviations.*

Table 3.5. Usual Clinical Significance of AEROBIC Isolates Pending Susceptibility Testing (cont'd)

GRAM-NEGATIVE BACILLI				
Isolate	**Isolate Significance**	**Preferred Therapy**	**Alternate Therapy**	**Comments**
Enterobacter agglomerans, aerogenes, cloacae	• CSF = C*, P (from NS procedure) • Blood = C*, P (from IV line/urinary tract infection) • Sputum = C (not a cause of pneumonia) • Urine = C, P (post-urologic instrumentation) • Stool = NP • Wound = C, P (rarely in compromised hosts)	Any carbapenem (IV)	Any quinolone (IV/PO) Aztreonam (IV) Piperacillin (IV) Cefepime (IV)	Not a cause of community-acquired or nosocomial pneumonia. Common colonizer of respiratory secretions and wound/urine specimens. Antibiotic resistance to E. cloacae > E. aerogenes > E. agglomerans. Treatment of Enterobacter colonizers with ceftazidime or ciprofloxacin may result in MDR/ESBL Enterobacter sp.
Escherichia coli	• CSF = P (ABM) • Blood = P (from GI/GU source) • Sputum = P (rarely CAP from urinary source, VAP) • Urine = C, P (CAB, cystitis, pyelonephritis) • Stool = C, P (diarrhea) • Wound = P (cellulitis)	Any 1st, 2nd, 3rd generation cephalosporin (IV/PO) Amoxicillin (PO) Any quinolone (IV/PO) Ceftriaxone (IV) Nitrofurantoin (PO) (UTIs only)	Aztreonam (IV) Gentamicin (IV) TMP–SMX (IV/PO)	Common pathogen, usually from GI/GU source. Many strains are resistant to ampicillin and some to 1st generation cephalosporins. ESBL-producing E. coli may be treated with a carbepenem.
Francisella tularensis	• CSF = NP • Blood = P (isolation dangerous)	Doxycycline (IV/PO)	Chloramphenicol (IV/PO)	Six clinical tularemia syndromes. Alert microbiology laboratory of potentially biohazardous specimens. Do not culture.

	• Sputum = P (tularemic pneumonia; isolation dangerous) • Urine/Stool = NP • Wound = P (isolation dangerous)	Gentamicin (IV/IM) Streptomycin (IM)	Any quinolone (IV/PO)	Resistant to penicillins and cephalosporins. Bioterrorist tularemia is treated the same as naturally-acquired tularemia.
Hafnia alvei	• CSF = C, P (from NS procedure) • Blood = C*, P (from IV line/urinary tract infection) • Sputum = C (not pneumonia) • Urine = C, P (post-urologic instrumentation) • Stool = NP • Wound = C, P (rarely in compromised hosts)	Cefepime (IV) Any quinolone (IV/PO) Aztreonam (IV)	Piperacillin (IV) Imipenem (IV) Meropenem (IV)	Formerly Enterobacter hafniae. Uncommon nosocomial pathogen. Rarely pathogenic in normal hosts. Cause of UTIs in compromised hosts.
Helicobacter (Campylobacter) pylori	• CSF = NP • Blood = NP • Sputum = NP • Urine = NP • Stool = P (from upper GI tract biopsy specimens, not stool) • Wound = NP	Omeprazole (PO) + clarithromycin XL (PO) Omeprazole (PO) + amoxicillin (PO) Metronidazole (PO) + amoxicillin (PO) + bismuth subsalicylate (PO)	Doxycycline (PO) + metronidazole (PO) + bismuth subsalicylate (PO)	Optimal therapy awaits definition. Treat until cured. Some strains of resistant H. pylori may respond to treatment with a quinolone. TMP–SMX is ineffective.

C = colonizer; C = skin contaminant; NP = non-pathogen at site; P = pathogen at site; (IV/PO) = IV or PO. See p. xi for all other abbreviations.*

Table 3.5. Usual Clinical Significance of AEROBIC Isolates Pending Susceptibility Testing (cont'd)

GRAM-NEGATIVE BACILLI				
Isolate	**Isolate Significance**	**Preferred Therapy**	**Alternate Therapy**	**Comments**
Hemophilus influenzae, parainfluenzae, aphrophilus, paraphrophilus	• CSF = P (ABM) • Blood = P (from respiratory tract or cardiac source) • Sputum = C, P (CAP) • Urine = NP • Stool = NP • Wound = P	For all Hemophilus species Any 2nd, 3rd generation cephalosporin (IV/PO) Any quinolone (IV/PO) Doxycycline (IV/PO)	For all Hemophilus species Chloramphenicol (IV) TMP–SMX (IV/PO) Azithromycin (PO) Aztreonam (IV) Ampicillin-resistant H. influenzae Meropenem (IV) Imipenem (IV) Ertapenem (IV) Cefepime (IV) Aztreonam (IV)	1st generation cephalosporins, erythromycin, and clarithromycin have limited anti-H. influenzae activity; doxycycline and azithromycin are better. Hemophilus species are common colonizers of the respiratory tract. Rarely a cause of "culture-negative" SBE (H. parainfluenzae/aphrophilus are HACEK organisms). Growth enhanced with CO_2. 1st gen. cephalosporins and penicillin have little anti-H. influenzae activity.
Kingella (Moraxella) kingae	• CSF = NP • Blood = P (from skeletal or cardiac source) • Sputum = C • Urine = NP • Stool/wound = NP	Ampicillin (IV) + any aminoglycoside (IV)	Any 3rd generation (IV) cephalosporin + any aminoglycoside (IV) Imipenem (IV) Meropenem (IV) Any quinolone (IV/PO)	Common colonizer of respiratory tract, but rarely a respiratory pathogen. Causes septic arthritis/osteomyelitis in children and endocarditis in adults (one of HACEK organisms). Oxidase positive. Growth enhanced with CO_2.

Klebsiella pneumoniae, oxytoca	• CSF = P (ABM) • Blood = P (from respiratory, GI, GU source) • Sputum = C, P (CAP/VAP) • Urine = C (CAB), P • Stool = NP • Wound = C, P	Tigecycline (IV) Any carbapenem (IV)	Any 3rd generation cephalosporin (IV, PO) except ceftazidine Any quinolone (IV/PO) Aztreonam (IV) Cefepime (IV)	TMP–SMX may be ineffective in systemic infection. Anti-pseudomonal penicillins have limited anti-Klebsiella activity. Klebsiella usually susceptible to carbapenems. Carbapenem resistant MDR Klebisella usually susceptible to tigecycline, colistin, polymyxin B.
Klebsiella ozaenae, rhinoscleromatis	• CSF = NP • Blood = NP • Sputum = NP • Urine = NP • Stool = NP • Wound = P (rhinoscleromatis lesions)	Any quinolone (PO)	TMP–SMX (PO) + rifampin (PO)	Skin infection usually requires prolonged treatment for cure (weeks-to-months).
Legionella sp.	• CSF = NP • Blood = NP • Sputum = P (CAP or VAP) • Urine = NP • Stool = NP • Wound = NP	Any quinolone (IV/PO) Doxycycline (IV/PO) Tigacycline (IV) Azithromycin (IV/PO)	Clarithromycin XL (PO) Erythromycin (IV) Telithromycin (PO)	Anti-Legionella activity: quinolones > doxycycline > erythromycin. Erythromycin failures are not uncommon. Rarely a cause of culture-negative SBE/PVE.
Leptospira interrogans	• CSF = P (ABM) • Blood = P (1° bacteremia) • Sputum = NP • Urine = P (excreted in urine) • Stool = NP • Wound = NP	Doxycycline (IV/PO) Penicillin G (IV) Any 3rd generation cephalosporin (IV/PO)	Amoxicillin (PO)	Blood/urine cultures may be positive during initial/bacteremic phase, but are negative during immune phase. Relapse is common. Resistant to chloramphenicol.

C = colonizer; C = skin contaminant; NP = non-pathogen at site; P = pathogen at site; (IV/PO) = IV or PO. See p. xi for all other abbreviations.*

Table 3.5. Usual Clinical Significance of AEROBIC Isolates Pending Susceptibility Testing (cont'd)

GRAM-NEGATIVE BACILLI				
Isolate	**Isolate Significance**	**Preferred Therapy**	**Alternate Therapy**	**Comments**
Moraxella (Branhamella) catarrhalis	• CSF = NP • Blood = P (rarely from CAP) • Sputum = C, P (CAP) • Urine = NP • Stool = NP • Wound = NP	Any 2nd, 3rd generation cephalosporin (IV/PO) Any quinolone (IV/PO) Telithromycin (PO) Doxycycline (IV/PO)	Azithromycin (PO) Clarithromycin XL (PO) TMP–SMX (IV/PO) Amoxicillin/ clavulanic acid (PO)	Almost all strains are β-lactamase positive and resistant to penicillin/ampicillin. β-lactamase-resistant β-lactams are effective.
Morganella morganii	• CSF = NP • Blood = P (from GU source) • Sputum = NP • Urine = P (CAB, cystitis, pyelonephritis) • Stool = NP • Wound = P (cellulitis rare)	Any quinolone (IV/PO) Any 3rd generation cephalosporin (IV) Any carbapenem (IV)	Any aminoglycoside (IV) Aztreonam (IV) Cefepime (IV)	Common uropathogen. Causes bacteremia with urosepsis. Rare cause of wound infections.
Ochrobactrum anthropi (CDC group Vd)	• CSF = NP • Blood = P (from IV line infections) • Sputum = C • Urine = C • Stool/Wound = C	Any quinolone (IV/PO) TMP–SMX (IV/PO)	Any aminoglycoside (IV) Imipenem (IV) Meropenem (IV)	Pathogen in compromised hosts. Oxidase and catalase positive. Resistant to β-lactams.

Pasteurella multocida	• CSF = P (ABM) • Blood = P (from respiratory source, bite wound/abscess) • Sputum = C, P (CAP, bronchiectasis) • Urine = C, P (pyelonephritis) • Stool = NP • Wound = P (human/animal bites)	Amoxicillin (PO) Doxycycline (IV/PO) Penicillin G (IV)	Ampicillin/sulbactam (IV) Piperacillin (IV) Any quinolone (IV/PO)	Common cause of infection following dog/cat bites. Many antibiotics are effective, but erythromycin is ineffective.
Plesiomonas shigelloides	• CSF = NP • Blood = P (from GU source) • Sputum = NP • Urine = NP • Stool = P (diarrhea) • Wound = NP	Any quinolone (PO) TMP–SMX (PO)	Doxycycline (PO) Aztreonam (PO)	Infrequent cause of diarrhea, less commonly dysentery. Oxidase positive. β-lactamase strains are increasing. Resistant to penicillins.
Proteus mirabilis, vulgaris	• CSF = NP • Blood = P (from urinary source) • Sputum = C • Urine = C, P (from urologic instrumentation) • Stool = NP • Wound = C, P (wound infection)	P. mirabilis, indole (–) Ampicillin (IV) Any 1st, 2nd, 3rd gen. cephalosporin (IV/PO) P. vulgaris, indole (+) Any 3rd generation cephalosporin (IV/PO) Cefepime (IV) Any quinolone (IV/PO)	P. mirabilis, indole (–) TMP–SMX (IV/PO) Amoxicillin (PO) P. vulgaris, indole (+) Aztreonam (IV) Any carbapenem (IV) Any aminoglycoside (IV)	Usually a uropathogen. Most antibiotics are effective against P. mirabilis (indole-negative); P. penneri (indole-negative P. vulgaris) is resistant to ceftriaxone. Indole-positive Proteus sp. require potent antibiotics to treat non-UTIs. P. penneri (indole-negative P. vulgaris) resistant to 3rd gen. cephalosporins; use cefepime, carbapenem, or quinolone.

C = colonizer; C = skin contaminant; NP = non-pathogen at site; P = pathogen at site; (IV/PO) = IV or PO.* *See p. xi for all other abbreviations.*

Table 3.5. Usual Clinical Significance of AEROBIC Isolates Pending Susceptibility Testing (cont'd)

GRAM-NEGATIVE BACILLI				
Isolate	**Isolate Significance**	**Preferred Therapy**	**Alternate Therapy**	**Comments**
Providencia alcalifaciens, rettgeri, stuartii	• CSF = NP • Blood = C*, P (from GU source) • Sputum/Stool = NP • Urine = C, P • Wound = C, P (rare)	Any quinolone (IV/PO) Any 3rd generation cephalosporin (IV/PO) Cefepime (IV) Meropenem (IV) Ertapenem (IV)	Any aminoglycoside (IV) Aztreonam (IV) Piperacillin (IV) Imipenem (IV)	Almost always a uropathogen. Formerly classified as indole-positive Proteus.
Pseudomonas aeruginosa	• CSF = NP • Blood = P (from respiratory, GU source) • Sputum = C (usually), P (rarely indicates VAP) • Urine = C, P (from urologic instrumentation) • Stool = NP • Wound = C (almost always)	Monotherapy Meropenem (IV) Cefepime (IV) Combination therapy either meropenem (IV) or cefepime (IV) *plus* amikacin	Doripenem (IV) Colistin (IV) Polymyxin B (IV) Amikacin (IV) Aztreonam (IV)	For serious systemic P. aeruginosa infection, double-drug therapy preferred. All double anti-P. aeruginosa regimens are equally effective. Individual differences in activity (MICs) are unimportant if combination therapy is used. If MDR P. aeruginosa meropenem susceptible, treat with meropenem. If MDR P. aeruginosa meropenem resistant, treat with colistin, polymyxin B, or doripenem.
Pseudomonas (Chryseomonas) luteola (CDC group Ve-1)	• CSF = NP • Blood = P (from IV line infection) • Sputum = NP • Urine = NP • Stool = NP • Wound = NP	Imipenem (IV) Meropenem (IV) Cefepime (IV)	Piperacillin/ tazobactam (IV) Aztreonam (IV)	Opportunistic pathogen primarily in compromised hosts.

Pseudomonas (Flavimonas) oryzihabitans (CDC group Ve-2)	• CSF = P (NS procedures) • Blood = P (from IV line infection) • Sputum = NP • Urine = NP • Stool = NP • Wound = P (rare)	Imipenem (IV) Meropenem (IV) Cefepime (IV)	Any 3rd generation cephalosporin (IV) Piperacillin (IV) Aztreonam (IV)	Rare cause of central IV line infections in compromised hosts (usually in febrile neutropenics). Rare cause of peritonitis in CAPD patients. Oxidase negative, unlike other Pseudomonas species.
Salmonella typhi, non-typhi	• CSF = NP • Blood = P (from GI source) • Sputum = NP • Urine = P (only with enteric fever) • Stool = C (carrier), P (gastroenteritis, enteric fever) • Wound = NP	Any quinolone (IV/PO) Any 3rd generation cephalosporin (IV)	Chloramphenicol (IV) TMP–SMX (IV/PO) Doxycycline (IV/PO)	Carrier state is best eliminated by a quinolone or TMP–SMX. If drug therapy fails to eliminate carrier state, look for hepatic/bladder calculi for persistent focus. Many strains are resistant to ampicillin/amoxicillin.
Serratia marcescens	• CSF = P (from NS procedures) • Blood = P (from IV line or urinary source) • Sputum = C, P (rarely in VAP) • Urine = C, P (post-urologic instrumentation) • Stool = NP • Wound = C, P (rare)	Any 3rd generation cephalosporin (IV/PO) (except ceftazidime) Any quinolone (IV/PO) Cefepime (IV)	Any carbapenem (IV) Gentamicin (IV) Aztreonam (IV) Piperacillin (IV)	Enterobacteriaceae. Associated with water sources. Common colonizer of respiratory secretions/urine in ICU. Serratia nosocomial pneumonia and PVE are rare. Cause of septic arthritis, osteomyelitis, and SBE (IV drug abusers). Among the aminoglycosides, gentamicin has the greatest anti-Serratia activity.

C = colonizer; C = skin contaminant; NP = non-pathogen at site; P = pathogen at site; (IV/PO) = IV or PO. See p. xi for all other abbreviations.*

Table 3.5. Usual Clinical Significance of AEROBIC Isolates Pending Susceptibility Testing (cont'd)

GRAM-NEGATIVE BACILLI				
Isolate	**Isolate Significance**	**Preferred Therapy**	**Alternate Therapy**	**Comments**
Shigella boydii, sonnei, flexneri, dysenteriae	• CSF = NP • Blood = P (from GI source) • Sputum = NP • Urine = NP • Stool = P (Shigella dysentery) • Wound = NP	Any quinolone (IV/PO)	TMP–SMX (IV/PO) Azithromycin (IV/PO)	No carrier state. Severity of dysentery varies with the species: S. dysenteriae (most severe) > S. flexneri > S. sonnei/boydii (least severe).
Steno-trophomonas (Pseudomonas, Xanthomonas) maltophilia	• CSF = C, P (from NS procedures) • Blood = C*, P (from IV line infection, GU source) • Sputum = C (not VAP) • Urine = C, P (from urologic instrumentation) • Stool = NP • Wound = C, P (rarely in compromised hosts)	TMP–SMX (IV/PO) Minocycline (IV/PO)	Cefepime (IV) Any respiratory quinolone (IV/PO)	Potential pulmonary pathogen only in bronchiectasis/cystic fibrosis. Resistant to aminoglycosides and carbapenems. Susceptible to colistin, polymyxin B.
Streptobacillus moniliformis	• CSF = P (brain abscess) • Blood = P (from wound) • Sputum = P (lung abscess) • Urine = NP • Stool = NP	Penicillin (IV) Ampicillin (IV) Amoxicillin (PO)	Oxycycline (IV/PO) Erythromycin (IV) DClindamycin (IV/PO)	Cause of Haverhill fever and rat-bite fever, with abrupt onset of severe headache/arthralgias after bite wound has healed. No regional adenopathy. Morbilliform/petechial rash. Arthritis in 50%. May cause SBE.

	• Wound = P (from rat bite)			
Vibrio cholerae	• CSF = NP • Blood = P (from GI source) • Sputum = NP • Urine = NP • Stool = P (cholera) • Wound = NP	Doxycycline (IV/PO) Any quinolone (IV/PO)	TMP–SMX (IV/PO)	No carrier state. Treat for 3 days. Single-dose therapy is often effective. Resistant to ampicillin.
Vibrio parahaemolyticus	• CSF = NP • Blood = P (from GI source) • Sputum = NP • Urine = NP • Stool = P (diarrhea) • Wound = P	Doxycycline (IV/PO)	Any quinolone (IV/PO)	Most cases of gastroenteritis caused by V. parahaemolyticus are self-limited and require no treatment.
Vibrio vulnificus, alginolyticus	• CSF = NP • Blood = P (from GI/ wound source) • Sputum = NP • Urine = NP • Stool = P (diarrhea) • Wound = P (water-contaminated wound raw oysters, other shell fish ingestion)	Doxycycline (IV/PO) Any quinolone (IV/PO)	Piperacillin (IV) Ampicillin/ sulbactam (IV)	Causes necrotizing soft tissue infection resembling gas gangrene. Patients are critically ill with fever, bullous lesions, diarrhea, and hypotension. Treat wound infection, bacteremia. Aminoglycoside susceptibilities are unpredictable.
Yersinia enterocolitica	• CSF = NP • Blood = P (from GI source) • Sputum = NP • Urine = NP • Stool = P (diarrhea) • Wound = NP	Any quinolone (IV/PO) Gentamicin (IV) Doxycycline (IV/PO)	TMP–SMX (IV/PO) Any 3rd generation cephalosporin (IV/PO)	Cause of diarrhea with abdominal pain. If pain in is right lower quadrant, may be mistaken for acute appendicitis.

C = colonizer; C = skin contaminant; NP = non-pathogen at site; P = pathogen at site; (IV/PO) = IV or PO.* *See p. xi for all other abbreviations.*

Table 3.5. Usual Clinical Significance of AEROBIC Isolates Pending Susceptibility Testing (cont'd)

Isolate	Isolate Significance	Preferred Therapy	Alternate Therapy	Comments
GRAM-NEGATIVE BACILLI				
Yersinia pestis	• CSF = NP • Blood = P (septicemic plague; isolation required; dangerous) • Sputum = P (pneumonic plague; isolation required; dangerous) • Urine = NP • Stool = NP • Wound = P (lymph nodes, lymph node drainage; bubonic plague; isolation required; dangerous)	Doxycycline (IV/PO) Streptomycin (IM) Gentamicin (IV/IM) Any quinolone (IV/PO)	Chloramphenicol (IV/PO)	Cause of bubonic, septicemic, and pneumonic plague. Doxycycline or any quinolone may be used for prophylaxis. Alert microbiology laboratory of potentially biohazardous specimens. Do not culture. Bioterrorist plague is treated the same as naturally-acquired plague.
SPIROCHETES				
Borrelia burgdorferi	• CSF = P (neuroborreliosis) • Blood = P (rarely isolated; requires special media) • Sputum = NP • Urine = NP • Stool = NP • Wound = P (rarely isolated from erythema migrans lesions)	Doxycycline (PO) Amoxicillin (PO)	Any cephalosporin (PO) Azithromycin (PO) Erythromycin (PO)	Cause of Lyme disease. β-lactams and doxycycline are effective. Erythromycin least effective for erythema migrans. Minocycline may be preferred to doxycycline for neuroborreliosis.

Borrelia recurrentis	• CSF = P (ABM) • Blood = P (1° bacteremia) • Sputum = NP • Urine = NP • Stool = NP • Wound = NP	Doxycycline (IV/PO) Azithromycin (IV/PO)	Erythromycin (IV) Penicillin (IV) Ampicillin (IV) Any 1st, 2nd, 3rd generation cephalosporin (IV/PO)	Cause of relapsing fever. May be recovered from septic metastatic foci. Septic emboli may cause sacroiliitis, SBE, myositis, orchitis, or osteomyelitis.
Spirillum minus	• CSF = NP • Blood = P (from wound source, SBE) • Sputum = NP • Urine = NP • Stool = NP • Wound = P (from rat bite)	Penicillin (IV) Amoxicillin (PO)	Doxycycline (IV/PO) Any quinolone (IV/PO)	Cause of rat-bite fever. Bite wound heals promptly, but 1–4 weeks later becomes painful, purple and swollen, and progresses to ulceration and eschar formation. Painful regional adenopathy. Central maculopapular rash is common (rarely urticarial). Arthralgias/arthritis is rare compared to rat-bite fever from Streptobacillus moniliformis. Rarely causes SBE.

C = colonizer; C = skin contaminant; NP = non-pathogen at site; P = pathogen at site; (IV/PO) = IV or PO. See p. xi for all other abbreviations.*

Table 3.6. Clinical Significance of CAPNOPHILIC Isolates Pending Susceptibility Testing

GRAM-NEGATIVE BACILLI				
Isolate	**Isolate Significance**	**Preferred Therapy**	**Alternate Therapy**	**Comments**
Capnocytophaga canimorsus (group DF-2)	• CSF = NP • Blood = P (from GI source, bite wound) • Sputum = NP • Urine = NP • Stool = NP • Wound = P (from dog/cat bite)	Ampicillin/ sulbactam (IV) Piperacillin/ tazobactam (IV) Imipenem (IV) Meropenem (IV) Ertapenem (IV)	Clindamycin (IV/PO) Any quinolone (IV/PO) Doxycycline (IV/PO)	Associated with animal bites or cancer. May cause fatal septicemia in cirrhotics/asplenics. Resistant to aminoglycosides, metronidazole, TMP–SMX, and aztreonam.
Capnocytophaga ochraceus (group DF-1)	• CSF = NP • Blood = P (from GI, wound, abscess source) • Sputum = NP • Urine = NP • Stool = NP • Wound = P	Ampicillin/ sulbactam (IV) Piperacillin/ tazobactam (IV) Imipenem (IV) Meropenem (IV) Ertapenem (IV)	Clindamycin (IV/PO) Any quinolone (IV/PO) Doxycycline (IV/PO)	Thin, spindle-shaped bacilli resemble Fusobacteria morphologically. "Gliding motility" seen in hanging drop preparations. Cause of septicemia, abscesses, and wound infections. Resistant to aminoglycosides, metronidazole, TMP–SMX, and aztreonam.
Eikenella corrodens	• CSF = NP • Blood = P (SBE in IV drug abusers) • Sputum = NP • Urine = NP • Stool = NP • Wound = P (IV drug abusers)	Penicillin (IV) Ampicillin (IV) Imipenem (IV) Meropenem (IV) Ertapenem (IV)	Piperacillin (IV) Ampicillin/ sulbactam (IV) Doxycycline (IV/PO) Amoxicillin (PO)	Cause of "culture-negative" SBE (one of the HACEK organisms). Resistant to clindamycin and metronidazole.

C = colonizer; C = skin contaminant; NP = non-pathogen at site; P = pathogen at site; (IV/PO) = IV or PO. See p. xi for all other abbreviations.*

Table 3.7. Usual Clinical Significance of ANAEROBIC Isolates Pending Susceptibility Testing

Isolate	Isolate Significance	Preferred Therapy	Alternate Therapy	Comments
GRAM-POSITIVE BACILLI				
Peptococcus	• CSF = P (brain abscess) • Blood = P (from GI/pelvic source) • Sputum = C, P (aspiration pneumonia, lung abscess) • Urine/Stool = NP • Wound = P (rarely a sole pathogen)	Penicillin (IV) Ampicillin (IV) Amoxicillin (PO) Clindamycin (IV/PO)	Chloramphenicol (IV) Erythromycin (IV) Any carbapenem (IV) Moxifloxacin (IV/PO)	Normal flora of mouth, GI tract, and pelvis. Associated with mixed aerobic/anaerobic dental, abdominal, and pelvic infections, especially abscesses.
Peptostreptococcus	• CSF = P (brain abscess) • Blood = P (GI/pelvic source) • Sputum = C, P (aspiration pneumonia, lung abscess) • Urine/Stool = NP • Wound = P (rarely a sole pathogen)	Penicillin (IV) Ampicillin (IV) Amoxicillin (PO) Clindamycin (IV/PO)	Chloramphenicol (IV) Erythromycin (IV) Any carbapenem (IV) Moxifloxacin (IV/PO)	Normal flora of mouth, GI tract, and pelvis. Associated with mixed aerobic/anaerobic dental, abdominal, and pelvic infections, especially abscesses.
GRAM-POSITIVE BACILLI				
Actinomyces israelii, odontolyticus	• CSF = P (brain abscess) • Blood = NP	Amoxicillin (PO) Doxycycline (PO)	Erythromycin (PO) Clindamycin (PO)	Anaerobic and non-acid fast. Usually presents as cervical, facial, thoracic, or abdominal masses/fistulas. Prolonged

C = colonizer; C = skin contaminant; NP = non-pathogen at site; P = pathogen at site; (IV/PO) = IV or PO. See p. xi for all other abbreviations.*

Table 3.7. Clinical Significance of ANAEROBIC Isolates Pending Susceptibility Testing (cont'd)

GRAM-POSITIVE BACILLI				
Isolate	**Isolate Significance**	**Preferred Therapy**	**Alternate Therapy**	**Comments**
	• Sputum = C, P (lung abscess) • Urine = NP • Stool = NP • Wound = P (fistulas/ underlying abscess)			(6–12 month) treatment is needed for cure. Unlike Nocardia, Actinomyces rarely causes CNS infections. May be cultured from polymicrobial brain abscess of pulmonary origin. Quinolones, aminoglycosides, metronidazole, and TMP–SMX have little activity.
Arachnia propionica	• CSF = P (brain abscess) • Blood = P (from dental, GI, lung source) • Sputum = C, P (lung abscess) • Urine = NP • Stool = NP • Wound = NP	Clindamycin (IV/PO) Ampicillin (IV) + gentamicin (IV)	Erythromycin (IV)	Polymicrobial pathogen in dental, lung, and brain abscesses.
Bifidobacterium sp.	• CSF = P (brain abscess) • Blood = NP • Sputum = C, P (lung abscess) • Urine/Stool = NP • Wound = NP	Clindamycin (IV/PO) Ampicillin (IV) + gentamicin (IV)	Erythromycin (IV)	Usually part of polymicrobial infection.
Clostridium botulinum	• CSF = NP • Blood = NP • Sputum = NP	Penicillin (IV)	Clindamycin (IV/PO) Imipenem (IV) Meropenem (IV)	Give trivalent equine antitoxin (p. 165) as soon as possible. Antibiotic therapy is adjunctive.

	• Urine/Stool = NP • Wound = P (wound botulism)			
Clostridium difficile	• CSF = NP • Blood = P (rarely from GI source) • Sputum = NP • Urine = NP • Stool = C (normal fecal flora), P (antibiotic-associated diarrhea/colitis) • Wound = NP	C. difficile diarrhea Vancomycin (PO) Nitazoxanide (PO) C. difficile colitis Metronidazole (IV/PO) Nitazoxanide (PO)	C. difficile diarrhea Metronidazole (PO) C. difficile colitis Tigacycline (IV)	**C. difficile diarrhea** PO vancomycin preferred. *PO vancomycin more reliably effective than PO metronidazole*. Nitazoxanide also highly effective. PO metronidazole, not PO vancomycin, increases prevalence of VRE. **C. difficile colitis**, use IV or PO metronidazole (IV vancomycin ineffective). Nitazoxanide (PO) or tigacycline (IV) also highly effective. Diagnose C. difficile diarrhea by stool C. difficile toxin assay. Diagnose C. difficile pancolitis colitis by C. difficile + toxin assay plus abdominal CT scan/ colonoscopy.
Clostridium perfringens, septicum, novyi	• CSF = NP • Blood = P (from GI source/malignancy) • Sputum = NP • Urine = NP • Stool = NP • Wound = P (gas gangrene)	Penicillin (IV) Piperacillin/ tazobactam (IV) Meropenem (IV) Ertapenem (IV)	Clindamycin (IV) Chloramphenicol (IV) Imipenem (IV)	Usual cause of myonecrosis (gas gangrene). Surgical debridement is crucial; antibiotic therapy is adjunctive. Also causes emphysematous cholecystitis/cystitis.
Clostridium tetani	• CSF = NP • Blood = NP • Sputum = NP • Urine/Stool = NP • Wound = P (wound tetanus)	Penicillin (IV) Clindamycin (IV)	Imipenem (IV) Meropenem (IV)	Prompt administration of tetanus immune globulin is crucial (p. 166). Antibiotic therapy is adjunctive.

C = colonizer; C = skin contaminant; NP = non-pathogen at site; P = pathogen at site; (IV/PO) = IV or PO. See p. xi for all other abbreviations.*

Table 3.7. Usual Clinical Significance of ANAEROBIC Isolates Pending Susceptibility Testing (cont'd)

GRAM-POSITIVE BACILLI				
Isolate	**Isolate Significance**	**Preferred Therapy**	**Alternate Therapy**	**Comments**
Eubacterium sp.	• CSF = P (brain abscess) • Blood = P (from dental, GI, GU, lung source) • Sputum = P (lung abscess) • Urine/Stool = NP • Wound = NP	Clindamycin (IV/PO) Ampicillin (IV) + gentamicin (IV)	Erythromycin (IV)	Pathogen in lung/pelvic/brain abscesses, and chronic periodontal disease. Eubacterium bacteremias are associated with malignancies.
Lactobacillus sp.	• CSF = P (ABM) • Blood = P (1° bacteremia, SBE, or from endometritis) • Sputum = NP • Urine = P (rare) • Stool = NP • Wound = NP	Ampicillin (IV) + gentamicin (IV) Clindamycin (IV/PO)	Erythromycin (IV)	Uncommon pathogen in normal/compromised hosts. Rare cause of SBE. Variably resistant to cephalosporins and quinolones. Some clindamycin-resistant strains. Resistant to metronidazole and vancomycin.
Propionibacterium acnes	• CSF = C*, P (meningitis from NS shunts) • Blood = C*, P (from IV line infection, SBE) • Sputum = NP • Urine = NP • Stool = NP • Wound = C	Penicillin (IV) Clindamycin (IV/PO)	Doxycycline (IV/PO)	Common skin colonizer/blood culture contaminant. Rarely causes prosthetic joint infection, endocarditis, or CNS shunt infection. Resistant to metronidazole.

GRAM-NEGATIVE BACILLI				
Bacteroides fragilis group (B. distasonis, ovatus, thetaiotaomicron, vulgatus)	• CSF = P (meningitis from Strongyloides hyperinfection) • Blood = P (from GI/pelvic source) • Sputum = NP • Urine = NP, P (only from colonic fistula) • Stool = NP • Wound = NP	Tigecycline (IV) Piperacillin/tazobactam (IV) Any carbapenem (IV)	Moxifloxacin (IV/PO) Ampicillin/sulbactam (IV) Clindamycin (IV/PO) *or combination of* Metronidazole (IV/PO) *plus either* ceftriaxone (IV) or levofloxacin (IV/PO)	Major anaerobe below the diaphragm. Usually part of polymicrobial lower intra-abdominal and pelvic infections. Cefotetan is less effective against B. fragilis DOT strains (B. distasonis, B. ovatus, B. thetaiotaomicron). Resistant to penicillin.
Fusobacterium nucleatum	• CSF = P (brain abscess) • Blood = P (from lung, GI source) • Sputum = P (aspiration pneumonia, lung abscess) • Urine = NP • Stool = NP • Wound = P (rarely)	Clindamycin (IV/PO) Piperacillin/tazobactam (IV) Ampicillin/sulbactam (IV)	Chloramphenicol (IV) Metronidazole (IV/PO)	Mouth flora associated with dental infections and anaerobic lung infections. F. nucleatum is associated with jugular vein septic phlebitis and GI cancer.
Prevotella (Bacteroides) bivia	• CSF = NP • Blood = P (from dental, lung, pelvic source) • Sputum = P (lung abscess) • Urine = NP • Stool = NP • Wound = NP	Penicillin (IV/PO) Any β-lactam (IV/PO)	Any quinolone (IV/PO) Doxycycline (IV/PO) Clindamycin (IV/PO)	Cause of dental, oropharyngeal, and female genital tract infections.

C = colonizer; C = skin contaminant; NP = non-pathogen at site; P = pathogen at site; (IV/PO) = IV or PO. See p. xi for all other abbreviations.*

Table 3.7. Usual Clinical Significance of ANAEROBIC Isolates Pending Susceptibility Testing (cont'd)

GRAM-NEGATIVE BACILLI				
Isolate	**Isolate Significance**	**Preferred Therapy**	**Alternate Therapy**	**Comments**
Prevotella (Bacteroides) melaninogenicus, intermedius	• CSF = P (brain abscess) • Blood = P (from oral/ pulmonary source) • Sputum = P (from aspiration pneumonia, lung abscess) • Urine = NP • Stool = NP • Wound = NP	<u>Aspiration pneumonia/lung abscess</u> Any β-lactam (IV/PO) Any quinolone (IV/PO) <u>Brain abscess</u> Penicillin (IV)	<u>Aspiration pneumonia/lung abscess</u> Doxycycline (IV/PO) <u>Brain abscess</u> Chloramphenicol (IV)	Predominant anaerobic flora of mouth. Known as "oral pigmented" Bacteroides (e.g., B. melanogenicus). Antibiotics used to treat community-acquired pneumonia are effective against oral anaerobes (e.g., Prevotella) in aspiration pneumonia; does not require anti-B. fragilis coverage with clindamycin, metronidazole, or moxifloxacin.

C = colonizer; C = skin contaminant; NP = non-pathogen at site; P = pathogen at site; (IV/PO) = IV or PO.* *See p. xi for all other abbreviations.*

Table 3.8. Clinical Significance of YEAST/FUNGI Pending Susceptibility Testing

YEAST/FUNGI				
Isolate	****Usual Isolate Significance**	**Preferred Therapy**	**Alternate Therapy**	**Comments**
Aspergillus species	• CSF = P (only from disseminated infection) • Blood = C, P (1° fungemia or from pulmonary source) • Sputum = C, P (pneumonia) • Urine = NP • Stool = NP • Wound = NP, P (rarely, but possible with extensive wounds, e.g., burns)	See p. 54: Voriconazole (IV/PO) Amphotericin B lipid formulation (IV)	See p. 54: Posaconazole (PO); Amphotericin B deoxycholate (IV)	A. fumigatus is the usual cause of invasive aspergillosis. Growth of Aspergillus sp. from a specimen can represent airborne contamination, but repeated growth or growth from a significantly immunocompromised patient with a consistent syndrome should be considered as evidence of possible infection. Aspergillus pneumonia and disseminated aspergillosis are common in patients receiving chronic steroids or immuno-suppressive therapy (esp. organ transplants). Recovery of Aspergillus from Sputum or BAL is not diagnostic of Aspergillus pneumonia/or (increasingly available) detection of circulating galactomannan are used to confirm the diagnosis.

C = colonizer; C = skin contaminant; NP = non-pathogen at site; P = pathogen at site; (IV/PO) = IV or PO. See p. xi for all other abbreviations.*

** Fungi can produce disseminated infections that involve essentially any organ. Isolation of a fungus from any normal sterile site should be cause for a careful review of the patient's epidemiology, risk factors, and clinical presentation.

Table 3.8. Usual Clinical Significance of YEAST/FUNGI Pending Susceptibility Testing (cont'd)

YEAST/FUNGI				
Isolate	****Usual Isolate Significance**	**Preferred Therapy**	**Alternate Therapy**	**Comments**
Candida albicans	• CSF = P (only from disseminated infection) • Blood = P (1° candidemia or from IV line infection) • Sputum = C, P (only from disseminated infection) • Urine = C, P (from cystitis, pyelonephritis) • Stool = C (source of candiduria) • Wound = NP	Fluconazole (IV/PO) Micafungin (IV) Caspofungin (IV) Anidulafungin (IV) Posaconazole (PO)	Amphotericin B deoxycholate (IV/PO) Amphotericin B lipid formulation (IV) Itraconazole (IV/PO) Voriconazole (IV/PO)	Common colonizer of GI/GU tracts. Colonization common in diabetics, alcoholics, patients receiving steroids/antibiotics. Commonest cause of fungemia in hospitalized patients. Candidemia secondary to central IV lines should always be treated as possible disseminated disease even though this is not invariably the case. Repeated blood cultures and careful follow-up (including ophthalmoscopy) should be undertaken to exclude possible occult dissemination following even a single positive blood culture. Primary candidal pneumonia is rare.
Candida non-albicans	• CSF = P (only from disseminated infection) • Blood = P (1° candidemia or from IV line infection) • Sputum = NP • Urine = C (indwelling catheters), P (from cystitis, pyelonephritis) • Stool = C (source of candiduria) • Wound = NP	Micafungin (IV) Caspofungin (IV) Anidulafungin (IV) Posaconazole (PO) Voriconazole (IV/PO)	Fluconazole (IV/PO) Amphotericin B deoxycholate (IV/PO) Amphotericin B lipid formulation (IV) Itraconazole (IV/PO)	Non-albicans Candida cause the same spectrum of invasive disease as C. albicans. Fluconazole-susceptibility varies predictably by species. C. glabrata (usually) and C. krusei (almost always) are resistant to fluconazole. C. lusitaniae is often resistant to amphotericin B (deoxycholate and lipid-associated formulations). Other species are generally susceptible to all agents.

Cryptococcus neoformans	• CSF = P (meningitis, brain abscess) • Blood = P (from pulmonary source) • Sputum = P (pneumonia) • Urine = NP • Stool = NP • Wound = NP*	<u>CNS</u> Amphotericin B deoxycholate (IV) ± flucytosine (PO) <u>Non-CNS</u> Amphotericin B deoxycholate (IV) Amphotericin B lipid formulation (IV)	<u>CNS</u> Fluconazole (IV/PO) <u>Non-CNS</u> Itraconazole (IV/PO) Fluconazole (IV/PO)	C. neoformans meningitis may occur with or without dissemination. Cryptococcal pneumonia frequently disseminates to CNS. C. neoformans in blood cultures occurs in compromised hosts (e.g., HIV/AIDS) and indicates disseminated infection.
Histoplasma capsulatum	• CSF = P (from disseminated infection, pneumonia) • Blood = P (1° fungemia, rarely SBE) • Sputum = P (pneumonia, mediastinitis) • Urine = P • Stool = P • Wound = P	Itraconazole (IV/PO) Amphotericin B deoxycholate (IV)	Fluconazole (IV/PO) Amphotericin B lipid formulation (IV)	Histoplasma recovered from CSF/ blood cultures indicates dissemination. Disseminated (reactivated latent) histoplasmosis is most common in compromised hosts (e.g., HIV/AIDS). Itraconazole is ineffective for meningeal histoplasmosis, but is preferred for chronic suppressive therapy.

C = colonizer; C = skin contaminant; NP = non-pathogen at site; P = pathogen at site; (IV/PO) = IV or PO. See p. xi for all other abbreviations.*

* Cutaneous cryptococcus represents disseminated infection.

** Fungi can produce disseminated infections that involve essentially any organ. Isolation of a fungus from any normal sterile site should be Cause for a careful review of the patient's epidemiology, risk factors, and clinical presentation.

Table 3.8. Usual Clinical Significance of YEAST/FUNGI Pending Susceptibility Testing (cont'd)

YEAST/FUNGI				
Isolate	****Usual Isolate Significance**	**Preferred Therapy**	**Alternate Therapy**	**Comments**
Malassezia furfur	• CSF = NP • Blood = P (from IV line infection) • Sputum = NP • Urine = NP • Stool = NP • Wound = P (eosinophilic folliculitis)	Itraconazole (IV/PO) Ketoconazole (PO)	Fluconazole (IV/PO)	M. furfur IV line infections are associated with IV lipid hyperalimentation emulsions. Fungemia usually resolves with IV line removal. Morphology in blood is blunt buds on a broad base yeast. M. furfur requires long chain fatty acids for growth (overlay agar with thin layer of olive oil, Tween 80, or oleic acid).
Penicillium marneffei	• CSF = NP • Blood = P (usually from dissemination) • Sputum = P (pneumonia) • Urine = NP • Stool = NP • Wound = NP*	Amphotericin B deoxycholate (IV) Itraconazole (IV/PO)	Amphotericin B lipid formulation (IV)	Histoplasma-like yeast forms seen in lymph nodes, liver, skin, bone marrow, blood. Characteristic red pigment diffuses into agar. Causes granulomatous tissue reaction ± necrosis. Skin lesions indicate dissemination. Rash may be papular, or resembles molluscum contagiosum with central umbilication. Hepatosplenomegaly is common. Dissemination is common in HIV.

C = colonizer; C = skin contaminant; NP = non-pathogen at site; P = pathogen at site; (IV/PO) = IV or PO. See p. xi for all other abbreviations.*

* Cutaneous lesions represents disseminated infection.

** Fungi can produce disseminated infections that involve essentially any organ. Isolation of a fungus from any normal sterile site should be cause for a careful review of the patient's epidemiology, risk factors, and clinical presentation.

Table 3.9. Technique for Gram Stain and Giemsa Stain

GRAM STAIN

Clinical applications: CSF, sputum, urine

Technique:

1. Place specimen on slide.
2. Heat fix smear on slide by passing it quickly over a flame.
3. Place crystal violet solution on slide for 20 seconds.
4. Wash gently with water.
5. Apply Gram iodine solution to slide for 20 seconds.
6. Decolorize the slide quickly in solution of acetone/ethanol.
7. Wash slide gently with water.
8. Counterstain slide with safranin for 10 seconds.
9. Wash gently with water; air dry or blot dry with bibulous paper.

Interpretation: Gram-negative organisms stain red; gram-positive organisms stain blue. B fragilis stains weakly pink. Fungi stain deep blue. See Tables 3.10–3.12 for interpretation of Gram stain findings in CSF, urine, sputum, and feces, respectively.

GIEMSA STAIN

Clinical applications: Blood buffy coat, bone marrow

Technique:

1. Place specimen on slide.
2. Fix smear by placing slide in 100% methanol for 1 minute.
3. Drain methanol off slide.
4. Flood slide with Giemsa stain (freshly diluted 1:10 with distilled water) for 5 minutes.
5. Wash slide gently with water; air dry.

Interpretation: Fungi/parasites stain light/dark blue.

Table 3.10. Clinical Use of CSF Gram Stain, WBC Type, Glucose (see Color Atlas of CSF Gram stains)

Gram Stain	Organism/Condition	
Gram-positive bacilli	Pseudomeningitis (Bacillus, Corynebacteria)	Listeria
Gram-negative bacilli	H. influenzae (small, encapsulated, pleomorphic)	Non-enteric/enteric aerobic bacilli (larger, unencapsulated)
Gram-positive cocci	Gp A, B, D, streptococci (pairs/ chains) S. pneumoniae (pairs)	S. aureus (pairs/clusters) S. epidermidis (pairs/clusters)
Gram-negative diplococci	Neisseria meningitidis	

Table 3.10. Clinical Use of CSF Gram Stain, WBC Type, Glucose (cont'd)

Gram Stain	Organism/Condition	
Mixed organisms (polymicrobial)	Pseudomeningitis Anaerobic organisms (brain abscess with meningeal leak)	Neonatal meningitis Meningitis 2° to penetrating head trauma
WBC Type/Glucose	**Organism/Condition**	
Purulent CSF, no organisms	Neisseria meningitidis	Listeria
Clear CSF, no organisms	Viral meningitis Viral encephalitis TB/fungal meningitis Sarcoidosis meningitis Meningeal carcinomatosis Brain abscess Parameningeal infection Septic emboli 2° to SBE SLE cerebritis Lyme's disease	Lymphocytic choriomeningitis (LCM) Drug induced aseptic meningitis Listeria HIV Syphilis Leptospirosis Bacterial meningitis (very early/partially-treated) Meningitis (leukopenic host) Rocky Mountain Spotted Fever
Cloudy CSF, no WBCs	S. pneumoniae	
Predominantly PMNs, decreased glucose	Bacterial meningitis (partially-treated) Listeria HSV-1/2 encephalitis TB (early/beginning therapy) Sarcoidosis	Parameningeal infection Septic emboli 2° to SBE Amebic meningoencephalitis Syphilis (early) Posterior-fossa syndrome
Predominantly lymphocytes, normal glucose	Bacterial meningitis (partially-treated) Sarcoidosis Lyme's disease HIV Leptospirosis Rocky Mountain Spotted Fever	Viral meningitis Viral encephalitis Parameningeal infection TB/fungal meningitis Parasitic meningitis Meningeal carcinomatosis
Predominantly lymphocytes, decreased glucose	Bacterial meningitis (partially-treated) TB/fungal meningitis Sarcoidosis Lymphocytic choriomeningitis (LCM) Mumps	Enteroviral meningitis Listeria Leptospirosis Syphilis Meningeal carcinomatosis
Red blood cells	Traumatic tap CNS bleed/tumor Listeria Leptospirosis Herpes (HSV-1) encephalitis	TB meningitis Amebic (Naegeleria) meningoencephalitis Anthrax

Table 3.11. Clinical Use of the Sputum Gram Stain (see Color Atlas of Sputum Gram stains)

Gram Stain	Organism	Comments
Gram-positive diplococci	S. pneumoniae	Lancet-shaped encapsulated diplococci (not streptococci)
Gram-positive cocci (grape-like clusters)	S. aureus	Clusters predominant. Short chains or pairs may also be present
Gram-positive cocci (short chains or pairs)	Group A streptococci	Virulence inversely proportional to length of streptococci. Clusters not present
Gram-positive beaded/ filamentous branching organisms	Nocardia	Coccobacillary forms common
Gram-negative cocco-bacillary organisms	H. influenzae	Pleomorphic may be encapsulated. Gram negative cocci/bacilli. Lightly stained
Gram-negative bacilli	Klebsiella P. aeruginosa	Plump and encapsulated Thin and often arranged in end-to-end pairs
Gram-negative diplococci	Moraxella (Branhamella) catarrhalis Neisseria meningitidis	Kidney bean-shaped diplococci

Table 3.12. Clinical Use of the Urine Gram Stain (see Color Atlas of Urine Gram stains)

Gram Stain	Organism	Comments
Gram-positive cocci (clusters)*	S. aureus S. epidermidis S. saprophyticus	Skin flora contaminant Skin flora contaminant Uropathogen
Gram-positive cocci (chains)	Group B streptococci Group D streptococci E. faecalis E. faecium	Uropathogen Uropathogen May represent colonization or infection May represent colonization or infection
Gram-negative bacilli*	Coliform bacilli	Uropathogen; may represent colonization or infection
Gram-negative diplococci*	N. gonorrhoeae N. meningitidis	Gonococcal urethritis Rare cause of urethritis

* Staphylococci (except S. saprophyticus), S. pneumoniae, and B. fragilis are *not* uropathogens.

Table 3.13. Clinical Use of the Fecal Gram Stain

Gram Stain	Possible Organisms	
Fecal leukocytes present	Enteropathogenic E. coli (EPEC) Enteroinvasive E. coil (EIEC) Shigella Yersinia Campylobacter Salmonella Vibrio parahaemolyticus Vibrio vulnificus	Aeromonas hydrophila Chlamydia trachomatis Plesiomonas shigelloides Neisseria gonorrhoeae (proctitis) Herpes simplex virus (HSV-1) *Noninfectious:* Ulcerative colitis
No fecal leukocytes	Enterovirus Rotavirus Coronavirus Enterotoxigenic E. coli (ETEC) S. aureus Clostridium perfringens Adenovirus	Norwalk virus Vibrio cholerae Bacillus cereus (food poisoning) Giardia lamblia Isospora belli Cryptosporidia Strongyloides stercoralis
Fecal leukocytes variable	Clostridium difficile Enterohemorrhagic E. coli (EHEC)	Cytomegalovirus (CMV) Herpes simplex virus (HSV-1)
Red blood cells present	Shigella Salmonella Campylobacter EPEC EHEC Enteroinvasive E. coli (EIEC) Enterohemorrhagic E. coli (EHEC)	Clostridium difficile Cytomegalovirus (CMV) Yersinia Plesiomonas shigelloides *Noninfectious:* Ulcerative colitis

REFERENCES AND SUGGESTED READINGS

Aridan S, Paetznick V, Rex JH. Comparative evaluation of disk diffusion with microdilution assay in susceptibility of caspofungin against Aspergillus and fusarium isolates. Antimicrob Agents Chemother 46:3084–7, 2002.

Baldis MM, Keidich SD, Mukhejee PK, et al. Mechanisms of fungal resistance: an overview. Drugs 62:1025–40, 2002.

Bartlett JG. Antibiotic-associated diarrhea. N Engl J Med 346:334–9, 2002.

Bingen E, Leclercq R, Fitoussi F, et al. Emergence of group A streptococcus strains with different mechanisms of macrolide resistance. Antimicrob Agents Chemother 46:1199–203, 2002.

Bouza E, Cercenado E. Klebsiella and enterobacter: antibiotic resistance and treatment implications. Semin Respir Infect 17:215–30, 2002.

Boyce JM. Methicillin-resistant Staphylococcus aureus. Lancet Infect Dis 5:653–63, 2005.

Brueggemann AB, Coffmen SL, Rhomberg P, et al. Fluoroquinolone resistance in Streptococcus pneumoniae in United States. Antimicrob Agents Chemother 46:680–8, 2002.

Courvalin P. Vancomycin resistance in gram-positive cocci. Clin Infect Dis 42:S25–S34, 2006.

Cunha BA. Clinical relevance of penicillin-resistant Streptococcus pneumoniae. Semin Respir Infect 17:204–14, 2002.

Cunha BA. Pseudomonas aeruginosa: resistance and therapy. Semin Respir Infect 17:231–9, 2002.

Cunha BA. MRSA & VRE: In vitro susceptibility versus in vivo efficacy. Antibiotics for Clinicians 4:31–32, 2000.

Cunha BA. The significance of antibiotic false sensitivity testing with in vitro testing. J Chemother 9:25–35, 1997.

Daneman N, McGeer, Green K, Low DE. Macrolide Resistance in Bacteremic Pneumococcal Disease: Implications for Patient Management. Clin Infect Dis 43:432–8, 2006.

Doern GV. Macrolide and Ketolide Resistance with Streptococcus pneumoniae. Med Clin N Am 90:1109–24, 2006.

Espinel-Ingroff A, Chaturvedi V, Fothergill A, et al. Optimal testing conditions for determining MICs and minimum fungicidal concentrations of new and established antifungal agents for uncommon molds: NCCLS collaborative study. J Clin Microbiol 40:3776–81, 2002.

Falagas ME, Kasiakou SK. Colistin: the revival of polymyxins for the management of multidrug-resistant gram-negative bacterial infections. Clin Infect Dis 40:1333–41, 2005.

Fuchs PC, Barry AL, Brown SD. In vitro activity of telithromycin against Streptococcus pneumoniae resistant to other antibiotics, including cefotaxime. J Antimicrob Chemother 49:399–401, 2002.

Gould IM. The clinical significance of methicillin-resistant Staphylococcus aureus. J Hosp Infect 61:277–282, 2005.

Halstead DC, Abid J, Dowzicky MJ. Antimicrobial susceptibility among Acinetobacter calcoaceticus-baumannii complex and enterobacteriacae collected as part of the tigecycline evaluation and surveillance trial. Journal of Infection 55:49–57, 2007.

Holmes A, Ganner M, McGuane S, et al. Staphylococcus aureus isolates carrying Panton-Valentine leucocidin genes in England and Wales: frequency, characterization, and association with clinical disease. J Clin Microbiol 43:2384–90, 2005.

Jain R, Danziger LH. Multidrug-resistant Acinetobacter infections: an emerging challenge to clinicians. Ann Pharmacother 38:1449–59, 2004.

Jevitt LA, Thorne GM, Traczewski MM, et al. Multicenter evaluation of the Etest and disk diffusion methods for differentiating Daptomycin-susceptible from non-Daptomycin-susceptible Staphylococcus aureus isolates. J Clin Microbiol 44:3098–3104, 2006.

Jiang X, Zhang Z, Li M, et al. Detection of Extended-Spectrum B-Lactamases in Clinical Isolates of Pseudomonas aeruginosa. Antimicrobial Agents and Chemotherapy 50:2990–95, 2006.

King A, Bathgate T, Phillips I. Erythromycin susceptibility of viridans streptococci from the normal throat flora of patients treated with azithromycin or clarithromycin. Clin Microbiol Infect 8:85–92, 2002.

Kocazeybek B, Arabaci U, Erenturk S. Investigation of various antibiotic combinations using the E-Test method in multiresistant Pseudomonas aeruginosa strains. Chemotherapy 48:31–5, 2002.

Kontoyiannis DP, Lewis RE. Antifungal drug resistance of pathogenic fungi. Lancet 359:1135–44, 2002.

Kralovic SM, Danko LH, Roselle GA. Laboratory reporting of Staphylococcus aureus with reduced susceptibility to vancomycin in United States Department of Veterans Affairs facilities. Emerg Infect Dis 8:402–7, 2002.

Kremery V, Barnes AJ. Non-albicans Candida spp. causing fungaemia: pathogenicity and antifungal resistance. J Hosp Infect 50:243–60, 2002.

Laverdiere M, Hoban D, Restieri C, et al. In vitro activity of three new triazoles and one echinocandin against Candida bloodstream isolates from cancer patients. J Antimicrob Chemother 50:119–23, 2002.

Linden PK. Treatment options for vancomycin-resistant enterococcal infections. Drugs 62:425–41, 2002.

Linder JA, Stafford RS. Erythromycin-resistant group A streptococci. N Engl J Med 347:614–5, 2002.

Lonks JR, Garau J, Gomez L, et al. Failure of macrolide antibiotic treatment in patients with bacteremia due to erythromycin-resistant Streptococcus pneumoniae. Clin Infect Dis 35:556–64, 2002.

Metlay JP, Fishman NO, Joffe MM, et al. Macrolide Resistance in Adults with Bacteremic Pneumococcal Pneumonia. Emerging Infect Dis 12, 1223–30, 2006.

Midolo PD, Matthews D, Fernandez CD, et al. Detection of extended spectrum beta-lactamases in the routine clinical microbiology laboratory. Pathology 34:362–4, 2002.

Mollering RC Jr. Problems with antimicrobial resistance in gram-positive cocci. Clin Infect Dis 26:1177–8, 1998.

Naas T, Fortineau N, Spicq C, et al. Three-year survey of community-acquired methicillin-resistant Staphylococcus aureus producing Panton-Valentine leukocidin in a French university hospital. J Hosp Infect 61:321–9, 2005.

Paterson DL, Bonomo RA. Extended-spectrum β-lactamases: a clinical update. Clin Microbiol Rev 18:657–86, 2005.

Pelaez T, Alcala L, Alonso R, et al. Reassessment of Clostridium difficile susceptibility to metronidazole and vancomycin. Antimicrob Agents Chemother 46:1647–50, 2002.

Perri MB, Hershberger E, Ionescu M, et al. In vitro susceptibility of vancomycin-resistant enterococci (VRE) to fosfomycin. Diagn Microbiol Infect Dis 42:269–71, 2002.

Poole K. Aminoglycoside resistance in Pseudomonas aeruginosa. Antimicrob Agents Chemother 49:479–87, 2005.

Rex JH, Pfaller MA, Walsh TJ, et al. Antifungal susceptibility testing: practical aspects and current challenges. Clin Microbiol Rev 14:643–658, 2002.

Rex JH, Rinaldi MG, Pfaller MA. Resistance of Candida species to fluconazole. Antimicrob Agents Chemother 39:1–8, 1995.

Robinson DA, Sutcliffe JA, Tweodros W, et al. Evolution and Global Dissemination of Macrolide-Resistant Group A Streptococci. Antimicrobial Agents and Chemotherapy 50:2903–11, 2006.

Ruhe JJ, Monson T, Bradsher RW, et al. Use of long-acting tetracyclines for methicillin-resistant Staphylococcus aureus infections: case series and review of the literature. Clin Infect Dis 40:142–934, 2005.

Stratton CW. In Vitro Susceptibility Testing Versus In Vivo Effectiveness. Med Clin N Am 90:1077–88, 2006.

Suzuki S, Yamazaki T, Narita M, et al. Clinical Evaluation of Macrolide-Resistant Mycoplasm pneumoniae. Antimicrobial Agents and Chemotherapy 50:709–12, 2006.

Swenson JM, Killgore GE, Tenover FC. Antimicrobial susceptibility testing of Acinetobacter spp. by NCCLS broth microdilution and disk diffusion methods. J Clin Microbiol 42:5102–8, 2004.

Syndman DR, Jacobut NV, McDermott LA, et al. National survey on the susceptibility of Bacteroides fragilis: report and analysis of trends for 1997–2000. Clin Infect Dis 35(Suppl 1):S126–34, 2002.

Taccone FS, Rodriguez-Villalobos H, DeBacker D, et al. Successful treatment of septic shock due to pan-resistant Acinetobacter baumannii using combined antimicrobial therapy including tigecycline. Eur J Clin Microbiol Infect Dis 25:257–60, 2006.

Tenover FC, Moellering RC. The rationale for revising the clinical and laboratory standards institute vancomycin minimal inhibitory concentration interpretive criteria for Staphylococcus aureus. Clin Infect Dis 44:1208–1215, 2007.

Tomioka H, Sato K, Shimizu T, et al. Anti-Mycobacterium tuberculosis activities of new fluoroquinolones in combination with other antituberculous drugs. J Infect 44:160–5, 2002.

Turner PJ. Trends in antimicrobial susceptibilities among bacterial pathogens isolated from patients hospitalized in European medical centers: 6-year report of the MYSTIC Surveillance Study (1997–2002). Diagn Microbiol Infect Dis 51:281–9, 2005.

Wagenvoort JHT, Ciraci VE, Penders RJR, et al. Superior discriminative performance of ceftizoxime disk diffusion test for detecting methicillin-resistant Staphylococcus aureus. Eur J Clin Microbiol Infect Dis 25:405–6, 2006.

Walsh FM, Amyes SG. Microbiology and drug resistance mechanisms of fully resistant pathogens. Curr Opin Microbiol 7:439–44, 2004.

Yong D, Lee K, Yum JH, et al. Imipenem-EDTA disk method for differentiation of metallo-beta-lactamase-producing clinical isolates of Pseudomonas spp. and Acinetobacter spp. J Clin Microbiol 40:3798–801, 2002.

Yuan S, Astion ML, Shapiro J, et al. Clinical impact associated with corrected results in clinical microbiology testing. J Clin Microbiol 43:2188–93, 2005.

TEXTBOOKS

Anaissie EJ, McGinnis MR, Pfaller MA (eds). Clinical Mycology. Churchill Livingstone, New York, 2003.

Bottone EJ (ed). An Atlas of the Clinical Microbiology of Infectious Diseases, Volume 1. Bacterial Agents. The Parthenon Publishing Group, Boca Raton, 2004.

Bottone EJ (ed). An Atlas of the Clinical Microbiology of Infectious Diseases, Volume 2. Viral, fungal, and parasitic agents. Taylor and Francis, 2006.

Bryskier A (ed). Antimicrobial Agents. ASM Press, Washington, D.C., 2005.

de la Maza LM, Pezzlo MT, Shigei JT, et al. (eds). Color Atlas of Medical Bacteriology. ASM Press, Washington, D.C., 2004.

Forbes BA, Sahm DF, Weissfeld AS, et al. (eds). Bailey & Scott's Diagnostic Microbiology, 12th Edition. St. Louis, Mosby, 2007.

Gorbach SL, Bartlett JG, Blacklow NR (eds). Infectious Diseases, 3rd Edition. Philadelphia, Lippincott, Williams & Wilkins, 2004.

Janda JM, Abbott SL (eds). The Enterobacteria, 2nd Edition. ASM Press, Washington, D.C., 2006.

Koneman EW, Allen SD, Janda WM, et al. (eds). Color Atlas and Textbook of Diagnostic Microbiology, 5th Edition. Lippincott-Raven Publishers, Philadelphia, 1997.

Lorian V (ed). Antibiotics in Laboratory Medicine. 5th Edition. Lippincott Williams & Wilkins, Philadelphia, 2005.

Madigan MT, Martinko JM, Parker J (eds). Brock Biology of Microorganisms. 10th Edition. Prentice Hall, Upper Saddle River, NJ, 2003.

Mandell GL, Bennett JE, Dolin R (eds). Mandell, Douglas, and Bennett's Principles and Practice of infectious Diseases, 7th Edition. Philadelphia, Elsevier Churchill Livingstone, 2010.

Murray PR, Baron EJ, Phaller MA, et al. (eds). Manual of Clinical Microbiology, 9th Edition. Washington, DC, ASM Press, 2007.

Scholar EM Pratt WB (eds). The Antimicrobial Drugs, 2nd Edition, Oxford University Press, New York, 2000.

Chapter 4

Parasites, Fungi, Unusual Organisms*

Kenneth F. Wagner, DO, James H. McGuire, MD
Burke A. Cunha, MD, John H. Rex, MD
Edward J. Bottone, PhD

See Color Atlas of Fungal stains (see p. 345).

Parasites, Fungi, Unusual Organisms in Blood

Microfilaria in Blood

Subset	Pathogen	Preferred Therapy	Alternate Therapy
Filariasis	Brugia malayi	Diethylcarbamazine: day 1: 50 mg (PO) day 2: 50 mg (PO) q8h day 3: 100 mg (PO) q8h days 4–14: 2 mg/kg (PO) q8h	Ivermectin 200 mcg/kg (PO) × 1 dose ± albendazole 400 mg (PO) × 1 dose
	Wuchereria bancrofti	Albendazole 400 mg (PO) × 1 dose plus diethylcarbamazine: day 1: 50 mg (PO) day 2: 50 mg (PO) q8h day 3: 100 mg (PO) q8h days 4–14: 2 mg/kg (PO) q8h ± doxcycline 100 mg (PO) q12h × 6 weeks	Ivermectin 400 mcg/kg (PO) × 1 dose.

Brugia malayi

Clinical Presentation: May present as an obscure febrile illness, chronic lymphedema, lymphangitis, or cutaneous abscess. "Filarial fevers" usually last 1 week and spontaneously remit.

Diagnostic Considerations: Diagnosis by demonstrating microfilaria on Giemsa's stained thick blood smear or by using the concentration method; yield is increased by passing blood through a Millipore filter before staining. Several smears should be taken over 24 hours. Adult worms may be detected in scrotal lymphatics by ultrasound. Common infection in Southeast Asia (primarily China, Korea, India, Indonesia, Malaysia, Philippines, Sri Lanka). Most species have nocturnal periodicity (microfilaria in blood at night). Eosinophilia is most common during periods of acute inflammation.

Pitfalls: Genital manifestations—scrotal edema, epididymitis, orchitis, hydrocele—are frequent with W. bancrofti, but rare with B. malayi.

Prognosis: Related to state of health and extent of lymphatic obstruction. No satisfactory treatment is available. Single-dose ivermectin is effective treatment for microfilaremia, but does not kill the adult worm (although diethylcarbamazine kills some). If no microfilaria in blood, full-dose diethylcarbamazine (2 mg/kg q8h) can be started on day one. Antihistamines or corticosteroids may decrease allergic reactions from disintegration of microfilaria.

Wuchereria bancrofti

Clinical Presentation: May present as an obscure febrile illness, chronic lymphedema, lymphangitis, or cutaneous abscess. Genital (scrotal) lymphatic edema, groin lesions, epididymitis, orchitis, hydroceles are characteristic. Chyluria may occur. "Filarial fevers" usually last 1 week and spontaneously remit. Lymphedema worsened by cellulitis associated with Tinea pedis infections.

Diagnostic Considerations: Diagnosis by demonstrating microfilaria on Giemsa's stained thick blood smear or by using the concentration method; yield is increased by passing blood through a

Millipore filter before staining. Several smears should to be taken over 24 hours. W. bancrofti is the most common human filarial infection, particularly in Asia (China, India, Indonesia, Japan, Malaysia, Philippines), Southeast Asia, Sri Lanka, Tropical Africa, Central/South America, and Pacific Islands. Most species have nocturnal periodicity (microfilaria in blood at night). Eosinophilia is common.
Pitfalls: Differentiate from "hanging groins" of Loa Loa, which usually do not involve the scrotum.
Prognosis: Related to state of health and extent of lymphatic obstruction. No satisfactory treatment is available. Single-dose ivermectin is effective treatment for microfilaremia, but does not kill the adult worm (although diethylcarbamazine kills some). If no microfilaria in blood, full-dose diethylcarbamazine (2 mg/kg q8h) can be started on day one. Antihistamines or corticosteroids decrease allergic reactions from disintegration of microfilaria. Wolbachia bacteria are endosymbionts in W. bancrofti filariasis. Treatment with doxycycline effective against Wolbachia which are important in microfilarial reproduction.

Trypanosomes in Blood

Subset	Pathogen	Preferred Therapy	Alternate Therapy
Chagas' disease (American trypanosomiasis)	Trypanosoma cruzi	Nifurtimox 8–10 mg/kg/day (PO) in 3–4 divided doses × 30–90 days	Benznidazole 2.5–3.5 mg/kg (PO) q12h × 30–90 days
Loa Loa (Loiasis)	L. loa	Diethylcarbamazine 5–10 mg/kg in 3÷ doses (PO) × 3 weeks **or** Albendazole 200 mg (PO) q12h × 3 weeks	
Sleeping sickness *West African trypanosomiasis*	Trypanosoma brucei gambiense	Hemolymphatic stage Pentamidine 4 mg/kg (IM) q24h × 10 days Late disease with CNS involvement Consecutive 10-day melarsoprol-nifurtimox low-dose combination therapy—2 days of melarsoprol alone [0.6 mg/kg(IV) on day 1 and 1.2 mg/kg (IV) on day 2], followed by 8 days of oral nifurtimox 7.5 mg/kg (PO) q12h combined with melarsoprol at 1.2 mg/kg/day [total melarsoprol dose, 11.4 mg/kg; total nifurtimox dose, 120 mg/kg]	Hemolymphatic stage Suramin 200 mg test dose (IV), then 1 gm (IV) on days 1,3,7,14 and 21 Late disease with CNS involvemen Eflornithine 100 mg/kg (IV) q6h × 2 weeks

Trypanosomes in Blood (cont'd)

Subset	Pathogen	Preferred Therapy	Alternate Therapy
East African trypanosomiasis	Trypanosoma brucei rhodesiense	Hemolymphatic stage: Suramin 200 mg test dose (IV), then 1 gm (IV) on days 1,3,7,14 and 21 Late disease with CNS involvement Melarsoprol 2–3.6 mg/kg (IV) q24h × 3 days. After 1 week, give 3.6 mg/kg (IV) q24h × 3 days; repeat again in 10–21 days	Hemolymphatic stage: Eflornithine, pentamidine (see doses above) variably effective Late disease with CNS involvement None

Chagas' Disease (Trypanosoma cruzi) American Trypanosomiasis

Clinical Presentation: Presents acutely after bite of infected reduviid bug with unilateral painless edema of the palpebrae/periocular tissues (Romaña's sign), or as an indurated area of erythema and swelling with local lymph node involvement (chagoma). Fever, malaise, and edema of the face and lower extremities may follow. Generalized lymphadenopathy and hepatosplenomegaly occur. Patients with chronic disease may develop cardiac involvement (cardiomyopathy with arrhythmias, heart block, heart failure, thromboembolism), GI involvement (megaesophagus, megaduodenum, megacolon) or CNS involvment in HIV/immunosuppressed.

Diagnostic Considerations: Common in Central and South America. Acquired from infected reduviid bug, which infests mud/clay parts of primitive dwellings. Transmitted by blood transfusion (~10%), organ transplants, and congenitally. Diagnosis in acute disease by detecting trypanosomes in wet prep of anticoagulated blood or stained buffy coat smears. Amastigote forms present intracellularly in monocytes/histiocytes in Giemsa-stained smears, bone marrow or lymph node aspirates, or by xenodiagnosis. Screening test ELISA IFA; confirmatory test RIPA (radioimmuno precipitation assay).

Pitfalls: Do not overlook the diagnosis in patients from endemic areas with unexplained heart block ± apical ventricular aneurysms. May be transmitted by blood transfusion/organ transplantation.

Prognosis: Related to extent of cardiac GI, or CNS involvement.

Sleeping Sickness (T. brucei gambiense/rhodesiense) West African/East African Trypanosomiasis

Clinical Presentation: Sleeping sickness from T. brucei gambiense is milder than sleeping sickness from T. brucei rhodesiense, which is usually a fulminant infection. A few days to weeks after bite of tsetse fly, patients progress through several clinical stages:

- *Chancre stage*: Trypanosomal chancre occurs at bite site and lasts several weeks.
- *Blood/lymphatic stage*: Blood parasitemia is associated with intermittent high fevers, headaches and insomnia, followed by generalized adenopathy. Posterior cervical lymph node enlargement (Winterbottom's sign) is particularly prominent with T. brucei gambiense. Hepatosplenomegaly and transient edema/pruritus/irregular circinate rash are common. Myocarditis (tachycardia unrelated to fevers) occurs early (before CNS involvement) and is responsible for acute deaths from T. brucei rhodesiense.
- *CNS stage*: Occurs after a few months of non-specific symptoms, and is characterized by increasing lethargy, somnolence (sleeping sickness), and many subtle CNS findings. Coma and

death ensue without treatment. With melarsoprol, use prednisolone 1 mg/kg (PO) q24h (start steroid 1 day prior to first dose and continue to last dose).

Diagnostic Considerations: Diagnosis by demonstrating trypanosomes in blood, chancre, or lymph nodes aspirates by Giemsa-stained thin and thick preparations, light microscopy, or buffy coat concentrates with acridine orange. CSF determines early vs. late stage disease (> 20 WBCs/mm^3).

Pitfalls: Do not miss other causes of prominent bilateral posterior cervical lymph node enlargement (e.g., lymphoma, EBV).

Prognosis: Related to extent of cardiac/CNS involvement. Relapse may occur.

Loa Loa (Loiasis)

Clinical Presentation: Cutaneous swellings (Calabar swellings) with pruritus. Adults may be visible when migrations under the conjuctiva or under the skin. Disappear in 10 minutes. Calabar swellings are painless and appear on the extremeties. Eosinophilia prominent.

Diagnostic Considerations: Demonstrates of microfilariae in blood (at noon) or by demonstration of L. loa in skin/eye. Immunodiagnosis unhelpful.

Pitfalls: Calabar swellings occur one at time and may last for hours/days; may persist for years.

Prognosis: Poorest with CNS involvement.

Spirochetes in Blood

Subset	Pathogen	Preferred Therapy	Alternate Therapy
Relapsing fever *Louse-borne (LBRF)* *Tick-borne (TBRF)*	Borrelia recurrentis At least 15 Borrelia species (U.S. B. hermsi; Africa: B. duttonii; Africa/Middle East: B. crocidurae)	LBRF Erythromycin 500 mg (IV or PO) q6h × 7 days TBRF Doxycycline 200 mg (PO) × 3 days, then 100 mg (PO) q12h × 7 days	TBRF with CNS involvement Penicillin G 2 mu (IV) q4h × 2 weeks **or** Ceftriaxone 1 gm (IV) q12h × 2 weeks **or** Cefotaxime 3 gm (IV) q6h × 2 weeks
Rat bite fever	Spirillum minus	Penicillin G 4 mu (IV) q4h. Can switch to amoxicillin 1 gm (PO) q8h for total therapy of 2 weeks **or** Doxycycline 200 mg (IV or PO) q12h × 3 days, then 100 mg (IV or PO) q12h × 11 days	Erythromycin 500 mg (IV or PO) q6h × 2 weeks **or** Chloramphenicol 500 mg (IV) q6h × 2 weeks

Relapsing Fever, Louse-Borne (LBRF) / Tick-Borne (TBRF)

Clinical Presentation: Abrupt onset of "flu-like" illness with high fever, rigors, headache, myalgias, arthralgias, tachycardia, dry cough, abdominal pain after exposure to infected louse or tick. Truncal petechial rash and conjunctival suffusion are common. Hepatosplenomegaly/DIC may occur. Bleeding

complications are more common in LBRF. Fevers last ~ 1 week, remit for a week, and usually relapse only once in LBRF, but several times in TBRF. Relapses usually last 2–3 days. Fevers are often higher in TBRF.
Diagnostic Considerations: Borreliae are found in > 70% of infected febrile patients when wet blood smears are examined by dark field microscopy or by Giemsa or Wright-stained thick and thin peripheral blood smears. LBRF is endemic in South American Andes, Central and East Africa, and is associated with crowded, unhygienic conditions. TBRF is seen throughout the world, and is endemic in Western U.S., British Columbia, Mexico, Central/South America, Mediterranean, Central Asia, and Africa.
Pitfalls: Spirochetes are most likely to be seen during febrile periods. Some treatment failures occur in TBRF with single-dose therapy.
Prognosis: Good if treated early. Usually no permanent sequelae.

Rat Bite Fever (Spirillum minus)

Clinical Presentation: Infection develops 1–4 weeks following bite of wild rat. Healed rat bite becomes red, painful, swollen and ulcerated, with regional lymphangitis/adenopathy. Recurrent fevers occurs in 2–4 day fever cycles. Fevers are usually accompanied by chills, headache, photophobia, nausea, vomiting. Rash on palms/soles develops in > 50%. Arthritis, myalgias, and SBE are rare.
Diagnostic Considerations: Short thick spirochetes are seen in peripheral blood smears, exudate, or lymph node tissue examined by dark field microscopy or by Giemsa or Wright's stain. Mostly seen in Asia. Differential diagnosis includes Borrelia, malaria, and lymphoma. VDRL is positive.
Pitfalls: May be confused with syphilis, due to rash on palms/soles and false-positive syphilis serology in 50%. SBE occurs with Streptobacillus moniliformis, not S. minus (unless there is preexisting valvular disease). Bite wound ulcerates in S. minus, not Streptobacillus moniliformis.
Prognosis: Patients with arthritis have a protracted course.

Intracellular Inclusion Bodies in Blood

Subset	Pathogen	Preferred Therapy	Alternate Therapy
Babesiosis	Babesia microti	Azithromycin 500 mg (PO) × 1, then 250 mg (PO) q24h × 7 days **plus** Atovaquone (suspension) 750 mg (PO) q12h × 7 days	Clindamycin 600 mg (PO) q8h × 7 days **plus** Quinine 650 mg (PO) q8h × 7 days
Ehrlichiosis/ anaplasmosis *Human monocytic ehrlichiosis (HME)* *Human granulocytic anaplasmosis (HGA)*	 Ehrlichia chaffeensis, ewubguum Anaplasma (Ehrlichia) phagocytophilium	Doxycycline 200 mg (IV or PO) q12h × 3 days, then 100 mg (IV or PO) q12h × 1–2 weeks total	Any once-daily quinolone (IV or PO) × 1–2 weeks **or** Ciprofloxacin 400 mg (IV) q12h or 750 mg (PO) q12h × 1–2 weeks **or** Chloramphenicol 500 mg (IV or PO) q6h × 1–2 weeks

Intracellular Inclusion Bodies in Blood (cont'd)

Subset	Therapy
Malaria *Benign tertian* (Plasmodium ovale, Plasmodium vivax) *Malignant tertian* (Plasmodium falciparum)	*Chloroquine-sensitive strains:* Chloroquine phosphate 10 mg/kg base (PO) initially and at 24 hours, then 5 mg/kg base (PO) at 48 hours **with or without** artesunate 4 mg/kg (PO) q24h × 3 days. <u>For P. vivax or P. ovale, add</u> primaquine phosphate 26.3 mg (15 mg base) (PO) q24h × 2 weeks *Chloroquine-resistant strains* **<u>Mild/moderately ill:</u>** Quinine sulfate 650 mg (500 mg base) (PO) q8h × 7 days *plus* Doxycycline 200 mg (PO) q12h × 3 days, then 100 mg (PO) q12h × 4 days **or** Atovaquone/proguanil (250/100 mg PO tab) 4 tablets as single dose q24h or 2 tabs (PO) q12h × 3 days **or**
Subset	**Pathogen** **Preferred Therapy** **Alternate Therapy**
Quartan (Plasmodium malariae) *Monkey malaria* (P. knowlesi)	Artesunate 4 mg/kg/d (PO) × 3 days *plus* Mefloquine 25 mg/kg (PO) on day 1; 15 mg/kg (PO) on day 2; and 10 mg/kg (PO) on day 3 **or** Artemether/lumefantrine 4 tablets (20/120 mg tablets) (PO) q12h with fatty foods × 3 days **or** Dihydroartemisinin 40 mg plus piperaquine 320 mg (PO) q24h × 3 days <u>*Asia/Latin America:*</u> Artesunate/mefloquine (AS/MQ) 1 tab* (PO) q24h × 3 days <u>*Africa:*</u> Artesunate/amodiaquine (AS/AQ) 2 tabs† (PO) q24h × 3 days (age ≥ 7 years); 1 tab† (PO) q24h × 3 days (age < 7 years) **<u>Critically ill:</u>** Quinidine 10 mg/kg (IV) over 1–2 hours, followed by 1.2 mg/kg/hr constant (IV) infusion until parasitemia < 1%; complete 7 days total therapy with doxycycline or oral regimen (above) **or** Quinine 20 mg (salt)/kg (IV) over 4 hours (in D_5W), then 10 mg (salt)/kg (IV) over 2 hours q8h until able to take oral meds; complete 7 days total therapy with doxycycline or oral regimen (above) **or** Artemether 3.2 mg/kg (IM) × 1 dose, then 1.6 mg/kg (IM) q24h until able to take oral meds; complete 7 days total therapy with doxycycline or PO regimen **or** Artesunate 2.4 mg/kg (IV) initially and at 12 and 24 hours, then q24h until able to take oral meds; complete 7 days total therapy with doxycycline or PO regimen

* AS/MQ adult tablet (100 mg AS/220 mg MQ); pediatric tablet (25 mg AS/55 mg MQ).

† AS/AQ adult tablet (100 mg AS/270 mg AQ); pediatric tablet (50 mg AS/153 mg AQ).

Babesiosis (Babesia microti)

Clinical Presentation: "Malarial-like illness" with malaise, fever, shaking chills, myalgias, arthralgias, headaches, abdominal pain, relative bradycardia, and splenomegaly. Laboratory abnormalities include anemia, atypical lymphocytes in peripheral smear, lymphopenia, thrombocytopenia, mildly elevated LFTs, ↑ LDH, proteinuria, and hemoglobinuria. Transmitted by infected Ixodes ticks.

Diagnostic Considerations: Characteristic four merozoites (often pear shaped) arranged in "Maltese cross" formation (tetrads) when examined by Giemsa or Wright-stained thick and thin peripheral blood smears. IFA serology ≥ 1:256 is diagnostic of acute infection. Hyposplenic patients may have profound hemolytic anemia and life-threatening infection.

Pitfalls: Co-infection with Lyme disease may occur. No serological cross-reactivity between Babesia and Borrelia (Lyme disease). Merozoites only may be confused with P. falciparum malaria. Travel history is important. Doxycycline ineffective.

Prognosis: Severe/fatal if ↓/absent splenic function. Exchange transfusions may be life saving.

Ehrlichiosis (HME/HGA)

Clinical Presentation: Acute febrile illness with chills, headache, malaise, myalgias, leukopenia, atypical lymphocytes, thrombocytopenia, ↑ LFTs. No vasculitis. Resembles Rocky Mountain spotted fever (RMSF), but without rash.

Diagnostic Considerations: Characteristic "morulae" (spherical, basophilic, mulberry-shaped, cytoplasmic inclusion bodies) seen in peripheral blood neutrophils in HGA. PCR from blood is 86% sensitive and highly specific for early diagnosis. Obtain acute and convalescent IFA serology. HGA vector is Ixodes ticks clinical co-infection with B. burgdorferi (Lyme Disease) is rare, but may occur main HME vector Ambylomma americanum (lone star tick).

Pitfalls: Morula are not seen in HME, so blood smears are unhelpful. Rash occurs in > 90% in Rocky Mountain spotted fever, but is uncommon in HME and rare in HGA.

Prognosis: Good if treated early. Delayed response complications in co-infection.

Malaria (Plasmodium ovale/vivax/falciparum/malariae/knowlesi)

Clinical Presentation: Presents acutely with fever/chills, severe headaches, cough, nausea/vomiting, diarrhea, abdominal/back pain. Typical "malarial paroxysm" consists of chills, fever and profuse sweating, followed by extreme prostration. There are a paucity of physical findings, but most have tender hepatomegaly/splenomegaly and relative bradycardia. Anemia, thrombocytopenia, atypical lymphocytes, and ↑ LDH/LFTs are common.

Diagnostic Considerations: Diagnosis by visualizing Plasmodium on thick/thin Giemsa or Wright-stained smears.

Pitfalls: Be wary of diagnosing malaria without headache/anemia. Assume all P. falciparum are chloroquine-resistant. Chloroquine-resistant P. vivax are now seen in South America, New Guinea, and Oceania (Indonesia). Chloroquine-sensitive strains are acquired in Central America (north of Panama Canal), Haiti, and parts of the Middle East (although chloroquine-resistant strains have been reported in Yemen, Oman, Saudi Arabia, and Iran). Check for severe G6PD deficiency before starting therapy. P. knowlesi (monkey malaria emerging cause of human malaria. Resembles P. malariae (microscopically) but may be severe resembing P. falciparum (clinically). Treat P. knowlesi as chloroquine sensitive (P. vivax, P. ovale, P. malariae) malaria.

Prognosis: Related to species. P. falciparum with high-grade parasitemia is most severe, and may be complicated by coma, hypoglycemia, renal failure, or non-cardiogenic pulmonary edema. If parasitemia exceeds 15%, consider exchange transfusions.

Fungi/Mycobacterium in Blood

See histoplasmosis (p. 338), Mycobacterium tuberculosis (treat as pulmonary TB, pp. 323, 329), Mycobacterium avium-intracellulare (pp. 318, 339).

Parasites, Fungi, Unusual Organisms in CSF/Brain

Cysts/Mass Lesions in CSF/Brain

Subset	Pathogens	Preferred Therapy	Alternate Therapy
Cerebral nocardiosis	Nocardia sp.	Preferred IV Therapy: TMP–SMX (TMP 5 mg/kg, SMX 15 mg/kg) (IV) q6h until clinical improvement, then (PO) therapy Alternate IV PO Therapy: Minocycline or doxycycline 100 mg (IV) q12h until clinical improvement, then (PO) therapy	Preferred PO Therapy TMP–SMX 1 DS tablet (PO) q12h × 6 months Alternate PO Therapy Minocycline 100 mg (PO) q12h × 6 months **or** doxycycline 100 mg (PO) q12h × 6 months
Cerebral amebiasis	Entamoeba histolytica	Metronidazole 750 mg (PO) q8h × 10 days **or** Tinidazole 800 mg (PO) q8h × 5 days	
Primary amebic meningo-encephalitis	Naegleria fowleri	See p. 21	
Granulomatous amebic encephalitis	Acanthamoeba	See p. 22	
Cerebral echinococcosis (hydatid cyst disease)	Echinococcus granulosus or multilocularis	Surgical resection plus albendazole 400 mg* (PO) q12h until cured	Surgical resection plus mebendazole 50 mg/kg (PO) q24h until cured
Cerebral gnathostomiasis	Gnathostoma spinigerum	Surgical resection	Albendazole 400 mg (PO) q12h × 3 weeks **or** Ivermectin 200 mcg/kg/d × 2 days
Cerebral coenurosis	Taenia multiceps	Surgical resection	

* If < 60 kg, give albendazole 7.5 mg/kg.

Cysts/Mass Lesions in CSF/Brain (cont'd)

Subset	Pathogens	Preferred Therapy	Alternate Therapy
Neurocysticercosis	Taenia solium	Albendazole 400 mg* (PO) q12h × 2 weeks	Praziquantel 25 mg/kg (PO) q8h × 14 days ± cimetidine 400 mg (PO) q8h (to ↑ praziquantel levels)
Cerebral paragonimiasis (lung fluke)	Paragonimus westermani	Praziquantel 25 mg/kg (PO) q8h × 2 days	Bithionol 50 mg/kg (PO) q48h × 10–15 doses
Cerebral toxoplasmosis	Toxoplasma gondii	See pp. 326–327	
Cryptococcomas/ meningitis	Cryptococcus neoformans	See p. 325	
Chagas' disease (American trypanosomiasis)	Trypanosoma cruzi	Nifurtimox 2 mg/kg (PO) q6h × 4 months	Benznidazole 3.5 mg/kg (PO) q12h × 2 months

* If < 60 kg, give albendazole 7.5 mg/kg.

Cerebral Nocardiosis

Clinical Presentation: CNS mass lesion resembling brain tumor/abscess. Symptoms are highly variable, and result from local effects of granulomas/abscesses in CNS. Up to 40% of patients with systemic nocardiosis have associated mass lesions in CNS.

Diagnostic Considerations: Diagnosis by demonstrating Nocardia (gram positive, delicate, beaded, branching filaments) in brain biopsy specimens. Notify laboratory for modified acid fast specimen staining/aerobic cultures if suspect Nocardia. Nocardia are weakly acid-fast and aerobic.

Pitfalls: Usually not limited to brain. Look for Nocardia in skin, lungs or liver. Use in-vitro susceptibility data to guide therapy for refractory cases. IV regimens are recommended for critically ill patients. HIV/AIDS patients require life-long suppression with TMP–SMX.

Prognosis: Related to health of host, degree of immunosuppression, and extent of lesions.

Cerebral Amebiasis (Entamoeba histolytica)

Clinical Presentation: Rare cause of brain abscess. Onset is frequently abrupt with rapid progression. Suspect in patients with a history of amebiasis and altered mental status/focal neurologic signs. If present, meningeal involvement resembles acute bacterial meningitis. CT/MRI shows focal lesions.

Diagnostic Considerations: Diagnosis by demonstrating E. histolytica trophozoites in wet preps or by trichrome stain from aspirated brain lesions under CT guidance. Worldwide distribution. Mass lesions may be single or multiple, and more commonly involve the left hemisphere. Most patients have concomitant liver ± lung abscesses.

Pitfalls: Trophozoites/cysts in stool are not diagnostic of CNS disease. E. histolytica serology is often positive, but is nonspecific. E. histolytica trophozoites are not present in CSF.
Prognosis: Related to size/location of CNS lesions.

Primary Amebic Meningoencephalitis (Naegleria fowleri) (see p. 23)

Granulomatous Amebic Encephalitis (Acanthamoeba) (see p. 23)

Cerebral Echinococcosis (Echinococcus granulosus) Hydatid Cyst Disease

Clinical Presentation: Most cysts are asymptomatic. Mass lesions may cause seizures, cranial nerve abnormalities, other focal neurologic symptoms.
Diagnostic Considerations: CT/MRI typically shows a single large cyst without edema or enhancement. Multiple cysts are rare. Diagnosis by demonstrating protoscolices in "hydatid sand" in cysts. Usually associated with liver/lung hydatid cysts.
Pitfalls: E. granulosus serology lacks specificity.
Prognosis: Related to size/location of CNS cysts. CSF eosinophilia is not a feature of CNS involvement. Treatment consists of surgical removal of total cyst after instilling cysticidal agent (hypertonic saline, iodophor, ethanol) into cyst plus albendazole.

Cerebral Echinococcosis (Echinococcus multilocularis) Hydatid Cyst Disease

Clinical Presentation: Frequently associated with hydatid bone cysts (may cause spinal cord compression), liver/lung cysts. Peripheral eosinophilia occurs in 50%, but eosinophils are not seen in the CSF.
Diagnostic Considerations: E. multilocularis ELISA is sensitive and specific.
Pitfalls: Praziquantel is ineffective for CNS hydatid cyst disease. Imaging studies suggest carcinoma/sarcoma. Diagnosis is frequently not made until brain biopsy.
Prognosis: If treatment is effective, improvement of CNS lesions is evident in 8 weeks. Brain/bone cysts are difficult to cure.

Cerebral Gnathostomiasis (Gnathostoma spinigerum)

Clinical Presentation: Nausea, vomiting, increased salivation, skin flushing, pruritus, urticaria, and upper abdominal pain 1–6 days after exposure. Cerebral form presents as eosinophilic meningitis with radiculomyeloencephalitis, with headache and severe sharp/shooting pains in extremities often followed by paraplegia and coma. Any cranial nerve may be involved. The most characteristic feature is changing/migratory neurological findings. Intense peripheral eosinophilia occurs in 90% of patients. CSF has eosinophilic pleocytosis and may have RBCs.
Diagnostic Considerations: In cases with ocular involvement, the worm may be seen in the anterior chamber of eye. Specific Gnathostoma serology of CSF is helpful in establishing the diagnosis. Acquired from infected cat/dog feces. Most cases occur in Southeast Asia also Mexico, Peru, and Spain. Few other CNS infections have both RBCs and eosinophils in the CSF.
Pitfalls: Do not miss associated eye involvement or characteristic episodic non-pitting subcutaneous edema.
Prognosis: Related to invasion of medulla/brainstem.

Cerebral Coenurosis (Taenia multiceps)

Clinical Presentation: CNS mass lesion with seizures/cranial nerve abnormalities, often presenting as a posterior-fossa syndrome. Common sites of CNS involvement include paraventricular and basal subarachnoid spaces. Eosinophils not in CSF.

Diagnostic Considerations: Diagnosis by demonstrating protoscolices in brain cyst specimens. Worldwide distribution. Transmitted via dog feces.
Pitfalls: Do not miss associated ocular lesions, which mimic intraocular neoplasms/granulomas.
Prognosis: Related to size/extent of CNS lesions.

Neurocysticercosis (Taenia solium)

Clinical Presentation: Chronic eosinophilic meningitis/mass lesions with seizures. Hydrocephalus is common. Spinal involvement may result in paraplegia. Cerebral cysts are usually multiple.
Diagnostic Considerations: CT/MRI shows multiple enhancing and non-enhancing unilocular cysts. Diagnosis by specific T. solium serology of serum/CSF or excision of cyst. Neurocysticercosis is the most common CNS parasite. Worldwide in distribution; most common in Eastern Europe, Asia, Latin America.
Pitfalls: Cranial nerve abnormalities are uncommon.
Prognosis: Related to extent/location of CNS lesions. Adjunctive therapy includes corticosteroids, anti-epileptics, and shunt for hydrocephalus.

Cerebral Paragonimiasis (Paragonimus westermani) Lung Fluke

Clinical Presentation: Can resemble epilepsy, cerebral tumors, or brain embolism. Primary focus of infection is pulmonary, with pleuritic chest pain, cough, and night sweats. CNS findings are a manifestation of extrapulmonary (ectopic) organ involvement.
Diagnostic Considerations: Diagnosis by demonstrating operculated eggs in sputum, pleural fluid, or feces. Multiple sputum samples are needed to demonstrate P. westermani eggs. Charcot-Leyden crystals are seen in sputum. Endemic in Far East, India, Africa, and Central/South America.
Pitfalls: Extrapulmonary (ectopic) organ involvement (cerebral, subcutaneous, abdominal) is common. Up to 20% of patients have normal chest x-rays.
Prognosis: Related to size/location of CNS cysts and extent of lung involvement.

Cerebral Toxoplasmosis (T. gondii) (see pp. 326–327)

Cerebral Cryptococcosis (C. neoformans) (see p. 325)

Chagas' Disease (Trypanosoma cruzi) American Trypanosomiasis

Clinical Presentation: Acute unilateral periorbital cellulitis (Romaña's sign) or regional adenopathy and edema of extremity at site of infected reduviid bug (Chagoma). Chronic disease manifests as myocarditis/heart block or megaesophagus, megaduodenum, megacolon. Hepatosplenomegaly is common. Overt CNS signs are frequently absent. CNS Chagas' disease typically have hypodense ring enhancing lesions with surrounding edema on head CT/MRI scans. If meningoencephalitis develops, the prognosis is very poor. In immunosuppressed patients (especially AIDS), recrudescence of disease occurs with development of T. cruzi brain abscesses.
Diagnostic Considerations: Diagnosis in acute disease by demonstrating trypanosomes in wet prep of anticoagulated blood or stained buffy coat smears. Amastigote forms present intracellularly in monocytes/histiocytes in Giemsa-stained smear of bone marrow/lymph node aspirate, or by xenodiagnosis. Serology (mostly used for chronic disease) has limited value in endemic areas due to lack of specificity, but is useful in non-endemic areas. Common in Central/South America. Acquired from infected reduviid bugs, which infest mud/clay/stone parts of primitive dwellings. Infection in humans occurs in areas containing reduviids that defecate during or immediately after a blood meal.

Diagnostic Considerations: Screening test ELISA IFA; confirmatory test RIPA (radioimmuno precipitation assay).

Pitfalls: Do not overlook diagnosis in persons from endemic areas with unexplained heart block. For children ages 11–16 years, use nifurtimox 3.5 mg/kg (PO) q6h × 3 months. For children < 11 years, use nifurtimox 5 mg/kg (PO) q6h × 3 months.

Prognosis: Related to extent of GI cardiac or CNS involvement. The addition of gamma interferon to nifurtimox × 20 days may shorten the acute phase of the disease.

Parasites, Fungi, Unusual Organisms in Lungs

Pulmonary Cystic Lesions/Masses

Subset	Pathogens	Preferred Therapy	Alternate Therapy
Alveolar echinococcosis	Echinococcus multilocularis	Operable cases Wide surgical resection plus albendazole 400 mg* (PO) q12h or mebendazole 50 mg/kg (PO) q24h until cured	Inoperable cases: Albendazole 400 mg* (PO) q12h × 1 month, then repeat therapy after 2 weeks × 3 cycles (i.e., 4 total months of albendazole)
Pulmonary amebiasis	Entamoeba histolytica	Metronidazole 750 mg (PO) q8h × 10 days	Tinidazole 800 mg (PO) q8h × 5 days
Pulmonary paragonimiasis (lung fluke)	Paragonimus westermani	Praziquantel 25 mg/kg (PO) q8h × 2 days	Bithionol 50 mg/kg (PO) q48h × 4 weeks (14 doses)

* If < 60 kg, give albendazole 7.5 mg/kg.

Alveolar Echinococcosis (Echinococcus multilocularis)

Clinical Presentation: Slowly growing cysts remain asymptomatic for 5–20 years, until space-occupying effect elicits symptoms. Rupture/leak into bronchial tree can cause cough, chest pain, and hemoptysis.

Diagnostic Considerations: Diagnosis is suggested by typical "Swiss cheese calcification" findings on chest x-ray, and confirmed by specific E. multilocularis serology (which does not cross react with E. granulosus). Most common in Northern forest areas of Europe, Asia, North America, and Arctic. Acquired by ingestion of viable parasite eggs in food. Tapeworm-infected canines/cats or wild rodents are common vectors. Less common than infection with E.granulosus.

Pitfalls: Do not confuse central cavitary lesions with squamous cell carcinoma.

Prognosis: Related to size/location of cysts.

Pulmonary Amebiasis (Entamoeba histolytica)

Clinical Presentation: Cough, pelvic pain, fever, and right lung/pleural mass mimicking pneumonia or lung abscess. Bronchopleural fistulas may occur. Sputum has "liver-like" taste if cyst ruptures into bronchus. Bacterial co-infection is rare. Amebic lung lesions are associated with hepatic liver abscesses, and invariably involve the right lobe of lung/diaphragm.

Diagnostic Considerations: Diagnosis by aspiration of lungs cysts, which may be massive. Amebic serology is sensitive and specific. Worldwide distribution. Acquired by ingesting amebic cysts. Key to diagnosis is concomitant liver involvement; liver abscess presents years after initial diarrheal episode.

Pitfalls: Lung involvement is rarely the sole manifestation of amebic infection, and is usually due to direct extension of amebic liver abscess (10–20% of amebic liver abscesses penetrate through the diaphragm and into the lungs). Follow metronidazole with paromomycin 500 mg (PO) q8h × 7 days to eliminate intestinal focus.

Prognosis: Related to severity/extent of cysts.

Pulmonary Paragonimiasis (Paragonimus westermani) Lung Fluke

Clinical Presentation: Mild infection; may be asymptomatic. Acute phase of infection is accompanied by abdominal pain, diarrhea and urticaria, followed by pleuritic chest pain/eosinophilic pleural effusion. Chronic symptoms occur within 6 months after exposure, with dyspnea/dry cough leading to productive cough ± hemoptysis. Complications include lung abscess, bronchiectasis, cough, and night sweats. Eosinophilia may be present acutely.

Diagnostic Considerations: Oriental lung fluke acquired by ingestion of freshwater crayfish/crabs. After penetration of the gut/peritoneal cavity, the fluke migrates through the diaphragm/pleural space and invades lung parenchyma. Incubation period is 2–20 days. Diagnosis by demonstrating operculated eggs in sputum, pleural fluid, or feces. Multiple sputum samples are needed to demonstrate P. westermani eggs. Charcot-Leyden crystals are seen in sputum, and characteristic chest x-ray findings of ring-shaped/crescent infiltrates with "thin-walled" cavities are evident in ~ 60%. Endemic in Asia, Africa, and Latin America. Chest x-ray findings take months to resolve.

Pitfalls: May have extrapulmonary (ectopic) organ involvement (e.g., cerebral, subcutaneous, abdominal). Up to 20% have normal chest x-rays. Commonest cause of eosinophilic pleural effusions in endemic areas. Diagnosis should be questioned if pleural effusion fluid does not have eosinophils.

Prognosis: Related to degree of lung damage (e.g., bronchiectasis) and extrapulmonary organ involvement, especially CNS.

Pulmonary Coin Lesions

Subset	Pathogens	Preferred Therapy	Alternate Therapy
Dog heartworm	Dirofilaria immitis	No therapy necessary	
Aspergilloma	Aspergillus	No therapy if asymptomatic. Surgery for massive hemoptysis	Itraconazole 200 mg (PO) solution q24h × 3–6 months **or** Voriconazole (see "usual dose," p. 695) × 3–6 months

Dog Heartworm (Dirofilaria immitis)

Clinical Presentation: Asymptomatic "coin lesion" after bite of infected mosquito transmits parasite from dogs to humans. Differential diagnosis includes granulomas and malignancy.

Diagnostic Considerations: Diagnosis by specific serology or pathological demonstration of organism in granuloma, usually when a coin lesion is biopsied to rule out malignancy. Worldwide

distribution. Acquired from pet dogs. Dirofilariasis causes dog heartworm in carrier, but presents as a solitary lung nodule in humans.
Pitfalls: Often confused with malignancy.
Prognosis: Excellent.

Pulmonary Aspergilloma

Clinical Presentation: Coin lesion(s) ± productive cough, hemoptysis, wheezing. May be asymptomatic. Usually occurs in pre-existing cavitary lung lesions, especially TB with cavity > 2 cm.
Diagnostic Considerations: Diagnosis by chest x-ray appearance of fungus ball in cavity and Aspergillus precipitins/biopsy or by demonstrating Aspergillus hyphae and "fruiting bodies" (conidiophores) in respiratory specimens. May present with "crescent sign" on chest x-ray (white fungus ball silhouetted against black crescent of the cavity).
Pitfalls: Role of itraconazole or voriconazole as therapy is unclear.
Prognosis: Related to degree of hemoptysis.

Pulmonary Infiltrates/Mass Lesions¶

Subset	Pathogens	Preferred Therapy	Alternate Therapy
Pulmonary blastomycosis	Blastomyces dermatitidis	Mild illness: Itraconazole 200 (PO) TID × 3 days and then QD or BID for a total of 6–12 months (adequate serum levels should be confirmed). Moderately severe or severe illness: A lipid-associated formulation of amphotericin B for 1–2 weeks followed by itraconazole as for mild illness.	Fluconazole has been disappointing; its use is limited to specialized settings such as CNS blastomycosis. Amphotericin B deoxycholate 0.7–1 mg/kg may be used as initial therapy instead of a lipid-associated amphotericin.
Pulmonary histoplasmosis	Histoplasma capsulatum	Mild illness: Therapy is not always needed, but symptoms lasting more than a month may be treated with Itraconazole 200 (PO) TID × 3 days and then QD or BID for a total of 6–12 weeks. Moderately severe or severe illness: A lipid-associated formulation of amphotericin B for 1–2 weeks followed by itraconazole as for mild illness. Chronic cavity histoplasmosis requires at least a year of therapy & confirmation of adequate blood levels.	Strategies are complex (See Wheat LJ et al. Clin Infect Dis 45:807–825, 2007).

¶ See Color Atlas section.

Pulmonary Infiltrates/Mass Lesions (cont'd)

Subset	Pathogens	Preferred Therapy	Alternate Therapy
Pulmonary paracoccidioidomycosis (South American blastomycosis)	Paracoccidioides brasiliensis	Itraconazole 200 mg (PO) q24h × 6 months **or** Ketoconazole 400 mg (PO) q24h × 18 months	Amphotericin B 0.5 mg/kg (IV) q24h until 1.5–2.5 grams given
Pulmonary actinomycosis	Actinomyces israelii	Amoxicillin 1 gm (PO) q8h × 6 months **or** Doxycycline 100 mg (PO) q12h × 6 months	Clindamycin 300 mg (PO) q8h × 6 months **or** Chloramphenicol 500 mg (PO) q6h × 6 months
Pulmonary aspergillosis *BPA*	Aspergillus	Systemic oral steroids	Itraconazole 200 mg (PO) q12h × 8 months
Acute invasive pneumonia/ aspergillus	Aspergillus	See p. 320	
Chronic pneumonia aspergillus	Aspergillus	Treat the same as on p. 160	Treat the same as on p. 160
Pulmonary sporotrichosis	Sporothrix schenckii	Lipid-associated formulation of amphotericin B (p. 513) (IV) q24h × 3 weeks **or** 3 B deoxycholate 0.5 mg/kg (IV) q24h until 1–2 grams given	Itraconazole 200 mg (PO)* q12h until cured **or** Lipid-associated formulation of amphotericin B (p. 513) (IV) q24h until cured
Pulmonary coccidioidomycosis	Coccidioides immitis	Itraconazole 200 mg (PO)* q12h until cured **or** Fluconazole 800 mg (IV or PO) × 1 dose, then 400 mg (PO) q24h until cured	Amphotericin B deoxycholate 1 mg/kg (IV) q24h × 7 days† **or** Lipid-associated formulation of amphotericin B (p. 513) (IV) q24h × 7 days
Pulmonary nocardiosis	Nocardia asteroides	TMP–SMX 5–10 mg/kg/d (TMP) in 2–4 doses (IV) × 3–6 weeks, then 1 DS tablet (PO) q12h until cured	Minocycline 100 mg (PO) q12h until cured

* Initiate therapy with itraconazole 200 mg (IV) q12h × 7–14 days.

† Follow with itraconazole 200 mg (PO) solution q12h until cured.

Pulmonary Infiltrates/Mass Lesions (cont'd)

Subset	Pathogens	Preferred Therapy	Alternate Therapy
Pulmonary cryptococcosis	Cryptococcus neoformans	Fluconazole 800 mg (IV or PO) × 1 dose, then 400 mg (PO) q24h until cured	Amphotericin B deoxycholate 0.5 mg/kg (IV) q24h until 1–2 grams given **or** Lipid-associated formulation of amphotericin B (p. 513) (IV) q24h × 3 weeks
Pulmonary zygomycosis (mucor-mycosis)	Rhizopus/ Mucor/Absidia	Lipid-associated formulation of amphotericin B (p. 513)(IV) q24h × 1–2 weeks† *or* × 3 wks **or** Amphotericin B deoxycholate 1–1.5 mg/kg (IV) q24h × 1–2 wks† *or* until 2–3 grams given	Itraconazole 200 mg (PO)* q12h until cured
Pulmonary pseudall-escheriasis	Pseudallescheria boydii/ Scedosporium apiospermum	Voriconazole (see "usual dose," p. 695) until cured	Itraconazole 200 mg (PO)* q12h until cured

BPA = bronchopulmonary aspergillosis.

* Initiate therapy with itraconazole 200 mg (IV) q12h × 7–14 days.

† Follow with itraconazole 200 mg (PO) solution q12h until cured.

Pulmonary Blastomycosis (Blastomyces dermatitidis)

Clinical Presentation: Highly variable. May present as a chronic/non-resolving pneumonia with fever/cough and characteristic "right-sided perihilar infiltrate" ± small pleural effusion.

Diagnostic Considerations: May be recovered from sputum or demonstrated in lung tissue specimens. Usual sites of dissemination include skin, bones and prostate, not CNS or adrenals.

Pitfalls: Dissemination to extra-pulmonary sites may occur years after pneumonia.

Prognosis: Related to severity/extent of infection. One-third of cases are self-limited and do not require treatment.

Pulmonary Histoplasmosis (Histoplasma capsulatum)

Clinical Presentation: Acute primary infection presents as self-limiting flu-like illness with fever, headache, nonproductive cough, chills, and chest pain. Minority of patients become overtly ill with complicated respiratory or progressive pulmonary infection. Can cause arthralgias, E. nodosum, E. multiforme, or pericarditis. May occur in outbreaks. Chronic infection presents as chronic pneumonia resembling TB or chronic disseminated infection. Eosinophilia common.

Diagnostic Considerations: May be recovered from sputum or demonstrated in lung tissue specimens. Worldwide distribution, but most common in Central/South Central United States. Acute disseminated histoplasmosis suggests HIV/AIDS. Intracellular (PMNs/monocytes) organisms may be seen in Wright/Giema stained peripheral blood smears/buffy coat smears in disseminated infection. Acute histoplasmosis with immunodiffusion (ID) assay M band precipitins; chronic histoplasmosis with ID assay M band precipitins or CF ≥ 1:32. Histoplasma urinary antigen useful in diagnosis of acute/disseminated histoplasmosis. ↑ LDH.

Pitfalls: Pleural effusion is uncommon. Do not treat old/inactive/minimal histoplasmosis, histoplasmosis pulmonary calcification, or histoplasmosis fibrosing mediastinitis. Differentiate from TB and kala-azar. Resembles kala-azar histologically, but rod-shaped kinetoplasts (kala-azar) are absent extracellularly also in histoplasmosis.

Prognosis: Related to severity/extent of infection. No treatment is needed for self-limiting acute-histoplasmosis presenting as flu-like illness. HIV/AIDS patients should receive life-long suppressive therapy with itraconazole 200 mg (PO) solution q24h.

Pulmonary Paracoccidioidomycosis (South American Blastomycosis)

Clinical Presentation: Typically presents as a chronic pneumonia syndrome with productive cough, blood-tinged sputum, dyspnea, and chest pain. May also develop fever, malaise, weight loss, mucosal ulcerations in/around mouth and nose, dysphagia, changes in voice, cutaneous lesions on face/limbs, or cervical adenopathy. Can disseminate to prostate, epididymis, kidneys, or adrenals.

Diagnostic Considerations: Characteristic "pilot wheel" shaped yeast in sputum. Diagnosis by culture and stain (Gomori) of organism from clinical specimen. Found only in Latin American. One-third of cases have only pulmonary involvement. Skin test is non-specific/non-diagnostic.

Pitfalls: No distinguishing radiologic features. No clinical adrenal insufficiency, in contrast to TB or histoplasmosis. Hilar adenopathy/pleural effusions are uncommon.

Prognosis: Related to severity/extent of infection. HIV/AIDS require life-long suppression with TMP–SMX 1 DS tablet (PO) q24h or itraconazole 200 mg (PO) solution q24h.

Pulmonary Actinomycosis (Actinomyces israelii)

Clinical Presentation: Indolent, slowly progressive infiltrates involving the pulmonary parenchyma ± pleural space. Presents with fever, chest pain, weight loss. Cough/hemoptysis are less common. Chest wall sinuses frequently develop. Chest x-ray shows adjacent dense infiltrate. "Sulfur granules" are common in sinus drainage fluid.

Diagnostic Considerations: Diagnosis by stain/culture of drainage from sinuses or lung/bone biopsy specimens. Actinomyces are non-acid fast and anaerobic to microaerophilic.

Pitfalls: No CNS lesions, but bone erosion is common with chest lesions. Prior antibiotic therapy may interfere with isolation of organism.

Prognosis: Excellent when treated until lesions resolve. Use IV regimen in critically ill patients, then switch to oral regimen.

Bronchopulmonary Aspergillosis (BPA / ABPA)

Clinical Presentation: Migratory pulmonary infiltrates in chronic asthmatics. Eosinophilia is common, and sputum shows Charcot-Leyden crystals/brown flecks containing Aspergillus.

Diagnostic Considerations: Diagnosis by Aspergillus in sputum and high-titers of Aspergillus precipitins in serum. BPA is an allergic reaction in chronic asthmatics, *not* an infectious disease. Pulmonary infiltrates with peripheral eosinophilia in chronic asthmatics suggests the diagnosis.
Pitfalls: Correct diagnosis is important since therapy is steroids, not antifungals.
Prognosis: Related to severity/duration of asthma and promptness of steroid therapy.

Acute Invasive Aspergillus Pneumonia (see p. 320)

Chronic Aspergillus Pneumonia

Clinical Presentation: Occurs in patients with AIDS, chronic granulomatous disease, alcoholism, diabetes, and those receiving steroids for chronic pulmonary disease. Usual features include chronic productive cough ± hemoptysis, low-grade fever, weight loss, and malaise. Chronic Aspergillus pneumonia resembles TB, histoplasmosis, melioidosis.
Diagnostic Considerations: Diagnosis by lung biopsy demonstrating septate hyphae invading lung parenchyma. Aspergillus may be in sputum, but is not diagnostic of Aspergillus pneumonia.
Pitfalls: May extend into chest wall, vertebral column, or brachial plexus.
Prognosis: Related to severity/extent of infection. Cavitation is a favorable prognostic sign.

Pulmonary Sporotrichosis (Sporothrix schenckii)

Clinical Presentation: Usually presents as productive cough, low-grade fever, and weight loss. Chest x-ray shows cavitary thin-walled lesions with associated infiltrate. Hemoptysis is unusual. Differential diagnosis includes other thin-walled cavitary lung lesions (e.g., histoplasmosis, coccidioidomycosis, atypical TB, paragonimiasis).
Diagnostic Considerations: Diagnosis by lung biopsy demonstrating invasive lung disease, not broncho-alveolar lavage. Usually a history of puncture/traumatic wound involving an extremity. May be associated with septic arthritis/osteomyelitis.
Pitfalls: Sporotrichosis in lungs implies disseminated disease. May need repeated attempts at culture.
Prognosis: Related to extent of infection/degree of immunosuppression.

Pulmonary Coccidioidomycosis (Coccidioides immitis)

Clinical Presentation: Usually presents as a solitary, peripheral, thin-walled cavitary lesion in early or later stage of primary infection. May present as a solitary pulmonary nodule. E. nodosum and bilateral hilar adenopathy are common (in contrast to sporotrichosis). Hemoptysis is unusual.
Diagnostic Considerations: Diagnosis by demonstration of spherules with endospores in sputum/BAL or biopsy specimens/Coccidioides serology. Increased incidence of dissemination in Filipinos, Blacks, and American Indians. Eosinophils in CSF in disseminated infection with CNS involvement. May be associated with chronic meningitis/osteomyelitis. CF IgG titer ≥ 1:32 diagnostic of active disease.
Pitfalls: Dissemination is preceded by ↓ Coccidioides titers/disappearance of Erythema nodosum.
Prognosis: Related to extent of infection/degree of immunosuppression.

Pulmonary Nocardiosis (Nocardia asteroides)

Clinical Presentation: Usually presents as a dense lower lobe lung mass ± cavitation. May have associated mass lesions in CNS. Chest wall sinuses are more common with Actinomycosis.

Diagnostic Considerations: Diagnosis by demonstrating organisms by stain/culture of lung specimens. Nocardia are weakly acid-fast and aerobic.

Pitfalls: Use IV regimens in critically ill patients. HIV/AIDS patients require life-long suppressive therapy with TMP–SMX or minocycline.

Prognosis: Related to extent of infection/degree of immunosuppression.

Pulmonary Cryptococcosis (Cryptococcus neoformans)

Clinical Presentation: Individual focus of infection is usually inapparent/minimal when patient presents with disseminated cryptococcal infection. Pneumonia is typically a minor part of disseminated disease; CNS manifestations usually predominate (e.g., headache, subtle cognitive changes, occasional meningeal signs, focal neurological deficits).

Diagnostic Considerations: Diagnosis by serum cryptococcal antigen, by demonstrating encapsulated yeasts in sputum/lung specimens, or by culture of pulmonary specimens.

Pitfalls: Clinical presentation of isolated cryptococcal pneumonia is rare. HIV/AIDS patients require life-long suppressive therapy with fluconazole.

Prognosis: Related to extent of dissemination/degree of immunosuppression.

Pulmonary Zygomycosis (Mucormycosis) (Rhizopus/Mucor/Absidia/Cunninghamella)

Clinical Presentation: Progressive pneumonia with fever, dyspnea, hemoptysis and cough unresponsive to antibiotic therapy. Usually seen only in compromised hosts. Chest x-ray is not characteristic, but shows infiltrate with consolidation in > 50% of patients. Cavitation occurs in 40% as neutropenia resolves.

Diagnostic Considerations: Diagnosis by demonstrating branched non-septate "ribbon-like" hyphae with right angle branching in biopsy specimens in lung biopsy. Pleural effusion is not a feature of pulmonary mucormycosis.

Pitfalls: Causes rhinocerebral mucormycosis in diabetics, pneumonia in leukopenic compromised hosts.

Prognosis: Related to degree of immunosuppression and underlying disease. Angioinvasive with a propensity for dissemination.

Pulmonary Pseudallescheriasis (P. boydii/S. apiospermum)

Clinical Presentation: Progressive pulmonary infiltrates indistinguishable from Aspergillosis or Mucor. Usually seen only in compromised hosts (e.g., prolonged neutropenia, high-dose steroids, bone marrow or solid organ transplants, AIDS). Manifests as cough, fever, pleuritic pain, and often hemoptysis. No characteristic chest x-ray appearance.

Diagnostic Considerations: Diagnosis by culture of organisms in lung biopsy. Hemoptysis is common in patients with cavitary lesions. CNS involvement is rare.

Pitfalls: One of few invasive fungi unresponsive to amphotericin B deoxycholate. Cause of sinusitis in diabetics, and pneumonia in leukopenic compromised hosts.

Prognosis: Related to severity/extent of infection and degree of immunosuppression. Cavitary lesions causing hemoptysis often require surgical excision. Disseminated infection is often fatal.

Parasites, Fungi, Unusual Organisms in the Heart

Chagas' Disease (Trypanosoma cruzi) American Trypanosomiasis

Subset	Pathogens	Preferred Therapy	Alternate Therapy
Chagas' disease (American trypanosomiasis)	Trypanosoma cruzi	Nifurtimox 8–10 mg/kg/day (PO) in 3–4 divided doses × 30–90 days	Benznidazole 2.5–3.5 mg/kg (PO) q12h × 30–90 days

Parasites, Fungi, Unusual Organisms in Liver

Liver Flukes

Subset	Pathogens	Preferred Therapy	Alternate Therapy
Fascioliasis	Fasciola hepatica Fasciola gigantica	Triclabendazole 10 mg/kg (PO) × 1 or 2 doses	Bithionol 30–50 mg/kg (PO) q48h × 10–15 doses
Clonorchiasis/ Opisthorchiasis	Clonorchis sinensis Opisthorchis viverrini	Praziquantel 25 mg/kg (PO) q8h × 3 doses	C. sinensis: Albendazole 400 mg (PO) q12h × 7 days O. viverrini: None

Hepatic Fascioliasis (F. hepatica/F. gigantica)

Clinical Presentation: Frequently asymptomatic, but may present acutely with fever, right upper quadrant pain, nausea, diarrhea, wheezing, urticaria, hepatomegaly, eosinophilia, anemia. ELISA, IHA, CF, CIE serology helpful with acute diagnosis. Aspiration of biliary fluid may show flukes/eggs. Chronic disease is associated with gallstones, cholecystitis, cholangitis, liver abscess, generalized adenopathy. Subacute nodules, hydrocele, lung/brain abscess can be seen in ectopic forms.

Diagnostic Consideration: Diagnosis by F. hepatica/F. gigantica eggs in stool. Endemic in sheep-raising areas (sheep liver flukes). Acquired from freshwater plants (watercress). Not associated with cholangiocarcinoma.

Pitfalls: May present as Katayama syndrome resembling schistosomiasis, with high fever, eosinophilia, and hepatosplenomegaly. Unlike other trematodes, praziquantel is ineffective. Chronic F. hepatica often asymptomatic, but may present with intermittent biliary colic. No eosinophilia. Abdominal ultrasound/CT shows crescentic/leaf shaped defects in gallbladder/hepatic ducts.

Prognosis: Related to extent/location of liver damage.

Hepatic Clonorchiasis (C. sinensis) / Opisthorchiasis (O. viverrini)

Clinical Presentation: Frequently asymptomatic, but may present 2–4 weeks after ingestion of fluke with fever, tender hepatomegaly, rash, and eosinophilia. Chronically presents as recurrent cholangitis, chronic cholecystitis, or pancreatitis. Associated with cholangiocarcinoma (unlike fascioliasis).

Diagnostic Considerations: Diagnosis by visualizing C. sinensis/O. viverrini (operculated lemon-shaped) eggs in stool. Clonorchiasis is acquired from ingesting raw/inadequately cooked infected freshwater (Cyprinoid) fish in Southeast Asia. Opisthorchiasis is acquired from ingesting raw/inadequately cooked infected freshwater fish/crayfish from Laos, Cambodia, or Thailand.
Pitfalls: Cholecystitis with eosinophilia should suggest clonorchiasis.
Prognosis: Related to extent/location of hepatic damage. Associated with cholangiocarcinoma.

Cystic Masses in Liver

Subset	Pathogens	Preferred Therapy	Alternate Therapy
Hepatic amebiasis	Entamoeba histolytica	Metronidazole 750 mg (PO) q8h × 7–10 days	Tinidazole 2 gm/day (PO) in 3 divided doses × 3 days
Hepatic echinococcosis (hydatid cyst disease)	Echinococcus granulosus	Operable Surgical resection **plus** Albendazole 400 mg* (PO) q12h × 1–6 months	Inoperable Albendazole 400 mg* (PO) q12h × 1–6 months

* If < 60 kg, give albendazole 7.5 mg/kg.

Hepatic Amebiasis (Entamoeba histolytica)

Clinical Presentation: Presents insidiously with weight loss and night sweats, or acutely ill with fever, nausea, vomiting, right upper quadrant pain. Typically, amebic liver abscesses are single, affect the posterior right lobe of liver, and do not show air/fluid levels. (In contrast, bacterial liver abscesses are usually multiple, distributed in all lobes of liver, and often show air/fluid levels.) Amebic liver abscesses do not calcify like hydatid cysts.
Diagnostic Considerations: Diagnosis by E. histolytica serology/E. histolytica in abscess wall. Worldwide distribution. Acquired by ingesting amebic cysts. Amebic liver abscess usually presents years after initial mild amebic dysenteric episode.
Pitfalls: Amebic abscess fluid ("Anchovy paste") contains no PMNs or amebas; amebas are found only in abscess wall. Eosinophilia is not a feature of amebiasis.
Prognosis: Related to health of host/extrapulmonary spread.

Hepatic Echinococcosis (Echinococcus granulosus) Hydatid Cyst Disease

Clinical Presentation: Right upper quadrant pain/mass when cysts enlarge enough to cause symptoms. Hepatic cysts are unilocular in 70%, multilocular in 30%.
Diagnostic Considerations: Diagnosis by demonstrating E. granulosus scolices/hooklets in cyst/hydatid sand. Serology is unreliable. Worldwide distribution in sheep/cattle raising areas. Acquired by ingestion of eggs from dogs.
Pitfalls: Eosinophilia not a feature of hydatid cyst disease. Hydatid cysts are multifaceted, loculated, and calcified.
Prognosis: Related to location/extent of extrahepatic cysts. Large cysts are best treated by surgical removal after injection with hypertonic saline, alcohol, or iodophor to kill germinal layer/daughter cysts. Percutaneous drainage under ultrasound guidance plus albendazole may be effective.

Hepatomegaly

Subset	Pathogens	Preferred Therapy	Alternate Therapy
Visceral leishmaniasis (Kala-azar)	Leishmania donovani	Antimony stibogluconate 20 mg/kg (IV/IM) q24h × 28 days **or** Amphotericin B deoxycholate 1 mg/kg (IV) q48h × 30 days **or** AmBisome (L-Amb) 3 mg/kg (IV) × 5 days and on day 10*†	Miltefosine 50 mg (PO) q12h × 28 days **or** Paromomycin 15 mg/kg (IM) q24h × 21 days
Indian (Bihar state) visceral leishmaniasis (Kala-azar)	L. donovani	AmBisome (L-Amb) 5 mg/kg (IV) × 1 dose, then miltefosine 50 mg (PO with food) q12h × 7–14 days	
Schistosomiasis	Schistosoma mansoni	Praziquantel 20 mg/kg (PO) q12h × 2 doses	Oxamniquine 15 mg/kg (PO) × 1 dose¶
	Schistosoma japonicum	Praziquantel 20 mg/kg (PO) q8h × 3 doses	None

* For immunocompetent patients who do not achieve parasitic clearance, consider repeat course of therapy.
† Ultra short course therapy with AmBisome is 10 mg/kg (IV) × 2 days.
¶ In Africa, give 20 mg/kg (PO) q24h × 3 days.

Visceral Leishmaniasis (Leishmania donovani) Kala-azar

Clinical Presentation: Subacute or chronic systemic cases manifest months to years after initial exposure to Leishmania, most often with fever, weight loss, anemia, hepatosplenomegaly ± generalized adenopathy. Long eyelashes in some. Laboratory abnormalities include leukopenia, anemia, and polyclonal gammopathy on SPEP. Incubation period is usually 3–8 months. May have atypical presentation in HIV/AIDS (e.g., no splenomegaly). Acutely can mimic malaria with chills/temperature spikes. Post–Kala-azar dermatitis may resemble leprosy, and is persistent/common on face.

Diagnostic Considerations: Double quotidian fever (double daily temperature spike) in persons from endemic areas with hepatosplenomegaly suggests the diagnosis. Kala-azar in children may have ↑ triglycerides/↓ HDL. Diagnosis by liver/bone marrow. Histologically, Kala-azar resembles histoplasmosis. Key diagnostic finding in tissue biopsy specimens is intracellular amastigotes with adjacent rod-shaped kinetoplasts. L. donovani serology is specific; immunochromatographic Anti-K39 strip test is also useful. Most common in Southern Europe, Middle East, Asia, Africa, South America. Facial lesion is a clue to the diagnosis.

Pitfalls: In acute cases, can mimic malaria with chills and temperature spikes, but no thrombocytopenia or atypical lymphocytes. Antimony resistance is common in India (Bihar state).

Prognosis: Related to degree of liver/spleen involvement.

Hepatic Schistosomiasis (Schistosoma mansoni/japonicum)

Clinical Presentation: May present acutely with Katayama fever (serum sickness-like illness with wheezing and eosinophilia) 4–8 weeks after exposure. May be accompanied or followed by fever/chills, headache, cough, abdominal pain, diarrhea, generalized lymphadenopathy, or hepatosplenomegaly. Laboratory abnormalities include leukocytosis, eosinophilia, and polyclonal gammopathy on SPEP. Resolves spontaneously after 2–4 weeks. After 10–15 years, may present chronically as hepatosplenic schistosomiasis, with pre-sinusoidal portal hypertension, hepatomegaly (L > R lobe enlargement), no jaundice, and intact liver function.

Diagnostic Considerations: Diagnosis by S. mansoni/S. japonicum eggs in stool/liver biopsy. Serology is good for acute (not chronic) schistosomiasis. CT/MRI of liver shows "turtle back" septal calcifications. Rare complications include cor pulmonale and protein-losing enteropathy. Increased incidence of hepatitis B/C and chronic Salmonella infections. Renal complications include glomerulonephritis and nephrotic syndrome.

Pitfalls: Chronic schistosomiasis is not associated with eosinophilia. S. hematobium does not infect the liver/spleen. Oxamniquine is contraindicated in pregnancy.

Prognosis: Related to egg burden.

Parasites, Fungi, Unusual Organisms in Stool/Intestines

Intestinal Protozoa

Subset	Pathogens	Preferred Therapy	Alternate Therapy
Amebiasis	E. histolytica	See p. 86	
Giardiasis	Giardia lamblia	See p. 86	
Isosporiasis	Isospora belli	TMP–SMX 1 DS tablet (PO) q6h × 10 days, then q12h × 3 weeks. If immuno-compromised give TMP–SMX 1 DS tablet (PO) q6h × 3 weeks	Ciprofloxacin 500 mg (PO) q12h × 7 days **or** Pyrimethamine 75 mg (PO) q24h + folinic acid 10 mg (PO) q24h × 2 weeks
Dientamoebiasis	Dientamoeba fragilis	Doxycycline 100 mg (PO) q12h × 10 days	Iodoquinol 650 mg (PO) q8h × 20 days **or** Paromomycin 8–12 mg/kg (PO) q8h × 7 days **or** Metronidazole 500-750 mg (PO) q8h × 10 days
Blastocystis	Blastocystis hominis	Nitazoxanide 500 mg (PO) q12h × 3 days **or** Metronidazole 750 mg (PO) q8h × 10 days	Iodoquinol 650 mg (PO) q8h × 20 days **or** TMP–SMX 1 DS tablet (PO) q12h × 7 days
Cyclospora	Cyclospora	See p. 86	

Intestinal Protozoa (cont'd)

Subset	Pathogens	Preferred Therapy	Alternate Therapy
Cryptosporidiosis	Cryptosporidia	See p. 86 (for HIV/AIDS, see p. 330)	
Balantidiasis	Balantidium coli	Doxycycline 100 (PO) q12h × 10 days	Iodoquinol 650 mg (PO) q8h × 20 days **or** Metronidazole 750 mg (PO) q8h × 5 days

Amebiasis (Entamoeba histolytica) (see p. 89)

Giardiasis (Giardia lamblia) (see p. 88)

Isosporiasis (Isospora belli)

Clinical Presentation: Acute/subacute onset of diarrhea. Isospora belli is the only protozoa to cause diarrhea with eosinophils in stool.

Diagnostic Considerations: Diagnosis by demonstrating cysts in stool and organisms in intestinal biopsy specimen. Associated with HIV, immigration from Latin America, daycare centers, and mental institutions. If stool exam is negative, "string test"/duodenal aspirate and biopsy may be helpful.

Pitfalls: Difficult to eradicate; may last months. Multiple stool samples may be needed for diagnosis. Add folinic acid 10 mg (PO) q24 if pyrimethamine is used. In HIV/AIDS, may need life-long suppressive therapy with TMP–SMX 1–2 DS tablet (PO) q24h (pp. 326, 330).

Prognosis: Related to adequacy of treatment/degree of immunosuppression.

Dientamoebiasis (Dientamoeba fragilis)

Clinical Presentation: Acute/subacute onset of diarrhea. No cyst stage. Lives only as trophozoite.

Diagnostic Considerations: Diagnosis by demonstrating trophozoites in stool/intestinal by trichrome stain. Mucus in diarrheal stools, not blood. May have abdominal pain. Diarrhea may last for months/years.

Pitfalls: Frequently associated with pinworm (Enterobius vermicularis) infection.

Prognosis: Related to adequacy of fluid replacement/underlying health of host.

Blastocystis (Blastocystis hominis)

Clinical Presentation: Acute/subacute onset of diarrhea.

Diagnostic Considerations: Diagnosis by demonstrating cysts and trophozoites in stool by trichrome stain. Trichrome stain reveals characteristic "halo" (slime capsule) in stool specimens.

Pitfalls: Uncommon GI pathogen. Consider as cause of diarrhea only after other pathogens excluded.

Prognosis: Related to adequacy of fluid replacement/underlying health of host.

Cyclospora (see p. 89)

Cryptosporidiosis (see p. 88; for HIV/AIDS, see p. 330)

Balantidiasis (Balantidium coli)

Clinical Presentation: Acute/subacute onset of diarrhea. Fecal WBCs only with mucosal invasion. Largest intestinal protozoa and only ciliated protozoa to infect humans.

Diagnostic Considerations: Diagnosis by demonstrating organism in stool/intestinal biopsy specimen. Identifying features include darkly staining "kidney shaped" nucleus and large size. Fulminant dysentery seen only in debilitated/compromised hosts.

Pitfalls: Stools not bloody. Diarrhea may be intermittent.

Prognosis: Related to adequacy of fluid replacement/underlying health of host.

Intestinal Nematodes (Roundworms)

Subset	Pathogens	Preferred Therapy	Alternate Therapy
Capillariasis	Capillaria (Aonchotheca) philippinensis	Mebendazole 200 mg (PO) q12h × 20 days	Albendazole 400 mg (PO) q24h × 10 days
Angiostrongyliasis (rodent lung/ intestinal worm)	Angiostrongylus Cantonensis	Mebendazole 200–400 mg (PO) q8h × 10 days	Thiabendazole 25 mg/ kg (PO) × q8h × 3 days (max. 3 gm/day)
Hookworm	Necator americanus/ Ancylostoma duodenale	Albendazole 400 mg (PO) × 1 dose **or** Mebendazole 100 mg (PO) q12h × 3 days or 500 mg (PO) × 1 dose	Pyrantel pamoate 11 mg/kg (PO) q24h × 3 days (max. 1 gm/ day)
Strongyloidiasis	Strongyloides stercoralis	Ivermectin 200 mcg/kg (PO) q24h × 2 days **or** Thiabendazole 25 mg/kg (PO) q12h × 2 days (max. 3 gm/day)	Albendazole 400 mg (PO) q24h × 3 days
Ascariasis	Ascaris lumbricoides	Albendazole 400 mg (PO) × 1 dose **or** Mebendazole 100 mg (PO) q12h × 3 days or 500 mg (PO) × 1 dose	Pyrantel pamoate 11 mg/kg (PO) × 1 dose (max. 1 gm)
Trichostrongyliasis	Trichostrongylus orientalis	Pyrantel pamoate 11 mg/kg (PO) × 1 dose (max. 1 gm)	Albendazole 400 mg (PO) × 1 dose **or** Mebendazole 100 mg (PO) q12h × 3 days

Intestinal Nematodes (Roundworms) (cont'd)

Subset	Pathogens	Preferred Therapy	Alternate Therapy
Pinworm	Enterobius vermicularis	Pyrantel pamoate 11 mg/kg (PO) × 1 dose (max. 1 gm); repeat in 2 weeks **or** Albendazole 400 mg (PO) × 1 dose; repeat in 2 weeks	Mebendazole 100 mg (PO) × 1 dose; repeat in 2 weeks
Whipworm	Trichuris trichiura	Mebendazole 100 mg (PO) q12h × 3 days, or 500 mg (PO) × 1 dose	Albendazole 400 mg (PO) q24h × 3 days **or** Ivermectin 200 mg/kg (PO) q24h × 3 days

Capillariasis (Capillaria philippinensis)

Clinical Presentation: Intermittent voluminous watery diarrhea ± malabsorption. Fever is uncommon.
Diagnostic Considerations: Diagnosis by demonstrating ova or parasite in stools. Resembles Trichuris, but C. philippinensis ova are larger and have a "pitted shell" with prominent polar plugs. Peripheral eosinophilia is uncommon until after therapy.
Pitfalls: Serology is positive in 85%, but cross-reacts with other parasites.
Prognosis: Related to severity of malabsorption/extra-intestinal disease.

Angiostrongyliasis (A. cantonensis) Rodent Lung/Intestinal Worm

Clinical Presentation: Presents as appendicitis (worm resides and deposits eggs in arteries/arterioles around ileocecum/appendix).
Diagnostic Considerations: Diagnosis by demonstrating organism in biopsied/excised tissue. May involve proximal small bowel, liver, CNS. When in CNS, a cause of eosinophilic meningitis.
Pitfalls: Can present as RLQ mass/fever resembling regional enteritis (Crohn's disease), but with eosinophilia and leukocytosis.
Prognosis: Related to severity of malabsorption and extra-intestinal disease.

Hookworm (Necator americanus/Ancylostoma duodenale)

Clinical Presentation: Pruritic, vesicular eruptions at site of filariform larval entry ("ground itch"). Pulmonary symptoms and transient eosinophilia may occur during migratory phase to intestines. Later, abdominal pain, diarrhea, weight loss, hypoalbuminemia, and anemia develop.
Diagnostic Considerations: Diagnosis by demonstrating eggs in stools. Larvae rare in fresh stool specimens (eggs may hatch if stools allowed to stand too long prior to examination). N. americanus can ingest 0.3 ml of blood/worm/day, much greater than A. duodenale. Anemia may be severe with heavy infestation (up to 100 mL/day).
Pitfalls: Eggs in fresh stool, not rhabditiform larvae. Eggs in hyperinfection syndrome.
Prognosis: Related to severity of anemia/malabsorption.

Strongyloidiasis (Strongyloides stercoralis)

Clinical Presentation: Pruritic, papular, erythematous rash. Pulmonary symptoms (cough, asthma) may occur during lung migration phase. May develop Loeffler's syndrome (pulmonary infiltrates with

eosinophilia) or ARDS in heavy infections. Intestinal phase associated with colicky abdominal pain, diarrhea, and malabsorption.
Diagnostic Considerations: Diagnosis by demonstrating larvae in stool specimens/duodenal fluid. Usually asymptomatic in normal hosts, but causes "hyperinfection syndrome" in compromised hosts. CNS strongyloides (part of hyperinfection syndrome) should suggest diagnosis of HIV in non-immunosuppressed patients. Diarrhea/abdominal pain mimics regional enteritis (Crohn's disease) or ulcerative colitis. Malabsorption is common and mimics tropical sprue. Anemia is usually mild.
Pitfalls: Usually rhabditiform larvae (not eggs) in stools.
Prognosis: Related to severity of malabsorption.

Ascariasis (Ascaris lumbricoides)

Clinical Presentation: Pulmonary symptoms (cough, asthma) may occur during larval lung migration phase. May develop Loeffler's syndrome (pulmonary infiltrates with eosinophilia), as with hookworm/Strongyloides. Intestinal symptoms develop late. Usually asymptomatic until intestinal/biliary obstruction occurs. Can obstruct the appendix/pancreatic duct.
Diagnostic Considerations: Diagnosis by demonstrating eggs in stool specimens. Abdominal ultrasound can detect obstruction from adult worms. Most infections are asymptomatic; symptoms are related to "worm burden"/ectopic migration. Each female worm may produce up to 250,000 eggs/day.
Pitfalls: Lung involvement (bronchospasm, bronchopneumonia, lung abscess) is prominent in HIV/AIDS.
Prognosis: Related to worm burden/extra-intestinal organ invasion.

Trichostrongyliasis (Trichostrongylus orientalis)

Clinical Presentation: Mild intestinal symptoms with persistent eosinophilia.
Diagnostic Considerations: Diagnosis by demonstrating eggs in stool specimens. Most prevalent in the Middle East and Asia. Mild anemia. Eosinophilia is usually > 10%.
Pitfalls: Must differentiate eggs from hookworm, and rhabditiform larvae from Strongyloides. T. orientalis eggs have "pointed ends."
Prognosis: Related to extent of disease/underlying health of host.

Pinworm (Enterobius vermicularis)

Clinical Presentation: Primarily affects children. Perianal pruritus (ectopic migration) is the main symptom. Worm lives in the cecum, but patients do not have intestinal symptoms.
Diagnostic Considerations: Scotch tape of anus at night can be used to detect eggs left by migrating female worms (Scotch tape test).
Pitfalls: Abdominal pain and diarrhea should prompt search for Dientamoeba fragilis, since co-infection is common.
Prognosis: Excellent.

Whipworm (Trichuris trichiura)

Clinical Presentation: May present as "chronic appendicitis." Severe infestation may cause bloody diarrhea/abdominal pain ("Trichuris dysentery syndrome"), rectal prolapse.
Diagnostic Considerations: Diagnosis by demonstrating large eggs with bile-stained, triple-layered eggshell walls and doubly operculated transparent plugs. Most patients are asymptomatic or mildly anemic.

Pitfalls: Commonly co-exists with Ascaris, hookworm, or E. histolytica.
Prognosis: Related to severity/extent of dysentery. May need retreatment if heavy infection.

Intestinal Cestodes (Tapeworms)

Subset	Pathogens	Preferred Therapy	Alternate Therapy
Beef tapeworm	Taenia saginata	Praziquantel 5–10 mg/kg (PO) × 1 dose	Niclosamide 2 gm (PO) × 1 dose
Pork tapeworm	Taenia solium	Praziquantel 5–10 mg/kg (PO) × 1 dose	Niclosamide 2 gm (PO) × 1 dose
Dwarf tapeworm	Hymenolepis nana	Praziquantel 25 mg/kg (PO) × 1 dose	Nitazoxanide 500 mg (PO) q12h × 3 days
Fish tapeworm	Diphyllobothrium latum	Praziquantel 10 mg/kg (PO) × 1 dose	Niclosamide 2 gm (PO) × 1 dose

Beef Tapeworm (Taenia saginata) / Pork Tapeworm (Taenia solium)

Clinical Presentation: Usually mild symptoms (weight loss, anemia), since most infections are caused by a single tapeworm.
Diagnostic Considerations: Diagnosis by demonstrating proglottids in stool. Taenia eggs in stool cannot be speciated; all are brown and spherical with a radially-striated inner shell. T. saginata may survive for 10 years, T. solium for 25 years.
Pitfalls: Severe cases may cause appendicitis, intestinal obstruction/perforation.
Prognosis: Related to severity of malabsorption/intestinal obstruction.

Dwarf Tapeworm (Hymenolepis nana)

Clinical Presentation: Usually asymptomatic.
Diagnostic Considerations: Diagnosis by demonstrating typical eggs in stool, with two shells enclosing inner oncosphere with hooklets. ELISA is positive in 85%, but cross-reacts with Taenia/Cysticercosis. GI symptoms develop with stool egg counts > 15,000/gm.
Pitfalls: Abdominal pain and diarrhea in heavy infestations.
Prognosis: Related to severity of malabsorption/underlying health of host.

Fish Tapeworm (Diphyllobothrium latum)

Clinical Presentation: Symptoms secondary to macrocytic anemia from vitamin B_{12} deficiency. Most infestations are asymptomatic.
Diagnostic Considerations: Diagnosis by demonstrating operculated eggs and proglottids in stool.
Pitfalls: Vitamin B_{12} deficiency anemia requires prolonged infection (> 3 years).
Prognosis: Related to severity of B_{12} deficiency anemia/underlying health of host.

Intestinal Trematodes (Flukes/Flatworms)

Subset	Pathogens	Preferred Therapy
Fasciolopsiasis	Fasciolopsis buski	Praziquantel 25 mg/kg (PO) q8h × 3 doses
Heterophyiasis	Heterophyes heterophyes Metagonimus yokogawai	Praziquantel 25 mg/kg (PO) q8h × 3 doses

Fasciolopsiasis (Fasciolopsis buski)

Clinical Presentation: Diarrhea with copious mucus in stool. Most cases are asymptomatic.

Diagnostic Considerations: Diagnosis by demonstrating eggs in stool. May have eosinophilia, low-grade fever ± malabsorption. Intestinal obstruction is the most serious complication.

Pitfalls: Mimics peptic ulcer disease with upper abdominal pain relieved by food.

Prognosis: Related to severity/extent of malabsorption/intestinal obstruction.

Heterophyiasis (Heterophyes heterophyes/Metagonimus yokogawai)

Clinical Presentation: Usually asymptomatic or mild intestinal symptoms. Embolization of eggs may result in myocarditis, myocardial fibrosis, or cerebral hemorrhage. Eosinophilia may be present.

Diagnostic Considerations: Diagnosis by demonstrating large operculated eggs in stool. Small intestine fluke.

Pitfalls: Difficult to differentiate from clonorchis sinensis.

Prognosis: Related to extent/severity of extra-intestinal dissemination to heart, lungs, CNS.

Other Intestinal Infections

Subset	Pathogen	Preferred Therapy
Whipple's disease	Tropheryma whippelii	Ceftriaxone 2 gm (IV) q24h × 2 weeks* **or** Penicillin G 6 mu (IV) q6h × 2 weeks plus Streptomycin 1 gm (IM) q24h × 2 weeks* **or** Ceftriaxone 1 gm (IV) q24h × 2 weeks plus Streptomycin 1 gm (IM) q24h × 2 weeks*

* Follow with TMP–SMX 1 DS tablet (PO) q12h × 1 year or doxycycline 100 mg (PO) q12h × 1 year.

Whipple's Disease (Tropheryma whippelii)

Clinical Presentation: Diarrhea, fever, encephalopathy/dementia, weight loss, polyarthritis, myocarditis, pericarditis, general lymphadenopathy ± malabsorption.

Diagnostic Considerations: Diagnosis by demonstrating organism by PAS staining macrophages in small bowel biopsy specimens.

Pitfalls: May present with dementia mimicking Alzheimer's disease, or FUO mimicking celiac disease or lymphoma. Optimum length of treatment is unknown. Relapses occur.

Prognosis: Related to severity/extent of extra-intestinal disease.

Parasites, Fungi, Unusual Organisms in Skin/Muscle

Infiltrative Skin/Subcutaneous Lesions

Subset	Pathogens	Preferred Therapy
Cutaneous leishmaniasis *Old World*	Leishmania major Leishmania tropica	Sodium stibogluconate 20 mg/kg (IV or IM) q24h × 20 days **or** Pentamidine 4 mg/kg (IM) q48h × 4 doses
New World	Leishmania mexicana Leishmania braziliensis	Sodium stibogluconate 20 mg/kg (IV or IM) q24h × 20–28 days **or** Pentamidine 4 mg/kg (IM) q48h × 4 doses
Leprosy *Lepromatous*	Mycobacterium leprae	Dapsone 100 mg (PO) q24h × 1–2 years + clofazimine 50 mg (PO) q24h × 1–2 years + rifampin 600 mg (PO) monthly × 1–2 years
Non-lepromatous (tuberculoid)	Mycobacterium leprae	Dapsone 100 mg (PO) q24h × 6 months + rifampin 600 mg (PO) monthly × 6 months
Loa Loa (Loiasis)	L. loa	Diethylcarbamazine 5–10 mg/kg in 3÷ doses (PO) × 3 weeks **or** Albendazole 200 mg (PO) q12h × 3 weeks
Erythrasma	Corynebacterium minutissimum	Erythromycin 250 mg (PO) q6h × 2 weeks

Cutaneous Leishmaniasis (Old World/New World)

Clinical Presentation: Variable presentation. Typically, a nodule develops then ulcerates, with a raised/erythematous outer border and a central area of granulation tissue. May be single or multiple. Usually non-pruritic/non-painful. Occurs weeks after travel to endemic areas (New World leishmaniasis: Latin America; Old World leishmaniasis: Central Asia).

Diagnostic Considerations: Diagnosis by demonstrating Leishmania amastigotes in biopsy specimen.

Pitfalls: Most skin lesions undergo spontaneous resolution. However, treatment is advisable for lesions caused by L. braziliensis or related species causing mucosal leishmaniasis.

Prognosis: Excellent.

Lepromatous Leprosy (Mycobacterium leprae)

Clinical Presentation: Diffuse, symmetrical, red or brown skin lesions presenting as macules, papules, plaques, or nodules. May also present as diffuse thickening of skin, especially involving ear lobes, face, and extremities. Loss of eyebrows/body hair may occur.

Diagnostic Considerations: Diagnosis by demonstrating organism in acid fast stain of tissue specimens. Afebrile bacteremia is frequent, and buffy coat smears positive for M. leprae. Erythema nodosum and polyclonal gammopathy on SPEP are common, and lepromin skin test/PPD are negative (anergic). When present, peripheral neuropathy is often symmetrical and acral in distribution.
Pitfalls: Differential diagnosis is large. Consider leprosy in patients with unexplained skin diseases.
Prognosis: Good if treated early.

Non-Lepromatous (Tuberculoid) Leprosy (Mycobacterium leprae)

Clinical Presentation: Small number of asymmetrical, hypopigmented skin lesions, which are often scaly with sharp borders and associated anesthesia. Asymmetric peripheral nerve trunk involvement is common.
Diagnostic Considerations: Diagnosis by demonstrating granulomas with few acid-fast bacilli. Differentiate from cutaneous leishmaniasis by skin biopsy. Lepromin skin test/PPD are positive and SPEP is normal (in contrast to lepromatous leprosy).
Pitfalls: Wide spectrum of presentations depending on immune status and duration of disease. Differential diagnosis is large. Consider leprosy in patients with unexplained skin diseases.
Prognosis: Good if treated early.

Erythrasma (Corynebacterium minutissimum)

Clinical Presentation: Reddened/raised skin lesions on face/trunk. Not hot or pruritic.
Diagnostic Considerations: Differentiated from Tinea versicolor by culture. C. minutissimum skin lesions fluoresce red under UV light.
Pitfalls: Resembles Tinea versicolor, but lesions primarily involve the face, not trunk.
Prognosis: Excellent.

Infiltrative Skin Lesions ± Ulcers/Sinus Tracts/Abscesses

Subset	Pathogens	Preferred Therapy
Cutaneous histoplasmosis	Histoplasma capsulatum	Treat as for disseminated histoplasmosis (Page 264) if part of systematic syndrome. If solely involves the skin, itraconazole 200 (PO) BID until resolution.
Cutaneous blastomycosis	Blastomyces dermatitidis	Treat the same as pulmonary infection (p. 264)
Cutaneous coccidioidomycosis	Coccidioides immitis	Treat the same as pulmonary infection (p. 265)
Cutaneous actinomycosis	Actinomyces israelii	Treat the same as pulmonary infection (p. 265)
Cutaneous nocardiosis	Nocardia sp.	Treat the same as pulmonary infection (p. 265)
Cutaneous amebiasis	Entamoeba histolytica	Treat the same as pulmonary infection (p. 262)

Infiltrative Skin Lesions ± Ulcers/Sinus Tracts/Abscesses (cont'd)

Subset	Pathogens	Preferred Therapy
Cutaneous mycobacteria *Scrofula*	Mycobacterium tuberculosis	INH 300 mg (PO) q24h + rifampin 600 mg (PO) q24h × 6 months
	M. scrofulaceum	Surgical excision is curative
M. haemophilum	M. haemophilum	Surgical excision/TMP–SMX 1 DS tablet (PO) q12h or minocycline 100 mg (PO) q12h or quinolone (PO) until cured
M. chelonae	M. chelonae	Surgical excision + clarithromycin 500 mg (PO) q12h × 6 months
M. fortuitum	M. fortuitum	Minocycline **or** doxycycline 100 mg (PO) q12h × 6–12 months **plus** TMP–SMX 1 DS tablet (PO) q12h × 6–12 months
Swimming pool granuloma	M. marinum	Clarithromycin XL 1 gm (PO) q24h × 3 months + rifampin 600 mg (PO) q24h × 3 months **or** TMP–SMX 1 DS tablet (PO) q12h × 3 months + ethambutol 15 mg/kg (PO) q24h × 3 months **or** Doxycycline 100 mg (PO) q12h × 3 months
Buruli ulcer	M. ulcerans	TMP–SMX 1 DS tablet (PO) q12h + ethambutol 15 mg/kg (PO) q24h × 6 weeks
Cutaneous MAI	Mycobacterium avium-intracellulare	Ethambutol 15 mg/kg (PO) q24h + azithromycin 1200 mg (PO) weekly × 6 months

Cutaneous Histoplasmosis (Histoplasma capsulatum)

Clinical Presentation: Chronic, raised, verrucous lesions.

Diagnostic Considerations: Diagnosis by demonstrating organism by culture/tissue staining.

Pitfalls: Skin nodules represent disseminated histoplasmosis, not isolated skin infection. Look for histoplasmosis elsewhere (e.g., lung, liver, bone marrow). Skin nodules (± chronic pneumonia) with osteolytic bone lesions suggests. African histoplasmosis due to H. capsulation var. duboisii.

Prognosis: Related to extent of infection/degree of immunosuppression.

Cutaneous Blastomyces (Blastomyces dermatitidis)

Clinical Presentation: Painless, erythematous, well-circumscribed, hyperkeratotic, crusted nodules or plaques that enlarge over time. Some may ulcerate and leave an undermined edge.

Diagnostic Considerations: Diagnosis by demonstrating organism by culture/tissue staining. Blastomyces dermatitidis affects many organs.

Pitfalls: When found in skin, look for Blastomyces elsewhere (e.g., lungs, prostate).
Prognosis: Related to extent of infection/degree of immunosuppression.

Cutaneous Coccidioidomycosis (Coccidioides immitis)

Clinical Presentation: Skin lesions take many forms, including raised verrucous lesions, cold subcutaneous abscesses, indolent ulcers, or small papules.
Diagnostic Considerations: Diagnosis by demonstrating organism by culture/tissue staining.
Pitfalls: Skin nodules represent disseminated coccidioidomycosis, not isolated skin infection. Look for Coccidioides elsewhere (e.g., CNS, bone, lungs).
Prognosis: Related to extent of infection/degree of immunosuppression.

Cutaneous Actinomycosis (Actinomyces israelii)

Clinical Presentation: Erythematous, uneven, indurated, woody, hard, cervicofacial tumor. Localized single/multiple sinus tracts in chest wall, abdominal wall, or inguinal/pelvic area may be present.
Diagnostic Considerations: Diagnosis by demonstrating organism by culture/tissue staining.
Pitfalls: Look for underlying bone involvement.
Prognosis: Good with early/prolonged treatment.

Cutaneous Nocardia (Nocardia brasiliensis)

Clinical Presentation: Subcutaneous abscesses may rupture to form chronically draining fistulas.
Diagnostic Considerations: Diagnosis by demonstrating organism by culture/tissue staining. May present as "Madura foot."
Pitfalls: Look for underlying immunosuppressive disorder.
Prognosis: Related to extent of infection/degree of immunosuppression.

Cutaneous Amebiasis (Entamoeba histolytica)

Clinical Presentation: Ulcers with ragged edges, sinus tracts, amebomas, and strictures may develop around the anus/rectum or abdominal wall.
Diagnostic Considerations: Diagnosis by demonstrating organism by tissue staining.
Pitfalls: If abdominal sinus tract is present, look for underlying ameboma and evidence of infection in other organs (e.g., CNS, lung, liver).
Prognosis: Related to extent of infection/degree of organ damage.

Scrofula (Mycobacterium tuberculosis)

Clinical Presentation: Cold, chronic, anterior cervical adenopathy ± sinus tracts. Usually in children.
Diagnostic Considerations: Diagnosis by acid-fast stain and culture of node/drainage.
Pitfalls: Cured by antibiotic therapy alone. No need for surgical excision.
Prognosis: Excellent with treatment.

Scrofula (Mycobacterium scrofulaceum)

Clinical Presentation: Cold, chronic, anterior cervical adenopathy ± sinus tracts. Usually in adults.
Diagnostic Considerations: Diagnosis by acid-fast stain and culture of node/drainage.
Pitfalls: Highly resistant to anti-TB therapy.
Prognosis: Excellent with surgical excision.

Cutaneous Mycobacterium haemophilum

Clinical presentation: Particularly common in immunosuppressed/HIV patients, presents as multiple, painful cutaneous ulcers/abscesses ± draining fistulas.

Diagnostic Considerations: Diagnose by PCR, RT-PCR assay.

Pitfalls: Suspect M. haemophilum if drainage from ulcer/abscess is AFB smear + but fails to grow on AFB media. M. haemophilus grows only on AFB media supplemented with ferric containing compounds i.e., hemin, hemoglobin, or ferric ammonium citrate. Susceptible to minocycline, TMP–SMX, or quinolones, but most strains resistant to INH, EMB, RIF, PZA.

Prognosis: Good with surgical excision/prolonged treatment.

Cutaneous Mycobacterium chelonae

Clinical presentation: Present as cold abscesses with draining fistulas.

Diagnostic Considerations: AF culture of wound drainage.

Pitfalls: Some strains clarithromycin resistant. May be susceptible to quinolones, doxycycline, or minocycline.

Prognosis: Good with effective therapy.

Cutaneous Mycobacterium fortuitum

Clinical Presentation: Usually associated with chronic foreign body infection, especially infected breast implants. Present as cold abscesses with draining fistulas.

Diagnostic Considerations: Diagnosis by demonstrating organism by acid fast smear are culture of drainage/infected prosthetic material.

Pitfalls: Highly resistant to anti-TB therapy, may be susceptible to quinolones or linezolid.

Prognosis: Good with surgical excision/prolonged treatment.

Swimming Pool Granuloma (Mycobacterium marinum)

Clinical Presentation: Begins as erythema with tenderness at inoculation site, followed by a papule or violaceous nodule that ulcerates and drains pus. May have sporotrichoid spread. Presents as a skin lesion unresponsive to antibiotics after abrasive water exposure (e.g., fish tank, swimming pool/lake).

Diagnostic Considerations: Diagnosis by demonstrating organism by acid-fast smear/culture.

Pitfalls: Resistant to INH/pyrazinamide. Surgical excision of isolated lesions may be needed.

Prognosis: Good with prolonged therapy.

Buruli Ulcer (Mycobacterium ulcerans)

Clinical Presentation: Begin as a firm, painless, movable, subcutaneous nodule. In 1–2 months, nodule becomes fluctuant, ulcerates, and develops an undermined edge. May have edema around lesion and in extremity (if involved).

Diagnostic Considerations: Diagnosis by acid-fast stain and culture of punch biopsy of ulcer rim. Patient is usually from Africa, but M. ulcerans also exists in Asia, Australia, and Central/South America.

Pitfalls: Steroids/skin grafting sometimes needed.

Prognosis: Good with surgical excision.

Cutaneous MAI (Mycobacterium avium-intracellulare)

Clinical Presentation: Nodules, abscesses, ulcers, plaques, ecthyma and draining sinuses can occur, but are uncommon in normal hosts and usually only seen in immunosuppressed patients.

Diagnostic Considerations: Diagnosis by demonstrating organism by acid-fast staining and culture (for species identification) of tissue biopsy specimens.

Pitfalls: Usually represents disseminated infection. Look for non-cutaneous evidence of infection (e.g., lungs, bone marrow, liver/spleen).

Prognosis: Related to extent of organ damage/degree of immunosuppression.

Skin Vesicles/Bullae

Subset	Pathogens	Preferred Therapy
Herpes simplex	Herpes simplex virus (HSV)	See p. 139 (for HIV/AIDS, see p. 337)
Herpes zoster	Varicella zoster virus (VZV)	See p. 139 (for HIV/AIDS, see pp. 316, 340)

Subcutaneous Serpiginous Lesions

Subset	Pathogens	Preferred Therapy
Cutaneous larva migrans (creeping eruption)	Ancylostoma braziliense	Ivermectin 150 mcg/kg (PO) q24h × 2 days **or** Albendazole 200 mg (PO) q12h × 3 days. Children may be treated topically with albendazole ointment (10%) q8h × 10 days
Guinea worm	Dracunculus medinensis	Surgical removal of worm near skin surface. Metronidazole 250 mg (PO) q8h × 10 days facilitates worm removal
Cutaneous gnathostomiasis	Gnathostoma spinigerum	Surgical removal **or** Albendazole 400 mg (PO) q24h × 3 weeks **or** Ivermectin 200 mcg/kg (PO) q24h × 2 days

Cutaneous Larva Migrans (Ancylostoma braziliense) Creeping Eruption

Clinical Presentation: Intensely pruritic, migratory, subcutaneous, raised serpiginous lesions.

Diagnostic Considerations: Diagnosis by clinical appearance.

Pitfalls: Must be differentiated from "swimmer's itch" caused by schistosomal cercariae.

Prognosis: Excellent with treatment.

Guinea Worm (Dracunculus medinensis)

Clinical Presentation: Serpiginous, raised, subcutaneous tract overlying worm.

Diagnostic Considerations: Diagnosis by demonstrating Dracunculus worm when surgically removed.

Pitfalls: Resembles cutaneous larva migrans, but worm is visible below the skin and lesions are serpiginous with Dracunculus. May be complicated by painful arthritis.

Prognosis: Excellent with treatment. Soaking extremity in warm water promotes emergence/removal of worm. Metronidazole can also be used to decrease inflammation and facilitate worm removal. Mebendazole 200–400 mg (PO) q12h × 6 days may kill worms directly.

Cutaneous Gnathostomiasis (Gnathostoma spinigerum)

Clinical Presentation: Painful, intermittent, subcutaneous swelling with local edema, intense pruritus, and leukocytosis with eosinophilia. Acquired by eating undercooked fish, frogs, and other intermediate larvae-containing hosts. May be complicated by eosinophilic meningitis.

Diagnostic Considerations: Diagnosis by demonstrating Gnathostoma in tissue specimens. Relatively common infection in Thailand and parts of Japan, South America, and Southeast Asia.

Prognosis: Good if limited to the skin and surgically removed. Poor with CNS involvement. Albendazole is preferred.

Skin Papules/Nodules/Abscesses

Subset	Pathogens	Preferred Therapy
Bacillary angiomatosis	Bartonella henselae Bartonella quintana	Doxycycline 100 mg (PO) q12h or azithromycin 250 mg (PO) q24h or any quinolone (PO) × 8 weeks
Cutaneous Alternaria	Alternaria alternata	Amphotericin B* 0.7–1.0 mg/kg (IV) q24h × 2–3 grams‡ Alternate therapy: Voriconazole, itraconazole, posaconazole, caspofungin. (See Drug Summaries (Chapter 11) for dosage) treat until cured
Entomophthoromycosis	E. basidiobolus E. conidiobolus	Amphotericin B* 0.7–1.0 mg/kg (IV) q24h × 1–2 grams‡ **or** TMP–SMX 1 DS tablet (PO) q24h until cured
Chromomycosis	Fonsecaea pedrosoi, compactum Phialophora verrucosa, others	Few small lesions: Wide/deep surgical excision or cryosurgery with liquid nitrogen Larger lesions: Itraconazole 200 mg (PO) solution q24h until lesions regress ± cryosurgery
Cutaneous Fusarium	Fusarium solani	Amphotericin B* 0.7–1.0 mg/kg (IV) q24h × 2–3 grams‡ **or** Voriconazole (see "usual dose," p. 695)
Cutaneous Penicillium	Penicillium marneffei	Amphotericin B* 0.6 mg/kg (IV) q24h × 14 days,‡ then itraconazole 200 mg (IV) q12 × 2 days followed by 200 mg (PO) q12h × 10 weeks. For HIV/AIDS, continue with itraconazole 200 mg (PO) q24h indefinitely
Cutaneous Prototheca	Prototheca wikermanii	Surgical excision. If excision is incomplete, add either amphotericin B* 0.7–1.0 mg/kg (IV) q24h × 2–3 grams‡ *or* itraconazole 200 mg (PO)† q12h until cured
Trichosporon	Trichosporon beigelii	Amphotericin B* 0.7–1.0 mg/kg (IV) q24h × 2–3 grams‡
Cutaneous aspergillosis	Aspergillus sp.	Voriconazole (see "usual dose," p. 695) **or**

* Amphotericin B deoxycholate.

‡ Lipid-associated formulation of amphotericin B (p. 513) may be a suitable alternative.

† Initiate therapy with itraconazole 200 mg (IV) q12h × 7–14 days.

Skin Papules/Nodules/Abscesses (cont'd)

Subset	Pathogens	Preferred Therapy
		Itraconazole 200 mg (IV) q12h × 7–14 days, then 200 mg (PO) solution q12h until cured
Cutaneous zygomycosis (mucormycosis)	Mucor/Rhizopus/ Absidia	Treat as for pulmonary zygomycosis, p. 266
Cutaneous coccidioidomycosis	Coccidioides immitis	Fluconazole 800 mg (PO) × 1 dose, then 400 mg (PO) q24h until cured **or** Itraconazole 200 mg (PO)† q12h until cured Alternate therapy Amphotericin B* 1 mg/kg (IV) q24h × 7 days, then 0.8 mg/kg (IV) q48h × 2–3 grams total dose‡
Cutaneous histoplasmosis	Histoplasma capsulatum	See p. 281
Cutaneous cryptococcosis	Cryptococcus neoformans	Amphotericin B* 0.5 mg/kg (IV) q24h × 1–2 grams‡ **or** Lipid-associated formulation of amphotericin B (p. 513) (IV) q24h × 3 weeks, **then follow with** Fluconazole 800 mg (PO) × 1 dose, then 400 mg (PO) q24h × 8–10 weeks
Cutaneous sporotrichosis	Sporothrix schenckii	Itraconazole 200 mg (PO). If HIV/AIDS, chronic suppressive therapy may be needed QD until 2–4 weeks after all lesions have resolved (typically 3–6 months in total). For alternative therapies see Kauffman CA et al. Clin Infect Dis 2007; 45: 1255–1265
Nodular/ pustular candidiasis	Candida sp.	Can be purely local syndrome if moisture or poor hygiene lead to local skin maceration. Therapy is then as for other forms mild cutaneous candidiasis (p. 282). But can also be a manifestation of disseminated disease and would be treated as for that syndrome (p. 288) (see p. 150)
Cutaneous onchocerciasis	Onchocerca volvulus	Ivermectin 150 mcg/kg (PO) × 1 dose, repeated q12 months until asymptomatic **plus** doxycycline 100 mg (PO) q12h × 6 weeks

* Amphotericin B deoxycholate.

† Initiate therapy with itraconazole 200 mg (IV) q12h × 7–14 days.

‡ Lipid-associated formulation of amphotericin B (p. 513) may be a suitable alternative.

Bacillary Angiomatosis (Bartonella henselae/quintana) Peliosis Hepatis

Clinical Presentation: Skin lesions resemble Kaposi's sarcoma. Liver lesions resemble CMV hepatitis in HIV/AIDS patients.

Diagnostic Considerations: Diagnosis by demonstrating organism by stain/culture of skin lesions or by blood culture after lysis-centrifugation.

Pitfalls: Requires life-long suppressive therapy.

Prognosis: Related to extent of infection/degree of immunosuppression.

Cutaneous Alternaria (Alternaria alternata)

Clinical Presentation: Bluish/purple papules that are often painful and non-pruritic. Usually seen only in leukopenic compromised hosts.

Diagnostic Considerations: Diagnosis by demonstrating organism by stain/culture in tissue specimen.

Pitfalls: Skin lesions usually represent disseminated disease in compromised hosts, not local infection. Fluconazole and micafungin ineffective.

Prognosis: Poor and related to degree of immunosuppression.

Cutaneous Entomophthoromycosis (E. basidiobolus / E. conidiobolus)

Clinical Presentation: E. conidiobolus infection presents as swelling of nose, paranasal tissues and mouth, accompanied by nasal stuffiness, drainage, and sinus pain. Begins as swelling of inferior nasal turbinates and extends until generalized facial swelling occurs. Subcutaneous nodules can be palpated in tissue. E. basidiobolus infection presents as a non-painful, firm, slowly progressive, subcutaneous nodule of the trunk, arms, legs, or buttocks.

Diagnostic Considerations: Diagnosis by demonstrating organism by stain/culture in tissue specimen. Skin lesions usually represent disseminated disease in compromised hosts, not localized infection.

Pitfalls: Unlike Mucor, E. basidiobolus does not usually invade blood vessels, although tissue infarction/necrosis is occasionally seen in diabetics and immunocompromised patients.

Prognosis: May spontaneously resolve. Surgical removal of accessible nodules and reconstructive surgery may be helpful for disfigurement.

Cutaneous Chromomycosis (F. pedrosoi/compactum, P. verrucosa, others)

Clinical Presentation: Warty papule/nodule that enlarges slowly to form a scarred, verrucous plaque. May also begin as a pustule, plaque, or ulcer. Over time, typical papule/nodule ulcerates, and the center becomes dry/crusted with raised margins. Lesions can be pedunculated/cauliflower-like.

Diagnostic Considerations: Diagnosis by demonstrating organism by stain/culture in tissue specimen. Chromomycosis remains localized within cutaneous/subcutaneous tissues.

Pitfalls: May resemble other fungal diseases. Sclerotic bodies in tissue and exudate distinguish chromomycosis from other related fugal diseases.

Prognosis: Related to degree of organ damage.

Cutaneous Fusarium (Fusarium solani)

Clinical Presentation: Presents in compromised hosts as multiple papules or painful nodules, initially macular with central pallor, which then become raised, erythematous, and necrotic. Seen mostly in leukopenic compromised hosts (especially acute leukemia and bone marrow transplants). Also a cause of mycetoma/onychomycosis.

Diagnostic Considerations: Diagnosis by demonstrating organism by stain/culture from blood/tissue.

Pitfalls: Skin lesions usually represent disseminated disease, not localized infection.

Prognosis: Poor/fair. Related to degree of immunosuppression. Amphotericin B lipid formulation (p. 513), colony-stimulating granulocyte factor, and granulocyte transfusions may be useful.

Cutaneous Penicillium (Penicillium marneffei)

Clinical Presentation: Papules, pustules, nodules, ulcers, or abscesses. Mostly seen in HIV/AIDS (requires life-long suppressive therapy with itraconazole).

Diagnostic Considerations: Diagnosis by demonstrating organism by stain/culture in tissue specimen. Affects residents/visitors of Southeast Asia/Southern China.

Pitfalls: Lesions commonly become umbilicated and resemble molluscum contagiosum. May present as disseminated infection.

Prognosis: Poor and related to degree of immunosuppression.

Cutaneous Prototheca (Prototheca wickermanii)

Clinical Presentation: Most common presentation is a single plaque or papulonodular lesion of the skin or subcutaneous tissue. Lesions are usually painless, slowly progressive (enlarge over weeks to months without healing), well-circumscribed, and may become eczematoid/ulcerated.

Diagnostic Considerations: Diagnosis by demonstrating organism by stain/culture in tissue specimen. Skin lesions in HIV/AIDS are not different from normal hosts.

Pitfalls: Lesions are usually painless and may resemble eczema.

Prognosis: Poor/fair. Related to degree of immunosuppression. Surgical excision has been successful.

Cutaneous Trichosporon (Trichosporon beigelii)

Clinical Presentation: Seen mostly in leukopenic compromised hosts (especially in acute leukemia, but also in HIV/AIDS, burn wounds, and organ transplants). Usually presents as multiple red-bluish/purple papules, which are often painful and non-pruritic.

Diagnostic Considerations: Diagnosis by demonstrating organism by stain/culture in tissue specimen.

Pitfalls: Skin lesions usually represent disseminated disease, not localized infection.

Prognosis: Related to extent of infection/degree of immunosuppression.

Cutaneous Aspergillosis (Aspergillus fumigatus)

Clinical Presentation: Seen at site of IV catheter insertion or adhesive dressing applied to skin in leukopenic, compromised hosts. Lesion is similar to pyoderma gangrenosum. May also invade burn wounds and cause rapidly progressive necrotic lesions.

Diagnostic Considerations: Diagnosis by demonstrating organism by stain/culture in tissue specimen.

Pitfalls: Infiltrative/ulcerative skin lesions usually represent disseminated disease in compromised hosts, not localized infection. May cause invasive dermatitis/skin lesions in HIV/AIDS.

Prognosis: Related to extent of infection/degree of immunosuppression.

Cutaneous Mucormycosis/Rhizopus/Absidia

Clinical Presentation: Necrotic skin lesion secondary to vascular invasion. Involves epidermis and dermis. Black eschars are evident.

Diagnostic Considerations: Diagnosis by demonstrating broad, non-septate hyphae with branches at right angles by stain/culture in tissue specimen.
Pitfalls: Skin lesions usually represent disseminated disease in compromised hosts, not localized infection. Contaminated elastic bandages have been associated with cutaneous Mucor.
Prognosis: Related to extent of infection/degree of immunosuppression.

Cutaneous Coccidioidomycosis (Coccidioides immitis)

Clinical Presentation: Skin lesions may take many forms, including verrucous granulomas, cold subcutaneous abscesses, indolent ulcers, or small papules.
Diagnostic Considerations: Diagnosis by demonstrating organism by stain/culture in tissue specimen.
Pitfalls: Skin lesions usually represent disseminated disease in compromised hosts, not local infection.
Prognosis: Related to extent of infection/degree of immunosuppression.

Cutaneous Histoplasmosis (Histoplasma capsulatum)

Clinical Presentation: Common cutaneous findings include maculopapular eruption, petechiae, and ecchymosis. Histopathology reveals necrosis around superficial dermal vessels.
Diagnostic Considerations: Diagnosis by demonstrating organism by stain/culture in tissue specimen.
Pitfalls: Skin lesions usually represent disseminated disease in compromised hosts, not local infection.
Prognosis: Related to extent of infection/degree of immunosuppression.

Cutaneous Cryptococcosis (Cryptococcus neoformans)

Clinical Presentation: May present as single or multiple papules, pustules, erythematous indurated plaques, soft subcutaneous masses, draining sinus tracts, or ulcers with undermined edges.
Diagnostic Considerations: Diagnosis by demonstrating spherules with endospores by stain/culture in tissue specimen.
Pitfalls: Skin lesions usually represent disseminated disease in compromised hosts, not localized infection. In AIDS patients, umbilicated papules resemble molluscum contagiosum. In organ transplants, cellulitis with necrotizing vasculitis may occur.
Prognosis: Related to extent of infection/degree of immunosuppression.

Cutaneous Sporotrichosis (Sporothrix schenckii)

Clinical Presentation: Primary cutaneous lymphatic sporotrichosis starts as a small, firm, movable, subcutaneous nodule, which then becomes soft and breaks down to form a persistent, friable ulcer. Secondary lesions usually develop proximally along lymphatic channels, but do not involve lymph nodes. Plaque form does not spread locally.
Diagnostic Considerations: Diagnosis by demonstrating organism by stain/culture in tissue specimen. Cutaneous disease arises at sites of minor trauma with inoculation of fungus into skin. Skin lesions usually represent disseminated disease in compromised hosts, not localized infection.
Pitfalls: HIV/AIDS patients with $CD_4 < 200$ may have widespread lymphocutaneous disease that ulcerates and is associated with arthritis. Unusual in axilla due to increased temperature.
Prognosis: Related to extent of infection/degree of immunosuppression.

Nodular/Pustular Candidiasis (see sepsis in chronic steroids, p. 155)

Cutaneous Onchocerciasis (Onchocerca volvulus)

Clinical Presentation: Early manifestation is pruritic, papular rash with altered pigmentation. Later, papules, scaling, edema, and depigmentation may develop. Nodules develop in deep dermis/subcutaneous tissue (especially over bony prominences) or in deeper sites near joints, muscles, bones. Endemic in Middle East, Central Africa, Central America.

Diagnostic Considerations: Diagnosis by serology/demonstration of microfilaria in thin snips of involved skin or in anterior chamber (by slit lamp) if eye involvement. Intradermal edema produces "peau d'orange" effect with pitting around hair follicles/sebaceous glands.

Pitfalls: Ivermectin is effective against microfilaria, not adult worms. Adults live ~ 18 years.

Prognosis: Related to location/extent of organ damage.

Rickettsia (Fever/Petechial Skin Rash)

Subset	Pathogens	Preferred Therapy	Alternate Therapy
Rocky Mountain spotted fever (RMSF)	Rickettsia rickettsii	Doxycycline 200 mg (IV or PO) q12h × 3 days, then 100 mg (IV or PO) × 4 days	Any quinolone (IV or PO) × 7 days **or** Chloramphenicol 500 mg (IV or PO) q6h × 7 days
Epidemic (louse-borne) typhus, flying squirrel typhus	Rickettsia prowazekii	Same as RMSF	Same as RMSF
Murine (flea-borne) typhus	Rickettsia typhi	Same as RMSF	Same as RMSF
Scrub (chigger mite-borne) typhus (Tsutsugamushi fever)	Rickettsia tsutsugamushi	Same as RMSF, or in mild cases azithromycin 500 mg (PO) × 1 dose	Rifampin 600–900 mg (PO) q24h × 7 days
Rickettsialpox	Rickettsia akari	Same as RMSF	Same as RMSF
Tick typhus fevers (Mediterranean spotted fever, Boutonneuse fever, Israeli spotted fever)	Rickettsia conorii Rickettsia parkeri	Same as RMSF	Same as RMSF
African tick bite fever	Rickettsia africae	Same as RMSF	Same as RMSF

Rocky Mountain Spotted Fever (Rickettsia rickettsia) RMSF

Clinical Presentation: Fever with relative bradycardia, severe frontal headache, severe myalgias of abdomen/back/legs 3–12 days after tick bite. Rash begins as erythematous macules on wrists and ankles 3–5 days after tick bite, and progresses to petechiae/palpable purpura with confluent areas of ecchymosis. Periorbital edema, conjunctival suffusion, acute deafness, and edema of the dorsum of the

hands/feet are important early signs. Abdominal pain can mimic acute abdomen, and meningismus and headache can mimic meningitis. Hepatosplenomegaly, cough, and coma may develop late. Laboratory findings include normal leukocyte count, thrombocytopenia, ↑ LFTs, and pre-renal azotemia. Hypotension/shock may occur secondary to myocarditis, which is the most common causes of death. Primary vector in United States is the Dermacentor tick; primary animal reservoir is small wild animals.
Diagnosis: Primarily a clinical diagnosis requiring a high index of suspicion and early empiric therapy. Early/rapid diagnosis can be made by DFA of biopsy specimen of rash. Specific R. rickettsii IFA, complement fixation, ELISA antibody titers are confirmatory. Include RMSF in differential diagnosis of any patient with fever and potential tick exposure, especially during the summer months.
Pitfalls: Most cases occur in eastern and southeastern United States, not Rocky Mountain area. Many cases go unrecognized due to nonspecific early findings. Early antibiotic therapy may blunt/eliminate serologic response. Patients with signs/symptoms of RMSF but without a rash should be considered as having ehrlichiosis ("spotless RMSF") until proven otherwise. Early therapy is essential; begin empiric therapy as soon as RMSF is suspected. Other adjunctive measures may be required.
Prognosis: Late (after day 5) initiation of treatment increases the risk of death by 5-fold. Adverse prognostic factors include myocarditis and severe encephalitis.

Epidemic (Louse-Borne) Typhus (Rickettsia prowazekii)

Clinical Presentation: High fever with relative bradycardia, chills, headache, conjunctival suffusion, and myalgias. A macular, rubella-like, truncal rash develops in most on the fifth febrile day, which may become petechial and involve the extremities, but spares the palms/soles. Facial swelling/flushing occurs at end of first week, along with CNS symptoms (e.g., tinnitus, vertigo, delirium) and GI complaints (diarrhea, constipation, nausea, vomiting, abdominal pain). Hypotension, pneumonia, renal failure, gangrene, cerebral infarction may develop late. Laboratory findings include normal leukocyte count, thrombocytopenia, and ↑ serum creatinine/LFTs. Primary vector is the human body louse; primary reservoir is humans.
Diagnosis: Primarily a clinical diagnosis requiring a high index of suspicion and early empiric therapy. Specific R. prowazekii antibody titers are confirmatory. Consider epidemic (louse-borne) typhus in febrile impoverished persons infested with lice, especially in Africa and parts of Latin America. Rarely seen in the United States. Milder recrudescent form (Brill-Zinsser disease) is also rare.
Pitfalls: Many cases go unrecognized due to nonspecific early findings. Early therapy is essential.
Prognosis: Gangrene of nose, ear lobes, genitalia, toes, and fingers may develop in severe cases. Death occurs in 10–50% of untreated patients.

Murine (Flea-Borne) Typhus (Rickettsia typhi)

Clinical Presentation: Similar to epidemic typhus but less severe, with fever in most, and headache, myalgias, and a macular rash in half. Laboratory findings include a normal leukocyte count, mild thrombocytopenia, and mildly ↑ LFTs. Primary vector is the Asian rat flea (Xenopsylla cheopis); primary reservoir is the commensal rat (Rattus genus). Uncommon in United States; most cases from Texas, California, Florida, Hawaii.
Diagnosis: Primarily a clinical diagnosis requiring a high index of suspicion. More common during summer and fall. Specific R. typhi antibody titers are confirmatory.
Pitfalls: Many cases go unrecognized due to nonspecific findings. Rash becomes maculopapular, compared to epidemic typhus, which remains macular. A similar illness is caused by R. felis.
Prognosis: Good if treated early. Death occurs in < 1%.

Scrub Typhus (Rickettsia tsutsugamushi) Tsutsugamushi Fever

Clinical Presentation: Fever, chills, headache, myalgias, arthralgias, GI symptoms, other nonspecific complaints. Eschar at mite bite site (tache noire) ± regional adenopathy. A macular, truncal rash develops in most, usually in the first week, and may progress to involve the extremities and face, but spares the palms/soles. Vasculitis may lead to cardiopulmonary, CNS, hematologic abnormalities during the second week. Hepatosplenomegaly is common. Primary vector/reservoir is the larval (chigger) trombiculid mite. Endemic areas include northern Australia, southeastern Asia, Indian subcontinent.

Diagnosis: Presumptive diagnosis is clinical. Specific R. tsutsugamushi serology is confirmatory.

Pitfalls: Incomplete therapy frequently results in relapse.

Prognosis: Excellent if treated early.

Rickettsialpox (Rickettsia akari)

Clinical Presentation: Milder illness than other rickettsioses, with initial eschar at bite site, high fever, and generalized rash (usually erythematous papules which become vesicular and spares the palms/soles). Fever peak is usually < 104°F, occurs 1–3 weeks after mite bite, and lasts ~ 1 week without therapy. Headache, photophobia, marked diaphoresis, sore throat, GI complaints (nausea/vomiting following initial headache) may occur. Most labs are normal, although leukopenia may be present. Primary vector is the mouse mite; primary animal reservoir is the house mouse. Rare in the United States.

Diagnosis: Presumptive diagnosis by clinical presentation. Specific R. akari serology is confirmatory.

Pitfalls: Do not confuse with African tick-bite fever, which may also have a vesicular rash.

Prognosis: Excellent even without therapy.

Tick Typhus Fevers (Rickettsia conorii, Rickettsia parkeri) Mediterranean Spotted Fever, Boutonneuse Fever, Israeli Fever

Clinical Presentation: Similar to RMSF with fever, chills, myalgias, but less severe. Unlike RMSF, an eschar is usually present at the site of the tick bite ± regional adenopathy. Leukocyte count is normal and thrombocytopenia is common. Transmitted by the brown dog tick, Rhipicephalus sanguineus.

Diagnosis: Presumptive diagnosis by clinical presentation. Specific R. conorii serology is confirmatory.

Pitfalls: Suspect in travelers from endemic areas with a RMSF-like illness. Consider different diagnosis in absence of an eschar.

Prognosis: Good with early treatment. Prostration may be prolonged even with proper therapy.

African Tick Bite Fever (Rickettsia africae)

Clinical Presentation: Similar to murine typhus with fever, chills, myalgias, but regional adenopathy and multiple eschars are common. Incubation period ~ 6 days. Amblyomma hebreum/variegatum tick vectors frequently bite humans multiple times.

Diagnosis: Presumptive diagnosis by clinical presentation. Specific R. africae serology is confirmatory.

Pitfalls: Rash is transient, and may be vesicular or absent.

Prognosis: Good even without therapy; excellent with therapy.

Other Skin Lesions

Subset	Pathogens	Topical Therapy	PO Therapy
Tinea versicolor (pityriasis)	Malassezia furfur (Pityrosporum orbiculare)	Clotrimazole cream (1%) or miconazole cream (2%) *or* ketoconazole cream (2%) daily × 7 days	Ketoconazole 200 mg (PO) q24h × 7 days **or** Itraconazole 200 mg (PO) q24h × 7 days **or** Fluconazole 400 mg (PO) × 1 dose
Eosinophilic folliculitis	Malassezia furfur (Pityrosporum orbiculare)	Preferred Therapy Ketoconazole cream (2%) topically × 2–3 weeks ± ketoconazole 200 mg (PO) q24h × 2–3 weeks	

Tinea Versicolor/Pityriasis (Malassezia furfur)

Clinical Presentation: Hyper- or hypopigmented scaling papules (0.5–1 cm), which may coalesce into larger plaques. Most commonly affects the upper trunk and arms. May be asymptomatic or pruritic.

Diagnostic Considerations: M. furfur also causes eosinophilic folliculitis in HIV/AIDS, and catheter-acquired sepsis mostly in neonates or immunosuppressed patients. Diagnosis is clinical.

Pitfalls: Skin pigmentation may take months to return to normal after adequate therapy.

Prognosis: Excellent.

Eosinophilic Folliculitis (Malassezia furfur)

Clinical Presentation: Intensely pruritic folliculitis, usually on lower extremities.

Diagnostic Considerations: Tissue biopsy shows eosinophilic folliculitis. Diagnosis by demonstrating organism by culture on Sabouraud's agar overlaid with olive oil.

Pitfalls: Resembles folliculitis, but lesions are concentrated on lower extremities (not on trunk as with cutaneous candidiasis).

Prognosis: Related to degree of immunosuppression. Use oral therapy if topical therapy fails.

Myositis

Subset	Pathogens	Preferred Therapy
Chromomycosis	Cladosporium/Fonsecaea	Itraconazole 200 mg (PO) q24h until cured **or** Terbinafine 250 mg (PO) q24h until cured
Trichinosis	Trichinella spiralis	Albendazole 400 mg (PO) q12h × 8–14 days **or** Mebendazole 5 mg/kg (PO) q12h × 2 weeks

Chromomycosis (Cladosporium/Fonsecaea)

Clinical Presentation: Subcutaneous/soft tissue nodules or verrucous lesions.
Diagnostic Considerations: Diagnosis by demonstrating organism by culture/tissue biopsy specimen.
Pitfalls: May resemble Madura foot or cause ulcerative lesions in muscle.
Prognosis: Related to degree of immunosuppression.

Trichinosis (Trichinella spiralis)

Clinical Presentation: Muscle tenderness, low-grade fevers, peripheral eosinophilia, conjunctival suffusion.
Diagnostic Considerations: Diagnosis by Trichinella serology or by demonstrating larvae in muscle biopsy.
Pitfalls: ESR is very low (near zero), unlike other causes of myositis, which have elevated ESRs.
Prognosis: Excellent with early treatment. Short-term steroids may be useful during acute phase. Therapy is ineffective against calcified larvae in muscle.

REFERENCES AND SUGGESTED READINGS

Adjei GO, Goka BQ, Kurtzhals AL. Neurotoxicity of Artemisinin Derivatives. Clin Infect Dis 43:1616–17, 2006.

Alexander BD, Pfaller MA. Contemporary Tools for the Diagnosis and Management of Invasive Mycoses. Clin Infect Dis 43:S15–S27, 2006.

Ansart S, Perez L, Vergely O, et al. Illnesses in travelers returning from the tropics: a prospective study of 622 patients. J Travel Med 12:312–18, 2005.

Avulunov A, Klaus S, Vardy D. Fluconazole for the treatment of cutaneous leishmaniasis. N Engl J Med 347:370–1, 2002.

Ayeh-Kumi PF, Petri Jr. WA. Amebiasis: An Update on Diagnosis and Treatment. Infections in Medicine 23:301–10, 2006.

Bisser S, N'Siesi FX, Lejon V, et al. Equivalence trial of melarsoprol and nifurtimox monotherapy and combination therapy for the treatment of second-stage Trypanosoma brucei gambiense sleeping sickness J Infect Dis 195:322–9, 2007.

Chayakulkeeree M, Ghannoum MA, Perfect JR. Zygomycosis: the re-emerging fungal infection. Clin Infect Dis 25:215–229, 2006.

Chen XM, Keithly JS, Paya CV, et al. Cryptosporidiosis. N Engl J Med 346:1723–1731, 2002.

Cheng AC, Currie BJ. Melioidosis: epidemiology, pathophysiology, and management. Clin Microbiol Rev 18:383–16, 2005.

Cisneros Herreros JM, Cordero Matia E. Therapeutic armamentarium against systemic fungal infections. Clin Microbiol and Infection 12:S53–64, 2006.

Croft SL, Yardley V. Chemotherapy of leishmaniasis. Curr Pharm Des 8:319–42, 2002.

Cunha BA. Malaria vs. Typhoid Fever: A Diagnostic Dilemma? Am J Med 118:1442–43, 2005.

DeGroote MA, Huitt G. Infections Due to Rapidly Growing Mycobacteria. Clin Infect Dis 42:1756–63, 2006.

Galgiani JN, Ampel NM, Blair JE, Catanzaro A, et al. Coccidioidomycosis. Clin Infect Dis 41: 1217–23, 2005.

Griffith, KS; Lewis, LS; Mali, S; Parise, ME. Treatment of Malaria in the United States. JAMA 297:2264–2277, 2007.

Haque R, Huston CD, Hughes M et al. Amebiasis. N Engl J Med 348:1565–73, 2003.

Herbrecht R, Natarajan A, Letscher-Bru V, et al. Invasive pulmonary aspergillosis. Semin Respir Crit Care Med 25:191–202, 2004.

International Artemisinin Study Group. Artesunate combinations for treatment of malaria: meta-analysis. Lancet 363:9–17, 2004.

Kremsner PG, Krishna S. Antimalarial combinations. Lancet 364:285–94, 2004.

Montoya JG, Liesenfeld O. Toxoplamosis. Lancet 363: 1965–76, 2004.

Munoz P, Guinea J, Bouza E. Update on invasive aspergillosis: clinical and diagnostic aspects. Clin Microbiol and Infection 12:S24–39, 2006.

Murray HW. Treatment of visceral leishmaniasis in 2004. Am J Trop Med Hyg 71:787–94, 2004.

Mushatt DM, Mihm LB, Dreisbach AW, et al. Antibiotic Dosing in Slow Extended Daily Dialysis. Clin Infect Dis 49:433–437, 2009.

Olliaro PL, Guerin PJ, Gerstl S, et al. Treatment options for visceral leishmaniasis: a systematic review of clinical studies done in India, 1980–2004. Lancet Infect Dis 5:763–4, 2005.

Ouellette M, Drummelsmith J, Papadopoulou B. Leishmaniasis: drugs in the clinic, resistance and new developments. Drug Resist Updat 7:257–66, 2004.

Perea S, Patterson TF. Invasive Aspergillus infections in hematologic malignancy patients. Semin Respir Infect 17:99–105, 2002.

Pirisi M, Salvador E, Bisoffi Z, et al. Unsuspected strongyloidiasis in hospitalized elderly patients with and without eosinophilia. Clin Microbiol Infect 12:787–92, 2006.

Ross AGP, Bartley PB, Sleigh AC, et al. Schistosomiasis. N Engl J Med 346:1212–1220, 2002.

Segal BH, WalshTJ.Current Approaches to Diagnosis and Treatment of Invasive Aspergillosis.Am J Respir Crit Care Med 173:707–17, 2006.

Sinha PK, Ranjan A, Singh VP, Das VNR, et al. Visceral leishmaniasis (kala-azar)—the Bihar (India) perspective. Journal of Infection 53:60–64, 2006.

Sobel JD.Combination therapy for invasive mycosis: evaluation of past clinical trial designs.Clin Infect Dis 15; 39 Suppl 4:S224–7, 2004.

Soto J. Miltefosine for new world cutaneous leishmaniasis. Clin Infect Dis 38:1266–72, 2004.

Tortoli E. Clinical Manifestations of nontuberculous mycobacteria infections. Clin Microbiol Infect 15:906–910, 2009.

Udall DN.Recent Updates on Onchocerciasis: Diagnosis and Treatment. Clin Infect Dis 44:53–60, 2007.

Vardakas KZ, Michalopoulos A, Kiriakidou KG, et al. Candidaemia: Incidence, risk factors, characteristics and outcomes in immunocompetent critically ill patients. Clinical Microbiology and Infectious Diseases 15:286–295, 2009.

White AC. New Developments in the Management of Neurocysticercosis. J of Infectious Diseases 199: 1261–1262.

Wormser GP, Dattwyler RJ, Shapiro ED, Halperin JJ, et al. The Clinical Assessment, Treatment, and Prevention of Lyme Disease, Human Granulocytic Anaplasmosis, and Babesiosis: Clinical Practice Guidelines by the Infectious Diseases Society of America. Clin Infect Dis 43:1089–134, 2006.

GUIDELINES

Chapman SW, Bradsher RW Jr, Campbell GD Jr, et al. Practice guidelines for the management of patients with blastomycosis. Infectious Diseases Society of America. Clin Infect Dis 30:679–83, 2000.

Galgiani JN, Ampel NM, Catanzaro A. et al. Practice guidelines for the treatment of coccidiomycosis. Infectious Diseases Society of America. Clin Infect Dis 30:658–61, 2000.

Hill DR, Ericsson CD, Pearson RD, Keystone JS, et al. The Practice of Travel Medicine: Guidelines by the Infectious Diseases Society of America. Clin Infect Dis 43: 1499–539, 2006.

Horn DL, Neofytos D, Anaissie EJ, et al. Epidemiology and Outcomes of Candidemia in 2019 Patients: Data from the Prospective Antifungal Therapy Alliance Registry. Clin Infect Dis 48:1695–1703, 2009.

Kauffman CA, Hajjeh R, Chapman SW.Practice guidelines for the management of patients with sporotrichosis. For the Mycoses Study Group.Infectious Diseases Society of America. Clin Infect Dis 30:684–7, 2000.

Pappas PG, Rex JH, Sobel JD, Filler SG, et al. Guidelines for the Treatment of Candidiasis. Clin Infect Dis 38: 161–89, 2004.

Perfect JR, Dismukes WE, Dromer F, et al. Clinical Practice Guidelines for the Management of Cryptococcal Disease: 2010 Update by the Infectious Disease Society of America. Clin Infect Disease 50:291–322, 2010

Saag MS, Graybill RJ, Larsen RA, Pappas PG, et al. Practice guidelines for the management of cryptococcal disease. Infectious Diseases Society of America. Clin Infect Dis 30:710–8, 2000.

Sobel JD. Practice guidelines for the treatment of fungal infections. For the Mycoses Study Group. Infectious Diseases Society of America. Clin Infect Dis 30:652, 2000.

Walsh TH, Anaissie EJ, Denning DW, et al. Treatment of Aspergillosis: Clinical Practice Guidelines of the Infectious Diseases Society of America. Clin Infect Dis 46: 327–60, 2008.

Wheat J, Sarosi G, McKinsey D, Hamill R, et al. Practice guidelines for the management of patients with histoplasmosis. Infectious Diseases Society of America. Clin Infect Dis 30:688–95, 2000.

TEXTBOOKS

Anaissie EJ, McGinnis MR. Pfaller MA (eds). Clinical Mycology.Churchill Livingston, New York, 2003.

Arikan S Rex JH. Antifungal Drugs. In: Manual of Clinical Microbiology, 8th Edition, ASM Press, Washington, D.C., 2003.

Bottone EJ (ed). An Atlas of the Clinical Microbiology of Infectious Diseases, Volume 1. Bacterial Agents. The Parthenon Publishing Group, Boca Raton, 2004.

Bottone EJ (ed). An Atlas of the Clinical Microbiology of Infectious Diseases, Volume 2. Viral, fungal, and parasitic agents. Taylor and Francis, 2006.

Bryskier A (ed). Antimicrobial Agents. ASM Press, Washington, D.C., 2005.

Calderone RA (ed). Candida and Candidiasis. Washington DC, ASM Press, 2002.

Cook GC (ed). Manson's Tropical Diseases, 23rd Edition. WB Saunders Company, Ltd., London, 2009.

Cunha BA (ed). Tick-Borne Infectious Diseases. Marcel Dekker, New York, 2000.

Despommier DD, Gwadz RW, Hotez PJ, Knirsch CA (eds). Parasitic Diseases, 4th Edition. Apple Trees Productions, LLC, New York, 2000.

Garcia LS (ed). Practical guide to Diagnostic Parasitology. ASM Press, Washington, DC, 2009.

Gorbach SL, Bartlett JG, Blacklow NR (eds). Infectious Diseases, 3rd Edition. Philadelphia, Lippincott, Williams & Wilkins, 2004.

Guerrant RL, Walker DH, Weller PF (eds). Tropical Infectious Disease: Principles, Pathogens & Practice 2nd Edition. Churchill Livingstone, Philadelphia, 2006.

Gutierrez Y (ed). Diagnostic Pathology of Parasitic Infections with Clinical Correlations, 2nd Edition. Oxford University Press, New York, 2000.

Howard DH (ed). Pathogenic Fungi in Humans and Animals. 2nd Edition. New York, Marcel Dekker, 2003.

Jong E, Sanford C. The Travel and Tropical Medicine Manual. 4th ed. Philadelphia: Saunders Elsevier, 2008.

Keystone JS, Kozarsky PE, Freedman DO, Nothdurft HO, Connor B. Travel Medicine 2nd ed. Philadelphia: Mosby Elsevier, 2008.

Knipe DM, Howley PM (eds). Fields Virology, 5th Edition. Lippincott Williams & Wilkins, Philadelphia, 2008.

Krauss H, Weber A, Appel M, (ed). Zoonoses. Infectious Diseases Transmissible from Animals to Humans, 3rd Edition. ASM Press, Washington, D.C. 2003.

Maertens JA, Marr KA. Diagnosis of Fungal Infections. Informa Healthcare, New York, 2007.

Mandell GL, Bennett JE, Dolin R (eds). Mandell, Douglas, and Bennett's Principles and Practice of infectious Diseases, 7th Edition. Philadelphia, Elsevier, 2010.

Porterfield JS (ed). Exotic Viral Infections. Chapman & Hall Medical, London, 1995.

Raoult D, Parola P. Rickettsial Diseases. Informa Healthcare, New York, 2007.

Rex JH. Approach to the Treatment of Systemic Fungal Infections. In: Kelley WN (ed). Kelley's Textbook of Internal Medicine, 4th Edition, 2000.

Richman DD, Whitley RJ, Hayden FG (eds). Clinical Virology, 2nd Edition. ASM Press, Washington, DC, 2002.

Scholssberg DM (ed). Current Therapy of Infectious Diseases, 3rd Edition, Mosby St. Louis, 2008.

Strickland GT (ed). Hunter's Tropical Medicine and Emerging Infectious Diseases, 8th Edition. W.B. Saunders Company, Philadelphia, 2000.

Sun T (ed). Parasitic Disorders: Pathology, Diagnosis, and Management, 2nd Edition. Williams & Wilkins, Baltimore, 1999.

Walker DH (ed). Biology of Rickettsial Diseases I/II. CRC Press, Boca Raton, 2000.

Warrell DA, Gilles HM. Essential Malariology, 4th Edition. Oxford University Press, New York, 2002.

Yu VL, Jr., Merigan TC, Jr., and Barriere SL (eds.). Antimicrobial Therapy & Vaccines 2nd Edition, Williams & Wilkins, Baltimore, MD, 2005.

Chapter 5
HIV Infection

Paul E. Sax, MD

HIV INFECTION OVERVIEW

Paul E. Sax, M.D.

Infection with Human Immunodeficiency Virus (HIV-1) leads to a chronic and without treatment usually fatal infection characterized by progressive immunodeficiency, a long clinical latency period, and opportunistic infections. The hallmark of HIV disease is infection and viral replication within T-lymphocytes expressing the CD_4 antigen (helper-inducer lymphocytes), a critical component of normal cell-mediated immunity. Qualitative defects in CD_4 responsiveness and progressive depletion in CD_4 cell counts increase the risk for opportunistic infections such as Pneumocystis (carinii) jiroveci pneumonia, and neoplasms such as lymphoma and Kaposi's sarcoma. HIV infection can also disrupt blood monocyte, tissue macrophage, and B-lymphocyte (humoral immunity) function, predisposing to infection with encapsulated bacteria. Direct attack of CD_4-positive cells in the central and peripheral nervous system can cause HIV meningitis, peripheral neuropathy, and dementia. More than 1 million people in the United States and 30 million people worldwide are infected with HIV. Without treatment, the average time from acquisition of HIV to an AIDS-defining opportunistic infection is about 10 years; survival then averages 1–2 years. There is tremendous individual variability in these time intervals, with some patients progressing from acute HIV infection to death within 1–2 years, and others not manifesting HIV-related immunosuppression for > 20 years after HIV acquisition. Antiretroviral therapy and prophylaxis against opportunistic infections have markedly improved the overall prognosis of HIV disease. The approach to HIV infection is shown in Figure 5.1.

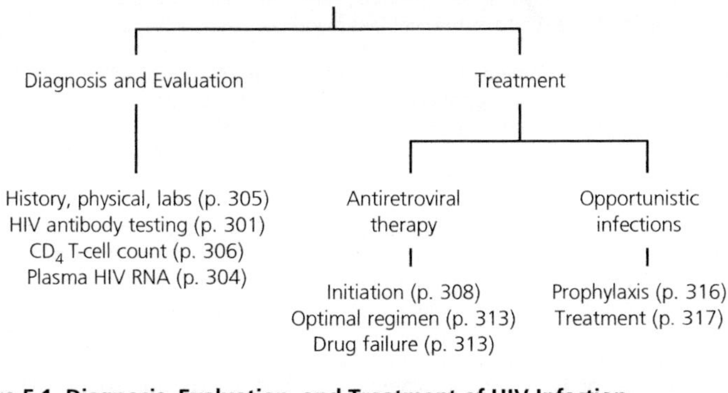

Figure 5.1. Diagnosis, Evaluation, and Treatment of HIV Infection

STAGES OF HIV INFECTION

A. **Viral Transmission.** HIV infection is acquired primarily by sexual intercourse (anal, vaginal, infrequently oral), exposure to contaminated blood (primarily needle transmission), or maternal-fetus (perinatal) transmission. Sexual practices with the highest risk of transmission include unprotected receptive anal intercourse (especially with mucosal tearing), unprotected receptive vaginal intercourse (especially during menses), and unprotected rectal/vaginal intercourse in the presence of genital ulcers (e.g., primary syphilis, genital herpes, chancroid). Lower risk sexual practices include insertive anal/vaginal intercourse and oral-genital contact. The risk of transmission after a single encounter with an HIV source has been estimated to be 1 in 150 with needle sharing, 1 in 300 with occupational percutaneous exposure, 1 in 300–1000 with receptive anal intercourse, 1 in 500–1250 with receptive vaginal intercourse, 1 in 1000–3000 with insertive vaginal intercourse, and 1 in 3000 with insertive anal intercourse. Transmission risk increases with the number of encounters and with higher HIV RNA plasma levels. The mode of transmission does not affect the natural history of HIV disease.

B. **Acute (Primary) HIV Infection (p. 301).** Acute HIV occurs 1–4 weeks after transmission, and is accompanied by a burst of viral replication with a decline in CD_4 cell count. Most patients manifest a symptomatic mononucleosis-like syndrome, which is often overlooked. Acute HIV infection is confirmed by a high HIV RNA in the absence of HIV antibody.

C. **Seroconversion.** Development of a positive HIV antibody test usually occurs within 4 weeks of acute infection, and invariably (with few exceptions) by 6 months.

D. **Asymptomatic HIV Infection** lasts a variable amount of time (average 8–10 years), and is accompanied by a gradual decline in CD_4 cell counts and a relatively stable HIV RNA level (sometimes referred to as the viral "set point").

E. **Symptomatic HIV Infection.** Previously referred to as "AIDS Related Complex (ARC)," findings include thrush or vaginal candidiasis (persistent, frequent, or poorly responsive to treatment), cervical dysplasia/carcinoma in-situ, herpes zoster (recurrent episodes or involving multiple dermatomes), oral hairy leukoplakia, peripheral neuropathy, diarrhea, or constitutional symptoms (e.g., low-grade fevers, weight loss).

F. **AIDS** is defined by a CD_4 cell count $< 200/mm^3$, a CD_4 cell percentage of total lymphocytes <14%, or one of several AIDS-related opportunistic infections. Common opportunistic infections include Pneumocystis (carinii) jiroveci pneumonia, cryptococcal meningitis, recurrent bacterial pneumonia, Candida esophagitis, CNS toxoplasmosis, tuberculosis, and non-Hodgkin's lymphoma. Other AIDS indicators in HIV-infected patients include candidiasis of the bronchi, trachea, or lungs; disseminated/extrapulmonary coccidiomycosis, cryptococcosis, or histoplasmosis; chronic (>1 month) intestinal cryptosporidiosis or isosporiasis; Kaposi's sarcoma; lymphoid interstitial pneumonia/pulmonary lymphoid hyperplasia; disseminated/extrapulmonary Mycobacterium (avium-intracellulare, kansasii, other species) infection; progressive multifocal leukoencephalopathy (PML); recurrent Salmonella septicemia; or HIV wasting syndrome.

G. **Advanced HIV Disease** is diagnosed when the CD_4 cell count is < 50/mm^3. Most AIDS-related deaths occur at this point. Common late stage opportunistic infections are caused by CMV disease (retinitis, colitis) or disseminated Mycobacterium avium-intracellulare (MAI).

ACUTE (PRIMARY) HIV INFECTION

A. **Description.** Acute clinical illness associated with primary acquisition of HIV, occurring 1–4 weeks after viral transmission (range: 6 days to 6 weeks). Symptoms develop in 50–90%, but are often mistaken for the flu, mononucleosis, or other nonspecific viral syndrome. More severe symptoms may correlate with a higher viral set point and more rapid HIV disease progression. Even without therapy, most patients recover, reflecting development of a partially effective immune response and depletion of susceptible CD_4 cells.

B. **Differential Diagnosis** includes **EBV, CMV**, viral hepatitis, enteroviral infection, 2° syphilis, toxoplasmosis, HSV with erythema multiforme, drug reaction, Behcet's disease, acute lupus.

C. **Signs and Symptoms** usually reflect hematogenous dissemination of virus to lymphoreticular and neurologic sites:
- Fever (97%).
- Pharyngitis (73%). Typically non-exudative (unlike EBV, which is usually exudative).
- Rash (77%). Maculopapular viral exanthem of the face and trunk is most common, but can involve the extremities, palms and soles.
- Arthralgia/myalgia (58%).
- Neurologic symptoms (12%). Headache is most common. Neuropathy, Bell's palsy, and meningoencephalitis are rare, but may predict worse outcome.
- Oral/genital ulcerations, thrush, nausea, vomiting, diarrhea, weight loss.

D. **Laboratory Findings**
1. **CBC.** Lymphopenia followed by lymphocytosis (common). Atypical lymphocytosis is variable, but usually low level (unlike EBV, where atypical lymphocytosis may be 20–30% or higher). Thrombocytopenia occurs in some.
2. **Elevated transaminases** in some but not all patients.
3. **Depressed CD_4 cell count.** Can rarely be low enough to induce opportunistic infections.
4. **HIV antibody.** Usually negative, although persons with prolonged symptoms of acute HIV may have positive antibody tests if diagnosed late during the course of illness.

E. Confirming the Diagnosis of Acute HIV Infection

1. **Obtain HIV antibody** after informed consent (if required by state law) to exclude prior disease.
2. **Order viral load test (HIV RNA PCR),** preferably RT-PCR. HIV RNA confirms acute HIV infection prior to seroconversion. Most individuals will have very high HIV RNA (>100,000 copies/mL). Be suspicious of a false-positive test if the HIV RNA is low (< 20,000 copies/mL). For any positive test, it is important to repeat HIV RNA and HIV antibody testing. p24 antigen can also be used to establish the diagnosis, but is less sensitive than HIV RNA PCR.
3. **Order other tests/serologies if HIV RNA test is negative.** Order throat cultures for bacterial/viral respiratory pathogens, EBV VCA IgM/IgG, CMV IgM/IgG, HHV-6 IgM/IgG, and hepatitis serologies as appropriate to establish a diagnosis for patient's symptoms.

F. Management of Acute HIV Infection

1. **Initiate antiretroviral therapy.** Patients with acute HIV infection should be referred to an HIV specialist, who ideally will enroll the patient into a clinical study. Most experts recommend antiretroviral therapy, although no long-term clinical studies comparing treatment vs. observation have been conducted. The optimal duration of therapy and role of intermittent treatment are under investigation.
2. **Obtain HIV resistance genotype (p. 314)** because of a rising background prevalence of transmission of antiretroviral therapy-resistant virus. A genotype resistance test is preferred; therapy can be started pending results of the test.
3. **Possible benefits for treatment of acute HIV infection.** Possible (but unproven) benefits include hastening symptom resolution, reducing viral transmission, lowering virologic "set point," and preserving virus-specific CD_4 responses.

APPROACH TO HIV TESTING (Figure 5.2)

A. Standard HIV Antibody Tests (see also Clin Infect Dis 2007;45:S221–S225). Most patients produce antibody to HIV within 6–8 weeks of exposure; half will have a positive antibody test in 3–4 weeks, and nearly 100% will have detectable antibody by 6 months.

1. **ELISA.** Usual screening test. All positives must be confirmed with Western blot or other more specific tests.
2. **Western blot.** CDC criteria for interpretation: **positive:** at least two of the following bands: p24, gp41, gp160/120; **negative:** no bands; **indeterminate:** any HIV band, but does not meet criteria for positivity.
3. **Test performance.** Standard method is ELISA screen with Western blot confirmation.
   - **a. ELISA negative:** Western blot is not required (ELISA sensitivity 99.7%, specificity 98.5%). Obtain HIV RNA if acute HIV infection is suspected.
   - **b. ELISA positive:** Confirm with Western blot. Probability that ELISA and Western blot are both false-positives is extremely low (< 1 per 140,000). Absence of p31 band could be a clue to a false positive Western blot.
   - **c. Unexpected ELISA/Western blot:** Repeat test to exclude clerical/computer error.

4. **Indeterminate Western Blot.** Common clinical problem, affecting 4–20% of reactive ELISAs. Usually due to a single p24 band or weak other bands. Causes include seroconversion in progress, advanced HIV disease with loss of antibody response,

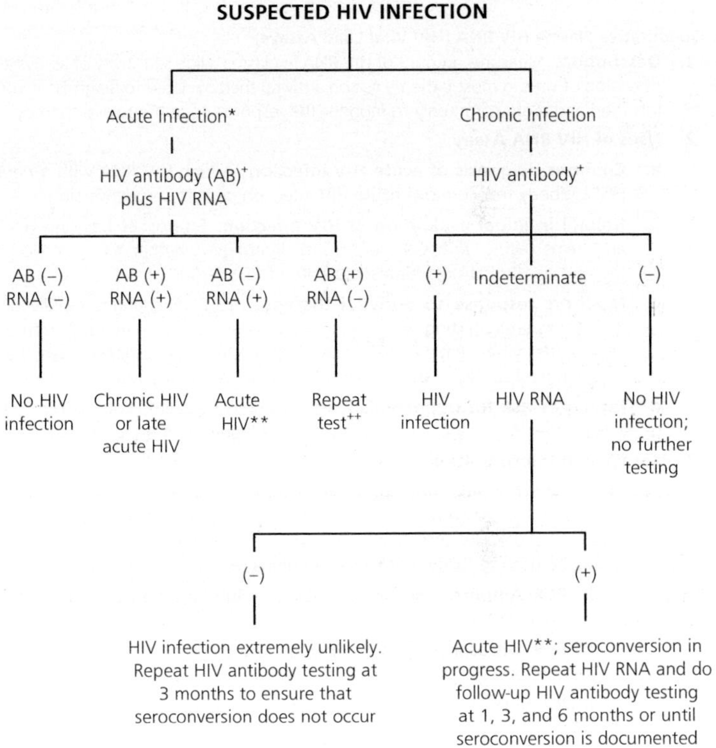

Figure 5.2. Approach to HIV Testing

(–) = negative test; (+) = positive test.

* Occurs 1–4 weeks after viral transmission. Most patients manifest a viral syndrome (fever, pharyngitis ± rash/arthralgias), which is often mistaken for the flu and therefore overlooked.

** HIV RNA in acute HIV infection should be very high (usually > 100,000 copies/mL).

\+ All positive ELISA tests must be confirmed by Western Blot; usually this is done automatically in clinical laboratories.

++ May be long-term non-progressor or laboratory error.

cross-reacting antibody from pregnancy, blood transfusions, organ transplantation, autoantibodies from collagen vascular disease, infection with HIV-2, influenza vaccination, or recipient of HIV vaccine. In low-risk patients, an indeterminate result almost never represents true HIV infection. Since seroconversion in progress is generally associated with high HIV RNA levels, the recommended approach is to order an HIV RNA test.

B. Quantitative Plasma HIV RNA (HIV Viral Load Assays)

1. **Description.** Measures amount of HIV RNA in plasma. High sensitivity of assays allows detection of virus in most patients not on antiviral therapy. Used to diagnose acute HIV infection and more commonly to monitor the response to antiretroviral therapy.
2. **Uses of HIV RNA Assay**
   a. **Confirms diagnosis of acute HIV infection.** A high HIV RNA with a negative HIV antibody test confirms acute HIV infection prior to seroconversion.

   b. **Helpful in initial evaluation of HIV infection.** Establishes baseline HIV RNA and helps (along with CD_4 cell count) determine whether to initiate or defer therapy, as HIV RNA correlates with rate of CD_4 decline.

   c. **Monitors response to antiviral therapy.** HIV RNA changes rapidly decline 2–4 weeks after starting or changing effective antiretroviral therapy, with slower decline thereafter. Patients with the greatest HIV RNA response have the best clinical outcome. No change in HIV RNA suggests therapy will be ineffective.

   d. **Estimates risk for opportunistic infection.** For patients with similar CD_4 cell counts, the risk of opportunistic infections is higher with higher HIV RNAs.
3. **Assays and Interpretation**
   a. **Tests, sensitivities, and dynamic range.** Three main assays, each with advantages and disadvantages, are widely used. Any assay can be used to diagnose acute HIV infection and guide/monitor therapy, but the same test should be used to follow patients longitudinally.

      1. **RT-PCR Amplicor** (Roche): Sensitivity = 400 copies/mL; dynamic range = 400–750,000 copies/mL.
      2. **RT-PCR Ultrasensitive 1.5** (Roche): Sensitivity = 50 copies/mL; dynamic range = 50–75,000 copies/mL.
      3. **bDNA Versant 3.0** (Bayer): Sensitivity = 75 copies/mL; dynamic range = 50–500,000 copies/mL.

   b. **Correlation between HIV RNA and CD_4.** HIV RNA assays correlate inversely with CD_4 cell counts, but do so imperfectly (e.g., some patients with high CD_4 counts have relatively high HIV RNA levels, and vice versa.) For any given CD_4, higher HIV RNA levels correlate with more rapid CD_4 decline. In response to antiretroviral therapy, changes in HIV RNA generally precede changes in CD_4 cell count.

   c. **Significant change in HIV RNA assay** is defined by at least a 2-fold (0.3 log) change in viral RNA (accounts for normal variation in clinically stable patients), or a 3-fold (0.5 log) change in response to new antiretroviral therapy (accounts for intra-laboratory and patient variability). For example, if a HIV RNA result = 50,000 copies/mL, then the range of possible actual values = 25,000–100,000 copies/mL, and the value needed to demonstrate antiretroviral activity is ≤ 17,000 copies/mL.

4. **Indications for HIV RNA Testing.** Usually performed in conjunction with CD_4 cell counts. Indicated for the diagnosis of acute HIV infection, and for initial evaluation of newly diagnosed HIV. Also recommended 2–8 weeks after initiation of antiretroviral therapy and every 3–4 months in all HIV patients.

5. **When to Avoid HIV RNA Testing**

   a. **During acute illnesses and immunizations.** Patients with acute infections (opportunistic infection, bacterial pneumonia, even HSV recurrences) may experience significant (> 5-fold) rises in HIV RNA, which return to baseline 1–2 months after recovery. Although data are conflicting, many studies show at least a transient increase in HIV RNA levels following influenza and other immunizations, which return to baseline after 1–2 months.

   b. **When results of test would not influence therapy.** Frequent scenario in patients with advanced disease who have no antiretroviral options or cannot tolerate therapy.

   c. **As a screening test for HIV infection,** except if acute (primary) HIV disease is suspected during the HIV antibody window (i.e., first 3–6 weeks after viral transmission).

INITIAL ASSESSMENT OF HIV-INFECTED PATIENTS

A. **Clinical Evaluation.** History and physical exam should focus on diagnoses associated with HIV infection. Compared to patients without HIV, the severity, frequency, and duration of these conditions are usually increased in HIV disease.

1. **Dermatologic:** Severe herpes simplex (oral/anogenital); herpes zoster (especially recurrent, cranial nerve, or disseminated); molluscum contagiosum; staphylococcal abscesses; tinea nail infections; Kaposi's sarcoma (from HHV-8 infection); petechiae (from ITP); seborrheic dermatitis; new or worsening psoriasis; eosinophilic pustular folliculitis; severe cutaneous drug eruptions (especially sulfonamides).

2. **Oropharyngeal:** Oral candidiasis; oral hairy leukoplakia (from EBV); Kaposi's sarcoma (most commonly on palate or gums); gingivitis/periodontitis; warts; aphthous ulcers (especially esophageal/perianal).

3. **Constitutional symptoms:** Fatigue, fevers, chronic diarrhea, weight loss.

4. **Lymphatic:** Persistent, generalized lymphadenopathy.

5. **Others:** Active TB (especially extrapulmonary); non-Hodgkin's lymphoma (especially CNS); unexplained leukopenia, anemia, thrombocytopenia (especially ITP); myopathy; miscellaneous neurologic conditions (cranial/peripheral neuropathies, Guillain-Barre syndrome, mononeuritis multiplex, aseptic meningitis, cognitive impairment).

B. Baseline Laboratory Testing (Table 5.1)

C. CD_4 Cell Count (lymphocyte subset analysis)

1. **Overview.** Acute HIV infection is characterized by a decline in CD_4 cell count, followed by a gradual rise associated with clinical recovery. Chronic HIV infection shows progressive declines (~ 50–80 cells/year) in CD_4 cell count without treatment, followed by more rapid decline 1–2 years prior to opportunistic infection (AIDS-defining diagnosis). Cell counts remain stable over 5–10 years in 5% of patients, while others may show rapid declines (> 300 cells/year). Since variability exists within individual patients and between laboratories, it is useful to *repeat any value before making management decisions.*

2. **Uses of CD_4 Cell Count**
   a. **Gives context of degree of immunosuppression** for interpretation of symptoms/signs (Table 5.2).
   b. **Used to guide therapy.** Guidelines support $CD_4 < 300/mm^3$ as a key threshold for initiating treatment, regardless of HIV RNA or symptoms; treatment should be considered for $CD_4 < 300–500/mm^3$. For prophylaxis against PCP, toxoplasmosis, and MAI/CMV infection, CD_4 cell counts of $200/mm^3$, $< 100/mm^3$, and $< 50/mm^3$ are used as threshold levels, respectively.
   c. **Provides estimate of risk of opportunistic infection or death.** CD_4 cell counts $< 50/mm^3$ are associated with a markedly increased risk of death (median survival 1 year), although some patients with low counts survive > 3 years even without antiretroviral therapy. Prognosis is heavily influenced by HIV RNA, presence/history of opportunistic infections or neoplasms, performance status, and the immune reconstitution response to antiretroviral therapy.

D. HIV RNA Assay (HIV RNA PCR) (p. 304)

Table 5.1. Baseline Laboratory Testing for HIV-Infected Patients

Test	Rationale
Repeat HIV serology (ELISA/confirmatory Western blot)	Indicated for patients unable to document a prior positive test, and for "low risk" individuals with a positive test (to detect computer/clerical error). Repeat serology is now less important since HIV RNA testing provides an additional means of confirming HIV infection.
CBC with differential, platelets	Detects cytopenias (e.g., ITP) seen in HIV. Needed to calculate CD_4 cell count.
Chemistry panel ("SMA 20") and fasting lipid panel	Detects renal dysfunction and electrolyte/LFT abnormalities, which may accompany HIV and associated infections (e.g., HIV nephropathy, HCV). Provides baseline lipid profile (many antiretroviral drugs can affect lipids).

Table 5.1. Baseline Laboratory Testing for HIV-Infected Patients (cont'd)

Test	Rationale
CD_4 cell count	Determines the need for antiretroviral therapy and opportunistic infection (OI) prophylaxis. Best test for defining risk of OIs and prognosis.
HIV RNA assay ("viral load")	Provides a marker for the pace of HIV disease progression. Determines indication for and response to antiretroviral therapy.
Tuberculin skin test (standard 5 TU of PPD)	Detects latent TB infection and targets patients for preventive therapy. Anergy skin tests are no longer indicated due to poor predictive value. HIV is the most powerful co-factor for the development of active TB.
PAP smear	Risk of cervical cancer is nearly twice as high in HIV-positive women compared to uninfected controls.
HLA-B*5701	Needed if abacavir therapy is planned, to assess risk for severe abacavir hypersensitivity reactions.
Toxoplasmosis serology (IgG)	Identifies patients at risk for subsequent cerebral/systemic toxoplasmosis and the need for prophylaxis. Those with negative tests should be counseled on how to avoid infection.
Syphilis serology (VDRL or RPR)	Identifies co-infection with syphilis, which is epidemiologically-linked to HIV. Disease may have accelerated course in HIV patients.
Hepatitis C serology (anti-HCV)	Identifies HCV infection and usually chronic carriage. If positive, follow with HCV genotype and HCV viral load assay. If the patient is antibody-negative and at high-risk for hepatitis, order HCV RNA to exclude a false-negative result.
Hepatitis B serologies (HBsAb, HBcAb, HBsAg)	Identifies patients who are immune to hepatitis B (HBsAb) or chronic carriers (HBsAg). If all three are negative, hepatitis B vaccine is indicated.
G6PD screen	Identifies patients at risk for dapsone or primaquine-associated hemolysis.
CMV serology (IgG)	Identifies patients who should receive CMV-negative or leukocyte-depleted blood if transfused.
VZV serology (IgG)	Identifies patients at risk for varicella (chickenpox), and those who should avoid contact with active varicella or herpes zoster patients. Serology-negative patients exposed to chickenpox should receive varicella-zoster immune globulin (VZIG).
Chest x-ray	Sometimes ordered as a baseline test for future comparisons. May detect healed granulomatous diseases/other processes. Indicated in all tuberculin skin test positive patients.

Table 5.2. Use of CD_4 Cell Count for Interpretation of Patient Signs/Symptoms

CD_4 Cell Count (cells/mm^3)	Associated Conditions
> 500	Most illnesses are similar to those in HIV-negative patients. Some increased risk of bacterial infections (pneumococcal pneumonia, sinusitis), herpes zoster, tuberculosis, skin conditions.
200–500*	Bacterial infections (especially pneumococcal pneumonia, sinusitis), cutaneous Kaposi's sarcoma, vaginal candidiasis, ITP.
50–200*	Thrush, oral hairy leukoplakia, classic HIV-associated opportunistic infections (e.g., P. [carinii] jiroveci pneumonia, cryptococcal meningitis, toxoplasmosis). For patients receiving prophylaxis, most opportunistic infection do not occur until CD_4 cell counts fall significantly below 100/mm^3.
< 50*	"Final common pathway" opportunistic infections (disseminated M. avium-intracellulare, CMV retinitis), HIV-associated wasting, neurologic disease (neuropathy, encephalopathy).

* Patients remain at risk for all processes noted in earlier stages.

ANTIRETROVIRAL THERAPY

Initiation of Antiretroviral Therapy (Figure 5.3). Combination antiretroviral therapy has led to dramatic reductions in HIV-related morbidity and mortality for patients with severe immunosuppression (CD_4 < 200) or a prior AIDS-defining illness. Treatment of asymptomatic patients is also now recommended for those with CD_4 cell counts between 200–350 cells/mm^3. Potential benefits of starting antiretroviral therapy with relatively high CD_4 cell counts include control of viral replication, reduction in HIV RNA, prevention of immunodeficiency, delayed time to onset of AIDS, decreased risk of drug toxicity, viral transmission, and selecting resistant virus. Potential risks of early antiretroviral therapy include reduced quality of life (from side effects/inconvenience), earlier development of drug resistance (with consequent transmission of resistant virus and limitation in future antiretroviral choices), unknown long-term toxicity of antiretroviral drugs, and unknown duration of effectiveness. The primary goals of therapy are prolonged suppression of viral replication to undetectable levels (HIV RNA < 50–75 copies/mL), restoration/preservation of immune function, and improved clinical outcome. Once initiated, antiretroviral therapy should be continued indefinitely.

DHHS Guidelines: Antiretroviral Therapy for Treatment-Naive Patients. Patients naïve to antiretroviral therapy should be started on a combination regimen that consists of either:

- **1-NNRTI + 2 NRTI or**
- **PI (preferably boosted with ritonavir) + 2NRTI**

This table includes antiretroviral component options for constructing a regimen for a treatment-naïve patient. Selection of a regimen should be individualized based on virologic efficacy, toxicities, pill burden, dosing frequency, drug-drug interaction potential, and comorbid conditions. Components are designated as preferred when clinical trial data suggest optimal and durable efficacy with acceptable tolerability and ease of use. Alternative components are those that clinical trial data show efficacy but that have disadvantages, such as antiviral activity or toxicities, compared with the preferred agent. In some cases, for an individual patient, a component listed as alternative may actually be the preferred component. When there is more than one component for a preferred or alternative option, the components are listed in alphabetical order. For management of an HIV-infected pregnant patient, please refer to http://www.aidsinfo.nih.gov/Guidelines/GuidelineDetail.aspx?MenuItem=Guidelines&Search=Off&GuidelineID=7&ClassID=1.

Table 5.3. DHHS Guidelines: Antiretroviral Therapy for Treatment-Naive Patients

SELECT NRTI PAIR PLUS EITHER NNRTI OR PI			
	NRTI Pair	**NNRTI**	**PI**
Preferred	• Tenofovir (TDF) + emtricitabine (FTC)[a]	• Efavirenz (EFV)[b]	• Atazanavir/ritonavir (ATV/r)[c] • Darunavir/ritonavir (DRV/r) • Fosamprenavir/ritonavir (FPV/r) • Lopinavir/ritonavir (LPV/r)[d]
Alternative	• Abacavir/lamivudine (ABC/3TC)[g] • Didanosine + lamivudine (3TC) (or emtricitabine) (FTC)[h] • Zidovudine (ZDV) + lamivudine (3TC)[i]	• Nevirapine (NVP)[f]	• Atazanavir (unboosted) (ATV)[e] • Fosamprenavir/ritonavir (FPV/r) – or fosamprenavir (unboosted) (FPV) • Saquinavir/ritonavir (SQV/r)

a Do not use in combination with unboosted atazanavir. Use with caution: with nevirapine due to reports of early virologic failure; in patients with underlying renal insufficiency.

b Do not use during 1st trimester of pregnancy or in those with high pregnancy potential. Use with caution in patients with unstable psychiatric disease.

c Do not use in patients who require high-dose (>20 mg omeprazole equivalent/day) proton pump inhibitors (PPIs). Use with caution in patients on PPIs (any dose), H2 blockers, or antacids.

d Do not use once-daily lopinavir/ritonavir in pregnant women.

e Do not use in combination with tenofovir or didanosine/lamivudine.

e Do not use in combination with tenofovir or didanosine/lamivudine.

f Do not use in patients with moderate to severe hepatic impairment (Child-Pugh score B or C). Do not use in women with pre-ARV CD4 >250 cells/mm^3 or in men with pre-ARV CD4 >400 cells/mm^3. Use with caution in patients on tenofovir/emtricitabine (or lamivudine)—early virologic failure has been reported with this combination.

Table 5.3. DHHS Guidelines: Antiretroviral Therapy for Treatment-Naive Patients (cont'd)

g Do not use in patients who test positive for HLA-B*5701. Use with caution in the presence of the following: HIV RNA >100,000 copies/mL—higher rate of virologic failure reported in ACTG 5202; or high risk for cardiovascular disease.

h Do not use in combination with unboosted atazanavir. Do not use in patients with a history of pancreatitis or peripheral neuropathy.

i Use with caution in the presence of pretreatment anemia and/or neutropenia (may improve or worsen with zidovudine).

Adapted from: Aberg JA, Kaplan JE, Libman H, et al. Primary care guidelines for the management of persons infected with human immunodeficiency virus: 2009 update by the HIV medicine Association of the Infectious Society of America. Clin Infect Dis. 49:651–681, 2009.

Table 5.4. IAS-USA Guidelines: Recommended Components of Initial Antiretroviral Therapy and Considerations for Choosing a Regimen

Component	Considerations for Choice	Major Toxic Effects and Cautions
	Nucleoside reverse transcriptase inhibitors[a]	
Tenofovir/ emtricitabine[b,c]	Well tolerated Efficacy superior to zidovudine/ lamivudine and similar to stavudine/ lamivudine Available as a once-daily fixed dose	Baseline renal function should be evaluated before initiating tenofovir Reduce dose or avoid in patients with renal dysfunction
Abacavir/ lamivudine[d]	Noninferior to tenofovir/emtricitabine in 1 trial May have less activity in patients with viral load ≥ 100000 HIV RNA copies/mL Available as a once-daily fixed dose	Hypersensitivity syndrome in 5% to 8% of persons (risk associated with HLA-B*5701 genotype) Risk reduced with HLA-B*5701 screening May be associated with increased risk of myocardial infarction
Efavirenz	Standard-of-care comparator in many trials Available as a once-daily fixed dose with tenofovir/emtricitabine	Central nervous system toxicity may be limiting Potentially teratogenic in first trimester of pregnancy Associated with lipoatrophy when given with thymidine reverse transcriptase inhibitors
Lopinavir	Substantial clinical trial data and phase 4 experience supporting efficacy Heat-stable tablet 1 or 2 doses per day for treatment-naive patients	Gastrointestinal adverse effects Hyperlipidemia, especially hypertriglyceridemia

Table 5.4. IAS-USA Guidelines: Recommended Components of Initial Antiretroviral Therapy and Considerations for Choosing a Regimen (cont'd)

Component	Considerations for Choice	Major Toxic Effects and Cautions
Ritonavir-boosted protease inhibitors[f]		
Atazanavir	Noninferior to ritonavir-boosted lopinavir Less hyperlipidemia and diarrhea Once-daily dosing	Hyperbilirubinemia (UGT1A1-28 alleles and T3435C polymorphism in *MDR1* gene) Occasionally associated with nephrolithiasis Acid-reducing agents decrease atazanavir concentrations; proton pump inhibitors should be used cautiously
Fosamprenavir	Noninferior to ritonavir-boosted lopinavir Once-daily or twice-daily dosing possible; more robust data with twice-daily dose	Similar adverse effect profile to ritonavir-boosted lopinavir Rash
Darunavir	Noninferior to ritonavir-boosted lopinavir and superior in those with viral load ≥ 100000 HIV RNA copies/mL Less nausea, lower triglyceride levels 800 mg + 100 mg ritonavir once daily	Rash
Saquinavir	Noninferior to ritonavir-boosted lopinavir, with lower triglyceride levels. Twice-daily dosing	High pill burden

Abbreviation: HIV, human immunodeficiency virus.

a Zidovudine/lamivudine is considered an alternative.

b A baseline urinalysis and estimation of creatinine clearance or glomerular filtration rate for assessment of renal function are recommended. All patients receiving tenofovir should be observed for development of renal dysfunction.

c Or lamivudine.

d Or emtricitabine.

e Nevirapine (in women with <250 CD4 cells/μL and men with <400 CD4 cells/μL) is considered an alternative (see "What to Start" section of text).

f Substantial clinical trial data exist for ritonavir-boosted lopinavir as initial antiretroviral therapy, including data on long-term outcomes. Each of the other ritonavir-boosted protease inhibitors has been compared with ritonavir-boosted lopinavir but not with one another. Choice of ritonavir-boosted protease inhibitor should be individualized.

Adapted from: Aberg JA, Kaplan JE, Libman H, et al. Primary care guidelines for the management of persons infected with human immunodeficiency virus: 2009 update by the HIV medicine Association of the Infectious Society of America. Clin Infect Dis. 49:651–681, 2009.

Table 5.5. Major Decisions in Selecting the Initial Antiretroviral Regimen*

Decision	Comment
What is the optimal NRTI to pair with 3TC or FTC?	Because of the availability of once-daily, fixed-dose formulations and a low risk of lipoatrophy, many clinicians are currently choosing either TDF (co-formulated with FTC as Truvada) or ABC (co-formulated with 3TC as Epzicom). ABC therapy should be preceded by testing for HLA-B*5701 to reduce the risk of ABC hypersensitivity. Some studies have suggested that ABC treatment is associated with an increased risk of myocardial infarction (Lancet 2008 Apr 26;371[9622]:1417–26; AIDS 2008 Sep 12; 22[14]:F17–24). Furthermore, ABC/3TC had a higher rate of virologic failure compared with TDF/FTC in patients with a baseline HIV RNA greater than 100,000 copies per mL (XVII International AIDS Conference. August 3–8, 2008. Mexico City. Abstract THAB0303.). Based on these data, the DHHS guidelines now list TDF/FTC as the preferred NRTI pair. The IAS-USA guidelines still list ABC/3TC but add these caveats.
Should the third drug be an NNRTI or a PI or raltegravir?	NNRTI-based regimens—in particular those containing EFV—are in general simpler to take than PI-based treatments. EFV-based regimens have also demonstrated superior antiviral activity in prospective clinical trials (N Engl J Med 2008 May 15;358[20]:2095–106), although interestingly, immunologic response was better with the boosted PI. While PI-based regimens have a somewhat higher pill burden and more drug-drug interactions, they confer a lower risk of resistance in the case of virologic failure. Raltegravir demonstrated comparable efficacy to EFV in a prospective clinical trial, with fewer drug-related adverse effects (Lancet 2009).
If an NNRTI-based regimen is chosen, which agent should be used?	In general, EFV is the preferred NNRTI due to comparable or superior antiviral activity to all comparators in prospective clinical trials. It is also available as a single-tablet triple regimen combined with TDF and FTC. However, EFV should be avoided in women of childbearing potential who may wish to become pregnant and may be difficult to tolerate for patients with psychiatric disease. In these contexts, NVP would be preferred, so long as the baseline CD4 cell count does not exceed 250/mm^3 in a woman or 400/mm^3 in a man.
If a PI-based regimen is chosen, which PI should be used?	There are more options for PI-based than for NNRTI-based therapy. In general, RTV-boosted PIs provide the best combination of simplicity and antiviral potency. Recent comparative clinical trials have suggested more favorable tolerability and efficacy with ATV/r + DRV/r over LPV/r (Lancet 2008;372:646–55 and AIDS 2008;22:1389–97).

* All recommended regimens consist of three active agents: an NRTI pair (containing 3TC or FTC as one of the drugs) plus either an NNRTI or a PI. information on adverse drug reactions and drug-drug interactions highlight important differences between available agents. Combinations not listed as "Preferred" or "Alternative" regimens in Tables 5.3 and 5.4 should in general be avoided.

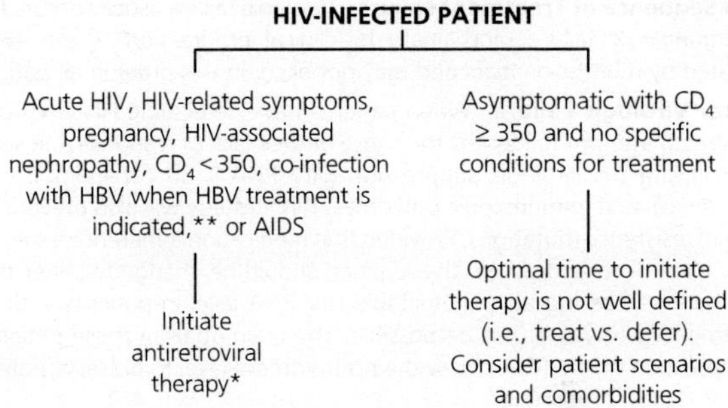

Figure 5.3. Indications for Initiating Antiretroviral Therapy

* See Tables 5.4 and 5.5.

** Treat with fully suppressive antiviral drugs active against both HIV and hepatitis B virus (HBV).

Selection of Optimal Antiretroviral Therapy. Selection of the optimal initial antiretroviral regimen must take into consideration antiviral potency, tolerability, and safety. In the DHHS and IAS-USA Guidelines (Tables 5.3 and 5.4).

ANTIRETROVIRAL TREATMENT FAILURE (Table 5.6)

Antiretroviral treatment failure can be defined in various ways, as described below. Causes of treatment failure include inadequate adherence, preexisting drug resistance, regimen complexity, side effects, and suboptimal pharmacokinetics. All of these factors can lead to persistent viral replication and evolution of drug resistance. Poor medication adherence is the most common cause of treatment failure.

A. Types of Treatment Failure

1. **Virologic Failure** is most strictly defined as the inability to achieve or maintain virologic suppression. In a treatment-naïve patient, the HIV RNA level should be < 400 copies/mL after 24 weeks or < 50 copies/mL by 48 weeks after starting therapy. Virologic rebound is seen when there is repeated detection of HIV RNA after virologic suppression in either treatment-naïve or treatment-experienced patients.
2. **Immunologic Failure** can occur in the presence or absence of virologic failure and is defined as a failure to increase the CD_4 cell count by 25–50 cells/mm^3 above baseline during the first year of therapy, or as a decrease in CD_4 cell count to below baseline count while on therapy.
3. **Clinical Failure** is the occurrence or recurrence of HIV-related events after at least 3 months on potent antiretroviral therapy, excluding events related to an immune reconstitution syndrome.

4. **Usual Sequence of Treatment Failure.** Virologic failure usually occurs first, followed by immunologic failure, and finally by clinical progression. These events may be separated by months or years and may not occur in this order in all patients.

B. **Goals After Virologic Failure.** When patients have detectable HIV RNA on treatment, clinicians should attempt to identify the cause of their lack of response and set a treatment goal of achieving full virologic suppression (HIV RNA < 50 copies/mL). In addition to improving clinical and immunologic outcomes, this strategy will also prevent the selection of additional resistance mutations. Provided that medication adherence issues and regimen tolerability have been addressed, the regimen should be changed sooner than later. On the other hand, achieving an undetectable HIV RNA level in patients with an extensive prior treatment history may not be possible. The main goals in these patients should be partial suppression of HIV RNA below the pretreatment level to preserve immune function and prevent clinical progression.

C. **Resistance Testing and Selection of New Antiretroviral Therapy.** Genotypic assays characterize nucleotide sequences of the reverse transcriptase/protease portions of the virus, and identify resistance mutations associated with various drugs. Phenotypic assays attempt to grow the virus in the presence of drugs, providing a more intuitively applicable measurement of resistance (similar to that done with bacteria). Compared to phenotypic assays, genotypic assays are faster (1–2 weeks vs. 2–4 weeks for results), less expensive ($400 vs. $1000), and have less inter-laboratory variability; however, mutations do not always correlate with resistance and results are difficult to interpret.

Table 5.6. Management of Antiretroviral Treatment Failure

Type of Failure	Recommended Approach	Comments
Virologic failure *Limited or intermediate prior treatment*	Assess for adherence and regimen tolerability. Obtain genotype resistance test. Select new regimen based on resistance test results and tolerability.	Usually associated with limited or no detectable resistance. If no resistance is found, consider re-testing for resistance 2–4 weeks after resuming antivirals. Stop NNRTI's if resistance is detected. Virologic suppression is likely if adherence is good.
Extensive prior treatment	Assess for adherence and regimen tolerability. Obtain resistance test – consider phenotype, "virtual phenotype," or phenotype-genotype combination if level of resistance is likely to be high. Obtain viral tropism assay to assess possible use of CCR5 antagonist. Select new regimen using at least 2 new active agents; if 2 new active agents not available, continue a "holding" regimen.	In patients with resistance to NRTI's, NNRTI's and PI's, the new regimen should generally contain at least: (1) at least one drug from a new drug class (integrase inhibitor, CCR5 antagonist, or fusion inhibitor); (2) a boosted PI with activity against resistant viruses (tipranavir or darunavir); and (3) one or two NRTI's, one of them 3TC or FTC. A holding regimen should always contain 3TC or FTC plus a boosted PI; NNRTI's should never be used.

Table 5.6. Management of Antiretroviral Treatment Failure (cont'd)

Type of Failure	Recommended Approach	Comments
Low-level HIV RNA (50–1000 copies)	Assess for adherence, drug-drug interactions, intercurrent illness, recent immunizations. Repeat test in 3–4 weeks.	For low-level viremia followed by undetectable HIV RNA ("blip"), no treatment change is necessary. If HIV RNA is persistently detectable at > 500 copies/mL, obtain resistance test as described above, and treat accordingly. If HIV RNA is persistently detectable at 50–500 copies/mL, consider regimen "intensification" with use of an additional agent.
Immunologic failure *Detectable HIV RNA*	Assess for adherence and tolerability. If non-adherent, resume treatment after barriers to adherence are addressed. If adherent, obtain resistance testing and alter therapy as described above.	If HIV RNA is back to pre-treatment baseline, non-adherence is the most likely explanation.
Suppressed HIV RNA	Investigate for modifiable conditions that may be associated with impaired CD_4 response (chronic HCV, treatment with ZDV, TDF + ddI). If no modifiable conditions found, continue current regimen.	Prognosis for patients with suppressed HIV RNA and immunologic failure better than for those with comparable CD_4 cell counts and detectable viremia.
Clinical failure *Detectable HIV RNA*	Treat OI with appropriate anti-infective therapy. Assess for antiretroviral adherence and tolerability. Send resistance test and choose new regimen based on results of test and other treatment options.	OI's (IRIS excluded) most commonly occur in those not on antiretroviral therapy due to poor compliance and/or regimen tolerability.
Suppressed HIV RNA	Continue current antiretrovirals. Treat OI with appropriate anti-infective therapy. If symptoms persist and IRIS is likely, use adjunctive corticosteroids.	IRIS most likely when baseline CD_4 cell count is low (< 200/mm^3); onset usually weeks-to-months after starting a potent regimen. IRIS been reported with virtually all OI's. True clinical progression with suppressed HIV RNA is unusual; IRIS should not be considered a sign of treatment failure.

IRIS = immune reconstitution inflammatory syndrome, OI = opportunistic infection.

OPPORTUNISTIC INFECTIONS IN HIV DISEASE (Tables 5.7, 5.8)

Patients with HIV disease are at risk for infectious complications not otherwise seen in immunocompetent patients. Such opportunistic infections occur in proportion to the severity of immune system dysfunction (reflected by CD_4 cell count depletion). While community acquired infections (e.g., pneumococcal pneumonia) can occur at any CD_4 cell count, "classic" HIV-related opportunistic infections (PCP, toxoplasmosis, cryptococcus, disseminated M. avium-intracellulare, CMV) do not occur until CD_4 cell counts are dramatically reduced. Specifically, it is rare to encounter PCP in HIV patients with CD_4 > 200/mm^3, and CMV and disseminated MAI occur at median CD_4 cell counts < 50/mm^3.

Table 5.7. Overview of Prophylaxis (See Table 5.8 for details)

Infection	Indication	Intervention
PCP	CD_4 < 200/mm^3	TMP–SMX
TB (M. tuberculosis)	PPD > 5 mm (current or past) or contact with active case	INH
Toxoplasma	IgG Ab (+) and CD_4 < 100/mm^3	TMP–SMX
MAI	CD_4 < 50/mm^3	Azithromycin or clarithromycin
S. pneumoniae	CD_4 > 200/mm^3	Pneumococcal vaccine
Hepatitis B (HBV)	Susceptible patients	Hepatitis B vaccine
Hepatitis A (HAV)	HCV (+) and HA Ab (–); HCV (–) and HA Ab (–) gay men and travelers to endemic areas, chronic liver disease	Hepatitis A vaccine
Influenza	All patients	Annual flu vaccine Swine influenza (H_1N_1) vaccine
VZV	Exposure to chickenpox or shingles; no prior history	VZIG

Abbreviations: Ab = antibody; HA = Hepatitis A; HCV = Hepatitis C virus; VZIG = varicella-zoster immune globulin; VZV = varicella- zoster virus; other abbreviations (p. xi).

Table 5.8. Prophylaxis of Opportunistic Infections in HIV

Infection	Indications and Prophylaxis	Comments
P. (carinii) jiroveci pneumonia (PCP)	Indications: CD_4 < 200/mm^3, oral thrush, constitutional symptoms, or previous history of PCP Preferred prophylaxis: TMP–SMX 1 DS tablet (PO) q24h or 1 SS tablet (PO) q24h. 1 DS tablet (PO) 3×/week is also effective, but daily dosing may be slightly more effective based on 1 comparative study Alternate prophylaxis: Dapsone 100 mg (PO) q24h (preferred as second-line by most; more effective than aerosolized pentamidine when CD_4 cell count < 100) **or** Atovaquone 1500 mg (PO) q24h (comparably effective to dapsone and aerosolized pentamidine; more GI toxicity vs. dapsone, but less rash) **or** Aerosolized pentamidine 300 mg via Respirgard II nebulizer once monthly (exclude active pulmonary TB first to avoid nosocomial transmission)	Without prophylaxis, 80% of AIDS patients develop PCP, and 60–70% relapse within one year after the first episode. Prophylaxis with TMP–SMX also reduces the risk for toxoplasmosis and possibly bacterial infections. Among patients with prior non-life-threatening reactions to TMP–SMX, 55% can be successfully rechallenged with 1 SS tablet daily, and 80% can be rechallenged with gradual dose escalation using TMP–SMX elixir (8 mg TMP + 40 mg SMX/mL) given as 1 mL × 3 days, then 2 mL × 3 days, then 5 mL × 3 days, then 1 SS tablet (PO) q24h. Macrolide-regimens for MAI (azithromycin, clarithromycin) add to efficacy of PCP prophylaxis. Primary and secondary prophylaxis may be discontinued if CD_4 cell counts increase to > 200 cells/mm^3 for 3 months or longer in response to antiretroviral therapy (i.e., immune reconstitution). Prophylaxis should be resumed if the CD_4 cell count decreases to < 200/mm^3.
Toxoplasmosis	Indications: CD_4 < 100/mm^3 with positive toxoplasmosis serology (IgG) Preferred prophylaxis: TMP–SMX 1 DS tablet (PO) q24h Alternate prophylaxis: Dapsone 50 mg (PO) q24h + pyrimethamine 50 mg (PO) weekly + folinic acid 25 mg (PO) weekly **or**	Incidence of toxoplasmosis in seronegative patients is too low to warrant chemoprophylaxis. Primary prophylaxis can be discontinued if CD_4 cell counts increase to > 200/mm^3 for at least 3 months in response to antiretroviral therapy. Secondary prophylaxis (chronic maintenance therapy) may be discontinued in patients who responded to initial therapy, remain asymptomatic, and whose CD_4 counts increase to > 200/mm^3 for 6 months or longer in response to

Table 5.8. Prophylaxis of Opportunistic Infections in HIV

Infection	Indications and Prophylaxis	Comments
	Dapsone 100 mg/pyrimethamine 50 mg twice weekly (no folinic acid) **or** Atovaquone 1500 mg (PO) q24h	antiretroviral therapy. Prophylaxis should be restarted if the CD_4 count decreases to < 200/mm^3. Some experts would obtain an MRI of the brain as part of the evaluation prior to stopping secondary prophylaxis.
M. tuberculosis (TB)	Indications: PPD induration ≥ 5 mm or history of positive PPD without prior treatment, or close contact with active case of TB. Must exclude active disease (chest x-ray mandatory). Indicated at any CD_4 cell count Preferred prophylaxis: INH 300 mg (PO) q24h × 9 months + pyridoxine 50 mg (PO) q24h × 9 months Alternate prophylaxis: Rifampin 600 mg (PO) q24h × 2 months + pyrazinamide 20 mg/kg (PO) q24h × 2 months. Rifampin should not be given to patients receiving PI's	Consider prophylaxis for skin test negative patients when the probability of prior TB exposure is > 10% (e.g., patients from developing countries, IV drug abusers in some cities, prisoners). However, a trial testing this strategy in the U.S. did not find a benefit for empiric prophylaxis. INH prophylaxis delayed progression to AIDS and prolonged life in Haitian cohort with positive PPD treated × 6 months. Rifampin plus pyrazinamide × 2 months was effective in a multinational clinical trial (but the combination may ↑ hepatotoxicity). Rifabutin may be substituted for rifampin in rifampin-containing regimens.
M. avium-intracellulare (MAI)	Indications: CD_4 < 50/mm^3 Preferred prophylaxis: Azithromycin 1200 mg (PO) once a week (fewest number of pills; fewest drug interactions; may add to efficacy of PCP prophylaxis) **or** Clarithromycin 500 mg (PO) q12h (more effective than rifabutin; associated with survival advantage; resistance detected in some breakthrough cases) Alternate prophylaxis: Rifabutin (less effective). See TB (p. 323) for dosing	Macrolide options (azithromycin, clarithromycin) preferable to rifabutin. Azithromycin is preferred for patients on protease inhibitors (fewer drug interactions). Primary prophylaxis may be discontinued if CD_4 cell counts increase to > 100/mm^3 and HIV RNA suppresses for 3–6 months or longer in response to antiretroviral therapy. Secondary prophylaxis may be discontinued for CD_4 cell counts that increase to > 100/mm^3 × 6 months or longer in response to antiretroviral therapy if patients have completed 12 months of MAI therapy and have no evidence of disease. Resume MAI prophylaxis for CD_4 < 100/mm^3.

Table 5.8. Prophylaxis of Opportunistic Infections in HIV (cont'd)

Infection	Indications and Prophylaxis	Comments
Pneumococcus (S. pneumoniae)	Indications: $CD_4 > 200/mm^3$ Preferred prophylaxis: Pneumococcal polysaccharide (23 valent) vaccine.* Re-vaccinate × 1 at 5 years	Incidence of invasive pneumococcal disease is > 100-fold higher in HIV patients. Efficacy of vaccine is variable in clinical studies.
Influenza (human seasonal)	Indications: Generally recommended for all patients Preferred prophylaxis: Influenza vaccine (inactivated whole virus and split virus vaccine)*	Give annually (optimally October- January). Some experts do not give vaccine if CD_4 is $< 100/mm^3$ (antibody response is poor). New intranasal live virus vaccine is contraindicated in immunosuppressed patients.
Hepatitis B (HBV)	Indications: All susceptible (anti-HBcAb negative and anti-HBsAg negative) patients Preferred prophylaxis: Hepatitis B recombinant DNA vaccine*	Response rate is lower than in HIV-negative controls. Repeat series if no response, especially if CD_4 was low during initial series and is now increased.
Hepatitis A (HAV)	Indications: All susceptible patients who are also infected with hepatitis C; HAV-susceptible seronegative gay men or travelers to endemic areas; chronic liver disease; illegal drug users Preferred prophylaxis: Hepatitis A vaccine*	Response rate is lower than in HIV-negative controls.
Measles, mumps, rubella	Indications: Patients born after 1957 and never vaccinated; patients vaccinated between 1963–1967 Preferred prophylaxis: MMR (measles, mumps, rubella) vaccine*	Single case of vaccine-strain measles pneumonia in severely immuno-compromised adult who received MMR; vaccine is therefore contraindicated in patients with severe immunodeficiency ($CD_4 < 200$).

* Same dose as for normal hosts (see pp. 362–365). If possible, give vaccines early in course of HIV infection, while immune system may still respond. Alternatively, to increase the likelihood of response in patients with advanced HIV disease, vaccines may be administered after 6–12 months of effective antiretroviral therapy. Vaccines should be given when patients are clinically stable, not acutely ill (e.g., give during a routine office visit, rather than during hospitalization for an opportunistic infection). Live vaccines (e.g., oral polio, oral typhoid, Yellow fever) are generally contraindicated, but measles vaccine is well-tolerated in children, and MMR vaccine is recommended for adults as described above.

Table 5.8. Prophylaxis of Opportunistic Infections in HIV (cont'd)

Infection	Indications and Prophylaxis	Comments
H. influenzae	Indications: Not generally recommended for adults Preferred prophylaxis: H. influenzae type B polysaccharide vaccine*	Incidence of H. influenzae disease is increased in HIV patients, but 65% are caused by non-type B strains. Unclear whether vaccine offers protection.
Travel vaccines*	Indications: Travel to endemic areas	All considered safe except oral polio, yellow fever, and live oral typhoid—each a live virus vaccine.

* Same dose as for normal hosts (see pp. 362–365). If possible, give vaccines early in course of HIV infection, while immune system may still respond. Alternatively, to increase the likelihood of response in patients with advanced HIV disease, vaccines may be administered after 6–12 months of effective antiretroviral therapy. Vaccines should be given when patients are clinically stable, not acutely ill (e.g., give during a routine office visit, rather than during hospitalization for an opportunistic infection). Live vaccines (e.g., oral polio, oral typhoid, Yellow fever) are generally contraindicated, but measles vaccine is well-tolerated in children, and MMR vaccine is recommended for adults as described above.

TREATMENT OF OPPORTUNISTIC INFECTIONS

Antiretroviral therapy (ART) and specific antimicrobial prophylaxis regimens have led to a dramatic decline in HIV-related opportunistic infections. Today, opportunistic infections occur predominantly in patients not receiving ART (due to undiagnosed HIV infection or nonacceptance of therapy), or in the period after starting ART (due to lack of immune reconstitution or from eliciting a previously absent inflammatory host response). Despite high rates of virologic failure in clinical practice, the rate of opportunistic infections in patients compliant with ART remains low, presumably due to continued immunologic response despite virologic failure, a phenomenon that may be linked to impaired "fitness" (virulence) of resistant HIV strains. For patients on or off ART, the absolute CD_4 cell count provides the best marker of risk for opportunistic infections.

Respiratory Tract Opportunistic Infections

Aspergillosis, Invasive Pulmonary

Pathogen	Preferred Therapy	Alternate Therapy
Aspergillus fumigatus (rarely other species)	Voriconazole 400 mg (IV or PO) q12h × 2 days, then 200 mg (IV or PO) q12h until cured (typically 6–18 months)	Amphotericin B deoxycholate 1 mg/kg (IV) q24h until 2–3 gm total dose given (optimal duration of therapy poorly defined) **or** Amphotericin B lipid formulations (Abelcet or Ambisome) 5 mg/kg/day (IV) until cured

Clinical Presentation: Pleuritic chest pain, hemoptysis, cough in a patient with advanced HIV disease. Additional risk factors include neutropenia and use of corticosteroids.
Diagnostic Considerations: Diagnosis by bronchoscopy with biopsy/culture. Open lung biopsy (usually video-assisted thorascopic surgery) is sometimes required. Radiographic appearance includes cavitation, nodules, sometimes focal consolidation. Dissemination to CNS may occur, and manifests as focal neurological deficits.
Pitfalls: Positive sputum culture for Aspergillus in advanced HIV disease should heighten awareness of possible infection.
Therapeutic Considerations: Decrease/discontinue corticosteroids, if possible. If present, treat neutropenia with granulocyte-colony stimulating factor (G-CSF) to achieve absolute neutrophil count > 1000/mm³. There are insufficient data to recommend chronic suppressive or maintenance therapy.
Prognosis: Poor unless immune deficits can be corrected.

Bacterial Pneumonia

Usual Pathogens	Preferred Therapy	Comments
Streptococcus pneumoniae (most common) Haemophilus influenzae Pseudomonas aeruginosa	**Monotherapy with** Levofloxacin 750 mg (PO/IV) q24h or moxifloxacin 400 mg (PO/IV) q24h × 7–14 days, depending on severity **or combination therapy with** Ceftriaxone 1–2 gm (IV) q24h (or cefotaxime 1 gm [IV] q8h) ***plus*** azithromycin 500 gm q24h × 7–14 days	For severe immunodeficiency (CD_4 < 100/mm³), neutropenia, or a prior history of pseudomonas infection, broaden coverage to include *P. aeruginosa* and other gram-negative bacilli by adding **either** ceftazidime 1 gm (IV) q8h **or** cefepime 1 gm (IV) q12h **or** ciprofloxacin 750 mg (PO) q12h or 400 mg (IV) q8h.

Clinical Presentation: HIV-infected patients with bacterial pneumonia present similar to those without HIV, with a relatively acute illness (over days) that is often associated with chills, rigors, pleuritic chest pain, and purulent sputum. Patients who have been ill over weeks to months are more likely have PCP, tuberculosis, or a fungal infection. Since bacterial pneumonia can occur at any CD_4 cell count, this infection is frequently the presenting symptom of HIV disease, prompting initial HIV testing and diagnosis.
Diagnostic Considerations: The most common pathogens are Streptococcus pneumoniae, followed by Haemophilus influenzae. The pathogens of atypical pneumonia (Legionella pneumophila, Mycoplasma pneumoniae, and Chlamydia pneumoniae) are rarely encountered, even with extensive laboratory investigation. A lobar infiltrate on chest radiography is a further predictor of bacterial pneumonia. Blood cultures should be obtained, as HIV patients have an increased rate of bacteremia compared to those without HIV.
Pitfalls: Sputum gram stain and culture are generally only helpful if collected prior to starting antibiotics, and only if a single organism predominates. HIV patients with bacterial pneumonia may rarely have a more subacute opportunistic infection concurrently, such as PCP or TB.
Therapeutic Considerations: Once improvement has occurred, a switch to oral therapy is generally safe. Patients with advanced HIV disease are at greater risk of bacteremic pneumonia due to gram-negative bacilli, and should be covered empirically for this condition.
Prognosis: Response to therapy is generally prompt and overall prognosis is good.

Pneumocystis (carinii) jiroveci Pneumonia (PCP)

Subset	Preferred Therapy	Alternate Therapy
Mild or moderate disease (pO_2 > 70 mmHg, A-a gradient < 35)	TMP–SMX DS 2 tablets (PO) q8h × 21 days	Dapsone 100 mg (PO) q24h × 21 days plus TMP 5 mg/kg (PO) q8h × 21 days (↓ leukopenia/hepatitis vs. TMP–SMX) **or** Primaquine 30 mg (PO) q24h × 21 days plus clindamycin 300–450 mg (PO) q6h-q8h × 21 days **or** Atovaquone 750 mg (PO) q12h with food × 21 days **or** Trimetrexate 45 mg/m² or 1.2 mg/kg (IV) q24h × 21 days plus leucovorin 20 mg/m² or 0.5 mg/kg (IV or PO) q6h (leucovorin must be continued for 3 days after the last trimetrexate dose)
Severe disease (pO_2< 70 mmHg, A-a gradient > 35)	TMP–SMX (5 mg/kg TMP) (IV) q6h × 21 days **plus** Prednisone 40 mg (PO) q12h on days 1–5, then 40 mg (PO) q24h on days 6–10, then 20 mg (PO) q24h on days 11–21. Methylprednisolone (IV) can be substituted at 75% of prednisone dose	Pentamidine 4 mg/kg (IV) q24h (infused over at least 60 minutes) × 21 days plus prednisone × 21 days. (Dose reduction of pentamidine to 3 mg/kg [IV] q24h may reduce toxicity)

Clinical Presentation: Fever, cough, dyspnea; often indolent presentation. Physical exam is usually normal. Chest x-ray is variable, but commonly shows a diffuse interstitial pattern. Elevated LDH and exercise desaturation are highly suggestive of PCP.

Diagnostic Considerations: Diagnosis by immunofluorescent stain of induced sputum or bronchoscopy specimen. Check ABG if O_2 saturation is abnormal or respiratory rate is increased.

Pitfalls: Slight worsening of symptoms is common after starting therapy, especially if not treated with steroids. Do not overlook superimposed bacterial pneumonia or other secondary infections, especially while on pentamidine. Patients receiving second-line agents for PCP prophylaxis—in particular aerosolized pentamidine–may present with atypical radiographic findings, including apical infiltrates, multiple small-walled cysts, pleural effusions, pneumothorax, or single/multiple nodules.

Therapeutic Considerations: Outpatient therapy is possible for mild disease, but only when close follow-up is assured. Adverse reactions to TMP–SMX (rash, fever, GI symptoms, hepatitis, hyperkalemia, leukopenia, hemolytic anemia) occur in 25–50% of patients, many of whom will need a second-line regimen to complete therapy (e.g., trimethoprim-dapsone or atovaquone). Unless an adverse reaction to TMP–SMX is particularly severe (e.g., Stevens-Johnson syndrome or other life-threatening problem), TMP–SMX may be considered for PCP prophylaxis, since prophylaxis requires a much lower dose (only

10–15% of treatment dose). Patients being treated for severe PCP with TMP–SMX who do not improve after one week may be switched to pentamidine, although there are no prospective data to confirm this approach. In general, patients receiving antiretroviral therapy when PCP develops should have their treatment continued, since intermittent antiretroviral therapy can lead to drug resistance. For newly-diagnosed or antiretroviral-naive HIV patients, treatment of PCP may be completed before starting antiretroviral therapy. Steroids should be tapered, not discontinued abruptly. Adjunctive steroids increase the risk of thrush/herpes simplex infection, but probably not CMV, TB, or disseminated fungal infection.

Prognosis: Usually responds to treatment. Adverse prognostic factors include ↑ A-a gradient, hypoxemia, ↑ LDH.

Pulmonary Tuberculosis (for isolates sensitive to INH and rifampin)

Pathogen	Patients NOT Receiving PI's or NNRTI's	Patients Receiving PI's or NNRTI's*
Mycobacterium tuberculosis (TB)	<u>Initial phase (8 weeks)</u> INH 300 mg (PO) q24h **plus** Rifampin† 600 mg (PO) q24h **plus** Pyrazinamide (PZA) 25 mg/kg (PO) q24h **plus** Ethambutol (EMB) 15–20 mg/kg (PO) q24h <u>Continuation phase (18 weeks)</u> INH 300 mg (PO) q24h **plus** Rifampin† 600 mg (PO) q24h	<u>Initial phase (8 weeks)</u> INH 300 mg (PO) q24h **plus** Rifabutin* **plus** PZA 25 mg/kg (PO) q24h **plus** EMB 15 mg/kg (PO) q24h × 8 weeks. <u>Continuation phase (18 weeks)</u> INH 300 mg (PO) q24h **plus** Rifabutin*

* Rifabutin dose: If PI is nelfinavir, indinavir, amprenavir or fosamprenavir, then rifabutin dose is 150 mg (PO) q24h. If PI is ritonavir, lopinavir/ritonavir or atazanavir, then rifabutin dose is 150 mg (PO) 2–3 times weekly. If NNRTI is efavirenz, then rifabutin dose is 450 mg (PO) q24h or 600 mg (PO) 2–3 times weekly. If NNRTI is nevirapine, then rifabutin dose is 300 mg (PO) q24h. Rifabutin is **contraindicated** in patients receiving delavirdine or hard-gel saquinavir. <u>Patients receiving PI's AND NNRTI's</u>: as above, except adjust rifabutin to 300 mg (PO) q24h.

† For patients receiving triple NRTI regimens, substitute rifabutin 300 mg (PO) q24h for rifampin.

Clinical Presentation: May present atypically. HIV patients with high (> 500/mm^3) CD_4 cell counts are more likely to have a typical pulmonary presentation, but patients with advanced HIV disease may have a diffuse interstitial pattern, hilar adenopathy, or a normal chest x-ray. Tuberculin skin testing (TST) is helpful if positive, but unreliable if negative due to anergy.

Diagnostic Considerations: In many urban areas, TB is one of the most common HIV-related respiratory illnesses. In other areas, HIV-related TB occurs infrequently except in immigrants or patients arriving from highly TB endemic areas. Maintain a high Index of suspicion for TB in HIV patients with unexplained fevers/pulmonary infiltrates.

Pitfalls: Extrapulmonary and pulmonary TB often coexist, especially in advanced HIV disease.
Therapeutic Considerations: Treatment by directly observed therapy (DOT) is strongly recommended for all HIV patients. If patients have cavitary disease or either positive sputum cultures or lack of clinical response at 2 months, total duration of therapy should be increased up to 9 months. If hepatic transaminases are elevated (AST > 3 times normal) before treatment initiation, treatment options include: (1) standard therapy with frequent monitoring; (2) rifamycin (rifampin or rifabutin) + EMB + PZA for 6 months; or (3) INH + rifamycin + EMB for 2 months, then INH + rifamycin for 7 months. Once-weekly rifapentine is not recommended for HIV patients. Non-severe immune reconstitution inflammatory syndrome (IRIS) may be treated with nonsteroidal anti-inflammatory drugs (NSAIDs); severe cases should be treated with corticosteroids. In all cases of IRIS, antiretroviral therapy should be continued if possible. Monitor carefully for signs of rifabutin drug toxicity (arthralgias, uveitis, leukopenia).
Prognosis: Usually responds to treatment. Relapse rates are related to the degree of immunosuppression and local risk of re-exposure to TB.

CNS Opportunistic Infections

CMV Encephalitis (or Polyradiculitis)

Pathogen	Preferred Therapy	Alternate Therapy
Cytomegalovirus (CMV)	Acute therapy Ganciclovir (GCV) 5 mg/kg (IV) q12h until symptomatic improvement (typically > 3 weeks). *For severe cases*, consider acute therapy with Ganciclovir 5 mg/kg (IV) q12h plus Foscarnet 60 mg/kg (IV) q8h or 90 mg/kg (IV) q12h until symptomatic improvement Follow with lifelong suppressive therapy Valganciclovir 900 mg (PO) q24h	Acute therapy Foscarnet 60 mg/kg (IV) q8h or 90 mg/kg (IV) q12h × 3 weeks Follow with lifelong suppressive therapy Valganciclovir 900 mg (PO) q24h

Clinical Presentation: Encephalitis presents as fever, mental status changes, and headache evolving over 1–2 weeks. True meningismus is rare. CMV encephalitis occurs in advanced HIV disease (CD_4 < 50/mm^3), often in patients with prior CMV retinitis. Polyradiculitis presents as rapidly evolving weakness/sensory disturbances in the lower extremities, often with bladder/bowel incontinence. Anesthesia in "saddle distribution" with ↓ sphincter tone possible.
Diagnostic Considerations: CSF may show lymphocytic or neutrophilic pleocytosis; glucose is often decreased. For CMV encephalitis, characteristic findings on brain MRI include confluent periventricular abnormalities with variable degrees of enhancement. Diagnosis is confirmed by CSF CMV PCR (preferred), CMV culture, or brain biopsy.
Pitfalls: For CMV encephalitis, a wide spectrum of radiographic findings are possible, including mass lesions (rare). Obtain ophthalmologic evaluation to exclude active retinitis. For polyradiculitis, obtain

sagittal MRI of the spinal cord to exclude mass lesions, and CSF cytology to exclude lymphomatous involvement (can cause similar symptoms).

Therapeutic Considerations: Ganciclovir plus foscarnet may be beneficial as initial therapy for severe cases. Consider discontinuation of valganciclovir maintenance therapy if CD_4 increases to > 100–150/mm^3 × 6 months or longer in response to antiretroviral therapy.

Prognosis: Unless immune reconstitution occurs, response to therapy is usually transient, followed by progression of symptoms.

Comments: Unless CD_4 cell count increases in response to antiretroviral therapy, response to anti-CMV treatment is usually transient, followed by progression of symptoms.

Cryptococcal Meningitis

Pathogen	Preferred Therapy	Alternate Therapy
Cryptococcus neoformans	Acute infection (induction therapy) Amphotericin B deoxycholate 0.7 mg/kg (IV) q24h × 2 weeks ± flucytosine (5-FC) 25 mg/kg (PO) q6h × 2 weeks **or** Amphotericin B lipid formulation 4 mg/kg (IV) q24h × 2 weeks ± flucytosine (5-FC) 25 mg/kg (PO) q6h × 2 weeks Consolidation therapy Fluconazole 400 mg (PO) q24h × 8 weeks or until CSF cultures are sterile Chronic maintenance therapy (secondary prophylaxis) Fluconazole 200 mg (PO) q24h	Acute infection (induction therapy) Amphotericin B 0.7 mg/kg/day (IV) × 2 weeks **or** Fluconazole 400–800 mg (IV or PO) q24h × 6 weeks (less severe disease) **or** Fluconazole 400–800 mg (IV or PO) q24h plus flucytosine (5-FC) 25 mg/kg (PO) q6h × 4–6 weeks Consolidation therapy Itraconazole 200 mg (PO) q12h × 8 weeks or until CSF cultures are sterile Chronic maintenance therapy Itraconazole 200 mg (PO) q24h for intolerance to fluconazole or failed fluconazole therapy

Clinical Presentation: Often indolent onset of fever, headache, subtle cognitive deficits. Occasional meningeal signs and focal neurologic findings, though non-specific presentation is most common.

Diagnostic Considerations: Diagnosis usually by cryptococcal antigen; India ink stain of CSF is less sensitive. Diagnosis is essentially excluded with a negative serum cryptococcal antigen (sensitivity of test in AIDS patients approaches 100%). If serum cryptococcal antigen is positive, CSF antigen may be negative in disseminated disease without spread to CNS/meninges. Brain imaging is often normal, but CSF analysis is usually abnormal with a markedly elevated opening pressure.

Pitfalls: Be sure to obtain a CSF opening pressure, since reduction of increased intracranial pressure is critical for successful treatment. Remove sufficient CSF during the initial lumbar puncture (LP) to reduce closing pressure to < 200 mm H_2O or 50% of opening pressure. Increased intracranial pressure requires repeat daily lumbar punctures until CSF pressure stabilizes; persistently elevated pressure should prompt placement of a lumbar drain or ventriculo-peritoneal shunting. Adjunctive corticosteroids are not recommended.

Therapeutic Considerations: Optimal total dose/duration of amphotericin B prior to fluconazole switch is unknown (2–3 weeks is reasonable if patient is doing well). Treatment with 5-FC is optional; however, since 5-FC is associated with more rapid sterilization of CSF, it is reasonable to start 5-FC and then discontinue it for toxicity (neutropenia, nausea). Fluconazole is preferred over itraconazole for life-long maintenance therapy. Consider discontinuation of chronic maintenance therapy in patients who remain asymptomatic with CD_4 >100–200/mm^3 for > 6 months due to ART.

Prognosis: Variable. Mortality up to 40%. Adverse prognostic factors include increased intracranial pressure, abnormal mental status.

Progressive Multifocal Encephalopathy (PML)

Pathogen	Therapy
Reactivation of latent papovavirus (JC strain most common)	Effective antiretroviral therapy with immune reconstitution

Clinical Presentation: Hemiparesis, ataxia, aphasia, other focal neurologic defects, which may progress over weeks to months. Usually alert without headache or seizures on presentation.

Diagnostic Considerations: Demyelinating disease caused by reactivation of latent papovavirus (JC strain most common). Diagnosis by clinical presentation and MRI showing patchy demyelination of white matter ± cerebellum/brainstem. JC virus PCR of CSF is useful for non-invasive diagnosis. In confusing or atypical presentation, biopsy may be needed to distinguish PML from other opportunistic infections, CNS lymphoma, or HIV encephalitis/encephalopathy.

Pitfalls: Primary HIV-related encephalopathy has a similar appearance on MRI.

Therapeutic Considerations: Most effective therapy is antiretroviral therapy with immune reconstitution. Some patients experience worsening neurologic symptoms once ART is initiated due to immune reconstitution induced inflammation. ART should be continued, with consideration of adjunctive steroids. Randomized controlled trials have evaluated cidofovir and vidarabine—neither is effective nor recommended.

Prognosis: Rapid progression of neurologic deficits over weeks to months is common. Best chance for survival is immune reconstitution in response to antiretroviral therapy, although some patients will have progressive disease despite immune recovery.

Toxoplasma Encephalitis

Pathogen	Preferred Therapy	Alternate Therapy
Toxoplasma gondii	<u>Acute therapy (× 6–8 weeks until good clinical response)</u> Pyrimethamine 200 mg (PO) × 1 dose, then 50 mg (< 60 kg body weight) or 75 mg (> 60 kg) (PO) q24h	<u>Acute therapy (× 6–8 weeks until good clinical response)</u> Pyrimethamine 200 mg (PO) × 1 dose, then 50 mg (< 60 kg body weight) or 75 mg (> 60 kg) (PO) q24h plus clindamycin 600 mg (IV or PO) q6h plus leucovorin 10 mg (PO) q24h

Toxoplasma Encephalitis (cont'd)

Pathogen	Preferred Therapy	Alternate Therapy
	plus Sulfadiazine 1000 mg (< 60 kg) or 1500 mg (> 60 kg) (PO) q6h **plus** Leucovorin 10 mg (PO) q24h *For severely ill patients who cannot take oral medications*, treat with TMP–SMX (5 mg/kg TMP and 25 mg/kg SMX) (IV) q12h Follow with lifelong suppressive therapy Sulfadiazine 0.5–1 gm (PO) q6h **plus** Pyrimethamine 50 mg (PO) q24h **plus** Leucovorin 10 mg (PO) q24h	**or** TMP–SMX (5 mg/kg TMP and 25 mg/kg SMX) (IV or PO) q12h **or** Atovaquone 1.5 gm (PO) q12h (with meals or nutritional supplement) plus pyrimethamine (as above) **or** Atovaquone 1.5 gm (PO) q12h (with meals or nutritional supplement) plus sulfadiazine 1.0–1.5 mg (PO) q6h **or** Atovaquone 1.5 gm (PO) q12h (with meals) **or** Pyrimethamine (see above) plus leucovorin 10 mg (PO) q24h plus azithromycin 900–1200 mg (PO) q24h Lifelong suppressive therapy Clindamycin 300–450 mg (PO) q6-8h plus pyrimethamine 50 mg (PO) q24h plus leucovorin 10 mg (PO) q24h (2nd choice regimen) **or** Atovaquone 750 mg (PO) q12h ± pyrimethamine 25 mg (PO) q24h and leucovorin 10 mg (PO) q24h (3rd choice regimen)

Clinical Presentation: Wide spectrum of neurologic symptoms, including sensorimotor deficits, seizures, confusion, ataxia. Fever/headache are common.

Diagnostic Considerations: Diagnosis by characteristic radiographic appearance and response to empiric therapy in a for T. gondii seropositive patient.

Pitfalls: Use leucovorin (folinic acid) 10 mg (PO) daily with pyrimethamine-containing regimens, not folate/folic acid. Radiographic improvement may lag behind clinical response.

Therapeutic Considerations: Alternate agents include atovaquone, azithromycin, clarithromycin, minocycline (all with pyrimethamine if possible). Decadron 4 mg (PO or IV) q6h is useful for edema/mass effect. Chronic suppressive therapy can be discontinued if patients are free from signs and symptoms of disease and have a CD_4 cell count > 200/mm^3 for > 6 months due to ART.

Prognosis: Usually responds to treatment if able to tolerate drugs. Clinical response is evident by 1 week in 70%, by 2 weeks in 90%. Radiographic improvement is usually apparent by 2 weeks. Neurologic recovery is variable.

Gastrointestinal Tract Opportunistic Infections

Campylobacter (C. jejuni) Enteritis

Subset	Preferred Therapy
Mild disease	Might withhold therapy unless symptoms persist for several days
Moderate disease	Ciprofloxacin 500 mg (PO) q12h × 1 week **or** Azithromycin 500 mg (PO) q24h × 1 week
Bacteremia	Ciprofloxacin 500 mg (PO) q12h × 2 weeks* **or** Azithromycin 500 mg (PO) q24h × 2 weeks*

* Consider addition of aminoglycoside in bacteremic patients.

Clinical Presentation: Acute onset of diarrhea, sometimes bloody; constitutional symptoms may be prominent.

Diagnostic Considerations: Diagnosis by stool culture; bacteremia may rarely occur, so blood cultures also indicated. Suspect campylobacter in AIDS patient with diarrhea and curved gram-negative rods in blood culture. Non-jejuni species may be more strongly correlated with bacteremia.

Therapeutic Considerations: Optimal therapy not well defined. Treat with quinolone or azithromycin; modify therapy based on susceptibility testing. Quinolone resistance can occur and correlates with treatment failure. Role of aminoglycoside is unclear.

Prognosis: Depends on underlying immune status; prognosis is generally good.

Clostridium difficile Diarrhea/Colitis

Pathogen	Preferred Therapy	Alternate Therapy
C. difficile	Metronidazole 500 mg (PO) q8h × 10–14 days. Avoid use of other C. difficile associated antibiotics if possible	Vancomycin 125 mg (PO) q6h × 10–14 days. Avoid use of difficile associated antibiotics if possible

Clinical Presentation: Diarrhea and abdominal pain following antibiotic therapy. Diarrhea may be watery or bloody. Proton pump inhibitors increase the risk. Among antibiotics, clindamycin and beta-lactams are most frequent. Rarely due to aminoglycosides, linezolid, doxycycline, TMP–SMX, carbapenems, daptomycin, vancomycin.

Diagnostic Considerations: Most common cause of bacterial diarrhea in U.S. among HIV patients. Watery diarrhea with positive C. difficile toxin in stool specimen. C. difficile stool toxin test is sufficiently sensitive/specific. If positive, no need to retest until negative (endpoint is end of diarrhea); if negative, no need to retest (repeat tests) will be negative). C. difficile colitis may be distinguished clinically from C. difficile diarrhea by temperature > 102°F, ↑ WBC, ↑ ESR, and/or abdominal pain.

C. difficile virulent epidemic strain is type B1 (toxinotype III), which produces 20-times the amount of toxin A/B compared to less virulent strains.

Pitfalls: In a patient with C. difficile diarrhea, C. difficile colitis is suggested by the presence of ↑ WBC, ↑ ESR, abdominal pain and temperature > 102°F; confirm diagnosis with CT of abdomen, which will show colonic wall thickening. New virulent strain of C. difficile may present with colitis with temperature ≤ 102°F, little/no ↑ WBC, and little/no abdominal pain; confirm diagnosis with CT/MRI of abdomen. C. difficile toxin may remain positive in stools for weeks following treatment; do not treat positive stool toxin unless patient has symptoms.

Therapeutic Considerations: Initiate therapy for mild disease with metronidazole; symptoms usually begin to improve within 2–3 days. For moderate or severe disease, or with evidence of colitis clinically (leukocytosis, fever, colonic thickening on CT scan), vancomycin has become the preferred agent in many centers due to concern for the more virulent strain, and based on the results of some observational studies suggesting vancomycin is more effective. The duration of therapy should be extended beyond 14 days if other systemic antibiotics must be continued. Relapse occurs in 10–25% of patients, and rates may be higher in patients with HIV due to the frequent need for other antimicrobial therapy. First relapses can be treated with a repeat of the initial regimen of metronidazole or vancomycin. For multiple relapses, a long-term taper is appropriate: week 1–125 mg 4x/day; week 2–125 mg 2x/day; week 3–125 mg once daily; week 4–125 mg every other day; weeks 5 and 6–125 mg every three days. Every effort should be made to resume a normal diet and to avoid other antibacterial therapies. Probiotic treatments (such as lactobacillus or Saccharomyces boulardii) have not yet been shown to reduce the risk of relapse in controlled clinical trials.

Prognosis: Prognosis with C. difficile colitis is related to severity of the colitis.

CMV Esophagitis/Colitis

Infection	Preferred Therapy	Alternate Therapy
Initial infection	Ganciclovir 5 mg/kg (IV) q12h × 3–4 weeks or until signs and symptoms have resolved. Valganciclovir 900 mg (PO) q12h can be used if able to tolerate oral intake. Maintenance therapy is generally not necessary but should be considered after relapses	Foscarnet 60 mg/kg (IV) q8h or 90 mg/kg (IV) q12h × 3–4 weeks or until signs and symptoms have resolved
Relapses	Valganciclovir 900 mg (PO) q24h indefinitely; consider discontinuation if CD_4 > 200/mm^3 for ≥ 6 months on ART	

Clinical Presentation: Localizing symptoms, including odynophagia, abdominal pain, diarrhea, sometimes bloody stools.

Diagnostic Considerations: Diagnosis by finding CMV inclusions on biopsy. CMV can affect the entire GI tract, resulting in oral/esophageal ulcers, gastritis, and colitis (most common). CMV colitis varies greatly in severity, but typically causes fever, abdominal cramping, and sometimes bloody stools.

Pitfalls: CMV colitis may cause colonic perforation and should be considered in any AIDS patient presenting with an acute abdomen, especially if radiography demonstrates free intraperitoneal air.

Therapeutic Considerations: Duration of therapy is dependent on clinical response, typically 3–4 weeks. Consider chronic suppressive therapy for recurrent disease. Screen for CMV retinitis.
Prognosis: Relapse rate is greatly reduced with immune reconstitution due to antiretroviral therapy.

Cryptosporidia Enteritis

Pathogen	Preferred Therapy	Alternate Therapy
Cryptosporidium sp.	Effective ART with immune reconstitution to CD_4 > 100/mm^3 can result in complete resolution of symptoms and clearance of infection	Nitazoxanide 500 mg (PO) q12h × 4–6 weeks **or** Paromomycin 1 gm (PO) q12h × 2–4 weeks

Clinical Presentation: High-volume watery diarrhea with weight loss and electrolyte disturbances, especially in advanced HIV disease.
Diagnostic Considerations: Spore-forming protozoa. Diagnosis by AFB smear of stool demonstrating characteristic oocyte. Malabsorption may occur.
Pitfalls: No fecal leukocytes; organisms are not visualized on standard ova and parasite exams (need to request special stains).
Therapeutic Considerations: Anecdotal reports of antimicrobial success. Newest agent nitazoxanide may be effective in some settings, but no increase in cure rate for nitazoxanide if CD_4 < 50/mm^3. Immune reconstitution in response to antiretroviral therapy is the most effective therapy, and may induce prolonged remissions and cure. Anti-diarrheal agents (Lomotil, Pepto-Bismol) are useful to control symptoms. Hyperalimentation may be required for severe cases.
Prognosis: Related to degree of immunosuppression/response to antiretroviral therapy.

Isospora (Isospora belli) Enteritis

Subset	Preferred Therapy	Alternate Therapy
Acute infection	TMP 160 mg and SMX 800 mg (IV or PO) q6h × 10 days **or** TMP 320 mg and SMX 1600 mg (IV or PO) q12h × 10–14 days	Pyrimethamine 50–75 mg (PO) q24h *plus* leucovorin 5–10 mg (PO) q24h **or** Ciprofloxacin 500 mg (PO) q12h or other fluoroquinolones
Chronic maintenance therapy for CD_4 < 200 (secondary prophylaxis)	TMP 320 mg plus SMX 1600 mg (PO) q24h*	Pyrimethamine 25 mg (PO) q24h plus leucovorin 5–10 mg (PO) q24h*

* Discontinuation of secondary prophylaxis may be considered if CD_4 > 200/mm^3 for > 3 months.

Clinical Presentation: Severe chronic diarrhea without fever/fecal leukocytes.
Diagnostic Considerations: Spore-forming protozoa (Isospora belli). Oocyst on AFB smear of stool larger that cryptosporidium (20–30 microns vs. 4–6 microns). More common in HIV patients from the tropics (e.g., Haiti). Less common than cryptosporidium or microsporidia. Malabsorption may occur.

Pitfalls: Multiple relapses are possible.
Therapeutic Considerations: Chronic suppressive therapy may be required if CD_4 does not increase.
Prognosis: Related to degree of immunosuppression/response to antiretroviral therapy.
Comments: Immune reconstitution with ART results in fewer relapses.

Microsporidia Enteritis

Pathogen	Therapy*
Microsporidia other than Enterocytozoon bienuesi	Albendazole 400 mg (PO) q12h (continue until $CD_4 > 200/mm^3$)
Enterocytozoon bienuesi	Fumagillin 60 mg (PO) q24h (not available in the U.S.)
Trachipleistophora or Brachiola	Itraconazole 400 mg (PO) q24h plus albendazole 400 mg (PO) q12h

* Regardless of species, ART with immune reconstitution is a critical component of treatment.

Clinical Presentation: Intermittent chronic diarrhea without fever/fecal leukocytes.
Diagnostic Considerations: Spore-forming protozoa (S. intestinalis, E. bieneusi). Diagnosis by modified trichrome or fluorescent antibody stain of stool. Microsporidia can rarely disseminate to sinuses/cornea. Severe malabsorption may occur.
Pitfalls: Microsporidia is too small for detection by routine microscopic examination of stool.
Therapeutic Considerations: Albendazole is less effective for E. bieneusi than S. intestinalis, but speciation is usually not possible. May consider treatment discontinuation for $CD_4 < 200/mm^3$ if patient remains asymptomatic (no signs or symptoms of microsporidiosis). If ocular infection is present, continue treatment indefinitely.
Prognosis: Related to degree of immunosuppression/response to antiretroviral therapy.

Oropharyngeal/Esophageal Candidiasis

Infection	Therapy	Fluconazole-Resistance
Oropharyngeal candidiasis (thrush)	Preferred therapy Fluconazole 100 mg (PO) q24h × 1–2 weeks Alternate therapy Itraconazole oral solution 200 mg (PO) q24h × 1–2 weeks **or** clotrimazole troches 10 mg (PO) 5x/day × 1–2 weeks **or** nystatin suspension 4–6 mL q6h or 1–2 flavored pastilles 4–5x/day × 1–2 weeks	Fluconazole at doses up to 800 mg (PO) q24h × 1–2 weeks **or** Caspofungin 70 mg (IV) on day 1, then 50 mg (IV) q24h × 1–2 weeks **or** Micafugin 150 mg (IV) q24h × 1–2 weeks **or**

Oropharyngeal/Esophageal Candidiasis (cont'd)

Infection	Therapy	Fluconazole-Resistance
Esophageal candidiasis	Preferred therapy Fluconazole 100 mg (up to 400 mg) (IV or PO) q24h × 1–2 weeks Alternate therapy Itraconazole oral solution 200 mg (PO) q24h × 2–3 weeks **or** voriconazole 200 mg (PO) q24h × 2–3 weeks **or** caspofungin 50 mg (IV) q24h × 2–3 weeks	Amphotericin B 0.3 mg/kg (IV) q24h × 1–2 weeks **or** Amphotericin liposomal or lipid complex 3–5 mg/kg (IV) q24h × 1–2 weeks

Oral Thrush (Candida)

Clinical Presentation: Dysphagia/odynophagia. More common/severe in advanced HIV disease.

Diagnostic Considerations: Pseudomembranous (most common), erythematous, and hyperplastic (leukoplakia) forms. Pseudomembranes (white plaques on inflamed base) on buccal muscosa/tongue/gingiva/palate scrape off easily, hyperplastic lesions do not. Diagnosis by clinical appearance ± KOH/gram stain of scraping showing yeast/pseudomycelia. Other oral lesions in AIDS patients include herpes simplex, aphthous ulcers, Kaposi's sarcoma, oral hairy leukoplakia.

Pitfalls: Patients may be asymptomatic.

Therapeutic Considerations: Fluconazole is superior to topical therapy in preventing relapses of thrush and treating Candida esophagitis. Continuous treatment with fluconazole may lead to fluconazole-resistance, which is best treated initially with itraconazole suspension and, if no response, with IV caspofungin or amphotericin. Chronic suppressive therapy is usually only considered for severely immunosuppressed patients.

Prognosis: Improvement in symptoms are often seen within 24–48 hours.

Candida Esophagitis

Clinical Presentation: Dysphagia/odynophagia, almost always in the setting of oropharyngeal thrush. Fever is uncommon.

Diagnostic Considerations: Most common cause of esophagitis in HIV disease. For persistent symptoms despite therapy, endoscopy with biopsy/culture is recommended to confirm diagnosis and assess azole-resistance.

Pitfalls: May extend into stomach. Other common causes of esophagitis include CMV, herpes simplex, and aphthous ulcers. Rarely, Kaposi's sarcoma, non-Hodgkin's lymphoma, zidovudine, dideoxycytidine, and other infections may cause esophageal symptoms.

Therapeutic Considerations: Systemic therapy is preferred over topical therapy. Failure to improve on empiric therapy mandates endoscopy to look for other causes, especially herpes viruses/aphthous ulcers. Consider maintenance therapy with fluconazole for frequent relapses, although the risk of fluconazole resistance is increased. Fluconazole-resistance is best treated initially with itraconazole suspension and, if no response, with IV caspofungin, micafungin, or amphotericin.

Prognosis: Relapse rate related to degree of immunosuppression.

Salmonella Gastroenteritis (non-typhi)

Subset	Preferred Therapy	Alternate Therapy
Mild disease	Ciprofloxacin 750 mg (PO) q12h × 1–2 weeks	TMP–SMX 1 DS (PO) q12h × 2 weeks **or**
CD_4 < 200	Ciprofloxacin 750 mg (PO) q12h × 4–6 weeks	Ceftriaxone 2 gm (IV) q24h × 2 weeks **or**
Bacteremia	Ciprofloxacin 750 mg (PO) q12h × 4–6 weeks, then 500 mg (PO) q12h indefinitely	Cefotaxime 1 gm (IV) q8h × 2 weeks

Clinical Presentation: Patients with HIV are at markedly increased risk of developing salmonellosis. Three different presentations may be seen: (1) self-limited gastroenteritis, as typically seen in immunocompetent hosts; (2) a more severe and prolonged diarrheal disease, associated with fever, bloody diarrhea, and weight loss; or (3) Salmonella septicemia, which may present with or without gastrointestinal symptoms.

Diagnostic Considerations: The diagnosis is established through cultures of stool and blood. Given the high rate of bacteremia associated with Salmonella gastroenteritis—especially in advanced HIV disease—blood cultures should be obtained in any HIV patient presenting with diarrhea and fever.

Pitfalls: A distinctive feature of salmonella bacteremia in patients with AIDS is its propensity for relapse (rate > 20%).

Therapeutic Considerations: The mainstay of treatment is a fluoroquinolone; greatest experience is with ciprofloxacin, but newer quinolones (moxifloxacin, levofloxacin) may also be effective. For uncomplicated salmonellosis in an HIV patient with CD_4 > 200/mm^3, 1–2 weeks of treatment is reasonable to reduce the risk of extraintestinal spread. For patients with advanced HIV disease (CD_4 < 200/mm^3) or who have salmonella bacteremia, at least 4–6 weeks of treatment is required. Chronic suppressive therapy, given for several months or until antiretroviral therapy-induced immune reconstitution ensues, is indicated for patients who relapse after cessation of therapy. Consider using ZDV as part of the antiretroviral regimen (ZDV is active against Salmonella).

Prognosis: Usually responds well to treatment. Relapse rate in AIDS patients with bacteremia is > 20%.

Shigella (Shigella sp.) Enteritis

Subset	Preferred Therapy	Alternate Therapy
No bacteremia	Fluoroquinolone (IV or PO) × 3–7 days	TMP–SMX 1 DS tablet (PO) q12h × 3–7 days **or** Azithromycin 500 mg (PO) on day 1, then 250 mg (PO) q24h × 4 days
Bacteremia	Extend treatment duration to 14 days	Extend treatment duration to 14 days

Clinical Presentation: Acute onset of bloody diarrhea/mucus.

Diagnostic Considerations: Diagnosis by demonstrating organism in stool specimens. Shigella ulcers in colon are linear, serpiginous, and rarely lead to perforation. More common in gay men.

Therapeutic Considerations: Shigella dysentery is more acute/fulminating than amebic dysentery. Shigella has no carrier state, unlike Entamoeba. Shigella infections acquired outside of United States have high rates of TMP–SMX resistance. Therapy is indicated to shorten the duration of illness and to prevent spread of infection. Shigella has no carrier state.

Prognosis: Good if treated early. Severity of illness related to Shigella species: S. dysenteriae (most severe) > S. flexneri > S. boydii/S. sonnei (mildest).

Other Opportunistic Infections

Candida Vaginitis

Pathogen	Therapy
Candida albicans	Intravaginal miconazole suppository 200 mg q24h × 3 days or miconazole 3% × 7 days **or** Nystatin vaginal tablet 100,000U q24h × 14 days **or** Itraconazole 200 mg (PO) q12h × 1 day (or 200 mg q24h × 3 days) **or** Fluconazole 150 mg (PO) × 1 dose

Clinical Presentation: White, cheesy, vaginal discharge or vulvar rash ± itching/pain. Local infection not a sign of disseminated disease.

Diagnostic Considerations: Local infection. Not a manifestation of disseminated disease.

Pitfalls: Women with advanced AIDS receiving fluconazole may develop fluconazole-resistant Candida.

Therapeutic Considerations: For recurrence, consider maintenance with fluconazole 100–200 mg (PO) weekly.

Prognosis: Good response to therapy. Relapses are common.

CMV (Cytomegalovirus) Retinitis

	Preferred Therapy	Alternate Therapy
Initial therapy	Initiate systemic CMV therapy* pending ophthalmology consult For immediate sight-threatening lesions Ganciclovir (GCV) intraocular implant plus valganciclovir 900 mg (PO) q12h for at least 21 days; can	Initiate systemic CMV therapy* pending ophthalmology consult Ganciclovir 5 mg/kg (IV) q12h × 2–3 weeks, then either 5 mg/kg (IV) q24h or valganciclovir 900 mg (PO) q24h **or**

* Length of high-dose induction therapy depends on rate of response to treatment, typically 2–4 weeks.

CMV (Cytomegalovirus) Retinitis (cont'd)

	Preferred Therapy	Alternate Therapy
	reduce dose to maintenance therapy (below) when retinitis deemed inactive by consulting ophthalmologist <u>For peripheral lesions</u> Valganciclovir 900 mg (PO) q12h × 21 days	Foscarnet 60 mg/kg (IV) q8h or 90 mg/kg (IV) q12h × 3 weeks, then 90–120 mg/kg (IV) q24h **or** Cidofovir 5 mg/kg (IV) × 2 weeks, then every 2 weeks. Give probenecid 2 gm (PO) 3 hours before and 1 gm (PO) 2 and 8 hours after cidofovir (total of 4 gm)
Maintenance therapy	Valganciclovir 900 mg (PO) q24h indefinitely **or** Foscarnet 90–120 mg/kg (IV) q24h indefinitely	Cidofovir 5 mg/kg (IV) every other week with probenecid as above **or** Fomivirsen 1 vial (330 mg) injected into vitreous, then repeated every 2–4 weeks

* Length of high-dose induction therapy depends on rate of response to treatment, typically 2–4 weeks.

Clinical Presentation: Blurred vision, scotomata, field cuts common. Often bilateral, even when initial symptoms are unilateral.

Diagnostic Considerations: Diagnosis by characteristic hemorrhagic ("tomato soup and milk") retinitis on funduscopic exam. Consult ophthalmology in suspected cases.

Pitfalls: May develop immune reconstitution vitreitis after starting antiretroviral therapy.

Therapeutic Considerations: Oral valganciclovir is the preferred option for initial and maintenance therapy. Life-long maintenance therapy for CMV retinitis is required for CD_4 counts < 100/mm^3, but may be discontinued if CD_4 counts increase to > 100–150/mm^3 for 6 or more months in response to antiretroviral therapy (in consultation with ophthalmologist). Patients with CMV retinitis who discontinue therapy should undergo regular eye exams to monitor for relapse. Ganciclovir intraocular implants might need to be replaced every 6–8 months for patients who remain immunosuppressed with CD_4 < 100–150/mm^3. Immune recovery uveitis (IRU) may develop in the setting of immune reconstitution due to ART and be treated by ophthalmologist with periocular corticosteroid ± systemic corticosteroid.

Prognosis: Good initial response to therapy. High relapse rate unless CD_4 improves with antiretroviral therapy.

Coccidioidomycosis (C. immitis) Infection

Infection	Therapy*
Nonmeningeal infection	<u>Acute therapy (diffuse pulmonary or disseminated disease)</u> Amphotericin B deoxycholate 0.5–1.0 mg/kg (IV) q24h until clinical improvement (usually 500–1000 mg total dose). Some specialists add an azole to amphotericin B therapy

* Therapy for meningeal infection should be lifelong with fluconazole 400–800 mg q24h. There are insufficient data to recommend discontinuation of chronic maintenance therapy in other settings.

Coccidioidomycosis (C. immitis) Infection (cont'd)

Infection	Therapy*
	Acute therapy (milder disease) Fluconazole 400–800 mg (PO) q24h or Itraconazole 200 mg (PO) q12h Chronic maintenance therapy (secondary prophylaxis) Preferred: Fluconazole 400 mg (PO) q24h indefinitely; alternative: or Itraconazole 200 mg capsule (PO) q12h indefinitely
Meningeal infection*	Acute therapy Fluconazole 400–800 mg (IV) or (PO) q24h. Intrathecal amphotericin B if no response to azole therapy Chronic maintenance therapy (secondary prophylaxis) Fluconazole 400 mg (PO) q24h or itraconazole 200 mg capsule (PO) q12h indefinitely

* Therapy for meningeal infection should be lifelong with fluconazole 400–800 mg q24h. There are insufficient data to recommend discontinuation of chronic maintenance therapy in other settings.

Clinical Presentation: Typically a complication of advanced HIV infection (CD_4 cell count < 200/mm^3). Most patients present with disseminated disease, which can manifest as fever, diffuse pulmonary infiltrates, adenopathy, skin lesions (multiple forms – verrucous, cold abscesses, ulcers, nodules), and/or bone lesions. Approximately 10% will have spread to the CNS in the form of meningitis (fever, headache, altered mental status).

Diagnostic Considerations: Consider the diagnosis in any patient with advanced HIV-related immunosuppression who has been in a C. immitis endemic area (Southwestern US, northern Mexico) and presents with a systemic febrile syndrome. Diagnosis can be made by culture of the organism, visualization of characteristic spherules on histopathology, or a positive complement-fixation antibody (≥ 1:16). In meningeal cases, CSF profile shows low glucose, high protein, and lymphocytic pleocytosis.

Pitfalls: Antibody titers often negative on presentation. CSF profile of meningitis can be similar to TB.

Prognosis: Related to extent of infection and degree of immunosuppression. Clinical response tends to be slow, especially with a high disease burden and advanced HIV disease. Meningeal disease is treated life-long regardless of CD_4 recovery.

Extrapulmonary Tuberculosis

Pathogen	Therapy
Mycobacterium tuberculosis	Treat the same as pulmonary TB (see p. 323). May require longer duration of therapy based on clinical response

Clinical Presentation: Multiple presentations possible (e.g., lymphadenitis, osteomyelitis, meningitis, hepatitis). Dissemination is more common in patients with low CD_4 cell counts (< 100/mm^3).

Diagnostic Considerations: Diagnosis by isolator blood cultures or tissue biopsy.

Pitfalls: Patients with disseminated disease frequently have pulmonary disease, which has implications for infection control.

Therapeutic Considerations: Response to therapy may be slower than in normal hosts.
Prognosis: Usually responsive to therapy.

Herpes Simplex Virus (HSV) Disease

Infection	Preferred Therapy	Alternate Therapy
Orolabial lesions or initial/recurrent genital HSV	Famciclovir 500 mg (PO) q12h × 1–2 weeks **or** valacyclovir 1 gm (PO) q12h × 1–2 weeks **or** acyclovir 400 mg (PO) q8h × 1–2 weeks	Acyclovir-resistant HSV Foscarnet 60–100 mg/kg (IV) q12h until clinical response **or** Cidofovir 5 mg/kg (IV) weekly until clinical response
Moderate-to-severe mucocutaneous HSV	Initial therapy: Acyclovir 5 mg/kg (IV) q8h × 2–7 days. If improvement, switch to famciclovir 500 mg (PO) q12h **or** valacyclovir 1 gm (PO) q12h **or** acyclovir 400 mg (PO) q8h to complete 7–10 days	Acyclovir-resistant HSV Foscarnet 60–100 mg/kg (IV) q12h until clinical response **or** Cidofovir 5 mg/kg (IV) weekly until clinical response
HSV keratitis	Trifluridine 1% ophthalmic solution, one drop onto cornea q2h, not to exceed 9 drops per day and no longer than 21 days. Treatment in conjunction with ophthalmology consultation	Acyclovir-resistant HSV Foscarnet 60–100 mg/kg (IV) q12h until clinical response **or** Cidofovir 5 mg/kg (IV) weekly until clinical response
HSV encephalitis	Acyclovir 10 mg/kg (IV) q8h × 2–3 weeks **or** Valacyclovir 1 gm (PO) q6h × 2–3 weeks	Acyclovir-resistant HSV Foscarnet 60–100 mg/kg (IV) q12h until clinical response **or** Cidofovir 5 mg/kg (IV) weekly until response
Multiple mucocutaneous (oral or anogenital) relapses (chronic suppressive therapy)	Acyclovir 400 mg (PO) q12h **or** Famciclovir 250 mg (PO) q12h **or** Valacyclovir 500 mg (PO) q12h	Patients may be able to titrate dose downward to maintain response

Herpes Simplex (genital/oral)

Clinical Presentation: Painful, grouped vesicles on an erythematous base that rupture, crust, and heal within 2 weeks. Lesions may be chronic, severe, ulcerative with advanced immunosuppression.
Diagnostic Considerations: Diagnosis by viral culture of swab from lesion base/roof of blister; alternative diagnostic techniques include Tzanck prep or immunofluorescence staining.
Pitfalls: Acyclovir prophylaxis is not required in patients receiving ganciclovir or foscarnet.

Therapeutic Considerations: In refractory cases, consider acyclovir resistance and treat with foscarnet. Topical trifluridine ophthalmic solution (Viroptic 1%) may be considered for direct application to small, localized areas of refractory disease; clean with hydrogen peroxide, then debride lightly with gauze, apply trifluridine, and cover with bacitracin/polymyxin ointment and nonadsorbent gauze; topical cidofovir (requires compounding) also may be tried. Chronic suppressive therapy with oral acyclovir, famciclovir, or valacyclovir may be indicated for patients with frequent recurrences, dosing similar to HIV-negative patients.
Prognosis: Responds well to treatment except in severely immunocompromised patients, in whom acyclovir resistance may develop. Prognosis for HSV meningitis is excellent.

Herpes Encephalitis (HSV-1)

Clinical Presentation: Acute onset of fever and change in mental status.
Diagnostic Considerations: EEG is abnormal early (< 72 hours), showing unilateral temporal lobe abnormalities. Brain MRI is abnormal before CT scan, which may require several days before a temporal lobe focus is seen. Definitive diagnosis is by CSF PCR for HSV-1 DNA. Profound decrease in sensorium is characteristic of HSV meningoencephalitis. CSF may have PMN predominance and low glucose levels, unlike other viral causes of meningitis. A different clinical entity is HSV meningitis, which is usually associated with HSV-2 and can recur with lymphocytic meningitis.
Pitfalls: Rule out non-infectious causes of encephalopathy. Surprisingly, HIV encephalitis is a relatively rare cause of encephalitis in patients with HIV.
Therapeutic Considerations: Treat as soon as possible since neurological deficits may be mild and reversible early on, but severe and irreversible later.
Prognosis: Related to extent of brain injury and early antiviral therapy. Prognosis for HSV meningitis is excellent.

Histoplasmosis (H. capsulatum), Disseminated

Subset	Preferred Therapy	Alternate Therapy
Acute phase (3–10 days or until clinically improved)	Liposomal amphotericin B 3 mg/kg × 1–2 weeks or other lipid associated formulations at 5 mg/kg	Amphotericin B doxycholate 0.7–1 mg/kg **or** Intravenous itraconazole (200 mg q12 × 4 doses then 200 mg q24)
Continuation phase	Itraconazole 200 (PO) TID × 3 days and then QD or BID for atleast 12 months (adequate serum levels should be confirmed). Immunosuppressed patients may require lifelong suppressive therapy.	Itraconazole oral solution 200 mg (PO) q12h × 12 weeks **or** Fluconazole 800 mg (PO) q24h × 12 weeks
Meningitis	Amphotericin B deoxycholate 0.7 mg/kg (IV) q24h × 12–16 weeks **or** Liposomal amphotericin B 4 mg/kg (IV) q24h × 12–16 weeks	Fluconazole 800 mg (PO) q24h × 12 weeks

* Duration of therapy dependent on response to therapy.

Clinical Presentation: Two general forms: Mild disease with fever/lymph node enlargement (e.g., cervical adenitis), or severe disease with fever, wasting ± diarrhea/meningitis/GI ulcerations.
Diagnostic Considerations: Diagnosis by urine/serum histoplasmosis antigen, sometimes by culture of bone marrow/liver or isolator blood cultures. May occur in patients months to years after having lived/moved from an endemic area.
Pitfalls: Relapse is common after discontinuation of therapy. Cultures may take 7–21 days to turn positive.
Therapeutic Considerations: Initial therapy depends on severity of illness on presentation. Extremely sick patients should be started on amphotericin B deoxycholate, with duration of IV therapy dependent on response to treatment. Mildly ill patients can be started on itraconazole. All patients require chronic suppressive therapy, with possible discontinuation for immune reconstitution with CD_4 counts > 100/mm^3 for at least 6 months. HIV patients with CD_4 > 500/mm^3 and acute pulmonary histoplasmosis might not require therapy, but a short course of itraconazole (4–8 weeks) is reasonable to prevent systemic spread.
Prognosis: Usually responds to treatment, except in fulminant cases.

Mycobacterium avium-intracellulare (MAI)

Pathogen	Preferred Therapy	Alternate Therapy
Mycobacterium avium-intracellulare (MAI)	<u>At least 2 drugs as initial therapy</u> Clarithromycin 500 mg (PO) q12h plus ethambutol 15 mg/kg (PO) q24h (usually 800 mg or 1200 mg daily). Consider adding third drug, rifabutin 300 mg (PO) q24h, for patients with CD_4 < 50/mm^3, high mycobacterial loads and severely symptomatic disease. Duration of therapy is **lifelong**, although consider discontinuation in asymptomatic patients with > 12 months therapy and CD_4 > 100/mm^3 for > 6 months in response to ART	<u>Alternative to clarithromycin</u> Azithromycin 500–600 mg (PO) q24h <u>Alternative 3rd or 4th drug for severe symptoms or disseminated disease</u> Ciprofloxacin 500–750 mg (PO) q12h **or** Levofloxacin 500 mg (PO) q24h **or** Amikacin 10–15 mg/kg (IV) q24h

Clinical Presentation: Typically presents as a febrile wasting illness in advanced HIV disease (CD_4 < 50/mm^3). Focal invasive disease is possible, especially in patients with advanced immunosuppression after starting antiretroviral therapy. Focal disease likely reflects restoration of pathogen-specific immune response to subclinical infection ("immune reconstitution inflammatory syndrome" [IRIS]), and typically manifests as lymphadenitis (mesenteric, cervical, thoracic) or rarely disease in the spine mimicking Pott's disease. Immune reconstitution syndrome usually occurs within weeks to months after starting antiretroviral therapy for the first time, but may occur a year or more later.
Diagnostic Considerations: Diagnosis by isolation of organism from a normally sterile body site (blood, lymph node, bone marrow, liver biopsy). Lysis centrifugation (DuPont isolator) is the preferred blood culture method. Anemia/↑ alkaline phosphatase are occasionally seen.

Pitfalls: Isolator blood cultures may be negative, especially in immune reconstitution inflammatory syndrome initially.

Therapeutic Considerations: Some studies suggest benefit for addition of rifabutin 300 mg (PO) q24h, others do not. Rifabutin may require dosage adjustment with NNRTI's and PI's (see p. 270). For concurrent use with nelfinavir, indinavir, or amprenavir, decrease rifabutin to 150 mg (PO) q24h. For concurrent use with ritonavir, decrease rifabutin to 150 mg (PO) 2–3x/week. For concurrent use with efavirenz, increase rifabutin to 450–600 mg (PO) q24h. The dose of PI's or NNRTI's may need to be increased by 20–25%. Monitor carefully for rifabutin drug toxicity (arthralgias, uveitis, leukopenia). Treat IRIS initially with NSAIDs; if symptoms persist, systemic corticosteroids (prednisone 20–40 mg daily) for 4–8 weeks can be used. Some patients will require a more prolonged course of corticosteroids with a slow taper over months. Azithromycin is often better tolerated than clarithromycin and has fewer drug-drug interactions. Optimal long-term management is unknown, though most studies suggest that treatment can be discontinued in asymptomatic patients with > 12 months of therapy and CD_4 > 100/mm^3 for > 6 months.

Prognosis: Depends on immune reconstitution in response to antiretroviral therapy. Adverse prognostic factors include high-grade bacteremia or severe wasting.

Varicella Zoster Virus (VZV)

Infection	Preferred Therapy
Primary VZV infection (chickenpox)	Acyclovir 10 mg/kg (IV) q8h × 7–10 days. Can start with or change to oral therapy with valacyclovir 1 gm (PO) q8h or famciclovir 500 mg (PO) q8h after defervescence if no evidence of visceral involvement exists
Local dermatomal herpes zoster	Famciclovir 500 mg (PO) q8h × 7–10 days **or** Valacyclovir 1 gm (PO) q8h × 7–10 days
Extensive cutaneous or visceral involvement	Acyclovir 10 mg/kg (IV) q8h until cutaneous and visceral disease has clearly resolved and the patient is clinically improved
Acute retinal necrosis	Acyclovir 10 mg/kg (IV) q8h until progression stops, then valacyclovir 1 gm (PO) q8h × 6 weeks. Treat in conjunction with close ophthalmologic consultation

Clinical Presentation: Primary varicella (chickenpox) presents as clear vesicles on an erythematous base that heal with crusting and sometimes scarring. Zoster usually presents as painful tense vesicles on an erythematous base in a dermatomal distribution. In patients with HIV, primary varicella is more severe/prolonged, and zoster is more likely to involve multiple dermatomes/disseminate. VZV can rarely cause acute retinal necrosis, which requires close consultation with ophthalmology.

Diagnostic Considerations: Diagnosis is usually clinical. In atypical cases, immunofluorescence can be used to distinguish herpes zoster from herpes simplex.

Pitfalls: Extend treatment beyond 7–10 days if new vesicles are still forming after initial treatment period. Corticosteroids for dermatomal zoster are not recommended in HIV-positive patients.

Therapeutic Considerations: IV therapy is generally indicated for severe disease/cranial nerve zoster.

Prognosis: Usually responds slowly to treatment.

Hepatitis Coinfection

Hepatitis C Infection

Pathogen	Therapy
Hepatitis C virus (HCV)	Peginterferon alfa-2b 1.5 mcg/kg (SQ) weekly* or Peginterferon alfa-2a 180 mcg (SQ) weekly* **plus** Ribavirin† (PO) (weight-based dosing: if < 75 mg, 400 mg in morning and 600 mg in evening; if > 75 kg, 600 mg q12h)

* Duration of therapy (all genotypes): 48 weeks for patients who demonstrate an early virologic response (> 2 log decrease in HCV viral load at 12 weeks); 12 weeks for patients who fail to achieve an early virologic response at 12 weeks (therapy beyond 12 weeks is almost always futile for achieving virologic cure).

† Monotherapy (peginterferon alfa-2b or alfa-2a) is indicated in patients with a contraindication to ribavirin (e.g., unstable cardiopulmonary disease, pre-existing anemia, hemoglobinopathy).

Clinical Presentation: Persistently elevated liver transaminases; usually asymptomatic.

Diagnostic Considerations: All HIV-positive patients should be tested for HCV antibody. If the antibody test is negative but the likelihood of HCV infection is high (IDU, unexplained increase in LFTs), obtain an HCV RNA since false-negative antibody tests may occur, especially in advanced HIV disease. Since LFT elevation does not correlate well with underlying HCV activity, a liver biopsy is the best way to assess the degree of fibrosis and inflammation.

Therapeutic Considerations:

Once Diagnosis is Established. Advise patients to abstain from alcohol and administer vaccinations for hepatitis A and B (if non-immune). Also obtain HCV RNA levels with genotype assessment. HCV RNA levels do not have prognostic significance for underlying degree of liver disease, but higher levels make treatment for cure less likely. Genotype results also correlate with cure rates (reported cure rates: 60–75% for genotypes 2 and 3; 15–25% for genotype 1). Some clinicians elect to treat HCV without a liver biopsy due to: the risks, costs, and discomfort of the test; the potential to underestimate the degree of HCV activity due to sampling error; and the high rate of treatment success for genotypes 2 and 3.

Optimal Patient Characteristics for HCV Treatment in HIV include no active psychiatric disease or substance abuse; stable HIV disease with undetectable HIV RNA and higher CD_4 cell count; receiving an antiretroviral regimen that does not contain ddI (in particular), d4T, or ZDV; and adherent to medications, follow-up visits, and blood test monitoring. Only a small proportion of patients will meet all these criteria; therefore, to maximize treatment effect, it is important to optimize clinical status prior to starting HCV therapy. Patients should be fully educated regarding the goals and risks of treatment, with provision of written information about side effects, local support groups, and whom to contact with questions. It is useful to administer the first dose of treatment in the office in order to provide instructions on injection techniques.

Choice of Drug Therapy. The treatment of choice for HCV infection is pegylated interferon plus ribavirin. All patients should also receive hepatitis A vaccine and counseling to avoid alcohol use. For further information, please consult other resources.

Monitoring. Monitoring consists of safety/efficacy evaluations. Results of HCV RNA testing are used to decide between completing 48 weeks of HCV therapy vs. discontinuing treatment at 12 or 24 weeks due to low probability of cure (Figure 5.4).

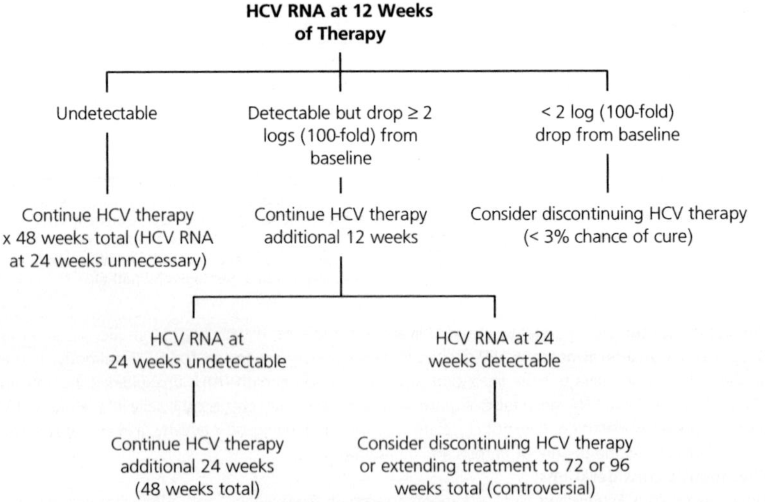

Figure 5.4. Management of HCV Infection Based on HCV RNA Testing

HCV RNA should be assessed at week 12. If the HCV viral load has not dropped by more than 2 logs (100-fold), then the likelihood of achieving a cure is extremely low. Many patients and providers will elect to discontinue therapy at this point, although theoretically low-dose peg-interferon may help improve liver fibrosis independent of its antiviral effect. (This strategy is being tested in clinical trials.) HCV RNA should be measured at weeks 24 and 48. If undetectable at week 48, additional measurements should be obtained at weeks 4, 12, and 24 after stopping treatment. An undetectable HCV RNA at week 24 post-treatment is the current standard for assessing a "sustained virologic response" (SVR), which can be equated with cure. Importantly, patients cured of HCV are susceptible to re-acquisition and should be cautioned about resuming high-risk behavior.

Internet Resources:

- HIV/HCV Co-infection Center of Excellence: www.uchsc.edu/mpaetc/coinfection
- AIDSinfo: www.aidsinfo.nih.gov
- Chronic Hepatitis C: Current Disease Management: www.niddk.nig.gov/
- Hep C Connection: www.hepc-connection.org
- Hepatitis Resource Network (HRN): www.h-r-n.org
- HIV and Hepatitis.com: www.hivandhepatitis.com
- Johns Hopkins Hepatitis C and HIV Coinfection Information: www.hopkins-hepc.org
- Management of Hepatitis C: 2002, NIH Consensus Statement: http://consensus.nih.gov/cons/cons.htm
- National HIV/AIDS Clinicians' Consultation Center: www.ucsf.ed/hivcntr

- The National AIDS Treatment Advocacy Project: www.natap.org
- Projects in Knowledge: www.projectsinknowledge.com

Hepatitis B Infection

HBV/HIV Status		
Need to Treat HIV	**Need to Treat HBV**	**Recommendation***
Yes	No	TDF plus either 3TC or FTC is the preferred NRTI backbone. Avoid monotherapy with TDF, 3TC, or FTC to reduce the risk of selecting HBV resistance.
Yes	Yes	TDF plus either 3TC or FTC is the preferred NRTI backbone. Avoid monotherapy with TDF, 3TC, or FTC to reduce the risk of selecting HBV resistance. If TDF cannot be used (e.g., underlying renal disease), add entecavir to reduce the risk of selecting for 3TC or FTC resistance.
No	Yes	Entecavir (NRTI without anti-HIV activity) is preferred in this setting as it will not select for HIV resistance. Recommended dose of entecavir is 0.5 mg qd if no prior treatment with 3TC or FTC, and 1.0 mg qd for prior treatment with 3TC or FTC. While adefovir 10 mg qd does not have appreciable HIV activity, there is a theoretical risk that long-term use will select for HIV resistance. Pegylated interferon alpha is another option, albeit with higher rates of adverse effects than entecavir.
Need to discontinue NRTI's (TDF, 3TC, or FTC) with anti-HBV activity		Consider starting entecavir prior to discontinuation to prevent flares of underlying liver disease.

* TDF, 3TC, and FTC should be administered at standard doses used for HIV infection (TDF 300 mg qd, 3TC 300 mg qd, FTC 200 mg qd).

Epidemiology: Hepatitis B virus (HBV) infection is relatively common in patients with HIV, with approximately 60% showing some evidence of prior exposure. Chronic hepatitis B infection interacts with HIV infection in several important ways: (1) HBV increases the risk of liver-related death and hepatotoxicity from antiretroviral therapy; (2) 3TC, FTC, and tenofovir each have anti-HBV activity. Thus selection of antiretroviral therapy for patients with HBV can have clinical and resistance implications for HBV as well as HIV. This is most notable with 3TC and FTC, as a high proportion of coinfected patients will develop HBV-associated resistance to these drugs after several years of therapy; (3) Cessation of anti-HBV therapy may lead to exacerbations of underlying liver disease, which have been fatal in some cases; and (4) Immune reconstitution may lead to worsening of liver status, presumably because HBV disease is immune mediated. This is sometimes associated with loss of HBEAg.

Diagnostic Consideration: Obtain HBSAb, HBSAg, and HBCAb at baseline in all patients. If negative, hepatitis B vaccination is indicated. If chronic HBV infection (positive HBSAg) is identified, obtain HBEAg, HBEAb, and HBV DNA levels. As with HCV infection, vaccination with hepatitis A vaccine and counseling to avoid alcohol are important components of preventive care.

Therapeutic Considerations: The optimal treatment for HBV infection is in evolution. Current guidelines suggest treatment of HBV in all patients with active HBV replication, defined as a detectable HBEAg or HBV DNA. Pending long-term studies defining optimal management, the recommendations set forth in the grid above are reasonable. Patients being treated with regimens for HBV should be monitored for ALT every 3–4 months. HBV DNA levels provide a good marker for efficacy of therapy and should be monitored. The goal of therapy is to reduce HBV DNA to as low a level as possible, preferably below the limits of detection. The duration of HBV therapy is not well established; with development of HBEAb, while some individuals without HIV can stop therapy after reversion of HBEAg to negative, there are no clear stopping rules for HIV-coinfected patients.

REFERENCES AND SUGGESTED READINGS

GUIDELINES

Aberg JA, Kaplan JE, Libman H, et al. Primary care guidelines for the management of persons infected with human immunodeficiency virus: 2009 update by the HIV medicine Association of the Infectious Society of America. Clin Infect Dis 49:651–681, 2009.

Antiretroviral Postexposure Prophylaxis After Sexual, Injection-Drug Use, or Other Nonoccupational Exposure to HIV in the United States. MMWR 2005;54(RR02): 1–20.

Guidelines for the Use of Antiretroviral Agents in Pediatric HIV Infection. www.hivatis.org guidelines. October 26, 2006.

Guidelines for Treating Opportunistic Infections Among HIV-Infected Adults and Adolescents. www.hivatis.org. January 29, 2008.

Management of Possible Sexual, Infection-Drug-Use, or Other Nonoccupational Exposure to HIV, Including Considerations Related to Antiretroviral Therapy - 2005. www.hivatis.org.

MMWR. Guidelines for the Prevention and Treatment of Opportunistic Infections Among HIV-Exposed and HIV-Infected Children. Recommendations from CDC, the National Institutes of Health, the HIV Medicine Association of the Infectious Diseases Society of America, the Pediatric Infectious Diseases Society, and the American Academy of Pediatrics. 58:1–166, 2009.

Panel on Antiretroviral Guidelines for Adults and Adolescents. Guidelines for the use of antiretroviral agents in HIV-1 infected adults and adolescents. Department of Health and Human Services. November 3, 2008; 1–139. Available at http://www.aidsinfor.nih.gov/ContentFiles/AdultandAdolescentGL.pdf.

Perfect JR, Dismukes WE, Dromer F, et al. Clinical Practice Guidelines for the Management of Cryptococcal Disease: 2010 Update by the Infectious Disease Society of America. Clin Infect Disease 50:291–322, 2010.

Public Health Service Task Force Recommendations for Use of Antiretroviral Drugs in Pregnant HIV-1–Infected Women for Maternal Health and Interventions to Reduce Perinatal HIV-1 Transmission in the United States www.hivatis.org. November 2, 2007.

Treatment of Tuberculosis - June 20, 2003. www.hivatis.org.

Updated Public Health Service Guidelines for the management of occupational exposures to HIV and recommendations for post-exposure prophylaxis. MMWR 54(RR-9):1–17, Sept. 30, 2005.

Updated U.S. Public Health Service Guidelines for the management of occupational exposures to HBV, HCV, and HIV and recommendations for postexposure prophylaxis. MMWR 50(RR-11); 1–42, June 29, 2001.

TEXTBOOKS

Bartlett JG, et al. A pocket guide to adult HIV/AIDS treatment, Health Resources and Service Administration, Fairfax, 2004.

Bartlett JG (ed). The Johns Hopkins Hospital 2005–06 Guide to Medical Care of Patients with HIV Infection, 10th edition, Lippincott Williams & Wilkins, Philadelphia, 2005.

Bartlett JG, Gallant JE (eds). 2007 Medical Management of HIV Infection. Baltimore MMHIV 2007.

Dolin R, Masur H, Saag MS (eds). AIDS Therapy, 2nd edition. Churchill Livingstone, New York, 2003.

Gorbach SL, Bartlett JG, Blacklow NR (eds). Infectious Diseases, 3rd edition. Philadelphia, Lippincott, Williams & Wilkins, 2004.

Mandell GL, Bennett JE, Dolin R (eds). Mandell, Douglas, and Bennett's Principles and Practice of Infectious Diseases, 7th edition. Philadelphia, Elsevier, 2010.

Sax PE, Cohen CJ, Kuritzkes DR (eds). HIV Essentials. 3rd edition. Jones & Bartlett, Sudbury, MA, 2010.

Wormser GP (ed). AIDS, 4th edition, Elsevier, Philadelphia, 2004.

Chapter 6
Antibiotic Prophylaxis and Immunizations*

Pierce Gardner, MD
Ronald L. Nichols, MD
Burke A. Cunha, MD

* For prophylaxis of opportunistic infections in HIV/AIDS, see Chapter 5, pp. 317–320.

ANTIBIOTIC PROPHYLAXIS

Antibiotic prophylaxis is designed to prevent infection for a defined period of time. **Prophylaxis is most likely to be effective when given for a short duration against a single pathogen with a known sensitivity pattern,** and least likely to be effective when given for a long duration against multiple organisms with varying/unpredictable sensitivity patterns (Table 6.1). It is a common misconception that antibiotics used for prophylaxis should not be used for therapy and vice versa. **The only difference between prophylaxis and therapy is the inoculum size and the duration of antibiotic administration:** In prophylaxis, there is no infection, so the inoculum is minimal/none and antibiotics are administered only for the duration of exposure/surgical procedure. With therapy, the inoculum is large (infection already exists), and antibiotics are continued until the infection is eradicated.

Table 6.1. Factors Affecting the Efficacy of Surgical Antibiotic Prophylaxis

Number of Organisms	Susceptibility Pattern	Duration of Protection	Efficacy of Prophylaxis
Single organism	Predictable	Short	Excellent
Multiple organisms	Predictable	Short	Excellent
Single organism	Unpredictable	Short	Good
Single organism	Predictable	Long	Good
Multiple organisms	Unpredictable	Long	Poor/none

SURGICAL PROPHYLAXIS

Antibiotic prophylaxis is designed to achieve effective antibiotic serum/tissue concentrations at the time of initial surgical incision, and is maintained throughout the "vulnerable period" of the procedure (i.e., time between skin incision and skin closure) (Table 6.2). If prophylaxis is given too early, antibiotic levels will be suboptimal/nonexistent when protection is needed. Properly timed pre-operative antibiotic prophylaxis is desirable for optimal effectiveness since **antibiotics given after skin closure are unlikely to be effective.** When no infection exists prior to surgery (clean/clean contaminated surgery), single-dose prophylaxis is preferred. When infection is present/likely prior to surgery ("dirty" surgery, e.g., perforated colon, TURP in the presence of positive urine cultures, repair of open fracture), antibiotics are given for > 1 day and represent early therapy, not true prophylaxis. Parenteral cephalosporins are commonly used for surgical prophylaxis, and ordinarily given as a bolus injection/rapid IV infusion 15–60 minutes prior to the procedure. Prophylaxis with vancomycin or gentamicin is given by slow IV infusion over 1–2 hours, starting ~1–2 hours prior to the procedure.

Table 6.2. Surgical Prophylaxis

Procedure	Usual Organisms	Preferred Prophylaxis	Alternate Prophylaxis	Comments
CNS shunt (VP/VA) placement, craniotomy, open CNS trauma	S. epidermidis (CoNS) S. aureus (MSSA)	MRSA/MRSE unlikely Ceftriaxone 1 gm (IV) × 1 dose MRSA/MRSE likely Linezolid 600 mg (IV) × 1 dose	MRSA/MRSE unlikely Cefotaxime 2 gm (IV) × 1 dose **or** Ceftizoxime 2 gm (IV) × 1 dose MRSA/MRSE likely Linezolid 600 mg (PO) × 1 dose **or** Vancomycin 1 gm (IV) × 1 dose **or** Minocycline 200 mg (IV) × 1 dose	Administer immediately prior to procedure. Vancomycin protects against wound infections, but may not prevent CNS infections. Give vancomycin slowly IV over 1 hour prior to procedure.
Thoracic (non-cardiac) surgery	S. aureus (MSSA)	Cefazolin 1 gm (IV) × 1 dose **or** Ceftriaxone 1 gm (IV) × 1 dose	Cefotaxime 2 gm (IV) × 1 dose **or** Ceftizoxime 2 gm (IV) × 1 dose	Administer immediately prior to procedure.
Cardiac valve replacement surgery	S. epidermidis (MSSE/MRSE) S. aureus (MSSA/ MRSA) Enterobacter	Vancomycin 1 gm (IV) × 1 dose **plus** Gentamicin 120 mg (IV) × 1 dose	Linezolid 600 mg (IV) × 1 dose **plus** Gentamicin 120 mg (IV) × 1 dose	Administer vancomycin and gentamicin slowly IV over 1 hour prior to procedure.
Coronary artery bypass graft (CABG) surgery	S. aureus (MSSA)	Cefazolin 2 gm (IV) × 1 dose **or** Ceftriaxone 1 gm (IV) × 1 dose	Cefotaxime 2 gm (IV) × 1 dose **or** Ceftizoxime 2 gm (IV) × 1 dose	Administer immediately prior to procedure. Except for ceftriaxone, repeat dose intraoperatively for procedures lasting > 3 hours.
Biliary tract surgery	E. coli Klebsiella E. faecalis (VSE)	Cefazolin 1 gm (IV) × 1 dose **or** Meropenem 1 gm (IV) × 1 dose	Ampicillin/ sulbactam 3 gm (IV) × 1 dose **or** Piperacillin 4 gm (IV) × 1 dose	Administer immediately prior to procedure (anaerobic coverage unnecessary).

Table 6.2. Surgical Prophylaxis (cont'd)

Procedure	Usual Organisms	Preferred Prophylaxis	Alternate Prophylaxis	Comments
Hepatic surgery	E. coli Klebsiella E. faecalis (VSE) B. fragilis	Ampicillin/ sulbactam 3 gm (IV) × 1 dose **or** Piperacillin 4 gm (IV) × 1 dose	Meropenem 1 gm (IV) × 1 dose **or** Moxifloxacin 400 mg (IV) × 1 dose	Administer immediately prior to procedure.
Stomach, upper small bowel surgery	S. aureus (MSSA) Group A streptococci	Ceftriaxone 1 gm (IV) × 1 dose **or** Cefazolin 1 gm (IV) × 1 dose	Cefotaxime 2 gm (IV) × 1 dose **or** Ceftizoxime 2 gm (IV) × 1 dose	Administer immediately prior to procedure (anaerobic coverage unnecessary).
Distal small bowel, colon surgery	E. coli Klebsiella B. fragilis	Oral Neomycin* **plus either** Erythromycin base* **or** Metronidazole* Parenteral Ertapenem 1 gm (IV) × 1 dose	Piperacillin 3 gm (IV) × 1 dose **or** Cefoxitin 2 gm (IV) × 1 dose **or combination therapy with** Metronidazole 1 gm (IV) × 1 dose **plus either** Ceftriaxone 1 gm (IV) × 1 dose **or** Levofloxacin 500 mg (IV) × 1 dose **or** Gentamicin 240 mg (IV) × 1 dose	Administer immediately prior to procedure. Give gentamicin slowly IV over 1 hour.
Pelvic (OB/GYN) surgery	Aerobic GNBs Anaerobic streptococci B. fragilis	Ceftriaxone 1 gm (IV) × 1 dose **plus** Metronidazole 1 gm (IV) × 1 dose	Cefotetan 2 gm (IV) × 1 dose **or** Cefoxitin 2 gm (IV) × 1 dose **or** Ceftizoxime 2 gm (IV) × 1 dose	Administer immediately prior to procedure.

* After appropriate diet and catharsis give either neomycin 1 gm (PO) plus erythromycin base 1 gm (PO) at 1 pm, 2 pm, and 11 pm, or give neomycin 2 gm (PO) plus metronidazole 2 gm (PO) at 7 pm and 11 pm the day before an 8 am operation.

COLOR ATLAS

CSF, Sputum, and Urine Gram Stains

Paul E. Schoch, PhD
Edward J. Bottone, PhD
Daniel Caplivski, MD

CSF GRAM STAINS

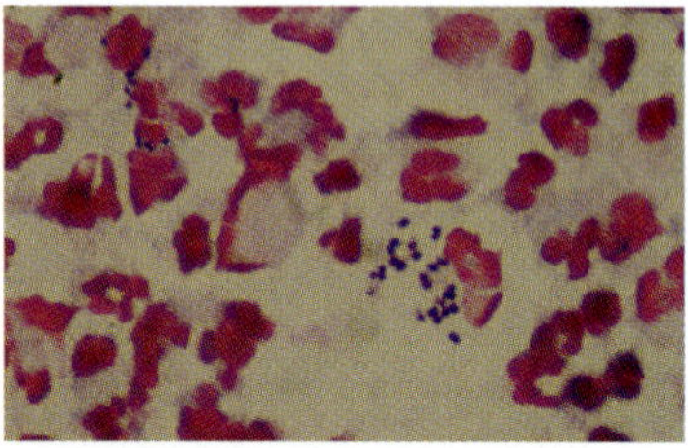

Staphylococcus aureus

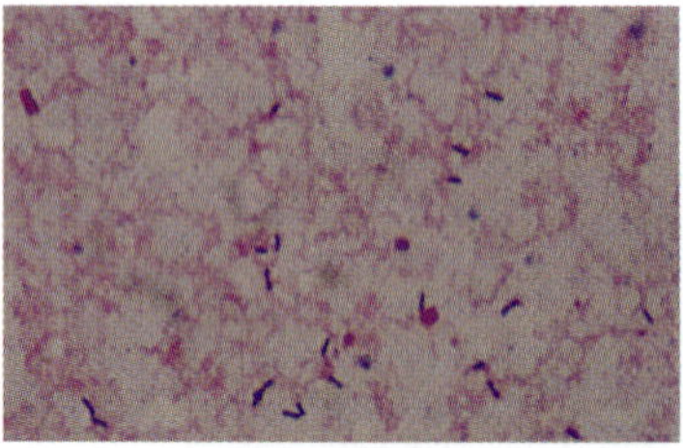

Listeria monocytogenes

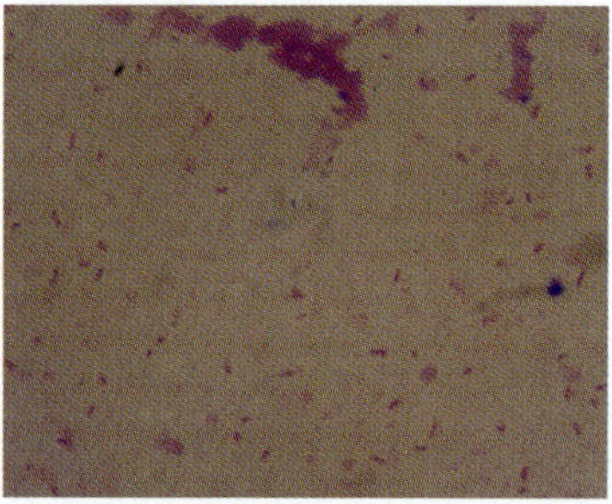

H. influenzae

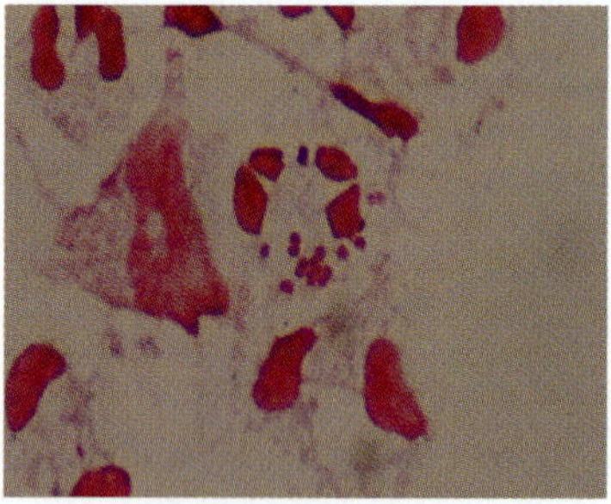

Neisseria meningitidis

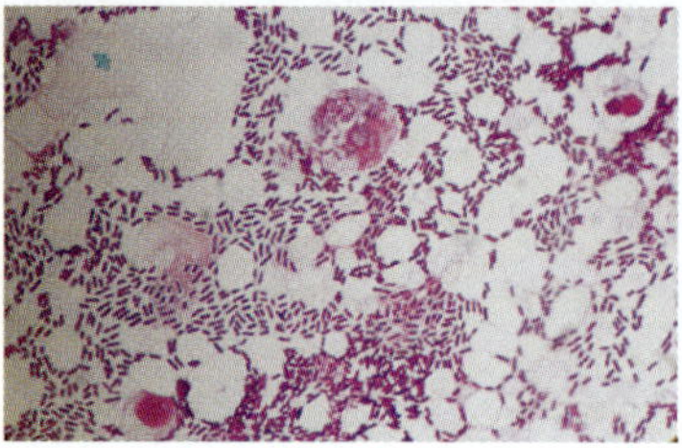

Klebsiella pneumoniae

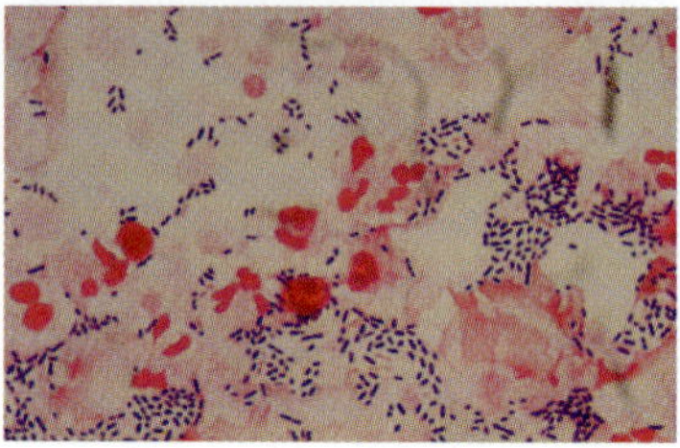

Streptococcus pneumoniae

SPUTUM GRAM STAINS

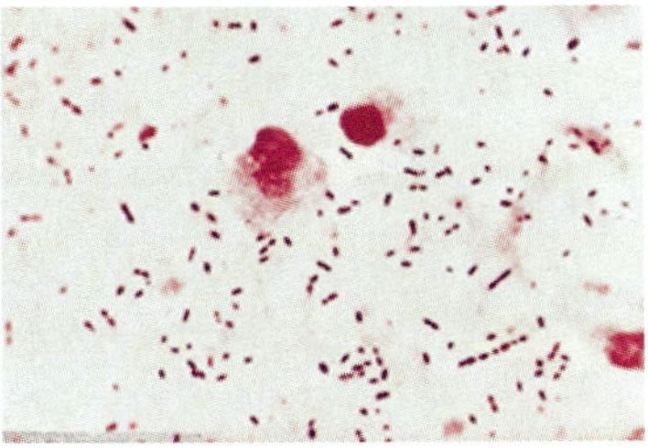

Streptococcus pneumoniae

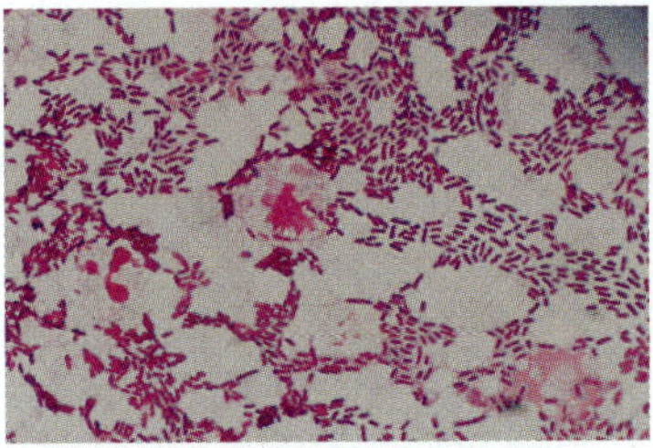

Klebsiella pneumoniae

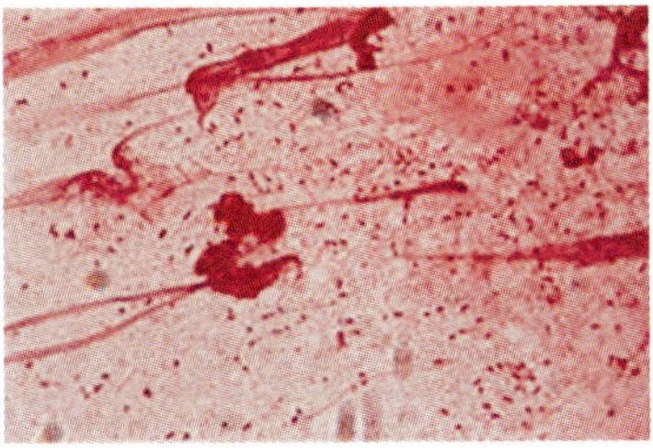

Hemophilus influenzae

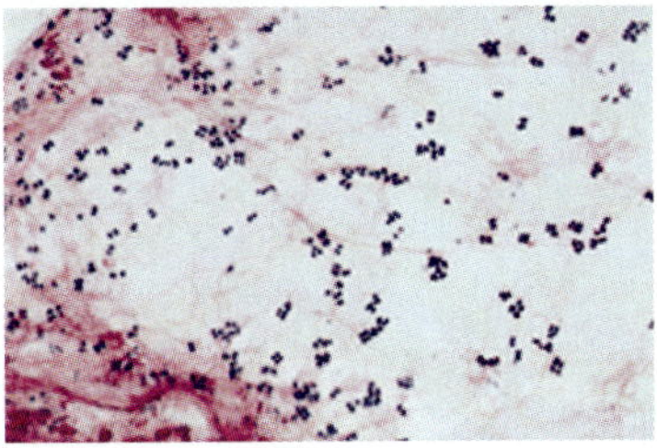

Staphylococcus aureus

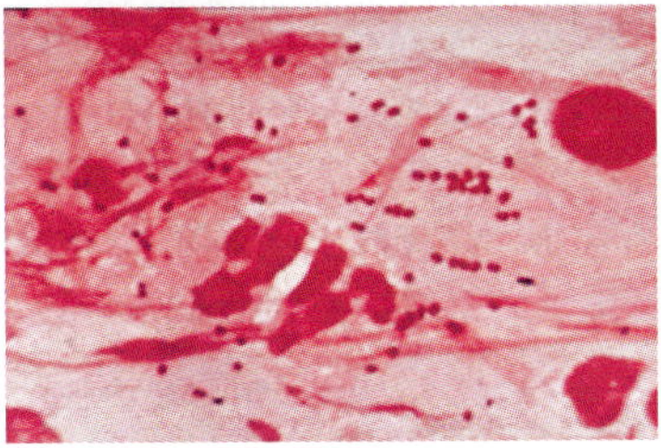

Moraxella catarrhalis

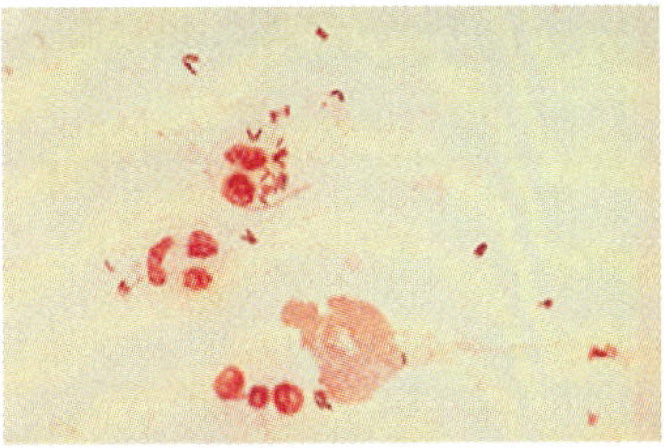

Pseudomonas aeruginosa

URINE GRAM STAINS

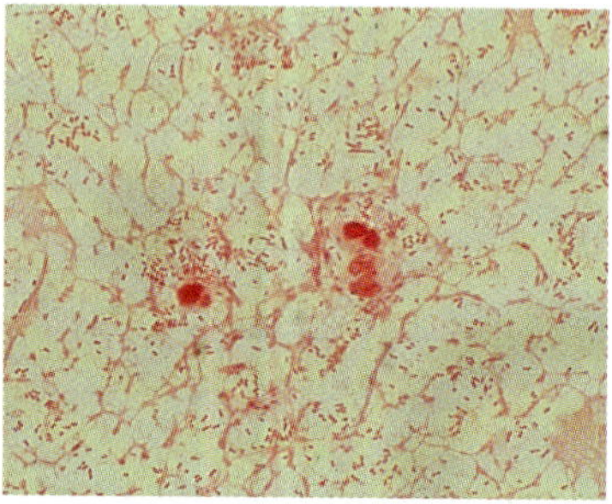

E. coli

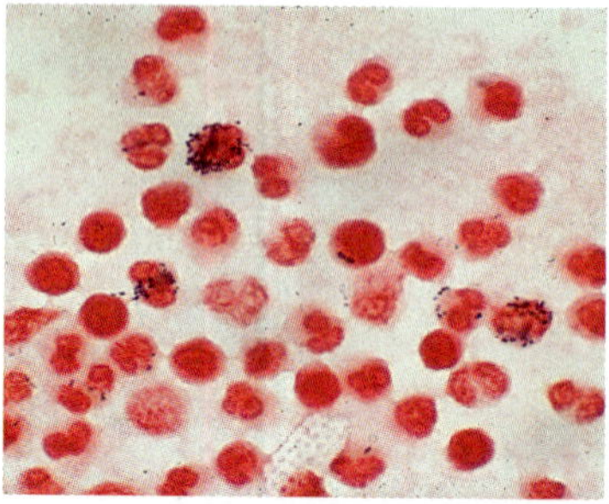

Group B streptococci

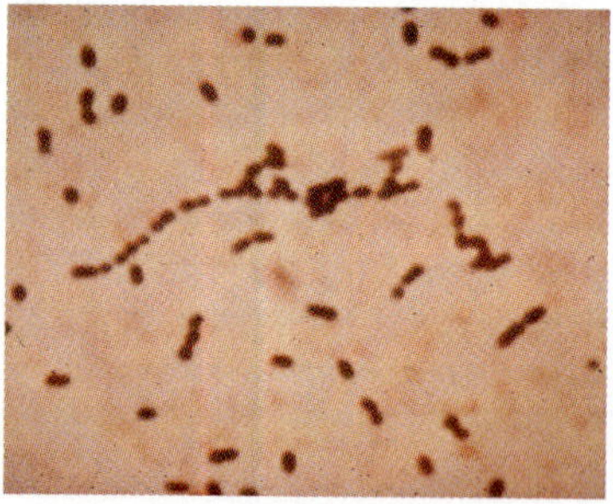

Enterococci

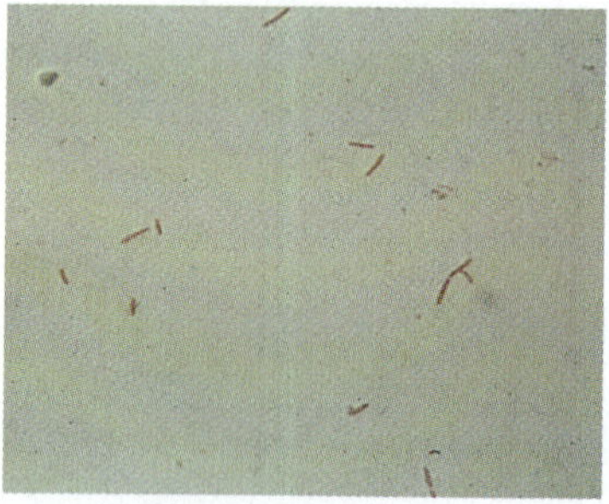

Pseudomonas aeruginosa

COLOR ATLAS

Fungal Stains

Daniel Caplivski, MD
Edward J. Bottone, PhD

FUNGAL STAINS

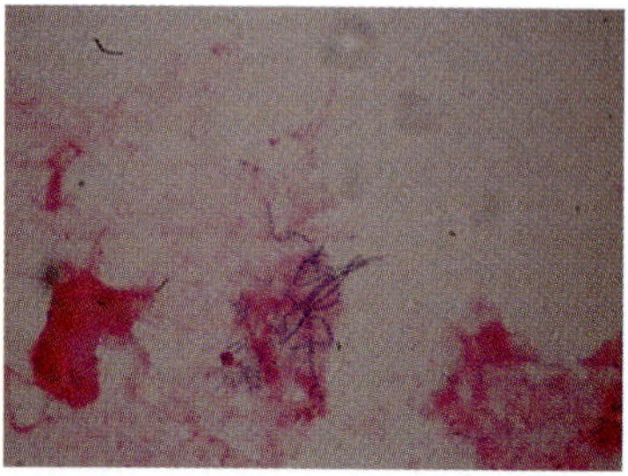 Actinomyces (lung biopsy)	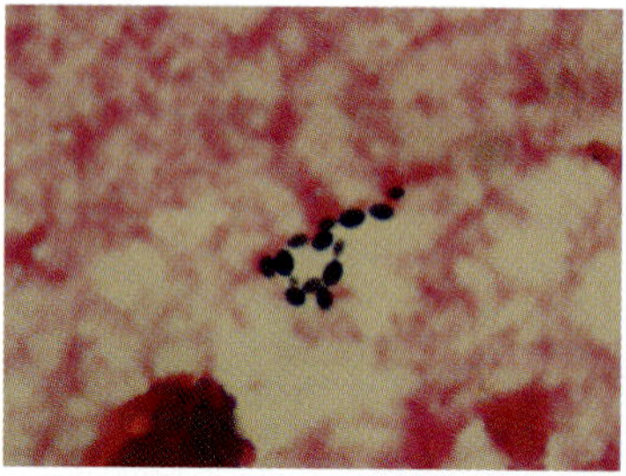 Candida albicans (blood)
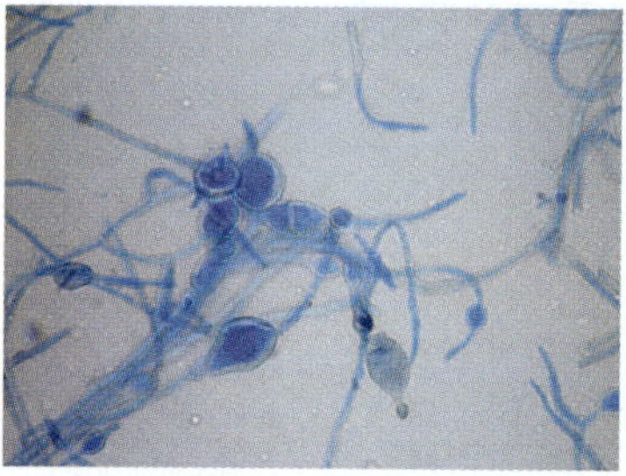 Alternaria (skin biopsy)	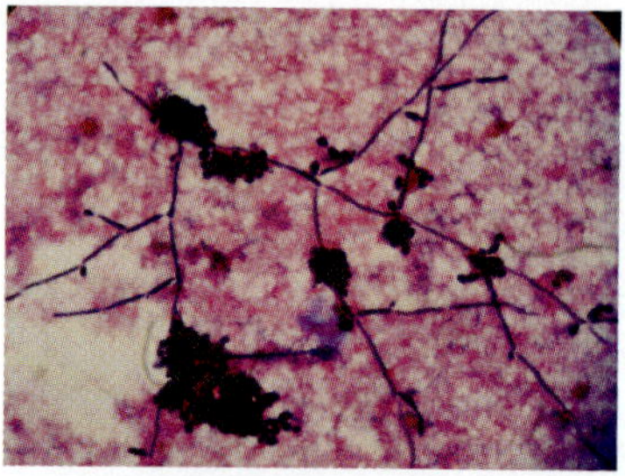 Candida albicans with pseudohyphae (blood)
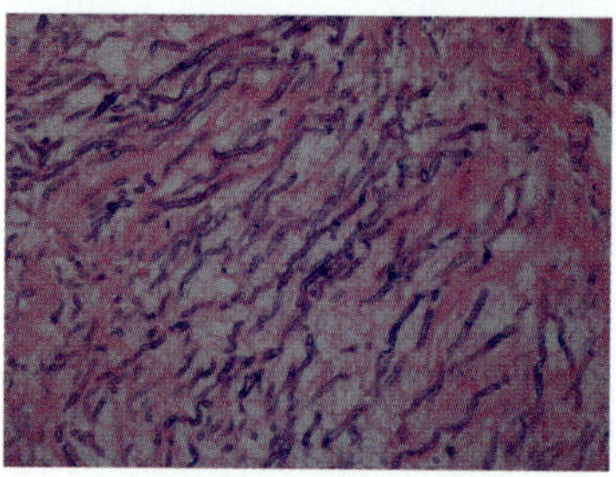 Aspergillus (lung biopsy)	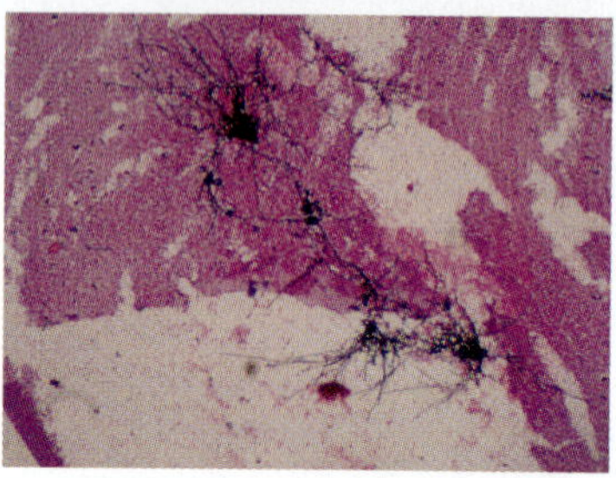 Candida as fungal ball (lung biopsy)

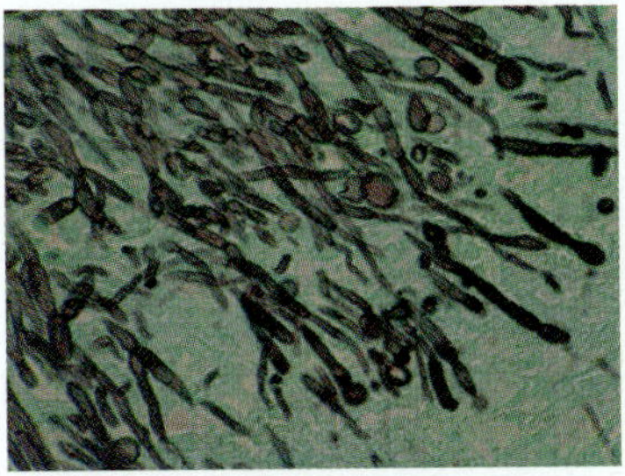

Candida (liver biopsy)

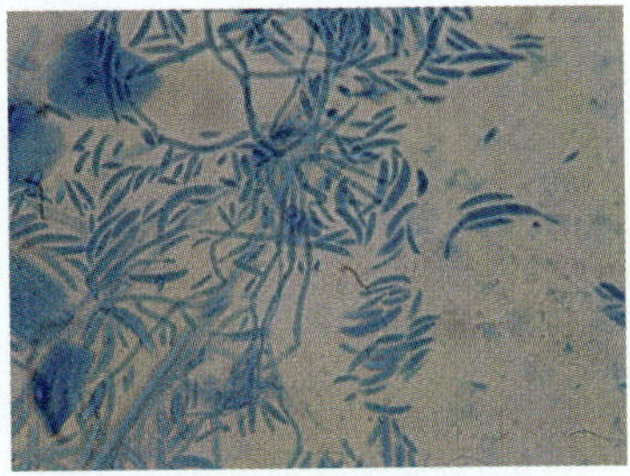

Fusarium (skin biopsy)

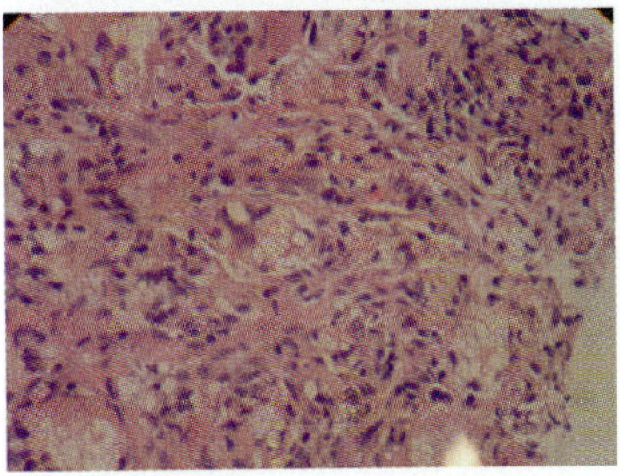

Cryptococcus (lung biopsy)

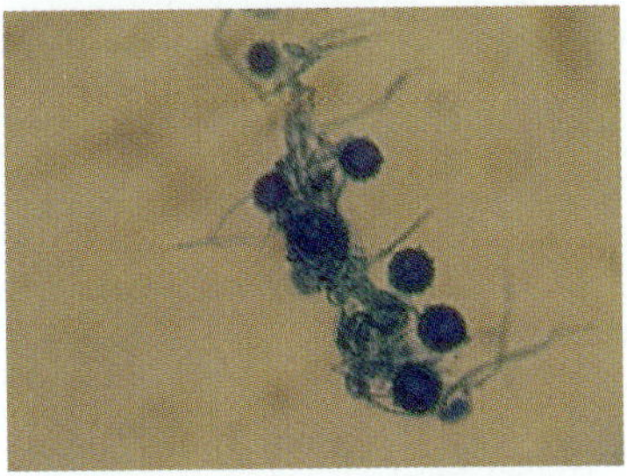

Histoplasma capsulatum (lung biopsy)

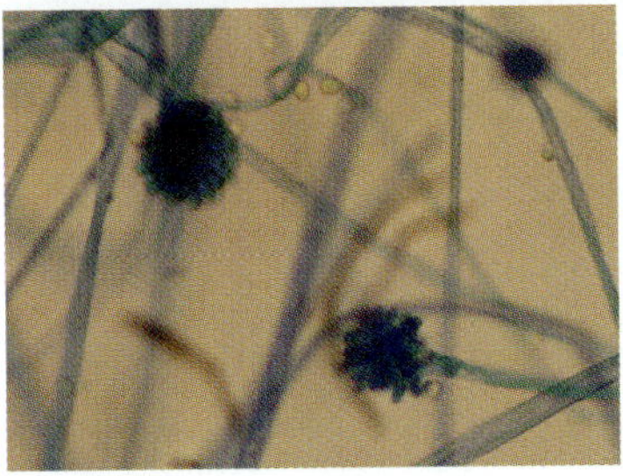

Cunninghamella (lung biopsy)

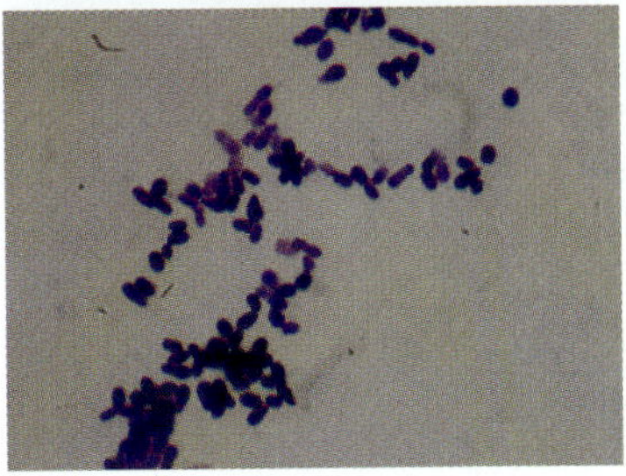

Malasezzia (blood)

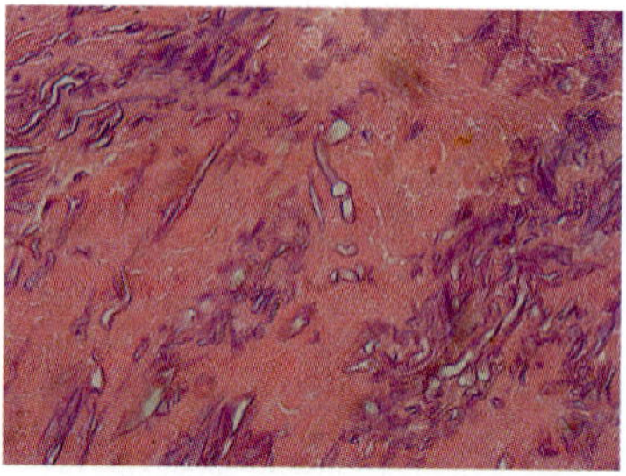

Mucormycosis (bone marrow)

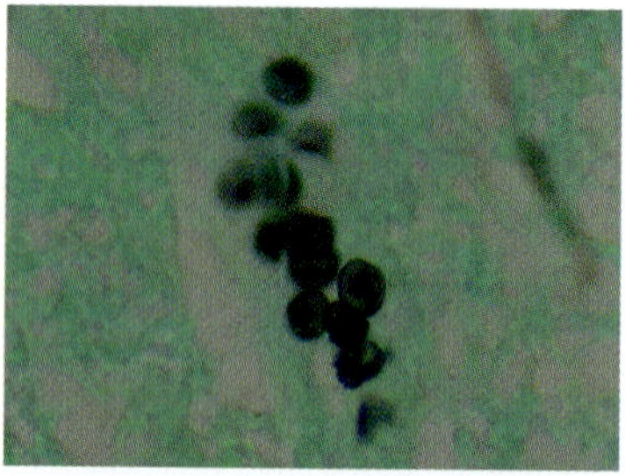

Pneumocystis (lung biopsy)

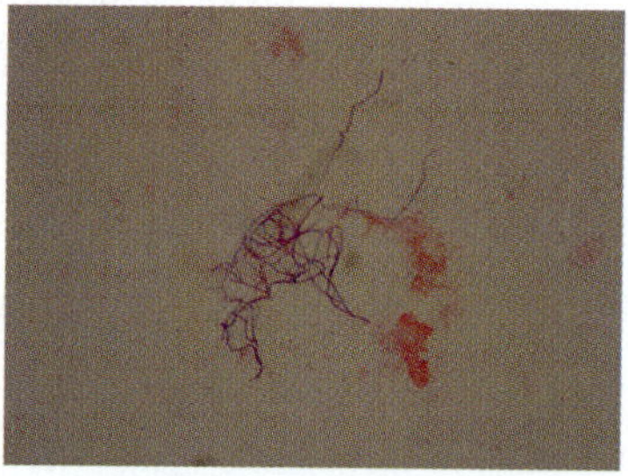

Nocardia (lung biopsy)

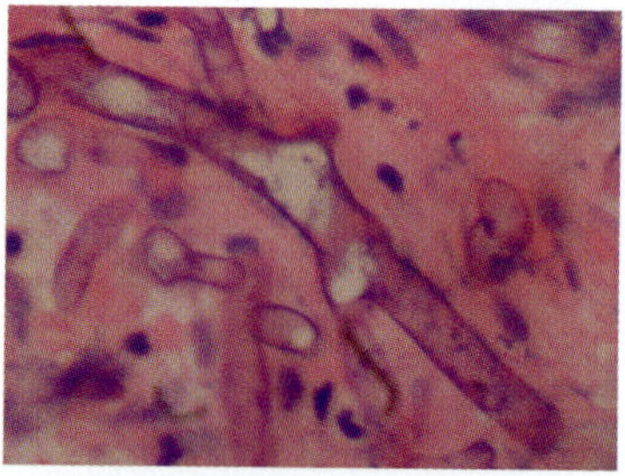

Rhizomucor (sinus biopsy)

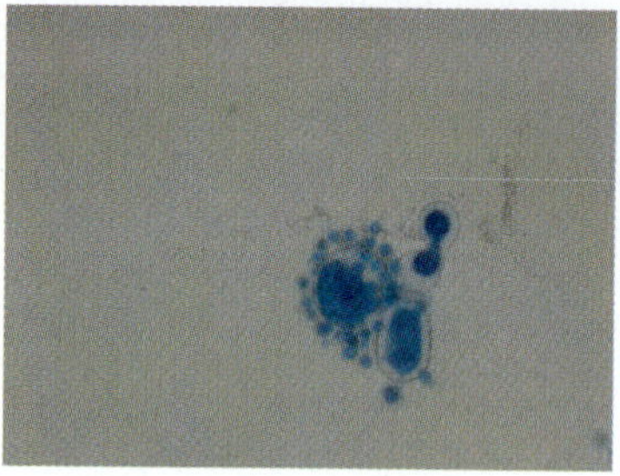

Paracoccidioidomycosis (bone biopsy)

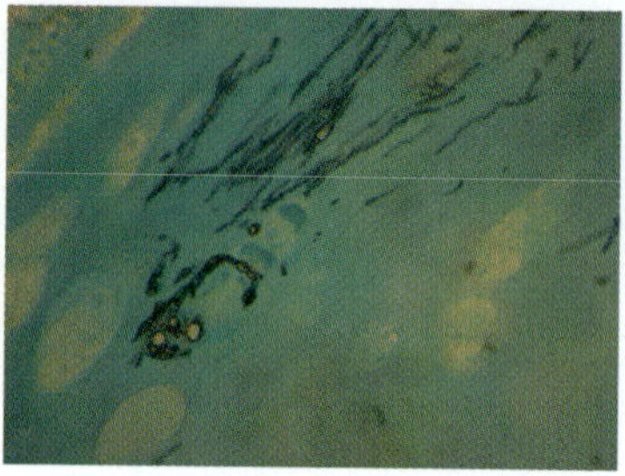

Scedosporium (lung biopsy)

Table 6.2. Surgical Prophylaxis (cont'd)

Procedure	Usual Organisms	Preferred Prophylaxis	Alternate Prophylaxis	Comments
Orthopedic prosthetic implant surgery (total hip/knee replacement)	S. epidermidis (CoNS) S. aureus (MSSA)	MRSA/MRSE unlikely Cefazolin 2 gm (IV) × 1 dose MRSA/MRSE likely Vancomycin 1 gm (IV) × 1 dose	MRSA/MRSE unlikely Ceftriaxone 1 gm (IV) × 1 dose MRSA/MRSE likely Linezolid 600 mg (IV) × 1 dose	Administer immediately prior to procedure. Post-operative doses are ineffective and unnecessary.
Arthroscopy	S. aureus (MSSA)	Cefazolin 1 gm (IV) × 1 dose **or** Ceftriaxone 1 gm (IV) × 1 dose	Cefotaxime 2 gm (IV) × 1 dose **or** Ceftizoxime 2 gm (IV) × 1 dose	Pre-procedure prophylaxis is usually unnecessary in clean surgical procedures.
Orthopedic surgery (open fracture)	S. aureus (MSSA) Aerobic GNBs	Ceftriaxone 1 gm (IV) × 1 week	Clindamycin 600 mg (IV) q8h × 1 week **plus** Gentamicin 240 mg (IV) q24h × 1 week	Represents early therapy, not true prophylaxis. Duration of post-op antibiotics depends on severity of infection.
Urological implant surgery	S. aureus (MSSA) Aerobic GNBs bacilli	Ceftriaxone 1 gm (IV) × 1 dose	Cefotaxime 2 gm (IV) × 1 dose **or** Ceftizoxime 2 gm (IV) × 1 dose	Administer immediately prior to procedure.
TURP, cystoscopy	P. aeruginosa P. cepacia P. maltophilia E. faecalis (VRE) Aerobic GNBs	Ciprofloxacin 400 mg (IV) × 1 dose **or** Piperacillin 4 gm (IV) × 1 dose	Levofloxacin 500 mg (IV) × 1 dose **or** Gatifloxacin 400 mg (IV) × 1 dose	Prophylaxis given to TURP patients with positive pre-op urine cultures. Represents early therapy, not true prophylaxis. No prophylaxis required for TURP if pre-op urine culture is negative.
	E. faecium (VRE)	Linezolid 600 mg (IV) × 1 dose	Quinupristin/dalfopristin 7.5 mg/kg (IV) × 1 dose	

MSSA/MRSA = methicillin-sensitive/resistant S. aureus; MSSE/MRSE = methicillin-sensitive/resistant S. epidermidis.

POST-EXPOSURE MEDICAL PROPHYLAXIS (Table 6.3)

Some infectious diseases can be prevented by post-exposure prophylaxis (PEP). To be maximally effective, PEP should be administered within 24 hours of the exposure, since the effectiveness of prophylaxis > 24 hours after exposure decreases. PEP is usually reserved for persons with close face-to-face/intimate contact with an infected individual. Casual contact does not warrant PEP.

Table 6.3. Post-Exposure Medical Prophylaxis

Exposure	Usual Organisms	Preferred Prophylaxis	Alternate Prophylaxis	Comments
Meningitis	N. meningitidis	Any quinolone (PO) × 1 dose	Minocycline 100 mg (PO) q12h × 2 days **or** Rifampin 600 mg (PO) q12h × 2 days	Must be administered within 24 hours of close face-to-face exposure to be effective. Otherwise, observe and treat if infection develops. Avoid tetracyclines in children ≤ 8 years.
	H. influenzae	Rifampin 600 mg (PO) q24h × 3 days	Any quinolone (PO) × 3 days	Must be administered within 24 hours of close face-to-face exposure to be effective. H. influenzae requires 3 days of prophylaxis.
Viral influenza (human seasonal)	Influenza virus, type A or B	Oseltamivir (Tamiflu) 75 mg (PO) q24h for duration of outbreak (or at least 7 days after close contact to an infected person). For CrCl 10–30 cc/min, give 75 mg (PO) q48h‡	Rimantadine 100 mg (PO) q12h* for duration of outbreak (or at least 7–10 days after close contact to infected person) **or** Amantidine 200 mg (PO) q24h† for duration of outbreak (or at least 7–10 days after close contact to infected person)	Give to non-immunized contacts and high-risk contacts even if immunized. Begin at onset of outbreak or within 3 days of close contact to an infected person. Oseltamivir is active against both influenza A and B; rimantadine and amantadine are only active against influenza A. Oseltamivir may be ineffective due to increased resistance.

Table 6.3. Post-Exposure Medical Prophylaxis (cont'd)

Exposure	Usual Organisms	Preferred Prophylaxis	Alternate Prophylaxis	Comments
Avian influenza	Influenza A (H_5N_1)	Oseltamivir (as for viral influenza, above)	Rimantadine **or** Amantadine[†] (as for viral influenza, above)	Oseltamivir may be ineffective due to increased resistance.
Swine influenza	Influenza A (H_1N_1)	Oseltamavir above (as for viral influenza, above)	Amantadine/ rimantadine ineffective	Continue PEP for swine influenza for 10 days after close contact exposure.[‡]
Pertussis	B. pertussis	Erythromycin 500 mg (PO) q6h × 2 weeks	TMP–SMX 1 SS tablet (PO) q12h × 2 weeks **or** Levofloxacin 500 mg (PO) q24h × 2 weeks	Administer as soon as possible after exposure. Effectiveness is greatly reduced after 24 hours.
Diphtheria	C. diphtheriae	Erythromycin 500 mg (PO) q6h × 1 week **or** Benzathine penicillin 1.2 mu (IM) × 1 dose	Azithromycin 500 mg (PO) q24h × 3 days	Administer as soon as possible after exposure. Effectiveness is greatly reduced after 24 hours.
TB	M. tuberculosis	INH 300 mg (PO) q24h × 9 months	Rifampin 600 mg (PO) q24h × 4 months	For INH, monitor SGOT/ SGPT weekly × 4, then monthly. Mild elevations are common and resolve spontaneously. INH should be stopped for SGOT/SGPT levels ≥ 5 × normal.

* For elderly, severe liver dysfunction, or CrCl < 10 cc/min, give 100 mg (PO) q24h.

† For age ≥ 65 years, give 100 mg (PO) q24h. For renal dysfunction, give 200 mg (PO) load followed by 100 mg q24h (CrCl 30–50 ml/min), 100 mg q48h (CrCl 15–29 ml/min), or 200 mg weekly (CrCl < 15 ml/min).

‡ ***Pediatric prophylaxis:*** < 15 kg: 30 mg PO qd for 10 days, > 15-24 kg: 45 mg PO qd for 10 days, 24-40 kg: 60 mg PO qd for 10 days, > 40 kg: same as adults.

Table 6.3. Post-Exposure Medical Prophylaxis (cont'd)

Exposure	Usual Organisms	Preferred Prophylaxis	Alternate Prophylaxis	Comments
Gonorrhea (GC)	N. gonorrhoeae	Ceftriaxone 125 mg (IM) × 1 dose	Spectinomycin 2 gm (IM) × 1 dose **or** Any oral quinolone × 1 dose	Administer as soon as possible after sexual exposure (≤ 72 hours). Ceftriaxone also treats incubating syphilis.
Syphilis	T. pallidum	Benzathine penicillin 2.4 mu (IM) × 1 dose	Doxycycline 100 mg (PO) q12h × 1 week	Administer as soon as possible after sexual exposure. Obtain HIV serology.
Chancroid	H. ducreyi	Ceftriaxone 250 mg (IM) × 1 dose	Azithromycin 1 gm (PO) × 1 dose **or** Any oral quinolone × 3 days	Administer as soon as possible after sexual exposure. Obtain HIV and syphilis serologies.
Non-gonococcal urethritis (NGU)	C. trachomatis U. urealyticum M. genitalium	Azithromycin 1 gm (PO) × 1 dose **or** Doxycycline 100 mg (PO) q12h × 1 week	Any oral quinolone × 1 week	Administer as soon as possible after sexual exposure. Also test for gonorrhea/Ureaplasma.
Varicella (chicken-pox)	VZV	Preferred: For exposure < 72 hours, give varicella-zoster immune globulin (VZIG) 625 mcg (IM) × 1 dose to immuno-compromised hosts and pregnant women (esp. with respiratory conditions). For others or exposure > 72 hours, consider acyclovir 800 mg (PO) 5x/day × 5–10 days Alternate: Varicella vaccine 0.5 mL (SC) × 1 dose. Repeat in 4 weeks		Administer as soon as possible after exposure (≤ 72 hours). Varicella vaccine is a live attenuated vaccine and should not be given to immunocompromised or pregnant patients. If varicella develops, start acyclovir treatment immediately.

Table 6.3. Post-Exposure Medical Prophylaxis (cont'd)

Exposure	Usual Organisms	Preferred Prophylaxis	Alternate Prophylaxis	Comments
Hepatitis B (HBV)	Hepatitis B virus	Unvaccinated Hepatitis B immune globulin (HBIG) 0.06 mL/kg (IM) × 1 dose **plus** HBV vaccine (40 mcg HBsAg/mL) deep deltoid (IM) at 0, 1, 6 months (can use 10-mcg dose in healthy adults < 40 years)	Previously vaccinated *Known responder* (anti-HBsAg antibody levels ≥ 10 IU/mL): No treatment. *Known non-responder* (anti-HBsAg antibody levels < 10 IU/mL): Treat as if unvaccinated. *Antibody status unknown:* Obtain HBsAg antibody levels to determine immunity status. If testing is not possible or results are not available within 24 hours of exposure, give HBIG plus 1 dose of HBV vaccine (booster).	
Hepatitis A (HAV)	Hepatitis A virus	HAV vaccine 1 mL (IM) × 1 dose	Immune serum globulin (IG) 0.02 mL/kg (IM) × 1 dose	Give HAV vaccine alone if within 14 days after exposure.
Rocky Mountain spotted fever	R. rickettsia	Doxycycline 100 mg (PO) q12h × 1 week	Any oral quinolone × 1 week	Administer prophylaxis after removal of Dermacentor tick.
Lyme disease	B. burgdorferi	Doxycycline 200 mg (PO) × 1 dose	Amoxicillin* 1 gm (PO) q8h × 3 days **or** Any oral 1st gen. cephalosporin* × 3 days **or** Azithromycin* 500 mg (PO) q24h × 3 days	If tick is in place ≥ 72 hours or is grossly engorged, prophylaxis may be given after tick is removed. Otherwise, prophylaxis is usually not recommended.

HDCV = human diploid cell vaccine, HRIG = human rabies immune globulin, PCEC = purified chick embryo cells, RVA = rabies vaccine absorbed.

* All or as much of the full dose of HRIG should be injected into the wound, and the remaining vaccine should be injected IM into the deltoid. Do not give HRIG at the same site or through the same syringe with PCEC, RVA, or HDCV.

Table 6.3. Post-Exposure Medical Prophylaxis (cont'd)

Exposure	Usual Organisms	Preferred Prophylaxis	Alternate Prophylaxis	Comments
		* Although experience is limited, single-dose prophylaxis with these agents is probably also effective.		
Zoonotic diseases (plague, anthrax)	B. anthracis Y. pestis	Doxycycline 100 mg (PO) q12h for duration of exposure	Any oral quinolone for duration of exposure	Continued for the duration of a naturally-acquired exposure/ outbreak. See p. 355 for bioterrorist plague/ anthrax recommendations.
Rabies	Rabies virus	No Previous Immunization HRIG 20 IU/kg* **plus either** PCEC 1 mL (IM) in deltoid **or** RVA 1 mL (IM) in deltoid **or** HDCV 1 mL (IM) in deltoid PCEC, RVA, HDCV given on days 0, 3, 7, 14, and 28 post-exposure	Previous Immunization PCEC 1 mL (IM) in deltoid on days 0 and 3 **or** RVA 1 mL (IM) in deltoid on days 0 and 3 **or** HDCV 1 mL (IM) in deltoid on days 0 and 3	Following unprovoked or suspicious dog or cat bite, immediately begin prophylaxis if animal develops rabies during a 10-day observation period. If dog or cat is suspected of being rabid, begin vaccination sequence immediately. Raccoon, skunk, bat, fox and most wild carnivore bites should be regarded as rabid, and bite victims should be vaccinated against rabies immediately (contact local health department regarding rabies potential of animals in your area). All potential rabies wounds should immediately be thoroughly cleaned with soap and water. Do not inject rabies vaccine IV (may cause hypotension/shock). Serum sickness may occur with HDCV.

HDCV = human diploid cell vaccine, HRIG = human rabies immune globulin, PCEC = purified chick embryo cells, RVA = rabies vaccine absorbed.

* All or as much of the full dose of HRIG should be injected into the wound, and the remaining vaccine should be injected IM into the deltoid. Do not give HRIG at the same site or through the same syringe with PCEC, RVA, or HDCV.

Table 6.3. Post-Exposure Medical Prophylaxis (cont'd)

Exposure	Usual Organisms	Preferred Prophylaxis	Alternate Prophylaxis	Comments
		BIOTERRORIST AGENTS		
Anthrax *Inhalation/ cutaneous*	B. anthracis	Doxycycline 100 mg (PO) q12h × 60 days **or** Ciprofloxacin 500 mg (PO) q12h × 60 days **or** Levofloxacin 500 mg (PO) q24h × 60 days	Amoxicillin 1 gm (PO) q8h × 60 days	Duration of anthrax PEP based on longest incubation period of inhaled spores in nares.
Tularemia pneumonia	F. tularensis	Doxycycline 100 mg (PO) q12h × 2 weeks	Ciprofloxacin 500 mg (PO) q12h × 2 weeks **or** Levofloxacin 500 mg (PO) q24h × 2 weeks	Duration of PEP for tularemia is 2 weeks, not 1 week as for plague.
Pneumonic plague	Y. pestis	Doxycycline 100 mg (PO) q12h × 7 days **or** Ciprofloxacin 500 mg (PO) q12h × 7 days **or** Levofloxacin 500 mg (PO) q24h × 7 days	Chloramphenicol 500 mg (PO) q6h × 7 days	Pneumonic plague should be considered bioterrorism since most natural cases of plague are bubonic plague.
Smallpox	Variola virus	Smallpox vaccine ≤ 4 days after exposure	None	Smallpox vaccine is protective when diluted 1:5.

CHRONIC MEDICAL PROPHYLAXIS/SUPPRESSION (Table 6.4)

Some infectious diseases are prone to recurrence/relapse and may benefit from intermittent or chronic suppressive therapy. The goal of suppressive therapy is to minimize the frequency/severity of recurrent infectious episodes.

Table 6.4. Chronic Medical Prophylaxis/Suppression

Disorder	Usual Organisms	Preferred Prophylaxis	Alternate Prophylaxis	Comments
Asplenia/ impaired splenic function	S. pneumoniae H. influenzae N. meningitidis	Amoxicillin 1 gm (PO) q24h indefinitely	Respiratory quinolone* (PO) q24h indefinitely	Long-term prophylaxis effective. Vaccines may be given but are not always protective. Use amoxicillin in children.
UTIs (recurrent)	Gram-negative bacilli Enterococci	Nitrofurantoin 100 mg (PO) q24h × 6 months	Amoxicillin 500 mg (PO) q24h × 6 mos **or** TMP–SMX 1 SS tablet (PO) q24h × 6 months	Prophylaxis for reinfection UTIs (≥ 3 per year). Relapse UTIs should be investigated for stones, abscesses, or structural problems.
Asymptomatic bacteriuria in pregnancy	Gram-negative bacilli	Nitrofurantoin 100 mg (PO) q24h × 1 week	Amoxicillin 1 gm (PO) q24h × 1 week	Prophylaxis prevents symptomatic infections.
Prophylaxis of CMV in organ transplants	CMV	Valganciclovir 900 mg (PO) q24h **or** Valacyclovir 2 gm (PO) q6h until CMV antigen levels ↓ to pre-flare levels		Begin prophylaxis when semi-quantitative CMV antigen levels ↑. Prevents CMV flare.
Prophylaxis of fungal infections in hemato-poeitic stem cell transplants	Candida albicans Non-albicans Candida	Micafungin 50 mg (IV) q24h **or** Posaconazole 200 mg (PO) q8h **or** Itraconazole 200 mg (PO) q12h		Prophylaxis given until neutropenia resolves (absolute neutrophil count ≥ 500 cells/ mm^3).
	Aspergillus	Posaconazole 200 mg (PO) q8h **or** Itraconazole 200 mg (PO) q12h		Prophylaxis given until neutropenia resolves (absolute neutrophil count ≥ 500 cells/mm^3).

* Levofloxacin 500 mg (PO) or gatifloxacin 400 mg (PO) q24h or moxifloxacin 400 mg (PO).

Table 6.4. Chronic Medical Prophylaxis/Suppression (cont'd)

Disorder	Usual Organisms	Preferred Prophylaxis	Alternate Prophylaxis	Comments
Prophylaxis of fungal infections in neutropenic patients†	Candida albicans Non-albicans Candida Aspergillus	Posaconazole 200 mg (PO) q8h **or** Itraconazole 200 mg (PO) q12h		Prophylaxis given until neutropenia resolves (absolute neutrophil count ≥ 500 cells/mm^3).
Recurrent genital herpes (< 6 episodes/ year)	H. simplex (HSV-2)	Famciclovir 125 mg (PO) q12h × 5 days **or** Valacyclovir 500 mg (PO) q24h × 5 days	Acyclovir 200 mg (PO) 5x/ day × 5 days	Begin therapy as soon as lesions appear. (For HIV disease, see Ch. 5.) Famciclovir 1 gm (PO) q12h × 1 day ↓ lesion progression by 2 days.
Recurrent genital herpes (> 6 episodes/ year)	H. simplex (HSV-2)	Famciclovir 250 mg (PO) q12h × 1 year **or** Valacyclovir 1 gm (PO) q24h × 1 year	Acyclovir 400 mg (PO) q12h × 1 year	Suppressive therapy is indicated for frequent recurrences. (For HIV disease, see Ch. 5.)
Acute exacerbation of chronic bronchitis (AECB)	S. pneumoniae H. influenzae M. catarrhalis	Moxifloxacin 400 mg or levofloxacin 500 mg or gatifloxacin 400 mg or gemifloxacin 320 mg (PO) q24h × 5 days **or** Amoxicillin/ clavulanic acid XR 2 tablets (PO) q12h × 5 days **or** Clarithromycin XL 1 gm (PO) q24h × 5 days **or** Doxycycline 100 mg (PO) q12h × 5 days **or** Azithromycin 500 mg (PO) × 3 days		Treat each episode individually.
Acute rheumatic fever (ARF)	Group A streptococci	Benzathine penicillin 1.2 mu (IM) monthly until age 30	Amoxicillin 500 mg (PO) q24h **or** Azithromycin 500 mg (PO) q72h until age 30	Group A streptococcal pharyngitis and acute rheumatic fever are uncommon after age 30.

† During induction chemotherapy for acute myelogenous leukemia (AML) or myelodysplastic syndrome (MDS).

Table 6.4. Chronic Medical Prophylaxis/Suppression (cont'd)

Disorder	Usual Organisms	Preferred Prophylaxis	Alternate Prophylaxis	Comments
Neonatal Group B streptococcal (GBS) infection (primary prevention)	Group B streptococci	Ampicillin 2 gm (IV) q4h at onset of labor until delivery	Clindamycin 600 mg (IV) q8h at onset of labor until delivery **or** Vancomycin 1 gm (IV) q12h at onset of labor until delivery	Indications: previous infant with GBS infection, maternal GBS colonization/ infection during pregnancy, vaginal/ rectal culture of GBS after week 35 of gestation, delivery ≤ week 37 of gestation without labor/ruptured membranes, ruptured membranes ≥ 12 hrs, or intrapartum temp ≥ 100.4°F.

Febrile neutropenia: Treat until neutropenia resolves (see p. 156).

ENDOCARDITIS PROPHYLAXIS (Tables 6.5–6.7)

Endocarditis prophylaxis is designed to prevent native/prosthetic cardiac valve infections by preventing procedure-related bacteremias due to cardiac pathogens. For procedures above-the-waist, usual pathogens are viridans streptococci from the mouth. For procedures below-the-waist, usual pathogens are enterococci. Since procedure-related bacteremias are usually asymptomatic and last less than 15 minutes, single-dose oral regimens prior to the procedure provide effective prophylaxis. Parenteral SBE prophylaxis is preferred for patients with previous endocarditis, shunts, or prosthetic heart valves. Regimens vary among the experts, and no regimen is fully protective. Since erythromycin-based regimens have had the highest failure rate in the past, macrolides have not been included in the recommendations.

Table 6.5. Indications for Infective Endocarditis (IE) Prophylaxis*

Subset	Prophylaxis Recommended (Column A)	Prophylaxis Not Recommended (Column B)
Cardiac conditions	• Ostium primum ASD • Prosthetic heart valves, including bioprosthetic and homograft valves • Previous infective endocarditis • Most congenital cardiac malformations • Rheumatic valve disease • Hypertrophic cardiomyopathy • MVP with valvular regurgitation	• Isolated ostium secundum ASD • Surgical repair without residue beyond 6 months of ostium secundum ASD or PDA • Previous coronary artery bypass surgery • MVP without valvular regurgitation • Physiologic, functional, or innocent murmurs • Previous Kawasaki's cardiac disease or rheumatic fever without valve disease
Procedures	• Dental procedures known to induce gingival/mucosal bleeding, including dental cleaning • Tonsillectomy or adenoidectomy • Surgical operations involving intestinal or respiratory mucosa • Rigid bronchoscopy • Sclerotherapy for esophageal varices • Esophageal dilation • Gallbladder surgery • Cystoscopy or urethral dilation • Urethral catheterization or urinary tract surgery if UTI is present • Prostate surgery • I & D of infected tissue • Vaginal hysterectomy • Vaginal delivery, D & C, IUD insertion/removal, or therapeutic abortion in the presence of infection	• Dental procedures not likely to induce gingival bleeding • Tympanostomy tube insertion • Flexible bronchoscopy ± biopsy • Endotracheal intubation • Endoscopy ± gastrointestinal biopsy • Cesarean section • D & C, IUD insertion/removal, or therapeutic abortion in the absence of infection • Cardiac pacemaker/defibrillator insertion • Coronary stent implantation • Percutaneous transluminal coronary angioplasty (PTCA) • Cardiac catheterization

ASD = atrial septal defect, D & C = dilatation and curettage, I & D = incision and drain, IUD = intrauterine device, MVP = mitral valve prolapse, PDA = patent ductus arteriosus, UTI = urinary tract infection.

* Prophylaxis is indicated for patients with cardiac conditions in Column A undergoing procedures in Column A. Prophylaxis is not recommended for patients or procedures in Column B. See Tables 6.6 and 6.7 for prophylaxis regimens for above-the-waist and below-the-waist procedures, respectively.

Table 6.6. Endocarditis Prophylaxis for Above-the-Waist (Dental, Oral, Esophageal, Respiratory Tract) Procedures*

Prophylaxis**	Reaction to Penicillin	Antibiotic Regimen
Oral prophylaxis	None	Amoxicillin 2 gm (PO) 1 hour pre-procedure†
	Non-anaphylactoid	Cephalexin 1 gm (PO) 1 hour pre-procedure
	Anaphylactoid	Clindamycin 300 mg (PO) 1 hour pre-procedure††
IV prophylaxis	None	Ampicillin 2 gm (IV) 30 minutes pre-procedure
	Non-anaphylactoid	Cefazolin 1 gm (IV) 15 minutes pre-procedure
	Anaphylactoid	Clindamycin 600 mg (IV) 30 minutes pre-procedure

* Endocarditis prophylaxis is directed against viridans streptococci, the usual SBE pathogen above the waist. Macrolide regimens are less effective than other regimens; clarithromycin/azithromycin regimens (500 mg PO 1 hour pre-procedure) are of unproven efficacy.

** Oral prophylaxis is preferred to IV prophylaxis, except in patients with previous endocarditis, shunts, or prosthetic heart valves.

† Some recommend a 3 gm dose of amoxicillin, which is excessive given the sensitivity of viridans streptococci to amoxicillin.

†† Some recommend a 600 mg dose of clindamycin, but a 300 mg dose gives adequate blood levels and is better tolerated (less diarrhea).

Table 6.7. Endocarditis Prophylaxis for Below-the-Waist (Genitourinary, Gastrointestinal) Procedures*†

Prophylaxis**	Reaction to Penicillin	Antibiotic Regimen
Oral prophylaxis	None	Amoxicillin 2 gm (PO) 1 hour pre-procedure
	Non-anaphylactoid, anaphylactoid	Linezolid 600 mg (PO) 1 hour pre-procedure
IV prophylaxis	None	Ampicillin 2 gm (IV) 30 minutes pre-procedure **plus** Gentamicin 80 mg (IM) or (IV) over 1 hour 60 minutes pre-procedure
	Non-anaphylactoid, anaphylactoid	Vancomycin 1 gm (IV) over 1 hour 60 minutes pre-procedure **plus** Gentamicin 80 mg (IM) or (IV) over 1 hour 60 minutes pre-procedure

* Endocarditis prophylaxis is directed against E. faecalis, the usual SBE pathogen below the waist.

** Oral prophylaxis is preferred to IV prophylaxis, except in patients with previous endocarditis, shunts, or prosthetic heart valves.

† Wilson W, et al. Prevention of Infective Endocarditis. Circulation 116:1736–1754, 2007.
Seto TB. The case for infectious endocarditis prophylaxis. Arch Intern Med 167:327–330, 2007.
Harrison JL, Hoen B, Prendergast BD. Antibiotic Prophylaxis for Infective Endocarditis. Lancet 371:1317–1319, 2008.

TRAVEL PROPHYLAXIS (Tables 6.8, 6.9)

Travelers may acquire infectious diseases from ingestion of fecally-contaminated water/food, exchange of infected body secretions, inhalation of aerosolized droplets, direct inoculation via insect bites, or from close contact with infected birds/animals. Recommendations to prevent infection in travelers consist of general travel precautions (Table 6.8), and specific travel prophylaxis regimens (Table 6.9).

Table 6.8. General Infectious Disease Travel Precautions

Exposure	Risk	Precautions
Unsafe water (fecally-contaminated)	Diarrhea/ dysentery, viral hepatitis (HAV)	• Avoid ingestion of unbottled/unpotable water. Be sure bottled water has an unbroken seal and has not been opened/refilled with tap water. • Avoid ice cubes made from water of uncertain of origin/handling, and drinking from unclean glasses. • Drink only pasteurized bottled drinks. Be sure bottles/cans are opened by you or in your presence. • Avoid drinking unpasteurized/warm milk; beer, wine, and pure alcoholic beverages are safe. • Eat only canned fruit or fresh fruit peeled by you or in your presence with clean utensils. • Avoid eating soft cheeses. • Avoid eating raw tomatoes/uncooked vegetables that may have been exposed to contaminated water. • Avoid using hotel water for tooth brushing/rinsing unless certain of purity. Many hotels use common lines for bath/sink water that is unsuitable for drinking. • Avoid wading/swimming/bathing in lakes or rivers.
Food-borne (fecally-contaminated)	Diarrhea/ dysentery	• Eat only seafood/poultry/meats that are freshly cooked and served hot. Avoid eating at roadside stands or small local restaurants with questionable sanitary practices. • "Boil it, peel it, or forget it."
Body fluid secretions	Viral hepatitis (HBV, HCV, etc.), STDs, HIV/other retroviruses	• Do not share utensils/glasses/straws or engage in "risky behaviors" involving body secretion exchange. • Avoid blood transfusion (use blood expanders instead). • Treat dental problems before travel.
Animal bite	Animal bite-associated infections	• Do not pet/play with stray dogs/cats. Rabies and other infections are common in wild (and some urban) animals.
Flying insects	Malaria, arthropod-borne infections	• Avoid flying/biting insects by wearing dark protective clothing (long sleeves/pants) and using insect repellent on clothes/exposed skin, especially during evening hours. • Minimize dawn-to-dusk outdoor exposure. • Use screens/mosquito nets when possible. • Do not use perfume, after shave, or scented deodorants/toiletries that will attract flying insects.

Table 6.9. Travel Prophylaxis Regimens

Exposure	Usual Pathogens	Prophylaxis Regimens	Comments
Traveler's diarrhea	E. coli Salmonella Shigella. Non-cholera vibrios V. cholerae Aeromonas Plesiomonas Rotavirus Norwalk virus Giardia lamblia Campylobacter Yersinia Cryptosporidium Cyclospora Enteroviruses Amebiasis	Doxycycline 100 mg (PO) q24h for duration of exposure **or** Any quinolone (PO) for duration of exposure **or** TMP–SMX 1 SS tablet (PO) q24h for duration of exposure	Observe without prophylaxis and treat mild diarrhea symptomatically with loperamide (2 mg). Persons with medical conditions adversely affected by dehydration caused by diarrhea may begin prophylaxis after arrival in country and continue for 1 day after returning home. Should severe diarrhea/dysentery occur, continue/switch to a quinolone, maximize oral hydration, and see a physician if possible. Anti-spasmodics may be used for symptomatic relief of mild, watery diarrhea. Bismuth subsalicylate is less effective than antibiotic prophylaxis. Traveler's diarrhea usually presents as acute watery diarrhea with low-grade fever after ingestion of fecally-contaminated water. Most cases are due to enterotoxigenic E. coli. TMP–SMX is active against some bacterial pathogens and Cyclospora, but not against E. histolytica or enteroviral pathogens (e.g., Rotavirus, Norwalk agent). Doxycycline is active against most bacterial pathogens and E. histolytica, but misses Campylobacter, Cryptosporidium, Cyclospora, Giardia, and enteroviral pathogens. Although emerging resistance is a problem, ciprofloxacin is active against most pathogens except Giardia, Cryptosporidium, Cyclospora, E. histolytica, and enteroviral pathogens. All antibiotics oftlineare inactive against viral/parasitic pathogens causing diarrhea.

Table 6.9. Travel Prophylaxis Regimens (cont'd)

Exposure	Usual Pathogens	Prophylaxis Regimens	Comments
Meningococcal meningitis	N. meningitidis	Pre-travel prophylaxis Meningococcal conjugate vaccine 0.5 mL (IM) ≥ 1 month prior to travel to outbreak area Post-exposure prophylaxis See p. 350	Acquired via close face-to-face contact (airborne aerosol/droplet exposure). Vaccine is highly protective against N. meningitidis serotypes A, C, Y, and W-135, but misses B serotype.
Hepatitis A (HAV)	Hepatitis A virus	HAV vaccine 1 mL (IM) prior to travel, then follow with a one-time booster 3, 6 months later	HAV vaccine is better than immune globulin for prophylaxis. Take care to avoid direct/indirect ingestion of fecally-contaminated water. HAV vaccine is recommended for travel to all developing countries. Protective antibody titers develop after 2 weeks.
Typhoid fever	S. typhi	ViCPS vaccine 0.5 mL (IM). Booster every 2 yrs for repeat travelers **or** Oral Ty21a vaccine 1 capsule (PO) q48h × 4 doses. Booster every 5 years for repeat travelers	For the oral vaccine, do not co-administer with antibiotics. Contraindicated in compromised hosts and children £ 6 years old. Take oral capsules with cold water. Degree of protective immunity is limited with vaccine. Some prefer chemoprophylaxis the same as for Traveler's diarrhea (p. 362).
Yellow fever	Yellow fever virus	Yellow fever vaccine 0.5 mL (SC). Booster every 10 years for repeat travelers	Vaccine is often required for travel to or from Tropical South America or Tropical Central Africa. Administer 1 month apart from other live vaccines. Contraindicated in children < 4 months old; caution in children £ 1 year old. Reactions may occur in persons with egg allergies. Immunity is probably life long, but a booster every 10 years is needed for vaccination certification by some countries.

Table 6.9. Travel Prophylaxis Regimens (cont'd)

Exposure	Usual Pathogens	Prophylaxis Regimens	Comments
Japanese encephalitis (JE)	Japanese encephalitis virus	JE vaccine 1 mL (SC) on days 0, 7, and 14 or 30. Booster schedule not established	Recommended for travelers planning prolonged (> 3 week) visits during the rainy season to rural, endemic areas of Asia (e.g., Eastern Russia, Indian subcontinent, China, Southeast Asia, Thailand, Korea, Laos, Cambodia, Vietnam, Malaysia, Philippines). Administer 3, 2 weeks before exposure. Children < 3 years may be given 0.5 mL (SC) on same schedule as adults.
Rabies	Rabies virus	HDCV, PCEC, or RVA 1 mL (IM) on days 0, 7, and 21 or 28 prior to travel **or** HDCV 0.1 mL (ID) on days 0, 7, and 21 or 28 prior to travel	Avoid contact with wild dogs/animals during travel. Dose of rabies vaccine for adults and children are the same. A booster dose prior to travel is recommended if antibody levels are measured and are low.
Tetanus Diphtheria Pertussis	C. tetani C. diphtheriae B. pertussis	Tdap 0.5 ml (IM)	Tdap preferred to Td since it also boosts pertussis immunity.
Malaria	P. vivax P. ovale P. malariae P. falciparum (chloroquine sensitive)	Chloroquine phosphate 500 mg (300 mg base) (PO) weekly **or** Malarone (atovaquone 250 mg + proguanil 100 mg) 1 tablet (PO) q24h **or** Mefloquine 250 mg (228 mg base) (PO) weekly **or** Doxycycline 100 mg (PO) q24h	Acquired from female Anopheles mosquito bites. Avoid mosquito exposure using long-sleeved shirts/long pants at dawn/dusk when mosquitoes feed. Screens/mosquito nets are the best natural protection. DEET/pyrethrin sprays on clothing is helpful. Begin chloroquine or mefloquine prophylaxis 1 week before travel to malarious areas (most of Africa, Latin America, Indian subcontinent, Southeast Asia), and continue for 4 weeks after returning home. Chemoprophylaxis reduces but does not eliminate the risk of malaria. Malarone or doxycycline

Table 6.9. Travel Prophylaxis Regimens (cont'd)

Exposure	Usual Pathogens	Prophylaxis Regimens	Comments
	P. falciparum (chloroquine resistant)	Doxycycline 100 mg (PO) q24h **or** Malarone (atovaquone 250 mg + proguanil 100 mg) 1 tablet (PO) q24h **or** Mefloquine 250 mg (228 mg base) (PO) weekly	prophylaxis may be given 1 day before travel, daily during malaria exposure, and for 1 week after returning home. Malarone is effective against sensitive/resistant P. falciparum strains, but not hepatic stages of P. vivax/P. ovale. Chloroquine-resistant P. falciparum is seen in sub-Saharan Africa, South America (except Chile, Argentina), Indian subcontinent, and Southern Asia (Burma, Thailand, Cambodia). Only areas without chloroquine-resistant P. falciparum are Middle East (except Saudi Arabia), Central America (west of Panama Canal), Haiti, and Dominican Republic. Fansidar resistance is common in chloroquine-resistant areas of Asia, Latin American, Africa. Mefloquine (but not doxycycline) resistance is seen in Thailand. Doxycycline is contraindicated in pregnancy, but chloroquine and proguanil are safe, and mefloquine is probably safe late in pregnancy. If pregnant, try to delay travel to malarial areas until after delivery.

HDCV = human diploid cell vaccine, PCEC = purified chick embryo cell vaccine, RVA = rabies vaccine absorbed, RIG = rabies immune globulin.

TETANUS PROPHYLAXIS (Table 6.10)

Current information suggests that immunity lasts for decades/life-time after tetanus immunization. A tetanus booster should not be routinely given for minor wounds, but is recommended for wounds with high tetanus potential (e.g., massive crush wounds, soil-contaminated wounds, or deep puncture wounds).

Table 6.10. Tetanus Prophylaxis in Routine Wound Management

History of Adsorbed Tetanus Toxoid	Wound Type	Recommendations
Unknown or < 3 doses	Clean, minor wounds	Td‡ or Tdap‡
	Tetanus-prone wounds†	(Td‡ or Tdap‡) plus TIG
≥ 3 doses	Clean, minor wounds	No prophylaxis needed
	Tetanus-prone wounds†	Td‡ if > 10 years since last dose*

DT = diphtheria and tetanus toxoids adsorbed (pediatrics), DTP = diphtheria and tetanus toxoids and pertussis vaccine adsorbed, Td = tetanus and diphtheria toxoids adsorbed (adult), TIG = tetanus immune globulin, Tdap = tetanus and diphtheria toxoids and pertussis vaccine absorbed.

† For example, massive crush wounds; wounds contaminated with dirt, soil, feces, or saliva; deep puncture wounds; or significant burn wounds or frostbite.

‡ For children < 7 years, DTP (DT if pertussis is contraindicated) is preferred to tetanus toxoid alone. For children ≥ 7 years old and adults, Tdap is preferred to Td or tetanus toxoid alone.

* More frequent booster doses are unnecessary and can increase side effects. Protection lasts > 20 yrs Adapted from: Centers for Disease Control and Prevention. MMWR Rep 40 (RR-10):1–28. 1991.

IMMUNIZATIONS (Table 6.11)

Immunizations are designed to reduce infections in large populations, and may prevent/decrease the severity of infection in non-immunized individuals. Compromised hosts with altered immune systems may not develop protective antibody titers to antigenic components of various vaccines. **Immunizations are not fully protective, but are recommended** (depending on the vaccine) for most normal hosts, since some protection is better than none. Post-exposure prophylaxis and travel prophylaxis are described on pp. 350 and 362–365.

Table 6.11. Adult Immunizations*

Vaccine	Indications	Dosage	Comments
Bacille Calmette Guérin (BCG)	Possibly beneficial for adults at high-risk of multiple-drug resistant tuberculosis	Primary: 1 dose (intradermal). Booster not recommended	Live attenuated vaccine. PPD remains positive for years/life. Contraindicated in immunocompromised hosts. Side effects include injection site infection or disseminated infection (rare).
Hemophilus influenzae (type B)	Consider for patients with splenic dysfunction	Primary: 0.5 mL dose (IM). Booster not recommended	Capsular polysaccharide conjugated to diphtheria toxoid. Benefit uncertain. Safety in pregnancy unknown. Mild local reaction in 10%.

Table 6.11. Adult Immunizations* (cont'd)

Vaccine	Indications	Dosage	Comments
Hepatitis A (HAV)	All children beginning age 12 to 23 months and adults at increased risk of HAV.	Primary: 1 mL dose (IM). One-time booster ≥ 6 months later. Booster not routinely recommended.	Inactivated whole virus. Pregnancy risk not fully evaluated. Mild soreness at injection site. Occasional headache/malaise.
Hepatitis B (HBV)	Household/sexual contact with carrier, IV drug use, multiple sex partners (heterosexual), homosexual male activity, blood product recipients, hemodialysis, occupational exposure to blood, residents/staff of institutions for developmentally disabled, prison inmates, residence ≥ 6 months in areas of high endemicity, others at high risk.	Primary (3 dose series): Recombivax 10 mcg (1 mL) or Engerix-B 20 mcg (1 mL) IM in deltoid at 0, 1, and 6 months. Alternate schedule for Engerix-B: 4 dose series at 0, 1, 2, and 12 months. Booster not routinely recommended.	Recombinant vaccine comprised of hepatitis B surface antigen. For compromised hosts (including dialysis patients), use specially packaged Recombivax 40-mcg doses (1 mL vial containing 40 mcg/mL). HBsAb titers should be obtained 6 months after 3-dose primary series. Those with non-protective titers (≤ 10 mIU/mL) should receive 1 dose monthly (with subsequent HbsAb testing) up to a maximum of 3 doses. Safety to fetus unknown; pregnancy not a contraindication in high-risk females. Mild local reaction in 10–20%. Occasional fever, headache, fatigue, nausea. Twinrix 1 mL (IM) (combination of Hepatitis A inactivated vaccine and Hepatitis B recombinant vaccine) is available for adults on a 0, 1, and 6-month schedule or 0, 7 days, 21–30 days, and 12 month schedules.
Herpes zoster (VZV)	Adults ≥ 60 years to reduce the frequency of shingles/ prevent post-herpetic neuralgia. Use in those with previous H. zoster is not yet defined. Protection best in 60–69 year group; efficacy decreases with increasing age.	Primary: 0.65 mL (SC). Need for revaccination not yet defined. Vaccine must be stored frozen and used within 30 minutes after thawing.	Duration of protection is at least 4 years. Injection site reactions in 48%. Contraindicated in immunocompromised hosts (with immunosuppressive disorder or receiving immunosuppressive drug) or untreated TB. Not indicated for therapy of H. zoster or post-herpetic neuralgia.

Table 6.11. Adult Immunizations* (cont'd)

Vaccine	Indications	Dosage	Comments
Influenza	Healthy persons ≥ 50 years, healthcare personnel, adults with high-risk conditions (e.g., heart disease, lung disease, diabetes, renal dysfunction, hemoglobinopathies, immunosuppression).	Annual vaccine. Single 0.5 mL dose (IM) between October and November (before flu season) is optimal, but can be given anytime during flu season.	Trivalent inactivated whole and split virus. Contraindications include anaphylaxis to eggs or sensitivity to thimerosal. Mild local reaction in up to 30%. Occasional malaise/myalgia beginning 6–12 hours after vaccination. Neurologic and allergic reactions are rare. For pregnancy, administer in 2nd or 3rd trimester during flu season. A nasally-administered live attenuated influenza vaccine has been approved for healthy individuals aged 5–49 years.
Measles	Adults born after 1956 without live-virus immunization or measles diagnosed by a physician or immunologic test. Also indicated for revaccination of persons given killed measles vaccine between 1963–67.	Primary: 0.5 mL dose (SC). A second dose (≥ 1 month later) is recommended for certain adults at increased risk of exposure (e.g., healthcare workers, travelers to developing countries). No routine booster.	Live virus vaccine (usually given in MMR). Contraindicated in compromised hosts, pregnancy, history of anaphylaxis to eggs or neomycin. Ineffective if given 3–11 months after blood products. Side effects include low-grade fever 5–21 days after vaccination (5–15%), transient rash (5%), and local reaction in 4–55% of persons previously immunized with killed vaccine (1963–67).
Meningococcus (invasive disease)	Patients with splenic dysfunction or defects in terminal complement; laboratory workers.	Meningococcal conjugate vaccine 0.5 mL (IM).	Also used in epidemic control of N. meningitides serogroups A, C, Y, and W-135.
Mumps	Non-immune adults.	Primary: 0.5 mL dose (SC). No routine booster.	Live attenuated vaccine (usually given in MMR). Contraindicated in immunocompromised hosts, pregnancy, history of anaphylaxis to eggs or neomycin. Side effects include mild allergic reactions (uncommon), parotitis (rare).

Table 6.11. Adult Immunizations* (cont'd)

Vaccine	Indications	Dosage	Comments
Papilloma (human) Virus (HPV)	Women up to 26 years of age. Contraindicated in pregnancy.	Primary: 0.5 mL (IM). Second dose: 2 months after 1st dose. Third dose: 6 months after 1st dose.	Quadrivalent vaccine used to prevent genital warts (Condyloma accuminata), cervical cancer, AIS, CIN, VIN, ValN due to HPV types 6, 11, 16, 18. Not indicated for therapy of active genital warts, cervical cancer, CIN, VIN, or ValN.
Pertussis	Use Tdap instead of Td in booster dose.	A Single Tdap booster dose 0.5 mL (IM). Schedule for subsequent boosters to be determined.	Recommended since adults may get pertussis or transmit it to susceptible infants.
Pneumococcus (S. neumoniae)	Immunocompetent hosts ≥ 65 years old, or > 2 years old with diabetes, CSF leaks, or chronic cardiac, pulmonary or liver disease. Also for immunocompromised hosts > 2 years old with functional/anatomic asplenia, leukemia, lymphoma, multiple myeloma, widespread malignancy, chronic renal failure, bone marrow/organ transplant, or on immunosuppressive/ steroid therapy.	Primary: 0.5 mL dose (SC or IM). A one-time booster at 5 years is recommended for immuno compromised hosts > 2 years old and for those who received the vaccine before age 65 for high-risk conditions.	Polyvalent vaccine against 23 strains. Studies are inadequate regarding routine reimmunization. Practitioners should decide their own policy.
Rubella	Non-immune adults, particularly women of childbearing age.	Primary: 0.5 mL dose (SC). No routine booster.	Live virus (RA 27/3 strain) vaccine (usually given in MMR). Contraindicated in immuno-compromised hosts, pregnancy, history of anaphylactic reaction to neomycin. Joint pains and transient arthralgias in up to 40%, beginning 3–25 days after vaccination and lasting 1–11 days; frank arthritis in < 2%.

Table 6.11. Adult Immunizations* (cont'd)

Vaccine	Indications	Dosage	Comments
Tetanus-diphtheria	Adults	Primary: Td two 0.5 mL doses (IM), 1–2 months apart; third dose 6–12 months after second dose Booster: a single Tdap 0.5 mL (IM) is recommended pending further evaluation regarding subsequent boosters.	Adsorbed toxoid vaccine. Contraindicated if hypersensitivity/neurological reaction or severe local reaction to previous doses. Side effects include local reactions, occasional fever, systemic symptoms, Arthus-like reaction in persons with multiple previous boosters, and systemic allergy (rare).
Varicella (VZV) chickenpox	Non-immune adolescents and adults, especially healthcare workers and others likely to be exposed.	Primary: Two 0.5 mL doses (SC), 4–8 weeks apart. Vaccine must be stored frozen and used within 30 minutes after thawing and reconstitution. No routine booster.	Live attenuated vaccine. Contraindications include pregnancy, active untreated TB, immunocompromised host, malignancy of bone marrow or lymphatic system, anaphylactic reaction to gelatin/neomycin, or blood product recipient within previous 6 months (may prevent development of protective antibody). Mild febrile illness in 10%. Injection site symptoms in 25–30% (local rash in 3%). Mild diffuse rash in 5%.

* For immunizations before organ transplantation or during pregnancy, please consult other resources.

REFERENCES AND SUGGESTED READINGS

Andrews WW, Kimberlin DF, Whitley R, Cliver S, Ramsey PS. Valacyclovir therapy to reduce recurrent genital herpes in pregnant women. Am J Obstet Gynecol 194:774–81, 2006.

Antrum RM, Solomkin JS. A review of antibiotic prophylaxis for open fractures. Orthop Rev 16:246–54, 1987.

Batiuk TD, Bodziak KA, Goldman M. Infectious disease prophylaxis in renal transplant patients: a survey of US transplant centers. Clin Transplant 16:1–8, 2002.

Baum SG. Oseltamivir and the Influenza Alphabet. Clin Infect Dis 43:445–6, 2006.

Bennett JE, Echinocandins for Candidemia in Adults without Neutropenia. New Engl J Med 355:1154–9, 2006.

Bow EJ, Rotstein C, Noskin GA, et al. A Randomized, Open-Label, Multicenter Comparative Study of the Efficacy and Safety of Piperacillin-Tazobactam and Cefepime for the Empirical Treatment of Febrile

Neutropenic Episodes in Patients with Hematologic Malignancies. Clin Infect Dis 43:447–59, 2006.

Brantley JS, Hicks L, Sra K, Tyring SK. Valacyclovir for the treatment of genital herpes. Expert Rev Anti-Infect Ther 4:367–76, 2006.

Burroughs, MH. Immunization in transplant patients. Pediatr Infect Dis J 21:158–60, 2002.

Caple J. Varicella-Zoster Virus Vaccine: A Review of its Use in the Prevention of Herpes Zoster in Older Adults. Drugs of Today 42:249–54, 2006.

Carratala J. Role of antibiotic prophylaxis for the prevention of intravascular catheter-related infection. Clin Microbiol Infect 7 (Suppl 4):83–90, 2001.

Chen LH, Wilson ME, Schlagenhauf P. Prevention of Malaria in Long-term Travelers. JAMA 296:2234–44, 2006.

Chattopadhyay B. Splenectomy pneumococcal vaccination and antibiotic prophylaxis. Br J Hosp Med 41:172–4, 1989.

Colizza S, Rossi S. Antibiotic prophylaxis and treatment of surgical abdominal sepsis. J Chemother 13:193–201, 2001.

Craig AS, Schaffner W. Prevention of hepatitis A with the hepatitis A vaccine. N Engl J Med 350:476–81, 2004.

Cullen M, Steven N, Billingham L, et al. Antibacterial prophylaxis after chemotherapy for solid tumors and lymphomas. N Engl J Med 353:988–98, 2005.

Cunha BA, Gossling HR, Nightingale CH, et al. Penetration of cefazolin and cefradine into bone in patients undergoing total knee arthroplasty. Infection 2: 80–84, 1984.

Cunha BA. Antibiotic tissue penetration. Bulletin of the New York Academy of Medicine 59:443–449, 1983.

Cunha BA, Ristuccia A, Jonas M, et al. Penetration of ceftizoxime and cefazolin into bile and gallbladder wall. Journal of Antimicrobial Chemotherapy 10: 117–120, 1982.

Cunha BA, Pyrtek LJ, Quintiliani R. Prophylactic antibiotics in cholecystectomy. Lancet 1:207–8, 1979.

Cunha BA, Gossling HR, Nightingale C, et al. Penetration characteristics of cefazolin, cephalothin, and cephradine into bone in patients undergoing total hip replacement. Journal of Bone and Surgery 59: 856–859, 1977.

Darouiche RG. Treatment of infections associated with surgical implants. N Engl J Med 350:1422–9, 2004.

De Lall F. Antibiotic prophylaxis in orthopedic prosthetic surgery. J Chemother 13 Spec No 1:48–53, 2001.

De la Camara R. Antifungal prophylaxis in haematology patients. 12:S65–76, 2006.

Diaz-Pedroche C, Lumbreras C, San Juan R, et al. Valganciclovir preemptive therapy for the prevention of cytomegalovirus disease in high-risk seropositive solid-organ transplant recipients. Transplantation 82:30–5, 2006.

Dietrich ES, Bieser U, Frank U, et al. Ceftriaxone versus other cephalosporins for perioperative antibiotic prophylaxis: a meta analysis of 43 randomized controlled trials. Chemotherapy 48:49–56, 2002.

Drew RH, Perfect JR.Use of Polyenes for Prophylaxis for Invasive Fungal Infections. Infections in Medicine 23:S12–24, 2006.

Eckart RE, Love SS, Atwood E, et al. Incidence and follow-up of inflammatory cardiac complications after smallpox vaccination. J Am Coll Cardiol 44:201–5, 2004.

Esposito S. Is single-dose antibiotic prophylaxis sufficient for any surgical procedure? J Chemother 11:556, 2000.

Faix, RG. Immunization during pregnancy. Clin Obstet Gynecol 45:42–58, 2002.

Farci P, Chessa L, et al. Treatment of chronic hepatitis D. J Viral Hepatitis 14(Suppl 1):58–63, 2007.

Fennessy BG, O'Sullivan MJ, Fulton GJ, et al. Prospective Study of Use of Perioperative Antimicrobial Therapy in General Surgery. Surgical Infections 7:355–60, 2006.

Gall SA. Immunology update: hepatitis B virus immunization today. Infect Dis Obstet Gynecol 9:63–4, 2001.

Gardner P, Eickhoff T. Immunization in adults in the 1990s. Curr Clin To Infect Dis 15:271–300, 1995.

Gardner P, Peter G. Recommended schedules for routine immunization of children and adults. Infect Dis Clin North Am 15:1–8, 2001.

Gardner P, Schaffner W. Immunization of adults. N Engl J Med 328:1252–8, 1993.

Grabe M. Perioperative antibiotic prophylaxis in urology. Curr Opin Urol 11:81–5, 2001.

Grandiere-Perez L, Ansart S, Paris, L, et al. Efficacy of Praziquantel During the Incubation and Invasive Phase of Schistosoma Haematobium Schistosomiasis in 18 Travelers. Am J Trop Med Hyg 74:814–18, 2006.

Guaschino S, De Santo D, De Seta F. New perspectives in antibiotic prophylaxis for obstetric and gynecological surgery. J Hosp Infect 50 (Suppl A):SS13–6, 2002.

Haines SJ. Antibiotic prophylaxis in neurosurgery. The controlled trials. Neurosurg Clin N Am 3:355–8, 1992.

Hartman BJ. Selective aspects of infective endocarditis: considerations on diagnosis, risk factors, treatment and prophylaxis. Adv Cardiol 39:195–202, 2002.

Hasin T, Davidovitch N, Cohen R, et al. Postexposure Treatment with Doxycycline for the Prevention of

Tick-Borne Relapsing Fever. N Engl J Med 355:147–55, 2006.

Hiemenz J, Cagnoni P, et al. Pharmacokinetic and maximum tolerated dose study of micafungin in combination with fluconazole versus fluconazole alone for prophylaxis of fungal infections in adult patients undergoing a bone marrow or peripheral stem cell transplant. Antimicrob Agents Chemother 49:1331–6, 2005.

Hill DR, Ericsson CD, Pearson RD, Keystone JS, et al. The Practice of Travel Medicine: Guidelines by the Infectious Diseases Society of America. Clin Infect Dis 43:1499–539, 2006.

Hoofnagle JH, Doo E, Liang TJ, et al. Management of hepatitis B: summary of a clinical research workshop. Hepatology 45:1056–1075, 2007.

Hoofnagle JH, Seeff LB. Peginterferon and ribavirin for chronic hepatitis C. N Engl J Med 355:2444–2451, 2006.

Hornberger H, Robertus K. Cost-Effectiveness of a Vaccine To Prevent Herpes Zoster and Postherpetic Neuralgia in Older Adults. 145:317–25, 2006.

Howdieshell TF, Heffernan D, Dipiro JT. Surgical Infection Society Guidelines for Vaccination after Traumatic Injury. Surgical Infections 7:275–303, 2006.

Itani KMF, Wilson SE, Awad SS, et al. Ertapenem versus Cefotetan Prophylaxis in Elective Colorectal Surgery. N Engl J Med 355:2640–51, 2006.

Jackson LA, Neuzil KM, Yu O et al. Effectiveness of pneumococcal polysaccharide vaccine in older adults. N Engl J Med 348:1747–55, 2003.

Jacobson RM. Vaccine safety. Immunol Allergy Clin North Am 23:589–603, 2003.

Jong EC, Nothdurft HD. Current drugs for antimalarial chemoprophylaxis: a review of efficacy and safety. J Travel Med 8(Supp. 3):S48–56, 2001.

Kain KC, Shanks GD, Keystone JS. Malaria chemoprophylaxis in the age of drug resistance. I. Currently recommended drug regimens. Clin Infect Dis 33: 226–34, 2001.

Kawai N, Ikematsu H, Iwaki N, et al. A Comparison of the Effectiveness of Oseltamivir for the Treatment of Influenza A and Influenza B: A Japanese Multicenter Study of the 2003–2004 and 2004–2005 Influenza Seasons. Clin Infect Dis 43:439–44, 2006.

Khoury JA, Storch GA, Bohl DL, et al. Prophylactic verus preemptive oral valganciclovir for the management of cytomegalovirus infection in adult renal transplant recipients. Am J Transplant 6:2134–43, 2006.

Leaper DJ, Melling AG. Antibiotic prophylaxis in clean surgery: clean non-implant wounds. J Chemother 13 (Spec No 1):96–101, 2001.

Lewis RT. Oral versus systemic antibiotic prophylaxis in elective colon surgery: a randomized study and meta-analysis send a message from the 1990s. Can J Surg 45:173–80, 2002.

Marcellin P, Lau GKK, Bonino F, et al. peginterferon alfa-2a alone, lamivudine alone, and two in combination in patients with HBeAg-negative chronic hepatitis B. N Engl J Med 351:1206–1217, 2004.

Musher DM, Rueda-Jaimes AM, Graviss EA, Rodriguez-Barradas MC. Effect of Pneumococcal Vaccination: A Comparison of Vaccination Rates in Patients with Bactermic and Nonbacteremic Pneumococcal Pneumonia. Clin Infect Dis 43:1004–08, 2006.

Paul M, Yahav D, Fraser A, et al. Empirical antibiotic monotherapy for febrile neutropenia: systematic review and meta-analysis of randomized controlled trials. J Antimicrob Chemother 57:176–89, 2006.

Peter G, Gardner P.Standards for immunization practice for vaccines in children and adults. Infect Dis Clin North Am 15:9–19, 2001.

Phillips P, Chan K, Hogg R, et al. Azithromycin prophylaxis for Mycobacterium avium complex during the era of highly active antiretroviral therapy: evaluation of a provincial program. Clin Infect Dis 34:371–8, 2002.

Pratesi C, Russo D, Dorigo W, et al. Antibiotic prophylaxis in clean surgery: vascular surgery. J Chemother 13 (Spec 1):123–8, 2001.

Rex JH, Sobel JD. Prophylactic antifungal therapy in the intensive care unit. Clin Infect Dis 32:1191–200, 2001.

Rolston KVI, Bodey GP. Comment on: Empirical antibiotic monotherapy for febrile neutropenia: systematic review and meta-analysis of randomized controlled trials. J Antimicrob Chemother 58:478–9, 2006.

Rupprecht CE, Gibbons RV. Prophylaxis against rabies. N Engl J Med 351:2626–35, 2004.

Ryan Et, Wilson ME, Kain KC. Illness after international travel. N Engl J Med 347:505–516, 2002.

Segreti J. Is antibiotic prophylaxis necessary for preventing prosthetic device infection. Infect Dis Clin North Am 13:871–7, 1999.

SetoT B. The case for infectious endocarditis prophylaxis. Arch Intern Med 167:327–330, 2007.

Seymour RA, Whitworth JM. Antibiotic prophylaxis for endocarditis, prosthetic joints, and surgery. Dent Clin North Am 46:635–51, 2002.

Sganga G. New perspectives in antibiotic prophylaxis for intra-abdominal surgery. J Hosp Infect 50 (Suppl A): S17–21, 2002.

Shiffman ML, Suter F, Bacon BR, et al. Peginterferon alfa-2a and ribavirin for 16 or 24 weeks in HCV genotype 2 or 3. N Engl J Med 357:124–134, 2007.

Siddiqui MA, Perry CM. Human papillomavirus quadrivalent (types 6, 11, 16, 18) recombinant vaccine (Gardasil). Drugs 66:1263–71, 2006.

Snydman DR. Prevention of cytomegalovirus (CMV) infection and CMV disease in recipients of solid organ transplants: the case for prophylaxis. Clin Infect Dis 40:709–12, 2005.

Sobel JD, Rex JH. Invasive candidiasis: Turning risk into a practical prevention policy? Clin Infect Dis 33: 187–190, 2001.

Spira AM. Yellow Fever: An Update on Risks, Presentation, and Prevention. Infections in Medicine 23: 385–89, 2006.

Taub DD, Ershler WB, Janowski M, et al. Immunity from Smallpox Vaccine Persists for Decades: A Longitudinal Study. Am J Med 121:1058–1064, 2008.

Thermidor M, Johnson DH, Cunha BA. Post-Yellow Fever Vaccine Encephalitis in an Elderly Adult. Infect Dis Practice 30:488–89, 2006.

Vazquez M, LaRussa PS, Gershon AA, et al. The effectiveness of the varicella vaccine in clinical practice. N Engl J Med 344:955–60, 2001.

Victor JC, Mourfi AS, Sundina TY, et al. Hepatitis A vaccine versus immune globulin for postexposure prophylaxis. N Engl J Med 357:1685–1694, 2007.

Wingard JR. Antifungal chemoprophylaxis after blood and marrow transplantation. Clin Infect Dis 34: 1386–90,2002.

Winston DJ, Busuttil RW. Randomized controlled trial of oral itraconazole solution versus intravenous/oral fluconazole for prevention of fungal infections in liver transplant recipients. Transplantation 74:688–95, 2002.

Wistrom J, Norrby R. Antibiotic prophylaxis of travellers' diarrhoea. Scand J Infect Dis Suppl70:111–29, 1990.

Zelenitsky SA, Ariano RE, Harding GK, et al. Antibiotic pharmacodynamics in surgical prophylaxis: an association between intraoperative antibiotic concentrations and efficacy. Antimicrob Agents Chemother 46:3026–30, 2002.

Zimmerman RK, Burns IT. Childhood immunization guidelines: current and future. Prim Care 21:693–715, 1994.

GUIDELINES

Advisory Committee on Immunization Practices. Recommended adult immunization schedule: United States. October 2007–September 2008. Ann Intern Med 147:725–729, 2007.

Antimicrobial prophylaxis for surgery. Medical Letter 4:83–88, 2006.

Dykewicz CA.Summary of the guidelines for preventing opportunistic infections among hematopoietic stem cell transplant recipients. Clin Infect Dis 33:139–44, 2001.

Hauser CJ, Adams CA, Eachempati SR. Prophylactic Antibiotic Use in Open Fractures: An Evidence-Based Guideline. Surgical Infections 7:379–405, 2006.

Lok AS, MacMahon BJ. Chronic hepatitis B. Hepatology 45:507–539, 2007.

National Centers for Infectious Diseases Travelers Health 2005. http://www.cdc.gov/travel/.

Prevention of Perinatal Group B Streptococcal Disease. Revised CDC guidelines. MMWR 51(11), August 12, 2002.

Recommended childhood & adolescent immunization schedule - United States. MMWR 55(51);Q1–Q4, January 5, 2007. www.cdc.gov/nip/recs/child-schedule-bw-print.pdf.

Strader DB, Wright T, Thomas DL, et al. Diagnosis, management, and treatment of hepatitis C. Hepatology 39:1147–1171, 2004.

Use of anthrax vaccine in response to terrorism: supplemental recommendations of the Advisory Committee on Immunization Practices. MMWR 51(No. 45);1024, November 15, 2002.

Yellow fever vaccine. Recommendations of the Advisory Committee on Immunization Practices (ACIP). MMWR 51(17), November 8, 2002.

TEXTBOOKS

Gorbach SL, Bartlett JG. Blacklow NR Infectious (eds). Diseases, 3rd edition. Lippincott, Williams & Wilkins, Philadelphia, 2004.

Hawker J, Begg N, Blairl, et al. Communicable Disease Control Handbook, 2nd edition. Malden, Massachusetts, Blackwell Publishing, 2005.

Keystone JS, Kozarski PE, Freedman DO, et al. Travel Medicine. Mosby, Edinburgh, 2004.

Mandell GL, Bennett JE, Dolin R. Mandell, Douglas, and Bennett's Principles and Practice of Infectious Diseases, 7th edition. Philadelphia, Elsevier, 2010.

Plotkin SA, Orenstein WA Vaccines 4th Edition. Philadelphia, W.B. Saunders, 2004.

Yu VL, Merigan Jr, TC, Barriere SL. Antimicrobial Therapy and Vaccines 2nd Edition. Williams & Wilkins, Baltimore, 2005.

Chapter 7

Pediatric Infectious Diseases and Pediatric Drug Summaries

Leonard R. Krilov, MD

George H. McCracken, Jr, MD

This chapter pertains to infectious diseases and antimicrobial agents in the pediatric population. It is organized by clinical syndrome, patient subset, and in some cases, specific organism. Clinical summaries immediately follow each treatment grid. Therapeutic recommendations are based on antimicrobial effectiveness, reliability, cost, safety, and resistance potential. Antimicrobial agents and duration of therapy are listed in the treatment grids; corresponding drug dosages are provided on pages 402–410 and represent the usual dosages for normal renal and hepatic function. Drug dosages in infants/children are generally based on weight, up to adult dosage as maximum. ***For any treatment category (i.e., preferred IV therapy, alternate IV therapy, PO therapy), recommended drugs are equally effective and not ranked by priority.*** Please refer to other pediatric drug references and the manufacturer's package inserts for dosage adjustments, side effects, drug interactions, and other important prescribing information.

"IV-to-PO Switch" in the last column of the shaded title bar in each treatment grid indicates the clinical syndrome can be treated either by IV therapy alone or IV followed by PO therapy, but *not* by PO therapy alone. "PO Therapy or IV-to-PO Switch" indicates the clinical syndrome can be treated by IV therapy alone, PO therapy alone, or IV followed by PO therapy (unless otherwise indicated in the footnotes under each treatment grid). Most patients on IV therapy able to take oral medications should be switched to PO equivalent therapy after clinical improvement. Chapters 1–6 and 8–9 in this handbook pertain to infectious diseases and antimicrobial agents in adults.

Empiric Therapy of CNS Infections

Acute Bacterial Meningitis

Subset (age)	Usual Pathogens	Preferred IV Therapy†	Alternate IV Therapy†
Neonate (0–30 days)	Group B streptococci E. coli Listeria monocytogenes Other gram-negatives (e.g., Citrobacter, Serratia) and gram-positives (e.g., Enterococci)	Ampicillin **plus** cefotaxime*	Ampicillin **plus** gentamicin*
1–3 months	Overlap neonate and > 3 months	Vancomycin **plus** **either** cefotaxime **or** ceftriaxone*	Ampicillin **plus** **either** cefotaxime **or** ceftriaxone*
> 3 months	S. pneumoniae N. meningitidis H. influenzae (very rare) Non-typeable H. influenzae (rare)	<u>Before culture results</u>: Vancomycin **plus** **either** ceftriaxone **or** cefotaxime* <u>After culture results</u> Discontinue vancomycin if penicillin-susceptible S. pneumoniae, N. meningitidis, or H. influenza is isolated	Meropenem* <u>Severe penicillin allergy</u> Vancomycin **plus** **either** rifampin **or** chloramphenicol*

Acute Bacterial Meningitis (cont'd)

Subset (age)	Usual Pathogens	Preferred IV Therapy†	Alternate IV Therapy†
CNS shunt infection (Treat initially for S. epidermidis; if later identified as MSSA, treat accordingly)	S. epidermidis S. aureus (MRSA)	Vancomycin **with or without** rifampin 10 mg/kg (IV or PO) q12h × 7–10 days after shunt removal	Linezolid × 7–10 days after shunt removal If MSSA isolated Nafcillin **with or without** rifampin 10 mg/kg (PO) q12h × 7–10 days after shunt removal
	S. aureus (MSSA)	Nafcillin × 7–10 days after shunt removal	Vancomycin × 7–10 days after shunt removal
	Enterobacteriaceae	Cefotaxime **or** ceftriaxone × 7–10 days after shunt removal	Meropenem × 7–10 days after shunt removal

MRSA/MSSA = methicillin-resistant/sensitive S. aureus. Duration of therapy represents total time IV or IV + PO. Most patients on IV therapy able to take PO meds should be switched to PO therapy after clinical improvement.

† **See pp. 402–410 for drug dosages.**

* Duration of therapy: Group B strep ≥ 14 days (with ventriculitis 4 weeks); E. coli, Citrobacter, Serratia ≥ 21 days; Listeria 10–14 days; Enterococcus ≥ 14 days; S. pneumoniae 10–14 days; H. influenza ≥ 10 days; N. meningitidis 4–7 days.

Acute Bacterial Meningitis (Normal Hosts)

Clinical Presentation: Fever, headache, stiff neck (or bulging anterior fontanelle in infants), irritability, vomiting, lethargy, evolving over hours to 1–2 days. The younger the child, the more nonspecific the presentation (e.g., irritability, lethargy, fever, poor feeding).

Diagnostic Considerations: Diagnosis by CSF chemistries, gram stain, culture. CSF findings are similar to those in adults: pleocytosis (100–5000 WBCs/mm^3; predominately PMNs), ↑ protein, ⇉ glucose. Normal CSF values differ by age:

	WBC/mm^3 (range); %PMNs	Protein, mg/dL (range)	Glucose, mg/dL (range)
Preterm	9 (0–25); 57% PMNs	115 (65–150)	50 (24–63)
Term newborn	8 (0–22); 61% PMNs	90 (20–170)	52 (34–119)
Child	0 (0–7); 0% PMNs	(5–40)	(40–80)

Modified from *The Harriet Lane Handbook*, 15th edition.

Pitfalls: The younger the child, the more nonspecific the presentation. With prior antibiotic use (e.g., oral therapy for otitis media), partially-treated meningitis is a concern; the addition of bacterial antigen or CIE tests may be of diagnostic value in this setting. Especially in the summer season, rapid viral diagnosis (especially enteroviral PCR) can exclude ABM and prevent unnecessary hospitalization and antibiotic use. HSV PCR can also be helpful in excluding ABM.

Therapeutic Considerations: Meningitic doses of antibiotics are required for the *entire* course of treatment. Repeat lumbar puncture (LP) is indicated at 24–48 hours if not responding clinically or in situations where a resistant organism is a concern (e.g., penicillin-resistant S. pneumonia, or neonate with gram-negative bacillary meningitis). Dexamethasone (0.3 mg/kg IV q12h × 2 days) may reduce neurologic sequelae (e.g., hearing loss) in children ≥ 6 weeks of age when given before/with the first dose of antibiotics.

Prognosis: Varies with causative agent and age at presentation. Overall mortality < 5% in US (higher in developing countries). Morbidity 30–35% with hearing loss the most common neurologic sequella. Incidence of neurologic sequelae: S. pneumoniae > H. influenzae > N. meningitidis. Use of H. influenzae (type B) and pneumococcal conjugate vaccines in routine childhood immunizations has reduced the incidence of meningitis caused by these pathogens, but recent emergence of pneumococcal serotype 19A is responsible for continued cases of meningococcal meningitis. Neonates are at increased risk of mortality and major neurologic sequelae, and there is a significant incidence of brain abscesses in neonates with gram-negative meningitis (especially Citrobacter and Serratia infections).

Acute Bacterial Meningitis (CNS Shunt Infections)

Clinical Presentation: Indolent (lethargy, irritability, vomiting) or acute (high fever, depressed mental status).

Diagnostic Considerations: Diagnosis by CSF gram stain/culture, often obtained by shunt tap.

Pitfalls: Blood cultures are usually negative for shunt pathogens and CSF WBCs may be low.

Therapeutic Considerations: High risk of nafcillin resistance with coagulase-negative staphylococcal infection. The addition of rifampin to vancomycin may improve clearance of bacteria. Removal of prosthetic material is usually necessary to achieve a cure.

Prognosis: Good with removal of prosthetic material.

Encephalitis

Subset	Usual Pathogens	IV Therapy†	IV-to-PO Switch†
Herpes	HSV-1	Acyclovir × 14–21 days	Treat IV only
Arbovirus	WNV, SLE, Powassan encephalitis, EEE, WEE, VEE, JE, CE	No specific therapy	
Mycoplasma	M. pneumoniae	Doxycycline **or** minocycline × 2–4 weeks	Doxycycline **or** minocycline × 2–4 weeks

Encephalitis (cont'd)

Subset	Usual Pathogens	IV Therapy†	IV-to-PO Switch†
Respiratory viruses	Influenza, Enteroviruses, Measles	No specific therapy	

Duration of therapy represents total time IV or IV + PO. Most patients on IV therapy able to take PO meds should be switched to PO therapy after clinical improvement. *WNV = West Nile Virus, SLE = St. Louis encephalitis, EEE = Eastern equine encephalitis, WEE = Western equine encephalitis, VEE = Venezuelan equine encephalitis, JE = Japanese encephalitis, CE = California encephalitis.*

† **See pp. 402–410 for drug dosages.**

Herpes Encephalitis (HSV-1)

Clinical Presentation: Acute onset of fever and mental status/behavioral changes. High fever with intractable seizures and profoundly depressed sensorium may dominate the clinical picture.

Diagnostic Considerations: Diagnosis by CSF PCR for HSV-1. CSF findings include ↑ RBC/WBC, ↓ glucose, and ↑↑ protein. Classic EEG changes with temporal lobe spikes may be present early. Brain biopsy is rarely, if ever, indicated.

Pitfalls: MRI/CT scan can be normal initially. Delays in diagnosis and therapy adversely affect outcome.

Therapeutic Considerations: HSV is the only treatable viral encephalitis in normal hosts.

Prognosis: Antiviral therapy improves survival, but based on level of consciousness at presentation, mortality is still 10–20%.

Arboviral Encephalitis

Clinical Presentation: Acute onset of fever, headache, altered mental status. Usually seasonal (more common in summer/fall), based on vector/travel history. Can be very severe with high mortality. Symptomatic West Nile encephalitis is rare in children.

Diagnostic Considerations: Serological studies are the primary means of diagnosis. PCR "encephalitis panels" are being developed for clinical use.

Therapeutic Considerations: No specific antiviral therapy. Supportive therapy is crucial.

Pitfalls: Be sure to elicit potential exposures/travel history in children with fever/altered mental status.

Prognosis: Varies with agent. Severe residual deficits and high mortality rates can occur, especially with Eastern Equine encephalitis.

Mycoplasma Encephalitis

Clinical Presentation: Acute onset of fever and mental status changes. Prodromal cough, sore throat, respiratory symptoms may occur.

Diagnostic Considerations: CSF shows mild pleocytosis with a predominance of mononuclear cells, normal or mildly ↓ glucose, and mildly ↑ protein. Mycoplasma IgG/IgM titers are elevated.

Pitfalls: CSF findings can be confused with viral encephalitis.

Therapeutic Considerations: Often self-limited illness even without antibiotic therapy. Doxycycline or minocycline penetrate CNS and can be used in children > 8 years of age. Macrolides may treat pulmonary infection but do not penetrate CNS.

Prognosis: Good. Neurologic sequelae are rare.

Respiratory Virus Encephalitis

Clinical Presentation: Encephalitis may occur during or immediately after an acute respiratory illness. Influenza encephalitis, although rare, may be especially severe with a number of deaths reported every year in previously healthy children and adolescents.

Diagnostic Considerations: Rarely, adenoviruses have been recovered from CSF or brain in cases of encephalitis. Encephalitis has also been described very rarely in association with RSV and parainfluenza infections as well.

Pitfalls: Most cases of encephalitis remain undiagnosed, in part due to failure to consider and test for respiratory viruses.

Therapeutic Considerations: No evidence to date suggests a benefit of anti-influenza therapy in influenza encephalitis.

Prognosis: Generally self-limited with recovery, but death has been reported with influenza encephalitis. Adenovirus encephalitis in immunocompromised hosts may also be severe.

Empiric Therapy of HEENT Infections

Periorbital (Preseptal) Cellulitis/Orbital Cellulitis

Subset	Usual Pathogens	Preferred IV Therapy†	Alternate IV Therapy†	IV-to-PO Switch†
Periorbital cellulitis	S. pneumoniae H. influenzae M. catarrhalis S. aureus	**Combination therapy with** Nafcillin **plus either** ceftriaxone **or** cefotaxime × 10–14 days	Ampicillin-sulbactam × 10–14 days	Amoxicillin-clavulanate **or** cefuroxime **or** cefpodoxime **or** cefdinir × 10–14 days
Orbital cellulitis	S. pneumoniae H. influenzae M. catarrhalis S. aureus Anaerobes Group A streptococci	**Combination therapy with** Nafcillin **plus** ceftriaxone × 10–14 days	Piperacillin-tazobactam **or** ampicillin-sulbactam **or** ticarcillin-clavulanate × 10–14 days	Amoxicillin-clavulanate **or** cefuroxime **or** cefpodoxime **or** cefdinir × 10–14 days

Duration of therapy represents total time IV or IV + PO. Most patients on IV therapy able to take PO meds should be switched to PO therapy after clinical improvement.

† **See pp. 402–410 for drug dosages.**

Clinical Presentation: Periorbital and orbital cellulitis are bacterial infections. Fever, lid swelling, and erythema around the eye often in conjunction with acute sinusitis. In periorbital cellulitis the infection is anterior to the orbital septum. Orbital cellulitis involves the orbit proper, extraocular muscles/nerves, and possibly the orbital nerve. Proptosis and limitation of ocular mobility define orbital cellulitis.

Diagnostic Considerations: CT scan is used to differentiate preseptal from periorbital cellulitis and identify the extent of orbital involvement when present.

Pitfalls: Failure to recognize orbital involvement leading to optic nerve damage or CNS extension/cavernous sinus thrombosis. CT scan cannot differentiate phlegmon from abscess.

Therapeutic Considerations: Orbital cellulitis is more emergent than periorbital cellulitis and should be treated with IV antibiotics initially. Surgical drainage may be indicated if a well defined abscess is present or in more severe disease.

Prognosis: Good with prompt antimicrobial therapy and ophthalmologic surgery if needed.

Sinusitis

Subset	Usual Pathogens	IV Therapy† (Hospitalized)	PO Therapy or IV-to-PO Switch† (Ambulatory)
Acute	S. pneumoniae H. influenzae M. catarrhalis	Ceftriaxone **or** cefuroxime × 1–2 weeks	Amoxicillin **or** amoxicillin/clavulanic acid **or** cephalosporin **or** clarithromycin* × 10–14 days **or** azithromycin* × 5 days
Chronic	Same as acute + oral anaerobes	Requires prolonged antimicrobial therapy (2–4 weeks)	

Duration of therapy represents total time IV, PO, or IV + PO. Most patients on IV therapy able to take PO meds should be switched to PO therapy soon after clinical improvement (usually < 72 hrs).

* Macrolides may be less effective and should be reserved for penicillin- and cephalosporin-allergic patients.

† **See pp. 402–410 for drug dosages.**

Clinical Presentation: Nasal discharge and cough frequently with headache, facial pain, and low-grade fever lasting > 10–14 days. Can also present acutely with high fever (≥ 104° F) and purulent nasal discharge ± intense headache for ≥ 3 days.

Diagnostic Considerations: Acute sinusitis is a clinical diagnosis. Imaging studies are not routinely indicated. Overlap with acute viral infection and allergic symptoms may make diagnosis difficult.

Pitfalls: Transillumination, sinus tenderness to percussion, and color of nasal mucus are not reliable indicators of sinusitis.

Therapeutic Considerations: Microbiology/antibiotics are similar to acute otitis media, but duration of therapy is 10–14 days. Failure to respond to initial antibiotic therapy suggests a resistant pathogen or an alternative diagnosis. There are insufficient data to support long-course antibiotic treatment. Quinolones not approved for sinusitis.

Prognosis: Good. For frequent recurrences, consider radiologic studies and ENT/allergy consultation.

Otitis Externa

Subset	Usual Pathogens	Topical Therapy
"Swimmer's ear"	Pseudomonas sp. Enterobacteriaceae S. aureus	Polymyxin B plus neomycin **plus** hydrocortisone (eardrops) q6h × 7–10 days **or** Ofloxacin (3% otic solution) q12h × 7–10 days

Clinical Presentation: Ear pain, itching, and sensation of fullness. Pain is exacerbated by tugging on the pinna or tragus of the outer ear. Purulent discharge may be visible in the external ear canal. Fever is generally absent.

Diagnostic Considerations: Otitis externa is a clinical diagnosis. A recent history of swimming or cleaning with cotton swabs is often elicited. Malignant otitis externa, as seen in elderly adults with diabetes mellitus, is extremely rare in children but may be seen in immunocompromised hosts.

Pitfalls: Failure to recognize a ruptured tympanic membrane may lead to a misdiagnosis of otitis externa based on purulence in the canal.

Therapeutic Considerations: Local cleansing (e.g., 2% acetic acid) and topical therapy with corticosporin-polymixin B-neomycin suspension is usually sufficient. Oral antibiotics should be considered for fever/cervical adenitis.

Prognosis: Excellent. Cleansing with 2% acetic acid drops after swimming prevents recurrences.

Acute Otitis Media

Subset	Usual Pathogens	IM Therapy†	PO Therapy†
Initial uncomplicated bacterial infection	S. pneumoniae H. influenzae M. catarrhalis	Ceftriaxone × 1 dose	Amoxicillin × 10 days **or** cefdinir × 10 days** **or** azithromycin (1-, 3-, or 5-day regimen) **or** erythromycin-sulfisoxazole × 10 days** **or** TMP–SMX × 10 days**
Treatment failure or resistant organism*	MRSP Beta-lactamase positive H. influenzae	Ceftriaxone q24h × 3 doses	Amoxicillin/clavulanic acid **or** ES-600†† × 10 days** or cephalosporin × 10 days‡*

DRSP = drug-resistant S. pneumoniae. Pediatric doses are provided; acute otitis media is uncommon in adults. For chronic otitis media, prolonged antimicrobial therapy is required.

† **See pp. 402–410 for drug dosages.**

* Treatment failure = persistent symptoms and otoscopy abnormalities 48–72 hours after starting initial antimicrobial therapy. For risk factors for DRSP, see Therapeutic Considerations, below. If still fails after recommended therapy, consider clindamycin for resistant S. pneumoniae or tympanocentesis for gram stain and culture.

** In children > 6 years of age with mild-moderate acute otitis media, a 5–7 day course of antimicrobial theory may be adequate.

†† ES-600 = 600 mg amoxicillin/5 mL.

‡ 10-day course with either cefuroxime axetil 15 mg/kg (PO) q12h or cefdinir 7 mg/kg (PO) q12h or 14 mg/kg (PO) q24h or cefpodoxime 5 mg/kg (PO) q12h may be used.

Clinical Presentation: Fever, otalgia, hearing loss. Nonspecific presentation is more common in younger children (irritability, fever). Key to diagnosis is examination of the tympanic membrane. Acute otitis media requires evidence of inflammation *and* effusion. Uncommon in adults.
Diagnostic Considerations: Diagnosis is made by finding an opaque, hyperemic, bulging tympanic membrane with loss of landmarks and decreased mobility on pneumatic otoscopy.
Pitfalls: Failure to remove cerumen (inadequate visualization of tympanic membrane) and reliance on history of ear tugging/pain are the main factors associated with overdiagnosis of otitis media. Otitis media with effusion (i.e., tympanic membrane retracted or in normal position with decreased mobility or mobility with negative pressure; fluid present behind the drum but normal in color) usually resolves spontaneously and should not be treated with antibiotics.
Therapeutic Considerations: Risk factors for infection with drug-resistant S. pneumoniae (DRSP) include antibiotic therapy in past 30 days, failure to respond within 48–72 hours of therapy, day care attendance, and antimicrobial prophylaxis. Macrolides and TMP–SMX may predispose to DRSP, and 25% of S. pneumoniae are naturally resistant to macrolides. Quinolones not approved for therapy.
Prognosis: Excellent, but tends to recur. Chronic otitis, cholesteatomas, mastoiditis are rare complications. Tympanostomy tubes/adenoidectomy for frequent recurrences of otitis media are the leading surgical procedures in children.

Mastoiditis

Subset	Usual Pathogens	Preferred IV Therapy†	Alternate IV Therapy†	PO Therapy or IV-to-PO Switch†
Acute	S. pneumoniae S. aureus Group A streptococci H. influenzae	Nafcillin **or** vancomycin (if MRSA suspected) **plus either** ceftriaxone **or** cefotaxime × 10–14 days	Ampicillin-sulbactam × 10–14 days	Amoxicillin-clavulanate **or** cefpodoxime **or** cefdinir × 10–14 days
Chronic	Polymicrobial, including P. aeruginosa, S. aureus, anaerobes, Enterobacteriaceae	Piperacillin **or** ticarcillin × 10–14 days	Meropenem **or** imipenem × 10–14 days	None

Duration of therapy represents total time IV, IV + PO, or PO. Most patients on IV therapy able to take PO meds should be switched to PO therapy after clinical improvement.
† **See pp. 402–410 for drug dosages.**

Clinical Presentation: Fever and otalgia with postauricular swelling/erythema pushing the ear superiorly and laterally. The presentation may be more subtle (e.g., less toxic, less swelling, Bell's palsy alone) in older children partially treated with antibiotics. Concomitant otitis media is rare.
Diagnostic Considerations: Acute mastoiditis is diagnosed clinically, but CT scan is definitive. Tympanocentesis through intact ear drum for aspirate and insertion of tympanostomy tube are helpful for microbiology and drainage, respectively. Chronic mastoiditis is often polymicrobial, including anaerobes and P. aeruginosa. Tuberculosis rarely presents as chronic mastoiditis.

Pitfalls: Do not overlook mastoiditis in older child with unresponsive otitis. Orbital involvement may lead to optic nerve damage or CNS extension/cavernous sinus thrombosis.
Therapeutic Considerations: Treatment is based on microbiology and requires at least 3 weeks of antibiotics.
Prognosis: Good with early treatment.

Pharyngitis

Subset	Usual Pathogens	IV or IM Therapy†	PO Therapy or IV-to-PO Switch†
Exudative (culture)	Group A streptococci	Benzathine penicillin IM × 1 dose	Penicillin V **or** amoxicillin × 10 days. *Alternate*: azithromycin 12 mg/kg/day × 5 days **or** cephalexin **or** cefadroxil **or** erythromycin **or** clarithromycin **or** clindamycin × 10 days
Asymptomatic carrier	Group A streptococci	No treatment indicated	No treatment indicated
Persistent/recurrent disease	Group A streptococci	Clindamycin	Amoxicillin-clavulanate × 10 days **or combination therapy with either** penicillin V **or** amoxicillin × 10 days plus rifampin added on days 7–10
Exudative, sexually active	N. gonorrhoeae	Ceftriaxone (IM) × 1 dose	Quinolone*
Lemierre's Syndrome (Jugular vein septic thrombophlebitis)‡	Fusobacterium necrophorum	Clindamycin (IV) **or** penicillin G (IV) × 4–6 weeks	Clindamycin **or** penicillin VK × 4–6 weeks
Vesicular, ulcerative	Enteroviruses HSV 1 or 2	Primary HSV: Acyclovir × 5–7 days	Primary HSV: Acyclovir **or** valacyclovir × 5–7 days

Duration of therapy represents total time IV, IM, IV + PO, or PO. Most patients on IV therapy able to take PO meds should be switched to PO therapy after clinical improvement.
† **See pp. 402–410 for drug dosages.**
* Likely okay in adolescent although licensed only for age > 18 years. See adult section for agents and dosages.
‡ Treat only IV or IV-to-PO switch.

Clinical Presentation: Acute sore throat and fever with tender cervical lymphadenitis. Primary clinical consideration is differentiating Group A streptococci (GAS) from viral/other causes (e.g., adenovirus, enterovirus, respiratory viruses, other strep groups [C, G], Arcanobacterium hemolyticum, M. pneumoniae, C. pneumoniae, EBV). GAS is less likely with concomitant coryza, conjunctivitis, hoarseness, cough, acute stomatitis, discrete oral ulcerations, or diarrhea–children with these manifestations should not be cultured routinely.

Diagnostic Considerations: Laboratory testing for GAS is recommended, since clinical differentiation of viral pharyngitis from GAS is not possible. Rapid tests for GAS antigens are reliable with excellent specificities, but due to variable sensitivities of the assays, a negative rapid test should be confirmed by a throat culture. The accuracy of antigen and culture tests is dependent on obtaining a good throat swab containing pharyngeal/tonsillar secretions.

Pitfalls: Be sure to obtain a good throat swab. Post-treatment testing is generally not recommended unless the patient is at high risk for rheumatic fever (e.g., family history, ongoing outbreak) or is still symptomatic after 10 days of therapy. Asymptomatic GAS carriers do not require antibiotic therapy, but identifying a "true carrier" may be difficult. Eradication of GAS carriage should be considered in the following situations: an outbreak of acute rheumatic fever or post-streptococcal glomerulonephritis; an outbreak of GAS in a closed community; a family history of rheumatic fever; multiple episodes of GAS infection within the family for many weeks despite therapy; family anxiety about the presence of GAS; or tonsillectomy is being considered based on persistent carriage. Eradication is achieved using the same antimicrobial regimen as for "persistent/recurrent disease" (see treatment grid).

Therapeutic Considerations: Penicillin V (or amoxicillin) is the drug of choice for GAS pharyngitis. Erythromycin is still considered the drug of choice for penicillin-allergic individuals, although macrolide-resistant GAS strains are being reported. First-generation cephalosporins are also useful alternatives. Broader spectrum agents, although likely effective, should not be used routinely. Tetracyclines and sulfonamides do not eradicate GAS pharyngitis. When eradication of carriage is indicated as noted above, clindamycin alone or penicillin plus rifampin may be useful.

Prognosis: Excellent. Rheumatic fever is rare in the US.

Empiric Therapy of Lower Respiratory Tract Infections

Community-Acquired Pneumonia

Subset (age)	Usual Pathogens	IV Therapy†	PO Therapy or IV-to-PO Switch†
Community-acquired pneumonia *Birth to 20 days*	Group B streptococci, Gram-negative enteric bacteria, CMV	Ampicillin **plus either** gentamicin **or** cefotaxime × 10–21 days	Not applicable

Duration of therapy represents total time IV or IV, PO, or IV + PO. Most patients on IV therapy able to take PO meds should be switched to PO therapy after clinical improvement.

† **See pp. 402–410 for drug dosages.**

Community-Acquired Pneumonia (cont'd)

Subset (age)	Usual Pathogens	IV Therapy[†]	PO Therapy or IV-to-PO Switch[†]
3 weeks to 3 months	RSV Parainfluenza Human metapneumovirus (hmpv)	None (supportive care)	None
	C. trachomatis S. pneumoniae B. pertussis S. aureus	Cefotaxime **or** ceftriaxone × 10–14 days*. Alternative: ampicillin **or** clindamycin*	Afebrile: Erythromycin × 14 days **or** azithromycin × 5–7 days. Lobar, febrile: Amoxicillin **or** amoxicillin/clavulanic acid **or** cefdinir **or** cefuroxime **or** cefpodoxime × 10–14 days
> 3 months to < 5 years	Viruses (RSV, parainfluenza, influenza, adenovirus, rhinoviruses)	RSV: consider ribavirin.[§] For infants at highest risk for severe RSV infection, consider palivizumab 15 mg/kg/month × 1–2 seasons for prevention. Influenza: Amantadine (influenza A) or oseltamivir (influenza A, B).[¶] Routine immunization for infants 6–23 months of age	
	S. pneumoniae H. influenzae M. pneumoniae	Ceftriaxone **or** cefotaxime **or** ertapenem × 10–14 days*	Amoxicillin **or** amoxicillin-clavulanate **or** clarithromycin **or** azithromycin × 10–14 days
5–15 years	M. pneumoniae C. pneumoniae S. pneumoniae	Ceftriaxone **or** cefotaxime **or** ertapenem × 10–14 days*	Erythromycin **or** clarithromycin **or** azithromycin **or** doxycycline (age > 8 years) × 10–14 days
Pertussis	Bordetella spp.[‡] certain Adenoviruses M. pneumoniae C. trachomatis C. pneumoniae	Azithromycin × 5 days **or** erythromycin × 14 days	Erythromycin estolate × 14 days **or** clarithromycin × 7 days **or** azithromycin × 5 days. If macrolide-intolerant: TMP–SMX × 14 days
Tuberculosis	M. tuberculosis	See p. 389	See p. 389

Duration of therapy represents total time IV or IV, PO, or IV + PO. Most patients on IV therapy able to take PO meds should be switched to PO therapy after clinical improvement.

† **See pp. 402–410 for drug dosages.**

* If chronic cough of more insidious onset, consider adding IV or PO macrolide (azithromycin, clarithromycin, erythromycin) to cover Pertussis/C. trachomatis (3 weeks–3 months of age), Mycoplasma (3 months–5 years of age), or Mycoplasma/C. pneumoniae (5–15 years of age).

‡ B. pertussis, B. parapertussis, B. bronchiseptica.

§ Use should be limited to the most severely ill with RSV, i.e., transplant patients.

¶ Amantadine resistance may limit use in influenza A.

Community-Acquired Pneumonia

Clinical Presentation: Fever ± dyspnea, cough, tachypnea with infiltrates on chest x-ray.

Diagnostic Considerations: Usual pathogens differ by age. In neonates, pneumonia is typically diffuse and part of early-onset sepsis. In young infants, there is significant overlap between signs and symptoms of bronchiolitis (primarily due to RSVU) and pneumonia. Severe pneumonia is usually due to bacterial infection, although the organism is frequently not isolated (e.g., blood cultures are positive in only 10–20% of children < 2 years of age with bacterial pneumonia). In young infants, Chlamydia trachomatis can be detected by antigen assay or culture of nasopharyngeal (NP) secretions. Mycoplasma pneumonia, diagnosed by cold agglutinins and IgG/IgM serologies, peaks at 5–15 years of age, although cases in children < 5 years have been reported. Respiratory viruses (RSV, influenza, adenoviruses, parainfluenza viruses, hmpv) can also be detected in NP secretions. If child lives in area with high prevalence of tuberculosis, consider tuberculosis in the differential diagnosis of primary pneumonia.

Pitfalls: Reliance on upper airway specimen for gram stain/culture leads to misdiagnosis and mistreatment, as true deep sputum specimen is rarely obtainable in children.

Therapeutic Considerations: Therapy is primarily empiric based on child's age, clinical/epidemiologic features and chest x-ray findings. Mycoplasma requires 2–3 weeks of treatment; C. pneumoniae may require up to 6 weeks of treatment. Routine use of conjugated pneumococcal vaccine (Prevnar) has decreased the incidence of pneumococcal pneumonia.

Prognosis: Varies with pathogen, clinical condition at presentation, and underlying health status. Prognosis is worse in children with chronic lung disease, congenital heart disease, immunodeficiency, neuromuscular disease, hemoglobinopathy.

Lower Respiratory Tract Infections due to Respiratory Viruses

Clinical Presentation: Viruses cause the majority of lower respiratory tract infections (LRTIs) in children. Respiratory syncytial virus (RSV) is the leading cause of LRTI in young infants, manifesting as bronchiolitis/viral pneumonia and causing annual mid-winter epidemics. The risk of secondary bacterial infection (other than possibly otitis media) is very low. Fever is typically low grade and usually improves over 3–5 days, even if hospitalized. Influenza viruses are another major cause of winter epidemic LRTIs in children of all ages. Hospitalization rates in infants under one year of age rival those in the > 65 year old population. Characteristic findings include high fever and diffuse inflammation of the airways. Young infants may have prominent GI symptoms as well. Secondary bacterial infection (otitis media, pneumonia, sepsis) are frequent complications of influenza. Primary influenza pneumonia, encephalopathy, and myocarditis are rare, severe complications. Other respiratory viruses associated with LRTIs in children include parainfluenza type 3 (viral pneumonia), parainfluenza types 1 and 2 (croup), adenoviruses, and the recently identified human metapneumovirus (hmpv). Swine influenza (H_1N_1) in children resembles that in adults with some important differences. In adults and children, leukocytosis rather than leukopenia is the role, otherwise unexplained relative lymphopenia is a cardinal finding in adults but is uncommon in children. In children, lymphocytosis is usual. Atypical lymphocytes are common in children, but are not present in adults with H_1N_1. Thrombocytopenia is common in both children and adults.

Diagnostic Considerations: Viral syndromes are often diagnosed based on clinical assessment alone. For confirmation or in more severe cases, rapid diagnosis by antigen detection (direct fluorescent antibody staining, ELISA, PCR) and/or viral culture are readily available.

Pitfalls: Routine use of corticosteroids or bronchodilators in RSV bronchiolitis are not supported by clinical evidence. Overuse of the diagnosis of "flu" (e.g., stomach flu, summer flu) has led to diluted appreciation for true influenza and its severity. Influenza vaccine has been traditionally underutilized in high-risk children with swine influenza (H_1N_1), as in adults, rapid influenza diagnostic tests (RIDTs) are falsely negative in > 30%.

Therapeutic Considerations: For most viral LRTIs treatment is primarily supportive (e.g., adequate hydration, fever control, supplemental oxygen for severe illness). Ribavirin is approved for RSV infection but is very rarely used due to uncertain clinical benefit, high cost, and cumbersome method of administration (prolonged aerosol). For infants at greatest risk of severe RSV disease (e.g., premature infants, infants with underlying chronic lung disease or congenital heart disease), monthly prophylaxis with palivizumab (Synagis) 15 mg/kg/month (IM) decreases RSV hospitalization rates. Per American Academy of Pediatrics guidelines, palivizumab is indicated for infants with chronic lung disease or congenital heart disease who are ≤ 24 months of age at start of RSV season. For premature infants, palivizumab is considered based on a combination of gestational age (GA) and chronological age (CA): GA ≤ 28 weeks plus CA ≤ 12 months; GA 29–32 weeks plus CA ≤ 6 months; GA 33–35 weeks plus CA ≤ 6 months plus 2 or more additional risk factors, including day care attendance, school-age siblings, cigarette smoke exposure, neuromuscular disease, or congenital airway anomalies. Annual influenza vaccination is indicated for high-risk children, including those > 6 months of age with asthma, metabolic disease, hemoglobinopathies, immunocompromised state, renal disease, or heart disease. Children who live with high-risk individuals (e.g., adult > 65 years of age, infant < 6 months of age, immunocompromised host) should also receive influenza vaccine. Additionally the ACIP, AAP, and AAFP recommend routine immunization for all children 6–59 months of age. The antiviral drugs amantadine (influenza A only) and oseltamivir (influenza A and B strains) have pediatric indications and can be used for treatment or prophylaxis as in adults. Some influenza A isolates may be amantadine resistant. Use Ostelamivir for swine influenza (H_1N_1) prophylaxis and therapy (Tables 7.1–7.3).

Table 7.1. Swine Influenza (H_1N_1) Antiviral Medication Dosing Recommendations

Antiviral		Treatment	Chemoprophylaxis
Oseltamivir			
Adults		75-mg capsule twice per day × 5 days	75-mg capsule once per day × 10 days
Children (age, 12 months or older), weight:	15 kg or less	60 mg per day divided into 2 doses	30 mg once per day
	15–23 kg	90 mg per day divided into 2 doses	45 mg once per day
	24–40 kg	120 mg per day divided into 2 doses	60 mg once per day
	> 40 kg	150 mg per day divided into 2 doses	75 mg once per day
Zanamivir			
Adults		Two 5-mg inhalations (10 mg total) twice per day	Two 5-mg inhalations (10 mg total) once per day
Children		Two 5-mg inhalations (10 mg total) twice per day (age, 7 years or older)	Two 5-mg inhalations (10 mg total) once per day (age, 5 years or older)

Table 7.2. Dosing Recommendations for Antiviral Treatment of Children Younger than 1 Year Using Oseltamivir

Age	Recommended Treatment Dose for 5 Days
< 3 months	12 mg twice daily
3–5 months	20 mg twice daily
6–11 months	25 mg twice daily

Table 7.3. Dosing Recommendations for Antiviral Chemoprophylaxis of Children Younger than 1 Year Using Oseltamivir

Age	Recommended Prophylaxis Dose for 10 Days
< 3 months	Not recommended unless situation judged critical due to limited data on use in this age group
3–5 months	20 mg once daily
6–11 months	25 mg once daily

Adapted from: http://www.journals.uchicago.edu/doi/full/10.1086/598513

Prognosis: Most children with viral LRTIs do well and recover without sequelae. Infants hospitalized with RSV infection have higher rates of wheezing episodes over the next 10 years. The highest rates of hospitalization from influenza occur in children < 2 years of age and in the elderly.

Pertussis

Clinical Presentation: Upper respiratory tract symptoms (congestion, rhinorrhea) over 1–2 weeks (catarrhal stage) progressing to paroxysms of cough (paroxysmal stage) lasting 2–4 weeks, often with a characteristic inspiratory whoop, followed by a convalescent stage lasting 1–2 weeks during which cough paroxysms decrease in frequency and severity. Fever is low grade or absent. In children < 6 months, whoop is frequently absent and apnea may occur. Duration of classic pertussis is 6–10 weeks. Older children and adults may present with persistent cough (without whoop) lasting 2–6 weeks. Complications include seizures, secondary bacterial pneumonia, encephalopathy, death; risk of complications is greatest in children < 1 year.

Diagnostic Considerations: Diagnosis is usually based on nature of cough and duration of symptoms. Laboratory diagnosis may be difficult. A positive culture for Bordetella pertussis from a nasopharyngeal swab inoculated on fresh selective media is diagnostic, but the organism is difficult to recover after 3–4 weeks of illness. Direct fluorescent antibody (DFA) staining of nasopharyngeal secretions is available, but sensitivities/specificities are variable to poor. Leukocytosis with lymphocytosis may be present in pertussis but can occur in response to other respiratory pathogens.

Pitfalls: Be sure to consider pertussis in older children and adults with prolonged coughing illness. Family contacts of index case should receive post-exposure antimicrobial prophylaxis. Virtually all children should be vaccinated against pertussis. A single booster dose of acellular pertussis is recommended at 11–12 years of age (additional guidelines for catch-up for older adolescents and adults up to 64 years of age). Rare contraindications to pertussis vaccination include anaphylaxis to a prior dose or encephalopathy within 7 days of a dose. Relative precautions to further pertussis immunization include: seizure within 3 days of a dose;

persistent, severe, inconsolable crying for ≥ 3 hours within 48 hours of a dose; collapse or shock-like state within 48 hours of a dose; or temperature of ≥ 40.5° C without other cause within 48 hours of a dose.

Therapeutic Considerations: Infants < 6 months frequently require hospitalization. By the paroxysmal stage, antibiotics have minimal effect on the course of the illness but are still indicated to decrease transmission. An association has been made between oral erythromycin and infantile hypertrophic pyloric stenosis in infants < 6 weeks of age; consider an alternative macrolide (azithromycin or clarithromycin) in these cases.

Prognosis: Good. Despite the prolonged course, long-term pulmonary sequelae have not been described after pertussis. Children < 1 year are at greatest risk of morbidity and mortality, although mortality rates remain very low.

Tuberculosis

Subset	Pathogen	PO or IM Therapy (see footnote for drug dosages)
Latent infection (positive PPD, clinically well, negative chest x-ray)	M. tuberculosis	INH × 9 months **or** rifampin × 6 months (if INH-resistant)
Pulmonary and extrapulmonary TB (except meningitis)	M. tuberculosis	INH **plus** rifampin **plus** PZA × 2 months followed by INH **plus** rifampin × 4 months†
Meningitis	M. tuberculosis	INH **plus** rifampin **plus** PZA **plus either** streptomycin (IM) **or** ethionamide × 2 months, followed by INH **plus** rifampin × 7–10 months (i.e., 9–12 months total therapy)‡
Congenital	M. tuberculosis	INH **plus** rifampin **plus** PZA **plus** streptomycin (IM)

Duration of therapy represents total time IV or IV, PO, or IV + PO. Most patients on IV therapy able to take PO meds should be switched to PO therapy after clinical improvement.

† If drug resistance is a concern, EMB or streptomycin (IM) is added (4-drug regimen in areas where MDR TB is prevalent) to the initial regimen until drug susceptibilities are determined.

‡ Plus steroids.

TB Drug	Daily dosage (mg/kg)	Twice weekly dosage (mg/kg)
Isoniazid (INH)	10–15	20–30
Rifampin	10–20	10–20
Ethambutol (EMB)	15–25	50
Pyrazinamide (PZA)	20–40	50
Streptomycin	20–40 (IM)	–
Ethionamide	15–20 (in 2–3 divided doses/day)	–

Alternative drugs (capreomycin, ciprofloxacin, levofloxacin, cycloserine, kanamycin, para-aminosalicylic acid) are used less commonly and should be administered in consultation with an expert in the treatment of tuberculosis.

Tuberculosis

Clinical Presentation: Most children diagnosed with tuberculosis have asymptomatic infection detected by tuberculin skin testing. Symptomatic disease typically presents 1–6 months after infection with fever, growth delay, weight loss, night sweats, and cough. Extrapulmonary involvement may present with meningitis, chronic mastoiditis, lymphadenopathy, bone, joint, or skin involvement. Renal tuberculosis and reactivation cavitary disease are rare in children but may be seen in adolescents.

Diagnostic Considerations: A positive tuberculin skin test indicates likely infection with M. tuberculosis. Tuberculin reactivity develops 2–12 weeks after infection. The definition of a positive skin test reaction is based on age, immune status, risk of exposure, and degree of suspicion of tuberculosis disease. Children < 8 years old cannot produce sputum for AFB smear and culture; specimens for analysis can be obtained by collecting 3 consecutive morning gastric aspirates.

Pitfalls: Tuberculosis may be missed if not considering the diagnosis in children at increased epidemiological risk for exposure. Tuberculous meningitis often presents insidiously with nonspecific irritability and lethargy weeks prior to the development of frank neurological defects.

Therapeutic Considerations: Choice of initial therapy depends on stage of disease and likelihood of resistant organisms (based on index case, geographical region of acquisition). For HIV-infected patients, duration of therapy is prolonged to ≥ 12 months. For tuberculosis meningitis and miliary disease, the addition of corticosteroids to anti-TB therapy is beneficial.

Prognosis: Varies with extent of disease, drug resistance and underlying immune status, but is generally good for pulmonary disease in children. Bone infection may result in orthopedic sequelae (e.g., Pott's disease of the spine with vertebral collapse). The prognosis for meningitis is guarded once focal neurological deficits and persistent depression of mental status occur.

Empiric Therapy of Vascular Infections

IV Catheter Infections (Broviac, Hickman, Mediport)

Subset	Usual Pathogens	Preferred IV Therapy†	Alternate IV Therapy†
Empiric; immunocompromised host	S. epidermidis S. aureus¶ Enterobacteriaceae Pseudomonas Viridans Streptococci Enterococcus	Meropenem **or** piperacillin/tazobactam **or** cefepime × 7–14 days	Piperacillin/tazobactam **plus** an aminoglycoside × 7–14 days
Isolate-based	S. aureus *MSSA*	Nafcillin **or** oxacillin for ≥ 2 weeks	Cefazolin **or** vancomycin (preferred if severe beta-lactam allergy) for ≥ 2 weeks

IV Catheter Infections (Broviac, Hickman, Mediport) (cont'd)

Subset	Usual Pathogens	Preferred IV Therapy†	Alternate IV Therapy†
	MRSA	Vancomycin **with or without** gentamicin (for potential synergy) for ≥ 2 weeks	Linezolid **or** quinupristindalfopristin for ≥ 2 weeks (addition of rifampin may be of benefit, for MRSA)
	Enterobacteriaceae Pseudomonas	Piperacillin **or** ticarcillin **with or without** an aminoglycoside* for ≥ 2 weeks	Meropenem **or** imipenem **with or without** an aminoglycoside* for ≥ 2 weeks
	ESBL-producing gram-negative bacilli	Meropenem **or** imipenem **with or without** an aminoglycoside* for ≥ 2 weeks	–
	Candida	Amphotericin B × 2–6 weeks‡	Fluconazole **or** caspofungin **or** liposomal amphotericin B (if renal dysfunction) × 2–6 weeks‡

MSSA/MRSA = methicillin-sensitive/resistant S. aureus. Duration of therapy represents total time IV.

† **See pp. 402–410 for drug dosages.**

* Gentamicin, tobramycin, or amikacin.

‡ Based on promptness of line removal, clearance of blood cultures, evidence of metastatic foci.

¶ If severely ill or suspicion of MRSA based on local epidemiology, include vancomycin in initial regimen pending culture results.

Clinical Presentation: Fever ± site tenderness, erythema.

Diagnostic considerations: Quantitative blood cultures from the peripheral blood/vascular catheter are best used to make the diagnosis. However in clinical practice these are not often obtained, and the diagnosis is based on culture results in conjunction with one or more of the following features: local phlebitis or inflammation at the catheter insertion site; embolic disease distal to the catheter; sepsis refractory to appropriate therapy; resolution of fever after device removal; or clustered infections caused by infusion-associated organisms.

Pitfalls: It may be difficult to differentiate infection from contamination in blood cultures, especially with coagulase-negative staphylococci. Multiple positive cultures with the same organism and/or clinical features noted above suggest infection, not colonization. Semiquantitative culture of the catheter tip yielding ≥ 15 colonies may also be useful in confirming the diagnosis but requires removal of the device.

Therapeutic Considerations: Indications for catheter removal include septic shock, tunnel infection, failure to respond to treatment within 48–72 hours, or infection with Candida, atypical mycobacteria, or possibly S. aureus. Otherwise attempt to retain the catheter while treating with antibiotics. Localized exit site infections (erythema, induration, tenderness, purulence) within 2 cm of the exit site should be treated topically (e.g., Neosporin, Bacitracin, Bactroban) in conjunction with systemic therapy.

Prognosis: Major complications (septic emboli, endocarditis, vasculitis) are rare with aggressive therapy. Recrudescent infection can occur after therapy/apparent clearance and can often be successfully treated with additional courses of antibiotics; persistence ultimately requires line removal.

Empiric Therapy of Gastrointestinal Infections

Acute Diarrheal Syndromes (Gastroenteritis)

Subset	Usual Pathogens	Preferred Therapy†	Alternate Therapy†
Community-acquired	Viruses (Rotavirus, Norwalk agent, enteric adenovirus, enteroviruses)	No specific therapy indicated	No specific therapy indicated
	Salmonella non-typhi	Ceftriaxone (IV) **or** cefotaxime (IV) × 10–14 days*	TMP–SMX (IV or PO) **or** amoxicillin (PO) **or** cefixime (PO) × 10–14 days
	Shigella	Ceftriaxone (IV) **or** azithromycin (PO) × 5 days	TMP–SMX (PO) **or** cefixime (PO) **or** ampicillin (PO) × 5 days
	Campylobacter	Erythromycin (PO) × 7 days **or** azithromycin (PO) × 5 days	Doxycycline (PO) (> 8 year old) × 7 days
	Yersinia enterocolitica	TMP–SMX (PO) × 5–7 days	Cefotaxime (IV) **or** tetracycline (PO) **or** doxycycline (PO) × 5–7 days
Traveler's diarrhea	E. coli	TMP–SMX (PO) × 3 days	Azithromycin (PO) × 3 days
Typhoid (Enteric) fever	Salmonella typhi	Ceftriaxone (IV) **or** cefotaxime (IV) × 10–14 days	TMP–SMX (IV or PO) **or** amoxicillin (PO) **or** cefixime (PO) × 10–14 days
Antibiotic-associated colitis	Clostridium difficile	Metronidazole (PO) × 7–10 days **or** nitazoxanide (PO) × 3 days	Vancomycin (PO) × 7–10 days
Chronic watery diarrhea	Giardia lamblia‡	Metronidazole (PO) × 5–7 days **or** nitazoxanide (PO) × 3 days	Tinidazole (PO) × 1 dose **or** furazolidone (PO) × 7–10 days **or** albendazole × 5–7 days

Acute Diarrheal Syndromes (Gastroenteritis) (cont'd)

Subset	Usual Pathogens	Preferred Therapy†	Alternate Therapy†
	Cryptosporidia‡	Nitazoxanide (PO) × 3 days	Human immunoglobulin (PO) **or** bovine colostrum (PO) for immunocompromised hosts
Acute dysentery	E. histolytica	Metronidazole (PO) × 10 days **followed by either** iodoquinol (PO) × 20 days **or** paromomycin (PO) × 7 days	Tinidazole (PO) × 3–5 days **followed by either** iodoquinol (PO) × 20 days **or** paromomycin (PO) × 7 days
	Shigella**	Ceftriaxone (IV) **or** azithromycin (PO) × 5 days	TMP–SMX (PO) **or** cefixime (PO) **or** ampicillin (PO) × 5 days

† **See pp. 402–410 for drug dosages.**

* Therapy only indicated in child < 3 to 6 months of age, immunocompromised host, or toxic appearing child.

** Mild cases acquire no antibiotic therapy. However, antibiotic therapy shortens durations of symptoms and by decreasing the duration of diarrhea limits potential syneral.

‡ May also present as acute watery diarrhea.

Acute Gastroenteritis (Community-Acquired)

Clinical Presentation: Typically presents with the acute onset of diarrhea with fever. This is not an indication for antibiotic therapy unless illness is severe (≥ 6 unformed stools/day, fever ≥ 102° F, bloody stools). Travel history regarding risk for potential E. coli and parasitic exposures is important.

Diagnostic Considerations: In the absence of blood in the stools viruses are the most common cause of acute community-acquired gastroenteritis. Rotaviruses are the most common cause of acute gastroenteritis in 4–24 month old children. Enteric adenoviruses, Norwalk-like virus, enteroviruses and astroviruses are common causes of gastroenteritis in older children. Commercially available antigen tests using ELISA or latex agglutination techniques are readily available to detect rotavirus. Testing for the other viral agents may not be as readily available. Inflammatory changes (presence of white blood cells and/or blood) in the stool are more consistent with bacterial infection. When requesting stool cultures, it may be necessary to order special conditions/media for the detection of yersinia or E. coli O157.

Pitfalls: Antimotility drugs may worsen the course of illness in children with colitis. Empiric therapy with antibiotics may prolong the carriage of Salmonella or increase the risk for developing hemolytic uremic syndrome (HUS) with E. coli O157 infection. The benefit of antibiotics in treating diarrhea caused by yersinia is also unproven. Thus, antibiotic therapy is not routinely indicated prior to culture results in most instances of diarrheal disease, especially as most such infections are self-limited.

Therapeutic Considerations: As above, pending cultures in the absence of severe symptoms or dysentery antibiotics may not be indicated. Overall, the fluoroquinolones have the most complete spectrum for pathogens causing bacterial diarrhea but are not presently approved for use in children < 18 years of age.

Prognosis: Good. Up to 5–10% of children with E. coli O157 are at risk for hemolytic-uremic syndrome.

Giardiasis (Giardia lamblia)

Clinical Presentation: Giardia lamblia is the most common parasite causing diarrheal illness in children. Giardiasis may present as acute watery diarrhea with abdominal pain and bloating or as a chronic, intermittent illness with foul smelling stools, abdominal distension, and anorexia.

Diagnostic Considerations: Trophozoites or cysts of Giardia lamblia can be identified in direct examination of infected stools with 75%–95% sensitivity on a single specimen. Testing 3 or more stools further increases sensitivity of detection. If giardiasis is suspected with negative stool tests, examination of duodenal contents (Entero- or string test) may be helpful.

Pitfalls: Asymptomatic infection is commonly seen in children in day care; therefore, indications to treat must take into account stool testing results *and* clinical findings.

Therapeutic Considerations: Treatment failures occur commonly, and retreatment with the same initial drug is recommended. Furazolidone is the only pediatric liquid available for treating giardiasis.

Prognosis: Good.

Cryptosporidiosis

Clinical Presentation: Usually presents as fever, vomiting, and non-bloody, watery diarrhea. Infection may also be asymptomatic. More severe and chronic infection is seen in immunocompromised patients (e.g., HIV infection). Cryptosporidia parasite is resistant to chlorine and maybe transmitted in swimming pools. Transmission can also occur from livestock, and a major outbreak through contamination of a public water supply has been reported.

Diagnostic Considerations: Cryptosporidium cysts are detected by microscopic examination of Kinyoun-stained stool specimens using a sucrose floatation method or formalin-ethyl acetate method to concentrate oocysts. This test is not part of routine stool ova and parasite examination and must be specifically requested. Shedding is intermittent; therefore, 3 stool samples should be submitted for optimal detection.

Pitfalls: The oocysts of cryptosporidium are small and may be missed by an inexperienced examiner. A commercially available ELISA test is available but may have false-positive and false-negative results.

Therapeutic Considerations: Treatment failures are frequent. In immunocompromised hosts oral human immune globulin and bovine colostrum are beneficial. Improvement in CD_4 counts with antiretroviral therapy in HIV-infected patients shortens the clinical illness.

Prognosis: Good. Recovery may take months.

Amebiasis (Entamoeba histolytica)

Clinical Presentation: E. histolytica can lead to a spectrum of clinical illnesses from asymptomatic infection to acute dysentery to fulminant colitis. Disseminated disease, primarily manifest as hepatic abscesses, can also occur. E. histolytica is most prevalent in developing countries and is transmitted by the fecal-oral route.

Diagnostic Considerations: Trophozoites or cysts of E. histolytica can be identified in stool specimens. In more severe disease (amebic colitis, hepatic abscesses), serum antibodies can be detected.
Pitfalls: Treatment with steroids or antimotility drugs can worsen symptoms and should not be used.
Therapeutic Considerations: Treatment is two-staged to eliminate tissue-invading trophozoites and organisms in the intestinal lumen. Surgical drainage of large hepatic abscesses may be beneficial.
Prognosis: Good.

Antibiotic-Associated Colitis (Clostridirim difficile)

Clinical Presentation: Classically occurs in a child receiving antibiotic therapy and presents as diarrhea, cramping, bloody/mucousy stools, abdominal tenderness, fever, and toxicity. It may also present weeks after a course of antibiotics.
Diagnostic Considerations: C. difficile toxin can be detected with commercially available immunoassays. Endoscopic finding of pseudomembranous colitis is the definitive method of diagnosis although rarely indicated.
Pitfalls: C. difficile may be normal flora in infants < 1 year of age and probably does not cause illness in this age group. The finding of C. difficile toxin in an infant should not be equated with cause and additional evaluations should be perused. Antimotility drugs may worsen symptoms and should be avoided.
Therapeutic Considerations: Cessation of antibiotics is recommended if possible in the presence of significant C. difficile colitis. Patients with severe symptoms or persistent diarrhea × 2–3 days after discontinuing antibiotics should then be treated with oral metronidazole or oral vancomycin. Up to 10–20% relapse after a single course; re-treatment using the same initial antibiotic is recommended.
Prognosis: Good.

Empiric Therapy of Bone and Joint Infections

Septic Arthritis

Subset	Usual Pathogens	Preferred IV Therapy†*	Alternate IV Therapy†*	IV-to-PO Switch†
Newborns (≤ 3 months)	S. aureus‡ Group B streptococci Enterobacteriaceae N. gonorrhea	**Combination therapy with** nafcillin **or** vancomycin **plus either** ceftriaxone **or** cefotaxime*	**Combination therapy with** vancomycin **or** clindamycin **plus either** ceftriaxone **or** cefotaxime **or** gentamicin **or** tobramycin*	Not applicable

† **See pp. 402–410 for drug dosages.**
* Total duration of therapy for non-gonococcal septic arthritis ≥ 3 weeks based on clinical response.
‡ If CA-MRSA is suspected based on clinical presentation/local epidemiology, consider empiric coverage for CA-MRSA with clindamycin, TMP–SMX, doxycycline, or vancomycin pending culture results.

Septic Arthritis (cont'd)

Subset	Usual Pathogens	Preferred IV Therapy†*	Alternate IV Therapy†*	IV-to-PO Switch†
Child (> 3 months to 14 years)	S. aureus‡ Group A streptococci S. pneumoniae Gram-negative bacilli N. meningitidis (H. influenza type b in prevaccine era) Kingella	**Combination therapy with** nafcillin **or** vancomycin **plus either** ceftriaxone **or** cefotaxime*	**Combination therapy with** vancomycin **or** clindamycin **plus either** ceftriaxone **or** cefotaxime*	Dicloxacillin **or** cephalexin **or** clindamycin (PO) after 1 week of IV therapy*
Adolescents (sexually active)	As above plus N. gonorrhoeae (typically 2 or 3 joints involved)	**Combination therapy with** nafcillin **or** vancomycin **plus either** ceftriaxone **or** cefotaxime*	<u>If GC isolated and penicillin allergy:</u> Ciprofloxacin **or** ofloxacin **or** spectinomycin	GC arthritis with prompt response to IV therapy may switch to ciprofloxacin **or** ofloxacin **or** cefixime to complete 7 days of total therapy

Duration of therapy represents total time IV or IV + PO. Most patients on IV therapy able to take PO meds should be switched to PO therapy after clinical improvement. Taper to individual drug therapy once organism isolated and sensitivities are available.

† **See pp. 402–410 for drug dosages**.

* Total duration of therapy for non-gonococcal septic arthritis ≥ 3 weeks based on clinical response.

‡ If CA-MRSA is suspected based on clinical presentation/local epidemiology, consider empiric coverage for CA-MRSA with clindamycin, TMP–SMX, doxycycline, or vancomycin pending culture results.

Clinical Presentation: Varies with age of the child. Presentation is often nonspecific in infants (i.e., fever, poor feeding, tachycardia). Physical exam findings can be subtle: asymmetrical tissue folds, unilateral swelling of an extremity, subtle changes in limb/joint position. In older children, signs and symptoms are more localized to the involved joint. Commonly affected joints: hips, elbows, knees.

Diagnostic Considerations: Joint aspiration (large-bore needle) shows 50,000–250,000 WBCs/mm^3 with a marked predominance of PMNs. Gram stain/culture of joint fluid confirm the diagnosis. Toxic synovitis, Lyme arthritis, rheumatoid arthritis, traumatic arthritis, and sympathetic effusion from adjacent osteomyelitis can mimic septic arthritis on presentation, but joint fluid has fewer WBCs and cultures are negative. Multiple joint involvement is more typical of rheumatic/Lyme disease. In young infants, persistence of the nutrient artery can lead to osteomyelitis and septic arthritis.

Pitfalls: Septic arthritis of the hip is an emergency concomitant condition requiring prompt joint aspiration and irrigation to minimize the risk of femoral head necrosis, which may occur within 24 hours. Toxic synovitis of the hip, which is treated with anti-inflammatory agents and observation, typically causes less fever, pain, and leukocytosis than septic arthritis; however, at times the two can not be differentiated and aspiration of the joint is indicated. In sexually active adolescents, consider N. gonorrhea and culture aspirate.

Therapeutic Considerations: IV therapy is recommended for at least 3–4 weeks, followed by oral therapy for a total antibiotic course of 4–6 weeks based on clinical response and laboratory parameters (WBC, ESR, CRP). Intra-articular therapy is not helpful. Empiric coverage is broader than for osteomyelitis in children.

Prognosis: Good with prompt joint aspiration and at least 3 weeks of antibiotics.

Acute Osteomyelitis, Osteochondritis, Diskitis

Subset	Usual Pathogens	Preferred IV Therapy†	Alternate IV Therapy†	IV-to-PO Switch or PO Therapy†
Acute osteomyelitis Newborn (0–3 months)	S. aureus§ Gram-negative bacilli Group B streptococci	**Combination therapy with** nafcillin **or** oxacillin **plus either** cefotaxime **or** ceftriaxone × 4–6 weeks	Vancomycin **plus either** cefotaxime **or** ceftriaxone × 4–6 weeks	Not applicable
> 3 months*	S. aureus§ Group A streptococci Gram-negative bacteria (rare) Salmonella (sickle cell disease)	Nafcillin **or** oxacillin **or** cefazolin × 4–6 weeks	Clindamycin **or** ampicillin-sulbactam **or** vancomycin × 4–6 weeks	Cephalexin **or** clindamycin **or** cefadroxil × 4–6 weeks
Osteochondritis	P. aeruginosa S. aureus§	Ticarcillin-clavulanate × 7–10 days after surgery **or combination therapy with** nafcillin plus ceftazidime × 7–10 days after surgery	Piperacillin **or** ciprofloxacin × 7–10 days after surgery	Ciprofloxacin** × 7–10 days after surgery
Diskitis	S. aureus, K. kingae Enterobacteriaceae S. pneumoniae S. epidermidis	PO Therapy: Cephalexin **or** cefadroxil **or** clindamycin × 3–4 weeks or ESR returns to normal††		

Duration of therapy represents total time IV, PO, or IV + PO. Most patients on IV therapy able to take PO meds should be switched to PO therapy soon after clinical improvement.

† **See pp. 402–410 for drug dosages.**

** Not approved for children but might consider in adolescent.

* Treat only IV or IV-to-PO switch.

†† Add gram-negative coverage only if culture proven.

§ If CA-MRSA is suspected based on clinical presentation/local epidemiology, consider empiric coverage for CA-MRSA with clindamycin, TMP–SMX, doxycycline, or vancomycin pending culture results.

Acute Osteomyelitis

Clinical Presentation: Acute onset of fever and pain/decreased movement around the infected area. Can be difficult to localize, especially in younger children. Occurs primarily via hematogenous spread (vs. direct inoculation) to metaphysis of long bones.

Diagnostic Considerations: Acute phase reactants are elevated (ESR, CRP, WBC). X-rays may not reveal osteolytic lesions for > 7 days, but soft tissue swelling and periosteal reaction may be seen as early as 3 days. Bone scan/MRI reveal changes in the first 24 hours, but bone scans are insensitive in neonates. Blood cultures may be positive, especially in younger children. Definitive diagnosis by bone aspirate for gram stain and culture, but empiric therapy is often initiated based on clinical history and the presence of an acute lytic lesion on MRI, bone scan, or x-ray.

Pitfalls: Bony changes on x-ray may not be present initially. It may be difficult to differentiate cellulitis from osteomyelitis, even on bone scan.

Therapeutic Considerations: Initiate empiric therapy by IV route. Treatment is required ≥ 4 weeks, but children with compliant families can complete therapy with high-dose oral antibiotics. With adequate treatment, CPR and ESR normalize over 2 weeks and 4 weeks, respectively.

Prognosis: Good with 4–6 weeks of total therapy. Long-term growth of affected bone may be impaired.

Osteochondritis of the Foot ("Puncture Wound Osteomyelitis")

Clinical Presentation: Tenderness, erythema, and swelling several days to weeks after a nail puncture wound through a sneaker/tennis shoe (Pseudomonas found in foam layer between sole and lining of shoe). Fever and other systemic complaints are rare. Develops in 1–2% of puncture wounds of foot.

Diagnostic Considerations: P. aeruginosa is the primary pathogen, although infection with S. aureus is also a concern.

Pitfalls: Antibiotics surgical of necrotic cartilage.

Therapeutic Considerations: With prompt debridement, 7–10 days of antibiotic therapy is usually sufficient.

Prognosis: Good with debridement and antibiotics.

Diskitis

Clinical Presentation: Typically involves the lumbar region and occurs in children < 6 years old. Presents with gradual onset (over weeks) of irritability and refusal to walk. Fever is low-grade or absent. Older children may be able to localize pain to back, hip, or abdomen. Pain is exacerbated by motion of the spine and can be localized by percussion of the vertebral bodies.

Diagnostic Considerations: ESR is elevated, but WBC count is normal. X-rays are usually normal initially, but later reveal disk space narrowing and sclerosis of the vertebrae. Increased disk space uptake can be seen on bone scan. MRI is very sensitive for assessing disk space involvement.

Therapeutic Considerations: Diskitis is probably a low-grade bacterial infection, but the role of antibiotic therapy is unclear. Bed rest and anti-inflammatory medications are the mainstays of treatment. Immobilization may be required for severe cases. Oral antibiotics are given for 3–4 weeks or until the ESR returns to normal.

Pitfalls: Difficult to isolate an organism, even with needle aspiration of disk space. S. aureus is the most common pathogen, but diskitis can also be caused by coagulase-negative staphylococcus, K. kingae, coliforms, S. pneumoniae.

Prognosis: Fusion of involved vertebrae may occur as the infection resolves. Otherwise, outcome is generally good.

Empiric Therapy of Skin and Soft Tissue Infections

Skin and Soft Tissue Infections

Subset	Usual Pathogens	Preferred IV Therapy†	Alternate IV Therapy†	PO Therapy or IV-to-PO Switch†
Cellulitis, impetigo	S. aureus Group A streptococci	Cefazolin **or** nafcillin **or** oxacillin × 7–10 days	Clindamycin‡ × 7–10 days	Cephalexin **or** cefadroxil **or** dicloxacillin **or** clindamycin **or** amoxicillin/clavulanate **or** erythromycin **or** azithromycin × 7–10 days
Severe pyodermas abscesses	CA-MRSA	Vancomycin **plus** Clindamycin × 7–14 days	Vancomycin or linezolid × 7–14 days	TMP–SMX or doxycycline × 7–14 days**
Animal bite wounds (dog/cat)	Group A streptococci P. multocida Capnocytophaga S. aureus	Ampicillin-sulbactam × 7–10 days	Piperacillin **or** ticarcillin × 7–10 days Penicillin allergy: Clindamycin **plus** TMP–SMX × 7–10 days (dog bites); doxycycline **or** cefuroxime × 7–10 days (cat bites)	Amoxicillin-clavulanate **or** doxycycline × 7–10 days
Human bite wounds	Oral anaerobes E. corrodens Group A streptococci S. aureus	Ampicillin-sulbactam × 5–7 days	Piperacillin **or** ticarcillin × 5–7 days Penicillin allergic patient: Clindamycin **plus** TMP–SMX × 5–7 days	Amoxicillin-clavulanate **or** doxycycline × 5–7 days
Cat scratch disease (CSD)*	Bartonella henselae	Gentamicin × 10–14 days	–	Azithromycin × 5 days **or** TMP–SMX **or** ciprofloxacin **or** rifampin × 10–14 days

† **See pp. 402–410 for drug dosages.**
** In children > 8 years of age.
* No well-controlled trials of antibiotic treatment for CSD to demonstrate benefit.
‡ Preferred therapy for patients in geographic regions with a high prevalence of MRSA or for those with penicillin/cephalosporin allergy.

Skin and Soft Tissue Infections (cont'd)

Subset	Pathogens	IV Therapy†	PO Therapy or IV-to-PO Switch†
Chicken pox *Immuno-compromised host*	VZV	Acyclovir × 7–10 days	Acyclovir **or** valacyclovir × 7–10 days
Immuno-competent host	VZV	Acyclovir × 5 days	Acyclovir **or** valacyclovir × 5 days
H. zoster (Shingles)	VZV	Same as for chicken pox	Acyclovir **or** valacyclovir × 10 days (for individuals ≥ 12 years of age)

Duration of therapy represents total time IV, PO, or IV + PO. Most patients on IV therapy able to take PO meds should be switched to PO therapy soon after clinical improvement.

† **See pp. 402–410 for drug dosages.**

Cellulitis

Clinical Presentation: Erythema, warmth, and tenderness of skin. Impetigo is characterized by a vesiculopapular rash with honey-colored discharge.

Diagnostic Considerations: Primarily a clinical diagnosis. Group A streptococci and Staphylococcus are primary pathogens in healthy children. Wound culture of discharge or leading edge of lesion and gram stain may be helpful.

Pitfalls: Differential diagnosis of cellulitis may include hypersensitivity to insect bites. Herpetic whitlow (HSV) may be mistaken for a bacterial skin or paronychial infection.

Therapeutic Considerations: First generation cephalosporin or semi-synthetic penicillin with anti-staphylococcal activity (i.e., dicloxacillin, nafcillin, oxacillin) are drugs of choice. Increasing incidence of community-acquired MRSA may affect treatment decisions.

Prognosis: Excellent. Impetigo may only require topical treatment/(mupirocin).

Bite Wounds

Clinical Presentation: 80% of animal bite wounds in children are from dogs, and 15%–50% of dog bites become infected. More than 50% of cat bites become infected, and due to their long teeth, there is an increased risk of inoculation into bone/joints with development of osteomyelitis/septic arthritis. Human bite wounds are most prone to infection, and 75%–90% of all human bites become infected.

Diagnostic Considerations: Clinical diagnosis. Culture of wound exudate may yield organism.

Pitfalls: Failure to assess depth of infection, especially with cat bites, may result in late identification of bone/joint infection. Macrolides are ineffective against P. multocida.

Therapeutic Considerations: It is important to cover oral anaerobes, S. aureus, and Group A streptococci in human bite wounds. P. multocida is an important pathogen in cat and dog bite wounds. Facial/hand lesions require plastic surgery. Recurrent debridement may be necessary, especially with human bite wound infections of hand. Assess tetanus immunization status for all bite wounds

(p. 364). For human bites consider the risk of HIV and hepatitis B. For dog bites consider the risk of rabies. Antimicrobial therapy initiated within 8 hours of a bite wound and administered for 2–3 days may decrease the rate of infection.

Prognosis: Good with early debridement and antibiotics.

Cat Scratch Disease (CSD)

Clinical Presentation: Classic presentation is a papular lesion at site of cat scratch with lymphadenitis in the draining region (axillary, epitrochlear, inguinal, cervical most commonly). Frequently associated with fever/malaise 1–2 weeks after scratch. Infection can present with conjunctivitis and ipsilateral preauricular lymph node (Parinaud oculoglandular syndrome). Unusual presentations in normal hosts include encephalitis, hepatitis, microabscesses in liver/spleen, fever of unknown origin, osteolytic lesions.

Diagnostic Considerations: Most often secondary to kitten scratch with Bartonella henselae. Diagnosed using specific serology for antibodies to B. henselae. CSD antigen skin test from pus obtained from aspirated CSD lymph nodes is unlicenced and should not be used.

Pitfalls: Failure to obtain history of kitten exposure. Surgical excision of lymph node is generally not necessary.

Therapeutic Considerations: Most lesions are self-limited and resolve over 2–4 months. There are no well-controlled studies, but antibiotic therapy may be helpful in severe cases with hepatosplenomegaly. Doxycycline, erythromycin, or azithromycin are helpful in immunocompromised hosts.

Prognosis: Very good with spontaneous resolution over 2–4 months.

Chicken Pox/Shingles (VZV)

Clinical Presentation: Primary illness is chicken pox, a generalized pruritic, vesicular rash with fever that erupts in crops of lesions over 3–5 days followed by crusting and recovery. Complications include bacterial superinfection of skin lesions, sepsis, cerebellar ataxia, thrombocytopenia, hepatitis, pneumonia and encephalitis. The disease tends to be more severe in adolescents and adults, particularly if immunocompromised. Primary infection early in pregnancy can rarely result in varicella embryopathy with imb atrophy and CNS malformations in the neonate. Reactivation disease (shingles) may occur in children and in normal hosts and remains localized to a single dermatome. Post-herpetic neuralgia occurs less often in children than adults. Reactivation disease in immunocompromised hosts can spread and re-disseminate.

Diagnostic Considerations: The characteristic eruption of chicken pox occurs in waves—multiple stages appear at the same time, from new papules and vesicles to more advanced larger and crusted lesions—and is unique to varicella. Direct fluorescent antibody staining of a scraped lesion can confirm the diagnosis.

Pitfalls: Initially lesions may be primarily papular, and if the diagnosis is not considered, exposure of others can occur.

Therapeutic Considerations: Antiviral therapy with acyclovir, if started within 24 hours of rash, should be considered for children > 12 years of age, those on steroid or salicylate therapy, and those with underlying chronic pulmonary, skin, or immunosuppressive states. Oral administration is acceptable, although IV therapy may be preferred for immunocompromised hosts at risk of disseminated disease. More severe varicella has been observed in individuals acquiring the infection from a household contact, presumable due to a higher innocuous with closer contact; household contacts may be considered for acyclovir therapy at onset of rash in child. Additionally, individuals ≥ 13 years may develop more extensive varicella than younger children. Immunocompromised children or pregnant women without a history of varicella or immunization may benefit from prophylaxis with varicella zoster immune globulin (VZIG) within 96 hours of varicella exposure. Newborns whose mothers develop chicken pox within 5 days before or 48 hours after delivery and exposed premature infants are also candidates for VZIG. A like-attenuated varicella vaccine has been licensed since 1995 for use in individuals ≥ 12 months of age who have not had chicken pox. A two-dose vaccine schedule is recommended for children ≥ 12 months of age.

Prognosis: Overall prognosis is good with complete recovery and minimal risk of scarring unless immunosuppressed host with disseminated disease. Although rare, Group A streptococcal toxic shock syndrome (manifest as cellulitis or in conjunction with necrotizing fasciitis complicating varicella skin lesions) and Group A streptococcal septicemia, which can occur in the absence of apparent secondarily infected skin lesions, may be fatal complications of varicella in normal children.

Common Pediatric Antimicrobial Drugs

Drug	Dosage in Neonates	Dosage in Infants/Children*
Acyclovir	20 mg/kg (IV) q8h × 14–21 days. Dosing interval may need to be increased for infants < 34 weeks post-maturational age (GA + CA) or if significant renal impairment or liver failure Chronic suppression: 75 mg/kg (PO) q12h	HSV encephalitis: 10 mg/kg (IV) q8h × 12–21 days Primary HSV infection: 10–20 mg/kg (PO) q6h × 5–10 days **or** 5 mg/kg/dose (IV) q8h × 5 days Varicella in immunocompromised hosts: 10 mg/kg (IV) q8h × 7–10 days Varicella in immunocompetent hosts: 20 mg/kg (PO) q6h × 5 days (maximum 800 mg/dose)
Albendazole	Not applicable	400 mg (PO) q24h
Amikacin**	*During first week of life* dosing is based on gestational age (administer IV dose over 30 min) • ≤ 27 weeks (or asphyxia, PDA, or indomethacin): 18 mg/kg (IV) q48h • 28–30 weeks: 18 mg/kg (IV) q36h • 31–33 weeks: 16 mg/kg (IV) q36h • ≥ 34 weeks: 15 mg/kg (IV) q24h	5–7.5 mg/kg (IV or IM) q8h

Drug	Dosage in Neonates			Dosage in Infants/Children*
	After first week of life: Initial dose of 15 mg/kg, then draw serum concentrations 30 min after end of infusion (peak) and 12–24 hours later (trough) to determine dosing interval. Aim for peak of 20–30 mcg/mL and trough of 2–5 mcg/mL			
Amoxicillin	Not indicated			22.5–45 mg/kg (PO) q12h
Amoxicillin-clavulanate	Not indicated			22.5–45 mg/kg (of amoxicillin component) (PO) q12h
Amphotericin B (conventional)	0.5–1 mg/kg (IV over 2–6 hours) q24-48h (Some authorities recommend an initial test dose of 0.1–0.5 mg/kg IV over 2–6 hours)			
Ampicillin	25–50 mg/kg/dose (IV or IM). Severe Group B streptococcal sepsis: 100 mg/kg/dose. Dosing interval is based on gestational age (GA) and chronological age (CA):			25–50 mg/kg (IV or IM) q6h
	GA + CA (weeks)	**CA (days)**	**Interval (hours)**	
	≤ 29	0–28 > 28	12 8	
	30–36	0–14 > 14	12 8	
	≥ 37	0–7 > 7	12 8	
Ampicillin-sulbactam	Not indicated			25–50 mg/kg (of ampicillin component) (IV) q6h
Azithromycin	Not indicated			Otitis media/sinusitis: 30 mg/kg (PO) × 1 dose **or** 10 mg/kg (PO) q24h × 3 days **or** 10 mg/kg (PO) on day 1 followed by 5 mg/kg (PO) q24h on days 2–5 Pharyngitis/tonsillitis: 12 mg/kg (PO) q24h × 5 days

* Dosages are generally based on weight (mg/kg), up to adult dose as maximum.

** Drug can be given IM but absorption may be variable.

Drug	Dosage in Neonates	Dosage in Infants/Children*
		Community-acquired pneumonia (not indicated for moderate or severe disease): 10 mg/kg (PO) × 5 days **or** 10 mg/kg (IV or PO) on day 1 followed by 5 mg/kg (IV or PO) q24h on days 2–5 Skin/soft tissue infections (including Cat Scratch Disease): 10 mg/kg (PO) on day 1 followed by 5 mg/kg (PO) q24h on days 2–5
Aztreonam	30 mg/kg (IV or IM). See *ampicillin* for dosing interval (p. 403)	30 mg/kg (IV or IM) q6-8h
Caspofungin	70 mg/m2 loading dose, then 50 mg/m2 (IV) q24h	70 mg/m2 loading dose, then 50 mg/m2 (IV) q24h
Cefadroxil	Not indicated	15 mg/kg (PO) q12h
Cefazolin	25 mg/kg (IV or IM). See *ampicillin* for dosing interval (above)	25–100 mg/kg/day (IV or IM) divided q8h
Cefdinir	Not indicated	7 mg/kg (PO) q12h or 14 mg/kg (PO) q24h
Cefepime	50 mg/kg (IV) q8-12h	33.3–50 mg/kg (IV or IM) q8h
Cefotaxime	50 mg/kg (IV or IM). (25 mg/kg/dose is adequate for gonococcal infection). See *ampicillin* for dosing interval	25–50 mg/kg (IV or IM) q6–8h
Cefotetan	Not indicated	20–40 mg/kg (IV or IM) q12h
Cefoxitin	25–33 mg/kg/dose (IV or IM). See *ampicillin* for dosing interval	80–160 mg/kg/day (IV or IM) divided q4–8h
Cefpodoxime	Not indicated	5 mg/kg (PO) q12h
Cefprozil	Not indicated	15 mg/kg (PO) q12h
Ceftazidime	30 mg/kg/dose (IV or IM). See *ampicillin* for dosing interval	25–50 mg/kg (IV or IM) q8h
Ceftibuten	Not indicated	9 mg/kg (PO) q24h
Ceftizoxime	Not indicated	50 mg/kg (IV or IM) q6–8h

* Dosages are generally based on weight (mg/kg), up to adult dose as maximum.

<table>
<tr><th>Drug</th><th colspan="3">Dosage in Neonates</th><th>Dosage in Infants/Children*</th></tr>
<tr><td>Ceftriaxone‡</td><td colspan="3">Sepsis and disseminated gonococcal infection: 50 mg/kg (IV or IM) q24h
Meningitis: 100 mg/kg loading dose followed by 80 mg/kg (IV or IM) q24h
Uncomplicated gonococcal ophthalmia:
50 mg/kg (maximum 125 mg) as a single dose (IV or IM)</td><td>50 mg/kg (IV or IM) q24h. Meningitis: 50 mg/kg (IV or IM) q12h or 100 mg/kg (IV or IM) q24h
Acute otitis media: 50 mg/kg (IM) × 1 dose (or 3 doses IM q24h in high-risk patients)</td></tr>
<tr><td>Cefuroxime</td><td colspan="3">Not indicated</td><td>10–15 mg/kg (PO) q12h
25–50 mg/kg (IV or IM) q8h</td></tr>
<tr><td>Cephalexin</td><td colspan="3">Not indicated</td><td>6.25–25 mg/kg (PO) q6h</td></tr>
<tr><td>Cephalothin</td><td colspan="3">Not indicated</td><td>25 mg/kg (IV or IM) q4-6h</td></tr>
<tr><td>Clarithromycin</td><td colspan="3">Not indicated</td><td>7.5 mg/kg (PO) q12h</td></tr>
<tr><td>Clindamycin</td><td colspan="3">5.0–7.5 mg (IV or PO). Dosing interval is based on gestational age (GA) and chronological age (CA)</td><td>5–10 mg/kg (IV or IM) q6-8h or 10–30 mg/kg/day (PO) divided q6-8h</td></tr>
<tr><td></td><td>GA + CA (weeks)</td><td>CA (days)</td><td>Interval (hours)</td><td></td></tr>
<tr><td></td><td>< 29</td><td>0–28
> 28</td><td>12
8</td><td></td></tr>
<tr><td></td><td>30–36</td><td>0–14
> 14</td><td>12
8</td><td></td></tr>
<tr><td></td><td>37–44</td><td>0–7
> 7</td><td>8
6</td><td></td></tr>
<tr><td>Dicloxacillin</td><td colspan="3">Not indicated</td><td>3.125–25 mg/kg (PO) q6h</td></tr>
<tr><td>Doxycycline</td><td colspan="3">Contraindicated</td><td>> 45 kg: 100 mg (PO) q12h
≤ 45 kg: 1.1–2.5 mg/kg (PO) q12h
Use only in children > 8 years (unless RMSF)
1–2 mg/kg (IV) q12–24h</td></tr>
</table>

* Dosages are generally based on weight (mg/kg), up to adult dose as maximum.

‡ Do not use in presence of hyperbilirubinemia.

Drug	Dosage in Neonates	Dosage in Infants/Children*
Erythromycin	Chlamydia pneumonitis/conjunctivitis or pertussis: 12.5 mg/kg (PO) q6h (E. estolate preferred) Other infections: E. estolate 10 mg/kg (PO) q8h **or** E. ethylsuccinate 10 mg/kg (PO) q6h Severe infections and PO not possible: 5–10 mg/kg (IV over ≥ 60 min) q6h	10–12.5 mg/kg (PO) q6–8h 5–12.5 mg/kg (IV) q6h
Ertapenem	Not indicated	15 mg/kg (IV) q12h (not to exceed 1 gm/day)
Ethambutol	See p. 389	See p. 389
Ethionamide	See p. 389	See p. 389
Fluconazole	Systemic infection or meningitis: 12 mg/kg (IV over 30 min or PO) × 1 dose, then 6 mg/kg/dose (IV or PO) with dosing interval based on gestational age (GA) and chronological age (CA) (below) Prophylaxis (e.g., extremely low birth weight infants in NICU with high rates of fungal disease): 3 mg/kg/dose (IV or PO) according to dosing interval grid (below) Thrush: 6 mg/kg (PO) × 1 dose, then 3 mg/kg (PO) q24h	10 mg/kg (IV or PO) loading dose followed by 3–6 mg/kg (IV or PO) q24h

GA + CA (weeks)	CA (days)	Interval (weeks)
≤ 29	0–14 > 14	72 48
30–36	0–14 > 14	48 24
37–44	0–7 > 7	48 24

* Dosages are generally based on weight (mg/kg), up to adult dose as maximum.

Drug	Dosage in Neonates	Dosage in Infants/Children*
Gentamicin**	*During first week of life* dosing is based on gestational age (administer IV dose over 30 min): • ≤ 29 weeks (or asphyxia, PDA, or indomethacin): 5 mg/kg (IV) q48h • 30–33 weeks: 4.5 mg/kg (IV) q48h • 34–37 weeks: 4 mg/kg (IV) q36h • ≥ 38 weeks: 4 mg/kg (IV) q24h *After first week of life:* Initial dose of 4 mg/kg, then draw serum concentrations 30 min after end of infusion (peak) and 12–24 hours later (trough) to determine dosing interval. Aim for peak of 5–12 mcg/mL and trough of 0.5–1 mcg/mL	2–2.5 mg/kg (IV or IM) q8h
Imipenem	20–25 mg/kg (IV) q12h	15–25 mg/kg (IV or IM) q6h
Iodoquinol	10–13.3 mg/kg (PO) q8h	10–13.3 mg/kg (PO) q8h
Isoniazid	See p. 389	See p. 389
Linezolid	10 mg/kg (IV) q12h	10 mg/kg (IV) q8h
Liposomal/lipid complex Amphotericin preparations	1–5 mg/kg (IV over 2 hours) q24h	3–6 mg/kg (IV) q24h
Meropenem	20 mg/kg (IV) q12h	10 mg/kg (IV) q8h (skin); 20 mg/kg (IV) q8h (intraabdominal); 40 mg/kg (IV) q8h (meningitis)
Methenamine mandelate	Not indicated	15–25 mg (PO) q6–8h
Metronidazole	15 mg/kg (IV or PO) × 1 dose, then 7.5 mg/kg/dose (IV or PO) with dosing interval based on gestational age (GA) and chronological age (CA):	5–12.5 mg/kg (PO) q8h 15 mg/kg (IV) × 1 dose followed by 7.5 mg/kg (IV) q6h

* Dosages are generally based on weight (mg/kg), up to adult dose as maximum.
** Drug can be given IM but absorption may be variable.

Drug	Dosage in Neonates			Dosage in Infants/Children*
	GA + CA (weeks)	CA (days)	Interval (hours)	
	≤ 29	0–28 > 28	24 48	
	30–36	0–14 > 14	24 12	
	37–44	0–7 > 7	24 12	
Micafungin	Not applicable			4–12 mg/kg (IV) q24 (higher dose for patients < 8 year of age
Mupirocin	Not indicated			Nasal cream: ½ of single use tube into nostril q12h × 5 days; Cream: apply q8h × 5–190 days
Nafcillin	25–50 mg/kg/dose (IV). See *ampicillin* for dosing interval (p. 403)			12.5–50 mg/kg (IV or IM) q6h
Nitazoxanide	Not applicable			Children 1–3 years old: 100 mg (PO) q12h; children 4–11 years old: 200 mg (PO) q12h
Nitrofurantoin	Not indicated			<u>UTI:</u> 1.25–1.75 mg/kg (PO) q6h <u>UTI prophylaxis:</u> 1–2 mg/kg (PO) q24h
Nystatin	<u>Oral:</u> 1 mL (preterm) to 2 mL (term) of 100,000 U/mL suspension applied with swab to each side of mouth q6h until 3 days after resolution of lesions <u>Topical:</u> Apply ointment or cream to affected area q6h until 3 days after resolution of lesions.			<u>Suspension:</u> 4–6 mL swish and swallow 4×/day <u>Troche:</u> 1–2 troches 4–5×/ day
Oxacillin	25–50 mg/kg/dose (IV). See *ampicillin* for dosing interval (above)			25–50 mg/kg (IV or IM) q6h
Paromomycin	Not applicable			10 mg/kg (PO) q8h
Penicillin G	25,000–50,000 IU/kg/dose (IV). See *ampicillin* for dosing interval <u>Meningitis:</u> 75,000–100,000 IU/kg			12,500–75,000 U/kg (IV or IM) q4-6h

* Dosages are generally based on weight (mg/kg), up to adult dose as maximum.

Drug	Dosage in Neonates	Dosage in Infants/Children*
	(IV) in meningitis (IV).† Q8-12h based on GA + CA, See ampicillin for dosing interval Crystalline penicillin G: IM: procaine penicillin G q24 hours. Congenital syphilis: Aqueous penicillin G 50,000 IU/kg (slow IV push) q12h × 7 days, then q8h to complete 10–14 days **or** procaine penicillin G 50,000 IU/kg (IM) q24h × 10–14 days	
Penicillin V	Not indicated	25–50 mg/kg (PO) q6-8h
Piperacillin	50–100 mg/kg/dose (IV or IM). See *ampicillin* for dosing interval (p. 403)	25–75 mg/kg (IV or IM) q6h; may increase to q4h in severe infection, especially with pseudomonas
Piperacillin-tazobactam	Not indicated	100–300 mg/kg/day (IV) (of piperacillin component) divided q6-8h
Pyrazinamide	See p. 389	See p. 389
Quinupristin-dalfopristin	7.5 mg/kg (IV) q12h	7.5 mg/kg (IV) q12h
Rifampin	10–20 mg/kg (PO) q24h **or** 5–10 mg/kg (IV) q24h	20 mg/kg (PO) q24h **or** 10 mg/kg (PO) q12h 10–20 mg/kg/day (IV) divided q12–24h
Streptomycin	See p. 389	See p. 389
Sulfisoxazole	Contraindicated	30–35 mg/kg (PO) q6h Otitis media prophylaxis: 37.5 mg/kg (PO) q12h
Tetracycline	Contraindicated	5–12.5 mg/kg (PO) q6h. Use only in children > 8 years
Ticarcillin	75–100 mg/kg/dose (IV). See *ampicillin* for dosing interval	25–75 mg/kg (IV or IM) q6h
Ticarcillin-clavulanate	75–100 mg/kg/dose (of ticarcillin component) (IV). See *ampicillin* for dosing interval (p. 403)	25–75 mg/kg (of ticarcillin component) (IV or IM) q6h
Tinidazole	Not applicable	50–60 mg/kg (PO) q24h
Tobramycin	Same as gentamicin	2–2.5 mg/kg (IV or IM) q8h

* Dosages are generally based on weight (mg/kg), up to adult dose as maximum.

<table>
<tr><th>Drug</th><th colspan="3">Dosage in Neonates</th><th>Dosage in Infants/Children*</th></tr>
<tr><td>Trimethoprim-sulfameth-oxazole (TMP–SMX)</td><td colspan="3">Contraindicated</td><td>UTI: 4–5 mg/kg (of trimethoprim component) (PO) q12h
Pneumocystis carinii pneumonia (PCP) 5 mg/kg (PO) q6h (typically after initial IV therapy)
UTI prophylaxis: 2–4 mg/kg (PO) q24h
IV dosing
PCP or severe infection: 5 mg/kg (of trimethoprim component) (IV) q6h
Minor infections: 4–6 mg/kg (of trimethoprim component) (IV) q12h</td></tr>
<tr><td>Vancomycin</td><td colspan="3">Bacteremia: 10 mg/kg/dose (IV)
Meningitis: 15 mg/kg/dose (IV). Administer IV dose over 60 min. Dosing interval is based on gestational age (GA) and chronological age (CA):</td><td>10–15 mg/kg (IV) q6h</td></tr>
<tr><td></td><td>GA + CA (weeks)</td><td>CA (days)</td><td>Interval (weeks)</td><td></td></tr>
<tr><td></td><td>≤ 29</td><td>0–14
> 14</td><td>18
12</td><td></td></tr>
<tr><td></td><td>30–36</td><td>0–14
> 14</td><td>12
8</td><td></td></tr>
<tr><td></td><td>37–44</td><td>0–7
> 7</td><td>12
8</td><td></td></tr>
<tr><td>Voriconazole</td><td colspan="3">Not applicable</td><td>7 mg/kg (IV) q12h
8 mg/kg (PO) q12h × 1 day, then 7 mg/kg (PO) q12h</td></tr>
</table>

* Dosages are generally based on weight (mg/kg), up to adult dose as maximum.

REFERENCES AND SUGGESTED READINGS

Betts R, Glasmacher A, Maertens J, et al. Efficacy of caspofungin against invasive Candida or invasive Aspergillus infections in neutropenic patients. Cancer 106:466–73, 2006.

Bisno AL, Kaplan EL. Strep Throat Over and Over: How Frequent? How Real? Mayo Clin Proc 81:1153–4, 2006.

CDC. Outbreak of Swine-Origin Influenza A (H_1N_1) Virus Infection—Mexico, March–April 2009, MMWR Dispatch 58:April 30, 2009.

CDC. Use of Rapid Influenza Diagnostic Tests for Patients with Influenza-like illness during the Novel H_1N_1 Influenza Virus (Swine Flu) Outbreak. Swine Influenza Bulletin June 12, 2009.

CDC. Recommended childhood and adolescent immunization schedule-United States, 2007. MMWR 55(51):Q1–Q4, January 5, 2007.

Cheng VCC, Lau Y-K, Lee K-I, et al. Fatal co-infection with swine origin influenza virus A/H_1N_1 and community-acquired methicillin resistant *Staphylococcus aureus*. J Infection (Epub ahead of print): 1–5, 2009.

Committee of Infectious Disease. Prevention of varicella: Recommendations for use of varicella vaccine in children, including a recommendation for a routine 2-dose varicella immunization schedule. Pediatrics 120:221–231, 2007.

Cunha BA. Influenza: historical aspects of epidemics and pandemics. Infect Dis Clin N Am 2004;18:141–155.

Cunha BA, Pherez FM, Schoch PE: The Diagnostic Importance of Relative Lymphopenia as a Marker of Swine Influenza (H_1N_1). Clinical Infectious Disease 47(1454–1456), 2009.

Dominguez-Cherit, G, Lapinsky, SE, Macias AE, et al. Critically I11 Patients with 2009 Influenza A (H_1N_1) in Mexico. JAMA 302:1872–1879, 2009.

Ellis JM, Kuti JL, Nicolau DP. Pharmacodynamic evaluation of meropenem and cefotaxime for pediatric meningitis: a report from the OPTAMA program. Pediatr Drugs 8:131–8, 2006.

Fox JW, Marcon MJ, Bonsu BK. Diagnosis of Streptococcal Pharyngitis by Detection of Streptococcus pyogenes in Posterior Pharyngeal vs Oral Cavity Specimens. Journal of Clin Microbiology 44:2593–94, 2006.

Groll AH, Attarbasehi A, Schuster FR, et al. Treatment with caspofungin in immunocompromised paediatric patients: a multicentre survey. A Antimicrob Chemother 57:527–35, 2006.

Hidron AI, Low CE, Honig EG, et al. Emergence of community-acquired methicillin-resistant Staphylococcus aureus strain USA300 as a cause of necrotizing community-onset pneumonia. Lancet Infect Dis 9:384–392, 2009.

Kaplan SL, Afghani B, Lopez P, et al. Linezolid for the treatment of methicillin-resistant Staphylococcus aureus infections in children. Pediatric Infect Disease 22:S178–185, 2003.

Lehtinen P, Jartti T, Virkki R, et al. Bacterial coinfections in children with viral wheezing. Eur J Clin Microbiol Infect Dis 25:463–9, 2006.

Lorente L, Lorenzo L, Martin MM, Jimenez A, Mora ML. Meropenem by continuous versus intermittent infusion in ventilator-associated pneumonia due to gram-negative bacilli. Ann Pharmacother 40:219–23, 2006.

Louie JK, Acosta M, Winter K, et al. Factors Associated with Death or Hospitalization Due to Pandemic 2009 Influenza (H_1N_1) Infection in California. JAMA 302: 1896–1902, 2009.

Mathys J, DeMeyere M. Acute pharyngitis: No Reliability of Rapid Streptococcal Tests and Clinical Findings. Arch Intern Med 166:2285–86, 2006.

MMWR. Hospitalized Patients with Novel Influenza A (H_1N_1) Infection—California, April–May, 2009. 58:536–541, 2009.

MMWR. Intensive-Care Patients with Severe Novel Influenza (H_1N_1) Virus Infection—Michigan, June 2009. 58:749–752, 2009.

Saiman L, Goldfarb J, Kaplan SL, et al. Safety and tolerability of linezolid in children. Pediatric Infect Disease 22:S193–200, 2003.

Solomkin JS, Mazuski JE, Bradley JS, et al. Diagnosis and Management of Complicated Intra-abdominal Infection in Adults and Children: Guidelines by the Surgical Infection Society and the Infectious Diseases Society of America. Clin Infect Dis 50:133–164, 2010.

TEXTBOOKS

Feigin RD, Cherry JD, Demmler GJ, Kaplan SL (eds). Textbook of Pediatric Infectious Diseases. 5th edition. Philadelphia, Saunders, 2004.

McMillan JA, DeAngelis CD, Feigin RD, Warshaw JB Oski's Pediatrics, Principles and Practice. 3rd edition. Lippincott, Williams & Wilkins, Philadelphia, 1999.

Pickering LK ed. Red Book: Report of the Committee on Infectious Diseases. American Academy of Pediatrics, 25th ed. Elk Grove Village, IL, 2006.

Remington JS, Klein JO (eds) Infectious Diseases of the Fetus and Newborn 6th edition. WB Saunders Co., Philadelphia, PA, 2006.

Shah S. Pediatric Infectious Disease Practice. New York: McGraw-Hill, 2009.

Siberry GK, Iannone R. The Harriet Lane Handbook. 18th edition. Mosby, St. Louis, MO, 2008.

Steele RW. Clinical Handbook of Pediatric Infectious Disease (3rd Ed.). Informa Healthcare, New York, 2007.

Chapter 8
CHEST X-RAY ATLAS

Burke A. Cunha, MD
Douglas S. Katz, MD
Robert Moore, MD
Daniel S. Siegal, MD

Chest X-Ray Patterns

This atlas has been developed to assist in the management of patients who present with respiratory symptoms and chest x-ray abnormalities. Eight common chest x-ray patterns are provided. Common infections and noninfectious etiologies are followed by usual clinical features, which can be used to identify the disorder and help guide empiric/specific therapy.

UNILATERAL FOCAL SEGMENTAL/LOBAR INFILTRATE WITHOUT EFFUSION

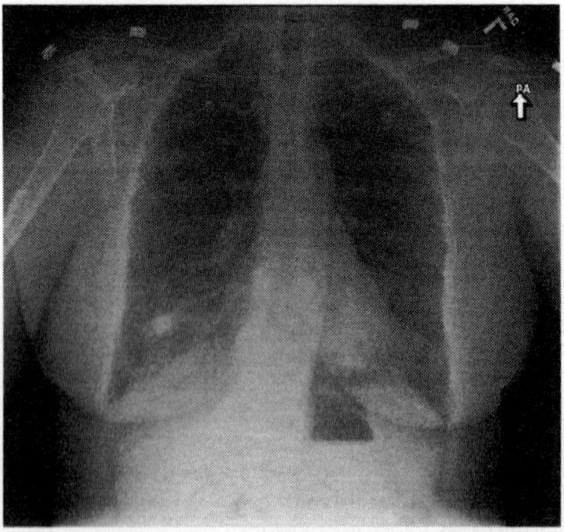

Infectious Causes

	Features (may have some, none, or all)			
Causes	**History**	**Physical**	**Laboratory**	**Chest X-Ray**
S. pneumoniae	Elderly, smokers, COPD, ↓ humoral immunity (multiple myeloma, SLE, CLL, hyposplenism).	Fever, chills, no relative bradycardia. Chest signs related to extent of consolidation.	↑ WBC, ↓ platelets (overwhelming infection/ hyposplenism), normal LFTs. Sputum with abundant PMNs and gram-positive diplococci. Blood cultures usually positive.	Consolidation usually limited to one lobe (RLL most common) ± air bronchogram. Pleural effusion very common. Empyema uncommon. No cavitation.
H. influenzae	Recent contact with H. influenzae URI.	Fever, chills.	↑ WBC. Sputum/ pleural effusion with gram-negative pleomorphic bacilli. Blood cultures often positive.	Usually RLL with small/moderate effusion. No empyema. No cavitation.

Infectious Causes (cont'd)

Causes	Features (may have some, none, or all)			
	History	Physical	Laboratory	Chest X-Ray
M. catarrhalis	Chronic/heavy smoker, COPD.	Nonspecific.	Sputum with gram-negative/variable diplococci. Blood cultures negative.	Usually lower lobe ± consolidation. No pleural effusion or cavitation.
K. pneumoniae	Nosocomial pneumonia or history of alcoholism in patient with community-acquired pneumonia.	Fever, chills, signs of alcoholic cirrhosis, signs of consolidation over involved lobe.	↑ WBC, ↑ platelets, ↑ SGOT/SGPT (2° to alcoholism). "Red currant jelly" sputum with PMNs and plump gram-negative encapsulated bacilli.	"Bulging fissure" sign secondary to expanded lobar volume. Empyema rather than pleural effusion. Cavitation in 5–7 days (thick walled).
Legionella	Recent contact with Legionella containing water. Usually elderly. May have watery diarrhea, abdominal pain, mental confusion.	Fever/chills, relative bradycardia. Hepatic/splenic enlargement goes against the diagnosis. ↓ breath sounds if consolidation or pleural effusion.	↑ WBC, ↑ SGOT/SGPT, ↓ PO_4^-, ↓ Na^+, ↑ CPK, ↑ ESR, ↑ CRP, ↑ ferritin levels, microscopic hematuria, L. pneumophila antigenuria (serotypes 01–06 only) may not be positive early. Mucoid/purulent sputum with few PMNs. Positive sputum DFA (before therapy) is diagnostic. ↑ Legionella titer ≥ 1:256 or ≥ 4-fold rise between acute and convalescent titers.	Rapidly progressive asymmetrical infiltrates clue to Legionella. Consolidation and pleural effusion not uncommon. Cavitation rare.

Infectious Causes (cont'd)

Causes	Features (may have some, none, or all)			
	History	Physical	Laboratory	Chest X-Ray
Psittacosis	Recent bird contact with psittacine birds. Severe headache.	Fever/chills, ± relative bradycardia, Horder's spots on face, epistaxis, ± splenomegaly. Signs of consolidation common.	↑/normal WBC, ↑ LFTs. Sputum with few PMNs. Positive C. psittaci serology.	Dense infiltrate. Consolidation common. Pleural effusion/ cavitation rare.
Q fever	Recent contact with sheep or parturient cats.	Fever/chills, ± relative bradycardia, splenomegaly, ± hepatomegaly.	↑/normal WBC, ↑ LFTs. Sputum with no bacteria/ few PMNs (caution–biohazard). Acute Q fever with ↑ in phase II ELISA antigens.	Dense consolidation. Cavitation/ pleural effusion rare.

Non-Infectious Causes

Causes	Features (may have some, none, or all)			
	History	Physical	Laboratory	Chest X-Ray
Atelectasis	Ineffectual moist recurrent cough characteristic of post-operative atelectasis.	Fevers ≤ 102°F. If large, signs of volume loss (↓ respiratory excursion, ↑ diaphragm, mediastinum shift toward affected side). If small, ↓ breath sounds over affected segment/lobe.	↑ WBC (left shift), normal platelets. Other lab results related to underlying cause of atelectasis.	Segmental infiltrate. RUL/RML atelectasis obscures right heart border. In LUL atelectasis, may be triangular infiltrate extending to upper anterior mediastinum mimicking malignancy. LLL atelectasis causes ↑ density of heart shadow. No cavitation or pleural effusion.

Non-Infectious Causes (cont'd)

Causes	Features (may have some, none, or all)			
	History	Physical	Laboratory	Chest X-Ray
Pulmonary embolus/ infarct	Acute onset dyspnea/ pleuritic chest pain. History of lower extremity trauma, stasis or hypercoagulable disorder.	↑ pulse/ respiratory rate.	↑ fibrin split products and D-dimers ± ↑ total bilirubin. Bloody pleural effusion. ECG with RV strain/P-pulmonale (large embolus). Positive V/Q scan and CT pulmonary angiogram.	Normal or show non-specific pleural-based infiltrates resembling atelectasis. Focal segmental/lobar hyperlucency (Westermark's sign) in some. "Hampton's hump" with infarct. Resolving infarcts ↓ in size but maintain shape/density ("melting ice cube").
Lymphoma	Fever, ↓ appetite with weight loss, night sweats, fatigue.	Adenopathy ± splenomegaly	Normal WBC, ↑ basophils, ↑ eosinophilia, ↓ lymphocytes, ↑ platelets, ↑ ESR, ↑ alkaline phosphatase, ↑$\propto_{1,2}$ globulins on SPEP.	Unilateral or asymmetrical bilateral hilar adenopathy. Lung infiltrate may appear contiguous with hilar adenopathy. No clear channel between mediastinum and hilar nodes. Small pleural effusions rare.
Alveolar cell carcinoma	Fever, ↑ appetite with weight loss, night sweats.	± dullness over lobe with large lower lobe lesions.	Positive cytology by BAL/lung biopsy.	Well/ill-defined circumscribed peripheral infiltrates ± air bronchograms. May be multifocal/ multilobar. Hilar adenopathy present. Stranding to the hilum ("pleural tail" sign). ± pleural effusion if lower lobe infiltrate. No cavitation.

Non-Infectious Causes (cont'd)

Causes	Features (may have some, none, or all)			
	History	Physical	Laboratory	Chest X-Ray
Aspiration pneumonia	Swallowing disorder 2° to CNS/GI disorder; impaired consciousness; recent aspiration 2° to dental, upper GI, or pulmonary procedure.	Unremarkable.	↑ WBC, ↑ ESR.	Infiltrate usually involves superior segments of lower lobes (or posterior segments of upper lobes if aspiration occurred supine). Focal infiltrate initially, which may be followed in 7 days by cavitation/lung abscess.

UNILATERAL FOCAL SEGMENTAL/LOBAR INFILTRATE WITH EFFUSION

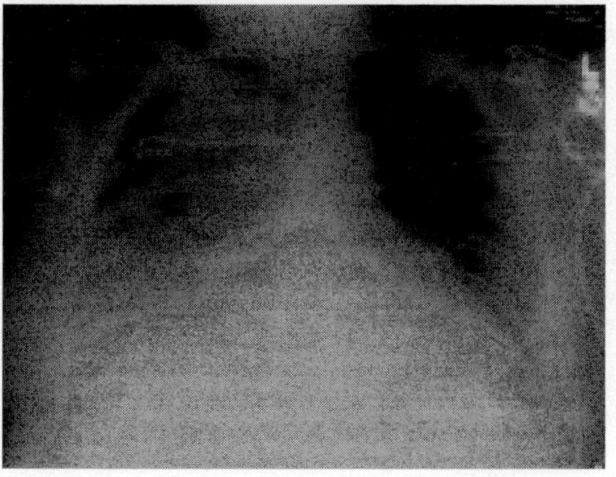

Infectious Causes

Causes	Features (may have some, none, or all)			
	History	Physical	Laboratory	Chest X-Ray
Klebsiella pneumoniae	Nosocomial pneumonia or history of alcoholism in patient with community-acquired pneumonia.	Fever, chills, signs of alcoholic cirrhosis, signs of consolidation over involved lobe.	↑ WBC, ↓ platelets, SGOT/SGPT (2° to alcoholism). "Red currant jelly" sputum with PMNs and plump gram-negative encapsulated bacilli.	"Bulging fissure" sign secondary to expanded lobar volume. Empyema rather than pleural effusion. Usually cavitation in 5–7 days (thick walled).
H. influenzae	Recent contact with H. influenzae URI.	Fever, chills.	↑ WBC. Sputum/pleural effusion with gram-negative pleomorphic bacilli. Blood cultures often positive.	Usually RLL with small/moderate effusion. No empyema. No cavitation.

Infectious Causes (cont'd)

Causes	Features (may have some, none, or all)			
	History	Physical	Laboratory	Chest X-Ray
TB (primary)	Recent TB contact.	Unilateral lower lobe dullness related to size of pleural effusion.	PPD (−)/anergic. Exudative pleural effusion (pleural fluid with ↑ lymphocytes, ↑ glucose, ± RBCs).	Lower lobe infiltrate with small/moderate pleural effusion. No cavitation or apical infiltrates. Hilar adenopathy asymmetrical when present.
Coccidio-mycosis (chronic)	Previous exposure in endemic coccidiomycosis areas. Asymptomatic.	± E. nodosum.	Normal WBC, no eosinophilia in chronic phase. Complement fixation IgG titer ≥ 1:32 indicates active disease.	Thick/thin-walled cavities < 3 cm ± calcifications. Air fluid level rare unless secondarily infected. Cavities usually in anterior segments of upper lobes (vs. posterior segments with TB). No surrounding tissue reaction. Pleural effusion common.
Tularemia	History of recent deer fly, rabbit, or tick exposure. Tularemia pneumonia may complicate any of the clinical presentations of tularemia.	Fever, chills, no relative bradycardia. Chest findings related to extent of infiltrate/consolidation and pleural effusion.	Normal/↑ WBC, normal LFTs. Sputum/pleural effusion with gram-negative coccobacilli (caution–biohazard). Bloody pleural effusion. Tularemia serology with ↑ microagglutination titer ≥ 1:160 acutely and ≥ 4-fold rise between acute and convalescent titers.	Pleural effusion ± hilar adenopathy.

Infectious Causes (cont'd)

Causes	Features (may have some, none, or all)			
	History	Physical	Laboratory	Chest X-Ray
Adenovirus	Recent URI.	Fever, chills, myalgias. Sore throat and conjunctivitis not associated with adenoviral pneumonia. Chest exam with signs of consolidation.	↑ adenoviral titers and positive adenoviral cultures of respiratory secretions.	Ill-defined infiltrate(s) without cavitation ± pleural effusion.
Legionella	Recent contact with Legionella containing water. Usually elderly. May have watery diarrhea, abdominal pain, mental confusion.	Fever/chills, relative bradycardia. Hepatic/ splenic enlargement goes against the diagnosis. ↓ breath sounds if consolidation or pleural effusion.	↑ WBC, ↑ SGOT/ SGPT, ↓ PO_4^-, ↓ Na^+, ↑ CPK, ↑ ESR, ↑ CRP, ↑ ferritin levels, microscopic hematuria, L. pneumophila antigenuria (serotypes 01–06 only) may not be positive early. Mucoid/purulent sputum with few PMNs. Positive sputum DFA (before therapy) is diagnostic. ↑ Legionella titer ≥ 1:256 or ≥ 4-fold rise between acute/ convalescent titers.	Rapidly progressive asymmetrical infiltrates clue to Legionella. Consolidation and pleural effusion not uncommon. Cavitation rare.
Group A streptococci	Recent exposure or recent blunt chest trauma ± chest pain.	Fever/chills. Physical signs related to size of pleural effusion.	↑ WBC. Pleural fluid is serosanguineous. Sputum/pleural fluid with gram-positive cocci in pairs/chains. Positive pleural fluid/ blood cultures.	Unilateral infiltrate may be obscured by large pleural effusion. No empyema. No cavitation.

Infectious Causes (cont'd)

Causes	Features (may have some, none, or all)			
	History	Physical	Laboratory	Chest X-Ray
Rhodococcus equi	Insidious onset of fever, dyspnea, chest pain, ± hemoptysis. Immuno-suppressed patients with ↓ cell-mediated immunity or exposure to cattle, horses, pigs.	Unremarkable.	Normal/↑ WBC. Sputum/pleural fluid with gram-positive pleomorphic weakly acid-fast bacilli. Sputum, pleural fluid, blood cultures positive for R. equi.	Segmental infiltrate with upper lobe predominance ± cavitation. Air-fluid levels and pleural effusion common.

Non-Infectious Causes

Causes	Features (may have some, none, or all)			
	History	Physical	Laboratory	Chest X-Ray
Pulmonary embolus/ infarct	Acute onset dyspnea/ pleuritic chest pain. History of lower extremity trauma, stasis or hypercoagulable disorder.	↑ pulse/ respiratory rate.	↑ fibrin split products and D-dimers ± ↑ total bilirubin. Bloody pleural effusion. ECG with RV strain/P-pulmonale (large embolus). Positive V/Q scan and CT pulmonary angiogram.	Normal or show non-specific pleural-based infiltrates resembling atelectasis. Focal segmental/ lobar hyperlucency (Westermark's sign) in some. "Hampton's hump" with infarct. Resolving infarcts ↓ in size but maintain shape/density ("melting ice cube").

Non-Infectious Causes (cont'd)

	Features (may have some, none, or all)			
Causes	**History**	**Physical**	**Laboratory**	**Chest X-Ray**
Lymphoma	Fever, ↓ appetite with weight loss, night sweats, fatigue.	Adenopathy ± splenomegaly.	Normal WBC, ↑ basophils, ↑ eosinophilia, ↓ lymphocytes, ↑ platelets, ↑ ESR, ↑ alkaline phosphatase, ↑$\propto_{1,2}$ globulins on SPEP.	Unilateral or asymmetrical bilateral hilar adenopathy. Lung infiltrate may appear contiguous with hilar adenopathy. No clear channel between mediastinum and hilar nodes. Small pleural effusions rare.
Alveolar cell carcinoma	Fever, ↑ appetite with weight loss, night sweats.	± dullness over lobe with large lower lobe lesions.	Positive cytology by BAL/lung biopsy.	Well/ill-defined circumscribed peripheral infiltrates ± air bronchograms. May be multifocal/ multilobar. Hilar adenopathy present. Stranding to the hilum ("pleural tail" sign). ± pleural effusion if lower lobe infiltrate. No cavitation.
Radiation pneumonitis	History of mantle radiation for lymphoma, lung cancer, or breast cancer.	Nonspecific.	Nonspecific.	Symmetrical infiltrates in the distribution of radiation therapy after 1 month. Infiltrates have "straight edges"± air bronchograms. Fibrosis common over radiation field after 9–12 months. Usually no pleural effusions (small, if present).

UNILATERAL ILL-DEFINED INFILTRATES WITHOUT EFFUSION

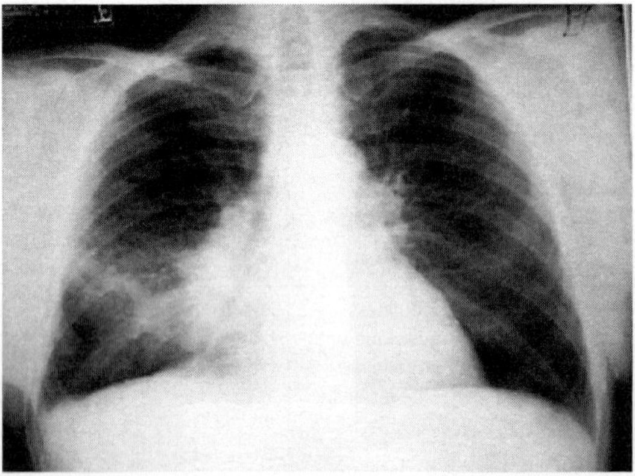

Infectious Causes

	Features (may have some, none, or all)			
Causes	**History**	**Physical**	**Laboratory**	**Chest X-Ray**
Mycoplasma pneumoniae	Prolonged dry/ nonproductive cough. No laryngitis. Mild sore throat/ear. Watery diarrhea.	Usually fevers ≤102 °F without relative bradycardia. Myalgias, bullous myringitis or otitis, non-exudative pharyngitis, E. multiforme. Chest exam with rales and no signs of consolidation or effusion.	Normal/↑ WBC; normal platelets, LFTs, PO_4^-, CPK. ↑ cold agglutinins (early). ↑ IgM (not IgG) Mycoplasma pneumoniae titers. Respiratory secretions culture positive for Mycoplasma pneumoniae.	Ill-defined usually lower lobe indistinct infiltrates. No consolidation or air bronchograms. Small/ no pleural effusion.

Infectious Causes (cont'd)

Causes	Features (may have some, none, or all)			
	History	Physical	Laboratory	Chest X-Ray
Chlamydophilia (Chlamydia) pneumoniae	Prolonged "mycoplasma-like" illness with laryngitis.	Low-grade fevers, myalgias, non-exudate pharyngitis, laryngitis. No relative bradycardia, ear findings, or rash. Chest exam without signs of consolidation or pleural effusion.	↑ WBC, normal platelets, normal LFTs. No cold agglutinins. ↑ IgM (not IgG) C. pneumoniae titers. Respiratory secretions culture positive for C. pneumoniae.	Ill-defined, usually lower lobe indistinct infiltrate(s). May be "funnel shaped." No consolidation, cavitation, or pleural effusion.
Adenovirus	Recent URI.	Fever, chills, myalgias. Sore throat and conjunctivitis not associated with adenoviral pneumonia. Chest exam with signs of consolidation.	↑ adenoviral titers and positive adenoviral cultures of respiratory secretions.	Ill-defined infiltrate(s) without cavitation ± pleural effusion.
Legionella	Recent contact with Legionella containing water. Usually elderly. May have watery diarrhea, abdominal pain, mental confusion.	Fever/chills, relative bradycardia. Hepatic/splenic enlargement goes against the diagnosis. ↓ breath sounds if consolidation or pleural effusion.	↑ WBC, ↑ SGOT/SGPT, ↓ PO_4^-, ↓ Na^+, ↑ CPK, ↑ ESR, ↑ CRP, ↑ ferritin levels, microscopic hematuria, L. pneumophila antigenuria (serotypes 01–06 only) may not be positive early. Mucoid/purulent sputum with few PMNs. Positive sputum DFA (before therapy) is diagnostic. ↑ Legionella titer ≥ 1:256 or ≥ 4-fold rise between acute/convalescent titers.	Rapidly progressive asymmetrical infiltrates clue to Legionella. Consolidation and pleural effusion not uncommon. Cavitation rare.

Infectious Causes (cont'd)

Causes	Features (may have some, none, or all)			
	History	Physical	Laboratory	Chest X-Ray
Psittacosis	Recent bird contact with psittacine birds. Severe headache.	Fever/chills, ± relative bradycardia, ± Horder's spots on face, epistaxis, ± splenomegaly. Signs of consolidation common.	↑/normal WBC, ↑ LFTs. Sputum with few PMNs. Positive C. psittaci serology.	Dense infiltrate. Consolidation common. Pleural effusion/ cavitation rare.
Q fever	Recent contact with sheep or parturient cats.	Fever/chills, ± relative bradycardia, splenomegaly, ± hepatomegaly.	↑/normal WBC, ↑ LFTs. Sputum with no bacteria/few PMNs (caution–biohazard). Acute Q fever with ↑ in phase II ELISA antigens.	Dense consolidation. Cavitation/ pleural effusion rare.
Nocardia	Fevers, night sweats, fatigue, ↓ cell-mediated immunity (e.g., HIV, organ transplant, immunosuppressive therapy).	Unremarkable.	Normal/↑ WBC, ↑ ESR. Sputum with gram-positive AFB.	Dense large infiltrates. May cavitate and mimic TB, lymphoma, or squamous cell carcinoma. No calcification ± pleural effusion.

Infectious Causes (cont'd)

Causes	Features (may have some, none, or all)			
	History	Physical	Laboratory	Chest X-Ray
Actinomycosis	Recent dental work.	± chest wall sinus tracts.	Normal/↑ WBC, ↑ ESR. Sputum with gram-positive filamentous anaerobic bacilli.	Dense infiltrates extending to chest wall. No hilar adenopathy. Cavitation rare. ± pleural effusion rare.
Cryptococcus neoformans	Exposure to air conditioner or pigeons.	Unremarkable.	Normal WBC. Cryptococcal serology with ↑ C. neoformans antigen levels.	Dense lower nodular mass lesions. No calcification or cavitation. ± pleural effusion.
Aspiration pneumonia	Swallowing disorder 2° to CNS/GI disorder; impaired consciousness; recent aspiration 2° to dental, upper GI, or pulmonary procedure.	Unremarkable.	↑ WBC, ↑ ESR.	Infiltrate usually involves superior segments of lower lobes (or posterior segments of upper lobes if aspiration occurred supine). Focal infiltrate initially, which may be followed in 7 days by cavitation/lung abscess.

Non-Infectious Causes

Causes	Features (may have some, none, or all)			
	History	Physical	Laboratory	Chest X-Ray
Bronchogenic carcinoma	Fever, ↓ appetite with weight loss, cough ± hemoptysis. Cough with copious clear/ mucoid sputum in large cell anaplastic carcinoma. Increased risk in smokers, aluminum/ uranium miners, cavitary lung disease (adeno-carcinoma), previous radiation therapy from lymphoma/ breast cancer.	Paraneoplastic syndromes especially with small (oat) cell/squamous cell carcinoma ± hypertrophic pulmonary osteoarthro-pathy.	Normal/↑ WBC, ↑ platelets, ↑ ESR, findings related to underlying malignancy, ± clubbing.	Small/squamous cell carcinomas present as central lesions/hilar masses. Adenocarcinoma/ large cell anaplastic carcinomas are usually peripheral initially. "Tumor tendrils" extending into surrounding lung tissue is characteristic. No calcifications (may be present on chest CT). Cavitation with squamous cell carcinoma. ± pleural effusions.
Lymphangitic metastases	History of breast, thyroid, pancreas, cervical, prostate, or lung carcinoma.	Findings related to underlying malignancy.	Normal/↑ WBC, ↑ ESR.	Interstitial indistinct pulmonary infiltrates (may be reticulonodular) with lower lobe predominance Usually unilateral but may be bilateral. No consolidation or cavitation ± pleural effusions.
Lung contusion	Recent closed chest trauma, chest pain.	Chest wall contusion over infiltrate.	↑ WBC (left shift).	Patchy ill-defined infiltrate(s) ± rib fractures/ pneumothorax in area of infiltrate. Infiltrate clears within 1 week.

Non-Infectious Causes (cont'd)

Causes	Features (may have some, none, or all)			
	History	Physical	Laboratory	Chest X-Ray
Congestive heart failure	Coronary heart disease, valvular heart disease, cardiomyopathy.	No/low-grade fevers ↑ pulse and respiratory rate, positive jugular venous distension and hepatojugular reflex, cardio-megaly, S_3, ascites, hepatomegaly, pedal edema.	↑ WBC (left shift), normal platelets, mildly ↑ SGOT/SGPT.	Cardiomegaly, pleural effusion (R > [R + L] > L). Kerley B lines with vascular redistribution to upper lobes. Typically bilateral rather than unilateral.
Alveolar cell carcinoma	Fever, ↑ appetite with weight loss, night sweats.	± dullness over lobe with large lower lobe lesions.	Positive cytology by BAL/lung biopsy.	Well/ill-defined circumscribed peripheral infiltrates ± air bronchograms. May be multifocal/ multilobar. Hilar adenopathy present. Stranding to the hilum ("pleural tail" sign). ± pleural effusion if lower lobe infiltrate. No cavitation.
Lymphoma	Fever, ↓ appetite with weight loss, night sweats, fatigue.	Adenopathy ± splenomegaly.	Normal WBC, ↑ basophils, ↑ eosinophilia, ↓ lymphocytes, ↑ platelets, ↑ ESR, ↑ alkaline phosphatase, ↑$\propto_{1,2}$ globulins on SPEP.	Unilateral or asymmetrical bilateral hilar adenopathy. Lung infiltrate may appear contiguous with hilar adenopathy. No clear channel between media-stinum and hilar nodes. Small pleural effusions rare.

Non-Infectious Causes (cont'd)

	Features (may have some, none, or all)			
Causes	**History**	**Physical**	**Laboratory**	**Chest X-Ray**
Pulmonary hemorrhage	History of closed chest trauma or hemorrhagic disorder.	↑ WBC (left shift), ↑ pulse rate, respiratory rate. Signs of closed chest trauma.	Anemia plus findings secondary to underlying hemorrhagic disorder.	Localized or diffuse fluffy alveolar infiltrate(s). No cavitation, consolidation, or effusion.
Systemic lupus erythematosus (SLE)	Fatigue, chest pain. History of SLE.	Fever/ myalgias, alopecia, malar rash, "cytoid bodies" in retina, painless oral ulcers, synovitis, splenomegaly, generalized adenopathy, Raynaud's phenomenon.	↑ ANA, ↑ DS-DNA, ↓ C_3, polyclonal gammopathy on SPEP, ↑ ferritin. Pleural fluids with ↑ ANA, ↓ C_3	Migratory ill-defined non-segmental infiltrates ± small pleural effusions. No consolidation or cavitation.
Aspiration pneumonia	Swallowing disorder 2° to CNS/GI disorder; impaired consciousness; recent aspiration 2° to dental, upper GI, or pulmonary procedure.	Unremarkable.	↑ WBC, ↑ ESR.	Infiltrate usually involves superior segments of lower lobes (or posterior segments of upper lobes if aspiration occurred supine). Focal infiltrate initially, which may be followed in 7 days by cavitation/lung abscess.

UNILATERAL ILL-DEFINED INFILTRATES WITH EFFUSION

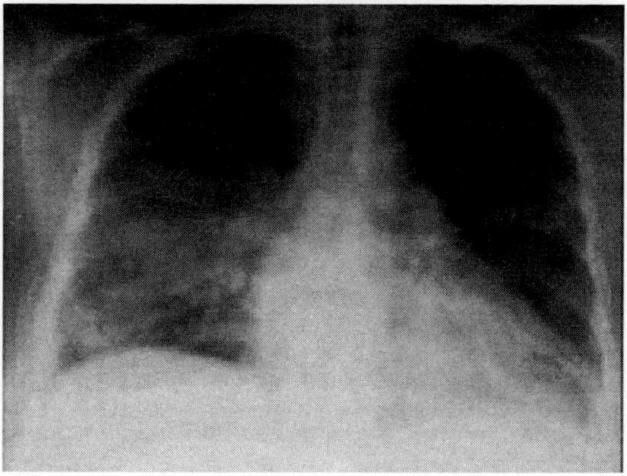

Infectious Causes

	Features (may have some, none, or all)			
Causes	History	Physical	Laboratory	Chest X-Ray
TB (primary)	Recent TB contact.	Unilateral lower lobe dullness related to size of pleural effusion.	PPD anergic. Exudative pleural effusion (pleural fluid with ↑ lymphocytes, ↑ glucose, ± RBCs).	Lower lobe infiltrate with small/moderate pleural effusion. No cavitation or apical infiltrates. Hilar adenopathy asymmetrical when present.
Nocardia	Fevers, night sweats, fatigue, ↓ cell-mediated immunity (e.g., HIV, organ transplant, immuno-suppressive therapy).	Unremarkable.	Normal/↑ WBC, ↑ ESR. Sputum with gram-positive AFB.	Dense large infiltrates. May cavitate and mimic TB, lymphoma, or squamous cell carcinoma. No calcification ± pleural effusion.

Infectious Causes (cont'd)

Causes	Features (may have some, none, or all)			
	History	Physical	Laboratory	Chest X-Ray
Legionella	Recent contact with Legionella containing water. Usually elderly. May have watery diarrhea, abdominal pain, mental confusion.	Fever/chills, relative bradycardia. Hepatic/splenic enlargement goes against the diagnosis. ↓ breath sounds if consolidation or pleural effusion.	↑ WBC, ↑ SGOT/SGPT, ↓ PO_4^-, ↓ Na^+, ↑ CPK, ↑ ESR, ↑ CRP, ↑ ferritin levels, microscopic hematuria, L. pneumophila antigenuria (serotypes 01–06 only) may not be positive early. Mucoid/purulent sputum with few PMNs. Positive sputum DFA (before therapy) is diagnostic. ↑ Legionella titer ≥ 1:256 or ≥ 4-fold rise between acute/convalescent titers.	Rapidly progressive asymmetrical infiltrates clue to Legionella. Consolidation and pleural effusion not uncommon. Cavitation rare.

Non-Infectious Causes

Causes	Features (may have some, none, or all)			
	History	Physical	Laboratory	Chest X-Ray
Lymphangitic metastases	History of breast, thyroid, pancreas, cervical, prostate, or lung carcinoma.	Findings related to underlying malignancy.	Normal/ ↑ WBC, ↑ ESR.	Interstitial indistinct pulmonary infiltrates (may be reticulonodular) with lower lobe predominance Usually unilateral but may be bilateral. No consoli-dation or cavitation ± pleural effusions.

Non-Infectious Causes (cont'd)

	Features (may have some, none, or all)			
Causes	**History**	**Physical**	**Laboratory**	**Chest X-Ray**
Pulmonary embolus/ infarct	Acute onset dyspnea/ pleuritic chest pain. History of lower extremity trauma, stasis or hypercoagulable disorder.	↑ pulse/ respiratory rate.	↑ fibrin split products and D-dimers ± ↑ total bilirubin. Bloody pleural effusion. ECG with RV strain/ P-pulmonale (large embolus). Positive V/Q scan and CT pulmonary angiogram.	Normal or show non-specific pleural-based infiltrates resembling atelectasis. Focal segmental/lobar hyperlucency (Westermark's sign) in some. "Hampton's hump" with infarct. Resolving infarcts ↓ in size but maintain shape/density ("melting ice cube").
Lymphoma	Fever, ↓ appetite with weight loss, night sweats, fatigue.	Adenopathy ± splenomegaly.	Normal WBC, ↑ basophils, ↑ eosinophilia, ↓ lymphocytes, ↑ platelets, ↑ ESR, ↑ alkaline phosphatase, $\uparrow\propto_{1,2}$ globulins on SPEP.	Unilateral or asymmetrical bilateral hilar adenopathy. Lung infiltrate may appear contiguous with hilar adenopathy. No clear channel between mediastinum and hilar nodes. Small pleural effusions rare.

Non-Infectious Causes (cont'd)

Causes	Features (may have some, none, or all)			
	History	Physical	Laboratory	Chest X-Ray
Bronchogenic carcinoma	Fever, ↓ appetite with weight loss, cough ± hemoptysis. Cough with copious clear/ mucoid sputum in large cell anaplastic carcinoma. Increased risk in smokers, aluminum/ uranium miners, cavitary lung disease (adeno-carcinoma), previous radiation therapy from lymphoma/ breast cancer.	Paraneoplastic syndromes especially with small (oat) cell/ squamous cell carcinoma ± hypertrophic pulmonary osteoarthropathy.	Normal/↑ WBC, ↑ platelets, ↑ ESR, findings related to underlying malignancy, ± clubbing.	Small/squamous cell carcinomas present as central lesions/ hilar masses. Adenocarcinoma/ large cell anaplastic carcinomas are usually peripheral initially. "Tumor tendrils" extending into surrounding lung tissue is characteristic. No calcifications (may be present on chest CT). Cavitation with squamous cell carcinoma. ± pleural effusions.
Alveolar cell carcinoma	Fever, ↑ appetite with weight loss, night sweats.	± dullness over lobe with large lower lobe lesions.	Positive cytology by BAL/lung biopsy.	Well/ill-defined circumscribed peripheral infiltrates ± air bronchograms. May be multifocal/ multilobar. Hilar adenopathy present. Stranding to the hilum ("pleural tail" sign). ± pleural effusion if lower lobe infiltrate. No cavitation.

Non-Infectious Causes (cont'd)

	Features (may have some, none, or all)			
Causes	**History**	**Physical**	**Laboratory**	**Chest X-Ray**
Metastatic carcinoma	History of breast, thyroid, renal cell, colon, pancreatic cancer or osteogenic sarcoma.	Findings related to underlying malignancy and, when present, to bone, hepatic, CNS metastases.	Secondary to effects of primary neoplasm, metastases, paraneoplastic syndrome.	Nodular lesions that vary in size. Metastatic lesions are usually well circumscribed with lower lobe predominance. Usually no bronchial obstruction (obstruction suggests colon, renal, or melanoma metastases). Usually no cavitation (except for squamous cell metastases). Calcification usually suggests osteosarcoma (rarely adenocarcinoma). Pleural effusion rare (except for breast cancer).

BILATERAL INFILTRATES WITHOUT EFFUSION

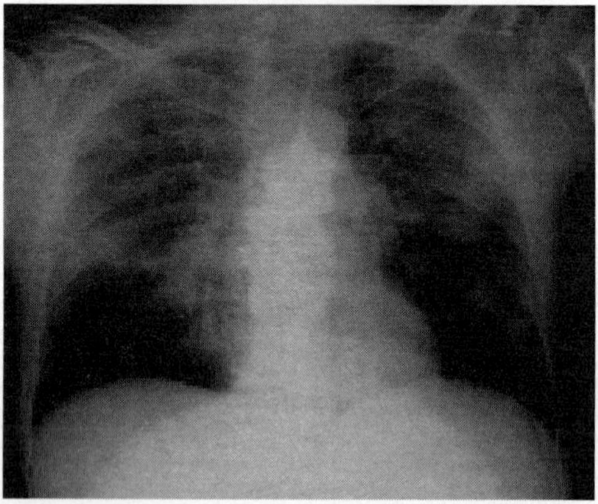

Infectious Causes

	Features (may have some, none, or all)			
Causes	**History**	**Physical**	**Laboratory**	**Chest X-Ray**
Influenza (human, avian, swine)	Acute onset of fever, myalgias, headache, fatigue, sore throat, rhinorrhea, dry cough, ± pleuritic chest pain.	↑ respiratory rate, cyanosis in severe cases.	↓ WBC, ↓ platelets, few/no atypical lymphocytes, ↑ A-a gradient. Influenza in respiratory secretions by culture/DFA. ↑ influenza titers.	Early normal/ near normal appearance. (< 48 hours) Later (> 48 hours) diffuse patchy bilateral interstitial infiltrates. No focal/segmental infiltrates unless secondary bacterial pneumonia present. ± small pleural effusions.

Infectious Causes (cont'd)

	Features (may have some, none, or all)			
Causes	**History**	**Physical**	**Laboratory**	**Chest X-Ray**
SARS	Acute onset of fever, myalgia, dry cough ± diarrhea.	↑ respiratory rate, cyanosis in severe cases.	N/↓ WBC, N/↓ platelets, ↓ pO_2, ↑ A-a gradient.	Culture of SARS – CoV from respiratory secretions.
HSV-1	Fever. Often presents in normal hosts as "failure to wean" from ventilator.	Unremarkable.	↑ WBC, ↓ pO_2, ↑ A-a gradient. HSV-1 in respiratory secretions by culture/DFA. Cytology with cytopathic changes of HSV.	Minimal bilateral diffuse infiltrates without cavitation or effusion.
RSV	Recent URI contact, dry cough, wheezing.	Mild lower respiratory tract infection in normal host. Moderate/ severe pneumonia in organ transplants.	Normal WBC; ↓ pO_2/↑ A-a gradient in severe RSV. RSV in respiratory secretions by culture/DFA.	Near normal chest x-ray or bilateral symmetrical patchy infiltrates. Consolidation uncommon. No cavitation or effusion.
VZV	VZV pneumonia occurs 2–3 days after rash. ↑ risk with pregnancy, smoking.	Healing vesicles, dry cough. Mild pneumonia in normal hosts. Moderate/ severe pneumonia in organ transplants.	↑ WBC, ↑ platelets, ↑ basophils; ↓ pO_2/↑ A-a gradient in severe chickenpox pneumonia. ↑ VZV titers.	Minimal diffuse fluffy interstitial infiltrates. Diffuse small calcifications may develop years later. No calcification of hilar nodes (in contrast to TB/ histoplasmosis).

Infectious Causes (cont'd)

Causes	Features (may have some, none, or all)			
	History	Physical	Laboratory	Chest X-Ray
CMV	↓ cell-mediated immunity (HIV, organ transplants, immunosuppressive therapy). Increasing dyspnea over 1 week	Fever ≤ 102 °F.	↓ pO_2, ↑ A-a gradient, ↑ LDH (PCP). PCP cysts or CMV "Cowdry Owl eye" inclusion bodies in respiratory secretions or transbronchial open lung biopsy.	Most HIV patients with PCP also have underlying CMV. Organ transplants with CMV usually do not have underlying PCP.
P (carinii) jiroveci (PCP)	↓ cell-mediated immunity (e.g., HIV, immuno-suppressive therapy). Increasing dyspnea over 1 week. Chest pain with shortness of breath suggests pneumothorax.	↓ breath sounds bilaterally. Other findings depend on size/location of pneumothorax (if present).	Normal/↑ WBC (left shift), ↑ lymphocytes, ↑ LDH. ↓ pO_2, ↓ DL_{CO}, ↑ A-a gradient. PCP cysts in sputum/ respiratory secretions.	Bilateral perihilar symmetrical patchy infiltrates ± pneumothorax. No calcification, cavitation, or pleural effusion.
TB (reactivation)	Fevers, night sweats, normal appetite with weight loss, cough ± hemoptysis.	± bilateral apical dullness.	Normal WBC, ↑ platelets, ↑ ESR (≤ 70 mm/h). Positive PPD. AFB in sputum smear/ culture.	Slowly progressive bilateral infiltrates. No pleural effusion. Usually in apical segment of lower lobes or apical/ posterior segments of upper lobes. Calcifications common.

Infectious Causes (cont'd)

Causes	Features (may have some, none, or all)			
	History	Physical	Laboratory	Chest X-Ray
Legionella	Recent contact with Legionella containing water. Usually elderly. May have watery diarrhea, abdominal pain, mental confusion.	Fever/chills, relative bradycardia. Hepatic/splenic enlargement goes against the diagnosis. ↓ breath sounds if consolidation or pleural effusion.	↑ WBC, ↑ SGOT/SGPT, ↑ pO_4^-, ↓ Na^+, ↑ CPK, ↑ ESR, ↑ CRP, ↑ ferritin levels, microscopic hematuria, L. pneumophila antigenuria (serotypes 01–06 only) may not be positive early. Mucoid/ purulent sputum with few PMNs. Positive sputum DFA (before therapy) is diagnostic. ↑ Legionella titer ≥ 1:256 or ≥ 4-fold rise between acute/ convalescent titers.	Rapidly progressive asymmetrical infiltrates clue to Legionella. Consolidation and pleural effusion not uncommon. Cavitation rare.
Psittacosis	Recent bird contact with psittacine birds. Severe headache.	Fever/chills, ± relative bradycardia, ± Horder's spots on face, epistaxis, ± splenomegaly. Signs of consolidation common.	↑/normal WBC, ↑ LFTs. Sputum with few PMNs. Positive C. psittaci serology.	Dense infiltrate. Consolidation common. Pleural effusion/ cavitation rare.

Infectious Causes (Cont'd)

Causes	Features (may have some, none, or all)			
	History	Physical	Laboratory	Chest X-Ray
Q fever	Recent contact with sheep or parturient cats.	Fever/chills, ± relative bradycardia, splenomegaly, ± hepato-megaly.	↑/normal WBC, ↑ LFTs. Sputum with no bacteria/few PMNs (caution–biohazard). Acute Q fever with ↑ in phase II ELISA antigens.	Dense consolidation. Cavitation/pleural effusion rare.
Nosocomial pneumonia (hema-togenous)	Fever/pulmonary symptoms ≥ 7 days in hospital. Increased risk with antecedent heart failure in previous 1–2 weeks.	Bilateral rales ± purulent respiratory secretions (tracheo-bronchitis).	↑ WBC (left shift). Normal pO_2/A-a gradient. Blood cultures positive for pulmonary pathogens. Respiratory secretions with WBCs ± positive culture of S. aureus, Enterobacter, P. aeruginosa, B. cepacia, Acinetobacter, Citrobacter, Klebsiella, or Serratia. Definitive diagnosis by lung biopsy/culture.	Bilateral symmetrical diffuse infiltrates. May be focal/segmental in aspiration nosocomial pneumonia. ↑ lung volumes (vs. ARDS). Klebsiella cavitation in 3–5 days; S. aureus and P. aeruginosa cavitation in 72 hours. No pleural effusion.

Non-Infectious Causes

	Features (may have some, none, or all)			
Causes	**History**	**Physical**	**Laboratory**	**Chest X-Ray**
Adult respiratory distress syndrome (ARDS)	Intubated on ventilator, multi-organ system failure.	± rales.	↑ WBC (left shift), normal ESR, ↓ pO_2, ↓ D_LCO, ↑ A-a gradient.	Bilateral fluffy infiltrates appearing ≥ 12 hours after profound hypoxemia. No cardiomegaly or pleural effusion. Reduced lung volumes (vs. nosocomial pneumonia or CHF). Bilateral consolidation ≥ 48 hours after appearance of infiltrates.
Goodpasture's Syndrome	Often preceded by a URI. Most common in 20–30 year old adults. Fever, weight loss, fatigue, cough, hemoptysis, hematuria.	Findings secondary to iron deficiency anemia.	↑ WBC, anemia, ↑ creatinine, urine with RBCs/RBC casts. Positive pANCA. Linear IgG pattern on alveolar/ glomerular basement membrane.	Bilateral fine reticulonodular infiltrates predominantly in lower lobes. No cavitation.
Wegener's granulo-matosis	Most common in middle-aged adults. Cough, fever, fatigue.	Findings of chronic sinusitis, bloody nasal discharge.	↑ WBC, anemia, ↑ platelets, ↑ ESR, ↑ RF, negative ANA, proteinuria, hematuria. Positive cANCA.	Bilateral asymmetrical nodular infiltrates of varying size with irregular margins. Cavitation common. Inner lining of cavities irregular. Air-fluid levels rare. ± pleural effusions. No calcifications.
Pulmonary hemorrhage	History of closed chest trauma or hemorrhagic disorder.	↑ WBC (left shift), ↑ pulse rate, ↑ respiratory rate. Signs of closed chest trauma.	Anemia plus findings secondary to underlying hemorrhagic disorder.	Localized or diffuse fluffy alveolar infiltrates. No cavitation, consolidation, or effusion.

Non-Infectious Causes (cont'd)

Causes	Features (may have some, none, or all)			
	History	Physical	Laboratory	Chest X-Ray
Chronic renal failure	Chronic renal failure on dialysis.	Findings related to uremia.	Normal/↑ WBC (left shift) plus findings related to renal failure.	Bilateral symmetrical fluffy perihilar infiltrates (butterfly pattern) ± pleural effusions. No cardiomegaly (unlike CHF), but large pericardial effusion can mimic cardiomegaly.
Lung contusion	Recent closed chest trauma, chest pain.	Chest wall contusion over infiltrate.	↑ WBC (left shift).	Patchy ill-defined infiltrate(s) ± rib fractures/pneumothorax in area of infiltrate. Infiltrate clears within 1 week.
Fat emboli	1–2 days post long bone fracture/ trauma.	↑ respiratory rate.	Urinalysis with "Maltese crosses."	Bilateral predominantly peripheral lower lobe infiltrates. Usually clears within 1 week.
Loeffler's Syndrome	Drug or parasitic exposure.	Unremarkable	Normal WBC, ↑ eosinophilia, ↑ ESR.	Characteristic "reversed bat-wing" pattern (i.e., peripheral infiltrates). Upper lobe predominance.
Sarcoidosis (Stage III)	Dyspena, fatigue, nasal stuffiness	Waxy/ yellowish papules on face/ upper trunk. Funduscopic exam with "candle wax drippings."	↑ ESR, normal LFTs, ↑ creatinine (if renal involvement), ↑ ACE levels, hypercalciuria, hypercalcemia, polyclonal gammopathy on SPEP. Anergic.	Bilateral nodular infiltrates of variable size without hilar adenopathy. Cavitation/ pleural effusion rare.

Non-Infectious Causes (cont'd)

Causes	Features (may have some, none, or all)			
	History	Physical	Laboratory	Chest X-Ray
Alveolar cell carcinoma	Fever, ↑ appetite with weight loss, night sweats.	± dullness over lobe with large lower lobe lesions.	Positive cytology by BAL/lung biopsy.	Well/ill-defined circumscribed peripheral infiltrates ± air bronchograms. May be multifocal/multilobar. Hilar adenopathy present. Stranding to the hilum ("pleural tail" sign). ± pleural effusion if lower lobe infiltrate. No cavitation.
Metastatic carcinoma	History of breast, thyroid, renal cell, colon, pancreatic cancer or osteogenic sarcoma.	Findings related to underlying malignancy and, when present, to bone, hepatic, CNS metastases.	Secondary to effects of primary neoplasm, metastases, paraneoplastic syndrome.	Nodular lesions that vary in size. Metastatic lesions are usually well circumscribed with lower lobe predominance. Usually no bronchial obstruction (obstruction suggests colon, renal, or melanoma metastases). Usually no cavitation (except for squamous cell metastases). Calcification usually suggests osteosarcoma (rarely adenocarcinoma). Pleural effusion rare (except for breast cancer).
Lymphoma	Fever, ↓ appetite with weight loss, night sweats, fatigue.	Adenopathy ± splenomegaly.	Normal WBC, ↑ basophils, ↑ eosinophilia, ↓ lymphocytes, ↑ platelets, ↑ ESR, ↑ alkaline phosphatase, ↑$\propto_{1,2}$ globulins on SPEP.	Unilateral or asymmetrical bilateral hilar adenopathy. Lung infiltrate may appear contiguous with hilar adenopathy. No clear channel between mediastinum and hilar nodes. Small pleural effusions rare.

Non-Infectious Causes (cont'd)

Causes	Features (may have some, none, or all)			
	History	Physical	Laboratory	Chest X-Ray
Leukostasis (AML)	Untreated acute myelogenous leukemia (AML).	Fever, sternal tenderness, petechiae, ecchymosis.	↑ WBC ($\geq$ 100 K/mm^3) with blasts in peripheral smear/bone marrow, ↓ platelets.	Diffuse symmetrical fluffy infiltrates without pleural effusion.
Drug-induced	Exposure to chemotherapeutic agents (e.g., BCNU, busulfan, methotrexate, cyclophosphamide, bleomycin) or other drugs (e.g., nitrofurantoin, sulfasalazine, amiodarone, opiates, cocaine).	Unremarkable.	Normal WBC ± ↑ eosinophilia, normal/↑ ESR/LFTs. Eosinophils in pleural effusion.	Bilateral coarse symmetrical patchy infiltrates/fibrosis ± pleural effusions. Hilar adenopathy only with drug-induced pseudolymphoma (secondary to dilantin). No cavitation.
Idiopathic pulmonary hemosiderosis (IPH)	Hemoptysis ± cough.	Findings of iron deficiency anemia.	Iron deficiency anemia. Hemosiderin in alveolar macrophages and urine.	Diffuse, bilateral ill-defined opacities or multiple "stellate" shaped infiltrates that clear between attacks. Recent hemorrhage may be superimposed on a fine reticular pattern that occurs after repeated bleeds.

Non-Infectious Causes (cont'd)

Causes	Features (may have some, none, or all)			
	History	Physical	Laboratory	Chest X-Ray
Bronchiolitis obliterans with organizing pneumonia (BOOP)	Fever, dyspnea, cough.	Unremarkable.	↑ WBC (left shift), ↑ LDH, ↓ pO_2, ↑ A-a gradient.	Classically bilateral patchy peripheral infiltrates. Often lower lobe predominance. No cavitation or pleural effusion.
Pulmonary alveolar proteinosis (PAP)	Asymptomatic if not infected with Nocardia.	Unremarkable.	Normal/↑ WBC, ↑ LDH	Bilateral granular or peripheral infiltrates in butterfly pattern. No hilar adenopathy, cardiomegaly, or pleural effusion.

BILATERAL INFILTRATES WITH EFFUSION

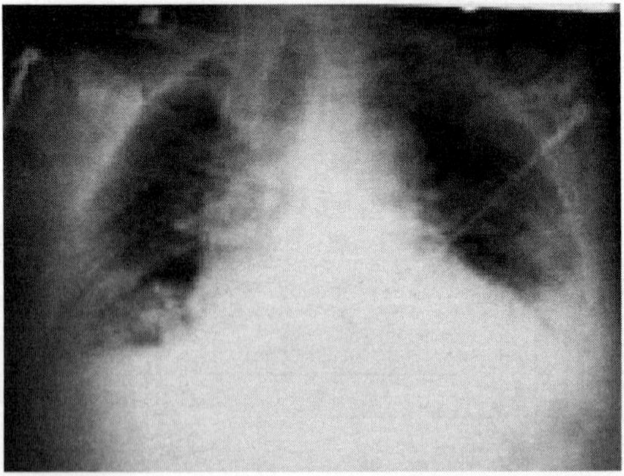

Infectious Causes

	Features (may have some, none, or all)			
Causes	**History**	**Physical**	**Laboratory**	**Chest X-Ray**
Legionella	Recent contact with Legionella containing water. Usually elderly. May have watery diarrhea, abdominal pain, mental confusion.	Fever/chills, relative bradycardia. Hepatic/ splenic enlargement goes against the diagnosis. ↓ breath sounds if consolidation or pleural effusion.	↑ WBC, ↑ SGOT/SGPT, ↑ PO_4^-, ↓ Na^+, ↑ CPK, ↑ ESR, ↑ CRP, ↑ ferritin levels, microscopic hematuria, L. pneumophila antigenuria (serotypes 01–06 only) may not be positive early. Mucoid/ purulent sputum with few PMNs. Positive sputum DFA (before therapy) is diagnostic. ↑ Legionella titer ≥ 1:256 or ≥ 4-fold rise between acute/convalescent titers.	Rapidly progressive asymmetrical infiltrates clue to Legionella. Consolidation and pleural effusion not uncommon. Cavitation rare.

Infectious Causes (cont'd)

	Features (may have some, none, or all)			
Causes	**History**	**Physical**	**Laboratory**	**Chest X-Ray**
Hantavirus (HPS)	Subacute onset, shortness of breath, substernal chest discomfort. Interim improvement followed by rapid deterioration.	↑ respiratory rate, cyanosis in severe cases.	↓ WBC, ↓ platelets ↓ pO_2, ↑ A-a gradient. ↑ hantavirus titers.	Large pleural effusions.
Measles	Recent airborne exposure.	Measles rash, Koplik's spots.	Normal/↑ WBC (left shift), normal/↓ platelets, ↑ LFTs, ↑ CPK, normal/↓ pO_2. If ↓ pO_2, then ↑ A-a gradient. ↑ IgM measles titer. Warthin-Finkeldey cells in respiratory secretions.	Bilateral diffuse fine reticulonodular infiltrates ± hilar adenopathy. Lower lobe predominance. Consolidation/ pleural effusion uncommon. No cavitation. Focal infiltrate indicates superimposed bacterial pneumonia.
Strongyl-oides	Strongyloides exposure. 1/3 asymptomatic; 2/3 with fever, dyspnea, cough. Hyperinfection syndrome with abdominal pain, diarrhea ± GI bleed.	With hyperinfection syndrome, fever, ↓ BP, abdominal tenderness ± rebound, ± meningitis.	↑ WBC (left shift), ↑ eosinophilia, ± anemia. Blood/CSF cultures positive for enteric gram-negative bacilli. Rhabditiform larvae in sputum/stool.	Diffuse hilar patchy infiltrates without consolidation or cavitation. Eosinophilic pleural effusion common.

Non-Infectious Causes

Causes	Features (may have some, none, or all)			
	History	Physical	Laboratory	Chest X-Ray
Congestive heart failure	Coronary heart disease, valvular heart disease, cardiomyopathy.	No/low grade fevers, ↑ pulse/ respiratory rate, positive jugular venous distension and hepatojugular reflex, cardiomegaly, S_3, ascites, hepatomegaly, pedal edema.	↑ WBC (left shift), normal platelets, mildly ↑ SGOT/ SGPT.	Cardiomegaly, pleural effusion (R > [R + L] > L). Kerley B lines with vascular redistribution to upper lobes. Typically bilateral rather than unilateral.
Chronic renal failure	Chronic renal failure on dialysis.	Findings related to uremia.	Normal/↑ WBC (left shift) plus findings related to renal failure.	Bilateral symmetrical fluffy perihilar infiltrates (butterfly pattern) ± pleural effusions. No cardiomegaly (unlike CHF), but large pericardial effusion can mimic cardiomegaly.
SLE	Fatigue, chest pain. History of SLE.	Fever/ myalgias, alopecia, malar rash, "cytoid bodies" in retina, painless oral ulcers, synovitis, splenomegaly, generalized adenopathy, Raynaud's phenomenon.	↑ ANA, ↑ DS-DNA, ↓ C_3, polyclonal gammopathy on SPEP, ↑ ferritin. Pleural fluids with ↑ ANA, ↓ C_3	Migratory ill-defined non-segmental infiltrates. No signs of consolidation or cavitation. ± small pleural effusions.

Non-Infectious Causes (cont'd)

Causes	Features (may have some, none, or all)			
	History	Physical	Laboratory	Chest X-Ray
Goodpasture's Syndrome	Often preceded by a URI. Most common in 20–30 year old adults. Fever, weight loss, fatigue, cough, hemoptysis, hematuria.	Findings secondary to iron deficiency anemia.	↑ WBC, anemia, ↑ creatinine, urine with RBCs/RBC casts. Positive pANCA. Linear IgG pattern on alveolar/ glomerular basement membrane.	Bilateral fine reticulonodular infiltrates predominantly in lower lobes. No cavitation.
Wegener's granulomatosis	Most common in middle-aged adults. Cough, fever, fatigue.	Findings of chronic sinusitis, bloody nasal discharge.	↑ WBC, anemia, ↑ platelets, ↑ ESR, ↑ RF, negative ANA, proteinuria, hematuria. Positive cANCA.	Bilateral asymmetrical nodular infiltrates of varying size with irregular margins. Cavitation common. Inner lining of cavities irregular. Air-fluid levels rare. ± pleural effusions. No calcifications.
Sarcoidosis (Stage III)	Dyspnea, fatigue, nasal stuffiness	Waxy/ yellowish papules on face/ upper trunk. Funduscopic exam with "candle wax drippings."	↑ ESR, normal LFTs, ↑ creatinine (if renal involvement), ↑ ACE levels, hypercalciuria, hypercalcemia, polyclonal gammopathy on SPEP. Anergic.	Bilateral nodular infiltrates of variable size without hilar adenopathy. Cavitation/pleural effusion rare.

Non-Infectious Causes (cont'd)

Causes	Features (may have some, none, or all)			
	History	Physical	Laboratory	Chest X-Ray
Lymphoma	Fever, ↓ appetite with weight loss, night sweats, fatigue.	Adenopathy ± splenomegaly.	Normal WBC, ↑ basophils, ↑ eosinophilia, ↓ lymphocytes, ↑ platelets, ↑ ESR, ↑ alkaline phosphatase, ↑$\alpha_{1,2}$ globulins on SPEP.	Unilateral or asymmetrical bilateral hilar adenopathy. Lung infiltrate may appear contiguous with hilar adenopathy. No clear channel between mediastinum and hilar nodes. Small pleural effusions rare.
Lymphangitic metastases	History of breast, thyroid, pancreas, cervical, prostate, or lung carcinoma.	Findings related to underlying malignancy.	Normal/ ↑ WBC, ↑ ESR.	Interstitial indistinct pulmonary infiltrates (may be reticulonodular) with lower lobe predominance Usually unilateral but may be bilateral. No consolidation or cavitation ± pleural effusions.
Drug-induced	Exposure to chemotherapeutic agents (e.g., BCNU, busulfan, methotrexate, cyclophosphamide, bleomycin) or other drugs (e.g., nitrofurantoin, sulfasalazine, amiodarone, opiates, cocaine).	Unremarkable.	Normal WBC ± ↑ eosinophilia, normal/↑ ESR/ LFTs. Eosinophils in pleural effusion.	Bilateral coarse symmetrical patchy infiltrates/ fibrosis ± pleural effusions. Hilar adenopathy only with drug-induced pseudolymphoma (secondary to dilantin). No cavitation.

CAVITARY INFILTRATES (THICK-WALLED)

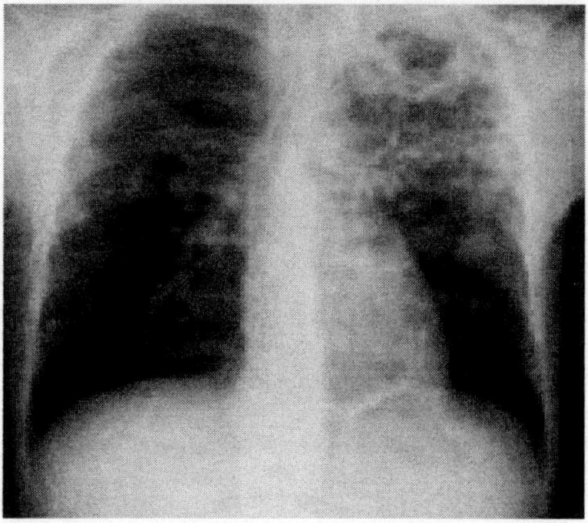

Infectious Causes Based on Speed of Cavitation

Speed of Cavitation	Causes
Very rapid cavitation (3 days)	S. aureus, P. aeruginosa
Rapid cavitation (5–7 days)	K. pneumoniae
Slow cavitation (> 7 days)	Pyogenic lung abscess, septic pulmonary emboli
Chronic cavitation	TB (reactivation), histoplasmosis (reactivation), sporotrichosis, melioidosis, nocardia, actinomycosis, Rhodococcus equi, amebic abscess, alveolar echinococcosis (hydatid cysts)

Infectious Causes

Causes	Features (may have some, none, or all)			
	History	Physical	Laboratory	Chest X-Ray
S. aureus	Fever, cough, dyspnea. Recent/concurrent influenza pneumonia.	↓ breath sounds ± cyanosis.	↑ WBC (left shift), ↓ pO_2, ↑ A-a gradient. Sputum positive for S. aureus. ↑ IgM influenza titers.	Multiple thick-walled cavitary lesions superimposed on normal looking lung fields or early minimal infiltrates of influenza.
P. aeruginosa	Nosocomial pneumonia usually on ventilator. Nearly always rapidly fatal.	Unremarkable.	↑ WBC (left shift). Respiratory secretions culture ± for P. aeruginosa. Blood cultures positive for P. aeruginosa (hematogenous nosocomial pneumonia).	Bilateral diffuse infiltrates with rapid cavitation (≤ 72 hours).
Klebsiella pneumoniae	Nosocomial pneumonia or history of alcoholism in patient with community-acquired pneumonia.	Fever, chills, signs of alcoholic cirrhosis, signs of consolidation over involved lobe.	↑ WBC, ↓ platelets, ↑ SGOT/SGPT (2° to alcoholism). "Red currant jelly" sputum with PMNs and plump gram-negative encapsulated bacilli.	"Bulging fissure" sign secondary to expanded lobar volume. Empyema rather than pleural effusion. Usually cavitation in 5–7 days (thick walled).
Pyogenic lung abscess	Recent aspiration. Fevers, chills, weight loss. Swallowing disorder secondary to CNS/GI disorder.	Foul (putrid lung abscess) breath.	↑ WBC, ↑ ESR. Sputum with normal oropharyngeal anaerobic flora in putrid lung abscess.	Thick-walled cavity in portion of lung dependent during aspiration (usually basilar segment of lower lobes if aspiration occurred supine). Cavitation occurs > 7 days.

Infectious Causes (cont'd)

Causes	Features (may have some, none, or all)			
	History	Physical	Laboratory	Chest X-Ray
Septic pulmonary emboli	Usually IV drug abuser with fever/chills. Tricuspid regurgitation murmur or recent OB/GYN surgical procedure.	Fever > 102 °F. Tricuspid valve regurgitant murmur with cannon A waves in neck.	Blood cultures positive for acute bacterial endocarditis pathogens.	Multiple peripheral nodules of varying size. Lower lobe predominance. Cavitation > 7 days characteristic of septic pulmonary emboli.
TB (reactivation)	Fevers, night sweats, normal appetite with weight loss, cough ± hemoptysis.	± bilateral apical dullness.	Normal WBC, ↑ platelets, ↑ ESR (≤ 70 mm/h). Positive PPD. AFB in sputum smear/culture.	Slowly progressive bilateral infiltrates. No pleural effusion. Usually in apical segment of lower lobes or apical/posterior segments of upper lobes. Calcifications common.
Histoplasmosis (reactivation)	Fever, night sweats, cough, weight loss, histoplasmosis exposure (River valleys of Central/Eastern United States).	± E. nodosum; otherwise unremarkable.	Normal WBC, normal/↑ eosinophilia, anemia, ↑ platelets, PPD negative. Immunodiffusion test with positive H precipitin band (diagnostic of active/chronic histoplasmosis).	Unilateral/bilateral multiple patchy infiltrates with upper lobe predilection. Bilateral hilar adenopathy uncommon. Calcifications common. No pleural effusion. Chest x-ray resembles reactivation TB.

Infectious Causes (cont'd)

Causes	Features (may have some, none, or all)			
	History	**Physical**	**Laboratory**	**Chest X-Ray**
Sporotrichosis	Fever, cough, weight loss. ± hemoptysis. Antecedent lympho-cutaneous or skeletal sporotrichosis, rare.	Only if secondary to residual of lympho-cutaneous sporotrichosis, ± E. nodosum.	Normal WBC. No eosinophilia.	Unilateral > bilateral upper lobe nodular densities. Thick or thin-walled cavities. No hilar adenopathy. No pleural effusion.
Melioidosis	Past travel to Asia (usually > 10 years). Fever, cough, hemoptysis.	Unremarkable.	↑ WBC (left shift), ↑ ESR, PPD negative. Sputum/blood cultures positive for B. (pseudomonas) pseudomallei.	Resembles reactivation TB, but lesions not apical and predominantly in middle/lower lung fields. No pleural effusion.
Nocardia	Fevers, night sweats, fatigue, ↓ cell-mediated immunity (e.g., HIV, organ transplant, immuno-suppressive therapy).	Unremarkable.	Normal/↑ WBC, ↑ ESR. Sputum with gram-positive AFB.	Dense large infiltrates. May cavitate and mimic TB, lymphoma, or squamous cell carcinoma. No calcification ± pleural effusion.
Actinomycosis	Recent dental work.	± chest wall sinus tracts.	Normal/↑ WBC, ↑ ESR. Sputum with Gram-positive filamentous anaerobic bacilli.	Dense infiltrates extending to chest wall. No hilar adenopathy. Cavitation ± pleural effusion rare.

Infectious Causes (cont'd)

Causes	Features (may have some, none, or all)			
	History	Physical	Laboratory	Chest X-Ray
Rhodococcus equi	Insidious onset of fever, dyspnea, chest pain, ± hemoptysis. Immuno-suppressed patients with ↓ cell-mediated immunity or exposure to cattle, horses, pigs.	Unremarkable.	Normal/↑ WBC. Sputum/pleural fluid with gram-positive pleomorphic weakly acid-fast bacilli. Sputum, pleural fluid, blood cultures positive for R. equi.	Segmental infiltrate with upper lobe predominance ± cavitation. Air-fluid levels and pleural effusion common.
Amebic cysts	Hepatic amebic abscess. Remote history of usually mild amebic dysentery.	± hepato-megaly.	Normal WBC and ESR. ↑ E. histolytica HI titers.	Well-circumscribed cavitary lesions adjacent to right diaphragm. ± calcifications. Sympathetic pleural effusion above hepatic amebic abscess.
Alveolar echinoco-ccosis (hydatid cysts)	Symptoms related to cyst size/ location: 1/3 asymptomatic; 2/3 with fever, malaise, chest pain ± hemoptysis. RUQ abdominal pain may occur.	Hepatomegaly common.	Normal/↑ WBC, no eosinophilia, ↑ alkaline phosphate/SGPT with hepatic cysts. Abdominal ultrasound/ CT with calcified hepatic irregularly shaped cysts ("Swiss cheese" calcification characteristic). ↑ E. multilocularis IHA titers.	RLL usual location (hepatic cysts penetrate diaphragm into RLL). Nodules are 70% solitary, 30% multiple. Pleural effusion rare. Endocyst membrane on surface of cyst fluid ("water lilly" sign) is characteristic.

Non-Infectious Causes

Causes	Features (may have some, none, or all)			
	History	Physical	Laboratory	Chest X-Ray
Wegener's granulomatosis	Most common in middle-aged adults. Cough, fever, fatigue.	Findings of chronic sinusitis, bloody nasal discharge.	↑ WBC, anemia, ↑ platelets, ↑ ESR, ↑ RF, negative ANA, proteinuria, hematuria. Positive cANCA.	Bilateral asymmetrical nodular infiltrates of varying size with irregular margins. Cavitation common. Inner lining of cavities irregular. Air-fluid levels rare. ± pleural effusions. No calcifications.
Squamous cell carcinoma	Long-term smoking history.	Clubbing, hypertrophic pulmonary osteoarthropathy ± findings 2° to superior vena caval syndrome and CNS/bone metastases.	↑ Ca^{++} (without bone metastases).	Unilateral perihilar mass lesion. Cavitation common. No pleural effusion.
Lymphoma	Fever, ↓ appetite with weight loss, night sweats, fatigue.	Adenopathy ± splenomegaly.	Normal WBC, ↑ basophils, ↑ eosinophilia, ↓ lymphocytes, ↑ platelets, ↑ ESR ↑ alkaline phosphatase, ↑$\alpha_{1,2}$ globulins on SPEP.	Unilateral or asymmetrical bilateral hilar adenopathy. Lung infiltrate may appear contiguous with hilar adenopathy. No clear channel between mediastinum and hilar nodes. Small pleural effusions rare.

Non-Infectious Causes (cont'd)

	Features (may have some, none, or all)			
Causes	**History**	**Physical**	**Laboratory**	**Chest X-Ray**
Metastatic carcinoma	History of breast, thyroid, renal cell, colon, pancreatic cancer or osteogenic sarcoma.	Findings related to underlying malignancy and, when present, to bone, hepatic, CNS metastases.	Secondary to effects of primary neoplasm, metastases, paraneoplastic syndrome.	Nodular lesions that vary in size. Metastatic lesions are usually well-circumscribed with lower lobe predominance. Usually no bronchial obstruction (obstruction suggests colon, renal, or melanoma metastases). Usually no cavitation (except for squamous cell metastases). Calcification usually suggests osteosarcoma (rarely adenocarcinoma). Pleural effusion rare (except for breast cancer).
Rheumatoid nodules	Usually in severe rheumatoid arthritis (RA); ± history of silicosis.	Findings secondary to RA. Rheumatoid nodules on exterior surfaces of arms.	Normal WBC, ↑ ESR, ↑ ANA, ↑ RF (high titer). Pleural fluid with ↓ glucose.	Lung nodules are round and well-circumscribed, predominantly in lower lobes and typically superimposed on interstitial lung disease ("rheumatoid lung"). Cavitation is common. ± pulmonary fibrosis, pleural effusion. Silicosis + RA nodules = Caplan's syndrome.

CAVITARY INFILTRATES (THIN-WALLED)

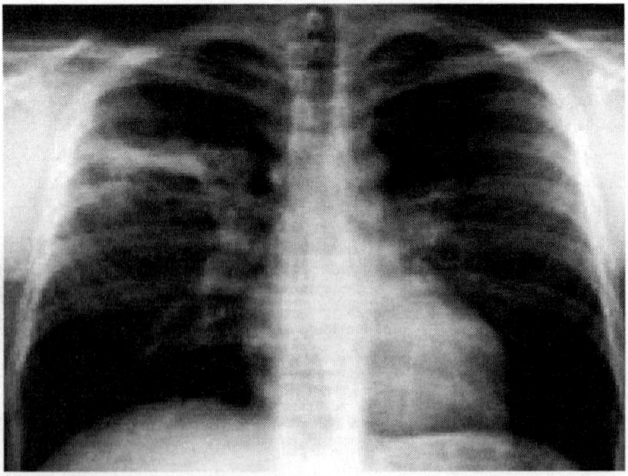

Infectious Causes

Causes	Features (may have some, none, or all)			
	History	Physical	Laboratory	Chest X-Ray
Atypical TB	Often occurs in setting of previous lung disease.	Unremarkable.	Normal WBC, ↑ ESR. Weakly positive PPD. Positive sputum AFB/ culture.	Multiple cavitary lesions ± calcifications usually involving both lungs. Resembles reactivation TB except that cavities are thin-walled. No pleural effusion.
Coccidiomycosis (reactivation)	Previous exposure in endemic coccidiomycosis areas (e.g., Southwest USA). Asymptomatic.	± E. nodosum.	Normal WBC. Eosinophilia acutely but not in chronic phase, and eosinophils in pleural fluid. CF IgG titer ≥ 1:32 indicates active disease.	Thick/thin walled cavities (< 3 cm) usually in anterior segments of lower lobes ± calcifications/ bilateral hilar adenopathy. Air-fluid levels rare unless secondarily infected. Pleural effusion rare.

Infectious Causes (cont'd)

Causes	Features (may have some, none, or all)			
	History	Physical	Laboratory	Chest X-Ray
Paragonimiasis	Ingestion of fresh-water crabs/ crayfish. Acute symptoms (< 6 months): fevers, abdominal pain, diarrhea followed by episodes of pleuritic chest pain. Chronic symptoms (> 6 months): fevers, night sweats, cough ± hemoptysis. Asymptomatic in some.	Wheezing, ± urticaria (acutely).	↑ WBC, eosinophilia. Eosinophils in pleural fluid. Sputum with Charot-Leyden crystals. Sputum/feces with operculated P. Westermani eggs.	Cavitary patchy or well-defined infiltrates predominantly in mid-lung fields. Hydropneumothorax common. Calcifications and pleural effusion common.
Sporotrichosis	Fever, cough, weight loss. ± hemoptysis. Antecedent lymphocutaneous or skeletal sporotrichosis, rare.	Only if secondary to residual of lympho-cutaneous sporotrichosis, ± E. nodosum.	Normal WBC. No eosinophilia.	Unilateral > bilateral upper lobe nodular densities. Thick or thin-walled cavities. No hilar adenopathy. No pleural effusion.
Pneumatoceles	Common in S. aureus pneumonia in children. Fever, cough, dyspnea. ± antecedent influenza.	Unremarkable unless pneumatocele ruptures, then signs of pneumothorax.	↑ WBC (left shift), ↓ pO_2 (secondary to influenza).	Multiple thin-walled cavities in areas of S. aureus pneumonia. Common in children; rare in adults.

Non-Infectious Causes

	Features (may have some, none, or all)			
Causes	**History**	**Physical**	**Laboratory**	**Chest X-Ray**
Emphysema (blebs/cyst)	Long history of smoking. Rupture of apical bleb common in males > 30 years. Pneumonia rare in severe emphysema (vs. chronic bronchitis) but may occur early in unaffected areas of lung.	Asthenic "pink puffers." Barrel chest. Diaphragmatic excursions < 2 cm.	Normal WBC, ↓ pO_2.	↓ lung markings ("vanishing lung") ± blebs. Hyperlucent lungs with upper lobe predominance. Flattened diaphragms, vertically elongated cardiac silhouette, ↑ retrocardiac and retrosternal airspaces. No infiltrates or pleural effusions. (In upper lobe emphysema, no vascular redistribution to upper lobes with CHF).
Bronchogenic cyst	Congenital anomaly. Usually asymptomatic. Cough if symptomatic.	Unremarkable unless secondarily infected, then signs 2° to mediastinal abscess.	Normal WBC/ ESR.	Circumscribed cystic lesion originates in lung but appears high in mediastinum. If filled with fluid, appears as solitary tumor. If near the trachea, may rupture into bronchus/trachea and cyst may contain air. If communicates openly with bronchus, appears as thin-walled cavitary nodule. If infected, presents as mediastinal abscess.
Cystic bronchiectasis	Recurrent pulmonary infections with purulent sputum ± hemoptysis.	Unremarkable unless dextrocardia with sinusitis (Kartagener's syndrome).	↑ WBC, normal ESR.	Bilateral large cystic lucencies at lung bases. Upper lobes relatively spared (unless secondary chronic aspiration). Thickened bronchial markings at bases. Bronchiectasis of cystic fibrosis predominantly involves upper lobes.

Non-Infectious Causes (cont'd)

Causes	Features (may have some, none, or all)			
	History	Physical	Laboratory	Chest X-Ray
Sequestered lung	Usually asymptomatic. Productive cough ± hemoptysis if communicates with bronchus or if infected.	Unremarkable.	Normal WBC, ↑ ESR.	Solid nodule unless communicates with bronchus, then thin-walled cavity ± air fluid levels. Usually posterior based segment of lower lobes (LLL > RLL). If > 3 cm, presents as mass lesion.
Histiocytosis X (eosinophilic granuloma, Langerhan's cell histiocytosis)	Patients usually 20–40 years. Usually asymptomatic. Fever, cough, dyspnea in some. Diabetes insipidus rare.	Hepato-splenomegaly, skin lesions, hemoptysis (rare).	Normal WBC, eosinophilia.	Pneumothorax superimposed on diffuse pulmonary fibrosis. Cystic bone lesions. Usually mid/upper lung fields with nodules/ thin-walled cysts or infiltrates. No hilar adenopathy or pleural effusion.

REFERENCES AND SUGGESTED READINGS

Burgener FA, Kormano M. Differential Diagnosis in Conventional Radiology, 2nd ed. Stuttgart, Georg Thieme Verlag, 1991.

Chapman S, Nakielny R. Aids to Radiological Differential Diagnosis, 2nd ed. London, Bailliere Tindall, 1990.

Conn RB, Borer WZ, Snyder JW. Current Diagnosis 9. Philadelphia, W. B. Saunders Company, 1997.

Crapo JD, Glassroth J, Karlinsky JB, King TE. Baum's Textbook of Pulmonary Diseases, 7th ed. Philadelphia, Lippincott Williams & Wilkins, 2004.

Cunha BA. Pneumonia Essentials, 3rd ed. Jones & Bartlett, Sudbury MA, 2010.

Eisenberg RL. Clinical Imaging. An Atlas of Differential Diagnosis, 2nd ed. Gaithersburg, Aspen Publishers, Inc., 1992.

Gorbach SL, Bartlett JG, Blacklow NR. Infectious Diseases, 3rd ed. Philadelphia, Lippincott Williams & Wilkins, 2004.

Karetzky M, Cunha BA, Brandstetter RD. The Pneumonias. New York, Springer-Verlag, 1993.

Kasper L, Braunwald E, Fauci AS, Hauser SL, Longo DL, Jameson JL. Harrison's Principles of Internal Medicine, 17th ed. New York, The McGraw Hill Companies, 2008.

Levison ME. The Pneumonias: Clinical Approaches to Infectious Diseases of the Lower Respiratory Tract. Boston, John Wright, PSG Inc., 1984.

Lillington GA, Jamplis RW. A Diagnostic Approach to Chest Diseases, 2nd ed. Baltimore, The Williams & Wilkins Company, 1977.

Mandell GL, Bennet JE, Dolin R. Mandell, Douglas, and Bennett's Principles and Practice of Infectious Diseases, 7th ed., Elsevier, 2010.

Murray JF, Nadel JA. Textbook of Respiratory Medicine, 3rd ed. Philadelphia, W.B. Saunders Company, 2000.

Teplick JE, Haskin ME. Roentgenologic Diagnosis, 3rd ed. Philadelphia, W. B. Saunders Company, 1976.

Wright FW. Radiology of the Chest and Related Conditions. London, Taylor & Francis, 2002.

Chapter 9

Infectious Disease Differential Diagnosis

Cheston B. Cunha, MD

Infectious diseases often present with important findings on physical diagnosis and laboratory evaluation. In this chapter, key findings of infectious diseases and noninfectious diseases likely to be considered in the differential diagnosis are presented. Tropical infections are also included since this book is also for international use.

Table 9.1. Fever Curves

Finding	Causes
Morning (am) temperature spikes	Infectious: TB, typhoid fever, Whipple's disease Noninfectious: PAN
Relative tachycardia	Infectious: gas gangrene, myocarditis (Coxsackie, RMSF, typhus, diptheria, trichinosis, VLM, influenza) Noninfectious: Hyperthyroidism, hypoxia, cardiac arrhythmias, pulmonary emboli
Relative bradycardia	Infectious: typhoid fever, typhus, leptospirosis, Legionnaire's disease, Q fever, psittacosis, RMSF, babesiosis, ehrlichiosis, yellow fever, dengue fever, arboviral hemorrhagic fevers Noninfectious: drug fever, CNS lesions, β-blockers, verapamil, diltiazem, lymphoma, factitious fever
Single fever spikes	Infectious: Transient bacteremia Noninfectious: Blood/blood product transfusions
Double quotidian fevers	Infectious: kala-azar, right sided GC ABE, miliary TB, mixed malarial infections Noninfectious: adult Still's disease, antipyretics
Camelback fever pattern	Infectious: Colorado tick fever, dengue fever, leptospirosis, brucellosis, LCM, yellow fever, poliomyelitis, smallpox, rat-bite fever (*Spirillum minus*), chikungunya fever, rift valley fever, african hemorrhagic fevers (Marburg, Ebola, Lassa, etc), echovirus (echo 9) Noninfectious: antipyretics

Table 9.2. General Appearance Abnormalities

Finding	Causes
Hypotension/ shock	Infectious: anthrax, plague, typhus, ***GI sources***: colon (perforation, colitis, abscess); ***GU sources***: cystitis (only in SLE, DM, alcoholism, multiple myeloma, Vibrio vulnificus, CLL, steroids); obstruction: relative (BPH), unilateral (partial), or bilateral/ureteral (partial/total); kidney (acute pyelonephritis, renal abscess, perinephric abscess, renal calculi); prostate (acute prostatitis, prostatic abscess). ***Other sources***: CVC infection, TSS (S. aureus, group A streptococci, C. sordellii), dengue fever, SARS, HPS, influenza (human, avian, swine), CAP (with decreased/absent splenic function), with severe cardiopulmonary disease or CA-MRSA (PVL+) with influenza/ILI Noninfectious: myocardial infarction, pulmonary embolism, acute pancreatitis, relative adrenal insufficiency, GI bleed, overzealous diuresis, inadequate volume replacement or hypotonic fluid replacement, aortic dissection, abdominal aneurysm rupture, rectus sheath hematoma
Soft tissue crepitance	Infectious: mixed aerobic/anaerobic infection* Noninfectious: subcutaneous emphysema, recent surgery in area of crepitance *Gas gangrene (minimal/no gas on auscultation)
Bullae	Infectious: gas gangrene (hemorrhagic), S. aureus > group A streptococci, V. vulnificus (hemorrhagic), necrotizing fasciitis, bullous impetigo Noninfectious: pemphigus, pemphigoid, dermatitis herpetiformis, TEN, porphyria, contact dermatitis, E. multiforme, DM, barbiturates
Generalized edema/nephrotic syndrome	Infectious: malaria (P. malariae), trichinosis, VZV, yellow fever, influenza A, HBV, HIV, EBV, CMV, 2° syphilis, leprosy Noninfectious: drugs, lymphomas, thiamine deficiency (wet beri-beri), kwashiorkor, post-streptococcal glomerulonephritis, DM, PAN, Henoch-Schönlein purpura, SLE, constrictive pericarditis, tricuspid regurgitation, IVC obstruction, myxedema, sickle cell disease, amyloidosis, alpha-1 antitrypsin deficiency, nail-patella syndrome, Wegener's granulomatosis, sarcoidosis, renal vein thrombosis
Erythroderma	Infectious: human T-cell leukemia virus 1 (HTLV-1), TSS, scarlet fever, dengue fever Noninfectious: psoriasis, lymphoma, atopic dermatitis, contact dermatitis, exfoliative dermatitis, drugs, ichthyosis, erythroleukemia, pityriasis, dermatomyositis, Kawasaki's disease
Hyper-pigmentation	Infectious: kala-azar, Whipple's disease, histoplasmosis Noninfectious: hemochromatosis, PBC, Addison's disease, drugs – brown (bleomycin), blue/gray (busulfan, fluorouracil, chlorpromazine), purple/gray (amiodarone), blue/gray (minocycline)

Table 9.2. General Appearance Abnormalities (cont'd)

Finding	Causes
Jaundice	Infectious: yellow fever, EBV, leptospirosis, ascariasis (in bile/pancreatic duct), viral hemorrhagic fevers, viral hepatitis Noninfectious: hepatobiliary malignancy, benign biliary obstruction, PBC, cirrhosis, hemolytic anemias, alcoholic hepatitis, drugs, Gilbert's syndrome, pancreatic carcinoma
Vitiligo	Infectious: leprosy, yaws, pinta, HIV Noninfectious: DM, hyperthyroidism, hypothyroidism, Hashimoto's thyroiditis
Lizard/elephant skin	Infectious: onchocerciasis Noninfectious: ichthyosis
Urticaria	Infectious: strongyloides, dracunculiasis, HBV, F. hepatica, schistosomal dermatitis Noninfectious: insect bites/stings, drugs, malignancies, cholinergic urticaria, serum sickness, urticarial vasculitis, cryoglobulinemia, systemic mastocytosis
Rash (below waist)	Infectious: Parvovirus B19 (stocking/glove) Noninfectious: Henoch-Schönlein Purpura (HSP)

Table 9.3. Head Abnormalities

Finding	Causes
Prematurely gray hair	Infectious: HIV Noninfectious: smoking, pernicious anemia
Temporal muscle wasting	Infectious: HIV Noninfectious: myotonic dystrophy
Facial swelling (edema)	Infectious: arboviral hemorrhagic fevers, trichinosis, leprosy, EEE, onchocerciasis Noninfectious: angioneurotic edema, nephrotic syndrome, acute glomerulonephritis, leukemic infiltrates, amyloidosis
Severe seborrheic dermatitis	Infectious: HIV Noninfectious: CGD
Facial red spots	Infectious: psittacosis (Horder's spots) Noninfectious: Campbell de Morgan spots

Table 9.3. Head Abnormalities (cont'd)

Finding	Causes
Localized alopecia	Infectious: leprosy, tinea capitis, smallpox, blastomycosis, VZV, TB (cutaneous) Noninfectious: SLE, DM, scleroderma, common variable immune deficiency (CVID)
Generalized alopecia	Infectious: post-malaria, post-typhoid fever, post-kala-azar, post-yellow fever, 2° syphilis, HIV Noninfectious: nutritional deficiencies, drugs, hyperthyroidism
Total/partial eyebrow loss	Infectious: leprosy, syphilis Noninfectious: iatrogenic, hereditary, hypothyroidism, hypopituitarism
Long eyelashes	Infectious: kala-azar, trypanosomiasis Noninfectious: hereditary, drugs, HIV drugs
Lacrimal gland enlargement *unilateral*	Infectious: Chagas' disease Noninfectious: malignancies
bilateral	Infectious: TB Noninfectious: Sjogren's syndrome, RA, SLE, sarcoidosis
Facial erythema	Infectious: facial cellulitis, erysipelas, TB (lupus vulgaris), arboviral hemorrhagic fevers Noninfectious: dermatomyositis, drugs, rosacea, carcinoid syndrome, SLE
Parotid enlargement	Infectious: mumps, Chagas' disease, rat bite fever (Streptobacillus moniliformis) Noninfectious: Sjogren's syndrome, sarcoidosis, cirrhosis
Scalp nodules	Infectious: myiasis, onchocerciasis Noninfectious: bony exostoses, malignancies, benign cysts, pyogenic granuloma, Kimura's disease

Table 9.4. Eye Abnormalities

Finding	Causes
Bilateral upper lid edema	Infectious: EBV (Hoagland's sign) Noninfectious: bilateral eye irritation
Bilateral lid edema	Infectious: trichinosis, meningococcemia, adenovirus Noninfectious: Wegener's granulomatosis

Table 9.4. Eye Abnormalities (cont'd)

Finding	Causes
Heliotrope eyelid discoloration	Infectious: cholera (early), influenza A (severe) Noninfectious: dermatomyositis
Periorbital edema *unilateral*	Infectious: Chagas' disease, loiasis, gnathostomiasis, sparganosis Noninfectious: insect bites, unilateral eye irritation
bilateral	Infectious: RMSF, trichinosis, tularemia, dengue fever Noninfectious: allergies, Insect bites, dermatomyositis
Argyll-Robertson pupils	Infectious: syphilis Noninfectious: sarcoidosis
Iritis	Infectious: onchocerciasis, 2° syphilis, relapsing fever, leprosy Noninfectious: SLE, dermatomyositis, Behçet's syndrome, Reiter's syndrome, RA
Conjunctivitis *unilateral*	Infectious: TB, HSV, tularemia, adult inclusion conjunctivitis, Chagas' disease, LGV, CSD, loiasis, ocular myiasis, diphtheria, adenovirus (types 8, 19) Noninfectious: SLE, eye irritation
bilateral	Infectious: TSS, measles, rubella, meningococcemia, gonorrhea, adenovirus (type 3), plague, RMSF, sparganosis, LGV, listeria, relapsing fever, pertussis, influenza, microsporidia, HHV-6, arboviral hemorrhagic fevers, dengue hemorrhagic fever Noninfectious: Kawasaki's disease, Reiter's syndrome, Steven-Johnson syndrome, adult Still's disease, eye irritation
Hemorrhagic conjunctivitis *unilateral*	Infectious: adenovirus (type 8, 19) Noninfectious: trauma
bilateral	Infectious: trichinosis, pertussis, leptospirosis, Coxsackie A (type 24), adenovirus (type 11), enterovirus (type 70), arboviral hemorrhagic fevers Noninfectious: trauma
Subconjunctival hemorrhage	Infectious: SBE, trichinosis, meningococcemia, pertussis, leptospirosis, RMSF Noninfectious: severe anemia, Kawasaki's disease
Conjunctival suffusion	Infectious: RMSF, leptospirosis, relapsing fever, ehrlichiosis, HPS, influenza (human, avian), arboviral hemorrhagic fevers Noninfectious: bilateral eye irritation

Table 9.4. Eye Abnormalities (cont'd)

Finding	Causes
Episcleritis	Infectious: TB, leprosy, 2° syphilis, Lyme disease Noninfectious: sarcoidosis, RA, adult Still's disease, SLE, PAN, TA, RE
Scleral nodules	Infectious: loiasis, sparganosis, leprosy, tularemia, TB Noninfectious: RA, vitamin A deficiency (Bitot's spots), sarcoidosis
Dry eyes	Infectious: measles Noninfectious: vitamin A deficiency, SLE, Sjogren's syndrome, RA, sarcoidosis
Watery eyes	Infectious: bacterial conjunctivitis, adenovirus Noninfectious: PAN, allergenic conjunctivitis
Uveitis	Infectious: TB, histoplasmosis, leprosy, 3° syphilis, malaria, HSV, VZV, EBV, TSS, typhus, LGV, CMV, African trypanosomiasis, brucellosis, leptospirosis, RMSF, CSD Noninfectious: adult Still's disease, SLE, PAN, sarcoidosis, Behçet's syndrome, Reiter's syndrome, RA, relapsing polychondritis, ankylosing spondylitis, Kawasaki's disease, Wegener's granulomatosis
Corneal haziness	Infectious: adenovirus, leprosy, trachoma, onchocerciasis Noninfectious: vitamin A deficiency, cataracts
Keratitis	Infectious: HSV, congenital syphilis, acanthamoeba, TB, toxoplasmosis, histoplasmosis, CMV, trachoma, microsporidia, nocardia, leprosy, onchocerciasis Noninfectious: Behçet's syndrome, Reiter's syndrome, Steven-Johnson syndrome, vitamin A deficiency
Corneal ulcers	Infectious: HSV, listeria, acanthamoeba, tularemia, shigella, RMSF Noninfectious: trauma, Wegener's granulomatosis
Endophthalmitis	Infectious: TB, candida, aspergillus, toxocara, serratia, S. pneumoniae Noninfectious: retinoblastoma
Chorioretinitis	Infectious: toxoplasmosis, CMV, onchocerciasis, congenital syphilis, histoplasmosis, TB, WNE, coccidiomycosis, leptospirosis Noninfectious: sarcoidosis, SLE, PAN
Cytoid bodies (cotton wool spots)	Infectious: CSD, HIV, CMV, SBE Noninfectious: SLE, adult Still's disease, PAN, atrial myxoma, Wegener's granulomatosis, TA

Table 9.4. Eye Abnormalities (cont'd)

Finding	Causes
Roth spots	Infectious: SBE, psittacosis, RMSF, malaria Noninfectious: PAN, SLE, DM, severe anemia, leukemia, cholesterol emboli syndrome, atrial myxoma, TA, Takayasu's arteritis
Periphlebitis (candle wax drippings)	Infectious: CMV, leptospirosis (Weil's syndrome) Noninfectious: sarcoidosis

Table 9.5. Ear Abnormalities

Finding	Causes
Acute deafness	Infectious: ABM, mumps (aseptic meningitis), RMSF, typhus, brucellosis, Lassa fever Noninfectious: sound/barotrauma
External ear lesions	Infectious: cutaneous leishmaniasis (Chiclero ulcer), leprosy, Kaposi's sarcoma Noninfectious: relapsing polychondritis, eczema, carcinoma, contact dermatitis, sarcoidosis, SLE, gout (tophi), keloids, actinic keratosis

Table 9.6. Nasal Abnormalities

Finding	Causes
Purple nose tip	Infectious: Kaposi's sarcoma, TB (Bazin's erythema induratum) Noninfectious: vasculitis, lymphoma, drugs, sarcoidosis
Nose tip gangrene	Infectious: Staphylococcus aureus ABE (emboli) Noninfectious: SLE, vasculitis
Epistaxis	Infectious: psittacosis, typhoid fever, nasal diphtheria, Colorado tick fever, TBRF, influenza, dengue hemorrhagic fever, arboviral hemorrhagic fevers, acute renal failure, leprosy, leptospirosis, VZV, TB, rhinosporidium, mucocutaneous leishmaniasis Noninfectious: Local trauma, sinus malignancies, von Willebrand's disease, polycythemia vera, Waldenstrom's macroglobulinemia, relapsing polychondritis
Nasal septal perforation	Infectious: leprosy, 2° syphilis, mucocutaneous leishmaniasis, blastomycosis, pinta, yaws Noninfectious: cocaine, lethal midline granuloma, Wegener's granulomatosis, miasis

Table 9.7. Mouth Abnormalities

Finding	Causes
Trismus	Infectious: tetanus Noninfectious: temporomandibular joint dislocation/arthritis, trigeminal neuralgia
Herpes labialis	Infectious: HSV, pneumococcal pneumonia, meningococcal meningitis, malaria Noninfectious: contact dermatitis (mimics H. labialis)
Angular chelitis	Infectious: 2° syphilis, HIV Noninfectious: riboflavin deficiency, trauma, contact dermatitis, anemia
Gingivitis	Infectious: trench mouth Noninfectious: Wegener's granulomatosis
Tongue tenderness	Infectious: relapsing fever Noninfectious: vitamin deficiencies, pernicious anemia
Tongue ulcers	Infectious: histoplasmosis, HSV, syphilis Noninfectious: aphthous ulcers, chemotherapy, radiation therapy
Leukoplakia	Infectious: HIV (hairy), syphilis Noninfectious: lichen planus
Oral ulcers *solitary*	Infectious: syphilis, CMV, histoplasmosis, TB Noninfectious: squamous cell carcinoma, Behçet's syndrome, Wegener's granulomatosis
multiple	Infectious: HSV, HFM disease, herpangina, brucellosis, Lassa fever Noninfectious: SLE, celiac disease, aphthous ulcers, squamous cell carcinoma, Behçet's syndrome, FAPA syndrome, hyper IgE (Job's) syndrome E. multiforme, RE, cyclic neutropenia, Sweet's syndrome
Frenal ulcer	Infectious: pertussis Noninfectious: trauma
Palatal petechiae	Infectious: Group A streptococci, EBV, CMV, HSV, VZV, toxoplasmosis, rubella, HIV, tularemia Noninfectious: thrombocytopenia (2° to any cause), platelet dysfunction disorders, DIC, Ehlers-Danlos syndrome, Marfan's syndrome

Table 9.7. Mouth Abnormalities (cont'd)

Finding	Causes
Palatal perforation	Infectious: congenital syphilis, myiasis Noninfectious: Post-surgical, midline granuloma, cocaine
Palatal vesicles	Infectious: ***Anterior*****:** HSV, VZV. ***Posterior*****:** herpangina (Coxsackie A), hand-foot-mouth disease (Coxsackie A) Noninfectious: bullous pemphigus, Steven-Johnson syndrome (drug-induced)
Uvular edema	Infectious: Group A streptococci Noninfectious: Franklin's disease, drugs, angioneurotic edema
Crimson crescents	Infectious: chronic fatigue syndrome (CFS), HIV Noninfectious: None
Tonsillar membranes	Infectious: diphtheria, Arcanobacterium hemolyticum Noninfectious: None
Tonsillar ulcers	Infectious: tularemia (oropharyngeal), 1° syphilis, Vincent's angina, TB Noninfectious: carcinoma, T-cell lymphoma, AML
Hoarseness	Infectious: laryngeal TB, C. pneumoniae, respiratory viruses, pertussis Noninfectious: recurrent laryngeal nerve paralysis

Table 9.8. Neck Abnormalities*

Finding	Causes
Enlarged greater auricular nerve	Infectious: leprosy Noninfectious: none
Bull neck	Infectious: diphtheria, mumps, Ludwig's angina, pertussis, group A streptococcal suppurative lymphangitis Noninfectious: angioneurotic edema, subcutaneous emphysema
Jugular vein tenderness	Infectious: suppurative jugular thrombophlebitis (Lemierre's syndrome) Noninfectious: thrombophlebitis
Neck sinus tract	Infectious: actinomycosis, TB, atypical TB Noninfectious: branchial cleft cyst, CGD
Superior vena cava syndrome	Infectious: actinomycosis Noninfectious: lymphoma, squamous cell carcinoma

* See Table 9.13 for Cervical adenopathy.

Table 9.9. Chest Abnormalities

Finding	Causes
Shoulder tenderness	Infectious: subdiaphragmatic abscess, septic arthritis (shoulder) Noninfectious: squamous cell carcinoma (Pancoast's tumor), bursitis
Sternal tenderness	Infectious: sternal osteomyelitis (post-open heart surgery) Noninfectious: metastatic carcinoma, pre-leukemia, acute leukemia, myeloproliferative disorder, trauma
Costochondral tenderness	Infectious: costochondritis (Coxsackie B) Noninfectious: trauma, plasmacytoma
Trapezius tenderness	Infectious: subdiaphragmatic abscess Noninfectious: fibromyalgia
Chest wall sinuses	Infectious: TB, actinomycosis, blastomycosis, abscess, M. fortuitum-chelonei (post-breast implant surgery), sternal osteomyelitis (post-sternotomy) Noninfectious: bronchogenic carcinoma
Spontaneous pneumothorax	Infectious: TB, PCP, Legionnaire's disease, lung abscess, pertussis Noninfectious: histiocytosis X (eosinophilic granuloma, Langerhan's cell histiocytosis), osteogenic sarcoma, emphysema, ARDS
Diffuse wheezing	Infectious: influenza, C. pneumoniae, M. pneumoniae Noninfectious: pulmonary emboli, LVF, asthma, Churg-Strauss granulomatosis, carcinoid syndrome, asthmatic bronchitis, angioedema
Chest dullness *consolidation*	Infectious: bacterial pneumonia, psittacosis, nocardia, Q fever Noninfectious: large cell carcinoma
pleural effusion	Infectious: group A streptococci, tularemia, H. influenzae, 1° TB Noninfectious: Meig's syndrome, pancreatitis, CHF, malignancies, pulmonary embolism

Table 9.10. Back Abnormalities

Finding	Causes
Spinal tenderness	Infectious: vertebral osteomyelitis, typhoid fever, TB, brucellosis, SBE Noninfectious: malignancies, multiple myeloma
D'espine's sign	Infectious: bilateral pneumonia (consolidation), TB Noninfectious: sarcoidosis, large cell carcinoma, lymphoma
Unilateral CVA tenderness	Infectious: pyelonephritis, renal/perinephric abscess Noninfectious: trauma

Table 9.11. Heart Abnormalities

Finding	Causes
Tachycardia	Infectious: myocarditis (Coxsackie, RMSF, typhus, diphtheria, trichinosis, Toxocara canis/cati (VLM), influenza dengue), gas gangrene Noninfectious: hypovolemia, hypoxia, MI, pulmonary embolism, CHF, Kawasaki's disease, substance withdrawl
Heart block *Acute*	Infectious: Lyme disease, ABE with paravalvular/septal abscess, diptheria Noninfectious: acute (inferior) MI, drugs
Chronic	Infectious: Chagas' disease Noninfectious: AV nodal ablation, sarcoidosis, Lev's/Lenegre's disease
Pericardial effusion (increased area of cardiac dullness)	Infectious: viral pericarditis, TB pericarditis Noninfectious: SLE, uremia, malignancy
Heart murmur	Infectious: SBE, 3° syphilis Noninfectious: valvular heart disease, severe anemia, Takayasu's arteritis, SLE (Libman-Sacks), endomyocardial fibroelastosis, atrial myxoma, marantic endocarditis

Table 9.12. Abdominal Abnormalities

Finding	Causes
Abdominal wall tenderness	Infectious: leptospirosis, abdominal wall cellulitis/abscess, trichinosis Noninfectious: trauma, rectus sheath hematoma
Abdominal wall sinus tract	Infectious: TB, abscess, ameboma, actinomycosis Noninfectious: carcinomas
Rose spots	Infectious: typhoid fever, shigella, trichinosis Noninfectious: Campbell de Morgan spots

Table 9.12. Abdominal Abnormalities (cont'd)

Finding	Causes
Right upper quadrant tenderness	Infectious: cholangitis, cholecystitis, pylephlebitis, splenic flexure diverticulitis, emphysematous cholecystitis (Clostridia sp.), hepatic abscess (amebic, echinococcal, bacterial), right lower lobe CAP, brucellosis, leptospirosis, typhoid fever, viral hepatitis Noninfectious: ptosed right kidney, acute pancreatitis, acalculous cholecystitis, Kawasaki's disease, cholesterol emboli syndrome, PAN, SLE, total parenteral nutrition, ceftriaxone (psuedocholelithiasis)
Right upper quadrant tympany	Infectious: peritonitis (2° to organ perforation) Noninfectious: post-abdominal surgery
Right upper quadrant mass	Infectious: bacterial abscess, echinococcal cysts, amebic abscess Noninfectious: ptosed right kidney, Reidel's lobe, hepatoma, malignancies, distended gallbladder (Couvoisier's sign)
Right lower quadrant tenderness	Infectious: shigella, typhoid fever, typhoidal EBV, typhoidal tularemia, parvovirus B19, TB, ameboma, typhlitis, actinomycetoma, pseudoappendicitis (scarlet fever), Legionnaires' disease, yersinia, campylobacter, measles (pre-eruptive), RMSF, PID, syphilis (luetic crisis), brucellosis Noninfectious: appendicitis, RE, ectopic pregnancy, diverticulitis, hyper IgE (Job's) syndrome, DM crisis, porphyria, pancreatitis, SLE
Left upper abdominal quadrant tenderness (splenic tenderness)	Infectious: SBE, brucellosis, typhoid fever, malaria, splenic abscess, EBV, CMV, HHV-6 Noninfectious: splenic infarct
Abdominal wall nodules	Infectious: leprosy Noninfectious: lipomas, panniculitis, metastatic disease, sarcoidosis
Perubilical purpura (thumbprint sign)	Infectious: strongyloides (hyperinfection syndrome) Noninfectious: retroperitoneal hemorrhage (Cullen's sign)

Table 9.12. Abdominal Abnormalities (cont'd)

Finding	Causes
Hepatomegaly	Infectious: viral hepatitis, bacterial liver abscess, amebic abscess, brucellosis, typhus Noninfectious: alcoholic cirrhosis, cholangiocarcinoma, carcinoma of pancreas, constrictive pericarditis, pericholangitis, veno-occlusive disease, autoimmune hepatitis, α-1antitrypsin deficiency, cystic fibrosis, fatty liver, hemangiomas, jejunoileal bypass, Reye's syndrome, multiple myeloma, hepatocellular carcinoma, metastatic carcinoma*, parenteral hyperalimentation (TPN)
Splenomegaly	Infectious: ***Mildly enlarged spleen:*** malaria, visceral leishmaniasis (kala-azar), SBE, ehrlichiosis, typhoid fever, typhus, brucellosis, viral hepatitis, EBV, CMV, relapsing fever, syphilis, toxoplasmosis, psitticosis, brucellosis, Q fever, CSD, schistosomiasis, trypanosomiasis, histoplasmosis, TB, splenic abscess, HIV, hydatid cysts, colorado tick fever; ***Moderately enlarged spleen:*** malaria, kala-azar; ***Massively enlarged spleen:*** malaria, kala-azar Noninfectious: ***Mildly enlarged spleen:*** SLE, sarcoidosis, Felty's syndrome, hemochromatosis, Wilson's disease, Budd-Chiari syndrome, megaloblastic anemia, iron deficiency anemia, systemic mastocytosis, angioblastic lymophadenopathy, splenic cysts, splenic trauma/hemorrhage, histiocytosis X (Langerhan's eosinophilic granuloma), hyperthyroidism, serum sickness, amyloidosis, berylliosis; Kawasaki's disease ***Moderately enlarged spleen:*** portal hypertension, hemolytic anemias, myeloproliferative disorders, CLL, Gaucher's disease, Niemann-Pick disease; ***Massively enlarged spleen:*** CML, hairy cell leukemia, lymphoma, myelofibrosis
Hepatosple-nomegaly	Infectious: malaria, typhoid fever, toxocara (visceral larval migrans), psittacosis, brucellosis, trypanosomiasis, kala-azar, 2° syphilis, EBV, CMV, schistosomiasis, toxoplasmosis, relapsing fever, RMSF, typhus, CSD, histoplasmosis, TB Noninfectious: hypernephroma, CGD, sarcoidosis
Ascites	Infectious: TB peritonitis, shistosomiasis, filariasis, spontaneous bacterial peritonitis Noninfectious: malignancies, Budd-Chiari syndrome, tricuspid regurgitation, constrictive pericarditis, inferior vena cava syndrome, Familial Mediterranean Fever, Henoch-Schönlein purpura, SLE, Whipple's disease, portal hypertension, pancreatic/bile ascites, CHF, Meig's syndrome

* Usually from lung, colon, pancreas, kidney, breast, stomach, or esophagus.

Table 9.13. Lymph Node Abnormalities

Finding	Causes
Preauricular adenopathy	Infectious: ipsilateral conjunctivitis, tularemia, anterior scalp infections, rat bite fever (Spirillum minus) Noninfectious: lymphoma
Occipital adenopathy	Infectious: posterior scalp infections, CSD, rubella Noninfectious: lymphoma
Anterior cervical adenopathy	Infectious: group A streptococcal pharyngitis, viral pharyngitis, mouth/dental infections, TB (scrofula), HHV-6, toxoplasmosis, CSD, brucellosis Noninfectious: head/neck cancer, Kawasaki's disease, lymphoma, SLE, Kikuchi's disease, Rosai-Dorfman disease
Posterior cervical adenopathy *unilateral*	Infectious: toxoplasmosis, African trypanosomiasis (Winterbottom's sign) Noninfectious: posterior scalp infection, Kawasaki's disease, lymphoma, Kikuchi's disease, Rosai-Dorfman disease
bilateral	Infectious: EBV, HHV-6, CMV, Chagas' disease Noninfectious: lymphoma, Kawasaki's disease, Rosai-Dorfman disease
Supraclavicular adenopathy	Infectious: TB, CSD Noninfectious: intra-abdominal malignancy (Virchow's sign), Kikuchi's disease
Infraclavicular adenopathy	Infectious: african trypanosomiasis, CSD Noninfectious: lymphoma
Epitrochlear adenopathy	Infectious: 2° syphilis, CSD, brucellosis Noninfectious: sarcoidosis, IVDA
Axillary adenopathy	Infectious: CFS (usually left), CSD, B. malayi, rat bite fever (Spirillum minus), brucellosis Noninfectious: lymphoma, CLL
Ulcer-node syndromes	Infectious: ***Ulcer > node:*** anthrax, rickettsial fevers (except RMSF), sporotrichosis, cutaneous leishmaniasis (new world). ***Node = ulcer:*** 1° syphilis, chancroid, tularemia (ulceroglandular), rat bite fever (Spirillum minus). ***Node > ulcer:*** syphilis, LGV, chancroid, HSV-2 Noninfectious: lymphoma
Periumbilical nodule	Infectious: intra-abdominal infection Noninfectious: malignancy (Sister Joseph's sign)

Table 9.13. Lymph Node Abnormalities (cont'd)

Finding	Causes
Inguinal adenopathy *unilateral*	Infectious: lower extremity infections, bubonic plague, rat bite fever (Spirillum minus), filariasis, leprosy, tularemia, CSD Noninfectious: intra-abdominal malignancy, bilateral lower extremity infection, IVDA
bilateral	Infectious: any infection causing generalized adenopathy, B. malayi, HSV-2, syphilis, LGV Noninfectious: any disorder causing generalized adenopathy
Generalized lymphadenopathy	Infectious: TB, EBV, HHV-6, CMV, rubella, measles, toxoplasmosis, CSD, LGV, brucellosis, group A streptococci, 2° syphilis, HIV, kala-azar (African), trypanosomiasis, arboviral hemorrhagic fevers Noninfectious: SLE, RA, CLL, adult Still's disease, Whipple's disease, pseudolymphoma (Dilantin), Kikuchi's disease, Gaucher's disease, sarcoidosis, serum sickness, hyperthyroidism, ALL, CLL, Kimura's disease

Table 9.14. Genitourinary Abnormalities

Finding	Causes
Epididymoorchitis	Infectious: mumps, TB, blastomycosis, melioidosis, brucellosis, leptospirosis, EBV, W. bancrofti, Coxsackie B, S. hematobium, LCM, GC, C. trachomatis (young adults), P. aeruginosa (elderly adults), Colorado tick fever, rat bite fever (Spirillum minus), relapsing fever Noninfectious: lymphoma, SLE, PAN, sarcoidosis, FMF, trauma, torsion, malignancy
Scrotal enlargement	Infectious: mumps, W. bancrofti (not B. malayi), Fournier's gangrene Noninfectious: hydrocele, testicular torsion
Groin mass	Infectious: onchocerciasis (hanging groins), TB, W. bancrofti, shistosomiasis Noninfectious: lymphoma
Perirectal fistula	Infectious: peri-rectal abscess, actinomycosis, LGV Noninfectious: RE, malignancies
Perirectal ulcer	Infectious: HSV, amebiasis cutis, 1° syphilis Noninfectious: malignancy
Prostate tenderness	Infectious: prostatitis, prostatic abscess Noninfectious: prostadynia

Table 9.15. Extremity Abnormalities

Finding	Causes
Digital gangrene	Infectious: SBE, S. aureus bacteremia/ABE (emboli), meningococcemia, RMSF, typhus Noninfectious: SLE, vasculitis, peripheral vascular disease
Splinter hemorrhages	Infectious: SBE, ABE, trichinosis Noninfectious: trauma, atrial myxoma, acute leukemia, RA, scurvy, mitral stenosis, severe anemia
Clubbing	Infectious: SBE, lung abscess, TB Noninfectious: ulcerative colitis (UC), Crohn's disease (RE), cirrhosis, cyanotic congenital heart disease, bronchogenic carcinoma, PBC, celiac disease, hyperthyroidism, hyperparathyroidism, bronchiectasis, hereditary
Dactylitis	Infectious: kala-azar, 2° syphilis Noninfectious: sarcoidosis, sickle cell disease
Tender fingertips	Infectious: SBE, typhoid fever Noninfectious: SLE, vasculitis, radial artery occlusion
Lymphangitis	Infectious: group A streptococci, B. malayi, onchocerciasis Noninfectious: IVDA
Nodular lymphangitis	Infectious: sporotrichosis, atypical TB, Erysipelothrix rhusiopathiae, kala-azar, coccidiomycosis, histoplasmosis, blastomycosis, nocardia, Pseudoallescheria boydii, cryptococcus, anthrax, group A streptococci, tularemia Noninfectious: ganglion cyst (wrist/hand only)
Painless purple palm/sole lesions	Infectious: ABE (Janeway lesions) Noninfectious: trauma
Carpal tunnel syndrome	Infectious: TB, leprosy Noninfectious: cirrhosis, RA, scleroderma, SLE, DM, hypothyroidism, sarcoidosis, multiple myeloma, amyloidosis
Verrucous hand/arm lesions	Infectious: TB, leprosy, syphilis, sporotrichosis, kala-azar, bartonellosis (verruga peruana) Noninfectious: squamous cell carcinoma, sarcoidosis

Table 9.15. Extremity Abnormalities (cont'd)

Finding	Causes
Edema of the dorsum of hand/foot	Infectious: RMSF, TSS, loiasis, dengue fever Noninfectious: trauma, PMR, Kawasaki's disease
Wrist swelling	Infectious: loiasis, septic arthritis Noninfectious: RA
Arthritis	Infectious: rat bite fever (Streptobacillus moniliformis), Lyme disease, LGV, brucellosis, GC, septic arthritis, parvovirus B19, shigella, yersinia, salmonella, mumps, chikungunya fever, dengue fever Noninfectious: FMF, RA, pseudogout, SLE, Whipple's disease, hyper IgD syndrome, Reiter's syndrome
Papular axillary lesions	Infectious: hydraadenitis suppurativa, 2° syphilis, yaws, blastomycosis Noninfectious: chronic contact dermatitis, acanthosis nigricans, Fox-Fordyce disease, seborrheic dermatitis
Tenosynovitis	Infectious: GC (acute), TB (chronic) Noninfectious: rheumatic diseases
Thigh tenderness (bilateral)	Infectious: gram-negative bacteremia (Louria's sign), leptospirosis, brucellosis, candidemia Noninfectious: myositis
Calf tenderness	Infectious: RMSF Noninfectious: myositis
Tender muscles	Infectious: trichinosis Noninfectious: myositis
Thrombophlebitis	Infectious: psittacosis, campylobacter Noninfectious: Behçet's disease, malignancy
Verrucous foot/leg lesions	Infectious: TB, cutaneous leishmaniasis, paracoccoidomycosis, sporotrichosis, leprosy, 2° syphilis, mycetoma Noninfectious: lichen planus, squamous cell carcinoma
Foot/leg ulcers	Infectious: M. ulcerans (Buruli ulcer may be anywhere), yaws, cutaneous diphtheria, cutaneous leishmaniasis, TB, rat bite fever (Spirillum minus) Noninfectious: sickle cell (medial malleolar ulcers), DM (only sole of foot/between toes), peripheral vascular disease

Table 9.15. Extremity Abnormalities (cont'd)

Finding	Causes
Leg edema *unilateral*	Infectious: onchocerciasis, B. malayi (below knee) Noninfectious: malignancy, Milroy's disease
bilateral	Infectious: elephantiasis (chronic recurrent erysipelas), Chagas' disease Noninfectious: lymphatic obstruction (2° to abdominal/pelvic malignancy), congenital yellow nail syndrome
Nodular arm/leg lesions	Infectious: TB (Bazin's erythema induratum), filariasis, sporotrichosis, cutaneous leishmaniasis, atypical TB, leprosy, HIV Noninfectious: erythema nodosum, PAN, thrombophlebitis, panniculitis, nodular vasculitis, Wegener's granulomatosis, Sweet's syndrome, myiasis
Palpable purpura	Infectious: meningococcemia, RMSF Noninfectious: vasculitis, cryoglobulinemia, Gardner-Diamond syndrome, Sweet's syndrome
Eschar	Infectious: ecthyma gangrenosum, typhus, rickettsial spotted fevers (except RMSF, rickettsial pox), anthrax, cutaneous diphtheria Noninfectious: burns, drugs, recluse spider bite
Scleroderma (wood hard skin lesions)	Infectious: actinomycosis Noninfectious: malignancies, DM
Hyperpigmented shins	Infectious: onchocerciasis Noninfectious: DM (dermopathy)
Cutaneous cold abscesses	Infectious: TB, atypical TB Noninfectious: hyper IgE (Job's) syndrome, CGD
Purple nodules	Infectious: disseminated cryptococcus, aspergillus, candida, trypanosomiasis, Kaposi's sarcoma, HIV Noninfectious: leukemia, lymphoma, melanoma
Painful leg nodules	Infectious: Kaposi's sarcoma Noninfectious: erythema nodosum, superficial thrombophlebitis, PAN, panniculitis, osteogenic sarcoma
Migratory rashes	Infectious: hookworms, dracunculiasis, loiasis, gnathostomiasis, strongyloidiasis, sparganosis Noninfectious: myiasis
Rash of palms/soles	Infectious: syphilis, RMSF, EBV, scarlet fever, echo 9, smallpox, monkeypox, chickenpox, rat bite fever (Streptobacillus moniliformis), HFM, orf Noninfectious: drug rashes

Table 9.15. Extremity Abnormalities (cont'd)

Finding	Causes
Erythema nodosum	Infectious: TB, group A streptococci, EBV, LGV, psittacosis, coccidiomycosis, blastomycosis, histoplasmosis, CSD, yersinia, campylobacter Noninfectious: UC, RE, drugs, sarcoidosis, lymphoma, SLE
Erythema multiforme	Infectious: HSV, M. pneumoniae, Coxsackie B Noninfectious: drugs
Plantar hyperkeratoses	Infectious: 3° syphilis, yaws, pinta, HIV, tungiasis Noninfectious: Reiter's syndrome, arsenic
Desquamation of hands/feet	Infectious: erysipelas, scarlet fever, TSS, severe infections, yaws, leptospirosis, influenza, measles, arboviral hemorrhagic fevers Noninfectious: Kawasaki's disease, post-edematous states, radiation therapy, vitamin A excess, pellagra, drugs
Nodules in compromised hosts	Infectious: fusaria (ulcerative with gray border), trichosporonosis, candida, cryptococcus Noninfectious: malignancies

Table 9.16. Neurological Abnormalities

Finding	Causes
Mental confusion/ encephalopathy (acute)	Infectious: Legionnaire's disease, HSV, HHV-6, RMSF, listeria, mycoplasma meningoencephalitis, amebic meningitis, trichinosis, brain abscess, anthrax, brucellosis, SBE, ABE, HIV, viral encephalitis, CSD, Whipple's disease, Q fever, Colorado tick fever, chikungunya fever Noninfectious: Wernicke's encephalopathy, toxic/metabolic disorders, Behçet's syndrome, SLE, alcoholism, drugs, CHF, chronic renal failure, hepatic encephalopathy, brain tumor, CNS metastases, meningeal carcinomatosis
Nuchal rigidity	Infectious: meningitis (bacterial, fungal, TB, viral) Noninfectious: meningismus, cervical arthritis
General muscle rigidity	Infectious: trichinosis, tetanus, rabies, viral encephalitis, brucellosis Noninfectious: malignancies, malignant neuroleptic syndrome, strychnine poisoning, Parkinson's disease
Transient deafness	Infectious: RMSF, mediterranean spotted fever, murine typhus, S. pneumoniae meningitis, H. influenzae meningitis, mumps, measles, VZV (Ramsey-Hunt Syndrome), EEE, congenital syphilis, brucellosis, Lassa fever Noninfectious: trauma, Susac's syndrome

Table 9.16. Neurological Abnormalities (cont'd)

Finding	Causes
Cranial nerve (CN) abnormalities *unilateral*	Infectious: 6th CN palsy (TB meningitis, N. meningitidis), 7th CN palsy (Lyme disease, N. meningitidis, CSD, mumps), 8th CN palsy (N. meningitidis), 5th, 6th, 7th CN palsies Noninfectious: 7th CN palsy (sarcoid meningitis, meningeal carcinomatosis), 2nd, 6th CN palsy (Wegener's granulomatosis)
bilateral	Infectious: 6th CN palsy (TB) Noninfectious: meningeal carcinomatosis
Optic nerve atrophy	Infectious: 3° syphilis, TB, toxoplasmosis, mumps, measles, rubella Noninfectious: sickle cell disease, severe anemia, polycythemia vera, drugs, sarcoidosis, TA, Behçet's syndrome, SLE, PAN, MS, glaucoma
Pupillary abnormalities *constricted pupil*	Infectious: neurosyphilis (Argyll Robertson), meningitis, encephalitis Noninfectious: drugs, cavernous sinus thrombosis, iritis, brain tumor, intracranial aneurysm
dilated pupil	Infectious: meningitis Noninfectious: drugs, alcohol, glaucoma, DM, chronic renal failure, brain tumor, brain herniation, intracranial aneurysm, CNS bleed, optic atrophy
Anisocoria	Infectious: TB, 3° syphilis, VZV, meningitis, encephalitis, botulism, diphtheria Noninfectious: DM, toxins, cavernous sinus thrombosis, glaucoma, brain tumor, intracranial aneurysm
Papilledema	Infectious: meningitis (bacterial, fungal, TB, viral, etc.) Noninfectious: pseudotumor cerebri, hypercarbia, brain tumor, DM, subarachnoid bleed, SLE, drugs, central retinal artery occlusion, cavernous sinus thrombosis, hypertensive encephalopathy
Mononeuritis multiplex	Infectious: leprosy, Lyme disease, HIV Noninfectious: DM, amyloidosis, sarcoidosis, lymphomatoid granulomatosis, vasculitis
Transverse myelitis	Infectious: HIV, HTLV-1, EBV, CMV, VZV, HSV, polio, rabies, TB, epidural abscess, typhus, brucellosis, shistosomiasis, Lyme disease, syphilis, toxoplasmosis Noninfectious: MS, malignancies, vaccines, SLE, sarcoidosis
Guillain-Barré syndrome	Infectious: influenza, Campylobacter jejuni, CMV, EBV, M. pneumoniae, brucellosis Noninfectious: influenza vaccine
Flaccid paralysis (acute)	Infectious: polio, WNE, CMV, VZV, rabies, botulism, JE, enterovirus (type 71), chikungunya fever, brucellosis Noninfectious: CVA, tick bite paralysis, hypocalcemic periodic paralysis

Table 9.16. Neurological Abnormalities (cont'd)

Finding	Causes
Hemiplegia/ hemiparesis	Infectious: SBE, subdural empyema, brain abscess, JE, brucellosis Noninfectious: TIA, CVA, malignancies, CNS vasculitis, migraine, GCA/TA, SLE, birth control pills, post-ictal

Table 9.17. WBC Abnormalities

Finding	Causes
Leukocytosis	Infectious: most acute infections Noninfectious: most acute non-infectious disease disorders, any major stress, steroids, drug fever, daptomycin
Leukopenia	Infectious: miliary TB, typhoid fever, malaria, tularemia, brucellosis, kala-azar, psittacosis, viral hepatitis, EBV, CMV, HHV-6, influenza, Colorado tick fever, histoplasmosis, relapsing fever, WNE, VEE, ehrlichiosis Noninfectious: drugs, pre/acute leukemias, Felty's syndrome, Gaucher's disease, splenomegaly, pernicious anemia, SLE, cyclic neutropenia, severe combined immunodeficiency disease (SCID), Chediak-Higashi syndrome, sarcoidosis
Lymphocytosis	Infectious: Whipple's disease, acute infection (convalescence), TB, brucellosis, pertussis, tularemia, 2° syphilis, histoplasmosis, EBV, CMV, HHV-6, mumps, viral hepatitis, rubella, VZV, kala-azar, toxoplasmosis, RMSF, chickungunya fever Noninfectious: ALL, CLL, lymphomas, carcinomas, multiple myeloma, RA, Hashimoto's thyroiditis, myxedema, adrenal insufficiency, thyrotoxicosis, vasculitis, Dilantin (DPH), p-aminosalicylic acid (PAS), serum sickness
Relative lymphopenia	Infectious: CMV, HHV-6, HHV-8, HIV, miliary TB, Legionella, typhoid fever, Q fever, brucellosis, SARS, malaria, babesiosis, influenza (human, avian, swine), RMSF, histoplasmosis, dengue fever, chickungunya fever, ehrlichiosis, parvovirus B19, HPS, WNE, viral hepatitis (early) Noninfectious: cytoxic drugs, steroids, sarcoidosis, SLE, lymphoma, RA, radiation, Wiskott-Aldrich syndrome, Whipple's disease, severe combine immunodeficiency disease (SCID), common variable immune deficiency (CVID), Di George's syndrome, Nezelof's syndrome, intestinal lymphangiectasia, ataxia-telangiectasia, constrictive pericarditis, tricuspid regurgitation, Kawasaki's disease, idiopathic CD_4 cytopenia, acute/ chronic renal failure, hemodialysis, myasthenia gravis, celiac disease alcoholic cirrhosis, coronary bypass, Wegener's granulomatosis, CHF, acute pancreatitis, carcinomas (terminal)

Table 9.17. WBC Abnormalities (cont'd)

Finding	Causes
Monocytosis	Infectious: TB, SBE, RMSF, diphtheria, histoplasmosis, brucellosis, kala-azar, 2° syphilis, malaria, babesiosis, recovery from chronic infection Noninfectious: sarcoidosis, myeloproliferative disorders, lymphomas, Gaucher's disease, RE, UC, celiac disease, RA, SLE, PAN, TA, post-splenectomy
Atypical lymphocytes†	Infectious: EBV*, CMV*, HHV-6, viral hepatitis, mumps, measles, rubella, VZV, toxoplasmosis, brucellosis, HSV, arboviral hemorrhagic fevers, malaria, dengue, babesiosis, ehrlichiosis Noninfectious: drug fever
Immunoblasts	Infectious: HPS Noninfectious: lymphomas
Eosinophilia	Infectious: trichinosis, echinococcosis, fascioliasis, paragonimiasis, taenia, Strongyloides stercoralis, hookworm, filariasis, schistosomiasis, Toxocara canis/cati (VLM), histoplasmosis, coccidioidomycosis, filariasis ascariasis, gnathostomiasis, angiostrongyliasis, cysticercosis, Isospora belli Noninfectious: dermatitis herpetiformis, pemphigus vulgaris, eczema, psoriasis, atopic dermatitis, mycosis fungoides, myeloproliferative disorders, polycythemia vera, CML, eosinophilic leukemia, eosinophilic gastritis, acute leukemias, sickle cell anemia, lymphomas, malignancies, Churg-Strauss granulomatosis, urticaria, hyper IgE syndrome (Job's syndrome), Sweet's syndrome, asthma, bronchopulmonary aspergillosis (BPA), angioneurotic edema, serum sickness, eosinophilia-myalgia syndrome, drug fever, dermatomyositis, PAN, allergic vasculitis, Loffler's syndrome, pulmonary infiltrates eosinophilia (PIE) syndrome, Loffler's endocarditis, Addison's disease, sarcoidosis, Wegener's granulomatosis, Goodpasture's syndrome, UC, RE, peritoneal dialysis, radiation, Wiskott-Aldrich syndrome, IgA deficiency, hay fever/allergic rhinitis, allergic vasculitis.
Basophilia	Infectious: smallpox, chickenpox (VZV) Noninfectious: pre-leukemias, acute leukemias, lymphomas, myeloproliferative disorders, postsplenectomy
WBC inclusions	Infectious: ehrlichiosis Noninfectious: staining artifacts

* May have > 20% atypical lymphocytes.

† Not seen with malignancies. Abnormal lymphocytes (morphologically monotonous) seen with acute leukemias.

Table 9.18. RBC Abnormalities

Finding	Causes
Schistocytes (microangiopathic hemolytic anemia)	Infectious: meningococcemia (DIC) Noninfectious: DIC (due to any cause), TTP, hemolytic uremic syndrome (HUS), "Waring Blender" syndrome (prosthetic valve), malignant hypertension
Spherocytes	Infectious: gas gangrene Noninfectious: autoimmune hemolytic anemias, hereditary spherocytosis, severe transfusion reactions, severe burns, cirrhosis
Target cells	Infectious: none Noninfectious: post-splenectomy, iron deficiency anemia, cirrhosis, hemoglobulin S or C, thalassemia
RBC inclusions	Infectious: malaria, babesiosis Noninfectious: artifacts, Cabot's rings (severe hemolytic anemia, pernicious anemia), Heinz bodies (GGPD deficiency, drug induced, hereditary anemias), Pappenheimer bodies (thalassemia, sideroblastic anemias, lead poisoning)
Howell-Jolly bodies†	Infectious: fulimant pneumococcal sepsis Noninfectious: asplenia/hyposplenism, congenital asplenia*, splenectomy, splenic infarcts, splenic neoplasms, megaloblastic anemias, thalassemia, steroids
Erythrophago-cytosis	Infectious: HIV, HSV, EBV, CMV, adenovirus, parvovirus B19, malaria, babesiosis, toxoplasmosis, kala-azar, histoplasmosis, cryptococcosis, disseminated candidiasis, typhoid fever, syphilis, listeria, SBE, Q fever, leprosy, TB, brucellosis Noninfectious: histiocytosis X (eosinophilic granuloma, Langerhans cell histiocytosis), myeloproliferative disorders, SLE, sarcoidosis, RA, lymphomas, acute leukemias, multiple myeloma, Chediak-Higashi syndrome, Dilantin, (DPH), familial hemophagocytic histiocytosis
Anemia (acute)	Infectious: Oroya fever, gas gangrene, malaria, babesiosis, CMV Noninfectious: ITP, "Waring blender" syndrome (prosthetic heart valve), hemorrhagic/necrotic pancreatitis, drug induced

* Chronic alcoholism, amyloidosis, chronic active hepatitis, IgA deficiency, intestinal lymphangectasia, myeloproliferative disorders, Waldenstrom's macroglobulinemia, NHL, celiac disease, RA, UC, thyroiditis, systemic mastocytosis, sickle cell disease, Fanconi's syndrome, Sezary's syndrome.

† Also "pitted/pocked" RBCs.

Table 9.19. Platelet Abnormalities

Finding	Causes
Thrombocytopenia	Infectious: acute/severe bacterial infections, measles, rubella, dengue, arboviral, hemorrhagic fevers, EBV, CMV, VZV, mumps, influenza (human, avian, swine), typhus, RMSF, WNE, ehrlichiosis, diphtheria, malaria, babesiosis, trypanosomiasis, TSS, histoplasmosis, kala-azar, HIV, miliary TB, relapsing fever, HPS, brucellosis Noninfectious: drugs, DIC, fat emboli syndrome, TTP, ITP, hemolytic uremic syndrome, pre/acute/leukemias, lymphomas, carcinomas, myeloproliferative disorders, multiple myeloma, Gaucher's disease, cirrhosis, hemodialysis
Thrombocytosis	Infectious: TB, chronic infections (e.g., osteomyelitis, abscess), SBE, Q fever, M. pneumoniae Noninfectious: Malignancies, myeloproliferative disorders, post-splenectomy, lymphomas, Wegener's granulomatosis, vasculitis, TA, PAN, Kawasaki's disease, fosfomycin, miconazole, ceftriaxone, oral cephalosporins, carbapenems, β-lactam/β-lactamase inhibitor combinations, iron therapy
Pancytopenia	Infectious: miliary TB, brucellosis, histoplasmosis, HBV, CMV, HIV Noninfectious: myeloproliferative disorders, drugs, malignancies, Chediak-Higashi syndrome, megaloblastic anemias, Gaucher's disease, hypersplenism, sarcoidosis, SLE, paroxysmal nocturnal hemoglobinuria (PNH), myelophistic anemias, leukemias, lymphoma

Table 9.20. Serum Test Abnormalities

Finding	Causes
Erythrocyte Sedimentation Rate (ESR) *highly elevated (≥100 mm/hr)*	Infectious: SBE, osteomyelitis, abscess Noninfectious: malignancies, rheumatic disorders, vasculitis, drug fever, PMR/GCA, uremia/chronic renal failure, cirrhosis, Kawasaki's disease, Sweet's syndrome
subnormal (~0 mm/hr)	Infectious: trichinosis, CFS Noninfectious: severe anemia, cachexia, massive hepatic necrosis, DIC, polycythemia vera, hypofibrinogenemia
SPEP (polyclonal gammopathy)	Infectious: HIV, malaria, kala-azar, LGV, rat bite fever, Toxocara canis/cati (VLM), Q fever (chronic) Noninfectious: SLE, PAN, cirrhosis, CAH, sarcoidosis, atrial myxoma, Takayasu's arteritis, Rosai-Dorfman disease

Table 9.20. Serum Test Abnormalities (cont'd)

Finding	Causes
Elevated ferritin levels (> 2 × normal)† *acute*	Infectious: Legionnaires' disease, WNE, EBV, CMV, MSSA/MRSA ABE Noninfectious: Kawasaki's disease, Rosai-Dorfman disease, hemophagocytic syndrome
chronic	Infectious: HIV, TB Noninfectious: Malignancies (preleukemias, lymphomas, multiple myeloma, hepatomas, liver/CNS metastases), myeloproliferative disorders, RA, adult Still's disease, SLE, TA, Kawasaki's disease, chronic renal failure; hemochromatosis, cirrhosis, α1 antitrypsin deficiency, CAH, cholestatic jaundice, sickle cell anemia, multiple blood transfusions, anemia of chronic disease
Elevated cold agglutinins	Infectious: Mycoplasma pneumoniae**, EBV, CMV, mumps, measles, malaria, Coxsackie, Q fever, HIV, HCV, influenza, adenovirus, trypanosomiasis Noninfectious: lymphomas, CLL, CML, multiple myeloma, Waldenstrom's macroglobulinemia, cold agglutinin disease, paroxysmal nocturnal hemoglobinuria, SLE, sinus histiocytosis
↑ Lactate dehydrogenase (LDH)	Infectious: malaria, babesiosis, viridans streptococcal SBE, PCP, disseminated histoplasmosis, disseminated TB/MAI, disseminated toxoplasmosis, HPS, oroya fever, gas gangrene, viral myocarditis, rubella, measles, viral hepatitis, CAP/NP, dengue hemorrhagic fever, trichinosis, SARS, adenovirus, CMV, ehrlichiosis, amebic liver abscess, influenza (human, avian, swine) Noninfectious: hemolyzed blood, hemolytic anemia, malignancies, pernicious anemia, megablastic anemia, pulmonary emboli, acute MI, renal infarction, muscle injury, liver injury, DIC, SLE pneumonitis, adult Still's disease, "Waring blender" syndrome (prosthetic heart valve), hemorrhagic/necrotic pancreatitis
↑ Procalcitonin levels (PCT)	Infectious: bacterial pneumonias (CAP, NHAP, NP), bacteremias (gram – > gram +), TB, ABM, fungal pneumonias, viral hepatitis, toxoplasmosis, osteomyelitis, SBE*, malaria (P. falciparum) Noninfectious: Renal insufficiency, alcoholic hepatitis, lung cancer (small cell), thyroid cancer, surgery, trauma, burns, cardiogenic shock, Goodpasture's syndrome shock, GVHD, peritoneal dialysis (PD), hypotension hemorrhagic/necrotic pancreatitis, normal variant (elderly) BMT, febrile neutropenia, drug fever, HD (not PD), immunosuppression/ steroids, OKT_3 therapy, tumor fever

* veridans streptococci.

** The higher the cold agglutinin titer above 1:64, the more likely the cold agglutinins are mycoplasmal in origin (in patients with CAP).

† Not an acute phase reactant when highly/persistently ↑ (> 2× normal).

Table 9.21. Liver Test Abnormalities

Finding	Causes
↑ Alkaline phosphatase (AP) *mildly elevated*	Infectious: Legionnaires' disease, viral hepatitis, liver abscess, EBV, CMV, Q fever, syphilis (2° or tertiary), TSS, hepatic candidiasis, clonorchiasis, ehrlichiosis, diphtheria, malaria, trypanosomiasis, histoplasmosis, HIV, miliary TB, relapsing fever, HPS Noninfectious: drugs, DIC, fat emboli syndrome, TTP, ITP, hemolytic uremic syndrome, pre/acute/leukemias, lymphomas, carcinomas, myeloproliferative disorders, multiple myeloma, Gaucher's disease, cirrhosis, posthepatic obstruction, alcoholic hepatitis, pregnancy, bone growth (children), osteomalacia, rickets, hyperthyroidism, UC, drug fever, hepatoma, liver metastases, lymphoma, normal variant (elderly)
moderately/highly elevated	Infectious: liver abscess Noninfectious: PBC, posthepatic obstruction, postnecrotic cirrhosis, Paget's disease, osteogenic sarcoma, hepatoma, bone fractures
↑ Serum transaminases (SGOT/SGPT) *mildly elevated*	Infectious: Legionella disease, psittacosis, Q fever, relapsing fever, brucellosis, TSS, RMSF, ehrlichiosis, liver abscess, syphilis (2° or tertiary), shigellosis, clonorchiasis, EBV, CMV, HSV-1, HHV-6, anicteric viral hepatitis, gonococcemia, malaria, gram-negative bacteremia, adenovirus Noninfectious: drug fever, cirrhosis, CHF, infarction (myocardial, cerebral, pulmonary), pancreatitis, intrahepatic cholestasis, sickle cell disease, amyloidosis, delirium tremens, intravascular hemolysis, UC, eosinophilia-myalgia syndrome, Kawasaki's disease
highly elevated	Infectious: viral hepatitis, yellow fever, arboviral hemorrhagic fevers, rhabdomyolysis (see infectious causes under myoglobulinuria p. 489) Noninfectious: shock liver, rhabdomyolysis (SGOT > SGPT) exercise, drugs (statins)
↑ Total bilirubin	Infectious: Legionnaires' disease, gonococcemia, liver abscess, EBV, CMV, pneumococcal bacteremia Noninfectious: hemolysis, Gilbert's syndrome, cirrhosis, alcoholic hepatitis, carcinoma (pancreatic, biliary), choledocholithiasis, amyloidosis, sickle cell disease
↑ GGT (GGTP)	Infectious: acute viral hepatitis Noninfectious: alcoholism, cirrhosis, alcoholic hepatitis, PBC, fatty liver, CAH, hepatoma, liver metastases, pancreatitis (acute), myocardial infarction (acute), breast cancer, lung cancer, prostate cancer, melanoma, hypernephroma, obstructive jaundice, cholestasis, CAH

Table 9.22. Rheumatic Test Abnormalities

Finding	Causes
↑ Rheumatoid factors (RF)	Infectious: SBE, TB, syphilis, kala-azar Noninfectious: cirrhosis, CAH, ITP, sarcoidosis, silicosis, asbestosis, RA, asthma, scleroderma, Behçet's disease, cryoglobulinemia, MCTD, SLE. Sjögren's, dermatomyositis, PBC, malignancy, normal variant (elderly)
↑ Anti-nuclear antibody titers (ANA)	Infectious: HIV, EBV, CMV, TB, SBE, leprosy, kala-azar, malaria Noninfectious: SLE, scleroderma, MCTD, CREST syndrome, RA, autoimmune (lupoid) hepatitis, CAH, dermatomyositis, autoimmune thyroiditis, ITP, PBC, multiple sclerosis, sarcoidosis, myasthenia gravis, ESRD on HD, normal variant (elderly)
↑ Double stranded DNA (DS-DNA)	Infectious: CMV, EBV Noninfectious: SLE, RA, CAH, PBC
↑ Angiotensin-converting enzyme levels (ACE)	Infectious: TB, leprosy, coccidiomycosis, viral hepatitis Noninfectious: sarcoidosis, allergic alveolitis, hyperparathyroidism, PBC, Gaucher's disease, DM, ESRD, hyperthyroidism, amyloidosis, myeloma, cirrhosis, psoriasis, silicosis, asbestosis, berylliosis
↑ c-ANCA	Infectious: viridans streptococcal SBE, chromomycosis, invasive aspergillosis, invasive amebiasis, Legionnaires' disease, leptospirosis, HIV Noninfectious: crescentic GMN, microscopic polyangitis (MPA), Sweet's syndrome, PAN, UC, RE, SLE, Churg-Strauss granulomatosis, Wegener's granulomatosis, HSP, TA, Kawasaki's disease
↑ Anti-smooth muscle antibodies (ASM)	Infectious: Q fever, HCV (chronic) Noninfectious: autoimmune (lupoid) hepatitis, Wilson's disease, PBC, normal variant (elderly)

Table 9.23. Urinary Abnormalities

Finding	Causes
Pyuria*§	Infectious: TB, leptospirosis, brucellosis, TSS, diphtheria, candida, GC, trichomonas, cystitis, pyelonephritis, prostatitis, acute urethral syndrome, partially treated UTI, medullary abscess, chlamydia/mycoplasma NGU, balanitis, acute appendicitis Noninfectious: interstitial nephritis, urethral irritation/inflammation, strenuous exercise, SLE, calculi, bladder tumors, chronic interstitial cystitis, RE, diverticulitis, Kawasaki's disease

* Gross pus suggests ruptured renal abscess.

§ WBC casts suggest SLE, nephritis, or acute pyelonephritis.

Table 9.23. Urinary Abnormalities (cont'd)

Finding	Causes
Hematuria *gross*	Infectious: ABE (renal septic emboli), malaria (P. falciparum), yellow fever, adenoviral cystitis (type 11) Noninfectious: renal malignancy, bladder malignancy, BPH, papillary necrosis, trauma
microscopic	Infectious: SBE, renal TB, schistosomiasis (S. hematobium), S. saprophyticus, HPS, Legionairre's disease, Q fever Noninfectious: trauma, prostatitis, malignancy, malignant hypertension, PAN, drug reactions, calculi, urethral stricture, renal vein thrombosis, hydronephrosis, polycystic kidney disease, malakoplakia, strenuous exercise, renal infarction
Proteinuria	Infectious: TB, HBV, syphilis, malaria (black water fever), brucellosis, SBE, chronic pyelonephritis, leprosy, shistosomiasis, any acute infection Noninfectious: strenuous exercise, post-streptococcal glomerulonephritis, malignant hypertension, ATN, amyloidosis, sickle cell disease, polycystic kidneys, scleroderma, PAN, Wegener's granulomatosis, Goodpasture's syndrome, multiple myeloma, lymphomas, renal neoplasm, renal trauma
Urinary pH *alkaline*	Infectious: Corynebacterium urealyticum, Klebsiella (rare), Proteus, Providencia, S. saprophyticus, Ureaplasma urealyticum Noninfectious: systemic alkalosis, postprandial "alkaline tide," alkalinization therapy, old urine, vegetarian diet
acidic	Infectious: TB Noninfectious: acidification therapy, systemic acidosis, ketosis
↓ Specific gravity (1.023 – 1.030)	Infectious: pyelonephritis† Noninfectious: diabetes insipidus, tubo-interstitial renal diseases, sickle cell disease
Nitrate positive	Infectious: most uropathogens** Noninfectious: none
Leukocyte esterase†‡	Infectious: acute cystitis, acute pyelonephritis Noninfectious: inflammation anywhere in the upper/lower GU tract

† Cystitis is associated with a normal specific gravity. The transient decrease in specific gravity of pyelonephritis corrects to normal following effective treatment.

** Negative urinary nitrate may occur with group B streptococci, group D enterococci, (VSE/VRE) S. saprophyticus, S. aureus, Acinetobacter sp., Gardnerella sp., Corynebacterium urealyticum, Burkholderia sp., Pseudomonas sp., Candida sp.

‡ ≥ 5 WBCs positive.

Table 9.23. Urinary Abnormalities (cont'd)

Finding	Causes
Eosinophiluria‡	Infectious: Shistosoma hematobium Noninfectious: cholesterol emboli syndrome, HSP, drug induced interstital nephritis, renal allograft rejection
Myoglobinuria	Infectious: Legionnaires' disease, gas gangrene, leptospirosis, Vibrio vulnificus, listeria, S. aureus, group A streptococci, group B streptococci, S. pneumoniae, tularemia, typhoid fever, echovirus, Coxsackie, influenza, adenovirus, EBV, CMV, HSV, VZV, HIV Noninfectious: crush injury, excessive exercise, MI, malignant neuroleptic syndrome, seizures, malignant hyperthermia, dermatomyositis, polymyositis, SLE, alcoholics, diabetic ketoacidosis, McArdle's syndrome, drugs (statins)
Chyluria	Infectious: W. bancrofti Noninfectious: abdominal or chest lymphatic obstruction

‡ ≥ 5 WBCs positive.

Table 9.24. Pleural Fluid Abnormalities

Pleural Fluid	Causes
Bloody*	Infectious: tularemia, anthrax Noninfectious: mesothelioma, pulmonary infarct, carcinoma (pulmonary/metastatic), lymphoma, trauma
Yellow/whitish	Infectious: empyema, hydatid cyst Noninfectious: chylous effusion
Brownish	Infectious: empyema, amebic cyst Noninfectious: parapneumonic effusion
Yellow-green	Infectious: None Noninfectious: rheumatoid lung
pH < 7.2	Infectious: empyema, TB Noninfectious: bronchogenic carcinoma (rarely), rheumatoid lung, SLE

* TB effusions are not grossly bloody, but often contain RBCs.

Table 9.24. Pleural Fluid Abnormalities (cont'd)

Pleural Fluid	Causes
↓ Glucose	Infectious: TB, bacterial, cryptococcosis, coccidiomycosis, mycoplasma, empyema Noninfectious: carcinoma, rheumatoid lung, lymphoma, esophageal rupture, parapneumonic effusion
↑ Protein	Infectious: TB Noninfectious: carcinoma, lymphoma, rheumatoid lung
↑ Amylase	Infectious: None Noninfectious: pancreatitis/pseudocyst, adenocarcinoma, esophageal rupture
Extracellular debris	Infectious: abscesses, anaerobic empyema Noninfectious: rheumatoid lung
PMNs	Infectious: bacteria, cryptococcosis, coccidiomycosis, empyema, TB (early) Noninfectious: pancreatitis, subdiaphragmatic abscess (sympathetic effusion), CHF, idiopathic
Lymphocytes	Infectious: TB Noninfectious: carcinoma, lymphoma, rheumatoid lung, SLE

Pleural Effusion Profiles in Various Diseases

Pleural Fluid	Infectious		Noninfectious		Rheumatoid Effusion	SLE
	TB	Empyema	Malignancy	Mesothelioma		
WBCs (per mm^3)	< 5000; lymphocyte predominance	> 10,000; PMN predominance	< 10,000; lymphocyte predominance	↑ PMNs/ lymphocytes	> 10,000; lymphocyte predominance	> 10,000; lymphocyte predominance
Eosinophils	–	–	+	±	–	–
RBCs (per mm^3)	< 10,000	–	> 100,000	–	–	–
pH	< 7.2	< 7.2	> 7.2	> 7.2	< 7.2	< 7.2
Glucose	↓↓	Normal/↓	↓	Normal/↓	↓↓↓	Normal

+ present; – absent; ± present or absent; ↑ increased; ↓ decreased.

Table 9.24. Pneumonia Clues Based on Pleural Effusion Characteristics (cont'd)

Pleural Fluid	Infectious		Noninfectious		Rheumatoid Effusion	SLE
	TB	Empyema	Malignancy	Mesothelioma		
Rheumatoid factor (RF)	↑	–	↑	–	↑	±
Other	< 1% meso-thelial cells; pleural biopsy/culture + for AFB	Purulent; foul odor (2° to anaerobic organisms)	↑ LDH_4/LDH_5; ↓ α-2 globulins; ↑ amylase; cytology + for malignant cells	Very viscous	Turbid greenish yellow; ↓ C_3; ↑↑ protein; epithelioid cells; degen-erated PMNs/amorphous cellular debris	↑ pleural fluid ANA is diagnostic; ↓ pleural fluid C_3

+ present; – absent; ± present or absent; ↑ increased; ↓ decreased.

Table 9.25. CSF Abnormalities

Finding	Causes
RBCs in CSF	Infectious: listeria, leptospirosis, TB, amebic meningoencephalitis, HSV, anthrax meningitis Noninfectious: traumatic tap, CNS bleed/tumor
Purulent CSF with negative gram Stain	Infectious: Neisseria meningitidis, Streptococcus pneumoniae Noninfectious: none
CSF with negative gram stain and predominantly PMNs/decreased glucose	Infectious: ABM (partially treated), listeria, HSV, TB (early), parameningeal infection, emboli secondary to SBE, amebic meningoencephalitis, CNS syphilis (early) Noninfectious: sarcoidosis, posterior-fossa syndrome/intracranial hemorrhage
CSF with negative gram stain and predominantly *lymphocytes/normal glucose*	Infectious: ABM (partially treated), viral meningitis, Lyme disease, HIV, leptospirosis, RMSF, parameningeal infection, TB, fungi, parasitic meningitis Noninfectious: sarcoidosis, meningeal carcinomatosis

Table 9.25. CSF Abnormalities (cont'd)

Finding	Causes
lymphocytes/ decreased glucose	Infectious: ABM (partially treated), TB, fungal, LCM, mumps, enteroviral meningitis, listeria, leptospirosis, syphilis Noninfectious: sarcoidosis, meningeal carcinomatosis
↑ CSF lactic acid levels	Infectious: **< 3 mMol/L**, viral meningitis, **< 4–6 mMol/L**, TB, HSV, meningitis (partially treated), parameningeal infection, cerebral malaria (mild); **> 6 mMol/L**, bacterial meningitis, cerebral malaria (severe) Noninfectious: **3–6 mMol/L**, sarcoidosis, SLE, cerebral anoxia, hepatic encephalopathy; meningeal carcinomatosis; CNS lymphomas, RBCs
Highly ↑ CSF Protein	Infectious: brain abscess, TB (with subarachnoid block), viral meningitis, viral encephalitis Noninfectious: brain tumor, MS, demyelinating CNS diseases
CSF eosinophils	Infectious: coccidioidomycosis, neurocysticercosis, gnathostomiasis, angiostrongyliasis, baylisascariasis, shistosomiasis, paragonamiasis, Toxocariasis canis/cati (VLM) Noninfectious: CNS lymphomas, CNS leukemias, V-A/VP shunts, myelography (contrast material), CNS vasculitis, drugs (NSAIDs, TMP–SMX), intrathecal drugs

Chapter 10

Antibiotic Pearls & Pitfalls

Burke A. Cunha, MD

PENICILLIN

- Penicillin is expensive because it is made by a single manufacturer.
- There are very few uses for parenteral penicillin therapy today.
- PRSP has been associated with TMP–SMX and macrolides, not penicillin.

AMPICILLIN

- Unless treating serious systemic infections due to E. faecalis (VSE), avoid using ampicillin. Ampicillin use results in increased E. coli resistance.
- Remember ampicillin is the preferred drug to treat serious systemic infections caused by VSE but is ineffective against E. faecium (VRE).
- Because susceptibility is in part "concentration dependent," do not assume that susceptibilities of ampicillin or amoxicillin are the same. On a same-dose basis, amoxicillin achieves twice the concentrations of ampicillin in body fluids (e.g., middle ear fluid, sinus fluid, bronchial fluid, urine).
- Remember that unlike ampicillin, amoxicillin is infrequently associated with oral thrush or irritative diarrhea.
- Amoxicillin 1 gm (PO) q8h can be used in ampicillin IV-to-PO switch programs since this dose provides levels comparable to parenteral (IM) ampicillin.

AMOXICILLIN/CLAVULANIC ACID

- Clavulanic acid is a beta-lactamase inhibitor which, when added to amoxicillin, restores its activity against beta-lactamase–producing strains of H. influenzae.
- The newer preparations of amoxicillin/clavulanic acid result in less gastrointestinal symptoms and diarrhea compared to older preparations with more clavulanate.
- Ineffective against PRSP due to alterations in PBPs which are not β-lactamase mediated.

ORAL ANTI-STAPHYLOCOCCAL PENICILLINS

- Do not rely on oral anti-staphylococcal penicillins such as dicloxacillin for methicillin-sensitive S. aureus (MSSA) infections since they are erratically/poorly absorbed and not consistently effective. When treating MSSA infections orally, a first generation cephalosporin (e.g., cephalexin) is preferable.
- Dicloxacillin is poorly tolerated due to its metallic taste and belching.

ORAL ANTI-PSEUDOMONAL PENICILLINS

- Avoid using indanyl carbenicillin for P. aeruginosa UTI's due to the rapid development of resistance with P. aeruginosa. Use other oral anti-P. aeruginosa agents for P. aeruginosa lower UTI's, e.g., doxycycline, levofloxacin, or fosfomycin.

PARENTERAL FIRST-GENERATION CEPHALOSPORINS

- IV cefazolin has limited activity against H. influenzae.
- Cefazolin remains useful for skin infections due to group A streptococci or MSSA.
- For treatment of biliary tract infections, cefazolin is active against E. coli and Klebsiella pneumoniae but is not active against E. faecalis (VSE).
- Cefazolin remains useful prophylaxis for cardiothoracic procedures in hospitals with low prevalence of MRSA.

ORAL FIRST-GENERATION CEPHALOSPORINS

- Cephalexin suboptimal for respiratory tract infections i.e., H. influenzae a likely pathogen (otitis media, sinusitis, AECB, community-acquired pneumonia) since 1st GCs have limited H. influenzae activity.
- For IV-to-PO switch programs and cephalexin 1gm (PO) q6h approximates the serum concentrations of parenteral (IM) cefazolin.
- Oral 3rd GCs do not have the same degree of anti-S. aureus MSSA activity as cephalexin.

PARENTERAL SECOND-GENERATION CEPHALOSPORINS

- Cefoxitin and cefotetan are useful for intra-abdominal infections.
- Cefuroxime offers no advantage for bacterial URIs over doxycycline, respiratory quinolones, or 3rd GCs and do not prevent CNS "seeding" by S. pneumoniae or H. influenzae bacteremia secondary to CAP.

ORAL SECOND-GENERATION CEPHALOSPORINS

- Oral second generation cephalosporins include cefaclor, cefprozil, and cefuroxime are used primarily to treat URIs.
- Cefaclor has limited ability to penetrate into respiratory secretions limiting its efficacy in URIs.
- Among the oral second generation cephalosporins, cefprozil has the greatest degree of penetration into respiratory secretions.

PARENTERAL THIRD-GENERATION CEPHALOSPORINS

- Except for cefoperazone, cephalosporins have no anti-E. faecalis (VSE) activity.
- Except for ceftriaxone, third generation cephalosporins predispose to C. difficile diarrhea. Ceftriaxone is associated with non-C. difficile diarrhea related to changes in colonic flora.
- Be aware that ceftriaxone is associated with pseudo-biliary lithiasis. Patients developing right upper quadrant pain on ceftriaxone should be suspected as having drug-induced pseudo/actual cholelithiasis.
- For CNS infections give third generation cephalosporins in "meningeal doses".
- The only third-generation cephalosporin associated with resistance is ceftazidime e.g., P. aeruginosa.
- Ceftazidime predisposes to MDR P. aeruginosa, and increases MRSA prevalence.
- Ceftazidime associated with ESBL K. pneumoniae, E. coli, or Enterobacter agglomerans.
- Ceftazidime little anti-MSSA activity.
- 3rd GCs *without* anti-B. fragilis activity are ceftazidime and ceftriaxone.
- 3rd GCs *without* significant anti-P. aeruginosa activity are cefotaxime, ceftizoxime, and ceftriaxone.

ORAL THIRD-GENERATION CEPHALOSPORINS

- Oral third generation cephalosporins, i.e., cefdinir, cefditoren, cefixime, cefpodoxime and ceftibuten are often used for their aerobic anti-GNB activity.
- Oral 3rd GCs do not have the same degree of activity against aerobic GNBs as their parenteral counterparts.
- Oral third generation cephalosporins have less anti-MSSA activity than their parenteral counterparts. The only 3rd GC with good anti-MSSA activity is cefpodoxime.

MONOBACTAMS

- Aztreonam has no gram-positive activity.
- Although structurally similar to the beta-lactams, aztreonam is safe in penicillin-allergic patients.

CARBAPENEMS

- Avoid imipenem in patients with seizures/CNS disorders since imipenem may cause seizures. Also, renal insufficiency increases imipenem's seizure potential.
- Imipenem predisposes to MDR P. aeruginosa and increases the prevalence of MRSA.
- All carbapenems have anti-pseudomonal activity except for ertapenem.
- Ertapenem has no anti-enterococcal activity, important in biliary/UTIs.
- Except for meropenem (meningeal dosed), carbapenems should not be used for meningitis.
- Avoid IV bolus injections/rapid infusions of doripenem, ertapenem or imipenem. Only meropenem may be administered as an IV bolus, important in septic shock.
- All carbapenems are active against ESBL-producing K. pneumoniae, E. coli, and Enterobacter aerogenes.
- Imipenem susceptibility breakpoints may overestimate imipenem's activity against Acinetobacter baumanni.

BETA-LACTAMASE INHIBITOR COMBINATIONS

- All beta-lactamase inhibitor combinations are active against Bacteroides fragilis.
- Piperacillin/tazobactam and sulbactam/ampicillin have the highest degree of anti-E. faecalis (VSE) activity among these antibiotics.
- Some strains of MDR Acinetobacter baumannii are susceptible only to sulbactam/ampicillin.
- Preferred for animal or human bites in penicillin-tolerant patients.
- Tazobactam does not enhance the anti-pseudomonal activity of piperacillin.
- Beta-lactamase inhibitors are not effective against PRSP strains (resistance mediated by alterations in PBPs, not beta-lactamases).

TETRACYCLINES

- There is virtually no clinical use for conventional tetracycline: doxycycline and minocycline, compared to tetracycline have a high degree of activity against key pathogens, e.g., *S. pneumoniae*, MSSA/MRSA, improved pharmacokinetics, and a low "resistance pontential".
- While MRSA may be susceptible to doxycycline *in vitro*, *in vivo* it frequently fails or the clinical response is delayed/incomplete. Minocycline IV/PO for treatment of MSSA/MRSA infections is clinically superior to doxycycline.
- Doxycycline has good CSF preparation and is often used for oral therapy of neuroborreliosis. Minocycline has even better CSF penetration and may be preferable to doxycycline for neuroborreliosis.
- At urinary concentrations, doxcycline is effective against *P. aeruginosa* CAB/lower UTIs, i.e., high urine levels > 300 mcg/ml. But, *in vitro* testing will report *P. aeruginosa* resistant to doxycycline.
- For non-viral zoonotic infections, doxycycline is effective therapy except for babesiosis. Although streptomycin/gentamicin preferred for tularemia, doxycycline is also effective.
- Minocycline is one of the few antibiotics active against VRE.
- Oral minocycline is useful to treat serious systemic infections i.e., MSSA/MRSA ABE or VRE.

CHLORAMPHENICOL

- Chloramphenicol is one of few drugs that can be given orally to treat acute bacterial meningitis due to susceptible organisms.
- Chloramphenicol is the only antibiotic that when given orally results in higher serum concentrations than when given at the same dose intravenously.
- Avoid chloramphenicol for the treatment of hepatobiliary infections and UTIs since chloram-phenicol is excreted into the bile as an inactivate metabolite, and urinary levels are low.
- Remember, aplastic anemia is a rare idiosyncratic side effect associated with oral/topical therapy but not IV therapy.
- Chloramphenicol-induced aplastic anemia is an idiosyncratic reaction and serial CBCs are unhelpful in predicting/avoiding aplastic anemia.
- Serial CBCs may be obtained to monitor dose-related side effects (anemia) not idiosyncratic side effects (aplastic anemia).
- Prolonged chloramphenicol therapy may cause sequential, dose-related suppression of bone marrow elements. Suppressed blood elements return in reverse sequence when chloramphenicol is discontinued.
- Chloramphenicol dose-related bone marrow suppression/toxicity is reversible and is not a harbinger of aplastic anemia.
- Vacuolization on bone marrow biopsy specimens in patients receiving chloramphenicol is a manifestation of chloramphenicol effect, not aplastic anemia.
- Chloramphenicol is effective for E. faecium (VRE) systemic infections.
- Avoid chloramphenicol in neonates (Gray Baby Syndrome) due to immature hepatic enzymes unable to metabolize chloramphenicol.

CLINDAMYCIN

- Clindamycin misses approximately 15% of coagulase-negative S. epidermidis (CoNS), the most common pathogen in foreign body/implant-related infections.
- Clindamycin is one of the few antibiotics able to penetrate/dissolve staphylococcal biofilms. Clindamycin may be useful adjunctively in treating foreign body associated infections when the prosthetic device cannot be removed.

- The incidence of C. difficile diarrhea is greater with PO > IV clindamycin.
- Clindamycin is active against most gram-positive cocci but not group D enterococci.
- Unless resistant, clindamycin is effective against CA-MRSA but not HA-MRSA/CO-MRSA (see Chapter 1, Table 1.11).
- With CA-MRSA, inducible clindamycin resistance (MLS(B)) should be suspected if erythromycin is resistant and clindamycin is susceptible. The "D test" will confirm clindamycin resistance.

AMINOGLYCOSIDES

- Among aminoglycosides, gentamicin has the most anti-gram-positive coccal activity.
- Amikacin has the highest degree of P. aeruginosa activity.
- Gentamicin and tobramycin have 6 loci that may be inactivated by acetylating, acetylating and phosphorylating enzymes. Amikacin has only 1 locus that may be attacked by these enzymes, making P. aeruginosa resistance less likely.
- Avoid aminoglycoside monotherapy in the treatment of nosocomial pneumonia since aminoglycoside activity is diminished in the presence of tissue hypoxia, WBC debris and local acidosis, which are prominent in nosocomial pneumonia.
- Avoid administering aminoglycosides via nebulizer since aerosolized aminoglycosides may predispose to resistance.
- Avoid administering aminoglycosides in split-daily doses. A single daily dose is optimal since aminoglycosides obey "concentration-dependent" killing kinetics.
- When aminoglycosides are given to patients with renal insufficiency, begin with the usual initial dose, then decrease the maintenance dose in proportion to the degree of renal dysfunction based on the creatinine clearance.
- If aminoglycosides are being used for synergy, use half the therapeutic dose (synergy dose).
- Aminoglycosides given on a once-daily basis optimize aminoglycoside antibacterial killing while minimizing nephrotoxic potential and eliminate the need for aminoglycoside levels.
- Aminoglycoside ototoxicity may occur with extremely high/prolonged peak levels. Episodic elevated peak levels are not associated with ototoxicity.
- When aminoglycosides are given on a once-daily basis, renal tubular cells have sufficient time between dosing intervals to decrease intracellular levels and thus avoid nephrotoxicity.

- Do not assess aminoglycoside nephrotoxicity based on the serum creatinine. Aminoglycoside nephrotoxicity is best assessed by indicators of renal tubular damage such as urinary renal cast counts.
- Limiting aminoglycoside therapy to 2 weeks with split-daily dosing minimizes the risk for aminoglycoside nephrotoxicity.
- Aminoglycosides are suboptimal for P. aeruginosa. Other antibiotics (e.g., meropenem, doripenem, cefepime) are preferred.
- Aminoglycosides appear to be active against streptococci in-vitro susceptibility testing, but aminoglycosides have no inherent activity against all streptococci, i.e., groups A, B, C, G, D.
- Aminoglycosides (e.g., gentamicin) are only active against group D enterococci (E. faecalis, VSE) when combined with penicillin or vancomycin.
- Avoid if possible using aminoglycosides for peritoneal lavage since the peritoneum provides a very large cross-sectional area for drug absorption, increasing the risk for neuromuscular blockade/respiratory arrest.
- For CNS infections, aminoglycosides must be administered intrathecally (I.T.) since they do not cross the blood brain barrier in sufficient concentrations to be therapeutic.

TMP–SMX

- Remember, TMP–SMX has the same spectrum as ceftriaxone (i.e., no P. aeruginosa coverage).
- Avoid using TMP–SMX to treat serious systemic K. pneumoniae infections. K. pneumoniae isolates that are sensitive to TMP–SMX in-vitro are often ineffective in-vivo.
- In patients with hypersensitivity reactions to TMP–SMX, it is always the sulfa component, not the TMP component, which is responsible. If continued treatment is desired with TMP–SMX, therapy may be completed with the TMP component alone.
- Although TMP–SMX is inactive against most streptococci, it is an excellent antibiotic against MSSA.
- TMP–SMX is active against CA-MRSA but only variably active against HA-MRSA and CO-MRSA (see Chapter 1, Table 1.11).

- For the treatment of hydradenitis suppurativa due to MSSA, TMP–SMX is a preferred antibiotic because of its ability to penetrate deep into infected sebaceous glands.
- For aerobic GNB bacteremias (other than P. aeruginosa), use TMP–SMX 10 mg/kg/day (IV/PO) given in 4 equally divided doses q6h.
- For CNS penetration and the treatment of unusual organisms (e.g., PCP), use TMP–SMX at dose of 20 mg/kg/day (IV/PO) given in 4 equally divided doses q6h.
- Avoid TMP–SMX in the treatment of respiratory tract infections since it is associated with PSRP/MDRSP.

QUINOLONES

- Using a dose of 750 mg IV/PO levofloxacin is preferred to ciprofloxacin for treatment of serious systemic *P. aeruginosa* infections.
- Quinolones do not lower the seizure threshold/cause seizures, with the exception of ciprofloxacin.
- Avelox is the only quinolone with a hepatobiliary mode of excretion; dose does not need to be modified and renal insufficiency but concentrations in the urine for lower UTIs may be suboptimal. For meningococcal prophylaxis, quinolones are equally effective (quinolones penetrate well into respiratory secretions/have a high degree of anti-meningococcal activity). The "respiratory quinolones", e.g., moxifloxacin, levofloxacin have a high degree of bioavailability which makes them ideal to treat systemic infections PO or as part of IV to PO switch therapy. Respiratory quinolones have anti-TB activity (an option in treating MDR TB).
- Ciprofloxacin has less activity against *S. pneumoniae* and *S. aureus* than moxifloxacin or levofloxacin.
- Quinolones have some degree of anti-*E. faecalis* (VSE) but have no *E. faecium* (VRE) activity. Among the quinolones, moxifloxacin has the highest degree of anti-VSE activity.

VANCOMYCIN

- If vancomycin is combined with a nephrotoxic drug and nephrotoxicity occurs, it should be ascribed to the nephrotoxic drug and not vancomycin.
- Vancomycin is a "concentration-dependent" drug (with MSSA/MRSA with MICs > 1 mcg/ml), but a "time dependent" drug (with MSSA/MRSA MICs < 1 mcg/ml).
- Since vancomycin obeys "concentration-dependent" killing kinetics for relatively resistant MSSA/MRSA and is not nephrotoxic, 30 mg/kg/day may be used for serious systemic infections.
- No need for vancomycin levels for usual vancomycin dosing. However, vancomycin levels may be useful in patients with unusually high volume of distribution (V_d) (e.g., edema/ascites, trauma, burns).
- Vancomycin "tolerance" is common among staphylococci and enterococci.
- Vancomycin is bacteriostatic against E. faecalis (VSE).
- Avoid vancomycin for empiric coverage of CVC infections. Treat potential CVC infection with cathether removal, not antibiotics.
- Vancomycin therapy may select out heteroresistant S. aureus (hVISA) due to cell wall thickening ("permeability-mediated" resistance).
- In CAP with PRSP bacteremia, avoid vancomycin for CNS coverage since CSF penetration is inadequate in the absence of meningeal inflammation.
- Because of its large molecular size, vancomycin does not penetrate well into most tissues (lung, bone, etc).
- Vancomycin IV predisposes to VRE, but PO vancomycin does not.

LINEZOLID

- Linezolid is highly active against the major gram-positive pathogens, including MSSA, MRSA, VSE, and VRE.
- Linezolid is equally efficacious when administered PO or IV.
- Unlike vancomycin, linezolid does not increase E. faecium (VRE) prevalence.

- Because linezolid is eliminated by hepatic mechanisms, no dosing adjustment is necessary in renal insufficiency.
- Linezolid is one of the few PO antibiotics that can be used to treat CNS infections.
- Linezolid is more cost effective than IV vancomycin when the total cost of IV vancomycin administration is calculated (cost of the PICC line + cost of the surgical procedure for PICC line insertion + cost of CXR to verify PICC line position + cost associated with home IV therapy + monitoring cost of vancomycin, e.g., serial creatinines + physician cost for PICC line removal + costs related to the diagnosis/consequence of vancomycin side effects).

QUINUPRISTIN/DALFOPRISTIN

- Quinupristin/dalfopristin is active against E. faecium (VRE) but not E. faecalis (VSE).
- Quinupristin/dalfopristin is highly effective against MSSA and MRSA and is a therapeutic alternative if other antibiotics fail/cannot be used to treat MSSA/MRSA infections.

DAPTOMYCIN

- Daptomycin is more active against MSSA/MRSA than Group D enterococci (VSE/VRE). If daptomycin is used to treat VSE/VRE, a higher dose may be required.
- Daptomycin is inactivated by calcium in alveolar surfactant fluid and should not be used for pneumonias.
- Following vancomycin therapeutic failures with MSSA/MRSA bacteremias/ABE, daptomycin resistance may occur during therapy.
- An initial dose of gentamicin may increase intracellular entry/effectiveness of daptomycin when treating MSSA/MRSA infections.

TIGECYCLINE

- Tigecycline may be given safely to patients with penicillin or sulfa drug allergy but avoid in patients with tetracycline allergy.
- Tigecycline (hepatobiliary elimination) does not need to be adjusted in renal insufficiency.

- Tigecycline is not a substrate or inhibitor of the cytochrome P450 system and is particularly useful in patients on multiple cardiac or HIV drugs.
- Tigecycline is highly active against MDR K. pneumoniae and may be the only antibiotic effective against such strains.

MACROLIDES

- Macrolides have been largely responsible for PRSP and MDRSP. Use instead doxycycline or a "respiratory quinolone".
- IV erythromycin lactobionate is the macrolide most likely to be associated with QTc prolongation. Macrolides with lower serum levels (e.g., azithromycin) are not associated with QTc prolongation.
- Macrolides may cause an "irritative" diarrhea but not C. difficile diarrhea.
- Erythromycin estolate may cause cholestatic jaundice in adults but not in children.
- Due to widespread group A streptococci and MSSA resistance to macrolides, avoid macrolides for the treatment of skin/soft tissue infections.

METRONIDAZOLE

- Metronidazole (IV) is preferred therapy for C. difficile *colitis*.
- Metronidazole (PO) frequently fails and is inferior to PO vancomycin for C. difficile *diarrhea*.
- A underecognized/untoward effect of metronidazole (PO) use for C. difficile *diarrhea* is increased VRE prevalence.
- Metronidazole has a long serum half life ($t_{1/2}$) of approximately 7 hr which permits once daily dosing, i.e., 1 g (IV) q24h. Except for C. difficile *colitis*, there is little rationale for dosing metronidazole 500 mg (IV) on a q6 or q8h basis.
- Metronidazole is one of the few hepatically eliminated antibiotics that requires a dosing adjustment in severe renal insufficiency (CrCl < 10 ml/min.)
- For cIAIs don't combine metronidazole and moxifloxacin (no rationale for double B. fragilis coverage).

TELAVANCIN

- Lipoglycopeptide with long $t_{½}$ (8 hrs) with normal renal function which permits once daily (q24h) dosing.
- Telavancin is not removed by HD (protein binding = 90%), but decreased efficacy with CrCl < 50 ml/min.
- Useful for cSSSIs due to MSSA, MRSA, VSE (*not* VRE), groups A, B streptococci and S. anginosus group.
- Falsely elevated INR, PT, PTT may occur with telavancin.
- Infuse telavancin 10 mg/kg (IV) slowly over 1 hour. Steady-state concentrations are achieved by the 3rd dose.

Chapter 11

Antimicrobial Drug Summaries

Burke A. Cunha, MD, Damary C. Torres, PharmD, David W. Kubiak, PharmD, Nardeen Mickail, MD, John H. Rex, MD, Mark H. Kaplan, MD

This section contains prescribing information pertinent to the clinical use of 153 antimicrobial agents in adults, as compiled from a variety of sources (p. 701). ***Antimicrobial agents for pediatric infectious diseases are described in Chapter 7***. The information provided is not exhaustive, and the reader is referred to other drug information references and the manufacturer's product literature for further information. Clinical use of the information provided and any consequences that may arise from its use are the responsibilities of the prescribing physician. The authors, editors, and publisher do not warrant or guarantee the information contained in this section, and do not assume and expressly disclaim any liability for errors or omissions or any consequences that may occur from such. **The use of any drug should be preceded by careful review of the package insert, which provides indications and dosing approved by the U.S. Food and Drug Administration. This information can be obtained on the website provided at the end of the reference list for each drug summary**.

Drugs are listed alphabetically by generic name; trade names follow in parentheses. To search by trade name, consult the index. Each drug summary contains the following information:

Usual dose. Represents the usual dose to treat most susceptible infections in adult patients with normal hepatic and renal function. Dosing for special situations is listed under the comments section; additional information can be found in Chapters 2, 4, 5 and the manufacturer's product literature. Loading doses for doxycycline, fluconazole, itraconazole, voriconazole, caspofungin, and other antimicrobials are described in either the usual dose or comments section. **Meningeal doses of antimicrobials used for CNS infection are described at the end of the comments section.**

Peak serum levels. Refers to the peak serum concentrations (mcg/ml) after the usual dose is administered. Peak serum level is useful in calculating the "kill ratios," the ratio of peak serum level to minimum inhibitory concentration (MIC) of the organism. **The higher the "kill ratio," the more effective the "dose dependent" antimicrobial is likely to be against a particular organism**.

Bioavailability. Refers to the percentage of the dose reaching the systemic circulation from the site of administration (PO or IM). **For PO antibiotics, bioavailability refers to the percentage of dose**

adsorbed from the GI tract. For IV antibiotics, "not applicable" appears next to bioavailability, since the entire dose reaches the systemic circulation. Antibiotics with high bioavailability (> 90%) are ideal for IV to PO switch therapy.

Excreted unchanged. Refers to the percentage of drug excreted unchanged, and **provides an indirect measure of drug concentration in the urine/feces. Antibiotics excreted unchanged in the urine in low concentration are unlikely to be useful for urinary tract infections.**

Serum half-life (normal/ESRD). The serum half-life ($T_{1/2}$) is the time (in hours) in which serum concentration falls by 50%. **Serum half-life is useful in determining dosing interval**. If the half-life of drugs eliminated by the kidneys is prolonged in end-stage renal disease (ESRD), then the total daily dose is reduced in proportion to the degree of renal dysfunction. If the half-life in ESRD is similar to the normal half-life, then the total daily dose does not change.

Plasma protein binding. Expressed as the **percentage of drug reversibly bound to serum albumin. It is the unbound (free) portion of a drug that equilibrates with tissues and imparts antimicrobial activity. Plasma protein binding is not typically a factor in antimicrobial effectiveness unless binding exceeds 95%**. Decreases in serum albumin (nephrotic syndrome, liver disease) or competition for protein binding from other drugs or endogenously produced substances (uremia, hyperbilirubinemia) will increase the percentage of free drug available for antimicrobial activity, and may require a decrease in dosage. Increases in serum binding proteins (trauma, surgery, critical illness) will decrease the percentage of free drug available for antimicrobial activity, and may require an increase in dosage.

Volume of distribution (V_d). Represents the apparent volume into which the drug is distributed, and is calculated as the amount of drug in the body divided by the serum concentration (in liters/kilogram). V_d is related to total body water distribution (V_d H_2O = 0.7 L/kg). Hydrophilic (water soluble) drugs are restricted to extracellular fluid and have a $V_d \leq 0.7$ L/kg. In contrast, **hydrophobic (highly lipid soluble) drugs penetrate most fluids/tissues of the body and have a large V_d**. Drugs that are concentrated in certain tissues (e.g., liver) can have a V_d greatly exceeding total body water. V_d is affected by organ profusion, membrane diffusion/permeability, lipid solubility, protein binding, and state of equilibrium between body compartments. **For hydrophilic drugs, increases in V_d may occur with burns, heart failure, dialysis, sepsis, cirrhosis, or mechanical ventilation**; decreases in V_d may occur with trauma, hemorrhage, pancreatitis (early), or GI fluid losses. Increases in V_d may require an increase in total daily drug dose for antimicrobial effectiveness; decreases in V_d may require a decrease in drug dose. **In addition to drug distribution, V_d reflects binding avidity to cholesterol membranes and concentration within organ tissues (e.g., liver).**

Mode of elimination. Refers to the primary route of inactivation/excretion of the antibiotic, which **impacts dosing adjustments in renal/hepatic failure.**

Dosage adjustments. Each grid provides dosing adjustments based on renal and hepatic function. **In renal insufficiency** (*for* ***renally eliminated antibiotics***), **the *initial dose* is the *same* as with normal renal function**; but the ***maintenance dose is decreased ~ ↓ CrCl*** (see antibiotic drug summaries for specific dosing recommendations). **Antimicrobial dosing for hemodialysis (HD)/peritoneal dialysis (PD) patients is the same as indicated for patients with a CrCl < 10 mL/min. Some antimicrobial agents require a supplemental dose immediately after hemodialysis (post–HD)/ peritoneal dialysis (post–PD)**; following the supplemental dose, antimicrobial dosing should once again resume as indicated for a CrCl < 10 mL/min. "No change" indicates no change from the usual dose. "Avoid" indicates the drug should be avoided in the setting described. "None" indicates no supplemental dose is required. "No information" indicates there are insufficient data from which to make a dosing recommendation. **Dosing recommendations are based on pharmacokinetic data, published studies, and experience**. CVVH dosing recommendations represent general guidelines, since antibiotic removal is dependent on area/type of filter, ultrafiltration rates, and sieving coefficients; replacement dosing should be individualized and guided by serum levels, if possible. **Creatinine clearance (CrCl) is used to gauge the degree of renal insufficiency, and can be estimated by the following calculation: CrCl (mL/min) = [(140 – age) × weight (kg)] / [72 × serum creatinine (mg/dL)]. The calculated value is multiplied by 0.85 for females**. It is important to recognize that due to age-dependent decline in renal function, elderly patients with "normal" serum creatinines may have low CrCls requiring dosage adjustments. (For example, a 70-year-old, 50-kg female with a serum creatinine of 1.2 mg/dL has an estimated CrCl of 34 mL/min.)

Slow extended daily dialysis (SLEDD) is now being used in some critical care patients. It is less likely to remove molecules > 1000 Daltons as compared to CVVH. Assuming a dialysate flow rate of 100 mL/min and a blood flow rate of 200 mL/min clearances during dialysis are about 82-98 mL/min using a Fresenius AV600 polysulfone hemodialyzer. However increasing the flow rate to 300 mL/min increases the clearance during dialysis to 170 mL/min. Therefore, doses during SLEDD may be the same as for normal renal function. **Clearances for SLEDD are comparable to CVVH except over a shorter period, so when no information is available, dosage adjustments can be made as for CVVH**. If needed, post-SLEDD doses should be given depending on the antibiotic.

"Antiretroviral Dosage Adjustment" grids indicate recommended dosage adjustments when protease inhibitors (PIs) and non-nucleoside reverse transcriptase inhibitor (NNRTIs) are combined or used in conjunction with rifampin or rifabutin.

Drug interactions. Refers to common/important drug-drug interactions, compiled from various sources. If a specific drug interaction is well-documented (e.g., antibiotic × with lovastatin), than other drugs from the same drug class (e.g., atorvastatin) may also be listed, based on theoretical considerations. Drug interactions may occur as a consequence of altered absorption (e.g., metal ion chelation of tetracycline), altered distribution (e.g., sulfonamide displacement of barbiturates from serum albumin), altered excretion (e.g., probenecid competition with penicillin for active transport in the kidney), altered metabolism (e.g., rifampin–induced hepatic P-450 metabolism of theophylline/warfarin; chloramphenicol inhibition of phenytoin metabolism).

Adverse side effects. Common/important side effects are indicated.

Allergic potential. Described as low or high. **Refers to the likelihood of a hypersensitivity reaction** to a particular antimicrobial.

Safety in pregnancy. Designated by the U.S. Food and Drug Administration's (USFDA) use-in-**pregnancy letter code** (Table 11.3).

Comments. Includes other useful information for each antimicrobial agent.

Cerebrospinal fluid penetration. Expressed as a **percentage relative to serum concentration**. If an antimicrobial is used for CNS infections, the meningeal dose is indicated directly above CSF penetration. No meningeal dose is given if CSF penetration is inadequate for treatment of meningitis due to susceptible organisms.

Biliary tract penetration. Expressed as a percentage relative to peak serum concentrations. Percentages > 100% reflect concentrations within the biliary system. This information is useful for estimating biliary tract concentrations.

Table 11.1 Selected Substrates, Inhibitors, and Inducers of Cytochrome P450 Isoenzymes

	Substrates	Inhibitors	Inducers
CYP1A2	Theophylline	Erythromycin	None
CYP2C9	Phenytoin, warfarin	Erythromycin, INH, metronidazole, amiodarone	TMX-SMX, RIF, phenobarbital, carbamazepine
CYP3A4	Cyclosporine, tacrolimus, simvastatin, diltiazem	Erythromycin, amiodarone	None
OATI	Oseltamivir, cidofovir	Probenecid	None
PGP	Quinolones, itraconazole, digoxin	Cyclosporine, tacrolimus	RIF

OAT-1 = organic anion transporter-1; TMP–SMX = trimethoprim sulfamethoxazole; RIF = rifampin; INH = isoniazid.

Table 11.2 Antibiotics and Cytochrome P450 Isoenzymes

Antibiotics that are not involved in CYP450 system	Antibiotics that are involved in CYP450 system either as inducer or inhibitor
Tigecycline, daptomycin, clindamycin, linezolid, vancomycin, minocycline, cephalosporins, carbapenems, nitrofurantoin, colistin, penicillins, oxacillin, aztreonam, moxifloxacin, aminoglycosides	Nafcillin, quinupristin/dalfopristin, macrolides, telithromycin, fluoroquinolones (except moxifloxacin), all azoles, rifampin, INH, TMP–SMX, tetracycline, doxycycline, metronidazole, chloramphenicol

Table 11.3 USFDA Use-in-Pregnancy Letter Code

Category	Interpretation
A	**Controlled studies show no risk.** Adequate, well-controlled studies in pregnant women have not shown a risk to the fetus in any trimester of pregnancy.
B	**No evidence of risk in humans.** Adequate, well-controlled studies in pregnant women have not shown increased risk of fetal abnormalities despite adverse findings in animals, or, in the absence of adequate human studies, animal studies show no fetal risk. The chance of fetal harm is remote, but remains a possibility.
C	**Risk cannot be ruled out.** Adequate, well-controlled human studies are lacking, and animal studies have shown a risk to the fetus or are lacking. There is a chance of fetal harm if the drug is administered during pregnancy, but potential benefit from use of the drug may outweigh potential risk.
D	**Positive evidence of risk.** Studies in humans or investigational or post-marketing data have demonstrated fetal risk. Nevertheless, potential benefit from use of the drug may outweigh potential risk. For example, the drug may be acceptable if needed in a life-threatening situation or serious disease for which safer drugs cannot be used or are ineffective.

Table 11.3 USFDA Use-in-Pregnancy Letter Code

Category	Interpretation
X	**Contraindicated in pregnancy.** Studies in animals or humans or investigational or post-marketing reports have demonstrated positive evidence of fetal abnormalities or risk which clearly outweigh any possible benefit to the patient.

Lipid-Associated Formulations of Amphotericin B. There are 3 licensed lipid-associated formulations of amphotericin B (LFAB) (Table 11.4). Although closely related in some ways, these formulations have distinct properties and must be understood separately. The principal advantage of the LFAB over amphotericin B deoxycholate (AMBD) is greater safety. In general, the rates of both acute infection-related toxicities (fever, chills, etc.) and chronic therapy-associated toxicities (principally nephrotoxicity) are reduced with LFAB. However, the LFAB can produce all of the toxicities of AMBD (and in selected patients, LFAB have been more toxic than AMBD). Overall, (L-Amb) (AmBisome) and ABLC (Abelcet) appear to be safer than ABCD (Amphotec, Amphocil). Whichever formulation is selected for therapy, it is important to specify its name carefully when prescribing. The phrase "lipid amphotericin B" should be avoided due to its imprecision. Patients who are tolerating one formulation may develop all the standard infusion-related toxicities if switched inadvertently to a new formulation. In general (and in contrast to the usual preference for generic names), use of trade names is the clearest way to specify the choice of drug in this category. In this handbook, the phrase "lipid-associated formulation of amphotericin B" suggests use of any of the 3 formulations. The issues surrounding the selection of an LFAB for an individual patient are summarized in Table 11.4 (see comments).

Table 11.4 Lipid-Associated Formulations of Amphotericin B

Generic name (abbreviation)	Trade names	Licensed (IV) dosages in the United States	Comments
Amphotericin B lipid complex (ABLC)	Abelcet	5 mg/kg/d	Reliable choice; long history of use.
Liposomal amphotericin B (L-Amb)	AmBisome	3 mg/kg/d (empiric therapy) 3–5 mg/kg/d (systemic fungal infections) 6 mg/kg/d (cryptococcal meningitis in HIV patients)	Reliable choice; best studied (L-Amb); well-supported dosing recommendations by indication; probably the least nephrotoxic; good data to support increasing the dose safely.
Amphotericin B colloidal dispersion, amphotericin B cholesteryl sulfate complex (ABCD)	Amphotec, Amphocil	3–4 mg/kg/d	Infusion-related toxicities have limited its use.

Abacavir (Ziagen) ABC

Drug Class: Antiretroviral NRTI (nucleoside reverse transcriptase inhibitor).

Usual Dose: 300 mg (PO) q12h.

Pharmacokinetic Parameters:

Peak serum level: 3 mcg/mL

Bioavailability: 83%

Excreted unchanged (urine): 1.2%

Serum half-life (normal/ESRD): 1.5/8 hrs

Plasma protein binding: 50%

Volume of distribution (V_d): 0.86 L/kg

Primary Mode of Elimination: Hepatic

Dosage Adjustments*

CrCl 50–80 mL/min	No change
CrCl 10–50 mL/min	No change
CrCl < 10 mL/min	No change
Post–HD dose	None
Post–PD dose	None
CVVH dose	No change
Mild hepatic insufficiency	200 mg (PO) q12h
Moderate or severe hepatic insufficiency	Avoid

Drug Interactions: Methadone (↑ methadone clearance with abacavir 600 mg bid); ethanol (↑ abacavir serum levels/half-life and may ↑ toxicity).

Adverse Effects: ***Abacavir may cause severe hypersensitivity reactions which may be fatal (see comments); usually during the first 4–6 weeks of therapy;* Patients who carry the HLA-B*5701 allele are at high risk for experiencing a hypersensitivity reaction to abacavir. Discontinue ZIAGEN as soon as a hypersensitivity reaction is suspected. Regardless of HLA-B*5701 status, permanently discontinue ZIAGEN if hypersensitivity cannot be ruled out, even when other diagnoses are possible. Following a hypersensitivity reaction to abacavir, NEVER restart ZIAGEN or any other abacavir-containing product**. Report cases of hypersensitivity syndrome to Abacavir Hypersensitivity Registry at 1-800-270-0425. Drug fever/rash, abdominal pain/diarrhea, nausea, vomiting, anorexia, bad dreams/sleep disorders, weakness, headache, ↑ SGOT/SGPT, hyperglycemia, hypertriglyceridemia, lactic acidosis with hepatic steatosis (rare, but potentially life-threatening toxicity with use of NRTI's).

Allergic Potential: High (~5%)

Safety in Pregnancy: C

Comments: Discontinue abacavir and ***do not restart in patients with signs/symptoms of hypersensitivity reaction***, which may include fever, rash, fatigue, nausea, vomiting, diarrhea, abdominal pain, anorexia, respiratory symptoms. Ethanol increases abacavir levels by 41%. When combined with didanosine rapid emergence of cross resistance via mutations to K65R, L74V, Y11F, and M184V occurs leading to failure of drug efficacy. Use with caution in patients with serious risk of coronary heart disease.

Cerebrospinal Fluid Penetration: 27–33%

REFERENCES:

Carr A, Workman C, Smith DE, et al. Abacavir substitution for nucleoside analogs in patients with HIV lipoatrophy. A randomized trial. JAMA 288:207–15, 2002.

Katalama C, Clotet B, Plettenberg A, et al. The role of abacavir (AVC, 1592) in antiretroviral therapy-experiences patients: results from randomized, double-blind, trial. CNA3002 European Study Team. AIDS 14:781–9, 2000.

Keating MR. Antiviral agents. Mayo Clin Proc 67:160–78, 1992.

"Usual dose" assumes normal renal/hepatic function. * For renal insufficiency, give usual dose × 1 followed by maintenance dose per CrCl. For dialysis patients, dose the same as for CrCl < 10 mL/min and give supplemental (post-HD/PD dose) immediately after dialysis. CrCl = creatinine clearance; CVVH = continuous veno-venous hemofiltration; HD/PD = hemodialysis/peritoneal dialysis. See pp. 509–513 for explanations, pp. xi–xii for abbreviations; Linezolid (↑ risk of serotonin syndrome, see p. 620).

McDowell JA, Lou Y, Symonds WS, et al. Multiple-dose pharmacokinetics and pharmacodynamics of abacavir alone and in combination with zidovudine in human immunodeficiency virus-infected adults. Antimicrob Agents Chemother 44:2061–7, 2000.

Panel on Antiretroviral Guidelines for Adults and Adolescents. Guidelines for the use of antiretroviral agents in HIV-1 infected adults and adolescents. Department of Health and Human Services. November 3, 2008; 1–139. Available at http://www.aidsinfor.nih.gov/ContentFiles/AdultandAdolescentGL.pdf.

Staszewski S, Keiser P, Mantaner J, et al. Abacavir-lamivudine-zidovudine vs. indinavir-lamivudine-zidovudine in antiretroviral-naive HIV-infected adults: a randomized equivalence trial. JAMA 285:1155–63, 2001.

Website: www.TreatHIV.com

Abacavir + Lamivudine (Epzicom) ABC/3TC

Drug Class: Antiretroviral NRTI combination.

Usual Dose: Epzicom tablet = abacavir 600 mg + lamivudine 300 mg. Usual dose: 1 tablet q24h.

Pharmacokinetic Parameters:

Peak serum level: 4.06/2.04 mcg/L

Bioavailability: 86/86%

Excreted unchanged (urine): 1.2/71%

Serum half-life (normal/ESRD): (1.5/8)/(5-7/20) hrs

Plasma protein binding: 50/36%

Volume of distribution (V_d): 0.86/1.3 L/kg

Primary Mode of Elimination: Hepatic/Renal

Dosage Adjustments*

CrCl < 50 mL/min	Not recommended
Post–HD dose	Not recommended
Post–PD dose	Not recommended
CVVH dose	Not recommended
Mild hepatic insufficiency	Contraindicated
Moderate or severe hepatic insufficiency	Contraindicated

Drug Interactions: Methadone (↑ methadone clearance with abacavir 600 mg bid); ethanol (↑ abacavir serum levels/half-life; may ↑ toxicity); didanosine, zalcitabine (↑ risk of pancreatitis); TMP–SMX (↑ lamivudine levels); zidovudine (↑ zidovudine levels).

Adverse Effects: Abacavir may cause severe hypersensitivity reactions that may be fatal (see comments), usually during the first 4–6 weeks of therapy; Patients who carry the HLA-B*5701 allele are at high risk for experiencing a hypersensitivity reaction to abacavir. Discontinue Abacavir as soon as a hypersensitivity reaction is suspected. Regardless of HLA-B*5701 status, permanently discontinue Abacavir if hypersensitivity cannot be ruled out, even when other diagnoses are possible. Following a hypersensitivity reaction to abacavir, NEVER restart Abacavir or any other abacavir-containing product. Report cases of hypersensitivity reactions to Abacavir Hypersensitivity Registry at 1-800-270-0425. Drug fever, rash, abdominal pain, diarrhea, nausea, vomiting, anorexia, anemia, leukopenia, photophobia, depression, insomnia, weakness, headache, cough, nasal complaints, dizziness, peripheral neuropathy, myalgias, ↑ AST/ALT, hyperglycemia, hypertriglyceridemia, pancreatitis, lactic acidosis with hepatic steatosis (rare, but potentially life-threatening toxicity with the NRTI's). Immune reconstitution syndrome and redistribution/accumulation of body fat have been reported in patients treated with combination antiretrovital therapy.

Allergic Potential: High (~5%)/Low

Safety in Pregnancy: C

Comments: In patients with signs/symptoms of hypersensitivity reactions discontinue and do not restart, which may include fever, rash, fatigue, nausea, vomiting,

---

"Usual dose" assumes normal renal/hepatic function. * For renal insufficiency, give usual dose × 1 followed by maintenance dose per CrCl. For dialysis patients, dose the same as for CrCl < 10 mL/min and give supplemental (post-HD/PD dose) immediately after dialysis. CrCl = creatinine clearance; CVVH = continuous veno-venous hemofiltration; HD/PD = hemodialysis/peritoneal dialysis. See pp. 509–513 for explanations, pp. xi–xii for abbreviations; Linezolid (↑ risk of serotonin syndrome, see p. 620).

diarrhea, abdominal pain, anorexia, respiratory symptoms. **Potential cross resistance with didanosine.** When combined with didanosine rapid emergence of cross resistance via mutations to K65R, L74V, Y115F, and M184V occurs leading to failure of drug efficacy. Severe acute exacerbations of hepatitis B have been reported in patients who are co-infected with hepatitis B virus (HBV) and HIV and have discontinued epivir. Hepatic function should be monitored closely for at least several months in patients who discontinue epivir.

Cerebrospinal Fluid Penetration: 27–33/15%

REFERENCES:

No authors listed. Two once-daily fixed-dose NRTI combination for HIV. Med Lett Drugs Ther. 47:19–20, 2005.

Panel on Antiretroviral Guidelines for Adults and Adolescents. Guidelines for the use of antiretroviral agents in HIV-1 infected adults and adolescents. Department of Health and Human Services. November 3, 2008; 1–139. Available at http://www.aidsinfor.nih.gov/ContentFiles/AdultandAdolescentGL.pdf.

Sosa N, Hill-Zabala C, Dejesus E. et al. Abacavir and lamivudine fixed-dose combination tablet once daily compared with abacavir and lamivudine twice daily in HIV-infected patients over 48 weeks. J Acquir Immune Defic Syndr. 40:422–7, 2005.

Website: www.epzicom.com

Abacavir + Lamivudine + Zidovudine (Trizivir) ABC/3TC/AZT

Drug Class: Antiretroviral NRTI combination.

Usual Dose: Trizivir tablet = abacavir 300 mg + lamivudine 150 mg + zidovudine 300 mg. Usual dose = 1 tablet (PO) q12h.

Pharmacokinetic Parameters:

Peak serum level: 3/1.5/1.2 mcg/mL
Bioavailability: 86/86/64%
Excreted unchanged (urine): 1.2/90/16%
Serum half-life (normal/ESRD): [1.5/6/1.1]/8/20/2.2] hrs
Plasma protein binding: 50/36/20%
Volume of distribution (V_d): 0.86/1.3/1.6 L/kg

Primary Mode of Elimination: Hepatic/renal

Dosage Adjustments*

CrCl < 50 mL/min	Avoid
Post–HD or Post–PD	Avoid
CVVH dose	Avoid
Moderate or severe hepatic insufficiency	Not recommended

Drug Interactions: Amprenavir, atovaquone (↑ zidovudine levels); clarithromycin (↓ zidovudine levels); cidofovir (↑ zidovudine levels, flu-like symptoms); doxorubicin (neutropenia); stavudine (antagonistic to zidovudine; avoid combination); TMP–SMX (↑ lamivudine and zidovudine levels); zalcitabine (↓ lamivudine levels). May exacerbate neutropenia in combination with gangcyclovir.

Adverse Effects: ***Abacavir may cause severe/fatal rash/hypersensitivity reaction;* Patients who carry the HLA-B*5701 allere are at high risk for experiencing a hypersensitivity reaction to abacavir. Discontinue Abacavir as soon as a hypersensitivity reaction is suspected. Regardless of HLA-B*5701 status, permanently discontinue Abacavir if hypersensitivity cannot be ruled out, even when other diagnoses are possible. Following a hypersensitivity reaction to abacavir, NEVER restart Abacavir or any other abacavir-containing product.** Most common (> 5%): nausea, vomiting, diarrhea, anorexia, insomnia, fever/chills, headache, malaise/fatigue. Others (less common): peripheral neuropathy, myopathy, steatosis, pancreatitis. Lab abnormalities: anemia, leukopenia, mild

---

"Usual dose" assumes normal renal/hepatic function. * For renal insufficiency, give usual dose × 1 followed by maintenance dose per CrCl. For dialysis patients, dose the same as for CrCl < 10 mL/min and give supplemental (post-HD/PD dose) immediately after dialysis. CrCl = creatinine clearance; CVVH = continuous veno-venous hemofiltration; HD/PD = hemodialysis/peritoneal dialysis. See pp. 509–513 for explanations, pp. xi–xii for abbreviations; Linezolid (↑ risk of serotonin syndrome, see p. 620).

hyperglycemia, ↑ LFTs, ↑ CPK, ↑ aldolase, hypertriglyceridemia. Immune reconstitution syndrome and redistribution/accumulation of body fat have been reported in patients treated with combination antiretroviral therapy.

Allergic Potential: High (~5%)

Safety in Pregnancy: C

Comments: Avoid in patients with CrCl < 50 mL/min. HBV hepatitis may relapse if lamivudine is discontinued.

REFERENCES:

Havlir DV, Lange JM. New antiretrovirals and new combinations. AIDS 12(Suppl A):S165–74, 1998.

McDowell JA, Lou Y, Symonds WS, et al. Multiple-dose pharmacokinetics and pharmacodynamics of abacavir alone and in combination with zidovudine in human immunodeficiency virus-infected adults. Antimicrob Agents Chemother 44:2061–7, 2000.

Panel on Clinical Practices for Treatment of HIV Infection. Guidelines for the Use of Antiretroviral Agents in HIV-Infected Adults and Adolescents. Department of Health and Human Services. www.hivatis.org. January 29, 2008.

Three new drugs for HIV infection. Med Lett Drugs Ther 40:114–6, 1998.

Weverling GJ, Lange JM, Jurriaans S, et al. Alternative multidrug regimen provides improved suppression of HIV-1 replication over triple therapy. AIDS 12:117–22, 1998.

Website: www.TreatHIV.com

Acyclovir (Zovirax)

Drug Class: Antiviral HSV; (see comments).

Usual Dose:

HSV-1/2: Herpes labialis: 400 mg (PO) 5x/day × 5 days. Genital herpes: *Initial therapy.* 200 mg (PO) 5x/day × 10 days. *Recurrent/intermittent therapy* (< 6 episodes/year): 200 mg (PO) 5x/day × 5 days. *Chronic suppressive therapy* (> 6 episodes/year): 400 mg (PO) q12h × 1 year. Mucosal/genital herpes: 5 mg/kg (IV) q8h × 7 days or 400 mg (PO) 5x/day × 7 days. Nosocomial pneumonia 5 mg/kg (IV) q8h × 10 days. Meningitis/Encephalitis: 10 mg/kg (IV) q8h × 10 days or 800 mg (PO) 5x/day × 10 days.

VZV: Chickenpox: 800 mg (PO) q6h × 5 days or 10 mg/kg (IV) q8h × 5 days. VZV pneumonia (normal hosts) 5–10 mg/kg (IV) q8h × 10 days (compromised hosts) 10 mg/kg (IV) q8h × 10 days. Herpes zoster (shingles): *Dermatomal/localized:* 800 mg (PO) 5x/day × 7–10 days. *Disseminated*: 10 mg/kg (IV) q8h × 7–10 days.

Pharmacokinetic Parameters:

Peak serum level: 7.7 mcg/mL

Bioavailability: 30%

Excreted unchanged (urine): 70%

Serum half-life (normal/ESRD): 3/5 hrs

Plasma protein binding: 30%

Volume of distribution (V_d): 0.7 L/kg

Primary Mode of Elimination: Renal

Dosage Adjustments* for HSV/VZV

CrCl 10–25 mL/min	No change/ 800 mg (IV/PO) q8h
CrCl < 10 mL/min	200 mg (IV/PO)q12h/ 800 mg (IV/PO) q12h
Post–HD dose	200 mg (IV/PO)/ 800 mg (IV/PO)
Post–PD dose	None
CVVH dose	See CrCl 10–25 mL/min
Moderate or severe hepatic insufficiency	No change

Drug Interactions: Cimetidine, probenecid, theophylline (↑ acyclovir levels); nephrotoxic drugs (↑ nephrotoxicity); zidovudine (lethargy); theophylline (↑ levels).

"Usual dose" assumes normal renal/hepatic function. * For renal insufficiency, give usual dose × 1 followed by maintenance dose per CrCl. For dialysis patients, dose the same as for CrCl < 10 mL/min and give supplemental (post-HD/PD dose) immediately after dialysis. CrCl = creatinine clearance; CVVH = continuous veno-venous hemofiltration; HD/PD = hemodialysis/peritoneal dialysis. See pp. 509–513 for explanations, pp. xi–xii for abbreviations; Linezolid (↑ risk of serotonin syndrome, see p. 620).

Adverse Effects: Seizures/tremors (dose related), encephalopathy, crystalluria, ATN. HUS (only with HIV) Base dose on ideal body weight in the elderly to minimize adverse effects.
Allergic Potential: Low
Safety in Pregnancy: C
Comments: Na^+ content = 4 mEq/g. CSF levels may be increased with probenecid.
Meningeal dose = VZV/HSV encephalitis dose.
Highly active against HSV and VZV. Some activity against CMV. No activity against EBV, RSV or adenoviruses.
Cerebrospinal Fluid Penetration: 50%

REFERENCES:

De Clercq E. Antiviral drugs in current clinical use. J Clin Virol 30:115–33, 2004.

Geers TA, Isada CM. Update on antiviral therapy for genital herpes infection. Cleve Clinic J Med 67:567–73, 2000.

Gupta R, Wald A, Krantz E, et al. Valacyclovir and acyclovir for suppression of shedding of herpes simplex virus in the genital tract. J Infect Dis 190:1374–81, 2004.

Keating MR. Antiviral Agents. Mayo Clin Proc 67:160–78, 1992.

Owens RC, Ambrose PG. Acyclovir. Antibiotics for Clinicians 1:85–93, 1997.

Whitley RJ, Gnann JW Jr. Acyclovir: a decade later. N Engl J Med 327:782–3, 1992.

Website: www.pdr.net

Adefovir dipivoxil (Hepsera)

Drug Class: Antihepatitis B drug
Usual Dose: 10 mg (PO) q24h.
Pharmacokinetic Parameters:
Peak serum level: 18 ng/mL
Bioavailability: 59%
Excreted unchanged (urine): 45%
Serum half-life (normal/ESRD): 7.5/9 hrs
Plasma protein binding: 4%
Volume of distribution (V_d): 0.4 L/kg
Primary Mode of Elimination: Renal

Dosage Adjustments*

CrCl ≥ 50 mL/min	10 mg (PO) q24h
CrCl 20–50 mL/min	10 mg (PO) q48h
CrCl 10–20 mL/min	10 mg (PO) q72h
Hemodialysis	10 mg (PO) q7d
Post–HD or PD dose	No information
CVVH dose	No information
Moderate or severe hepatic insufficiency	No change

Drug Interactions: No significant interaction with lamivudine, TMP–SMX, acetaminophen, ibuprofen.
Adverse Effects: Asthenia, headache, abdominal pain, nausea, flatulence, diarrhea, dyspepsia.
Allergic Potential: Low
Safety in Pregnancy:
Comments: May be taken with or without food. Does not inhibit CP450 isoenzymes. Do not discontinue abruptly to avoid exacerbation of HBV hepatitis.
Cerebrospinal Fluid Penetration: No data

REFERENCES:

Buti M, Esteban R. Adefovir dipivoxil. Drugs of Today 39:127–35, 2003.

Cundy KC, Burditch-Crovo P, Walker RE, et al. Clinical pharmacokinetics of adefovir in human HIV-1 infected patients. Antimicrob Agents Chemother 35:2401–2405, 1995.

Davis GL. Update on the management of chronic hepatitis B. Rev Gastroenterol Disord 2:106–15, 2002.

Hadziyannis SJ, Tassopoulos NC, Heathcote E, et al. Adefovir dipivoxil for the treatment of hepatitis B e antigen-negative chronic hepatitis B. N Engl J Med 348:800–7, 2003.

Perrillo R, Schiff E, Yoshida E, et al. Adefovir for the treatment of lamivudine-resistant hepatitis B mutants. Hepatology 32:129–34, 2000.

"Usual dose" assumes normal renal/hepatic function. * For renal insufficiency, give usual dose × 1 followed by maintenance dose per CrCl. For dialysis patients, dose the same as for CrCl < 10 mL/min and give supplemental (post-HD/PD dose) immediately after dialysis. CrCl = creatinine clearance; CVVH = continuous veno-venous hemofiltration; HD/PD = hemodialysis/peritoneal dialysis. See pp. 509–513 for explanations, pp. xi–xii for abbreviations; Linezolid (↑ risk of serotonin syndrome, see p. 620).

Peters MG, Hann Hw H, Martin P, et al. Adefovir dipivoxil alone or in combination with lamivudine in patients with lamivudine-resistant chronic hepatitis B. Gastroenterology 126:90–101, 2004.

Treatment of Hepatitis B e Antigen-Positive chronic hepatitis with telbivudine or adefovir. Annals of Intern Med 147:745–746, 2007.

Website: www.hepsera.com

Amantadine (Symmetrel)

Drug Class: Antiviral (influenza A).
Usual Dose: 200 mg (PO) q24h.
Pharmacokinetic Parameters:
Peak serum level: 0.5 mcg/mL
Bioavailability: 90%
Excreted unchanged (urine): 90%
Serum half-life (normal/ESRD): 16/192 hrs
Plasma protein binding: 67%
Volume of distribution (V_d): 6.6 L/kg
Primary Mode of Elimination: Renal
Dosage Adjustments*

CrCl > 30 mL/min	100 mg (PO) q24h
CrCl 15–30 mL/min	100 mg (PO) q48h
CrCl < 15 mL/min	200 mg (PO) qweek
Post–HD	200 mg (PO) qweek
Post–PD	None
CVVH dose	100 mg (PO) q48h
Moderate or severe hepatic insufficiency	No change

Drug Interactions: Alcohol (↑ CNS effects); benztropine, trihexyphenidyl (↑ interacting drug effect: dry mouth, ataxia); CNS stimulants (additive stimulation); digoxin (↑ digoxin levels); trimethoprim (↑ amantadine and trimethoprim levels); scopolamine (↑ scopolamine effect: blurred vision, slurred speech, toxic psychosis).

Adverse Effects: Confusion/delusions, insomnia, dysarthria, ataxia, anticholinergic effects (blurry vision, dry mouth, orthostatic hypotension, urinary retention, constipation), livedo reticularis, may ↑ QT_c interval.
Allergic Potential: Low
Safety in Pregnancy: C
Comments: May precipitate heart failure. Avoid co-administration with anticholinergics, MAO inhibitors, or antihistamines. Resistant to amantadine, widespread may improve peripheral airway function/oxygenation in ventilated patients with severe influenza (human, avian, swine). ***Highly active against influenza A. No activity against other viruses.***
Cerebrospinal Fluid Penetration:
Non-inflamed meninges = 15%
Inflamed meninges = 20%

REFERENCES:

Cunha BA, Amantadine may be lifesaving in severe influenza A. Clin Infect Dis 43:1372–3, 2006.

Douglas RG, Jr. Prophylaxis and treatment of influenza. N Engl J Med 322:443–50, 1990.

Geskey JM, Thomas NJ. Amantadine penetration into cerebrospinal fluid of a child with influenza A encephalitis. Pediatr Infect Dis J 23:270–2, 2004.

Gubareva LV, Kaiser L, Hayden FG. Influenza virus neuraminidase inhibitors. Lancet 355:827–5, 2000.

Keyers LA, Karl M, Nafziger AN, et al. Comparison of central nervous system adverse effects of amantadine and rimantadine used as sequential prophylaxis of influenza A in elderly nursing home patients. Arch Intern Med 160:1485–8, 2000.

Kawai N, Ikematsu H, Iwaki N, et al. Factors influencing the effectiveness of oseltamivir and amantadine for the treatment of influenza: A multicenter study from Japan of the 2002–2003 influenza season. Clin Infect Dis 40:1309–16, 2005.

Website: www.pdr.net

"Usual dose" assumes normal renal/hepatic function. * For renal insufficiency, give usual dose × 1 followed by maintenance dose per CrCl. For dialysis patients, dose the same as for CrCl < 10 mL/min and give supplemental (post-HD/PD dose) immediately after dialysis. CrCl = creatinine clearance; CVVH = continuous veno-venous hemofiltration; HD/PD = hemodialysis/peritoneal dialysis. See pp. 509–513 for explanations, pp. xi–xii for abbreviations; Linezolid (↑ risk of serotonin syndrome, see p. 620).

Amikacin (Amikin)

Drug Class: Aminoglycoside.

Usual Dose: 15 mg/kg or 1 gm (IV) q24h (preferred to q12h dosing).

Spectrum: (see ***Susceptibility Profiles*** pp. 194–199).

Pharmacokinetic Parameters:

Peak serum level: 20–30 mcg/mL (q12h dosing); 65–75 mcg/mL (q24h dosing)

Bioavailability: Not applicable

Excreted unchanged (urine): 95%

Serum half-life (normal/ESRD): 2/50 hrs

Plasma protein binding: < 5%

Volume of distribution (V_d): 0.25 L/kg

Primary Mode of Elimination: Renal

Dosage Adjustments*

CrCl 50–80 mL/min	7.5 mg/kg (IV) q24h or 500 mg (IV) q24h
CrCl 10–50 mL/min	7.5 mg/kg (IV) q48h or 500 mg (IV) q48h
CrCl < 10 mL/min	3.75 mg/kg (IV) q48h or 250 mg (IV) q48h
Post–HD dose	7.5 mg/kg (IV) or 500 mg (IV)
Post–HFHD dose	7.5 mg/kg (IV) or 500 mg (IV)
Post–PD dose	3.75 mg/kg (IV) or 250 mg (IV)
CVVH dose	7.5 mg/kg (IV) or 500 mg (IV) q12h
Moderate or severe hepatic insufficiency	No change

Drug Interactions: Amphotericin B, cephalothin, cyclosporine, enflurane, methoxyflurane, NSAIDs, polymyxin B, radiographic contrast, vancomycin (↑ nephrotoxicity); cis-platinum (↑ nephrotoxicity, ↑ ototoxicity); loop diuretics (↑ ototoxicity); neuromuscular blocking agents (↑ apnea, prolonged paralysis); non-polarizing muscle relaxants (↑ apnea).

Adverse Effects: Neuromuscular blockade with rapid infusion/absorption. Nephrotoxicity only with prolonged/extremely high serum trough levels; may cause reversible non–oliguric renal failure (ATN). Ototoxicity associated with prolonged/extremely high peak serum levels (usually irreversible): Cochlear toxicity (1/3 of ototoxicity) manifests as decreased high frequency hearing, but deafness is unusual. Vestibular toxicity (2/3 of ototoxicity) develops before ototoxicity (typically manifests as tinnitus).

Allergic Potential: Low

Safety in Pregnancy: D

Comments: Synergy dose: 7.5 mg/kg (IV) q24h or 500 mg (IV) q24h. **Single daily dosing virtually eliminates nephrotoxic/ototoxic potential**. Incompatible with solutions containing β-lactams, erythromycin, chloramphenicol, furosemide, sodium bicarbonate. IV infusion should be given slowly over 30 minutes. May be given IM. Intraperitoneal infusion ↑ risk of neuromuscular blockade. Avoid intratracheal/aerosolized intrapulmonary instillation, which may predispose to antibiotic resistance. V_d increases with edema/ascites, trauma, burns, cystic fibrosis; may require ↑ dose. V_d decreases with dehydration, obesity; may require ↓ dose. **Renal cast counts are the best indicator of aminoglycoside nephrotoxicity, not serum creatinine**. Dialysis removes ~ 50% of amikacin from serum. **CAPD dose:** 10–20 mg/L in dialysate (IP) with each exchange.

Therapeutic Serum Concentrations (for therapeutic efficacy, *not toxicity*): Peak (q24h/q12h dosing): 65–75/20–30 mcg/mL Trough (q24h/q12h dosing): 0/4–8 mcg/mL

"Usual dose" assumes normal renal/hepatic function. * For renal insufficiency, give usual dose × 1 followed by maintenance dose per CrCl. For dialysis patients, dose the same as for CrCl < 10 mL/min and give supplemental (post-HD/PD dose) immediately after dialysis. CrCl = creatinine clearance; CVVH = continuous veno-venous hemofiltration; HD/PD = hemodialysis/peritoneal dialysis. See pp. 509–513 for explanations, pp. xi–xii for abbreviations; Linezolid (↑ risk of serotonin syndrome, see p. 620).

Intrathecal (IT) dose: 10–40 mg (IT) q24h.
Cerebrospinal Fluid Penetration:
Non-Inflamed meninges = 15%
Inflamed meninges = 20%
Bile Penetration: 30%
(also see ***Antibiotic Pearls & Pitfalls*** pp. 502–503).

REFERENCES:

Bacopoulou F, Markantonis SL, Pavlou E, et al. A study of once-daily amikacin with low peak target concentrations in intensive care unit patients: pharmacokinetics and associated outcomes. J Crit Care. 18:107–13, 2003.

Cunha BA. New uses for older antibiotics: nitrofurantoin, amikacin, colistin, polymyxin B, doxycycline, and minocycline revisited. Med Clin North Am. 90:1089–107, 2006.

Cunha BA. Pseudomonas aeruginosa: Resistance and therapy. Semin Respir Infect 17:231–9, 2002.

Cunha BA. Aminoglycosides: Current role in antimicrobial therapy. Pharmacotherapy 8:334–50, 1988.

Edson RS, Terrel CL. The Aminoglycosides. Mayo Clin Proc 74:519–28, 1999.

Fulnecky E, Wright D, Scheld WM, et al. Amikacin and colistin for treatment of Acinetobacter baumanni meningitis. Journal of Infection 51;e249–e251, 2005.

Furin J, Nardell EA. Multidrug-resistant tuberculosis: An update on the best regimens. J Respir Dis 27:172–82, 2006.

Giamarellos-Bourboulis E, Kentepozidis N, Antonopoulou A, et al. Postantibiotic effect of antimicrobial combinations on multidrug-resistant Pseudomonas aeruginosa. Diagnostic Microbiology and Infectious Disease 51:113–117, 2005.

Karakoc B, Gerceker AA. In-vitro activities of various antibiotics, alone and in combination with amikacin against Pseudomonas aeruginosa. Int J Antimicrob Agents 18:567–70, 2001.

Poole K. Aminoglycoside resistance in Pseudomonas aeruginosa. Antimicrobial Agents and Chemotherapy 49:479–487, 2005.

Amoxicillin (Amoxil, A-cillin, Polymox, Trimox, Wymox)

Drug Class: Aminopenicillin.
Usual Dose: 1 gm (PO) q8h.
Spectrum: (see ***Susceptibility Profiles*** pp. 183–187).
Pharmacokinetic Parameters:
Peak serum level: 14 mcg/mL
Bioavailability: 90%
Excreted unchanged (urine): 60%
Serum half-life (normal/ESRD): 1.3/16 hrs
Plasma protein binding: 20%
Volume of distribution (V_d): 0.26 L/kg
Primary Mode of Elimination: Renal
Dosage Adjustments*

CrCl 50–80 mL/min	500 mg (PO) q8h
CrCl 10–50 mL/min	500 mg (PO) q12h
CrCl < 10 mL/min	500 mg (PO) q24h
Post–HD or post–PD	500 mg
CVVH dose	500 mg (PO) q12h
Moderate or severe hepatic insufficiency	No change

Drug Interactions: Allopurinol (↑ risk of rash).
Adverse Effects: Drug fever/rash, ↑ SGOT/SGPT.
Allergic Potential: High
Safety in Pregnancy: B
Comments: ↑ risk of rash with EBV infectious mononucleosis. No irritative diarrhea with 1 gm (PO) q8h dose due to nearly complete proximal GI absorption. Na^+ content = 2.7 mEq/g.
Cerebrospinal Fluid Penetration:
Non-inflamed/Inflamed meninges = 1%/8%
Bile Penetration: 3000%
(also see ***Antibiotic Pearls & Pitfalls*** pp. 495–508).

"Usual dose" assumes normal renal/hepatic function. * For renal insufficiency, give usual dose × 1 followed by maintenance dose per CrCl. For dialysis patients, dose the same as for CrCl < 10 mL/min and give supplemental (post-HD/PD dose) immediately after dialysis. CrCl = creatinine clearance; CVVH = continuous veno-venous hemofiltration; HD/PD = hemodialysis/peritoneal dialysis. See pp. 509–513 for explanations, pp. xi–xii for abbreviations; Linezolid (↑ risk of serotonin syndrome, see p. 620).

REFERENCES:

[No authors listed]. Acute otitis media in children: amoxicillin remains the standard antibiotic, but justified in certain situations only. Prescrire Int. 12:184–9, 2003.

Addo-Yobo E, Chisaka N, Hassan M, et al. Oral amoxicillin versus injectable penicillin for severe pneumonia in children age 3 to 59 months: a randomized multicentre equivalency study. Lancet 364:1141–48, 2004.

Abgueguen P, Azoulay-Dupuis E, Noel V, et al. Amoxicillin is ineffective against penicillin-resistant Streptococcus pneumoniae strains in a mouse pneumonia model simulating human pharmacokinetics. Antimicrob Agents Chemother 51:208–214, 2007.

Camacho MT, Casal J, AGuilar L, et al. Very High Resistance to Amoxicillin in Streptococcus pneumoniae: an Epidemiological Fact or a Technical Issue? Journal of Chemotherapy. 18:303–06, 2006.

Cunha BA. Oral Antibiotic Therapy of Serious Systemic Infections. Med Clin N Am 90:1197–1222, 2006.

Cunha BA. The aminopenicillins. Urology 40:186–190, 1992.

Curtin-Wirt C, Casey JR, Murray PC, et al. Efficacy of penicillin vs. amoxicillin in children with group A beta hemolytic streptococcal tonsillopharyngitis. Clin Pediatr (Phila). 42:219–24, 2003.

Dhaon NA. Amoxicillin tablets for oral suspension in the treatment of acute otitis media: a new formulation with improved convenience. Adv Ther 21:87–95, 2004.

Diaz-Pedroche C, Lumbreras C, San Juan R, et al. Valganciclovir preemptive therapy for the prevention of cytomegalovirus disease in high-risk seropositive solid-organ transplant recipients. Transplantation. 82:30–5, 2006.

Donowitz GR, Mandell GL. Beta-lactam antibiotics. N Engl J Med 318:419–26 and 318:490–500, 1993.

File Jr. TM; Clinical implications and treatment of multiresistant Streptococcus pneumoniae pneumonia. Clin Microbiol Infect. 12:31–41, 2006.

Moreillon P, Wilson WR, Leclercq R, et al. Single-dose oral amoxicillin or linezolid for prophylaxis of experimental endocarditis due to vancomycin-susceptible and vancomycin-resistant Enterococcus faecalis. Antimicrob Agents Chemother 51: 1661–1665, 2007.

Piglansky L, Leibovitz E, Raiz S, et al. Bacteriologic and clinical efficacy of high dose amoxicillin for therapy of acute otitis media in children. Pediatr Infect Dis J. 22:405–13, 2003.

Ready D, Lancaster H, Qureshi F, et al. Effect of amoxicillin use on oral microbiota in young children. Antimicrob Agents Chemother 48:2883–7, 2004.

Website: www.pdr.net

Amoxicillin/Clavulanic Acid (Augmentin)

Drug Class: Aminopenicillin/β-lactamase inhibitor combination.

Usual Dose: 500/125 mg (PO) q8h or 875/125 mg (PO) q12h for severe infections or respiratory tract infections.

Spectrum: (see ***Susceptibility Profiles*** pp. 183–187).

Pharmacokinetic Parameters:

Peak serum level: 10.0/2.2 mcg/mL

Bioavailability: 90/60%

Excreted unchanged (urine): 80/40%

Serum half-life (normal/ESRD): [1.3/16]/[½] hrs

Plasma protein binding: 18/25%

Volume of distribution (V_d): 0.26/0.3 L/kg

Primary Mode of Elimination: Renal

Dosage Adjustments* (based on 500 mg q8h):

CrCl 50–80 mL/min	500/125 mg (PO)q12h
CrCl 10–50 mL/min	500/125 mg (PO)q24h
CrCl < 10 mL/min	250/125 mg (PO)q24h
Post–HD dose	250/125 mg (PO)
Post–PD dose	None
CVVH dose	500/125 mg (PO)q24h
Moderate or severe hepatic insufficiency	No change

"Usual dose" assumes normal renal/hepatic function. * For renal insufficiency, give usual dose × 1 followed by maintenance dose per CrCl. For dialysis patients, dose the same as for CrCl < 10 mL/min and give supplemental (post-HD/PD dose) immediately after dialysis. CrCl = creatinine clearance; CVVH = continuous veno-venous hemofiltration; HD/PD = hemodialysis/peritoneal dialysis. See pp. 509–513 for explanations, pp. xi–xii for abbreviations; Linezolid (↑ risk of serotonin syndrome, see p. 620).

Drug Interactions: Allopurinol (↑ risk of rash).
Adverse Effects: Drug fever/rash, diarrhea, ↑ SGOT/SGPT. Rash potential same as ampicillin.
Allergic Potential: High
Safety in Pregnancy: B
Comments: ↑ risk of rash with EBV infectious mononucleosis. **875/125 mg formulation should not be used in patients with CrCl < 30 mL/min.**
Cerebrospinal Fluid Penetration:
Non-Inflamed meninges = 1%
Inflamed meninges = 1%
Bile Penetration: 3000%
(also see ***Antibiotic Pearls & Pitfalls*** p. 496).

REFERENCES:

Cunha BA. Amoxicillin/clavulanic acid in respiratory infections: microbiologic and pharmacokinetic considerations. Clinical Therapeutics 14:418–25, 1992.

Donowitz GR, Mandell GL. Beta-lactam antibiotics. N Engl J Med 318:419–26 and 318:490–500, 1993.

Easton J, Noble S, Perry CM. Amoxicillin/clavulanic acid: a review of its use in the management of paediatric patients with acute otitis media. Drugs. 63:313–40, 2003.

Fernandez-Sabe N, Carratala J, Dorca J, et al. Efficacy and safety of sequential amoxicillin-clavulanate in the treatment of anaerobic lung infections. Eur J Clin Microbiol Infect Dis 22:185–7, 2003.

File TM Jr, Lode H, Kurz H, et al. Double-blind, randomized study of the efficacy and safety of oral pharmacokinetically enhanced amoxicillin-clavulanic (2,000/125 milligrams) versus those of amoxicillin-clavulanic (875/125 milligrams), both given twice daily for 7 days, in treatment of bacterial community-acquired pneumonia adults. Antimicrob Agents Chemother 48:3323–31, 2004.

Klein JO. Amoxicillin/clavulanate for infections in infants and children: past, present and future. Pediatr Infect Dis J. 22:S139–48, 2003.

Malingoni MA, Song J, Herrington J, et al. Randomized controlled trial of moxifloxacin compared with piperacillin-tazobactam and amoxicillin-clavulanate for the treatment of complicated intra-abdominal infections. Ann Surg. 244:204–11, 2006.

Scaglione F, Caronzolo D, Pintucci JP, et al. Measurement of cefaclor and amoxicillin-clavulanic acid levels in middle-ear fluid in patients with acute otitis media. Antimicrob Agents Chemother 47:2987–9, 2003.

Wright AJ, Wilkowske CJ. The penicillins. Mayo Clin Proc 66:1047–63, 1991.

Website: www.augmentin.com

Amoxicillin/Clavulanic Acid ES-600 (Augmentin ES-600)

Drug Class: Aminopenicillin/β-lactamase inhibitor combination.
Usual Dose: 90 mg/kg/day oral suspension in 2 divided doses (see comments).
Spectrum: (see ***Susceptibility Profiles*** pp. 183–187).
Pharmacokinetic Parameters:
Peak serum level: 15.7/1.7 mcg/mL
Bioavailability: 90/60%
Excreted unchanged (urine): 70/40%
Serum half-life (normal/ESRD): [1.4/16]/[1.1/2] hrs
Plasma protein binding: 18%/25%
Volume of distribution (V_d): 0.26/0.3 L/kg
Primary Mode of Elimination: Renal
Dosage Adjustments*

CrCl < 30 mL/min	Avoid
Moderate or severe hepatic insufficiency	Use with caution

Drug Interactions: Allopurinol (↑ risk of rash).
Adverse Effects: Drug fever/rash, diarrhea, ↑ SGOT/SGPT. Rash potential same as ampicillin.
Allergic Potential: High
Safety in Pregnancy: B
Comments: 5 mL contains 600 mg amoxicillin and 42.9 mg clavulanatic acid. Take at start of meal to minimize GI upset. **Do not substitute 400 mg or 200 mg/5 mL formulation for ES-600.** Not

"Usual dose" assumes normal renal/hepatic function. * For renal insufficiency, give usual dose × 1 followed by maintenance dose per CrCl. For dialysis patients, dose the same as for CrCl < 10 mL/min and give supplemental (post-HD/PD dose) immediately after dialysis. CrCl = creatinine clearance; CVVH = continuous veno-venous hemofiltration; HD/PD = hemodialysis/peritoneal dialysis. See pp. 509–513 for explanations, pp. xi–xii for abbreviations; Linezolid (↑ risk of serotonin syndrome, see p. 620).

for children < 3 months or > 40 kg. Contains phenylalanine.

Volume of ES-600 to provide 90 mg/kg/day:

Weight	Volume (q12h)	Weight	Volume (q12h)
8 kg	3.0 mL	24 kg	9.0 mL
12 kg	4.5 mL	28 kg	10.5 mL
16 kg	6.0 mL	32 kg	12.0 mL
20 kg	7.5 mL	36 kg	13.5 mL

Cerebrospinal Fluid Penetration:
Non-Inflamed meninges = 1%
Inflamed meninges = 1%
Bile Penetration: 3000%
(also see ***Antibiotic Pearls & Pitfalls*** pp. 495–508).

REFERENCES:

Dagan R, Hoberman A, Johnson C, et al. Bacteriologic and clinical efficacy of high dose amoxicillin/clavulanate in children with acute otitis media. Pediatr Infect Dis J 20:829–37, 2001.

Easton J, Noble S, Perry CM. Amoxicillin/clavulanic acid: a review of its use in the management of paediatric patients with acute otitis media. Drugs 63:311–40, 2003.

Ghaffar F, Muniz LS, Katz K, et al. Effects of large dosages of amoxicillin/clavulanate or azithromycin on nasopharyngeal carriage of Streptococcus pneumoniae, Haemophilus influenzae, nonpneumococcal alpha-hemolytic streptococci, and Staphylococcus aureus in children with acute otitis media. Clin Infect Dis 34:1301–9, 2002.

Website: www.augmentin.com

Amoxicillin/Clavulanic Acid XR (Augmentin XR)

Drug Class: Aminopenicillin/β-lactamase inhibitor combination.
Usual Dose: 2000/125 mg (2 tablets) (PO) q12h (see comments).
Spectrum: (see ***Susceptibility Profiles*** pp. 183–187).
Pharmacokinetic Parameters:
Peak serum level: 17/2 mcg/mL
Bioavailability: 90/60%
Excreted unchanged (urine): 70/40%
Serum half-life (normal/ESRD): [1.3/16]/[½] hrs
Plasma protein binding: 18/25%
Volume of distribution (V_d): 0.26/0.3 L/kg
Primary Mode of Elimination: Renal
Dosage Adjustments*

CrCl > 30 mL/min	No change
CrCl < 30 mL/min	Avoid
Post–HD/PD dose	Avoid
CVVH dose	Avoid
Moderate or severe hepatic insufficiency	Use with caution

Drug Interactions: Allopurinol (↑ risk of rash); may ↓ effectiveness of oral contraceptives.
Adverse Effects: Drug fever, rash, diarrhea, ↑ SGOT/SGPT, nausea, abdominal pain.
Allergic Potential: High
Safety in Pregnancy: B
Comments: Amoxicillin/clavulanic acid XR is a time-released formulation. Do not crush tablets. XR formulation contains a different ratio of amoxicillin/clavulanic acid so other formulations cannot be interchanged. 2 tablets (1000/62.5 mg per tablet) = 2000/125 mg per dose. **2 gm amoxicillin effective against most strains of PRSP**. Take with food (not high fat meal) to increase absorption.
Cerebrospinal Fluid Penetration:
Non-Inflamed meninges = 1%
Inflamed meninges = 1%
Bile Penetration: 3000%
(also see ***Antibiotic Pearls & Pitfalls*** p. 496).

"Usual dose" assumes normal renal/hepatic function. * For renal insufficiency, give usual dose × 1 followed by maintenance dose per CrCl. For dialysis patients, dose the same as for CrCl < 10 mL/min and give supplemental (post-HD/PD dose) immediately after dialysis. CrCl = creatinine clearance; CVVH = continuous veno-venous hemofiltration; HD/PD = hemodialysis/peritoneal dialysis. See pp. 509–513 for explanations, pp. xi–xii for abbreviations; Linezolid (↑ risk of serotonin syndrome, see p. 620).

REFERENCES:

Augmentin XR. Med Lett Drugs Ther. 45:5–6, 2003.

Benninger MS. Amoxicillin/clavulanate potassium extended release tablets: a new antimicrobial for the treatment of acute bacterial sinusitis and community-acquired pneumonia. Expert Opin Pharmacother. 4:1839–46, 2003.

File Jr TM, Jacobs M, Poole M, et al. Outcome of treatment of respiratory tract infections due to Streptococcus pneumoniae, including drug-resistant strains, with pharmacokinetically enhanced amoxicillin/clavulatate. International J Antimicrobial Agents 20:235–247, 2002.

Kaye C, Allen A, Perry S, et al. The clinical pharmacokinetics of a new pharmacokinetically enhanced formulation of amoxicillin/clavulatate. Clin Therapeutics 23:578–584, 2001.

Website: www.augmentin.com

Amphotericin B (Fungizone)

Drug Class: Antifungal.
Usual Dose: 0.5–0.8 mg/kg (IV) q24h.
Pharmacokinetic Parameters:
Peak serum level: 1–2 mcg/mL
Bioavailability: Not applicable
Excreted unchanged (urine): 5%
Serum half-life (normal/ESRD): 15/48 days
Plasma protein binding: 90%
Volume of distribution (V_d): 4 L/kg
Primary Mode of Elimination: Metabolized
Dosage Adjustments*

CrCl 50–80 mL/min	No change
CrCl 10–50 mL/min	No change
Post–HD or post–PD	None
Post–HFHD dose	No change
CVVH dose	None
Moderate or severe hepatic insufficiency	No change

Drug Interactions: Adrenocorticoids (hypokalemia); aminoglycosides, cyclosporine, polymyxin B (↑ nephrotoxicity); digoxin (↑ digitalis toxicity due to hypokalemia); flucytosine (↑ flucytosine levels if amphotericin B produces renal dysfunction); neuromuscular blocking agents (↑ neuromuscular blockade due to hypokalemia).
Adverse Effects: Fevers/chills, flushing thrombophlebitis, bradycardia, seizures, hypotension, distal renal tubular acidosis (↓ K^+/↓ Mg^{++}), anemia, pancreatitis. If renal insufficiency is secondary to amphotericin, either ↓ daily dose by 50%, give dose every other day, or switch to an amphotericin lipid formulation.
Allergic Potential: Low
Safety in Pregnancy: B
Comments: Higher doses (1–1.5 mg/kg q24h) may be needed in life-threatening situations but are nephrotoxic and should only be administered under expert supervision. Do not co-administer in same IV with other drugs. Give by slow IV infusion over 2 hours initially. Aggressive hydration (1–2 liters/d) may reduce nephrotoxicity. **Test dose unnecessary.** Amphotericin B with granulocyte colony stimulating factor (GCSF) may result in ARDS. Amphotericin B with pentamidine may cause acute tubular necrosis in HIV/AIDS patients. **Fevers/chills may be reduced by meperidine, aspirin, NSAIDs, hydrocortisone or acetaminophen, if given 30–60 minutes before infusion. Bladder irrigation dose:** 50 mg/L until cultures are negative.
Highly active against Candida, Cryptococcus, Histoplasmosis, Blastomycosis, Sporotrichosis, Penicillum marneffei, Paracoccidiomycosis, Coccidiomycosis.
Some activity against Fusarium, Naegleria, Leishmania, or Mucor.
No activity against C. lusitaniae, Pseudoallescheria, or Trichosporon.

"Usual dose" assumes normal renal/hepatic function. * For renal insufficiency, give usual dose × 1 followed by maintenance dose per CrCl. For dialysis patients, dose the same as for CrCl < 10 mL/min and give supplemental (post-HD/PD dose) immediately after dialysis. CrCl = creatinine clearance; CVVH = continuous veno-venous hemofiltration; HD/PD = hemodialysis/peritoneal dialysis. See pp. 509–513 for explanations, pp. xi–xii for abbreviations; Linezolid (↑ risk of serotonin syndrome, see p. 620).

Meningeal dose = usual dose plus 0.5 mg 3–5x/week (IT) via Ommaya reservoir.
Cerebrospinal Fluid Penetration: < 10%

REFERENCES:

Arikan S, Lozano-Chiu M, Paetznick V, et al. In vitro synergy of caspofungin and amphotericin B against Aspergillus and Fusarium spp. Antimicrob Agents Chemother 46:245–7, 2002.

Barchiesi F, Maracci M, Baldassarri I, et al. Tolerance to amphotericin B in clinical isolates of Candida tropicalis. Diagn Microbiol Infect Dis 50:179–85, 2004.

Boucher HW, Groll AH, Chiou CC, et al. Newer systemic antifungal agents: pharmacokinetics, safety and efficacy. Drugs 64:1997–2020, 2004.

Cagnoni PJ. Liposomal amphotericin B versus conventional amphotericin B in the empirical treatment of persistently febrile neutropenic patients. J Antimicrob Chemother 49 Suppl 1:81–6, 2002.

Chocarro Martinez A, Gonzalez A, Garcia I. Caspofungin versus amphotericin B for the treatment of Candidal esophagtis. Clin Infect Dis 35:107; discussion 107–8, 2002.

Cruz JM, Peacock JE Jr., Loomer L, et al. Rapid intravenous infusion of Amphotericin B: A pilot study. Am J Med 93:123–30, 1992.

Deray G. Amphotericin B nephrotoxicity. J Antimicrob Chemother 49 Suppl 1:37–41, 2002.

Dupont B. Overview of the lipid formulations of amphotericin B. J Antimicrob Chemother 49 Suppl 1:31–6, 2002.

Ellis D. Amphotericin B: spectrum and resistance. J Antimicrob Chemother 49 Suppl 1:7–10, 2002.

Gallis HA, Drew RH, Pickard WW. Amphotericin B: 30 years of clinical experience. Rev Infect Dis 12:308–29, 1990.

Grim SA, Smith KM, Romanelli F, et al. Treatment of azole-resistant oropharyngeal candidiasis with topical amphotericin B. Ann Pharmacother 36:1383–6, 2002.

Lewis, RE, Wiederhold NP, Klepser ME. In vitro pharmacodynamics amphotericin B, itraconazole, and voriconazole against aspergillus, fusarium, and scedosporium spp. Antimicrobial Agents and Chemotherapy 49:945–951, 2005.

Lyman CA, Walsh TJ. Systemically administered antifungal agents: A review of their clinical pharmacology and therapeutic applications. Drugs 44:9–35, 1992.

Menzies D, Goel K, Cunha BA. Amphotericin B. Antibiotics for Clinicians 2:73–6, 1998.

Moosa MY, Alangaden GJ, Manavathu E. Resistance to amphotericin B does not emerge during treatment for invasive aspergillosis. J Antimicrob Chemother 49:209–13, 2002.

Nivoix Y, Zamfir A, Lutun P, Kara F, et al. Combination of caspofungin and an azole or an amphotericin B formulation in invasive fungal infections. J Infect. 52:67–74, 2006.

Pappas PG, Chetchotisakd P, Larsen RA, et al. A Phase II Randomized Trial of Amphotericin B Alone or Combined with Fluconazole in the Treatment of HIV-Associated Cryptococcal Meningitis. Clin Infect Dis 48:1775–1784, 2009.

Peleg AY, Woods ML. Continuous and 4 h infusion of amphotericin B: a comparative study involving high-risk hematology patients. J Antimicrob Chemother 54:803–8, 2004.

Perfect JR. "Amphoterrible": In the Era of Broad-Spectrum Zoles and Candins. Infections in Medicine. 23:S2, 2006.

Perfect JR, Dismukes WE, Dromer F, et al. Clinical Practice Guidelines for the Management of Cryptococcal Disease: 2010 Update by the Infectious Disease Society of America. Clin Infect Dis 50:291–322, 2010.

Yun-Sun H, Alexander BD, Lortholary O, et al. Lipid Formulations of Amphotericin B Significantly Improve Outcome in Solid Organ Transplant Recipients with Central Nervous System Cryptococcosis. Clin Infect Dis 49:1721–1728, 2009.

Website: www.pdr.net

Amphotericin B Lipid Complex (Abelcet) ABLC

Drug Class: Antifungal (see p. 513).
Usual Dose: 5 mg/kg (IV) q24h.
Pharmacokinetic Parameters:
Peak serum level: 1.7 mcg/mL
Bioavailability: Not applicable
Excreted unchanged (urine): 5%
Serum half-life (normal/ESRD): 173/173 hrs
Plasma protein binding: 90%
Volume of distribution (V_d): 131 L/kg

"Usual dose" assumes normal renal/hepatic function. * For renal insufficiency, give usual dose × 1 followed by maintenance dose per CrCl. For dialysis patients, dose the same as for CrCl < 10 mL/min and give supplemental (post-HD/PD dose) immediately after dialysis. CrCl = creatinine clearance; CVVH = continuous veno-venous hemofiltration; HD/PD = hemodialysis/peritoneal dialysis. See pp. 509–513 for explanations, pp. xi–xii for abbreviations; Linezolid (↑ risk of serotonin syndrome, see p. 620).

Primary Mode of Elimination: Metabolized

Dosage Adjustments*

CrCl 50–80 mL/min	No change
CrCl < 50 mL/min	No change
Post–HD/PD dose	None
Post–HFHD dose	No change
CVVH dose	None
Moderate or severe hepatic insufficiency	No change

Drug Interactions: Adrenocorticoids (hypokalemia); aminoglycosides, cyclosporine, polymyxin B (↑ nephrotoxicity); digoxin (↑ digitalis toxicity due to hypokalemia); flucytosine (↑ flucytosine effect); neuromuscular blocking agents (↑ neuromuscular blockade due to hypokalemia.)

Adverse Effects: Fevers/chills, flushing thrombophlebitis, bradycardia, seizures, hypotension, distal renal tubular acidosis (↓ K^+/↓ Mg^{++}), anemia. Fewer/less severe side effects and less nephrotoxicity than amphotericin B. Renal toxicity is dose-dependent (use caution).

Allergic Potential: Low

Safety in Pregnancy: B

Comments: See p. 511. Useful in patients unable to tolerate amphotericin B or in patients with amphotericin B nephrotoxicity. Infuse at 2.5 mg/kg/hr.

Highly active against Candida, Cryptococcus, Histoplasmosis, Blastomycosis, Sporotrichosis, Penicillum marneffei, Paracoccidiomycosis, Coccidiomycosis. Some activity against Fusarium, Naegleria, Leishmania, or Mucor.

No activity against C. lusitaniae, Pseudoallescheria, or Trichosporon.

Cerebrospinal Fluid Penetration: < 10%

REFERENCES:

Arikan S, Rex JH. Lipid-based antifungal agents: current status. Curr Pharm Des 7:393–415, 2001.

Dupont B. Overview of the lipid formulations of amphotericin B. J Antimicrob Chemother 49 Suppl 1:31–6, 2002.

Hiemenz JW, Walsh TJ. Lipid formulations of Amphotericin B: Recent progress and future directions. Clin Infect Dis 2:133–44, 1996.

Kauffman CA, Carver PL. Antifungal agents in the 1990s: Current status and future developments. Drugs 53:539–49, 1997.

Slain D. Lipid-based Amphotericin B for the treatment of fungal infections. Pharmacotherapy 19:306–23, 1999.

Trouet A. The amphotericin B lipid complex or abelcet: its Belgian connection, its mode of action and specificity: a review. Acta Clin Belg 57:53–7, 2002.

Website: www.pdr.net

Amphotericin B Liposomal (AmBisome)

Drug Class: Antifungal (see p. 513).

Usual Dose: 3–6 mg/kg (IV) q24h (see comments)

Pharmacokinetic Parameters:

Peak serum level: 17–83 mcg/mL

Bioavailability: Not applicable

Excreted unchanged (urine): 5%

Serum half-life (normal/ESRD): 153 hrs/no data

Plasma protein binding: 90%

Volume of distribution (V_d): 131 L/kg

Primary Mode of Elimination: Metabolized

Dosage Adjustments*

CrCl 50–80 mL/min	No change
CrCl < 50 mL/min	No change
Post–HD/PD dose	None
Post–HFHD dose	No change
CVVH dose	None
Moderate or severe hepatic insufficiency	No change

"Usual dose" assumes normal renal/hepatic function. * For renal insufficiency, give usual dose × 1 followed by maintenance dose per CrCl. For dialysis patients, dose the same as for CrCl < 10 mL/min and give supplemental (post-HD/PD dose) immediately after dialysis. CrCl = creatinine clearance; CVVH = continuous veno-venous hemofiltration; HD/PD = hemodialysis/peritoneal dialysis. See pp. 509–513 for explanations, pp. xi–xii for abbreviations; Linezolid (↑ risk of serotonin syndrome, see p. 620).

Drug Interactions: Adrenocorticoids (hypokalemia); aminoglycosides, cyclosporine, polymyxin B (↑ nephrotoxicity); digoxin (↑ digitalis toxicity due to hypokalemia); flucytosine (↑ flucytosine effect); neuromuscular blocking agents (↑ neuromuscular blockade due to hypokalemia).

Adverse Effects: Fevers/chills, flushing, thrombophlebitis, bradycardia, seizures, hypotension, distal renal tubular acidosis (↓ K^+/↓ Mg^{++}), anemia.

Allergic Potential: Low

Safety in Pregnancy: B

Comments: See p. 513. Less nephrotoxicity than amphotericin B and other amphotericin lipid preparations. **Empiric therapy of fungemia dose:** 3 mg/kg (IV) q24h can be used. **Suspected/ known Aspergillus dose:** 5 mg/kg (IV) q24h. **Cryptococcal meningitis dose:** 6 mg/kg (IV) q24h. ***Highly active against Candida, Cryptococcus, Histoplasmosis, Blastomycosis, Sporotrichosis, Penicillum marneffei, Paracoccidiomycosis, Coccidiomycosis. Some activity against Fusarium, Naegleria, Leishmania, or Mucor. No activity against C. lusitaniae, Pseudoallescheria, or Trichosporon.***

Cerebrospinal Fluid Penetration: < 10%

REFERENCES:

Adler-Moore J, Proffitt RT. AmBisome: liposomal formulation, structure, mechanism of action and preclinical experience. J Antimicrob Chemother 49 Suppl 1:211–30, 2002.

Chopra R. AmBisome in the treatment of fungal infections: the UK experience. J Antimicrob Chemother 49 Suppl 1:43–7, 2002.

De Marie S. Clinical use of liposomal and lipid-complexed amphotericin-B. J Antimicrob Chemother 33:907–16, 1994.

Hiemenz JW, Walsh TJ. Lipid formulations of amphotericin B: Recent progress and future directions. Clin Infect Dis 2:133–44, 1996.

Kuse ER, Chetchotisakd P, da Cunha CA, et al. Micafungin versus liposomal amphotericin B for candidaemia and invasive candidosis: a phase III randomised double-blind trial. Lancet 369:1519–1527, 2007.

Lequaglie C. Liposomal amphotericin B (AmBisome): efficacy and safety of low-dose therapy in pulmonary fungal infections. J Antimicrob Chemother 49 Suppl 1:49–50, 2002.

Slain D. Lipid-based amphotericin B for the treatment of fungal infections. Pharmacotherapy 19:306–23, 1999.

Website: www.ambisome.com

Amphotericin B Cholesteryl Sulfate Complex (Amphotec), ABCD (amphotericin B colloidal dispersion)

Drug Class: Antifungal (see p. 513).

Usual Dose: 3–4 mg/kg (IV) q24h.

Pharmacokinetic Parameters:

Peak serum level: 2.9 mcg/mL

Bioavailability: Not applicable

Excreted unchanged (urine): 5%

Serum half-life (normal/ESRD): 39/29 hrs

Plasma protein binding: 90%

Volume of distribution (V_d): 4 L/kg

Primary Mode of Elimination: Metabolized

Dosage Adjustments*

CrCl 50–80 mL/min	No change
CrCl < 50 mL/min	No change
Post–HD/PD dose	None
Post–HFHD dose	No change
CVVH dose	None
Moderate or severe hepatic insufficiency	No change

Drug Interactions: Adrenocorticoids (hypokalemia); aminoglycosides, cyclosporine, polymyxin B (↑ nephrotoxicity); digoxin

"Usual dose" assumes normal renal/hepatic function. * For renal insufficiency, give usual dose × 1 followed by maintenance dose per CrCl. For dialysis patients, dose the same as for CrCl < 10 mL/min and give supplemental (post-HD/PD dose) immediately after dialysis. CrCl = creatinine clearance; CVVH = continuous veno-venous hemofiltration; HD/PD = hemodialysis/peritoneal dialysis. See pp. 509–513 for explanations, pp. xi–xii for abbreviations; Linezolid (↑ risk of serotonin syndrome, see p. 620).

(↑ digitalis toxicity due to hypokalemia); flucytosine (↑ flucytosine effect); neuromuscular blocking agents (↑ neuromuscular blockade due to hypokalemia).

Adverse Effects: Fevers/chills, flushing, thrombophlebitis, bradycardia, seizures, hypotension, distal renal tubular acidosis (↓ K^+/↓ Mg^{++}), anemia. Fewer/less severe side effects/less nephrotoxicity vs. amphotericin B.

Allergic Potential: Low

Safety in Pregnancy: B

Comments: See p. 513. Reconstitute in sterile water, not dextrose, saline or bacteriostatic water. Do not co-administer with in same IV line with other drugs. Give by slow IV infusion over 2 hours (1 mg/kg/hr). Test dose unnecessary. ***Highly active against Candida, Cryptococcus, Histoplasmosis, Blastomycosis, Sporotrichosis, Penicillum marneffei, Paracoccidiomycosis, Coccidiomycosis. Some activity against Fusarium, Naegleria, Leishmania, or Mucor. No activity against C. lusitaniae, Pseudoallescheria, or Trichosporon.***

Cerebrospinal Fluid Penetration: < 10%

REFERENCES:

De Marie S. Clinical use of liposomal and lipid-complexed amphotericin B. J Antimicrob Chemother 33:907–16, 1994.

Kline S, Larsen TA, Fieber L, et al. Limited toxicity of prolonged therapy with high doses of amphotericin B lipid complex. Clin Infect Dis 21:1154–8, 1995.

Rapp RP, Gubbins PO, Evans ME. Amphotericin B lipid complex. Ann Pharmacother 31:1174–86, 1997.

Website: www.pdr.net

Ampicillin (various)

Drug Class: Aminopenicillin.

Usual Dose: 2 gm (IV) q4h, 500 mg (PO) q6h.

Spectrum: (see ***Susceptibility Profiles*** pp. 183–187.)

Pharmacokinetic Parameters:

Peak serum level: 48 (IV)/5 (PO) mcg/mL

Bioavailability: 50%

Excreted unchanged (urine): 90%

Serum half-life (normal/ESRD): 0.8/10 hrs

Plasma protein binding: 20%

Volume of distribution (V_d): 0.25 L/kg

Primary Mode of Elimination: Renal

Dosage Adjustments*

CrCl 50–80 mL/min	1 gm (IV) q4h 500 mg (PO) q6h
CrCl 10–50 mL/min	1 gm (IV) q8h 250 mg (PO) q8h
CrCl < 10 mL/min	1 gm (IV) q12h 250 mg (PO) q12h
Post–HD dose	1 gm (IV) 500 mg (PO)
Post–PD dose	1 gm (IV) 250 mg (PO)
CVVH dose	1 gm (IV) q8h 250 mg (PO) q12h
Moderate or severe hepatic insufficiency	No change

Drug Interactions: Allopurinol (↑ frequency of rash); warfarin (↑ INR).

Adverse Effects: Drug fever/rash, nausea, GI upset, irritative diarrhea, ↑ SGOT/SGPT, ↑ incidence of rash vs. penicillin (in patients with EBV, HIV, lymphocytic leukemias, or allopurinol), C. difficile diarrhea/colitis.

Allergic Potential: High

Safety in Pregnancy: B

Comments: Incompatible in solutions containing amphotericin B, heparin,

"Usual dose" assumes normal renal/hepatic function. * For renal insufficiency, give usual dose × 1 followed by maintenance dose per CrCl. For dialysis patients, dose the same as for CrCl < 10 mL/min and give supplemental (post-HD/PD dose) immediately after dialysis. CrCl = creatinine clearance; CVVH = continuous veno-venous hemofiltration; HD/PD = hemodialysis/peritoneal dialysis. See pp. 509–513 for explanations, pp. xi–xii for abbreviations; Linezolid (↑ risk of serotonin syndrome, see p. 620).

corticosteroids, erythromycin, aminoglycosides, or metronidazole. Na^+ content = 2.9 mEq/g.
Meningeal dose = 2 gm (IV) q4h.
Cerebrospinal Fluid Penetration:
Non-Inflamed meninges = 1%
Inflamed meninges = 10%
Bile Penetration: 3000%
(also see ***Antibiotic Pearls & Pitfalls*** p. 496).

REFERENCES:
Donowitz GR, Mandell GL. Beta-lactam antibiotics. N Engl J Med 318:419–26, 490–500, 1993.
Wright AJ. The penicillins. Mayo Clin Proc 74:290–307, 1999.
Wright AJ, Wilkowske CJ. The penicillins. Mayo Clin Proc 66:1047–63, 1991.

Ampicillin/sulbactam (Unasyn)

Drug Class: Aminopenicillin/β-lactamase inhibitor combination.
Usual Dose: 1.5–3 gm (IV) q6h (see comments).
Spectrum: (see ***Susceptibility Profiles*** pp. 183–187).
Pharmacokinetic Parameters:
Peak serum level: 109-150/48-88 mcg/mL
Bioavailability: Not applicable
Excreted unchanged (urine): 80/80%
Serum half-life (normal/ESRD): [1/9]/[1/9] hrs
Plasma protein binding: 28/38%
Volume of distribution (V_d): 0.25/0.38 L/kg
Primary Mode of Elimination: Renal/hepatic
Dosage Adjustments* (based on 3 gm q6h):

CrCl 50–80 mL/min	1.5 gm (IV) q6h
CrCl 10–50 mL/min	1.5 gm (IV) q12h
CrCl < 10 mL/min	1.5 gm (IV) q24h
Post–HD dose	1.5 gm (IV)
Post–PD dose	None
CVVH dose	1.5 gm (IV) q12h
Moderate or severe hepatic insufficiency	No change

Drug Interactions: Probenecid (↑ ampicillin/sulbactam levels); allopurinol (↑ rash).
Adverse Effects: Drug fever/rash, ↑ SGOT/SGPT, C. difficile diarrhea/colitis.
Allergic Potential: High
Safety in Pregnancy: B
Comments: **Mild/moderate infection dose:** 1.5 gm (IV) q6h. Pseudoresistance with E. coli/Klebsiella. **Meningeal dose** (for susceptible strains of MDR Acinetobacter baumanii meningitis): 4.5 gm (IV) q6h.
Na^+ content = 4.2 mEq/g.
Cerebrospinal Fluid Penetration: 30%
Bile Penetration: 900%
(also see ***Antibiotic Pearls & Pitfalls*** pp. 495–508).

REFERENCES:
Itokazu GS, Danziger LH. Ampicillin-sulbactam and ticarcillin-clavulanic acid: A comparison of their in vitro activity and review of their clinical efficacy. Pharmacotherapy 11:382–414, 1991.
Jain R, Danziger LH. Multidrug-resistant Acinetobacter infections: an emerging challenge to clinicians. Ann Pharmacother 38:1449–59, 2004.
Krol V, Hamid NS, Cunha BA. Neurosurgically Related Nosocomial Acinetobacter baumannii Meningitis in ICU. Journal of Hospital Infection 71:176–188, 2008.
Sensakovic JW, Smith LG. Beta-lactamase inhibitor combinations. Med Clin North Am 79:695–704, 1995.
Swenson JM, Killgore GE, Tenover FC. Antimicrobial susceptibility testing of Acinetobacter spp. by NCCLS broth microdilution and disk diffusion methods. J Clin Microbiol 42:5102–8, 2004.

"Usual dose" assumes normal renal/hepatic function. * For renal insufficiency, give usual dose × 1 followed by maintenance dose per CrCl. For dialysis patients, dose the same as for CrCl < 10 mL/min and give supplemental (post-HD/PD dose) immediately after dialysis. CrCl = creatinine clearance; CVVH = continuous veno-venous hemofiltration; HD/PD = hemodialysis/peritoneal dialysis. See pp. 509–513 for explanations, pp. xi–xii for abbreviations; Linezolid (↑ risk of serotonin syndrome, see p. 620).

Wood GC, Hanes SD, Croce MA, et al. Comparison of ampicillin-sulbactam and imipenem-cilastatin for the treatment of Acinetobacter ventilator-associated pneumonia. Clin Infect Dis 34:1425–30, 2002.

Wright AJ. The penicillins. Mayo Clin Proc 73:290–307, 1999.

Website: www.pdr.net

Amprenavir (Agenerase) APV

Drug Class: Antiretroviral protease inhibitor.
Usual Adult Dose: 1200 mg (PO) q12h (capsules) or 1400 mg (PO) q12h (solution); age 13–16 years < 50 kg or pediatrics 4–12 years: 20 mg/kg (PO) q12h (capsules) or 1.5 ml/kg (PO) q12h (15 mg/mL solution). Maximum dose 2400 mg/d (capsules), 2800 mg/d (oral solution)
Pharmacokinetic Parameters:
Peak serum level: 7.6 mcg/mL
Bioavailability: No data
Excreted unchanged (urine): 1%
Serum half-life (normal/ESRD): 7-10/7-10 hrs
Plasma protein binding: 90%
Volume of distribution (V_d): 6.1 L/kg
Primary Mode of Elimination: Hepatic
Dosage Adjustments*

CrCl > 10 mL/min	No change
CrCl < 10 mL/min	No change (avoid solution)
Post-HD/PD dose	No information
CVVH dose	No information
Moderate hepatic insufficiency	450 mg (PO) q12h (capsules)
Severe hepatic insufficiency	300 mg (PO) q12h (capsules)

Antiretroviral Dosage Adjustments:

Delavirdine	Avoid
Didanosine buffered solution	Take amprenavir 1 hour before or after
Efavirenz	No information
Indinavir	No information
Lopinavir/ritonavir	May ↓ lopinavir levels
Nelfinavir	No information
Nevirapine	No information
Ritonavir	Limited data for amprenavir 600 mg q12h + ritonavir 100 mg q12h (or amprenavir 1200 mg q24h + ritonavir 200 mg q24h)
Saquinavir	No information
Rifampin	Avoid combination
Rifabutin	Rifabutin 150 mg q24h or 300 mg 2–3x/week

Drug Interactions: Antiretrovirals, rifabutin, rifampin (see dose adjustment grid, above); bepridil, cisapride, ergotamine, statins, benzodiazepines, St. John's wort, pimozide, sildenafil, methadone (avoid if possible); carbamazepine, phenobarbital, phenytoin (may ↓ amprenavir levels, monitor anticonvulsant levels); H_2 blockers, proton pump inhibitors (↓ amprenavir levels).
Adverse Effects: Rash, Stevens-Johnson syndrome (rare), GI upset, headache, depression, taste perversion, diarrhea, perioral

"Usual dose" assumes normal renal/hepatic function. * For renal insufficiency, give usual dose × 1 followed by maintenance dose per CrCl. For dialysis patients, dose the same as for CrCl < 10 mL/min and give supplemental (post-HD/PD dose) immediately after dialysis. CrCl = creatinine clearance; CVVH = continuous veno-venous hemofiltration; HD/PD = hemodialysis/peritoneal dialysis. See pp. 509–513 for explanations, pp. xi–xii for abbreviations; Linezolid (↑ risk of serotonin syndrome, see p. 620).

paresthesias, hyperglycemia (including worsening diabetes, new-onset diabetes, DKA), ↑ cholesterol/triglycerides (evaluate risk for coronary disease/pancreatitis), fat redistribution, ↑ SGOT/SGPT, possible increased bleeding in hemophilia.

Allergic Potential: High. Amprenavir is a sulfonamide; use with caution in sulfa allergy

Safety in Pregnancy: C

Comments: Can be taken with or without food, but avoid high fat meals (may ↓ absorption). High vitamin E content. Capsules and solution are not interchangeable on a mg per mg basis. Decrease dosage in moderate or severe liver disease; use with caution. Oral solution contains propylene glycol: avoid in pregnancy, hepatic/renal failure, patients taking disulfiram or metronidazole, or children < 4 years old. Effective antiretroviral therapy consists of three antiretrovirals (same/different classes) GlaxoSmithKline discontinued production and sale of amprenavir in the United States in order to focus on production of the amprenavir prodrug, fosamprenavir. This action was not taken because of concerns about safety or efficacy of amprenavir. Amprenavir may continue to be available in some countries outside the United States.

REFERENCES:

Adkins JC, Faulds D. Amprenavir. Drugs 55:837–42, 1998.

Go J, Cunha BA. Amprenavir. Antibiotics for Clinicians 4:49–55, 2000.

Kappelhoff BS, Crommentuyn KM, de Maat MM, et al. Practical guidelines to interpret plasma concentrations of antiretroviral drugs. Clin Pharmacokinet 43:845–53, 2004.

Kaul DR, Cinti SK, Carver PL, et al. HIV protease inhibitors: Advances in therapy and adverse reactions, including metabolic complications. Pharmacotherapy 19:281–98, 1999.

Panel on Antiretroviral Guidelines for Adults and Adolescents. Guidelines for the use of antiretroviral agents in HIV-1 infected adults and adolescents. Department of Health and Human Services. November 3, 2008; 1–139. Available at http://www.aidsinfor.nih.gov/ContentFiles/AdultandAdolescentGL.pdf

Website: www.TreatHIV.com

Anidulafungin (Eraxis) (Ecalta)

Drug Class: Echinocandin antifungal.

Usual Dose: 200 mg (IV) × 1 dose, then 100 mg (IV) q24h.

Pharmacokinetic Parameters:

Peak serum level: 4.2 mg/L (100/50 mg dose)/7.2 mg/L (200/100 mg dose)

Bioavailability: Not applicable

Excreted unchanged (urine): < 1%

Serum half-life (normal/ESRD): 40–50 hours/ 40–50 hours

Plasma protein binding: 99%

Volume of distribution (V_d): 30–50L

Primary Mode of Elimination: Fecal (30%)

Dosage Adjustments*

CrCl < 50 mL/min	No change
Post–HD dose	None
Post–PD dose	None
CVVH dose	None
Moderate or severe hepatic insufficiency	No change

Drug Interactions: No significant interactions.

Adverse Effects: ↑ SGOT/SGPT/GGTP/alkaline phosphatase. Histamine-related reactions (rash, urticaria, pruritus, fever, dyspnea and hypotension) if infusion > 1.1 mg/min.

Allergic Potential: Histamine-related symptoms

Safety in Pregnancy: C

"Usual dose" assumes normal renal/hepatic function. * For renal insufficiency, give usual dose × 1 followed by maintenance dose per CrCl. For dialysis patients, dose the same as for CrCl < 10 mL/min and give supplemental (post-HD/PD dose) immediately after dialysis. CrCl = creatinine clearance; CVVH = continuous veno-venous hemofiltration; HD/PD = hemodialysis/peritoneal dialysis. See pp. 509–513 for explanations, pp. xi–xii for abbreviations; Linezolid (↑ risk of serotonin syndrome, see p. 620).

Comments: Not an inducer, inhibitor, or substrate of CYP450 system. Rate of infusion should not exceed 1.1 mg/min. Incompatible with other drugs. Do not infuse with other medications. Use reconstituted vials within 24 hours. Infusion solution should be stored at 25°C/77°F.

Highly active against Candida albicans, non-albicans Candida.

Some activity against Aspergillus.

No activity against Cryptococcus, Fusarium, Pseudoallescheria, Trichosporon, or Mucor.

Cerebrospinal Fluid Penetration: No data

REFERENCES:

Bennett JE, Echinocandins for candidemia in adults without neutropenia. N Engl J Med 355:1154–9, 2006.

Cohen-Wolkowiez M, Benjamin Jr. DK, Steinbach WJ, Smith PB. Anidulafungin: A new Echinocandin for the Treatment of Fungal Infections. Drugs of Today. 42:533–44, 2006.

Cota J, Carden M, Graybill JR, et al. In Vitro Pharmacodynamics of Anidulafungin and Caspofungin against Candida glabrata Isolates, Including Strains with Decreased Caspfungin Susceptibility. Antimicrob Agents Chemother 50:3926–28, 2006.

de la Torre P, Reboli AC. Anidulafungin: a new echinocandin for candidal infections. Expert Rev Anti Infect Ther. 5:45–52, 2007.

Dowell JA, Stogniew M, Krause D, et al. Anidulafungin does not require dosage in subjects with varying degrees of hepatic or renal impairment. J Clin Pharmacol 47:461–470, 2007.

Dowell JA, Stogniew M, Krause D, et al. Lack of pharmacokinetic interaction between anidulafungin and tacrolimus. J Clin Pharmacol 47:305–314, 2007.

Dowell JA, Schranz J, Baruch A, Foster G. Safety and pharmacokinetics of coadministered voriconazole and andigulafungin. J Clin Pharmacol. 45:1373–82, 2005.

Garber G, Laverdiere M, Libman M, et al. Anidulafungin versus fluconazole for invasive candidiasis. N Engl J Med 356:2472–2482, 2007.

Krause DS, Reinhardt J, Vazquez JA, et al. Phase 2, Randomized, Dose-Ranging Study Evaluating the Safety and Efficacy of Anidulafungin in Invasive Candidiasis and Candidemia. Antimicrob Agents Chemother 48:2021–24, 2004.

Morrison VA. Echinocandin antifungals: review and update. Expert Rev Anti Infect Ther. 4:325–42, 2006.

Nir-Paz R, Moses AE. Anidulafungin and fluconazole for candidiasis. N Engl J Med 357:1347–1348, 2007.

Paderu P, Garcia-Effron G, Balashov S, et al. Serum differentially alters the antifungal properties of echinocandin drugs. Antimicrob Agents Chemother 51:2253–2256, 2007.

Pappas PG, Rotstein CMF, Betts RF, et al. Micafungin versus caspofungin for treatment of candidemia and other forms of invasive candidiasis. Clin Infect Dis 45:883–893, 2007.

Patel PN, Charneski L. Anidulafungin (Eraxis) for Fungal Infections. Pharmacy and Therapeutics. 31:644–53, 2006.

Pfaller MA, Diekema DJ, Boyken L. Effectiveness of Anidulafungin in Eradicating Candida Species in Invasive Candidiasis. Antimicrob Agents Chemother 49:4795–97, 2005.

Raasch RH. Anidulafungin: review of a new echinocandin antifungal agent. Expert Rev Anti Infect Ther 2:499–508, 2004.

Reboli AC, Rotstein C, Pappas PG, et al. Anidulafungin versus fluconazole for invasive candidiasis. N Engl J Med 356:2472–2482, 2007.

Theuretzbacher U. Pharmacokinetics/pharmacodynamics of echinocandins. Eur J Clin Microbiol Infect Dis 23:805–12, 2004.

Turner MS, Drew RH, Perfect JR. Emerging echinocandins for treatment of invasive fungal infections. Expert Opin Emerg Drugs 11:231–50, 2006.

Vazquez JA, Sobel JD. Anidulafungin: A Novel Echinocandin. Clin Infect Dis 43:215–22, 2006.

Wiederhold NP, Lewis RE. The echinocandin antifungals: an overview of the pharmacology, spectrum and clinical efficacy. Expert Opin Investig Drugs 12:1313–33, 2003.

Website: www.eraxisrx.com

Atazanavir (Reyataz) ATV

Drug Class: Antiretroviral protease inhibitor.
Usual Dose: 400 mg (PO) q24h with food; 300 mg (PO) q24h when given with tenofovir 100 mg (PO) q24h with ritonavir.
Treatment Experienced Patients: 300 mg with ritonavir 100 mg once daily with food.
Pharmacokinetic Parameters:
Peak serum level: 3152 ng/mL; with ritonavir: 5233 ng/mL
Bioavailability: No data
Excreted unchanged (urine) (urine/feces): 7%/20%
Serum half-life (normal/ESRD): 6.5 hrs; with ritonavir: 8.6 hrs/no data
Plasma protein binding: 86%
Volume of distribution (V_d): No data
Primary Mode of Elimination: Hepatic
Dosage Adjustments*

CrCl < 50 mL/min	No data
Post–HD or PD dose	No data
CVVH dose	No data
Moderate hepatic insufficiency	300 mg (PO) q24h
Severe hepatic insufficiency	Avoid

Antiretroviral Dosage Adjustments:

Delavirdine	No information
Didanosine	Give atazanavir 2 hrs before didanosine with food
Efavirenz	Atazanavir 300 mg + ritonavir 100 + efavirenz 600 mg as single daily dose with food
Indinavir	Avoid combination
Lopinavir/ ritonavir	No information
Nelfinavir	No information
Nevirapine	No information
Ritonavir	Atazanavir 300 mg/d + ritonavir 100 mg/d as single daily dose with food
Saquinavir	↑ saquinavir (soft-gel) levels; no information
Rifampin	Avoid combination
Rifabutin	150 mg q48h or 3x/week

Drug Interactions: Antacids or buffered medications (↓ atazanavir levels; give atazanavir 2 hours before or 1 hour after); H_2-receptor blockers (↓ atazanavir levels. In treatment-naive patients taking an H_2-receptor antagonist, give either atazanavir 400 mg once daily with food at least 2 hours before and at least 10 hours after the H_2-receptor antagonist, or give atazanavir 300 mg once daily with ritonavir 100 mg once daily with food, without the need for separation from the H_2-receptor antagonist. In treatment-experienced patients, give atazanavir 300 mg once daily with ritonavir 100 mg once daily with food at least 2 hours before and at least 10 hours after the H_2-receptor antagonist); antiarrhythmics (↑ amiodarone, systemic lidocaine, quinidine levels; prolongs PR interval; monitor antiarrhythmic levels); antidepressants (↑ tricyclic antidepressant levels; monitor levels); calcium channel blockers (↑ calcium channel blocker levels, ↑ PR interval; ↓ diltiazem dose by 50%; use with caution; consider ECG monitoring); clarithromycin (↑ clarithromycin

---

"Usual dose" assumes normal renal/hepatic function. * For renal insufficiency, give usual dose × 1 followed by maintenance dose per CrCl. For dialysis patients, dose the same as for CrCl < 10 mL/min and give supplemental (post-HD/PD dose) immediately after dialysis. CrCl = creatinine clearance; CVVH = continuous veno-venous hemofiltration; HD/PD = hemodialysis/peritoneal dialysis. See pp. 509–513 for explanations, pp. xi–xii for abbreviations; Linezolid (↑ risk of serotonin syndrome, see p. 620).

and atazanavir levels; consider 50% dose reduction; consider alternate agent for infections not caused by MAI); cyclosporine, sirolimus, tacrolimus (↑ immunosuppressant levels; monitor levels); ethinyl estradiol, norethindrone (↑ oral contraceptive levels; use lowest effective oral contraceptive dose); lovastatin, simvastatin (↑ risk of myopathy, rhabdomyolysis; avoid combination); sildenafil (↑ sildenafil levels; do not give more than 25 mg q48h); tadalafil (max. 10 mg/72 hours); vardenafil (max. 2.5 mg/72 hours); St. John's wort (avoid combination); warfarin (↑ warfarin levels; monitor INR); tenofovir (tenofovir reduces systemic exposure to atazanavir). *Drugs that should not be co-administered with atazanavir* include cisapride, pimozide, rifampin, irinotecan, midazolam, triazolam, lovastatin, simvastatin, bepridil, some ergot derivatives, indinavir, proton pump inhibitors, St. John's wort.

Adverse Effects: Abdominal pain, nausea, vomiting, headache, diarrhea, asthenia, anorexia, and dizziness.

Allergic Potential: Low

Safety in Pregnancy: B

Comments: Monitor LFTs in patients with HBV, HCV. Take 400 mg (two 200-mg capsules) once daily with food. Bioavailability is enhanced with food. Monitor LFTs in patients with HBV, HCV. In moderate liver disease reduce dose to 200 mg once daily. It is not recommended in patients with severe liver impairment.

REFERENCES:

Colonno RJ, Thiry A, Limoli K, Parkin N. Activities of atazanavir (BMS-232632) against a large panel of Human Immunodeficiency Virus Type 1 clinical isolates resistant to one or more approved protease inhibitors. Antimicrob Agents Chemother 47:1324–33, 2003.

Haas DW, Zala C, Schrader S, et al. Therapy with atazanavir plus saquinavir in patients failing highly active antiretroviral therapy: a randomized comparative pilot trial. AIDS 17:1339–1349, 2003.

Havlir DV, O'Marro SD. Atazanavir: new option for treatment of HIV infection. Clin Infect Dis 38:1599–604, 2004.

Jemsek JG, Arathoon E, Arlotti M, et al. Body fat and other metabolic effects of atazanavir and efavirenz, each administered in combination with zidovudine plus lamivudine, in antiretroviral-naive HIV-infected patients. Clin Infect Dis 42:273–80, 2006.

Panel on Antiretroviral Guidelines for Adults and Adolescents. Guidelines for the use of antiretroviral agents in HIV-1 infected adults and adolescents. Department of Health and Human Services. November 3, 2008; 1–139. Available at http://www.aidsinfor.nih.gov/ContentFiles/AdultandAdolescentGL.pdf

Piliero PJ. Atazanavir: a novel HIV-1 protease inhibitor. Expert Opin Investig Drugs 11:1295–301, 2002.

Sanne I, Piliero P, Squires K, et al. Results of a phase 2 clinical trial at 48 weeks (AI424-007): a dose-ranging, safety, and efficacy comparative trial of atazanavir at three doses in combination with didanosine and stavudine in antiretroviral-naive subjects. J Acquir Immune Defic Syndr 32:18–29, 2003.

Wang F, Ross J. Atazanavir: a novel azapeptide inhibitor of HIV-1 protease. Formulary 38:691–702, 2003.

Website: www.reyataz.com

Atovaquone (Mepron)

Drug Class: Antiprotozoal.

Usual Dose: PCP treatment dose: 750 mg (PO) q12h with food. **PCP prophylaxis dose:** 1500 mg (PO) q24h with food.

Pharmacokinetic Parameters:

Peak serum level: 12–24 mcg/mL
Bioavailability: 30% (47% with food; food ↑ bioavailability by 2-fold)
Excreted unchanged (feces): 94%
Serum half-life (normal/ESRD): 2.9/2.9 days
Plasma protein binding: 99.9%
Volume of distribution (V_d): 0.6 L/kg

"Usual dose" assumes normal renal/hepatic function. * For renal insufficiency, give usual dose × 1 followed by maintenance dose per CrCl. For dialysis patients, dose the same as for CrCl < 10 mL/min and give supplemental (post-HD/PD dose) immediately after dialysis. CrCl = creatinine clearance; CVVH = continuous veno-venous hemofiltration; HD/PD = hemodialysis/peritoneal dialysis. See pp. 509–513 for explanations, pp. xi–xii for abbreviations; Linezolid (↑ risk of serotonin syndrome, see p. 620).

Primary Mode of Elimination: Hepatic

Dosage Adjustments*

CrCl < 80 mL/min	No change
Post–HD/PD dose	No information
CVVH dose	No information
Moderate or severe hepatic insufficiency	No information

Drug Interactions: Rifabutin, rifampin (↓ atovaquone effect); zidovudine (↑ zidovudine levels). Rifampin decreases atovaquone levels by 50%.

Adverse Effects: Rash, nausea, diarrhea, headache, fever, cough, anemia, leukopenia, ↑ SGOT/SGPT, ↑ amylase.

Allergic Potential: Low

Safety in Pregnancy: C

Comments: Active against T. gondii, PCP, Plasmodia, and Babesia. Take with food.

Cerebrospinal Fluid Penetration: < 1%

REFERENCES:

Artymowicz RJ, James VE. Atovaquone: A new anti-pneumocystis agent. Clin Pharmacol 12:563–70, 1993.

Baggish AL, Hill DR. Antiparasitic agent atovaquone. Antimicrob Agents Chemother 46:1163–73, 2002.

Bonoan JT, Johnson DH, Schoch PE, Cunha BA. Life threatening babesiosis treated by exchange transfusion with azithromycin and atovaquone. Heart & Lung 27:42–8, 1998.

Chan C, Montaner J, LeFebvre BA, et al. Atovaquone suspension compared with aerosolized pentamidine for prevention of Pneumocystis carinii pneumonia in human immunodeficiency virus infected subsets intolerant of trimethoprim or sulfamethoxazole. J Infect Dis 180:369–376, 1999.

Haile LG, Flaherty JF. Atovaquone: A review. Ann Pharmacother 27:1488–94, 1993.

Van Riemsdijk MM, Sturkenboom MC, Ditters JM, et al. Atovaquone plus chloroguanide versus mefloquine for malaria prophylaxis: A focus on neuropsychiatric adverse events. Clin Pharmacol Ther 72:294–301, 2002.

Wormser GP, Prasad A, Neuhaus E, et al. Emergence of Resistance to Azithromycin-Atovaquone in Immunocompromised Patients with Babesia microti Infection. Clin Infect Dis 50:381–386, 2010.

Atovaquone + Proguanil (Malarone)

Drug Class: Antimalarial.

Usual Dose: Malaria prophylaxis: 1 tablet (250 mg/100 mg) (PO) q24h for 2 days before entering endemic area, daily during exposure, and daily × 1 week post-exposure. Malaria treatment: 4 tablets (1000 mg/400 mg) (PO) as single dose × 3 days.

Pharmacokinetic Parameters:

Peak serum level: 38 mcg/mL

Bioavailability: 23/90%

Excreted unchanged (feces): 94/50%

Serum half-life (normal/ESRD): [60/60]/[21/no data] hrs

Plasma protein binding: 99/75%

Volume of distribution (V_d): 3.5/42 L/kg

Primary Mode of Elimination: Metabolized

Dosage Adjustments*

CrCl > 30 mL/min	No change
CrCl 10–30 mL/min	Avoid
CrCl < 10 mL/min	Avoid
Post–HD/PD dose	No information
CVVH dose	No information
Moderate or severe hepatic insufficiency	No change

Drug Interactions: Chloroquine (↑ incidence of mouth ulcers); metoclopramide, rifabutin, rifampin,

"Usual dose" assumes normal renal/hepatic function. * For renal insufficiency, give usual dose × 1 followed by maintenance dose per CrCl. For dialysis patients, dose the same as for CrCl < 10 mL/min and give supplemental (post-HD/PD dose) immediately after dialysis. CrCl = creatinine clearance; CVVH = continuous veno-venous hemofiltration; HD/PD = hemodialysis/peritoneal dialysis. See pp. 509–513 for explanations, pp. xi–xii for abbreviations; Linezolid (↑ risk of serotonin syndrome, see p. 620).

tetracycline (↓ atovaquone + proguanil effect); ritonavir (↑ or ↓ atovaquone + proguanil effect); typhoid vaccine (↓ typhoid vaccine effect).

Adverse Effects: Headache, dizziness, nausea, vomiting, diarrhea, abdominal pain, anorexia, myalgias, fever.

Allergic Potential: Low

Safety in Pregnancy: C

Comments: Malarone tablet = 250 mg atovaquone + 100 mg proguanil. **Effective against chloroquine sensitive/resistant strains of P. falciparum, but not P. ovale, P. vivax, or P. malariae**. Dosage may be decreased in patients with diarrhea. Take with food/milk.

Cerebrospinal Fluid Penetration: < 1%

REFERENCES:

Atovaquone/proguanil (Malarone) for malaria. Med Lett Drugs Ther 42:109–11, 2000.

Camus D, Djossou F, Schithuis HJ, et al. Atovaquone-proguanil versus chloroquine-proguanil for malaria prophylaxis in nonimmune pediatric travelers: results of an international, randomized, open-label study. Clin Infect Dis 38:1716–23, 2004.

Looareesuwan S, Chulay JD, Canfield CJ. Malarone (atovaquone and proguanil hydrochloride): a review of its clinical development for treating malaria. Malarone clinical trials study group. Am J Trop Med Hyg 60:533–41, 1999.

Marra F, Salzman JR, Ensom MH. Atovaquone-proguanil for prophylaxis and treatment of malaria. Ann Pharmacother. 37:1266–75, 2003.

McKeage K, Scott L. Atovaquone/proguanil: a review of its use for the prophylaxis of Plasmodium falciparum malaria. Drugs. 63:597–623, 2003.

Thapar MM, Ashton M, Lindegardh N, et al. Time-dependent pharmacokinetics and drug metabolism of atovaquone plus proguanil (Malarone) when taken as chemoprophylaxis. Eur J Clin Pharmacol 15:19–27, 2002.

Website: www.pdr.net

Azithromycin (Zithromax)

Drug Class: Macrolide (Azolide).

Usual Dose: 500 mg (IV/PO) × 1 dose, then 250 mg (IV/PO) q24h (see comments).

Spectrum: (see ***Susceptibility Profiles*** pp. 183–187).

Pharmacokinetic Parameters:

Peak serum level: 1.1 (IV)/0.2 (PO) mcg/mL
Bioavailability: 35%
Excreted unchanged (urine): 6%
Serum half-life (normal/ESRD): 68/68 hrs
Plasma protein binding: 50%
Volume of distribution (V_d): 31 L/kg

Primary Mode of Elimination: Hepatic

Dosage Adjustments*

CrCl 50–80 mL/min	No change
CrCl 10–50 mL/min	No change
CrCl < 10 mL/min	Use caution
Post–HD/PD dose	None
CVVH dose	None
Moderate or severe hepatic insufficiency	No change

Drug Interactions: Amiodarone, carbamazepine, cisapride, clozapine, corticosteroids, midazolam, triazolam, valproic acid (not studied/not reported); cyclosporine (↑ cyclosporine levels with toxicity); digoxin (↑ digoxin levels); pimozide (may ↑ QT interval, torsade de pointes).

Adverse Effects: Nausea, GI upset, Non-C. difficile diarrhea.

Allergic Potential: Low

Safety in Pregnancy: B

Comments: May ↑ QT_c interval. Bioavailability is decreased by food. **C. trachomatis urethritis**

"Usual dose" assumes normal renal/hepatic function. * For renal insufficiency, give usual dose × 1 followed by maintenance dose per CrCl. For dialysis patients, dose the same as for CrCl < 10 mL/min and give supplemental (post-HD/PD dose) immediately after dialysis. CrCl = creatinine clearance; CVVH = continuous veno-venous hemofiltration; HD/PD = hemodialysis/peritoneal dialysis. See pp. 509–513 for explanations, pp. xi–xii for abbreviations; Linezolid (↑ risk of serotonin syndrome, see p. 620).

dose: 1 gm (PO) × 1 dose. **N. gonorrhoea urethritis dose:** 2 gm (PO) × 1 dose. **MAI prophylaxis dose:** 1200 mg (PO) weekly. **MAI therapy dose:** 600 mg (PO) q24h.
Cerebrospinal Fluid Penetration: < 10%
Bile/serum ratio: > 3000%
(also see ***Antibiotic Pearls & Pitfalls*** pp. 495–508).

REFERENCES:

Alvarez-Elcoro S, Enzler MJ. The macrolides: Erythromycin, clarithromycin and azithromycin. Mayo Clin Proc 74:613–34, 1999.

Amsden GW, Gregory TB, Michalak CA, et al. Pharmacokinetics of azithromycin and the combination of ivermecting and albendazole when administered alone and concurrently in healthy volunteers. Am J Trop Med Hyg 76:1153–1157, 2007.

Bergman M, Huikko S, Huovinen P, et al. Macrolide and azithromycin use are linked to increased macrolide resistance in *Streptococcus pneumoniae*. Antimicrob Agents Chemother 50:3646–3650, 2006.

Chandra R, Liu P, Breen JD, et al. Clinical pharmacokinetics and gastrointestinal tolerability of a novel extended-release microsphere formulation of azithromycin. Clin Pharmacokinet 46:247–259, 2007.

Cochereau I, Goldschmidt P, Goepogui A, et al. Efficacy and safety of short duration azithromycin eye drops versus azithromycin single oral dose for the treatment of trachoma in children: a randomized, controlled, double-masked clinical trial. Br J Ophthalmol 91:667–672, 2007.

Cunha BA. Macrolides, doxycycline, and fluoroquinolones in the treatment of Legionnaires' Disease. Antibiotics for Clinicians 2:117–8, 1998.

Daneman N, McGeer A, Green K, et al. Macrolide resistance in bacteremic pneumococcal disease.: Implications for patient management. Clin Infect Dis 43:432–438, 2006.

DuPont HL. Azithromycin for the self-treatment of traveler's diarrhea. Clin Infect dis 44:347–349, 2007.

Frenck RW, Mansour A, Nakhla I, et al. Short-course azithromycin for the treatment of uncomplicated typhoid fever in children and adolescents. Clin Infect Dis 38:951–7, 2004.

Geisler WM. Management of uncomplicated Chlamydia trachomatis infections in adolescents and adults: evidence reviewed for the 2006 Centers for Disease Control and Prevention sexually transmitted diseases treatment guidelines. Clin Infect Dis 44(S3):S77–S83, 2007.

Haggerty CL, Ness RB. Newest approaches to treatment of pelvic inflammatory disease: a review of recent randomized clinical trials. Clin Infect Dis 44(S3):S953–S960, 2007.

Ioannidis JP, Contopoulos-Ioannidis DG, Chew P, Lau J. Meta-analysis of randomized controlled trials on the comparative efficacy and safety of azithromycin against other antibiotics for upper respiratory tract infections. J Antimicrob Chemother 48:677–89, 2001.

Jain R, Danzinger LH. The macrolide antibiotics: a pharmacokinetic and pharmacodynamic overview. Curr Pharm Des 10:3045–53, 2004.

Jenkins SG, Farrell DJ. Increase in Pneumococcus Macrolide Resistance, United States. Emerging Infect Dis 15:1260–1264, 2009.

Kim Y-S, Yun H-J, Shim SK, et al. A comparative trial of a single dose of azithromycin versus doxycycline for the treatment of mild scrub typhus. Clin Infect Dis 39:1329–35, 2004.

Magbanua JP, Goh BT, Michel CE, et al. Chlamydia trachomatis variant not detected by plasmid based nucleic acid amplification tests: molecular characterization and failure of single dose azithromycin. Sex Transm Infect 83:339–343, 2007.

Malhotra-Kumar S, Lammens C, Coenen S, et al. Effect of azithromycin and clarithromycin therapy on pharyngeal carriage of macrolide-resistant streptococci in healthy volunteers: a randomized, double-blind, placebo-controlled study. Lancet 369:482–490, 2007.

Mandell LA, Wunderdink RG, Anzuetto A, et al. Infectious Diseases Society of America/American Thoracic Society consensus guidelines on the management of community-acquired pneumonia in adults. Clin Infect Dis 44:S27–72, 2007.

"Usual dose" assumes normal renal/hepatic function. * For renal insufficiency, give usual dose × 1 followed by maintenance dose per CrCl. For dialysis patients, dose the same as for CrCl < 10 mL/min and give supplemental (post-HD/PD dose) immediately after dialysis. CrCl = creatinine clearance; CVVH = continuous veno-venous hemofiltration; HD/PD = hemodialysis/peritoneal dialysis. See pp. 509–513 for explanations, pp. xi–xii for abbreviations; Linezolid (↑ risk of serotonin syndrome, see p. 620).

McLean CA, Stoner BP, Workowski KA. Treatment of lymphogranuloma venereum. Clin Infect Dis 44(S3):S147–S152, 2007.

McMillan A, Young H. The treatment of pharyngeal gonorrhoea with a single oral dose of cefixime. Int J STD AIDS 18:253–254, 2007.

Mena LA, Mroczkowski TF, Nsuami M, et al. A Randomized Comparison of Azithromycin and Doxycycline for the Treatment of *Mycoplasma* genitalium – positive Urethritis in Men. Clin Infect Dis 48:1649–1654, 2009.

Nguyen D, Emond MJ, Mayer-Hamblett N, et al. Clinical response to azithromycin in cystic fibrosis correlates with in vitro effects on Pseudomonas aeruginosa phenotypes. Pediatr Pulmonol 42:533–541, 2007.

Paradisi F, Corti G. Azithromycin. Antibiotics for Clinicians 3:1–8, 1999.

Phillips P, Chan K, Hogg R, et al. Azithromycin prophylaxis for Mycobacterium avium complex during the era of highly active antiretroviral therapy: evaluation of a provincial program. Clin Infect Dis 34:371–8, 2002.

Pichichero ME, Hoeger WJ, Casey JR. Azithromycin for the treatment of pertussis. Pediatr Infect Dis J. 22:847–9, 2003.

Plouffe JF, Breiman RF, Fields BS, et al. Azithromycin in the treatment of Legionella pneumonia requiring hospitalization. Clin Infect Dis 37:1475–80, 2003.

Saiman L, Marshall BC, Mayer-Hamblett N, et al. Azithromycin in patients with cystic fibrosis chronically infected with Pseudomonas aeruginosa: a randomized controlled trial. JAMA. 290:1749–5, 2003.

Savaris RF, Teixeira LM, Torres TG, et al. Comparing ceftriaxone plus azithromycin or doxycycline for pelvis inflammatory disease: a randomized controlled trial Obstet Gynecol 110:53–60, 2007.

Schlossberg D. Azithromycin and clarithromycin. Med Clin N Amer 79:803–816, 1995.

Southern KW, Barker PM. Azithromycin for cystic fibrosis. Eur Respir J 24:834–8, 2004.

Suzuki S, Yamazaki T, Narita M. Clinical Evaluation of Macrolide-Resistant Mycoplasma pneumoniae. Antimocrobial Agents and Chemotherapy. 50:709–12, 2006.

Stoner BP. Current controversies in the management of adult syphilis. Clin Infect Dis 44(S3):S77–S83, 2007.

Swainston Harrison T, Keam SJ. Azithromycin extended release: a review of its use in the treatment of acute bacterial sinusitis and community-acquired pneumonia in the US. Drugs 773–79, 2007.

Toltzis P, Dul M, Blumer J. Change in pneumococcal susceptibility to azithromycin during treatment for acute otitis media. Pediatr Infect Dis 26:647–649, 2007.

Topic A, Skerk V, Puntaric A, et al. Azithromycin: 1.0 or 3.0 Gram Dose in the Treatment of Patients with Asymptomatic Urogenital Chlamydial Infections. Journal of Chemotherapy. 18:115–16, 2006.

Wolter J, Seeney S, Bell S, et al. Effect of long term treatment with azithromycin on disease parameters in cystic fibrosis: a randomised trial. Thorax 57:212–6, 2002.

Wormser GP, Prasad A, Neuhaus E, et al. Emergence of Resistance to Azithromycin-Atovaquone in Immunocompromised Patients with Babesia microti Infection. Clin Infect. Dis 50:381–386, 2010.

Website: www.zithromax.com

Aztreonam (Azactam)

Drug Class: Monobactam.

Usual Dose: 2 gm (IV) q8h (see comments).

Spectrum: (see ***Susceptibility Profiles*** pp. 194–199).

Pharmacokinetic Parameters:

Peak serum level: 204 mcg/mL

Bioavailability: Not applicable

Excreted unchanged (urine): 60–70%

Serum half-life (normal/ESRD): 1.7/7 hrs

Plasma protein binding: 56%

Volume of distribution (V_d)*: 0.2 L/kg*

Primary Mode of Elimination: Renal

Dosage Adjustments* (based on 2 gm IV q8h):

CrCl 50–80 mL/min	2 gm (IV) q8h
CrCl 10–50 mL/min	1 gm (IV) q8h
CrCl < 10 mL/min	500 mg (IV) q8h

"Usual dose" assumes normal renal/hepatic function. * For renal insufficiency, give usual dose × 1 followed by maintenance dose per CrCl. For dialysis patients, dose the same as for CrCl < 10 mL/min and give supplemental (post-HD/PD dose) immediately after dialysis. CrCl = creatinine clearance; CVVH = continuous veno-venous hemofiltration; HD/PD = hemodialysis/peritoneal dialysis. See pp. 509–513 for explanations, pp. xi–xii for abbreviations; Linezolid (↑ risk of serotonin syndrome, see p. 620).

Post–HD dose	250 mg (IV)
Post–PD dose	500 mg (IV)
CVVH dose	1 gm (IV) q8h
Moderate hepatic insufficiency	No change
Severe hepatic insufficiency	No change

Drug Interactions: None.
Adverse Effects: None.
Allergic Potential: Low
Safety in Pregnancy: B
Comments: Incompatible in solutions containing vancomycin or metronidazole. **No cross allergenicity with penicillins, β-lactams; safe to use in penicillin allergic patients. CAPD dose:** 1 gm (IP), then 250 mg/L of dialysate (IP) with each exchange. Meningeal dose = 2 gm (IV) q6h.
Cerebrospinal Fluid Penetration:
Non-Inflamed meninges = 1%
Inflamed meninges = 40%
Bile Penetration: 300%
(also see ***Antibiotic Pearls & Pitfalls*** pp. 495–508).

REFERENCES:

Brogden RN, Heal RC. Aztreonam: A review of its antibacterial activity, pharmacokinetic properties, and therapeutic use. Drugs 31:96–130, 1986.

Critchley IA, Sahm DF, Kelly LJ, et al. In vitro synergy studies using aztreonam and fluoroquinolone combinations against six species of Gram-negative bacilli. Chemotherapy. 49:44–8, 2003.

Cunha BA. Aztreonam: A review. Urology 41:249–58, 1993.

Cunha BA. Cross allergenicity of penicillin with carbapenems and monobactams. J Crit Illness 13:344, 1998.

Espedido BA, Thomas LC, Iredell JR. Metallo-beta-lactamase or extended-spectrum beta-lactamase: a wolf in sheep's clothing. J Clin Microbiol 45:2034–2036, 2007.

Fleming DR, Ziegler C, Baize T, et al. Cefepime versus ticarcillin and clavulanate potassium and aztreonam for febrile neutropenia therapy in high-dose chemotherapy patients. Am J Clin Oncol. 26:285–8, 2003.

Gasink LB, Neil OF, Nachamkin I, et al. Risk factors for the impact of infection or colonization with aztreonam-resistant Pseudomonas aeruginosa. Infection Com and Hospital Epidemiology 28:1175–1180, 2007.

Hellinger WC, Brewer NS. Carbapenems and monobactams: Imipenem, meropenem, and aztreonam. Mayo Clin Proc 74:420–34, 1999.

Johnson, Cunha BA. Aztreonam. Med Clin North Am 79:733–43, 1995.

Jordan EF, Nye MB, Luque AE. Successful treatment of Pasteurella multocida meningitis with aztreonam. Scand J Infect Dis 39:72–74, 2007.

Panagiotakopoulou A, Daikos GL, Miriagou V, et al. Comparative in vitro killing of carbapenems and aztreonam against Klebsiella pneumoniae producing VIM-1 metallo-beta-lactamase. Int J Antimicrob Agents 29:360–362, 2007.

Pendland SL, Messick CR, Jung R. In vitro synergy testing of levofloxacin, ofloxacin, and ciprofloxacin in combination with aztreonam, ceftazidime, or piperacillin against Pseudomonas aeruginosa. Diagn Microbiol Infect Dis 42:75–8, 2002.

Sader HS, Huynh HK, Jones RN. Contemporary in vitro synergy rates for aztreonam combined with newer fluoroquinolones and beta-lactams tested against gram-negative bacilli. Diagn Microbiol Infect Dis 47(3):547–50, 2003.

Website: www.elan.com/Products/

Capreomycin (Capastat)

Drug Class: Anti–TB drug.
Usual Dose: 1 gm (IM) q24h.
Pharmacokinetic Parameters:
Peak serum level: 30 mcg/mL
Bioavailability: Not applicable
Excreted unchanged (urine): 50%

"Usual dose" assumes normal renal/hepatic function. * For renal insufficiency, give usual dose × 1 followed by maintenance dose per CrCl. For dialysis patients, dose the same as for CrCl < 10 mL/min and give supplemental (post-HD/PD dose) immediately after dialysis. CrCl = creatinine clearance; CVVH = continuous veno-venous hemofiltration; HD/PD = hemodialysis/peritoneal dialysis. See pp. 509–513 for explanations, pp. xi–xii for abbreviations; Linezolid (↑ risk of serotonin syndrome, see p. 620).

Serum half-life (normal/ESRD): 5/30 hrs
Plasma protein binding: No data
Volume of distribution (V_d): 0.4 L/kg
Primary Mode of Elimination: Renal
Dosage Adjustments*

CrCl 50–80 mL/min	500 mg (IM) q24h
CrCl 10–50 mL/min	500 mg (IM) q48h
CrCl < 10 mL/min	500 mg (IM) q72h
Post–HD dose	500 mg (IM)
Post–PD dose	None
CVVH dose	500 mg (IM) q48h
Moderate hepatic insufficiency	No change
Severe hepatic insufficiency	No change

Drug Interactions: None.
Adverse Effects: Eosinophilia, leukopenia, drug fever/rash, ototoxicity (vestibular), nephrotoxicity (glomerular/tubular).
Allergic Potential: Moderate
Safety in Pregnancy: C
Comments: Pain/phlebitis at IM injection site. Additive toxicity with aminoglycosides/viomycin.
Cerebrospinal Fluid Penetration: < 10%

REFERENCES:

Davidson PT, Le HQ. Drug treatment of tuberculosis - 1992. Drugs 43:651–73, 1992.
Drugs for tuberculosis. Med Lett Drugs Ther 35:99–101, 1993.
Furin J, Nardell EA. Multidrug-resistant tuberculosis: An update on the best regimens. J Respir Dis 27:172–82, 2006.
Iseman MD. Treatment of multidrug resistant tuberculosis. N Engl J Med 329:784–91, 1993.
Website: www.pdr.net

Caspofungin (Cancidas)

Drug Class: Echinocandin antifungal.
Usual Dose: 70 mg (IV) × 1 dose, then 50 mg (IV) q24h (see comments).
Pharmacokinetic Parameters:
Peak serum level:
70 mg: 12.1 (single dose)*/14.83 mcg/mL* (multiple dose)
50 mg: 7.6/8.7 mcg/mL (multiple dose)
Bioavailability: Not applicable
Excreted unchanged (urine): 1.4%
Serum half-life (normal/ESRD): 10/10 hrs
Plasma protein binding: 97%
Volume of distribution (V_d): No data
Primary Mode of Elimination: Hepatic
Dosage Adjustments*

CrCl 50–80 mL/min	No change
CrCl 10–50 mL/min	No change
CrCl < 10 mL/min	No change
Post–HD/PD dose	None
CVVH dose	None
Moderate hepatic insufficiency	35 mg (IV) q24h (maintenance dose)
Severe hepatic insufficiency	No information

Drug Interactions: Carbamazepine, rifampin, dexamethasone, efavirenz, nelfinavir, nevirapine, phenytoin (↓ caspofungin levels; ↑ caspofungin maintenance dose to 70 mg/day); cyclosporine (↑ caspofungin levels, ↑ SGOT/SGPT; co-administration is discouraged unless careful monitoring can be ensured and unless the benefit of caspofungin outweighs the risk of hepatotoxicity); tacrolimus (↓ tacrolimus levels, ↑ SGOT/SGPT).

"Usual dose" assumes normal renal/hepatic function. * For renal insufficiency, give usual dose × 1 followed by maintenance dose per CrCl. For dialysis patients, dose the same as for CrCl < 10 mL/min and give supplemental (post-HD/PD dose) immediately after dialysis. CrCl = creatinine clearance; CVVH = continuous veno-venous hemofiltration; HD/PD = hemodialysis/peritoneal dialysis. See pp. 509–513 for explanations, pp. xi–xii for abbreviations; Linezolid (↑ risk of serotonin syndrome, see p. 620).

Adverse Effects: Drug fever/rash.
Allergic Potential: Low
Safety in Pregnancy: C
Comments: Administer by slow IV infusion over 1 hour; do not give IV bolus. Do not mix/co-infuse with glucose solutions. If co-administered with drugs that ↓ caspofungin levels or for highly-resistant organisms, then 70 mg (IV) q24h dosing may be used. For esophageal candidiasis, therapy is initiated with 50 mg (70 mg loading dose has not been studied).
Highly active against Candida albicans and non-*albicans *Candida.
Some activity against Aspergillus.
No activity against Cryptococcus, Fusarium, Pseudoallescheria, Trichosporon, or Mucor.
Cerebrospinal Fluid Penetration: < 1%

REFERENCES:

Arathoon EG, Gotuzzo E, Noriega LM, et al. Randomized, double-blind, multicenter study of caspofungin versus amphotericin B for treatment of oropharyngeal and esophageal candidiasis. Antimicrob Agents Chemother 46:451–7, 2002.

Bachmann SP, VandeWalle K, Ramage G, et al. In vitro activity of caspofungin against Candida albicans biofilms. Antimicrob Agents Chemother 46:3591–3596, 2002.

Barchiesi F, Schimizzi AM, Fothergill AW, et al. In vitro activity of the new echinocandin antifungal against common and uncommon clinical isolates of Candida species. Eur J Clin Microbiol Infect Dis 18:302–4, 1999.

Barchiesi F, Spreghini E, Tomassetti S, et al. Efficacy of caspofungin against invasive Candida or invasive Aspergillus infections in neutropenic patients. Antimicrob Agents Chemother 50:2719–27, 2006.

Bennett JE, Echinocandins for candidemia in adults without neutropenia. N Engl J Med 355:1154–9, 2006.

Betts RF, Nucci M, Talwar D, et al. A Multicenter, Double-Blind Trial of a High-Dose Caspofungin Treatment Regimen versus a Standard Caspofungin Treatment Regimen for Adult Patients with Invasive Candidiasis. Clin Infect Dis 48:1676–1684, 2009.

Betts R, Glasmacher A, Maertens J, et al. Efficacy of caspofungin against invasive Candida or invasive Aspergillus infections in neutropenic patients. Cancer. 106:466–73, 2006.

Black KE, Baden LR. Fungal infections of the CNS: treatment strategies for the immunocompromised patient. CNS Drugs 21:293–318, 2007.

Deresinski SC, Stevens DA. Caspofungin. Clin Infect Dis 36:1445–57, 2003.

Dominguez-Gil A, Martin I, Garcia Vargas M, et al. Economic evaluation of voriconazole versus caspofungin for the treatment of aspergillosis in Spain. Clin Drug Investig 27:197–205, 2007.

Falagas ME, Ntziora F, Betsi GI, et al. Caspofungin for the treatment of fungal infections: a systematic review of randomized controlled trials. Int J Animicrob Agents 29:136–143, 2007.

Gallagher JC, MacDougall C, Ashley ES, et al. Recent advances in antifungal pharmacotherapy for invasive fungal infections. Expert Rev Anti Infect Ther 2:253–68, 2004.

Glasmacher A, Cornely OA, Orlopp K, et al. Caspofungin treatment in severely ill, immunocompromised patients: a case-documentation study of 118 patients. J Antimicrob Chemother 57:127–34, 2006.

Grau S, Mateu-De Antonio J. Caspofungin acetate for treatment of invasive fungal infections. Ann Pharmacother. 37:1919, 2003.

Groll AH, Attarbasehi A, Schuster FR, et al. Treatment with caspofungin in immunocompromised paediatric patients: a multicentre survey. A Antimicrob Chemother 57:527–35, 2006.

Hope WW, Shoham S, Walsh TJ. The pharmacology and clinical use of caspofungin. Expert Opin Drug Metab Toxicol 3:263–274, 2007.

Ikeda F, Tanaka S, Ohki H, et al. Role of micafungin in the antifungal armamentarium. Curr Med Chem 14:1263–1275, 2007.

Keating G, Figgitt D. Caspofungin: a review of its use in esophageal candidiasis, invasive candidiasis and invasive aspergillosis. Drugs 63:2235–63, 2003.

Lomaestro BM. Caspofungin. Hospital Formulary 36:527–36, 2001.

"Usual dose" assumes normal renal/hepatic function. * For renal insufficiency, give usual dose × 1 followed by maintenance dose per CrCl. For dialysis patients, dose the same as for CrCl < 10 mL/min and give supplemental (post-HD/PD dose) immediately after dialysis. CrCl = creatinine clearance; CVVH = continuous veno-venous hemofiltration; HD/PD = hemodialysis/peritoneal dialysis. See pp. 509–513 for explanations, pp. xi–xii for abbreviations; Linezolid (↑ risk of serotonin syndrome, see p. 620).

Maertens J, Raad I, Petrikkos G, et al. Efficacy and safety of caspofungin for treatment of invasive aspergillosis in patients refractory to or intolerant of conventional antifungal therapy. Clin Infect Dis 39:1563–71, 2004.

Mattiuzzi GN, Alvarado G, Giles FJ, et al. Open-label, randomized comparison of itraconazole versus caspofungin for prophylaxis in patients with hematologic malignancies. Antimicrob Agents Chemother 50:143–7, 2006.

Mistry GC, Migoya E, Deutsch PJ, et al. Single- and multiple-dose administration of caspofungin in patients with hepatic insufficiency: implications for safety and dosing recommendations. J Clin Pharmacol 47:951–961, 2007.

Mora-Duarte J, Betts R, Rotstein C, et al. Comparison of caspofungin and amphotericin B for invasive candidiasis. N Engl J Med 347:2020–9, 2002.

Morrison VA. Echinocandin antifungals: review and update. Expert Rev Anti Infect Ther. 4:325–42, 2006.

Mullane K, Toor AA, Kalnicky C, et al. Posaconazole salvage therapy allows successful allogeneic hematopoietic stem cell transplantation in patients with refractory invasive mold infections. Transpl Infect Dis 9:89–96, 2007.

Nevado J, De Alarcon A, Hernandez A. Caspofungin: a new therapeutic option for fungal endocarditis. Clin Microbiol Infect. 11:248, 2005.

Nguyen TH, Hoppe-Tichy T, Geiss HK, et al. Factors influencing caspofungin plasma concentrations in patients of a surgical intensive care unit. J Antimicrob Chemother 60:100–106, 2007.

Nivoix Y, Zamfir A, Lutun P, Kara F, et al. Combination of caspofungin and an azole or an amphotericin B formulation in invasive fungal infections. J Infect. 52:67–74, 2006.

Pacetti SA, Gelone SP. Caspofungin acetate for treatment of invasive fungal infections. Ann Pharmacother 37:90–8, 2003.

Pappas PG, Rotstein CM, Betts RF, et al. Micafungin versus caspofungin for treatment of candidemia and other forms of invasive candidiasis. Clin Infect Dis 45:883–893, 2007.

Pfaller MA, Boyken L, Hollis RJ, et al. In vitro susceptibilities of Candida spp. to Caspofungin: four years of global surveillance. J Clin Microbiol. 44:760–3, 2006.

Pfaller MA, Messer SA, Boyken L, et al. Caspofungin activity against clinical isolates of fluconazole-resistant Candida. J Clin Microbiol. 41:5729–31, 2003

Rubin MA, Carroll KC, Cahill BC. Caspofungin in combination with itraconazole for the treatment of invasive aspergillosis in humans. Clin Infect Dis 34:1160–1, 2002.

Sobel JD, Bradshaw SK, Lipka CJ, et al. Caspofungin in the treatment of symptomatic candiduria. Clin Infect Dis 44:e46–e49, 2007.

Stone EA, Fung HB, Hirschenbaum HL. Caspofungin: an echinocandin antifungal agent. Clin Ther 24:351–77, 2002.

Walsh TJ, Adamson PC, Seibel NL, et al. Pharmacokinetics, safety, and tolerability of caspofungin in children and adolescents. Antimicrobial Agents and Chemotherapy 49: 4536–45,2005.

Walsh TJ, Teppler H, Donowitz GR, et al. Caspofungin versus liposomal amphotericin B for empirical antifungal therapy in patients with persistent fever and neutropenia. N Engl J Med 351:1391–402, 2004.

Website: www.cancidas.com

Cefaclor (Ceclor)

Drug Class: 2nd generation oral cephalosporin.
Usual Dose: 500 mg (PO) q8h.
Spectrum: (see ***Susceptibility Profiles*** pp. 188–193).
Pharmacokinetic Parameters:
Peak serum level: 13 mcg/mL
Bioavailability: 80%
Excreted unchanged (urine): 60–85%
Serum half-life (normal/ESRD): 0.8/3 hrs
Plasma protein binding: 25%
Volume of distribution (V_d): 0.30 L/kg
Primary Mode of Elimination: Renal
Dosage Adjustments*

"Usual dose" assumes normal renal/hepatic function. * For renal insufficiency, give usual dose × 1 followed by maintenance dose per CrCl. For dialysis patients, dose the same as for CrCl < 10 mL/min and give supplemental (post-HD/PD dose) immediately after dialysis. CrCl = creatinine clearance; CVVH = continuous veno-venous hemofiltration; HD/PD = hemodialysis/peritoneal dialysis. See pp. 509–513 for explanations, pp. xi–xii for abbreviations; Linezolid (↑ risk of serotonin syndrome, see p. 620).

CrCl > 50 mL/min	No change
CrCl < 50 mL/min	No change
Post–HD dose	500 mg (PO)
Post–PD dose	No change
CVVH dose	No change
Moderate or severe hepatic insufficiency	No change

Drug Interactions: None.
Adverse Effects: Drug fever/rash, C. difficile diarrhea/colitis.
Allergic Potential: High
Safety in Pregnancy: B
Comments: Limited penetration into respiratory secretions. **Ceclor CD 500 mg (PO) q12h is equivalent to cefaclor 250 mg (PO) q8h, not cefaclor 500 mg (PO) q8h. Ceclor CD 500 mg (PO) q12h is equivalent to 250 mg (PO) q8h of cefaclor**. Give with food.
Cerebrospinal Fluid Penetration: < 10%
Bile Penetration: 60%
(also see ***Antibiotic Pearls & Pitfalls*** pp. 495–508).

REFERENCES:
Cazzola M, Di Perna F, Boveri B. Interrelationship between the pharmacokinetics and pharmacodynamics of cefaclor advanced formulation in patients with acute exacerbation of chronic bronchitis. J Chemother 12:216–22, 2000.
Mazzei T, Novelli A, Esposito S, et al. New insight into the clinical pharmacokinetics of cefaclor: Tissue penetration. J Chemother 12:53–62, 2000.
Meyers BR. Cefaclor revisited. Clin Ther 22:154–66, 2000.
Website: www.pdr.net

Cefadroxil (Duricef, Ultracef)

Drug Class: 1st generation oral cephalosporin.
Usual Dose: 1000 mg (PO) q12h.
Spectrum: (see ***Susceptibility Profiles*** pp. 188–193).
Pharmacokinetic Parameters:
Peak serum level: 16 mcg/mL
Bioavailability: 99%
Excreted unchanged (urine): 85%
Serum half-life (normal/ESRD): 0.5/22 hrs
Plasma protein binding: 20%
Volume of distribution (V_d): 0.31 L/kg
Primary Mode of Elimination: Renal
Dosage Adjustments*

CrCl 50–80 mL/min	500 mg (PO) q12h
CrCl 10–50 mL/min	500 mg (PO) q24h
CrCl < 10 mL/min	500 mg (PO) q36h
Post–HD dose	500 mg (PO)
Post–PD dose	250 mg (PO)
CVVH dose	500 mg (PO) q24h
Moderate hepatic insufficiency	No change
Severe hepatic insufficiency	No change

Drug Interactions: None.
Adverse Effects: Drug fever/rash, C. difficile diarrhea/colitis.
Allergic Potential: High
Safety in Pregnancy: B
Comments: Penetrates oral/respiratory secretions well.
Cerebrospinal Fluid Penetration: < 10%

"Usual dose" assumes normal renal/hepatic function. * For renal insufficiency, give usual dose × 1 followed by maintenance dose per CrCl. For dialysis patients, dose the same as for CrCl < 10 mL/min and give supplemental (post-HD/PD dose) immediately after dialysis. CrCl = creatinine clearance; CVVH = continuous veno-venous hemofiltration; HD/PD = hemodialysis/peritoneal dialysis. See pp. 509–513 for explanations, pp. xi–xii for abbreviations; Linezolid (↑ risk of serotonin syndrome, see p. 620).

Bile Penetration: 20%
(also see ***Antibiotic Pearls & Pitfalls*** pp. 495–508).

REFERENCES:

Bucko AD, Hunt BJ, Kidd SL, et al. Randomized, double-blind, multicenter comparison of oral cefditoren 200 or 400 mg BID with either cefuroxime 250 mg BID or cefadroxil 500 mg BID for the treatment of uncomplicated skin and skin-structure infections. Clin Ther 24:1134–47, 2002.

Cunha BA. Antibiotics selection for the treatment of sinusitis, otitis media, and pharyngitis. Infect Dis Pract 7:S324–S326, 1998.

Gustaferro CA, Steckelberg JM. Cephalosporins: Antimicrobic agents and related compounds. Mayo Clin Proc 66:1064–73, 1991.

Website: www.pdr.net

Cefamandole (Mandol)

Drug Class: 2nd generation cephalosporin.
Usual Dose: 2 gm (IV) q6h.
Pharmacokinetic Parameters:
Peak serum level: 240 mcg/mL
Bioavailability: Not applicable
Excreted unchanged (urine): 85%
Serum half-life (normal/ESRD): 1/11 hrs
Plasma protein binding: 76%
Volume of distribution (V_d): 0.29 L/kg
Primary Mode of Elimination: Renal
Dosage Adjustments* (based on 2 gm q6h):

CrCl 50–80 mL/min	1 gm (IV) q6h
CrCl 10–50 mL/min	1 gm (IV) q6h
CrCl < 10 mL/min	1 gm (IV) q12h
Post–HD dose	1 gm (IV)
Post–PD dose	1 gm (IV)
CVVH dose	1 gm (IV) q6h
Moderate or severe hepatic insufficiency	No change

Drug Interactions: Alcohol (disulfiram-like reaction); antiplatelet agents, heparin, thrombolytics, warfarin (↑ risk of bleeding).
Adverse Effects: Drug fever/rash, ↑ INR.
Allergic Potential: High
Safety in Pregnancy: B
Comments: Incompatible in solutions with Mg^{++} or Ca^{++}. **Contains MTT side chain, but no increase in clinical bleeding**. Na^+ content = 3.3 mEq/g.
Cerebrospinal Fluid Penetration: < 10%
Bile Penetration: 300%

REFERENCES:

Cunha BA, Klimek JJ, Qunitiliani R. Cefamandole nafate in respiratory and urinary tract infections. Curr Ther Res 25:584–9, 1971.

Gentry LO, Zeluff BJ, Cooley DA. Antibiotic prophylaxis in open-heart surgery: A comparison of cefamandole, cefuroxime, and cefazolin. Ann Thorac Surg 46:167–71, 1988.

Peterson CD, Lake KD, Arom KV. Antibiotic prophylaxis in open-heart surgery patients: Comparison of cefamandole and cefuroxime. Drug Intell Clin Pharmacol 21:728–32, 1987.

Cefazolin (Ancef, Kefzol)

Drug Class: 1st generation cephalosporin.
Usual Dose: 1 gm (IV) q8h.
Spectrum: (see ***Susceptibility Profiles*** pp. 188–193).
Pharmacokinetic Parameters:
Peak serum level: 185 mcg/mL
Bioavailability: Not applicable
Excreted unchanged (urine): 96%

"Usual dose" assumes normal renal/hepatic function. * For renal insufficiency, give usual dose × 1 followed by maintenance dose per CrCl. For dialysis patients, dose the same as for CrCl < 10 mL/min and give supplemental (post-HD/PD dose) immediately after dialysis. CrCl = creatinine clearance; CVVH = continuous veno-venous hemofiltration; HD/PD = hemodialysis/peritoneal dialysis. See pp. 509–513 for explanations, pp. xi–xii for abbreviations; Linezolid (↑ risk of serotonin syndrome, see p. 620).

Serum half-life (normal/ESRD): 1.8/40 hrs
Plasma protein binding: 85%
Volume of distribution (V_d): 0.2 L/kg
Primary Mode of Elimination: Renal
Dosage Adjustments*

CrCl 50–80 mL/min	No change
CrCl 10–50 mL/min	500 mg (IV) q12h
CrCl < 10 mL/min	500 mg (IV) q24h
Post–HD dose	1 gm (IV)
Post–HFHD dose	1.5 gm (IV)
Post–PD dose	500 mg (IV)
CVVH dose	500 mg (IV) q12h
Moderate or severe hepatic insufficiency	No change

Drug Interactions: None.
Adverse Effects: Drug fever/rash, AIHA.
Allergic Potential: High
Safety in Pregnancy: B
Comments: Incompatible in solutions containing erythromycin, aminoglycosides, cimetidine, theophylline.
Cerebrospinal Fluid Penetration: < 10%
Bile Penetrations: 300%
(also see ***Antibiotic Pearls & Pitfalls*** pp. 495–508).

REFERENCES:

Cunha BA, Hamid N, Kessler H, Parchuri S. Daptomycin cure after cefazolin treatment failure of Methicillin-sensitive Staphylococcus aureus (MSSA) tricuspid valve acute bacterial endocarditis from a peripherally inserted central catheter (PICC) line. Heart & Lung. 34:442–7, 2005.

Cunha BA, Gossling HR, Pasternak HS, et al. Penetration of cephalosporins into bone. Infection 12:80–4, 1984.

Gentry LO, Zeluff BJ, Cooley DA. Antibiotic prophylaxis in open-heart surgery: A comparison of cefamandole, cefuroxime, and cefazolin. Ann Thorac Surg 46:167–71, 1988.

Kelkar PS, Li JTC. Cephalosporin allergy. N Engl J Med 345:804–809, 2001.

Khairullah Q, Provenzano R, Tayeb J, et al. Comparison of vancomycin versus cefazolin as initial therapy for peritonitis in peritoneal dialysis patients. Perit Dial Int 22:339–44, 2002.

Marshall WF, Blair JE. The cephalosporins. Mayo Clin Proc 74:187–95, 1999.

Nightingale CH, Klimek JJ, Quintiliani R. Effect of protein binding on the penetration of nonmetabolized cephalosporins into atrial appendage and pericardial fluids in open-heart surgical patients. Antimicrob Agents Chemother 17:595–8, 1980.

Quintiliani R, Nightingale CH. Cefazolin. Ann Intern Med 89:650–6, 1978.

Cefdinir (Omnicef)

Drug Class: 3rd generation oral cephalosporin.
Usual Dose: 600 mg (PO) q24h.
Spectrum: (see ***Susceptibility Profiles*** pp. 188–193).
Pharmacokinetic Parameters:
Peak serum level: 2.9 mcg/mL
Bioavailability: 16% (tab) / 25%(suspension)
Excreted unchanged (urine): 11–18%
Serum half-life (normal/ESRD): 1.7/3 hrs
Plasma protein binding: 70%
Volume of distribution (V_d): 0.35 L/kg
Primary Mode of Elimination: Renal
Dosage Adjustments*

CrCl > 30 mL/min	No change
CrCl < 30 mL/min	300 mg (PO) q24h
Post–HD dose	300 mg (PO)
Post–PD dose	None
CVVH dose	600 mg (PO) q24h
Moderate or severe hepatic insufficiency	No change

"Usual dose" assumes normal renal/hepatic function. * For renal insufficiency, give usual dose × 1 followed by maintenance dose per CrCl. For dialysis patients, dose the same as for CrCl < 10 mL/min and give supplemental (post-HD/PD dose) immediately after dialysis. CrCl = creatinine clearance; CVVH = continuous veno-venous hemofiltration; HD/PD = hemodialysis/peritoneal dialysis. See pp. 509–513 for explanations, pp. xi–xii for abbreviations; Linezolid (↑ risk of serotonin syndrome, see p. 620).

Drug Interactions: Probenecid (↑ cefdinir levels).
Adverse Effects: Drug fever/rash, C. difficile diarrhea/colitis.
Allergic Potential: High
Safety in Pregnancy: B
Comments: Good activity against bacterial respiratory pathogens. Available as capsules or suspension. **CAP dose:** 300 mg (PO) q12h; **Other respiratory infections dose:** 600 mg (PO) q24h.
Cerebrospinal Fluid Penetration: No data (also see ***Antibiotic Pearls & Pitfalls*** pp. 495–508).

REFERENCES:

Cefdinir: A new oral cephalosporin. Med Lett Drugs Therap 40:85–7, 1998.

Fogarty CM, Bettis RB, Griffin TJ, et al. Comparison of a 5 day regimen of cefdinir with a 10 day regimen of cefprozil for treatment of acute exacerbations of chronic bronchitis. J Antimicrob Chemother 45:851–8, 2000.

Guay DR. Cefdinir: an advanced-generation, broad-spectrum oral cephalosporin. Clin Ther 24:473–89, 2002.

Nemeth MA, Gooche WM 3rd, Hedrick J, et al. Comparison of cefdinir and penicillin for the treatment of pediatric streptococcal pharyngitis. Clin Ther 21:1525–32, 1999.

Perry CM, Scott LJ. Cefdinir: a review of its use in the management of mild-to-moderate bacterial infections. Drugs 64:1433–64, 2004.

Website: www.omnicef.com

Cefditoren (Spectracef)

Drug Class: 3rd generation oral cephalosporin.
Usual Dose: 400 mg (PO) q12h.
Spectrum: (see ***Susceptibility Profiles*** pp. 188–193).
Pharmacokinetic Parameters:
Peak serum level: 1.8 mcg/mL
Bioavailability: 16%
Excreted unchanged (urine): 20%
Serum half-life (normal/ESRD): 1.5/5 hrs
Plasma protein binding: 88%
Volume of distribution (V_d): 0.13 L/kg
Primary Mode of Elimination: Renal
Dosage Adjustments*

CrCl 50–80 mL/min	No change
CrCl 30–50 mL/min	200 mg (PO) q12h
CrCl < 30 mL/min	200 mg (PO) q24h
Post–HD dose	200 mg (PO)
Post–PD dose	No information
CVVH dose	No information
Moderate or severe hepatic insufficiency	No change

Drug Interactions: H_2 receptor antagonists, Al^{++}, Mg^{++}) antacids (↓ absorption of cefditoren); Probenecid (↓ elimination of cefditoren).
Adverse Effects: Drug fever/rash, C. difficile diarrhea/colitis.
Allergic Potential: Low
Safety in Pregnancy: B
Comments: Serum concentrations increased ~ 50% if taken without food. ↑ elimination of carnitine; do not use in carnitine deficiency or hereditary carnitine metabolism disorder. **Contains Na+ caseinate; avoid in patients with casein hypersensitivity.**
Cerebrospinal Fluid Penetration: No data (also see ***Antibiotic Pearls & Pitfalls*** pp. 495–508).

REFERENCES:

Alvarez-Sala JL, Kardos P, et al. Martinez-Beltran, et al. Clinical and Bacteriological Efficacy in Treatment of Acute Exacerbations of Chronic Bronchitis with Cefditoren-Pivoxil versus Cefuroxime-Axetil.

"Usual dose" assumes normal renal/hepatic function. * For renal insufficiency, give usual dose × 1 followed by maintenance dose per CrCl. For dialysis patients, dose the same as for CrCl < 10 mL/min and give supplemental (post-HD/PD dose) immediately after dialysis. CrCl = creatinine clearance; CVVH = continuous veno-venous hemofiltration; HD/PD = hemodialysis/peritoneal dialysis. See pp. 509–513 for explanations, pp. xi–xii for abbreviations; Linezolid (↑ risk of serotonin syndrome, see p. 620).

Antimicrob Agents and Chemother 50:1762–67, 2006.
Balbisi EA. Cefditoren, a new aminothiazolyl cephalosporin. Pharmacotherapy 22:1278–93, 2002.
Cafini F, Aguilar L, Alou L, et al. Cidal activity of oral third-generation to cephalosporins against *Streptococcus pneumoniae* in relation to ceftotaxime intrinsic activity. Eur J Clin Microbiol Infect Dis 27:679–683, 2008.
Chow J, Russel M, Bolk S. et al. Efficacy of cefditoren pivoxil vs. amoxicillin-clavulanic in acute maxillary sinusitis. Presented at the 40th Interscience Conference on Antimicrobial Agents and Chemotherapy; Abstract 835, Toronto, ON 2000.
Clark CL, Nagai K, Dewasse BE, et al. Activity of cefditoren against respiratory pathogens. J Antimicrob Chemother 50:33–41, 2002.
Darkes MJ, Plosker GL. Cefditoren pivoxil. Drugs 62:319–36, 2002.
Guay DR. Review of cefditoren, an advanced-generation, broad-spectrum oral cephalosporin. Clin Ther 23:1924–37, 2002.
Wellington K, Curran MP. Cefditoren pivoxil: a review of its use in the treatment of bacterial infections. Drugs 64:2597–618, 2004.
Website: www.pdr.net

Cefepime (Maxipime)

Drug Class: 4th generation cephalosporin.
Usual Dose: 2 gm (IV) q12h (see comments).
Spectrum: (see ***Susceptibility Profiles*** pp. 188–193).
Pharmacokinetic Parameters:
Peak serum level: 163 mcg/mL
Bioavailability: Not applicable
Excreted unchanged (urine): 80%
Serum half-life (normal/ESRD): 2.2/18 hrs
Plasma protein binding: 20%
Volume of distribution (V_d): 0.29 L/kg
Primary Mode of Elimination: Renal
Dosage Adjustments* (based on 2 gm q12h):

CrCl 50–80 mL/min	2 gm (IV) q24h
CrCl 10–50 mL/min	2 gm (IV) q48h
CrCl < 10 mL/min	500 mg (IV) q24h
Post–HD dose	2 gm (IV)
Post–HFHD dose	2 gm (IV)
Post–PD dose	1 gm (IV)
CAPD	2 gm (IV) q48h
CVVH dose	1 gm (IV) q24h
Moderate or severe hepatic insufficiency	No change

Drug Interactions: None.
Adverse Effects: Drug fever/rash, C. difficile diarrhea/colitis.
Allergic Potential: Moderate
Safety in Pregnancy: B
Comments: For proven serious systemic P. aeruginosa infections, febrile neutropenia, or cystic fibrosis, use 2 gm (IV) q8h. **Effective against some strains of ceftazidime-resistant P. aeruginosa**. For aerobic GNB bacteremias use 2 gm (IV) q12h. Meningeal dose: 2 gm (IV) q8h.
Cerebrospinal Fluid Penetration:
Non-Inflamed meninges = 1%
Inflamed meninges = 15%
Bile Penetration: 10%
(also see ***Antibiotic Pearls & Pitfalls*** pp. 495–508).

REFERENCES:

Ambrose PF, Owens RC Jr, Garvey MJ, et al. Pharmacodynamic considerations in the treatment of moderate to severe pseudomonal infections with cefepime. J Antimicrob Chemother 49:445–53, 2002.
Badaro R, Molinar F, Seas c, et al. A multicenter comparative study of cefepime versus broad-spectrum

"Usual dose" assumes normal renal/hepatic function. * For renal insufficiency, give usual dose × 1 followed by maintenance dose per CrCl. For dialysis patients, dose the same as for CrCl < 10 mL/min and give supplemental (post-HD/PD dose) immediately after dialysis. CrCl = creatinine clearance; CVVH = continuous veno-venous hemofiltration; HD/PD = hemodialysis/peritoneal dialysis. See pp. 509–513 for explanations, pp. xi–xii for abbreviations; Linezolid (↑ risk of serotonin syndrome, see p. 620).

antibacterial therapy in moderate and severe bacterial infections. Braz J Infect Dis 6:206–18, 2002.

Boselli E, Breilh D, Duflo F, et al. Steady-state plasma and intrapulmonary concentrations of cefepime administered in continuous infusion in critically ill patients with severe nosocomial pneumonia. Crit Care Med 31:2102–6, 2003.

Bow EJ, Rotstein C, Noskin GA, et al. A Randomized, Open-Label, Multicenter Comparative Study of the Efficacy and Safety of Piperacillin-Tazobactam and Cefepime for the Empirical Treatment of Febrile Neutropenic Episodes in Patients with Hematologic Malignancies. Clin Infect Dis 43:447–59, 2006.

Chapman TM, Perry CM. Cefepime: a review of its use in the management of hospitalized patients with pneumonia. Am J Respir Med 2:75–107, 2003.

Cornely OA, Bethe U, Seifert H, et al. A randomized monocentric trial in febrile neutropenic patients: ceftriaxone and gentamicin vs cefepime and gentamicin. Ann Hematol 81:37–43, 2002.

Cunha BA. Pseudomonas aeruginosa: Resistance and therapy. Semin Respir Infect 17:231–9, 2002.

Cunha BA, Gill MV. Cefepime. Med Clin North Am 79:721–32, 1995.

Ellis JM, Rivera L, Reyes G, et al. Cefepime cerebrospinal fluid concentrations in neonatal bacterial meningitis. Ann Pharmacother 41:900–901, 2007.

Fleming DR, Ziegler C, Baize T, et al. Cefepime versus ticarcillin and clavulanate potassium and aztreonam for febrile neutropenia therapy in high-dose chemotherapy patients. Am J Clin Oncol 26:285–8, 2003.

Fritsche TR, Sader HS, Jones RN. Comparative activity and spectrum of broad-spectrum beta-lactams (cefepime, ceftazidime, ceftriaxone, piperacillin/tazobactam) tested against 12,295 staphylococci and streptococci: report from the SENTRY antimicrobial surveillance program (North America: 2001–2002). Diagn Microbiol Infect Dis 47:435–40, 2003.

Grover SS, Sharma M, Chattopadhya D, Kapoor H, et al. Phenotypic and genotypic detection of ESBL mediated cephalosporin resistance in Klebsiella pneumoniae: Emergence of high resistance against cefepime, the fourth generation. Journal of Infection. 53:279–88, 2006.

Hoban DJ, Bouchillon SK, Dowzicky MJ. Antimicrobial susceptibility of extended-spectrum beta-lactamase producers and multidrug-resistant Acinetobacter baumannii throughout the United States and comparative in vitro activity of tigecycline, a new glycylcycline antimicrobial. Diagn Microbiol Infect Dis 57:423–428, 2007.

Huang SS, Lee SC, Lee N, et al. Comparison of in vitro activities of levofloxacin, ciprofloxacin, ceftazidime, cefepime, imipenem, and piperacillin-tazobactam against aerobic bacterial pathogens from patients with nosocomial infections. J Microbiol Immunol Infect 40:134–140, 2007.

Lee SY, Kuti JL, Nicolau DP. Cefepime pharmacodynamics in patients with extended spectrum beta-lactamase (ESBL) and non-ESBL infections. J Infect 54:463–468, 2007.

Montalar J, Segura A, Bosch C, et al. Cefepime monotherapy as an empirical initial treatment of patients with febrile neutropenia. Med Oncol 19:161–6, 2002.

Moreno E, Davila I, Laffond E, et al. Selective immediate hypersensitivity to cefepime. J Investig Allergol Clin Immunol 17:52–54, 2007.

Nguyen TD, Williams B, Trang E. Cefepime Therapy and All-Cause Mortality. Clin Infect Dis 48:902–904, 2009.

Paradisi F, Corti G, Strohmeyer M. Cefepime. Antibiotics for Clinicians 3:41–50, 1999.

Ramphal R. Developing Strategies to Minimize the Impact of Extended Spectrum B-Lactamases: Focus on Cefepime. Clin Infect Dis 42:S151–2, 2006.

Spriet I, Meersseman W, De Troy E, et al. Meropenem–valproic acid interaction in patients with cefepime-associated status epilepticus. Am J Health Syst Pharm 64:54–58, 2007.

Tam VH, McKinnon PS, Akins RL, et al. Pharmacodynamics of cefepime in patients with gram-negative infections. J Antimicrob Chemother 50:425–8, 2002.

Tam VH, McKinnon PS, Akins RL, et al. Pharmacokinetics and pharmacodynamics of cefepime in patients with various degrees of renal function. Antimicrob Agents Chemother 47:1853–61, 2003.

Toltzis P, Dul M, O'Riordan MA, et al. Cefepime use in a pediatric intensive care unit reduces colonization with resistant bacilli. Pediatr Infect Dis J. 22:109–14, 2003.

Yahave D, Paul M, Fraser A, et al. Efficacy and safety of cefepime: a systematic review and meta-analysis. Lancet Infect Dis 7:338–348, 2007.

Yang K, Guglielmo BJ. Diagnosis and treatment of extended-spectrum and AmpC beta-lactamase-producing organisms. Ann Pharmacother 41:1427–1435, 2007.

Website: www.elan.com/Products/

Cefixime (Suprax)

Drug Class: 3rd generation oral cephalosporin.
Usual Dose: 400 mg (PO) q12h or 200 mg (PO) q12h.
Spectrum: (see ***Susceptibility Profiles*** pp. 188–193).
Pharmacokinetic Parameters:
Peak serum level: 3.7 mcg/mL
Bioavailability: 50%
Excreted unchanged (urine): 50%
Serum half-life (normal/ESRD): 3.1/11 hrs
Plasma protein binding: 65%
Volume of distribution (V_d): 0.1 L/kg
Primary Mode of Elimination: Renal
Dosage Adjustments*

CrCl 10–50 mL/min	300 mg (PO) q24h
CrCl < 10 mL/min	200 mg (PO) q24h
Post–HD dose	300 mg (PO)
Post–PD dose	200 mg (PO)
CVVH dose	200 mg (PO) q12h
Moderate hepatic insufficiency	No change
Severe hepatic insufficiency	No change

Drug Interactions: Carbamazepine (↑ carbamazepine levels).
Adverse Effects: Drug fever/rash, C. difficile diarrhea/colitis.
Allergic Potential: High
Safety in Pregnancy: B
Comments: **PRNG dose:** 400 mg (PO) × 1 dose. Also useful for quinolone-resistant GC. **Little/no activity against S. aureus (MSSA).**
Cerebrospinal Fluid Penetration: < 10%
Bile Penetration: 800%
(also see ***Antibiotic Pearls & Pitfalls*** pp. 495–508).

REFERENCES:

Markham A, Brogden RN. Cefixime: A review of its therapeutic efficacy in lower respiratory tract infections. Drugs 49:1007–22, 1995.

Marshall WF, Blair JE. The cephalosporins. Mayo Clin Proc 74:187–95, 1999.

Quintiliani R. Cefixime in the treatment of patients with lower respiratory tract infections: Results of US clinical trials. Clinical Therapeutics 18:373–90, 1996.

Update to CDC's Sexually Transmitted Diseases Treatment Guidelines, 2006: Fluoroquinolones no longer recommended for treatment of gonococcal infections. MMWR 56:332–336, 2007.

Website: www.pdr.net

Cefoperazone (Cefobid)

Drug Class: 3rd generation cephalosporin.
Usual Dose: 2 gm (IV) q12h.
Spectrum: (see ***Susceptibility Profiles*** pp. 188–193).
Pharmacokinetic Parameters:
Peak serum level: 240 mcg/mL
Bioavailability: Not applicable
Excreted unchanged (urine): 20%
Serum half-life (normal/ESRD): 2.4/2.4 hrs
Plasma protein binding: 90%
Volume of distribution (V_d): 0.17 L/kg

"Usual dose" assumes normal renal/hepatic function. * For renal insufficiency, give usual dose × 1 followed by maintenance dose per CrCl. For dialysis patients, dose the same as for CrCl < 10 mL/min and give supplemental (post-HD/PD dose) immediately after dialysis. CrCl = creatinine clearance; CVVH = continuous veno-venous hemofiltration; HD/PD = hemodialysis/peritoneal dialysis. See pp. 509–513 for explanations, pp. xi–xii for abbreviations; Linezolid (↑ risk of serotonin syndrome, see p. 620).

Primary Mode of Elimination: Hepatic

Dosage Adjustments*

CrCl 50–80 mL/min	No change
CrCl 10–50 mL/min	No change
CrCl < 10 mL/min	No change
Post–HD dose	None
Post–PD dose	None
CVVH dose	None
Moderate hepatic insufficiency	No change
Severe hepatic insufficiency	1 gm (IV) q12h

Drug Interactions: Alcohol (disulfiram-like reaction); antiplatelet agents, heparin, thrombolytics, warfarin (↑ risk of bleeding).

Adverse Effects: Drug fever/rash. **↑ INR due to MTT side chain, but no increase in clinical bleeding. Prophylactic vitamin K unnecessary.**

Allergic Potential: Low

Safety in Pregnancy: B

Comments: One of the few antibiotics to penetrate into an obstructed biliary tract. May be administered IM. **Concentration dependent serum half life**. Na^+ content = 1.5 mEq/g. Meningeal dose = 2 gm (IV) q8h.

Cerebrospinal Fluid Penetration:

Non-Inflamed meninges = 1%

Inflamed meninges = 10%

Bile Penetration: 1200%

(also see ***Antibiotic Pearls & Pitfalls*** pp. 495–508).

REFERENCES:

Cunha BA. 3rd generation cephalosporins: A review. Clin Ther 14:616–52, 1992.

Klein NC, Cunha BA. Third-generation cephalosporins. Med Clin North Am 79:705–19, 1995.

Marshall WF, Blair JE. The cephalosporins. Mayo Clin Proc 74:187–95, 1999.

Oie S, Uematsu T, Sawa A, et al. In vitro effects of combinations of antipseudomonal agents against seven strains of multidrug-resistant Pseudomonas aeruginosa. J Antimicrob Chemother 52:911–4, 2004.

Website: www.pdr.net

Cefotaxime (Claforan)

Drug Class: 3rd generation cephalosporin.

Usual Dose: 2 gm (IV) q6h.

Spectrum: (see ***Susceptibility Profiles*** pp. 188–193).

Pharmacokinetic Parameters:

Peak serum level: 214 mcg/mL

Bioavailability: Not applicable

Excreted unchanged (urine): 20–36%; 15–25% excreted as active metabolite

Serum half-life (normal/ESRD): 1/15 hrs

Plasma protein binding: 37%

Volume of distribution (V_d): 0.25 L/kg

Primary Mode of Elimination: Renal

Dosage Adjustments*

CrCl 50–80 mL/min	No change
CrCl 10–50 mL/min	1 gm (IV) q6h
CrCl < 10 mL/min	1 gm (IV) q12h
Post–HD dose	1 gm (IV)
Post–PD dose	1 gm (IV)
CVVH dose	2 gm (IV) q8h
Moderate hepatic insufficiency	No change
Severe hepatic insufficiency	No change

"Usual dose" assumes normal renal/hepatic function. * For renal insufficiency, give usual dose × 1 followed by maintenance dose per CrCl. For dialysis patients, dose the same as for CrCl < 10 mL/min and give supplemental (post-HD/PD dose) immediately after dialysis. CrCl = creatinine clearance; CVVH = continuous veno-venous hemofiltration; HD/PD = hemodialysis/peritoneal dialysis. See pp. 509–513 for explanations, pp. xi–xii for abbreviations; Linezolid (↑ risk of serotonin syndrome, see p. 620).

Drug Interactions: None.
Adverse Effects: Drug fever/rash, C. difficile diarrhea/colitis.
Allergic Potential: Moderate
Safety in Pregnancy: B
Comments: Incompatible in solutions containing sodium bicarbonate, metronidazole, or aminoglycosides. **Desacetyl metabolite** ($t_{1/2}$ = 1.5 hrs) **synergistic with cefotaxime against S. aureus/B. fragilis**. Na^+ content = 2.2 mEq/g. Meningeal dose = 3 gm (IV) q6h.
Cerebrospinal Fluid Penetration:
Non-Inflamed meninges = 1%
Inflamed meninges = 10%
Bile Penetration: 75%
(also see ***Antibiotic Pearls & Pitfalls*** pp. 495–508).

REFERENCES:
Brogden RN, Spencer CM. Cefotaxime: A reappraisal of its antibacterial activity and pharmacokinetic properties and a review of its therapeutic efficacy when administered twice daily for the treatment of mild to moderate infections. Drugs 53:483–510, 1987.
File Jr. TM, Clinical implications and treatment of multiresistant Streptococcus pneumoniae pneumonia. Clin Microbiol Infect. 12:31–41, 2006.
Klein NC, Cunha BA. Third-generation cephalosporins. Med Clin North Am 79:705–19, 1995.
Marshall WF, Blair JE. The cephalosporins. Mayo Clin Proc 74:187–95, 1999.
Patel KB, Nicolau DP, Nightingale CH, et al. Comparative serum bactericidal activities of ceftizoxime and cefotaxime against intermediately penicillin-resistant Streptococcus pneumoniae. Antimicrob Agents Chemother 40:2805–8, 1996.
Website: www.pdr.net

Cefotetan (Cefotan)

Drug Class: 2nd generation cephalosporin (Cephamycin).
Usual Dose: 2 gm (IV) q12h.
Spectrum: (see ***Susceptibility Profiles*** pp. 188–193).
Pharmacokinetic Parameters:
Peak serum level: 237 mcg/mL
Bioavailability: Not applicable
Excreted unchanged (urine): 50–80%
Serum half-life (normal/ESRD): 4/10 hrs
Plasma protein binding: 88%
Volume of distribution (V_d): 0.17 L/kg
Primary Mode of Elimination: Renal
Dosage Adjustments* (based on 2 gm q12h):

CrCl 50–80 mL/min	2 gm (IV) q12h
CrCl 10–50 mL/min	2 gm (IV) q24h
CrCl < 10 mL/min	2 gm (IV) q48h
Post–HD dose	1 gm (IV)
Post–PD dose	1 gm (IV)
CVVH dose	1 gm (IV) q12h
Moderate or severe hepatic insufficiency	No change

Drug Interactions: Alcohol (disulfiram-like reaction); antiplatelet agents, heparin, thrombolytics, warfarin (↑ risk of bleeding).
Adverse Effects: Drug fever/rash, AIHA, C. difficile diarrhea/colitis. **↑ INR due to MTT side chain, but no increase in clinical bleeding.**
Allergic Potential: Low
Safety in Pregnancy: B
Comments: Less effective than cefoxitin against B. fragilis D.O.T strains. Na^+ content = 3.5 mEq/g.
Cerebrospinal Fluid Penetration: < 10%
Bile Penetration: 20%
(also see ***Antibiotic Pearls & Pitfalls*** pp. 495–508).

"Usual dose" assumes normal renal/hepatic function. * For renal insufficiency, give usual dose × 1 followed by maintenance dose per CrCl. For dialysis patients, dose the same as for CrCl < 10 mL/min and give supplemental (post-HD/PD dose) immediately after dialysis. CrCl = creatinine clearance; CVVH = continuous veno-venous hemofiltration; HD/PD = hemodialysis/peritoneal dialysis. See pp. 509–513 for explanations, pp. xi–xii for abbreviations; Linezolid (↑ risk of serotonin syndrome, see p. 620).

REFERENCES:

Moes GS, MacPherson BR. Cefotetan-induced hemolytic anemia: A case report and a review of the literature. Arch Pathol Lab Med 124:1344–6, 2000.

Ray EK, Warkentin TE, O'Hoski PL. Delayed onset of life-threatening immune hemolysis after perioperative antimicrobial prophylaxis with cefotetan. Can J Surg 43:461–2, 2000.

Stroncek D, Procter JL, Johnson J. Drug-induced hemolysis: Cefotetan-dependent hemolytic anemia mimicking an acute intravascular immune transfusion reaction. Am J Hematol 64:67–70, 2000.

Website: www.pdr.net

Cefoxitin (Mefoxin)

Drug Class: 2nd generation cephalosporin (Cephamycin).

Usual Dose: 2 gm (IV) q6h.

Spectrum: (see ***Susceptibility Profiles*** pp. 188–193).

Pharmacokinetic Parameters:

Peak serum level: 221 mcg/mL

Bioavailability: Not applicable

Excreted unchanged (urine): 85%

Serum half-life (normal/ESRD): 1/21 hrs

Plasma protein binding: 75%

Volume of distribution (V_d): 0.12 L/kg

Primary Mode of Elimination: Renal

Dosage Adjustments*

CrCl 50–80 mL/min	1 gm (IV) q8h
CrCl 10–50 mL/min	1 gm (IV) q12h
CrCl < 10 mL/min	1 gm (IV) q24h
Post–HD dose	1 gm (IV)
Post–PD dose	1 gm (IV)
CVVH dose	2 gm (IV) q12h
Moderate hepatic insufficiency	No change
Severe hepatic insufficiency	No change

Drug Interactions: None.

Adverse Effects: Drug fever/rash, C. difficile diarrhea/colitis.

Allergic Potential: Low

Safety in Pregnancy: B

Comments: Effective against B. fragilis, including D.O.T. strains (B. distasonis, B. ovatus, B. thetaiotaomicron) Na^+ content = 2.3 mEq/g.

Cerebrospinal Fluid Penetration: < 10%

Bile Penetration: 250%

(also see ***Antibiotic Pearls & Pitfalls*** pp. 495–508).

REFERENCES:

da Costa Darini AL, Palazzo IC. Cefoxitin does not include production of penicillin binding protein 2a in methicillin-susceptible Staphylococcus aureus strains. J Clin Microbiol 42:4412, 2004.

Donowitz GR, Mandell GL. Beta-lactam antibiotics. N Engl J Med 318:419–26 and 318:490–500, 1993.

Hansen EA, Cunha BA. Cefoxitin. Antibiotics for Clinicians 5:33–41, 2001.

Marshall WF Blair JE. The cephalosporins. Mayo Clin Proc 74:187–95, 1999.

Website: www.pdr.net

Cefpodoxime (Vantin)

Drug Class: 3rd generation oral cephalosporin.

Usual Dose: 200 mg (PO) q12h (see comments).

Spectrum: (see ***Susceptibility Profiles*** pp. 188–193).

"Usual dose" assumes normal renal/hepatic function. * For renal insufficiency, give usual dose × 1 followed by maintenance dose per CrCl. For dialysis patients, dose the same as for CrCl < 10 mL/min and give supplemental (post-HD/PD dose) immediately after dialysis. CrCl = creatinine clearance; CVVH = continuous veno-venous hemofiltration; HD/PD = hemodialysis/peritoneal dialysis. See pp. 509–513 for explanations, pp. xi–xii for abbreviations; Linezolid (↑ risk of serotonin syndrome, see p. 620).

Pharmacokinetic Parameters:
Peak serum level: 2.3 mcg/mL
Bioavailability: 50%
Excreted unchanged (urine): 30%
Serum half-life (normal/ESRD): 2.3/9.8 hrs
Plasma protein binding: 21–33%
Volume of distribution (V_d): 0.9 L/kg
Primary Mode of Elimination: Renal
Dosage Adjustments*

CrCl 50–80 mL/min	No change
CrCl 10–50 mL/min	200 mg (PO) q24h
CrCl < 10 mL/min	200 mg (PO) q24h
Post–HD dose	200 mg (PO)
Post–PD dose	200 mg (PO)
CVVH dose	200 mg (PO) q12h
Moderate hepatic insufficiency	No change
Severe hepatic insufficiency	No change

Drug Interactions: None.
Adverse Effects: Drug fever/rash, C. difficile diarrhea/colitis pulmonary infiltrates with eosinophilia, ↑ SGOT/SGPT.
Allergic Potential: High
Safety in Pregnancy: B
Comments: Only oral 3rd generation cephalosporin active against S. aureus (MSSA).
PPNG dose: 400 mg (PO) × 1 dose.
cSSSI dose: 400 mg (PO) q12h.
Cerebrospinal Fluid Penetration: < 10%
Bile Penetration: 100%
(also see ***Antibiotic Pearls & Pitfalls*** pp. 495–508).

REFERENCES:

Adam D, Bergogne-Berezin E, Jones RN. Symposium on cefpodoxime proxetil: A new third generation oral cephalosporin. Drugs 42:1–66, 1991.
Cohen R. Clinical efficacy of cefpodoxime in respiratory tract infection. J Antimicrob Chemother 50(Suppl):23–7, 2002.
Cohen R. Clinical experience with cefpodoxime proxetil in acute otitis media. Pediatr Infect Dis J 14:S12–8, 1995.
Liu P, Muller M, Grant M, et al. Interstitial tissue concentrations of cefpodoxime. J Antimicrob Chemother 50(Suppl):19–22, 2002.
Schatz BS, Karavokiros KT, Taeubel MA, et al. Comparison of cefprozil, cefpodoxime proxetil, loracarbef, cefixime, and ceftibuten. Ann Pharmacother 30:258–68, 1996.
Website: www.pdr.net

Cefprozil (Cefzil)

Drug Class: 2nd generation oral cephalosporin.
Usual Dose: 500 mg (PO) q12h.
Spectrum: (see ***Susceptibility Profiles*** pp. 188–193).
Pharmacokinetic Parameters:
Peak serum level: 10 mcg/mL
Bioavailability: 95%
Excreted unchanged (urine): 60%
Serum half-life (normal/ESRD): 1.3/5.9 hrs
Plasma protein binding: 36%
Volume of distribution (V_d): 0.23 L/kg
Primary Mode of Elimination: Renal
Dosage Adjustments*

CrCl 50–80 mL/min	No change
CrCl 10–50 mL/min	250 mg (PO) q12h
CrCl < 10 mL/min	250 mg (PO) q12h
Post–HD dose	500 mg (PO)

"Usual dose" assumes normal renal/hepatic function. * For renal insufficiency, give usual dose × 1 followed by maintenance dose per CrCl. For dialysis patients, dose the same as for CrCl < 10 mL/min and give supplemental (post-HD/PD dose) immediately after dialysis. CrCl = creatinine clearance; CVVH = continuous veno-venous hemofiltration; HD/PD = hemodialysis/peritoneal dialysis. See pp. 509–513 for explanations, pp. xi–xii for abbreviations; Linezolid (↑ risk of serotonin syndrome, see p. 620).

Post–PD dose	250 mg (PO)
CVVH dose	500 mg (PO) q24h
Moderate hepatic insufficiency	No change
Severe hepatic insufficiency	No change

Drug Interactions: None.
Adverse Effects: Drug fever/rash, C. difficile diarrhea/colitis.
Allergic Potential: Low
Safety in Pregnancy: B
Comments: Penetrates oral/respiratory secretions well. No resistance.
Cerebrospinal Fluid Penetration: < 10% (also see ***Antibiotic Pearls & Pitfalls*** pp. 495–508).

REFERENCES:
Cunha BA. New antibiotics for the treatment of acute exacerbations of chronic bronchitis. Adv Ther 13:313–23, 1996.
Gainer RB 2nd. Cefprozil: A new cephalosporin; its use in various clinical trials. South Med J 88:338–46, 1995.
Marshall WF Blair JE. The cephalosporins. Mayo Clin Proc 74:187–95, 1999.
Schatz BS, Karavokiros KT, Taeubel MA, et al. Comparison of cefprozil, cefpodoxime, proxetil, loracarbef, cefixime, and ceftibuten. Ann Pharmacother 30:258–68, 1996.
Website: www.pdr.net

Ceftazidime (Fortaz, Tazicef, Tazidime)

Drug Class: 3rd generation cephalosporin.
Usual Dose: 2 gm (IV) q8h (see comments).
Spectrum: (see ***Susceptibility Profiles*** pp. 188–193).
Pharmacokinetic Parameters:
Peak serum level: 170 mcg/mL
Bioavailability: Not applicable
Excreted unchanged (urine): 80–90%
Serum half-life (normal/ESRD): 1.9/21 hrs
Plasma protein binding: 10%
Volume of distribution (V_d): 0.36 L/kg
Primary Mode of Elimination: Renal
Dosage Adjustments*

CrCl 50–80 mL/min	1 gm (IV) q12h
CrCl 10–50 mL/min	1 gm (IV) q24h
CrCl < 10 mL/min	500 mg (IV) q24h
Post–HD dose	1 gm (IV)
Post–PD dose	500 mg (IV)
CVVH dose	1 gm (IV) q12h
Moderate hepatic insufficiency	No change
Severe hepatic insufficiency	No change

Drug Interactions: None.
Adverse Effects: Phlebitis, Drug fever/rash, C. difficile diarrhea/colitis.
Allergic Potential: High
Safety in Pregnancy: B
Comments: Incompatible in solutions containing vancomycin or aminoglycosides. ***Use increases MRSA prevalence and P. aeruginosa resistance. Potent inducer of Klebsiella/Enterobacter/E. coli ESBLs.*** Na^+ content = 2.3 mEq/g. **CAPD dose:** 125 mg/L of dialysate (I.P.) with each exchange.
Meningeal dose = 2 gm (IV) q8h.
Cerebrospinal Fluid Penetration:
Non-Inflamed meninges = 1%
Inflamed meninges = 20%

"Usual dose" assumes normal renal/hepatic function. * For renal insufficiency, give usual dose × 1 followed by maintenance dose per CrCl. For dialysis patients, dose the same as for CrCl < 10 mL/min and give supplemental (post-HD/PD dose) immediately after dialysis. CrCl = creatinine clearance; CVVH = continuous veno-venous hemofiltration; HD/PD = hemodialysis/peritoneal dialysis. See pp. 509–513 for explanations, pp. xi–xii for abbreviations; Linezolid (↑ risk of serotonin syndrome, see p. 620).

Bile Penetration: 50%
(also see ***Antibiotic Pearls & Pitfalls*** pp. 495–508).

REFERENCES:

Berkhout J, Visser LG, van den Broek PJ, et al. Clinical pharmacokinetics of cefamandole and ceftazidime administered by continuous intravenous infusion. Antimicrob Agents Chemother 47:1862–6, 2003.

Briscoe-Dwyer L. Ceftazidime. Antibiotics for Clinicians 1:41–8, 1997.

Fortaleza CM, Freire MP, de Carvalho Ramos M. Risk Factors for Recovery of Imipenem- or Ceftazidime-Resistant Pseudomonas aeruginosa Among Patients Admitted to a Teaching Hospital in Brazil. Infection Control and Hosp Epidemiol. 27:901–06, 2006.

Klein NC, Cunha BA. Third-generation cephalosporins. Med Clin North Am 79:705–19, 1995.

Marshall WF, Blair JE. The cephalosporins. Mayo Clin Proc 74:187–95, 1999.

Nicolau DP, Nightingale CH, Banevicius MA, et al. Serum bactericidal activity of ceftazidime: Continuous infusion versus intermittent injections. Antimicrob Agents Chemother 40:61–4, 1996.

Owens JC, Jr, Ambrose PG, Quintiliani R. Ceftazidime to cefepime formulary switch: Pharmacodynamic rationale. Conn Med 61:225–7, 1997.

Rains CP, Bryson HM, Peters DH. Ceftazidime: An update of its antibacterial activity, pharmacokinetic properties, and therapeutic efficacy. Drugs 49:577–617, 1995.

Website: www.pdr.net

Ceftibuten (Cedax)

Drug Class: 3rd generation oral cephalosporin.
Usual Dose: 400 mg (PO) q24h.
Spectrum: (see ***Susceptibility Profiles*** pp. 188–193).
Pharmacokinetic Parameters:
Peak serum level: 18 mcg/mL
Bioavailability: 80%
Excreted unchanged: 56% (urine); 39% (fecal)
Serum half-life (normal/ESRD): 2.4/22 hrs
Plasma protein binding: 65%
Volume of distribution (V_d): 0.2 L/kg
Primary Mode of Elimination: Renal
Dosage Adjustments*

CrCl 50–80 mL/min	400 mg (PO) q24h
CrCl 10–50 mL/min	200 mg (PO) q24h
CrCl < 10 mL/min	100 mg (PO) q24h
Post–HD dose	400 mg (PO)
Post–PD dose	200 mg (PO)
CVVH dose	200 mg (PO) q24h
Moderate hepatic insufficiency	No change
Severe hepatic insufficiency	No change

Drug Interactions: None.
Adverse Effects: Drug fever/rash
Allergic Potential: High
Safety in Pregnancy: B
Comments: Little/no activity against S. aureus/S. pneumoniae.
Cerebrospinal Fluid Penetration: < 10%
(also see ***Antibiotic Pearls & Pitfalls*** pp. 495–508).

REFERENCES:

Guay DR. Ceftibuten: A new expanded-spectrum oral cephalosporin. Ann Pharmacother 31:1022–33, 1997.

Owens RC Jr, Nightingale CH, Nicolau DP. Ceftibuten: An overview. Pharmacother 17:707–20, 1997.

Wiseman LR, Balfour JA. Ceftibuten: A review of its antibacterial activity, pharmacokinetic properties and clinical efficacy. Drugs 47:784–808, 1994.

Website: www.pdr.net

Ceftizoxime (Cefizox)

Drug Class: 3rd generation cephalosporin.
Usual Dose: 2 gm (IV) q8h (see comments).
Spectrum: (see ***Susceptibility Profiles*** pp. 188–193).
Pharmacokinetic Parameters:
Peak serum level: 132 mcg/mL
Bioavailability: Not applicable
Excreted unchanged (urine): 90%
Serum half-life (normal/ESRD): 1.7/35 hrs
Plasma protein binding: 30%
Volume of distribution (V_d): 0.32 L/kg
Primary Mode of Elimination: Renal
Dosage Adjustments*

CrCl 50–80 mL/min	1 gm (IV) q8h
CrCl 10–50 mL/min	1 gm (IV) q12h
CrCl < 10 mL/min	1 gm (IV) q24h
Post–HD dose	1 gm (IV)
Post–PD dose	1 gm (IV)
CVVH dose	1 gm (IV) q12h
Moderate hepatic insufficiency	No change
Severe hepatic insufficiency	No change

Drug Interactions: None.
Adverse Effects: Drug fever/rash, C. difficile diarrhea/colitis.
Allergic Potential: High
Safety in Pregnancy: B
Comments: Na^+ content = 2.6 mEq/g. **PRNG dose: 500 mg (IM) × 1 dose**. Meningeal dose = 3 gm (IV) q6h.
Cerebrospinal Fluid Penetration:
Non-Inflamed meninges = 1%
Inflamed meninges = 10%
Bile Penetration: 50%
(also see ***Antibiotic Pearls & Pitfalls*** pp. 495–508).

REFERENCES:

Klein NC, Cunha BA. Third-generation cephalosporins. Med Clin North Am 79:705–19, 1995.

Donowitz GR, Mandell GL. Beta-lactam antibiotics. N Engl J Med 318:419–26 and 318:490–500, 1993.

Marshall WF, Blair JE. The cephalosporins. Mayo Clin Proc 74:187–95, 1999.

Website: www.pdr.net

Ceftriaxone (Rocephin)

Drug Class: 3rd generation cephalosporin.
Usual Dose: 1–2 gm (IV) q24h (see comments).
Spectrum: (see ***Susceptibility Profiles*** pp. 188–193).
Pharmacokinetic Parameters:
Peak serum level: 151–257 mcg/mL
Bioavailability: Not applicable
Excreted unchanged (urine/feces): 33–67%
Serum half-life (normal/ESRD): 8/16 hrs
Plasma protein binding: 90%
Volume of distribution (V_d): 0.08–0.3 L/kg
Primary Mode of Elimination: Renal/hepatic
Dosage Adjustments*

CrCl 50–80 mL/min	No change
CrCl 10–50 mL/min	No change
CrCl < 10 mL/min	No change
Post–HD dose	None
Post–HFHD dose	No change
Post–PD dose	None

"Usual dose" assumes normal renal/hepatic function. * For renal insufficiency, give usual dose × 1 followed by maintenance dose per CrCl. For dialysis patients, dose the same as for CrCl < 10 mL/min and give supplemental (post-HD/PD dose) immediately after dialysis. CrCl = creatinine clearance; CVVH = continuous veno-venous hemofiltration; HD/PD = hemodialysis/peritoneal dialysis. See pp. 509–513 for explanations, pp. xi–xii for abbreviations; Linezolid (↑ risk of serotonin syndrome, see p. 620).

CVVH dose	No change
Moderate hepatic insufficiency	No change
Severe hepatic insufficiency	No change (max dose: 2 gm/d)

Drug Interactions: May cause intravascular precipitation when co-administered with calcium-containing solutions/products.

Adverse Effects: Drug fever/rash, non-C. difficle diarrhea, biliary lithiasis, may interfere with platelet aggregation, thrombocytosis.

Allergic Potential: High

Safety in Pregnancy: B. **Avoid near term in 3rd trimester** (↑ incidence of kernicterus in newborns)

Comments: Useful to treat PRSP/MDRSP in CAP/CNS. May be given IV or IM. Incompatible in solutions containing vancomycin. Na^+ content = 2.6 mEq/g. Meningeal dose = 2 gm (IV) q12h.

Warning: ***Do not administer with calcium-containing solutions/products within 48 hours of last administration of ceftriaxone.***

Cerebrospinal Fluid Penetration:
Non-Inflamed meninges = 1%
Inflamed meninges = 10%

Bile Penetration: 500%

(also see ***Antibiotic Pearls & Pitfalls*** pp. 495–508).

REFERENCES:

Araz N, Okan V, Demirci M, et al. Pseudolithiasis due to ceftriaxone treatment for meningitis in children: report of 8 cases. Tohoku J Exp Med 211:285–290, 2007.

Borg R, Dotevall L, Hagberg L, et al. Intravenous ceftriaxone compared with oral doxycycline for the treatment of Lyme neuroborreliosis. Scand J Infect Dis 37:449–454, 2005.

Cunha BA, Klein NC. The selection and use of cephalosporins: A review. Adv Ther 12:83–101, 1995.

Dietrich ES, Bieser U, Frank U, et al. Ceftriaxone versus other cephalosporins for perioperative antibiotic prophylaxis: a meta analysis of 43 randomized controlled trials. Chemotherapy 48:49–56, 2002.

Faella F, Pagliano P, Fusco U, Attanasio V, Conte M. Combined treatment with ceftriaxone and linezolid of pneumococcal meningitis: a case series including penicillin-resistant strains. Clin Micrbiol Infect. 12:391–4, 2006.

File Jr. TM, Clinical implications and treatment of multiresistant Streptococcus pneumoniae pneumonia. Clin Microbiol Infect. 12:31–41, 2006.

Freeman CD, Nightingale CH, Nicolau DP, et al. Serum bactericidal activity of ceftriaxone plus metronidazole against common intra-abdominal pathogens. Am J Hosp Pharm 51:1782–7, 1994.

Grassi C. Ceftriaxone. Antibiotics for Clinicians 2:49–57, 1998.

Karlowsky JA, Jones ME. Importance of using current NCCLS breakpoints to interpret cefotaxime and ceftriaxone MICs for Streptococcus pneumoniae. J Antimicrob Chemother 51:467–8, 2003.

Klein NC, Cunha BA. Third -generation cephalosporins. Med Clin North Am 79:705–19, 1995.

Knoll B, Tleyjeh IM, Steckelber JM, et al. Infective endocarditis due to penicillin-resistant viridans group streptococci. Clin Infect Dis 44:1585–1592, 2007.

Lamb HM, Ormrod D, Scott LJ, et al. Ceftriaxone: an update of its use in the management of community-acquired and nosocomial infections. Drugs 62:1041–89, 2002.

Marshall WF, Blair JE. The cephalosporins. Mayo Clin Proc 74:187–95, 1999.

Mohkam M, Karimi A, Gharib A, et al. Ceftriaxone associated nephrolithiasis: a prospective study in 284 children. Pediatr Nephrol 22:690–694, 2007.

Pichichero ME. Use of selected cephalosporins in penicillin-allergic patients: a paradigm shift. Diagn Microbiol Infect Dis 57:13S–18S, 2007.

Roberts JA, Boots R, Rickard CM, et al. Is continuous infusion ceftriaxone better than once-a-day dosing in intensive care? A randomized controlled pilot study. J Antimicrob Chemother 59:285–291, 2007.

Savaris RF, Teixeria LM, Torres TG, et al. Comparing ceftriaxone plus azithromycin or doxycycline for pelvic inflammatory disease: a randomized controlled trial. Obstet Gynecol 110:53–60, 2007.

Schaad UB, Suter S, Gianella-Borradori A, et al. A comparison of ceftriaxone and cefuroxime for the treatment of bacterial meningitis in children. N Engl J Med 322:141–7, 1990.

Shelburne SA 3rd, Greenburg SB, Aslam S, et al. Successful ceftriaxone therapy of endocarditis due to penicillin non-susceptible viridans streptococci. J Infect 54:e108–e110, 2007.

Tamm M, Todisco T, Feldman C, et al. Clinical and bacteriological outcomes in hospitalized patients with community-acquired pneumoniae treatment with azithromycin plus ceftriaxone, or ceftriaxone plus clarithromycin or erythromycin: a prospective, randomized, multicenter study. Clin Microbiol Infect 13:162–171, 2007.

Woodfield JC, Van Rij AM, Pettigrew RA, et al. A comparison of the prophylactic efficacy of ceftriaxone and cefotaxime in abdominal surgery. Am J Surg 185:45–9, 2003.

Website: www.rocheusa.com/products/rocephin

Cefuroxime (Kefurox, Zinacef, Ceftin)

Drug Class: 2nd generation IV/oral cephalosporin.

Usual Dose: 1.5 gm (IV) q8h; 500 mg (PO) q12h (see comments).

Spectrum: (see ***Susceptibility Profiles*** **p**p. 188–193).

Pharmacokinetic Parameters:

Peak serum level: 100 (IV)/7 (PO) mcg/mL

Bioavailability: 52%

Excreted unchanged (urine): 89%

Serum half-life (normal/ESRD): 1.2/17 hrs

Plasma protein binding: 50%

Volume of distribution (V_d): 0.15 L/kg

Primary Mode of Elimination: Renal

Dosage Adjustments*

CrCl 50–80 mL/min	No change
CrCl 10–50 mL/min	750 mg (IV) q12h 500 mg (PO) q12h
CrCl < 10 mL/min	750 mg (IV) q24h 250 mg (PO) q24h
Post–HD dose	750 mg (IV) 250 mg (PO)
Post–PD dose	750 mg (IV) 250 mg (PO)
CVVH dose	1.5 gm (IV) q12h 500 mg (PO) q12h
Moderate hepatic insufficiency	No change
Severe hepatic insufficiency	No change

Drug Interactions: None.

Adverse Effects: Drug fever/rash, C. difficile diarrhea/colitis.

Allergic Potential: High

Safety in Pregnancy: B

Comments: Oral preparation penetrates oral/respiratory secretions well. **PPNG dose:** 1 gm (IM) × 1 dose. **Ineffective for H. influenzae meningitis prophylaxis or therapy.**

Cerebrospinal Fluid Penetration: < 10% (also see ***Antibiotic Pearls & Pitfalls*** pp. 495–508).

"Usual dose" assumes normal renal/hepatic function. * For renal insufficiency, give usual dose × 1 followed by maintenance dose per CrCl. For dialysis patients, dose the same as for CrCl < 10 mL/min and give supplemental (post-HD/PD dose) immediately after dialysis. CrCl = creatinine clearance; CVVH = continuous veno-venous hemofiltration; HD/PD = hemodialysis/peritoneal dialysis. See pp. 509–513 for explanations, pp. xi–xii for abbreviations; Linezolid (↑ risk of serotonin syndrome, see p. 620).

REFERENCES:

Alvarez-Sala JL, Kardos P, Martinez-Beltran, et al. Clinical and Bacteriological Efficacy in Treatment of Acute Exacerbations of Chronic Bronchitis with Cefditoren-Pivoxil versus Cefuroxime-Axetil. Antimicrob Agents and Chemother 50:1762–67, 2006.

Bucko AD, Hunt BJ, Kidd SL, et al. Randomized, double-blind, multicenter comparison of oral cefditoren 200 or 400 mg BID with either cefuroxime 250 mg BID or cefadroxil 500 mg BID for the treatment of uncomplicated skin and skin-structure infections. Clin Ther 24:1134–47, 2002.

Gentry LO, Zeluff BJ, Cooley DA. Antibiotic prophylaxis in open-heart surgery: A comparison of cefamandole, cefuroxime, and cefazolin. Ann Thorac Surg 46:167–71, 1988.

Marshall WF, Blair JE. The cephalosporins. Mayo Clin Proc 74:187–95, 1999.

Perry Cm, Brogden RN. Cefuroxime axetil. A review of its antibacterial activity, pharmacokinetic properties, and therapeutic efficacy. Drugs 52:125–58, 1996.

Website: www.pdr.net

Cephalexin (Keflex)

Drug Class: 1st generation oral cephalosporin.
Usual Dose: 500 mg (PO) q6h.
Spectrum: (see ***Susceptibility Profiles*** pp. 188–193).
Pharmacokinetic Parameters:
Peak serum level: 18 mcg/mL
Bioavailability: 99%
Excreted unchanged (urine): > 90%
Serum half-life (normal/ESRD): 0.7/16 hrs
Plasma protein binding: 10%
Volume of distribution (V_d): 0.35 L/kg
Primary Mode of Elimination: Renal
Dosage Adjustments*

CrCl 50–80 mL/min	No change
CrCl 10–50 mL/min	250 mg (PO) q8h
CrCl < 10 mL/min	250 mg (PO) q12h
Post–HD dose	500 mg (PO)
Post–PD dose	250 mg (PO)
CVVH dose	250 mg (PO) q8h
Moderate hepatic insufficiency	No change
Severe hepatic insufficiency	No change

Drug Interactions: None.
Adverse Effects: Drug fever/rash, C. difficile diarrhea/colitis.
Allergic Potential: High
Safety in Pregnancy: B
Comments: Highly active against S. aureus (MSSA) and Group A streptococci. **Limited activity against H. influenzae.**
Cerebrospinal Fluid Penetration: < 10%
Bile Penetration: 200%
(also see ***Antibiotic Pearls & Pitfalls*** pp. 495–508).

REFERENCES:

Chow M, Quintiliani R, Cunha BA, et al. Pharmacokinetics of high dose oral cephalosporins. J Pharmacol 19:185–194, 1979.

Cunha BA. Cephalexin Remains Preferred Oral Antibiotic Therapy for Uncomplicated Cellulitis. Am J Med 121:e11–15, 2008.

Cunha BA. Oral Antibiotic Therapy of Serious Systemic Infections. Med Clin N Am 90:1197–1222, 2006.

Marshall WF Blair JE. The cephalosporins. Mayo Clin Proc 74:187–95, 1999.

"Usual dose" assumes normal renal/hepatic function. * For renal insufficiency, give usual dose × 1 followed by maintenance dose per CrCl. For dialysis patients, dose the same as for CrCl < 10 mL/min and give supplemental (post-HD/PD dose) immediately after dialysis. CrCl = creatinine clearance; CVVH = continuous veno-venous hemofiltration; HD/PD = hemodialysis/peritoneal dialysis. See pp. 509–513 for explanations, pp. xi–xii for abbreviations; Linezolid (↑ risk of serotonin syndrome, see p. 620).

Smith GH. Oral cephalosporins in perspective. DICP 24:45–51, 1990.
Website: www.pdr.net

Chloramphenicol (Chloromycetin)

Drug Class: No specific class.
Usual Dose: 500 mg (IV/PO) q6h.
Spectrum: (see ***Susceptibility Profiles*** pp. 183–187).
Pharmacokinetic Parameters:
Peak serum level: 9 mcg/mL
Bioavailability: 90%
Excreted unchanged (urine): 10%
Serum half-life (normal/ESRD): 2.5/3 hrs
Plasma protein binding: 50%
Volume of distribution (V_d): 1 L/kg
Primary Mode of Elimination: Hepatic
Dosage Adjustments*

CrCl 50–80 mL/min	No change
CrCl < 50 mL/min	No change
Post–HD dose	500 mg (IV/PO)
Post–PD dose	None
CVVH dose	No change
Moderate or severe hepatic insufficiency	No change

Drug Interactions: Barbiturates (↑ barbiturate effect, ↓ chloramphenicol effect); cyclophosphamide (↑ cyclophosphamide toxicity); cyanocobalamin, iron (↓ response to interacting drug); warfarin (↑ INR); phenytoin (↑ phenytoin toxicity); rifabutin, rifampin (↓ chloramphenicol levels); sulfonylureas (↑ sulfonylurea effect, hypoglycemia).
Adverse Effects:
Dose–related bone marrow suppression
Reversible. Bone marrow aspirate shows vacuolated WBCs ("chloramphenicol effect," not toxicity). Does not precede aplastic anemia
Idiosyncratic bone marrow toxicity
Irreversible aplastic anemia. May occur after only one dose; monitoring with serial CBCs is useless. Very rare. Usually associated with IM, intraocular, or oral administration. Rarely, if ever, with IV chloramphenicol.
Allergic Potential: Low
Safety in Pregnancy: C
Comments: Incompatible in solutions containing diphenylhydantoin, methylprednisone, aminophylline, ampicillin, gentamicin, erythromycin, vancomycin. **Dose-related marrow suppression is common, and reversible**. Hepatic toxicity related to prolonged/high doses (> 4 gm/d). **Oral administration results in higher serum levels than IV administration**. Do not administer IM. Chloramphenicol is inactivated in bile. **Urinary concentrations are therapeutically ineffective**. Na^+ content = 2.25 mEq/g. Meningeal dose = usual dose.
Cerebrospinal Fluid Penetration:
Non-Inflamed meninges = 90%
Inflamed meninges = 90%
Bile Penetration: 0%
(also see ***Antibiotic Pearls & Pitfalls*** p. 501).

REFERENCES:

Bouza E. New therapeutic choices for infections caused by methicillin-resistant *Staphylococcus aureus*. Clin Microbiol Infect Dis 15:44–52, 2009.
Cunha BA. Oral Antibiotic Therapy of Serious Systemic Infections. Med Clin N Am 90:1197–1222, 2006.
Cunha BA. New uses of older antibiotics. Postgrad Med 100:68–88, 1997.
Feder HM Jr, Osier C, Maderazo EG. Chloramphenicol: A review of its use in clinical practice. Rev Infect Dis 3:479–91, 1981.

"Usual dose" assumes normal renal/hepatic function. * For renal insufficiency, give usual dose × 1 followed by maintenance dose per CrCl. For dialysis patients, dose the same as for CrCl < 10 mL/min and give supplemental (post-HD/PD dose) immediately after dialysis. CrCl = creatinine clearance; CVVH = continuous veno-venous hemofiltration; HD/PD = hemodialysis/peritoneal dialysis. See pp. 509–513 for explanations, pp. xi–xii for abbreviations; Linezolid (↑ risk of serotonin syndrome, see p. 620).

Kasten MJ. Clindamycin, metronidazole, and chloramphenicol. Mayo Clin Proc 74:825–33, 1999.
Safdar A, Bryan CS, Stinson S, et al. Prosthetic valve endocarditis due to vancomycin-resistant Enterococcus faecium: treatment with chloramphenicol plus minocycline. Clin Infect Dis 34:61–3, 2002.
Smilack JD, Wilson WE, Cocerill FR 3rd. Tetracycline, chloramphenicol, erythromycin, clindamycin, and metronidazole. Mayo Clin Proc 66:1270–80, 1991.
Wareham DW, Wilson P. Chloramphenicol in the 21st century. Hosp Med 63:157–61, 2002.
Website: www.pdr.net

Cidofovir (Vistide)

Drug class: CMV antiviral (see comments).
Usual dose: 5 mg/kg (IV) weekly for 2 weeks, then 5 mg/kg every 2 weeks (for CMV retinitis in HIV patients, patients must have all of the following: SrCr < 1.5 mg/dL, CrCl > 55 mL/min, urine protein < 100 mg/dL).
Pharmacokinetic Parameters:
Peak serum level: 19.6 mcg/mL
Bioavailability: not applicable
Excreted unchanged: 1%
Serum half-life (normal/ESRD): 2.2 h/no data
Plasma protein binding: 6%
Volume of distribution (V_d): 0.54 l/kg
Primary Mode of Elimination: Renal
Dosage Adjustments*

SrCr increase of 0.3–0.4 mg/dL above baseline	3 mg/kg
SrCr increase of 0.5 mg/dL or greater	Discontinue cidofovir
Post–HD dose	No data
Post–PD dose	No data
CVVH dose	No data
Moderate or severe hepatic insufficiency	None

Drug Interactions: Contraindicated with other nephrotoxic drugs.
Adverse Effects: Nephrotoxicity; neutropenia; nausea, vomiting associated with probenecid, take with food; metabolic acidosis; decreased intraocular pressure; anterior uveitis and iritis acute renal failure requiring dialysis and contributing to death reported.
Allergic Potential: Low for cidofovir, high for probenecid.
Safety in Pregnancy: C
Comments: All patients must receive probenecid (2 g (PO) 3 hours before infusion start, then 1 g at 2 and again at 8 hours after completion of cidofovir infusion, take with food to minimize nausea and vomiting) and hydration with at least 1 L of normal saline with each dose of cidofovir; monitor neutrophils, growth factor support may be needed; contraindicated in severe hypersensitivity to probenecid or other sulfa drugs; direct ocular injection is contraindicated; effective contraception required for male and female patients; infuse over 1 hour; available as 375 mg / 5 mL single-use vial. ***Highly active against CMV and HSV. Some activity against BK virus, JC virus, VZV and adenoviruses. No activity against HHV-6, EBV, RSV, or influenza viruses.***

REFERENCES:

Lalezari JP, Stagg RJ, Kupperman BD, et al. Intravenous Cidofovir for Peripheral Cytomegalovirus Retinitis in Patients with AIDS. A Randomized, Controlled Trial. Ann Intern Med 126:257–63, 1997.

"Usual dose" assumes normal renal/hepatic function. * For renal insufficiency, give usual dose × 1 followed by maintenance dose per CrCl. For dialysis patients, dose the same as for CrCl < 10 mL/min and give supplemental (post-HD/PD dose) immediately after dialysis. CrCl = creatinine clearance; CVVH = continuous veno-venous hemofiltration; HD/PD = hemodialysis/peritoneal dialysis. See pp. 509–513 for explanations, pp. xi–xii for abbreviations; Linezolid (↑ risk of serotonin syndrome, see p. 620).

Lalezari JP, Randomized, controlled study of the safety and efficacy of intravenous cidofovir for the treatment of relapsing cytomegalovirus retinitis in patients with AIDS. J Acquir Immune Defic Syndr Hum Retrovirol. 17:339–44, 1998.
The Studies of Ocular Complications of AIDS Research Group in Collaboration with the AIDS Clinical Trials Group. Cidofovir (HPMPC) for the Treatment of Cytomegalovirus Retinitis in Patients with AIDS: the HPMPC Peripheral Cytomegalovirus Retinitis Trial. Ann Intern Med 126:264–74, 1997.

Ciprofloxacin (Cipro)

Drug Class: Fluoroquinolone.
Usual Dose: 400 mg (IV) q8-12h; 500–750 mg (PO) q12h (see comments).
Spectrum: (see ***Susceptibility Profiles*** pp. 194–199).
Pharmacokinetic Parameters:
Peak serum level: 4.6 (IV)/2.9 (PO) mcg/mL
Bioavailability: 70%
Excreted unchanged (urine): 70%
Serum half-life (normal/ESRD): 4/8 hrs
Plasma protein binding: 20–40%
Volume of distribution (V_d): 2.5 L/kg
Primary Mode of Elimination: Renal
Dosage Adjustments*

CrCl 50–80 mL/min	No change
CrCl 10–50 mL/min	400 mg (IV) q12h 500 mg (PO) q12h
CrCl < 10 mL/min	400 mg (IV) q24h 500 mg (PO) q24h
Post–HD dose	200–400 mg (IV) 250–500 mg (PO)
Post–PD dose	200–400 mg (IV) 250–500 mg (PO)
CVVH dose	200 mg (IV) q12h 250 mg (PO) q12h
Moderate hepatic insufficiency	No change
Severe hepatic insufficiency	No change

Drug Interactions: Al^{++}, Ca^{++}, Fe^{++}, Mg^{++}, Zn^{++} antacids, citrate/citric acid, dairy products (↓ absorption of ciprofloxacin only if taken together); caffeine, cyclosporine, theophylline (↑ interacting drug levels); cimetidine (↑ ciprofloxacin levels); foscarnet (↑ risk of seizures); oral hypoglycemics (slight ↑ or ↓ in blood glucose); NSAIDs (may ↑ risk of seizures/ CNS stimulation); phenytoin (↑ or ↓ phenytoin levels); probenecid (↑ ciprofloxacin levels); warfarin (↑ INR).
Adverse Effects: Drug fever/rash, C. difficile diarrhea/colitis, headache, dizziness, insomnia, malaise, seizures. FQ use has an increased risk of tendinitis/tendon rupture. Risk in highest in the elderly, those on steroids, and those with heart, lung or renal transplants.
Allergic Potential: Low
Safety in Pregnancy: C
Comments: Enteral feeding decreases ciprofloxacin absorption ≥ 30%. Use with caution in patients with severe renal insufficiency or seizure disorder. Administer 2 hours before or after H_2 antagonists, omeprazole, sucralfate, calcium, iron, zinc, multivitamins, or aluminum/magnesium containing medications. Administer ciprofloxacin (IV) as an intravenous infusion over 1 hour. **Nosocomial pneumonia dose:** 400 mg (IV) q8h.
↑ incidence of C. difficile diarrhea/colitis with PPIs (for patients on PPIs during FQ

"Usual dose" assumes normal renal/hepatic function. * For renal insufficiency, give usual dose × 1 followed by maintenance dose per CrCl. For dialysis patients, dose the same as for CrCl < 10 mL/min and give supplemental (post-HD/PD dose) immediately after dialysis. CrCl = creatinine clearance; CVVH = continuous veno-venous hemofiltration; HD/PD = hemodialysis/peritoneal dialysis. See pp. 509–513 for explanations, pp. xi–xii for abbreviations; Linezolid (↑ risk of serotonin syndrome, see p. 620).

therapy, switch to H_2 blocker for duration of FQ therapy).

Cerebrospinal Fluid Penetration:

Non-Inflamed meninges = 10%

Inflamed meninges = 26%

Bile Penetration: 3000%

(also see ***Antibiotic Pearls & Pitfalls*** pp. 495–508).

REFERENCES:

Bellmann R, Egger P, Gritsch W, et al. Pharmacokinetics of ciprofloxacin in patients with acute renal failure undergoing continuous venovenous haemofiltration: influence of concomitant liver cirrhosis. Acta Med Austriaca 29:112–6, 2002.

Davis R, Markham A, Balfour JA. Ciprofloxacin: An updated review of its pharmacology, therapeutic efficacy, and tolerability. Drugs 51:1019–74, 1996.

Debon R, Breilh D, Boselli E, et al. Pharmacokinetic parameters of ciprofloxacin (500 mg/5mL) oral suspension in critically ill patients with severe bacterial pneumonia: a comparison of two dosages. J Chemother 14:175–80, 2002.

Fantin B, Duval X, Massias L, et al. Ciprofloxacin Dosage and Emergence of Resistance in Human Commensal Bacteria. Journal of Infect Dis 200:390–398, 2009.

Pankey GA, Ashcraft DS. In vitro synergy of ciprofloxacin and gatifloxacin against ciprofloxacin-resistant pseudomonas aeruginosa. Antimicrobial Agents and Chemotherapy 49:2959–2964, 2005.

Peacock JE, Herrington DA, Wade JC, et al. Ciprofloxacin plus piperacillin compared with tobramycin plus piperacillin as empirical therapy in febrile neutropenic patients. A randomized, double-blind trial. Ann Intern Med 137:77–87, 2002.

Sanders CC. Ciprofloxacin: In vitro activity, mechanism of action, resistance. Rev Infect Dis 10:516–27, 1998.

Talan DA, Stamm WE, Hooton TM, et al. Comparison of ciprofloxacin (7 days) and trimethoprim-sulfamethoxazole (14 days) for acute uncomplicated pyelonephritis in women: a randomized trial. JAMA 283:1583–90, 2000.

Wacha H, Warren B, Bassaris H, et al. Comparison of Sequential Intravenous/Oral Ciprofloxacin Plus Metronidazole with Intravenous Ceftriaxone Plus Metronidazole for Treatment of Complicated Intra-Abdominal Infections. Surgical Infections. 7:341–54, 2006.

Walker RC, Wright AJ. The fluoroquinolones. Mayo Clin Proc 66:1249–59, 1991.

Website: www.cipro.com

Ciprofloxacin Extended-Release (Cipro XR)

Drug Class: Fluoroquinolone

Usual Dose: 500 mg or 1000 mg (PO) q24h (see comments).

Spectrum: (see ***Susceptibility Profiles*** pp. 194–199).

Pharmacokinetic Parameters (500/1000 mg):

Peak serum level: 1.59/3.11 mcg/mL

Bioavailability: 70%

Excreted unchanged (urine): 50–70%; 22% excreted as active metabolite

Serum half-life: 6.6/6.3 hrs

Plasma protein binding: 20–40%

Volume of distribution (V_d): 2.5 L/kg

Primary Mode of Elimination: Renal

Dosage Adjustments*

CrCl > 30 mL/min	No change
CrCl < 30 mL/min	No change for 500 mg dose; reduce 1000 mg dose to 500 mg (PO) q24h
Post–HD/PD dose	500 mg (PO)
CVVH dose	see CrCl < 30 mL/min
Moderate or severe hepatic insufficiency	No change

"Usual dose" assumes normal renal/hepatic function. * For renal insufficiency, give usual dose × 1 followed by maintenance dose per CrCl. For dialysis patients, dose the same as for CrCl < 10 mL/min and give supplemental (post-HD/PD dose) immediately after dialysis. CrCl = creatinine clearance; CVVH = continuous veno-venous hemofiltration; HD/PD = hemodialysis/peritoneal dialysis. See pp. 509–513 for explanations, pp. xi–xii for abbreviations; Linezolid (↑ risk of serotonin syndrome, see p. 620).

Drug Interactions: Al^{++}, Ca^{++}, Fe^{++}, Mg^{++}, Zn^{++} antacids, citrate/citric acid, dairy products, didanosine (↓ absorption of ciprofloxacin only if taken together); caffeine, cyclosporine, theophylline (↑ interacting drug levels); cimetidine (↑ ciprofloxacin levels); foscarnet (↑ risk of seizures); insulin, oral hypoglycemics (slight ↑ or ↓ in blood glucose); NSAIDs (may ↑ risk of seizures/CNS stimulation); phenytoin (↑ or ↓ phenytoin levels); probenecid (↑ ciprofloxacin levels); warfarin (↑ INR).
Adverse Effects: Drug fever/rash, C. difficile diarrhea/colitis, seizures. FQ use has an increased risk of tendinitis/tendon rupture. Risk in highest in the elderly, those on steroids, and those with heart, lung or renal transplants.
Allergic Potential: Low
Safety in Pregnancy: C
Comments: Uncomplicated UTI (acute cystitis) dose: 500 mg (PO) q24h; **complicated UTI/acute uncomplicated pyelonephritis dose:** 1000 mg (PO) q24h. May be administered with or without food. Administer at least 2 hours before or 6 hours after H_2 antagonists, omeprazole, sucralfate, calcium, iron, zinc, multivitamins, or aluminum/magnesium containing medications.
↑ incidence of C. difficile diarrhea/colitis with PPIs (for patients on PPIs during FQ therapy, switch to H_2 blocker for duration of FQ therapy).
Cerebrospinal Fluid Penetration:
Non-Inflamed meninges = 10%
Inflamed meninges = 26%
Bile Penetration: 3000%
(also see ***Antibiotic Pearls & Pitfalls*** pp. 495–508).

REFERENCES:
Website: www.ciproxr.com

Clarithromycin (Biaxin)

Drug Class: Macrolide.
Usual Dose: 500 mg (PO) q12h.
Spectrum: (see ***Susceptibility Profiles*** pp. 183–187).
Pharmacokinetic Parameters:
Peak serum level: 1–4 mcg/mL
Bioavailability: 50%
Excreted unchanged (urine): 20%
Serum half-life (normal/ESRD): 3-7/4 hrs
Plasma protein binding: 70%
Volume of distribution (V_d): 3 L/kg
Primary Mode of Elimination: Hepatic
Dosage Adjustments*

CrCl 10–80 mL/min	No change
CrCl < 10 mL/min	250 mg (PO) q12h
Post–HD dose	500 mg (PO)
Post–PD dose	None
CVVH dose	No change
Moderate or severe hepatic insufficiency	No change

Drug Interactions: Amiodarone, procainamide, sotalol, astemizole, terfenadine, cisapride, pimozide (may ↑ QT interval, torsade de pointes); carbamazepine (↑ carbamazepine levels, nystagmus, nausea, vomiting, diarrhea); cimetidine, digoxin, ergot alkaloids, midazolam, triazolam, phenytoin, ritonavir, tacrolimus, valproic acid (↑ interacting drug levels); clozapine, corticosteroids (not studied); cyclosporine (↑ cyclosporine levels with toxicity); efavirenz (↓ clarithromycin levels); rifabutin, rifampin (↓ clarithromycin levels, ↑ interacting drug levels); statins (↑ risk of rhabdomyolysis); theophylline (↑ theophylline levels, nausea,

"Usual dose" assumes normal renal/hepatic function. * For renal insufficiency, give usual dose × 1 followed by maintenance dose per CrCl. For dialysis patients, dose the same as for CrCl < 10 mL/min and give supplemental (post-HD/PD dose) immediately after dialysis. CrCl = creatinine clearance; CVVH = continuous veno-venous hemofiltration; HD/PD = hemodialysis/peritoneal dialysis. See pp. 509–513 for explanations, pp. xi–xii for abbreviations; Linezolid (↑ risk of serotonin syndrome, see p. 620).

vomiting, seizures, apnea); warfarin (↑ INR); zidovudine (↓ zidovudine levels).
Adverse Effects: Nausea, vomiting, GI upset, **Non-C. difficile diarrhea,** abdominal pain. May ↑ QT_c; avoid with other medications that prolong the QT_c interval and in patients with cardiac arrhythmias/heart block.
Allergic Potential: Low
Safety in Pregnancy: C
Comments: Peculiar "aluminum sand" taste sensation on swallowing.
Cerebrospinal Fluid Penetration: < 10%
Bile Penetration: 7000%
(also see ***Antibiotic Pearls & Pitfalls*** pp. 495–508).

REFERENCES:

Alcaide F, Calatayud L, Santin M, et al. Comparative in vitro activities of linezolid, telithromycin, clarithromycin, levofloxacin, moxifloxacin and four conventional antimycobacterial drugs against mycobacterium kansasii. Antimicrob Agents Chemother 48:4562–5, 2004.

Alvarez-Elcoro S, Enzler MJ. The macrolides: Erythromycin, clarithromycin and azithromycin. Mayo Clin Proc 4:613–34, 1999.

Benson CA, Williams PL, Cohn DL, and the ACTG 196/CPCRA 009 Study Team. Clarithromycin or rifabutin alone or in combination for primary prophylaxis of Mycobacterium avium complex disease in patients with AIDS: A randomized, double-blinded, placebo-controlled trial. J Infect Dis 181:1289–97, 2000.

Berg HF, Tjhie JH, Scheffer GJ, et al. Emergence and persistence of macrolide resistance in oropharyngeal flora and elimination of nasal carriage of Staphylococcus aureus after therapy with slow-release clarithromycin: a randomized, double-blind, placebo-controlled study. Antimicrob Agents Chemother 48:4138–8, 2004.

Bergman M, Huikko S, Huovinen P, et al. Macrolide and azithromycin use are linked to increased macrolide resistance in *Streptococcus pneumoniae*. Antimicrob Agents Chemother 50:3646–3650, 2006.

Chaisson RE, Keiser P, Pierce M, et al. Clarithromycin and ethambutol with or without clofazimine for the treatment of bacteremic Mycobacterium avium complex disease in patients with HIV infection. AIDS 11:311–317, 1997.

Daneman N, McGeer A, Green K, et al. Macrolide resistance in bacteremic pneumococcal disease.: Implications for patient management. Clin Infect Dis 43:432–438, 2006.

Dean NC, Sperry P, Wikler M, et al. Comparing Clarithromycin in Pneumonia Symptom Resolution and Process of Care. Antimicrob Agents Chemother 50:1164–69, 2006.

Jain R, Danzinger LH. The macrolide antibiotics: a pharmacokinetic and pharmacodynamic overview. Curr Pharm Des 10:3045–53, 2004.

Jenkins SG, Farrell DJ. Increase in Pneumococcus Macrolide Resistance, United States. Emerging Infect Dis 15:1260–1264, 2009.

Kafetzis DA, Chantzi F, Tigaani G, et al. Safety and tolerability of clarithromycin administered to children at higher-than-recommended doses. Eur J Clin Microbiol Infect Dis 26:99–103, 2007.

Kraft M, Cassell AGH, Jpak J, et al. Mycoplasma pneumoniae and Chlamydia pneumoniae in asthma: effect of clarithromycin. Chest 121:1782–8, 2002.

Mandell LA, Wunderdink RG, Anzuetto A, et al. Infectious Diseases Society of America/American Thoracic Society consensus guidelines on the management of community-acquired pneumonia in adults. Clin Infect Dis 44:S27–72, 2007.

McConnell SA, Amsden GW. Review and comparison of advanced-generation macrolides clarithromycin and dirithromycin. Pharmacotherapy 19:404–15, 1999.

Ozsoylar G, Sayin A, Bolay H. Clarithromycin monotherapy-induced delirium. J Antimicrob Chemother 59:331, 2007.

Periti P, Mazzei T. Clarithromycin: Pharmacokinetic and pharmacodynamic interrelationships and dosage regimen. J Chemother 11:11–27, 1999.

Portier H, Filipecki J, Weber P, et al Five day clarithromycin modified release versus 10 day penicillin V for group A streptococcal pharyngitis: a multi-centre, open-label, randomized study. J Antimicrob Chemother 49:337–44, 2002.

"Usual dose" assumes normal renal/hepatic function. * For renal insufficiency, give usual dose × 1 followed by maintenance dose per CrCl. For dialysis patients, dose the same as for CrCl < 10 mL/min and give supplemental (post-HD/PD dose) immediately after dialysis. CrCl = creatinine clearance; CVVH = continuous veno-venous hemofiltration; HD/PD = hemodialysis/peritoneal dialysis. See pp. 509–513 for explanations, pp. xi–xii for abbreviations; Linezolid (↑ risk of serotonin syndrome, see p. 620).

Rodvold KA. Clinical pharmacokinetics of clarithromycin. Clin Pharmacokinet 37:385–98, 1999.

Schlossberg D. Azithromycin and clarithromycin. Med Clin North Am 79:803–16, 1995.

Stein GE, Schooley S. Serum bactericidal activity of extended-release clarithromycin against macrolide-resistant strains of Streptococcus pneumoniae. Pharmacotherapy 22:593–6, 2002.

Svensson M, Strom M, Nelsson M et al. Pharmacodynamic effects of nitroimidazoles alone and in combination with clarithromycin on Helicobacter pylori. Antimicrob Agents Chemother 46:2244–8, 2002.

Tartaglione TA. Therapeutic options for the management and prevention of Mycobacterium avium complex infection in patients with acquired immunodeficiency syndrome. Pharmacotherapy 16:171–82, 1996.

Website: www.biaxin.com

Clarithromycin XL (Biaxin XL)

Drug Class: Macrolide.

Usual Dose: 1 gm (PO) q24h.

Spectrum: (see ***Susceptibility Profiles*** pp. 183–187).

Pharmacokinetic Parameters:

Peak serum level: 3 mcg/mL

Bioavailability: 50%

Excreted unchanged (urine): 20%; 10–15% excreted as active metabolite

Serum half-life (normal/ESRD): 4/4 hrs

Plasma protein binding: 70%

Volume of distribution (V_d): 3 L/kg

Primary Mode of Elimination: Hepatic

Dosage Adjustments*

CrCl 30–60 mL/min	No change
CrCl < 30 mL/min	500 mg (PO) q24h
Post–HD dose	None
Post–PD dose	None
CVVH dose	No change
Moderate hepatic insufficiency	No change
Severe hepatic insufficiency	No change

Drug Interactions: Amiodarone, procainamide, sotalol, astemizole, terfenadine, cisapride, pimozide (may ↑ QT interval, torsade de pointes); carbamazepine (↑ carbamazepine levels, nystagmus, nausea, vomiting, diarrhea); cimetidine, digoxin, ergot alkaloids, midazolam, triazolam, phenytoin, ritonavir, tacrolimus, valproic acid (↑ interacting drug levels); clozapine, corticosteroids (not studied); cyclosporine (↑ cyclosporine levels with toxicity); efavirenz (↓ clarithromycin levels); rifabutin, rifampin (↓ clarithromycin levels, ↑ interacting drug levels); statins (↑ risk of rhabdomyolysis); theophylline (↑ theophylline levels, nausea, vomiting, seizures, apnea); warfarin (↑ INR); zidovudine (↓ zidovudine levels).

Adverse Effects: Nausea, vomiting **Non-C. difficile diarrhea.** May ↑ QT_c; avoid with other medications that prolong the QT_c interval and in patients with cardiac arrhythmias/heart block.

Allergic Potential: Low

Safety in Pregnancy: C

Comments: Two 500 mg tablets of XL preparation permits once daily dosing and decreases GI intolerance.

Cerebrospinal Fluid Penetration: < 10%

Bile Penetration: 7000%

(also see ***Antibiotic Pearls & Pitfalls*** pp. 495–508).

REFERENCES:

Adler JL, Jannetti W, Schneider D, et al. Phase III, randomized, double-blind study of clarithromycin extended-release and immediate-release formulations

"Usual dose" assumes normal renal/hepatic function. * For renal insufficiency, give usual dose × 1 followed by maintenance dose per CrCl. For dialysis patients, dose the same as for CrCl < 10 mL/min and give supplemental (post-HD/PD dose) immediately after dialysis. CrCl = creatinine clearance; CVVH = continuous veno-venous hemofiltration; HD/PD = hemodialysis/peritoneal dialysis. See pp. 509–513 for explanations, pp. xi–xii for abbreviations; Linezolid (↑ risk of serotonin syndrome, see p. 620).

in the treatment of patients with acute exacerbation of chronic bronchitis. Clin Ther 22:1410–20, 2000.

Anzueto A, Fisher CL Jr, Busman T. Comparison of the efficacy of extended-release clarithromycin tablets and amoxicillin/clavulanate tablets in the treatment of acute exacerbation of chronic bronchitis. Clin Ther 23:72–86, 2000.

Bergman M, Huikko S, Huovinen P, et al. Macrolide and azithromycin use are linked to increased macrolide resistance in *Streptococcus pneumoniae*. Antimicrob Agents Chemother 50:3646–3650, 2006.

Daneman N, McGeer A, Green K, et al. Macrolide resistance in bacteremic pneumococcal disease.: Implications for patient management. Clin Infect Dis 43:432–438, 2006.

Gotfried HM. Clarithromycin (Biaxin) extended-release tablet: a therapeutic review. Expert Rev Anti Infect Ther 1:9–20, 2004.

Jenkins SG, Farrell DJ. Increase in Pneumococcus Macrolide Resistance, United States. Emerging Infect Dis 15:1260–1264, 2009.

Laine L, Estrada R, Trujillo M, et al. Once-daily therapy for H. pylori infection: Randomized comparison of four regimens. Am J Gastroenterol 94:962–6, 1999.

Mandell LA, Wunderdink RG, Anzuetto A, et al. Infectious Diseases Society of America/American Thoracic Society consensus guidelines on the management of community-acquired pneumonia in adults. Clin Infect Dis 44:S27–72, 2007.

Nalepa P, Dobryniewska M, Busman T, et al. Short-course therapy of acute bacterial exacerbation of chronic bronchitis: a double-blind, randomized, multicenter comparison of extended-release versus immediate-release clarithromycin. Curr Med Res Opin 19:411–20, 2003.

Website: biaxinxl.com

Clindamycin (Cleocin)

Drug Class: Lincosamide.
Usual Dose: 600–900 mg (IV) q8h; 150–300 mg (PO) q6h.
Spectrum: (see ***Susceptibility Profiles*** pp. 183–187).

Pharmacokinetic Parameters:
Peak serum level: 2.5–10 mcg/mL
Bioavailability: 90%
Excreted unchanged (urine): 10%; 3.6% excreted as active metabolite
Serum half-life (normal/ESRD): 2.4/4 hrs
Plasma protein binding: 90%
Volume of distribution (V_d): 1 L/kg
Primary Mode of Elimination: Hepatic
Dosage Adjustments*

CrCl < 10 mL/min	No change
Post–HD/PD dose	None
CVVH dose	No change
Moderate or severe hepatic insufficiency	No change

Drug Interactions: Muscle relaxants, neuromuscular blockers (↑ apnea, respiratory paralysis); kaolin (↓ clindamycin absorption); theophylline (↑ theophylline levels, seizures).
Adverse Effects: C. difficile diarrhea/colitis, neuromuscular blockade.
Allergic Potential: Low
Safety in Pregnancy: B
Comments: C. difficile diarrhea more common with PO vs. IV clindamycin. *Anti-spasmodics contraindicated in C. difficile diarrhea.*
Cerebrospinal Fluid Penetration: < 10%
Bile Penetration: 300%
(also see ***Antibiotic Pearls & Pitfalls*** p. 501).

REFERENCES:

Coyle EA, Cha R, Rybak MJ. Influences of linezolid, penicillin, and clindamycin, alone and in combination, on streptococcal pyrogenic exotoxin a release. Antimicrob Agents Chemother 47:1752–5, 2003.

"Usual dose" assumes normal renal/hepatic function. * For renal insufficiency, give usual dose × 1 followed by maintenance dose per CrCl. For dialysis patients, dose the same as for CrCl < 10 mL/min and give supplemental (post-HD/PD dose) immediately after dialysis. CrCl = creatinine clearance; CVVH = continuous veno-venous hemofiltration; HD/PD = hemodialysis/peritoneal dialysis. See pp. 509–513 for explanations, pp. xi–xii for abbreviations; Linezolid (↑ risk of serotonin syndrome, see p. 620).

Corpelet C, Vacher P, Coudor F, et al. Role of quinine in life-threatening Babesia divergens infection successfully treated with clindamycin. Eur J Clin Microbiol Infect Dis 24:74–75, 2005.

Cunha BA. Oral Antibiotic Therapy of Serious Systemic Infections. Med Clin N Am 90: 1197–1222, 2006.

Falagas ME, Gorbach SL. Clindamycin and metronidazole. Med Clin North Am 79:845–67, 1995.

Kadowaki M, Demura Y, Mizuno S, et al. Reappraisal of clindamycin IV monotherapy for treatment of mild-to-moderate aspiration pneumonia in elderly patients. Chest 127:1276–1282, 2005.

Kasten MJ. Clindamycin, metronidazole, and chloramphenicol. Mayo Clin Proc 74:825–33, 1999.

Klepser ME, Nicolau DP, Quintiliani R, et al. Bactericidal activity of low-dose clindamycin administered at 8- and 12-hour intervals against Streptococcus pneumoniae and Bacteroides fragilis. Antimicrob Agents Chemother 41:630–5, 1997.

Lell B, Dremsner PG. Clindamycin as an antimalarial drug: review of clinical trials. Antimicrob Agents Chemother 46:2315–20, 2002.

Levin TP, Suh B, Axelrod P, et al. Potential clindamycin resistance in clindamycin-susceptible, erythromycin-resistant staphylococcus aureus: Report of a clinical failure. Antimicrob Agents Chemother 49:1222–24, 2005

Patel M, Waites KB, Moser SA, Cloud GA, Hoesley CJ. Prevalence of Inducible Clindamycin Resistance among Community- and Hospital-Associated Staphylococcus aureus Isolates. Journal of Clinical Microbiology. 44:2481–84, 2006.

Website: www.pdr.net

Colistin/ Colistin methanesulfonate (Coly-Mycin M)

Drug Class: Cell membrane altering antibiotic.
Usual Dose: 1.7 mg/kg (IV) q8h.

Pharmacokinetic Parameters:
Peak serum level: 5 mcg/mL
Bioavailability: Not applicable
Excreted unchanged (urine): 90%
Serum half-life (normal/ESRD): 3.5/48–72 hrs
Plasma protein binding: < 10%
Volume of distribution (V_d): 15.8 L/kg
Primary Mode of Elimination: Renal
Dosage Adjustments*

CrCl 40–60 mL/min	2.5 mg/kg (IV) q12h
CrCl 10–40 mL/min	2.5 mg/kg (IV) q24h
CrCl < 10 mL/min	1.5 mg/kg (IV) q36h
Post–HD dose	None
Post–PD dose	None
CVVH dose	2.5 mg/kg (IV) q24h
Mild hepatic insufficiency	No change
Moderate or severe hepatic insufficience	No change

Drug Interactions: Neuromuscular blocking agents (↑ neuromuscular blockade); nephrotoxic drugs (↑ nephrotoxic potential).
Adverse Effects: Dose dependent/reversible nephrotoxic potential (acute tubular necrosis). Paresthesias, vertigo, dizziness, slurred speech, blurry vision, respiratory arrest.
Allergic Potential: Low
Safety in Pregnancy: B
Comments: 1 mg = 12,500 U. Colistin (Polymyxin E) has **less nephrotoxic potential than previously thought. Useful for MDR P. aeruginosa and Acinetobacter species**. Colistin is more active against P. aeruginosa than polymyxin B. For P. aeruginosa or Acinetobacter meningitis also give amikacin

"Usual dose" assumes normal renal/hepatic function. * For renal insufficiency, give usual dose × 1 followed by maintenance dose per CrCl. For dialysis patients, dose the same as for CrCl < 10 mL/min and give supplemental (post-HD/PD dose) immediately after dialysis. CrCl = creatinine clearance; CVVH = continuous veno-venous hemofiltration; HD/PD = hemodialysis/peritoneal dialysis. See pp. 509–513 for explanations, pp. xi–xii for abbreviations; Linezolid (↑ risk of serotonin syndrome, see p. 620).

10–40 mg (IT) q24h or colistin 10 mg (IT) q24h. **Intrathecal colistin dose:** 10 mg (IT) Q24h. Nebulizer dose: 80 mg in saline q8h; for recurrent infection use 160 mg q8h (freshly prepare solution and use within 24 hours). If possible, avoid aerosolized colistin, which may result in pulmonary/systemic toxicity due to the polymyxin E1 metabolite. Continuous infusion dose: give ½ of daily dose (IV) over 5–10 min, then give remaining ½ dose (in D5W or NS) 1 hour after initial dose over next 24 hours. **Cerebrospinal Fluid Penetration:** 25% (also see ***Antibiotic Pearls & Pitfalls*** pp. 495–508).

REFERENCES:

Berlana D, Llop JM, Fort E, et al. Use of colistin in the treatment of multidrug resistant gram-negative infections. Am J Health Syst Pharm 62:39–47, 2005.

Biancofiore G, Tascini C, Bisa M, et al. Colistin, meropenem and rifampin in a combination therapy for multi-drug resistant Acinetobacter baumannii multifocal infection. A case report. Minerva Anestesiol 73:181–185, 2007.

Canton R, Cobos N, de Gracia J, et al. Antimicrobial therapy for pulmonary pathogenic colonization and infection by Pseudomonas aeruginosa in cystic fibrosis patients. Clin Microbiol Infect 11:690–703, 2005.

Cunha BA. New uses for older antibiotics: nitrofurantoin, amikacin, colistin, polymyxin B, doxycycline, and minocycline revisited. Med Clin North Am. 90:1089–1107, 2006.

Evans ME, Feola DJ, Rapp RP. Polymyxin B sulfate and colistin: old antibiotics for emerging multiresistant gram-negative bacteria. Ann Pharmacother 33:960–7, 1999.

Falagas ME, Rafailidis PI. When to include polymyxins in the empirical antibiotic regimen in critically ill patients with fever? A decision analysis approach. Shock 27:605–609, 2007.

Falagas ME, Rafailidis PI, Kasiakou SK, et al. Effectiveness and nephrotoxicity of colistin monotherapy vs colistin-meropenem combination therapy for multidrug-resistant Gram-negative bacterial infections. Clin Micrbiol Infect. 12:1227–30, 2006.

Falagas ME, Kasiakou SK. Colistin: The revival of polymyxins for the management of multidrug-resistant gram-negative bacterial infections. Clin Infect Dis 40:1333–41, 2005.

Falagas ME, Rafailidis PI. Nephrotoxicity of Colistin: New Insight into an Old Antibiotic. Clin Infect Dis 48:1729–1731, 2009.

Fulnecky EJ, Wright D, Scheld M, et al. Amikacin and colistin for treatment of Acinetobacter baumannii meningitis. J Infect 51:e249–e251, 2005.

Goodwin NJ, Friedman EA. The effects of renal impairment, peritoneal dialysis, and hemodialysis on serum sodium colistimethate levels. Ann Intern Med 68:984–94, 1968.

Guevara RE, Terarshita D, English L, et al. An outbreak of multi-drug resistant Elizabethkingia meningoseptica associated with colistin use. #197. Presented at the Annual Interscience Conference on Antimicrobial Agents and Chemotherapy, Sept 2007.

Gump WC, Walsh JW. Intrathecal colistin for treatment of highly resistant Pseudomonas ventriculitis. Case report and review of the literature. J Neurosurg 102:915–7, 2005.

Hachem RY, Chemaly RF, Ahmar CA, et al. Colistin is effective in treatment of infections caused by multidrug-resistant Pseudomonas aeruginosa in cancer patients. Antimicrob Agents Chemother 51:1905–1911, 2007.

Hartzell JD, Neff R, Ake J, et al. Nephrotoxicity Associated with Intravenous Colistin (Colistimethate Sodium) Treatment at a Tertiary Care Medical Center. Clin Infect Dis 48:1724–1728, 2009.

Horton J, Pankey GA. Polymyxin B, colistin, and sodium colistimethate. Med Clin North Am 66:135–42, 1982.

Jimenez-Mejias ME, Pichardo-Guerrero C, Marquez-Rivas FJ, et al. Cerebrospinal fluid penetration and pharmacokinetic/pharmacodynamic parameters of intravenously administered colistin in a case of multidrug-resistant Acinetobacter baumannii meningitis. Eur J Clin Microbiol Infect Dis 21:212–4, 2002.

"Usual dose" assumes normal renal/hepatic function. * For renal insufficiency, give usual dose × 1 followed by maintenance dose per CrCl. For dialysis patients, dose the same as for CrCl < 10 mL/min and give supplemental (post-HD/PD dose) immediately after dialysis. CrCl = creatinine clearance; CVVH = continuous veno-venous hemofiltration; HD/PD = hemodialysis/peritoneal dialysis. See pp. 509–513 for explanations, pp. xi–xii for abbreviations; Linezolid (↑ risk of serotonin syndrome, see p. 620).

Koch-Weser G, Sidel VW, Federman EB, et al. Adverse effects of sodium colistimethate. Ann Intern Med 72:857–68, 1970.

Krol V, Hamid NS, Cunha BA. Neurosurgically Related Nosocomial Acinetobacter baumannii Meningitis in ICU. Journal of Hospital Infection 71:176–188, 2008.

Levin AS, Baron AA, Penco J, et al. Intravenous colistin as therapy for nosocomial infections caused by multidrug resistant Pseudomonas aeruginosa and Acinetobacter baumannii. Clin Infect Dis 28:1008–11, 1999.

Li J, Rayner CR, Nation RL, Owen RJ, Spelman D, Tan KE, Liolios L. Heteroresistance to Colistin in Multidrug-Resistant Acinetobacter baumannii. Antimicrobial Agents and Chemotherapy. 50:2946–50, 2006.

Li J, Nation RL, Turnidge JD. Defining the Dosage Units for Colistin Methanesulfonate: Urgent Need for International Harmonization. 50:4231–32, 2006.

Li J, Rayner CR, Nation RL, et al. Pharmacokinetics of colistin methanesulfonate and colistin in a critically ill patient receiving continuous venovenous hemodiafiltration. Antimicrob Agents Chemother 49:4814–5, 2005.

Li H, Turnidge J, Milne R, et al. In vitro pharmacodynamic properties of colistin and colistin methanesulfonate against Pseudomonas aeruginosa isolates from patients with cystic fibrosis. Antimicrob Agents Chemother 45:781–5, 2001.

Linden PK, Kusne S, Coley K, et al. Use of parenteral colistin for the treatment of serious infection due to antimicrobial-resistant Pseudomonas aeruginosa. Clin Infect Dis 37:154–60, 2003.

Markou N, Apostolakos H, Koumoudiou C, et al. Intravenous colistin in the treatment of sepsis from multi resistant gram-negative bacilli in critically ill patients. Crit Care 7:78–83, 2003.

Michalopoulos AS, Tsiodras S, Rellos K, et al. Colistin treatment in patients with ICU-acquired infections caused by multiresistant gram-negative bacteria: the renaissance of an old antibiotic. Clin Microbiol Infect 11:115–121, 2005.

Michalopoulos A, Kasiakou SK, Evangelos S, et al. Cure of multidrug-resistant Acinetobacter baumannii bacteraemia with continuous intravenous infusion of colistin. Clin Microbiol Infect 11:119–21, 2005.

Michalopoulos A, Kasiakou S, Rosmarakis E, et al. Cure of multidrug-resistance Acinetobacter baumannii bacteraemia with continuous intravenous infusion of colistin. Scand J Infect Dis 37:142–5, 2005.

Obritsch MD, Fish DN, MacLaren R, et al. Nosocomial infections due to multidrug-resistant Pseudomonas aeruginosa: epidemiology and treatment options. Pharmacotherapy 25:1353–64, 2005.

Owen RJ, Li J, Nation RL, et al. In vitro pharmacodynamics of colistin against Acinetobacter baumannii clinical isolates. J Antimicrob Chemother 59:473–477, 2007.

Papagelopoulos PJ, Mavrogenis AF, Giannitsioti E, et al. Management of a multidrug-resistant Pseudomonas aeruginosa infected knee arthroplasty using colistin. A care report and review of the literature. J Arthroplasty 22:457–463, 2007.

Paterson DL, Lipman J. Returning to the pre-antibiotic era in the critically ill: the XDR problem. Crit Care Med 35:1789–1791, 2007.

Plachouras D, Giamerllos-Bourboulis EJ, Kentepozidis N, et al. In vitro postantibiotic effect of colistin on multidrug-resistant Acinetobacter baumannii. Diagn Microbiol Infect Dis 57:419–422, 2007.

Reed MD, Stern RC, O'Riordan MA, et al. The pharmacokinetics of colistin in patients with cystic fibrosis. J Clin Pharmacol 41:645–54, 2001.

Rynn C, Wooton M, Bowker KE, et al. In vitro assessment of colistin's antipseudomonal antimicrobial interactions with other antibiotics. Clin Microbiol Infect 5:32–6, 1999.

Santamaria C, Mykietiuj A, Temporiti E, et al. Nephrotoxivity associated with the use of intravenous COLISTIN. Scand J Infect Dis 41:767–769, 2009.

Stein A, Raoult D. Colistin: an antimicrobial for the 21st century? Clin Infect Dis 35:901–2, 2002.

Steinfort DP, Steinfort C. Effect of long-term nebulized colistin on lung function and quality of life in patients with chronic bronchial sepsis. Intern Med J 37:495–498, 2007.

"Usual dose" assumes normal renal/hepatic function. * For renal insufficiency, give usual dose × 1 followed by maintenance dose per CrCl. For dialysis patients, dose the same as for CrCl < 10 mL/min and give supplemental (post-HD/PD dose) immediately after dialysis. CrCl = creatinine clearance; CVVH = continuous veno-venous hemofiltration; HD/PD = hemodialysis/peritoneal dialysis. See pp. 509–513 for explanations, pp. xi–xii for abbreviations; Linezolid (↑ risk of serotonin syndrome, see p. 620).

Tan TY, Ng SY. Comparison of Etest, Viteck and agar dilution for susceptibility testing of colistin. Clin Microbiol Infect 13:541–544, 2007.

Tarchini G. Nephrotoxicity associated with intravenous colistin. Clin Infect Dis 49:1773, 2009.

Wang S, Kwok M, McNamara JK, Cunha BA. Colistin for Multi-Drug Resistant (MDR) Gram-Negative Bacillary Infections. Antibiotics for Clinicans 11:389–396, 2007.

Wood GC, Swanson JM. Aerosolized antibacterials for the prevention and treatment of hospital-acquired pneumonia. Drugs 67:903–914, 2007.

Cycloserine (Seromycin)

Drug Class: Anti-TB drug.
Usual Dose: 250 mg (PO) q12h.
Pharmacokinetic Parameters:
Peak serum level: 20 mcg/mL
Bioavailability: 90%
Excreted unchanged (urine): 65%
Serum half-life (normal/ESRD): 10–25 hrs/no data
Plasma protein binding: No data
Volume of distribution (V_d): 0.2 L/kg
Primary Mode of Elimination: Renal
Dosage Adjustments*

CrCl 50–80 mL/min	No change
CrCl 10–50 mL/min	250 mg (PO) q12-24h
CrCl < 10 mL/min	250 mg (PO) q24h
Post–HD dose	None
Post–PD dose	250 mg (PO)
CVVH dose	No change
Moderate or severe hepatic insufficiency	No change

Drug Interactions: Alcohol (seizures); ethambutol, ethionamide (drowsiness, dizziness); phenytoin (↑ phenytoin levels).

Adverse Effects: Peripheral neuropathy, seizures (dose related), psychosis/delirium.
Allergic Potential: Low
Safety in Pregnancy: C
Comments: Avoid in patients with seizures. Ethambutol, ethionamide, or ethanol may increase CNS toxicity.
Meningeal dose = usual dose.
Cerebrospinal Fluid Penetration:
Non-Inflamed meninges = 90%
Inflamed meninges = 90%

REFERENCES:

Davidson PT, Le HQ. Drug treatment of tuberculosis 1992. Drugs 43:651–73, 1992.

Drugs for tuberculosis. Med Lett Drugs Ther 35:99–101, 1993.

Furin J, Nardell EA. Multidrug-resistant tuberculosis: An update on the best regimens. J Respir Dis 27:172–82, 2006.

Iseman MD. Treatment of multidrug resistant tuberculosis. N Engl J Med 329:784–91, 1993.

Dapsone

Drug Class: Antiparasitic, anti-leprosy, anti-PCP drug (PABA antagonist).
Usual Dose: 100 mg (PO) q24h (see comments).
Pharmacokinetic Parameters:
Peak serum level: 1.8 mcg/mL
Bioavailability: 85%
Excreted unchanged (urine): 10%
Serum half-life (normal/ESRD): 25/30 hrs
Plasma protein binding: 80%
Volume of distribution (V_d): 1.2 L/kg
Primary Mode of Elimination: Hepatic/renal
Dosage Adjustments*

CrCl 50–80 mL/min	No change
CrCl 10–50 mL/min	No change

"Usual dose" assumes normal renal/hepatic function. * For renal insufficiency, give usual dose × 1 followed by maintenance dose per CrCl. For dialysis patients, dose the same as for CrCl < 10 mL/min and give supplemental (post-HD/PD dose) immediately after dialysis. CrCl = creatinine clearance; CVVH = continuous veno-venous hemofiltration; HD/PD = hemodialysis/peritoneal dialysis. See pp. 509–513 for explanations, pp. xi–xii for abbreviations; Linezolid (↑ risk of serotonin syndrome, see p. 620).

CrCl < 10 mL/min	No change
Post–HD dose	None
Post–PD dose	None
CVVH dose	No change
Moderate hepatic insufficiency	No change
Severe hepatic insufficiency	No information

Drug Interactions: Didanosine (↓ dapsone absorption); oral contraceptives (↓ oral contraceptive effect); pyrimethamine, zidovudine (↑ bone marrow suppression); rifabutin, rifampin (↓ dapsone levels); trimethoprim (↑ dapsone and trimethoprim levels, methemoglobinemia).

Adverse Effects: Drug fever/rash, nausea, vomiting, hemolytic anemia in G6PD deficiency, methemoglobinemia.

Allergic Potential: High

Safety in Pregnancy: C

Comments: Useful in sulfa (SMX) allergic patients. Avoid, if possible, in G6PD deficiency or hemoglobin M deficiency. **PCP prophylaxis dose**: 100 mg (PO) q24h. **PCP therapy dose**: 100 mg (PO) q24h.

Cerebrospinal Fluid Penetration: < 50%

REFERENCES:

El-Sadr WM, Murphy RI, Yurik TM, et al. Atovaquone compared with dapsone to the prevention of Pneumocystis carinii in patients with HIV infection who cannot tolerate trimethoprim, sulfonamides, or both. N Engl J Med 339:1889–95, 1998.

Medina I, Mills J, Leoung G, et al. Oral therapy for Pneumocystis carinii pneumonia in the acquired immunodeficiency syndrome. A controlled trial of trimethoprim-sulfamethoxazole versus trimethoprim-dapsone. N Engl J Med 323:776–82, 1990.

Podzamczer D, Salazar A, Jiminez J, et al. Intermittent trimethoprim-sulfamethoxazole compared with dapsone-pyrimethamine for the simultaneous primary prophylaxis of Pneumocystis pneumonia and toxoplasmosis in patients infected with HIV. Ann Intern Med 122:755–61, 1995.

Website: www.pdr.net

Daptomycin (Cubicin)

Drug Class: Lipopeptide.

Usual Dose: Complicated skin/skin structure infections: 4 mg/kg (IV) q24h. Bacteremia, endocarditis: 6 mg/kg (IV) q24h.

Spectrum: (see ***Susceptibility Profiles*** pp. 194–199).

Pharmacokinetic Parameters:

Peak serum level:

4 mg/kg = 58 mcg/mL; 6 mg/kg = 99 mcg/mL

Bioavailability: Not applicable

Excreted unchanged (urine): 80%

Serum half-life (normal/ESRD): 8.1/29.8 hrs

Plasma protein binding: 92%

Volume of distribution (V_d): 0.096 L/kg

Primary Mode of Elimination: Renal

Dosage Adjustments*

CrCl > 30 mL/min	No change
CrCl < 30 mL/min	4 mg/kg (IV) q48h; 6 mg/kg (IV) q48h for bacteremia/ endocarditis
Post–HD dose	None
Post–PD dose	None
CVVH dose	None
Moderate or severe hepatic insufficiency	No change

Drug Interactions: Warfarin/statin (no significant interaction in small number of

"Usual dose" assumes normal renal/hepatic function. * For renal insufficiency, give usual dose × 1 followed by maintenance dose per CrCl. For dialysis patients, dose the same as for CrCl < 10 mL/min and give supplemental (post-HD/PD dose) immediately after dialysis. CrCl = creatinine clearance; CVVH = continuous veno-venous hemofiltration; HD/PD = hemodialysis/peritoneal dialysis. See pp. 509–513 for explanations, pp. xi–xii for abbreviations; Linezolid (↑ risk of serotonin syndrome, see p. 620).

volunteers; consider temporary suspension of statins during daptomycin use).

Adverse Effects: Constipation, nausea, headache. Rarely, ↑ CPK; in clinical trials, same or less (0.2%) than comparators; monitor for muscle pain/weakness and CPK weekly. False-positive ↑ INR.

Allergic Potential: No data

Safety in Pregnancy: B

Comments: Administer IV over 30 minutes in 0.9% a 50 mL bag with NaCl. Not compatible with dextrose-containing diluents. Cannot be given IM. Exhibits concentration-dependent killing. **High-dose daptomycin 12 mg/kg (IV) q24h has been used for MSSA/MRSA bacteremias/ABE unresponsive to other antistaphylococcal drugs without toxicity**. Post-antibiotic effect (PAE) up to 6 hours.

Cerebrospinal Fluid Penetration: ~ 5% (also see ***Antibiotic Pearls & Pitfalls*** p. 506).

REFERENCES:

Alder JD. Daptomycin: a new drug class for the treatment of gram-positive infections. Drugs Today 41:81–90, 2005.

Arias CA, Torres HA, Singh KV, et al. Failure of daptomycin monotherapy for endocarditis caused by enterococcus faecium strain with vancomycin-resistant and vancomycin-susceptible subpopulations and evidence of in vivo loss of a vanA gene cluster. Clin Infect Dis 45:1343–1346, 2007.

Baltch AL, Ritz WJ, Bopp LH, et al. Antimicrobial activities of daptomycin, vancomycin, and oxacillin in human monocytes and of daptomycin in combination with gentamicin and/or rifampin in human monocytes and in broth against Staphylococcus aureus. Antimicrob Agents Chemother 51:1559–1562, 2007.

Benevuto M, Benziger DP, Yankelev S, Vigliani G. Pharmacokinetics and Tolerability of Daptomycin at Doses up to 12 Milligrams per Kilogram of Body Weight Once Daily in Healthy Volunteers. Antimicrobial Agents and Chemotherapy. 50:3245–49, 2006.

Bouza E. New therapeutic choices for infections caused by methicillin-resistant *Staphylococcus aureus*. Clin Microbiol Infect Dis 15:44–52, 2009.

Cunha BA, Mickail N, Eisenstein L. E. faecalis vancomycin-sensitive enterococcal bacteremia unresponsive to a vancomycin tolerant strain successfully treated with high-dose daptomycin. Heart Lung. 36:456-461, 2007.

Cunha BA, Mickail N, Eisenstein L. E. faecalis Vancomycin Sensitive Enterococci (VSE) Bacteremia Unresponsive to Vancomycin Successfully Treated with High Dose Daptomycin. Heart & Lung 36:456–461, 2007.

Cunha BA, Eisenstein LE, Hamid NS. Pacemaker-induced Staphylococcus aureus mitral valve acute bacterial endocarditis complicated by persistent bacteremia from a coronary stent: Cure with prolonged/high-dose daptomycin without toxicity. Heart & Lung. 35:207–11, 2006.

Cunha BA. Persistent S. aureus Bacteremia: Clinical Pathway for Diagnosis and Treatment. Antibiotics for Clinicians. 10:S39–46, 2006.

Cunha BA. Staphylococcal aureus Acute Bacterial Endocarditis (ABE): Clinical Pathway for Diagnosis and Treatment. Antibiotics for Clinicians. 10:S29–33, 2006.

Cunha BA, Hamid N, Kessler H, Parchuri S. Daptomycin cure after cefazolin treatment failure of Methicillin-sensitive Staphylococcus aureus (MSSA) tricuspid valve acute bacterial endocarditis from a peripherally inserted central catheter (PICC) line. Heart & Lung. 34:442–7, 2005.

Dretler R, Branch T. MRSA knee infection treated successfully with daptomycin after two failed prolonged high-dose courses of vancomycin. Infect Dis Clin Pract 13:327–329, 2005.

Falagas ME, Giannopoulou KP, Ntziora F, et al. Daptomycin for endocarditis and/or bacteremia: a systematic review of the experimental and clinical evidence. J Antimicrob Chemother 60:7–19, 2007.

Fowler VG, Jr., Boucher HW, Corey GR, et al. Daptomycin versus standard therapy for bacteremia and endocarditis caused by Staphylococcus aureus. NEJM 355:653–665, 2006.

"Usual dose" assumes normal renal/hepatic function. * For renal insufficiency, give usual dose × 1 followed by maintenance dose per CrCl. For dialysis patients, dose the same as for CrCl < 10 mL/min and give supplemental (post-HD/PD dose) immediately after dialysis. CrCl = creatinine clearance; CVVH = continuous veno-venous hemofiltration; HD/PD = hemodialysis/peritoneal dialysis. See pp. 509–513 for explanations, pp. xi–xii for abbreviations; Linezolid (↑ risk of serotonin syndrome, see p. 620).

Hair PI, Keam SJ. Daptomycin: a review of its use in the management of complicated skin and soft-tissue infections and Staphylococcus aureus bacteremia. Drugs 67:1483–1512, 2007.

Hayes D Jr, Anstead MI, Kuhn RJ. Eosinophilic pneumonia induced by daptomycin. J Infect 54:e211–e213, 2007.

Holtom PD, Zalavras CG, Lamp KC, et al. Clinical experience with daptomycin treatment of foot or ankle osteomyelitis: a preliminary study. Clin Orthop Relat Res 461:35–39, 2007.

Jevitt LA, Thorne GM, Traczewski MM, et al. Multicenter Evaluation of the Etest and Disk Diffusion Methods for Differentiating Daptomycin-Susceptible from Non-Daptomycin-Susceptible Staphylococcus aureus Isolates. J of Clin Microbiology. 44:3098–104, 2006.

Kanafani ZA, Corey GR. Daptomycin: a rapidly bactericidal lipopeptide for the treatment of gram-positive infections. Expert Rev Anti Infect Ther 5:177–184, 2007.

Mohan S, McDermott BP, Cunha BA. Methicillin-resistant Staphylococcus aureus (MRSA) prosthetic valve endocarditis (PVE) with paravalvular abscess treated with daptomycin. Heart & Lung 34:69–71, 2005.

Patel JB, Jevitt LA, Hageman J, et al. An association between reduced susceptibility to daptomycin and reduced susceptibility to vancomycin in Staphylococcus aureus. Clin Infect Dis 42:1652–3, 2006.

Pfaller MA, Sader HS, Jones RN. Evaluation of the in vitro activity of daptomycin against 19615 clinical isolates of gram-positive cocci collected in North American hospitals (2002–2005). Diagn Microbiol Infect Dis 57:459–465, 2007.

Raad I, Hanna H, Jiang Y, et al. Comparative activities of daptomycin, linezolid, and tigecycline against catheter-related methicillin-resistant Staphylococcus bacteremia isolates embedded in biofilm. Antimicrob Agents Chemother 51:1656–1660, 2007.

Rouse MS, Steckelber MJ, Patel R. In vitro activity of ceftobiprole, daptomycin, linezolid, and vancomycin against methicillin-resistant staphylococci associated with endocarditis and bone and joint infection. Diagn Microbiol Infect Dis 58:363–365, 2007.

Rybak MJ, Bailey EM, Lamp KC, et al. Pharmacokinetics and bactericidal rates of daptomycin and vancomycin in intravenous drug abusers being treated for gram-positive endocarditis and bacteremia. Antimicrob Agents Chemother 36:1109–14, 1992.

Rybak, MJ, The efficacy and safety of daptomycin: first in a new class of antibiotics for Gram-positive bacteria. 12:24–32, 2006.

Sader HS, Fritsche TR, Jones RN. Daptomycin Bactericidal Activity and Correlation between Disk and Broth Microdilution Method Results in Testing of Staphylococcus aureus Strains with Decreased Susceptibility of Vancomycin. Antimicrob Agents Chemother 50:2330–36, 2006.

Samra Z, Ofir O, Shmuely H. In vitro susceptibility of methicillin-resistant Staphylococcus aureus and vancomycin-resistant Enterococcus faecium to daptomycin and other antibiotics. Eur J Clin Microbiol Infect Dis 26:363–365, 2007.

Vaudaux P, Francois P, Bisognano C, et al. Comparative efficacy of daptomycin and vancomycin in the therapy of experimental foreign body infection due to Staphylococcus aureus. J Antimicrob Chemother 52:89–95, 2003.

Weis F, Beiras-Fernandez A, Kaczmarek I, et al. Daptomycin for eradication of a systemic infection with a methicillin-resistant –Staphylococcus aureus in a biventricular assist device recipient. Ann Thorac Surg 84:269–270, 2007.

Website: www.cubist.com

Darunavir (Prezista) DRV

Drug Class: Antiretroviral protease inhibitor.

Usual Dose: 600 mg (two 300-mg tablets) of darunavir (PO) q12h plus 100 mg of ritonavir (PO) q12h.

Pharmacokinetic Parameters:

Peak serum level: 3578 ng/mL

Bioavailability: 37% (alone) 82% (with ritonavir)

Excreted unchanged: 41.2% (feces), 7.7% (urine)

"Usual dose" assumes normal renal/hepatic function. * For renal insufficiency, give usual dose × 1 followed by maintenance dose per CrCl. For dialysis patients, dose the same as for CrCl < 10 mL/min and give supplemental (post-HD/PD dose) immediately after dialysis. CrCl = creatinine clearance; CVVH = continuous veno-venous hemofiltration; HD/PD = hemodialysis/peritoneal dialysis. See pp. 509–513 for explanations, pp. xi–xii for abbreviations; Linezolid (↑ risk of serotonin syndrome, see p. 620).

Serum half-life (normal/ESRD): 15/15 hrs
Plasma protein binding: 95%
Volume of distribution (V_d): not studied
Primary Mode of Elimination: Fecal/renal
Dosage Adjustments*

CrCl 50–80 mL/min	No change
CrCl 10–50 mL/min	No change
CrCl < 10 mL/min	No change
Post–HD dose	No change
Post–PD dose	No change
CVVH dose	No change
Mild hepatic insufficiency	Not studied
Moderate or severe hepatic insufficiency	Not studied

Antiretroviral Dosage Adjustments:

Efavirenz	No information
Nevirapine	No change
Didanosine	1 hour before or 1 hour after darunavir
Tenofovir	No change
Fosamprenavir	No change
Indinavir	No information
Lopinavir/ritonavir	Avoid
Saquinavir	Avoid
Rifabutin	150 mg qod

Drug Interactions: Indinavir, ketaconazole, nevirapine, tenofovir (↑ darunavir levels); lopinavir/ritonavir, saquinavir, efavirenz (↓ darunavir levels); concomitant administration of darunavir/ritonavir with agents highly-dependent on CYP3A for clearance, astemizole, cisapride, dihydroergotamine, ergonovine, ergotamine, methylergonovine, midazolam, pimozide, terfenadine, midazolam, triazolam (may ↓ darunavir levels and ↓ effectiveness); sildenafil, vardenafil, tadalafil (↑ PDE-5 inhibitors; sildenafil do not exceed 25 mg in 48 hrs, vardenafil do not exceed 2.5 mg in 72 hrs, or tadalafil do not exceed 10 mg in 72 hrs).

Adverse Effects: Rash, diarrhea, nausea, headache, nasopharyngitis drug induced hepatitis. Use with caution in patients with preexisting liver disease. New-onset or exacerbations of pre-exisiting diabetes mellitus and hyperglycemia, and increased bleeding in hemophiliacs (class effect). Immune reconstitution syndrome.
Allergic Potential: High (see comments)
Safety in Pregnancy: B
Comments: Always take with food (increases AUC, Cmax by approximately 30%). Must be given with ritonavir to boost bioavailability. Darunavir contains a sulfonamide moiety (as do fosamprenavir and tipranavir); use with caution in patients with sulfonamide allergies. Astemizole, Terfenadine, Ergot Derivatives Dihydroergotamine, Ergonovine, Ergotamine, Methylergonovine, Cisapride, Pimozide, Midazolam, Triazolam, are contraindicated with darunavir. Phenobarbital, phenytoin, carbamazepine, or products containing St. John's wort, rifampin. Lovostatin and simavastatin may be taken with caution.
Cerebrospinal Fluid Penetration: No data

REFERENCES:

De Meyer S, Azijn H, Surleraux D, et al. TMC114, a novel human immunodeficiency virus type 1 protease inhibitor active against protease inhibitor-resistant

---

"Usual dose" assumes normal renal/hepatic function. * For renal insufficiency, give usual dose × 1 followed by maintenance dose per CrCl. For dialysis patients, dose the same as for CrCl < 10 mL/min and give supplemental (post-HD/PD dose) immediately after dialysis. CrCl = creatinine clearance; CVVH = continuous veno-venous hemofiltration; HD/PD = hemodialysis/peritoneal dialysis. See pp. 509–513 for explanations, pp. xi–xii for abbreviations; Linezolid (↑ risk of serotonin syndrome, see p. 620).

viruses, including a broad range of clinical isolates. Antimicrob Agents Chemother 49:2314–2321, 2005.
Dominique L. N. G, Surleraux T, Abdellah Tahri T, et al. Discovery and selection of TMC114, a next generation HIV-I protease inhibitor. J. Med Chem. 48:1813–1822, 2005.
Grinsztejn, B. TMC114/r is well tolerated in 3-class-experienced patients: week 24 of POWER 1 (TMC114-C213). Tibotec Pharmaceuticals. Rio de Janerio, Brazil. Available from URL: http://www.tibotec.com/content/congresses/www.tibotec.com/TMC114_SafetyPoster_ Dr_Grinsztein_IAS_FINAL.pdf
Katlama C. TMC114/r outperforms investigator-selected PI(s) in 3-class-experienced patients: week 24 primary efficacy analysis of POWER 1 (TMC114-C213). Tibotec Pharmaceuticals. Rio de Janerio, Brazil. Available from URL: http://www.tibotec.com/content/congresses/ www.tibotec.com/TMC114_EfficacyPoster_ProfKatlama_Finalias2005.pdf
Panel on Antiretroviral Guidelines for Adults and Adolescents. Guidelines for the use of antiretroviral agents in HIV-1 infected adults and adolescents. Department of Health and Human Services. November 3, 2008; 1–139. Available at http://www.aidsinfor.nih.gov/ContentFiles/AdultandAdolescentGL.pdf
Sorbera LA, Castaner J, Bayes M. Darunavir: Anti-HIV agent HIV protease inhibitor. Drugs of the Future. 30:441–449, 2005.
Website: www.prezista.com

Delavirdine (Rescriptor) DLV

Drug Class: Antiretroviral NNRTI (non-nucleoside reverse transcriptase inhibitor).
Usual Dose: 400 mg (PO) q8h.
Pharmacokinetic Parameters:
Peak serum level: 35 mcg/mL
Bioavailability: 85%
Excreted unchanged (urine): 5%
Serum half-life (normal/ESRD): 5.8 hrs/no data
Plasma protein binding: 98%
Volume of distribution (V_d): 0.5 L/kg

Primary Mode of Elimination: Hepatic
Dosage Adjustments*

CrCl 50–80 mL/min	No change
CrCl 10–50 mL/min	No change
CrCl < 10 mL/min	No change
Post–HD dose	None
Post–PD dose	None
CVVH dose	No change
Moderate hepatic insufficiency	No information
Severe hepatic insufficiency	No information

Antiretroviral Dosage Adjustments:

Amprenavir	Increased agenerase levels
Efavirenz	No information
Indinavir	Indinavir 600 mg q8h
Lopinavir/ritonavir	No information
Nelfinavir	No information (monitor for neutropenia)
Nevirapine	No information
Ritonavir	Delavirdine: no change; ritonavir: No information
Saquinavir soft-gel	Saquinavir soft-gel 800 mg q8h (monitor transaminases)
Rifampin, rifabutin	Avoid combination
Statins	Not recommended

"Usual dose" assumes normal renal/hepatic function. * For renal insufficiency, give usual dose × 1 followed by maintenance dose per CrCl. For dialysis patients, dose the same as for CrCl < 10 mL/min and give supplemental (post-HD/PD dose) immediately after dialysis. CrCl = creatinine clearance; CVVH = continuous veno-venous hemofiltration; HD/PD = hemodialysis/peritoneal dialysis. See pp. 509–513 for explanations, pp. xi–xii for abbreviations; Linezolid (↑ risk of serotonin syndrome, see p. 620).

Drug Interactions: With antiretrovirals adjust according to table above. Avoid in combination with rifabutin rifampin. Contraindicated with astemizole, terrenadine, Dihydroergotamine, ergonovine, ergotamine, methylergonovine, Cisapride, Pimozide, Alprazolam, midazolam, triazolam. Phenytoin may decrease delaviridine levels. Clarithromycin, dapsone nefedipine, warfarin cause increase in interacting drug levels. Sildenaril (do not exceed 25 mg in 48 hrs, tadalafil (max 10mg/72 hrs; vardenafil (max 2.5 mg/72hrs. St. John's wort substantially reduces delaviridine levels.

Adverse Effects: Drug fever/rash, Stevens–Johnson syndrome (rare), headache, nausea/vomiting, diarrhea, ↑ SGOT/SGPT. May cause immune reconstitution syndrome.

Allergic Potential: High

Safety in Pregnancy: C

Comments: May be taken with or without food, but food decreases absorption by 20%. May disperse four 100-mg tablets in > 3 oz. water to produce slurry; 200-mg tablets should be taken as intact tablets and not used to make an oral solution. Separate dosing with ddI or antacids by 1 hour.

Cerebrospinal Fluid Penetration: 0.4%

REFERENCES:

Been-Tiktak AM, Boucher CA, Brun-Vezinet F, et al. Efficacy and safety of combination therapy with delavirdine and zidovudine: A European/Australian phase II trial. Intern J Antimicrob Agents 11:13–21, 1999.

Conway B. Initial therapy with protease inhibitor-sparing regimens: Evaluation of nevirapine and delavirdine. Clin Infect Dis 2:130–4, 2000.

Demeter LM, Shafer RW, Meehan PM, et al. Delavirdine susceptibilities and associated reverse transcriptase mutations in human immunodeficiency virus type 1 isolates from patients in a phase I/II trial of delavirdine monotherapy (ACTG260). Antimicrob Agents Chemother 44:794–7, 2000.

Justesen US, Klitgaard NA, Brosen K, et al. Dose-dependent pharmacokinetics of delavirdine in combination with amprenavir in healthy volunteers. J Antimicrob Chemother 54:206–10, 2004.

Panel on Antiretroviral Guidelines for Adults and Adolescents. Guidelines for the use of antiretroviral agents in HIV-1 infected adults and adolescents. Department of Health and Human Services. November 3, 2008; 1–139. Available at http://www.aidsinfor.nih.gov/ContentFiles/AdultandAdolescentGL.pdf

Website: rescriptor.com

Didanosine EC (Videx) ddI

Drug Class: Antiretroviral NRTI (nucleoside reverse transcriptase inhibitor).

Usual Dose: 400 mg q24h for weight > 60 kg; 250 q24h for < 60 kg.

Pharmacokinetic Parameters:

Peak serum level: 29 mcg/mL

Bioavailability: 42%

Excreted unchanged (urine): 60%

Serum half-life (normal/ESRD): 1.6/4.1 hrs

Plasma protein binding: ≤ 5%

Volume of distribution (V_d): 1.1 L/kg

Primary Mode of Elimination: Renal

Dosage Adjustments*: > 60 kg/[< 60 kg]:

CrCl 30–59 mL/min	200 mg (PO) q24h [125 mg (PO) q24h]
CrCl 10–29 mL/min	125 mg (PO) q24h [125 mg (PO) q24h]
CrCl < 10 mL/min	125 mg (PO) q24h [not recommended]
Post–HD dose	No information
Post–PD dose	100 mg (PO)
CVVH dose	150 mg (PO) q24h

"Usual dose" assumes normal renal/hepatic function. * For renal insufficiency, give usual dose × 1 followed by maintenance dose per CrCl. For dialysis patients, dose the same as for CrCl < 10 mL/min and give supplemental (post-HD/PD dose) immediately after dialysis. CrCl = creatinine clearance; CVVH = continuous veno-venous hemofiltration; HD/PD = hemodialysis/peritoneal dialysis. See pp. 509–513 for explanations, pp. xi–xii for abbreviations; Linezolid (↑ risk of serotonin syndrome, see p. 620).

Moderate hepatic insufficiency	No change
Severe hepatic insufficiency	No change

Drug Interactions: Alcohol, lamivudine, pentamidine and valproic acid increase the risk of pancreatitis. Patients on tenofovir should have didanosine dose reduced to 250 mg/24 hrs. Concomitant use with tenofovir increases risk of virologic failure. The appropriate dose of didanosine when taken with tenofovir has not been determined in patients with creatinine clearance of ≤ 60 ml/min. Peripheral neuropathy is enhanced by stavudine, INH, metronidazole, ntirofuantoin, vincristine and zalcitabine. Dapsone levels are dramatically reduced by powder form especially and increase risk of pneumocystis. Decreases levels of cipro floxacin delavirdine, indinavir. Methadone will decrease didanosine levels. Coadministration of didanosine with ribavirin is not recommended.

Adverse Effects: Fatal and non-fatal pancreatitis have occured during therapy with didanosine used alone or in combination regimens. Tenofovir can increase this risk as well. Lactic acidosis and severe hepatomegaly with steatosis can also occur especially in pregnant women. Combination with stavuidine potentiates this risk and should be avoided especially in pregnancy and in patients with concomitant HCV/HBV. Other effects include diarrhea, peripheral neuropathy, rash and abdominal pain, anemia, leukopenia, alopecia. Depigmentation and optic neuritis have occured. Patients with underlying liver disease are at increased risk of hepatic toxicity.

Allergic Potential: Low

Safety in Pregnancy: B; should be avoided in pregnancy as it may cause fatal pancreatitis

Comments: Available as buffered powder for oral solution and enteric-coated extended-release capsules (Videx EC 400 mg PO q24h). Take 30 minutes before or 2 hours after meal (food decreases serum concentrations by 49%). Avoid in patients with alcoholic cirrhosis/history of pancreatitis. Use with caution in combination with tenofovir, which can potentiate risk of pancreatitis and require a significant dose reduction of ddI. Avoid use with ribavirin. Na^+ content = 11.5 mEq/g. Buffered tablets discontinued by U.S. manufacturer in February 2006.

Cerebrospinal Fluid Penetration: 20%

REFERENCES:

Barreiro P, Corbaton A, Nunez M, et al. Tolerance of didanosine as enteric-coated capsules versus buffered tablets. AIDS Patient Care STDS 18:329–31, 2004.

Hirsch MS, D'Aquila RT. Therapy for human immunodeficiency virus infection. N Engl J Med 328:1686–95, 1993.

HIV Trialists' Collaborative Group. Zidovudine, didanosine, and zalcitabine in the treatment of HIV infection: Meta-analyses of the randomised evidence. Lancet 353:2014–2025, 1999.

Montaner JS, Reiss P, Cooper D, et al. A randomized, double-blind trial comparing combinations of nevirapine, didanosine, and zidovudine for HIV-infected patients: The INCAS trial. Italy, the Netherlands, Canada and Australia Study. J Am Med Assoc 279:930–937, 1998.

Negredo E, Molto J, Munoz-Moreno JA, et al. Safety and efficacy of once-daily didanosine, tenofovir and nevirapine as a simplification antiretroviral approach. Antivir Ther 9:335–42, 2004.

Panel on Antiretroviral Guidelines for Adults and Adolescents. Guidelines for the use of antiretroviral agents in HIV-1 infected adults and adolescents. Department of Health and Human Services. November 3, 2008; 1–139. Available at http://www.aidsinfor.nih.gov/ContentFiles/AdultandAdolescentGL.pdf

Perry CM, Balfour JA. Didanosine: An update on its antiviral activity, pharmacokinetic properties, and therapeutic efficacy in the management of HIV disease. Drugs 52:928–62, 1996.

Rathbun RC, Martin ES 3rd. Didanosine therapy in patients intolerant of or failing zidovudine therapy. Ann Pharmacother 26:1347–51, 1992.

Website: www.pdr.net

Doripenem (Doribax)

Drug Class: Carbapenem.
Usual Dose: 500 mg–1 gm (IV) q8h.
Spectrum: (see ***Susceptibility Profiles*** pp. 194–199).
Pharmacokinetic Parameters:
Peak serum level: 23 mcg/mL
Bioavailability: Not applicable
Excreted unchanged (urine): 40%
Serum half-life (normal/ESRD): 1/6.20hrs
Plasma protein binding: 8.1%
Volume of distribution (V_d): 16.8 L/kg
Primary Mode of Elimination: Renal
Dosage Adjustments* (based on 1 gm dose; for 500 mg dosing use half of dose shown in grid)

CrCl 25–50 mL/min	1 gm (IV) q12h
CrCl 10–25 mL/min	500 mg (IV) q12h
CrCl < 10 mL/min	500 mg (IV) q24h
Post–HD dose	500 mg (IV)
Post–HFHD dose	500 mg (IV)
Post–PD dose	500 mg (IV)
CVVH dose	1 gm (IV) q12h
SLEDD dose	1 gm (IV) q12h
Moderate hepatic insufficiency	No change
Severe hepatic insufficiency	No change

Drug Interactions: Valproic acid (↓ valproic acid levels).
Adverse Effects: Most common (≥ 5%): headache, nausea, diarrhea, rash, phlebitis, pneumonitis if administered by inhalation (do not give by inhalation).
Allergic Potential: Anaphylaxis has been reported
Safety in Pregnancy: B
Comments: cSSSIs, cIAIs, or UTIs dose: 500 mg (IV) q8h. Administer over 1 hour. ***MDR P. aeruginosa, MDR Acinetobacter baumannii/nosocomial pneumonia dose:*** 1 gm (IV) q8h. **For NP/VAP, infuse IV over 4 hours.**
Cerebrospinal Fluid Penetration: None
Bile Penetration: 117%
(also see ***Antibiotic Pearls & Pitfalls*** pp. 495–508).

REFERENCES:

Anderson DL. Doripenem. Drugs for Today 42:399–404, 2006.

Chastra J, Wunderink R, Prokocimer P, et al. Efficacy and safety of doripenem vs. imipenem for ventilator-associated pneumonia. Presented at the 47th Annual Interscience Conference on Antimicrobial Agents and Chemotherapy; Chicago, IL, 2007.

Chen Y, Garber E, Zhao Q, et al. In vitro activity of doripenem (S-4661) against multidrug-resistance isolated from patients with cystic fibrosis. Antimicrob Agents Chemother 49:2510–2511, 2005.

Credito KL, Ednie LM, Appelbaum PC. Comparative anti-anaerobic activity of doripenem by MIC and time-kill analysis. Antimicrob Agents Chemother 15:epub, 2007.

"Usual dose" assumes normal renal/hepatic function. * For renal insufficiency, give usual dose × 1 followed by maintenance dose per CrCl. For dialysis patients, dose the same as for CrCl < 10 mL/min and give supplemental (post-HD/PD dose) immediately after dialysis. CrCl = creatinine clearance; CVVH = continuous veno-venous hemofiltration; HD/PD = hemodialysis/peritoneal dialysis. See pp. 509–513 for explanations, pp. xi–xii for abbreviations; Linezolid (↑ risk of serotonin syndrome, see p. 620).

Lister PD. Carbapenems in the USA: focus on doripenem. Expert Rev Anti Infect Ther 5:793–809, 2007.

Lucasti C, Jasovich A, Umeh O, et al. Treatment of complicated intra-abdominal infections: doripenem versus meropenem. Presented at the 17th European Congress of Clinical Microbiology and Infectious Diseases; Munich, Germany, 2007.

Mesaros N, Nordman P, Plesiat P, et al. Pseudomonas aeruginosa: resistance and therapeutic options at the turn of the new millennium. Clin Microbiol Infect 13:560–578, 2007.

Naber K, Redman R, Kotey P, et al. Intravenous therapy with doripenem versus levofloxacin with an option for oral step-down therapy in the treatment of complicated urinary tract infection and pyelonephritis. Presented at the 17th European Congress of Clinical Microbiology and Infectious Diseases; Munich, Germany, 2007.

Paterson DL, DePestel DD. Doripenem. Clin Infect Dis 49:291–298, 2009.

Rea-Neto. Efficacy and safety of intravenous doripenem vs. piperacillin/tazobactam in nosocomial pneumonia. Oral presentation at the 47th Annual Interscience Conference on Antimicrobial Agents and Chemotherapy; Chicago, IL, 2007.

Traczewski MM, Brown SD. In vitro activity of doripenem against Pseudomonas aeruginosa and Burkholderia cepacia isolates from both cystic fibrosis and non-cystic fibrosis patients. Antimicrob Agents Chemother 50:819–821, 2006.

Wexler HM, Engel AE, Glass D, et al. In vitro activities of doripenem and comparator agents against 364 anaerobic clinical isolates. Antimicrob Agents Chemother 49:4413–4417, 2005.

Zhanel GG, Wiebe R, Dilay L, et al. Comparative review of the carbapenems. Drugs 67:1027–1052, 2007.

Doxycycline (Vibramycin, Vibra-tabs)

Drug Class: 2nd generation IV/PO tetracycline.

Usual Dose: 100–200 mg (IV/PO) q12h or 200 mg (IV/PO) q24h. For serious systemic infection, begin therapy with a loading dose of 200 mg (IV/PO) q12h × 3 days, then continue at same dose or decrease to 100 mg (IV/PO) q12h to complete therapy (see comments).

Spectrum: (see ***Susceptibility Profiles*** pp. 183–187).

Pharmacokinetic Parameters:

Peak serum level: 100/200 mg = 4/8 mcg/mL
Bioavailability: 93%
Excreted unchanged (urine): 40%
Serum half-life (normal/ESRD): 18-22/18-22 hrs
Plasma protein binding: 93%
Volume of distribution (V_d): 0.75 L/kg

Primary Mode of Elimination: Hepatic

Dosage Adjustments*

CrCl < 10 mL/min	No change
Post–HD or PD dose	None
CVVH dose	No change
Moderate or severe hepatic insufficiency	No change

Drug Interactions: Antacids, Al^{++}, Ca^{++}, Fe^{++}, Mg^{++}, Zn^{++}, multivitamins, sucralfate (↓ doxycycline absorption); barbiturates, carbamazepine, phenytoin (↓ doxycycline half-life); bicarbonate (↓ doxycycline absorption, ↑ doxycycline clearance); warfarin (↑ INR).

Adverse Effects: Nausea if not taken with food. Phlebitis if given IV in inadequate volume. Avoid in pregnancy and children < 8 years.

Allergic Potential: Low

Safety in Pregnancy: D

Comments: Minimal potential for Candida overgrowth/diarrhea. Photosensitivity rare. Tablets better tolerated than capsules. **Absorption minimally effected** by iron, bismuth, milk, or antacids containing Ca^{++}, Mg^{++}, or Al^{++}. Serum half-life increases

"Usual dose" assumes normal renal/hepatic function. * For renal insufficiency, give usual dose × 1 followed by maintenance dose per CrCl. For dialysis patients, dose the same as for CrCl < 10 mL/min and give supplemental (post-HD/PD dose) immediately after dialysis. CrCl = creatinine clearance; CVVH = continuous veno-venous hemofiltration; HD/PD = hemodialysis/peritoneal dialysis. See pp. 509–513 for explanations, pp. xi–xii for abbreviations; Linezolid (↑ risk of serotonin syndrome, see p. 620).

with multiple doses. **GC dose** (not PPNG/TRNG): 100 mg (PO) q12h × 7 days. Meningeal dose = 200 mg (IV/PO) q12h.

Cerebrospinal Fluid Penetration:
Non-Inflamed meninges = 25%
Inflamed meninges = 25%

Bile Penetration: 3000%

(also see ***Antibiotic Pearls & Pitfalls*** pp. 495–508).

REFERENCES:

Berman B, Perez OA, Zell D. Update on rosacea and anti-inflammatory-dose doxycycline. Drugs Today 43:27–34, 2007.

Bernadino ALF, Kaushal D, Philipp MT. The Antibiotics Doxycycline and Minocycline Inhibit the Inflammatory Responses to the Lyme Disease Spirochete *Borrelia burgdorferi*. Journal of Infectious Diseases. 199:1379–1388, 2009.

Borg R, Dotevall L, Hagberg L, et al. Intravenous ceftriaxone compared with oral doxycycline for the treatment of Lyme neuroborreliosis. Scand J Infect Dis 37:449–454, 2005.

Colmenero JD, Munoz-Roca NL, Bermudez P, et al. Clinical findings, diagnostic approach, and outcome of Brucelloa melitensis epididymoorchitis. Diagn Microbiol Infect Dis 57:367–372, 2007.

Cunha BA. Doxycycline for Nursing Home Acquired Pneumonia (NHAP). Scandinavian Journal of Infectious Disease 41:77–78, 2009.

Cunha BA. New uses for older antibiotics: nitrofurantoin, amikacin, colistin, polymyxin B, doxycycline, and minocycline revisited. Med Clin North Am. 90:1089–107, 2006.

Cunha BA. Oral Antibiotic Therapy of Serious Systemic Infections. Med Clin N Am 90:1197–1222, 2006.

Cunha BA. Doxycycline for community-acquired pneumonia. Clin Infect Dis 37:870, 2003.

Cunha BA, Domenico PD, Cunha CB. Pharmacodynamics of doxycycline. Clin Micro Infect Dis 6:270–3, 2000.

Cunha BA. Doxycycline. Antibiotics for Clinicians 3:21–33, 1999.

Cunha BA. Doxycycline re-revisited. Arch Intern Med 159:1006–7, 1999.

Del Rosso JQ, Webster GF, Jackson M, et al. Two randomized phase III clinical trials evaluating anti-inflammatory dose doxycycline (40-mg doxycycline, USP capsules) administered` once daily for treatment of rosacea. J Am Acad Dermatol 56:791–802, 2007.

Haggerty CL, Ness RB. Newest approaches to treatment of pelvic inflammatory disease: a review of recent randomized clinical trials. Clin Infect Dis 44:953–960, 2007.

Hasin T, Davidovitch N, Cohen R, et al. Postexposure Treatment with Doxycycline for the Prevention of Tick-Borne Relapsing Fever. N Engl J Med 355:147–55, 2006.

Hoerauf A, Mand S, Fischer K, et al. Doxycycline as a novel strategy against bancroftian filariasis-depletion of Wolbachia endosymbionts from Wuchereria bancrofti and stop of microfilaria production. Med Microbiol Immunol (Berl). 192:211–6, 2003.

Johnson JR. Doxycycline for treatment of community-acquired pneumonia. Clin Infect Dis 35:632, 2002.

Jones RN, Sader HS, Fritsche TR. Doxycycline use for community-acquired pneumonia: contemporary in vitro spectrum of activity against Streptococcus pneumoniae. Diagn Microbiol Infect Dis 49:147–9, 2004.

Karkkonen K, Stiernstedt SH, Karisson M. Follow-up of patients treated with oral doxycycline for Lyme neuroborreliosis. Scand J Infect Dis 33:259–262, 2001.

Kim YS, Yun HJ, Shim SK, et al. A comparative trial of a single dose of azithromycin versus doxycycline for the treatment of mild scrub typhus. Clin Infect Dis 39:1329–35, 2004.

Lalloo DG, Shingadia D, Pasvol G, et al. UK malaria treatment guidelines. J Infect 54:111–121, 2007.

Mena LA, Mroczkowski TF, Nsuami M, et al. A Randomized Comparison of Azithromycin and Doxycycline for the Treatment of *Mycoplasma* genitalium – positive Urethritis in Men. Clin Infect Dis 48:1649–1654, 2009.

Mouratidis PX, Colston KW, Dalgleish AG. Doxycycline induces caspase-dependent apoptosis in human pancreatic cancer cells. Int J Cancer 120:743–752, 2007.

Naini AE, Harandi AA, Morghtaderi J, et al. Doxycycline: a pilot study to reduce diabetic proteinuria. Am J Nephrol 27:269–273, 2007.

Pappas G, Siozopoulou V, Akritidis N, et al. Doxycycline-rifampicin: physicians' inferior choice in brucellosis or how convenience reigns over science. J Infect 54:459–462, 2007.

Preshaw PM, Grainger P, Bradshaw MH, et al. Subantimicrobial dose doxycycline in the treatment of recurrent oral aphthous ulceration: a pilot study. J Oral Pathol Med 36:235–240, 2007.

Ranjbar M, Keramat F, Mamani M, et al. Comparison between doxycycline-rifampin-amikacin and doxycycline regimens in the treatment of brucellosis. Int J Infect Dis 11:152–156, 2007.

Roushan MRH, Mohraz M, Hajiahmadi M, et al. Efficacy of Gentamycin plus Doxycycline versus Streptomycin plus Doxycycline in the Treatment of Brucellosis in Humans. Clin Infect Dis 42:1075–80, 2006.

Schwartz BS, Graber CJ, Diep BA, et al. Doxycycline, not Minocycline, Induces Its Own Resistance in Multidrug-Resistant Community-Associated Methicillin-Resistant Staphylococcus aureus Clone USA300. Clin Infect Dis 48:1483–1484, 2009.

Shea KW, Ueno Y, Abumustafa F, Cunha BA. Doxycycline activity against Streptococcus pneumoniae. Chest 107:1775–6, 1995.

Solera J, Geijo P, Largo J, et al. A randomized, double-blind study to assess the optimal duration of doxycycline treatment for human brucellosis. Clin Infect Dis 39:1776–82, 2004.

Turner JD, Mand S, Debrah AY, et al. A Randomized, Double-Blind Clinical Trial of a 3-Week Course of Doxycycline plus Albendazole and Ivermectin for the Treatment of Wuchereria bancrofti Infection. Clin Infect Dis 42:1081–9, 2006.

Volovitz B, Shkap R, Amir J, et al. Absence of tooth staining with doxycycline treatment in young children. Clin Pediatr 46:121–126, 2007.

Wormser GP, Hallperin JJ. Oral doxycline for neuroborreliosis. The Lancet Neurology. 7: 2008.

Efavirenz (Sustiva) EFV

Drug Class: Antiretroviral NNRTI (non-nucleoside reverse transcriptase inhibitor).

Usual Dose: 600 mg (PO) q24h.

Pharmacokinetic Parameters:

Peak serum level: 12.9 mcg/mL
Bioavailability: Increased with food
Excreted unchanged (urine): 14–34%
Serum half-life (normal/ESRD): 40–55 hrs/no data
Plasma protein binding: 99%
Volume of distribution (V_d): No data

Primary Mode of Elimination: Hepatic

Dosage Adjustments*

CrCl < 60 mL/min	No change
Post–HD or PD dose	None
CVVH dose	No change
Moderate or severe hepatic insufficiency	No information

Antiretroviral Dosage Adjustments:

Delavirdine	No information
Indinavir	Indinavir 1000 mg q8h
Lopinavir/ritonavir (l/r)	Consider l/r 533/133 mg q12h in PI-experienced patients
Nelfinavir	No changes
Nevirapine	No information
Ritonavir	Ritonavir 600 mg q12h (500 mg q12h for intolerance)
Saquinavir	Avoid use as sole PI
Rifampin	No changes
Rifabutin	Rifabutin 450–600 mg q24h or 600 mg 2–3x/week if not on protease inhibitor

Drug Interactions: Antiretrovirals, rifabutin, rifampin (see dose adjustment grid,

---

"Usual dose" assumes normal renal/hepatic function. * For renal insufficiency, give usual dose × 1 followed by maintenance dose per CrCl. For dialysis patients, dose the same as for CrCl < 10 mL/min and give supplemental (post-HD/PD dose) immediately after dialysis. CrCl = creatinine clearance; CVVH = continuous veno-venous hemofiltration; HD/PD = hemodialysis/peritoneal dialysis. See pp. 509–513 for explanations, pp. xi–xii for abbreviations; Linezolid (↑ risk of serotonin syndrome, see p. 620).

above); astemizole, terfenadine, cisapride, ergotamine, midazolam, triazolam (avoid); carbamazepine, phenobarbital, phenytoin (monitor anticonvulsant levels; use with caution); caspofungin (↓ caspofungin levels, may ↓ caspofungin effect); methadone, clarithromycin (↓ interacting drug levels; titrate methadone dose to effect; consider using azithromycin instead of clarithromycin).

Adverse Effects: Drug fever/rash, CNS symptoms (nightmares, dizziness, neuropsychiatric symptoms, difficulty concentrating, somnolence), ↑ SGOT/SGPT, E. multiforme/Stevens-Johnson syndrome (rare), false positive cannabinoid test.

Allergic Potential: High

Safety in Pregnancy: D

Comments: Rash/CNS symptoms usually resolve spontaneously over 2–4 weeks. Take at bedtime. Avoid taking after high fat meals (levels ↑ 50%). 600-mg dose available as single tablet.

Cerebrospinal Fluid Penetration: 1%

REFERENCES:

Albrecht MA, Bosch RJ, Hammer SM, et al. Nelfinavir, efavirenz, or both after the failure of nucleoside treatment of HIV infection. N Engl J Med 345: 398–407, 2001.

Gallant JE, DeJesus D, Arribas JR, et al. Tenofovir DF, emtricitabine, and efavirenz vs. zidovudine, lamivudine, and efavirenz for HIV. N Engl J Med 354:251–60, 2006.

Go JC, Cunha BA. Efavirenz. Antibiotics for Clinicians 5:1–8, 2001.

Haas DW, Fessel WJ, Delapenha RA, et al. Therapy with efavirenz plus indinavir in patients with extensive prior nucleoside reverse-transcriptase inhibitor experience: A randomized, double-blind, placebo-controlled trial. J Infect Dis 183:392–400, 2001.

la Porte CJ, de Graaff-Teulen MJ, Colbers EP, et al. Effect of efavirenz treatment on the pharmacokinetics of nelfinavir boosted by ritonavir in healthy volunteers. Br J Clin Pharmacol 58:632–40, 2004.

Marzolini C, Telenti A, Decosterd LA, et al. Efavirenz plasma levels can predict treatment failure and central nervous system side effects in HIV-1-infected patients. AIDS 15:71–5, 2001.

Negredo E, Cruz L, Paredes R, et al. Virological, immunological, and clinical impact of switching from protease inhibitors to nevirapine or to efavirenz in patients with human immunodeficiency virus infection and long-lasting viral suppression. Clin Infect Dis 34:504–510, 2002.

Panel on Antiretroviral Guidelines for Adults and Adolescents. Guidelines for the use of antiretroviral agents in HIV-1 infected adults and adolescents. Department of Health and Human Services. November 3, 2008; 1–139. Available at http://www.aidsinfor.nih.gov/ContentFiles/AdultandAdolescentGL.pdf.

Website: www.sustiva.com

Efavirenz + Emtricitabine + Tenofovir disoproxil fumarate (Atripla) EVF/FTC/TDF

Drug Class: Antiretroviral agent.

Usual Dose: 1 tablet (efavirenz 600 mg/emtricitabine 200 mg/tenofovir 300 mg) (PO) q24h on an empty stomach.

Pharmacokinetic Parameters:

Peak serum level: 4.0/1.8 mcg/mL/296 ng/mL

Bioavailability: NR/93%/25%

Excreted unchanged: < 1% unchanged and 14–30% as metabolites/86%/32%

Serum half-life (normal/ESRD): (40–55 hrs/~10 hrs on hemodialysis)/(10 hrs/extended)/(17 hrs/no data)

Plasma protein binding: 99/< 4/< 0.7%

Volume of distribution (V_d): NR/NR/1.2 L/kg

Primary Mode of Elimination: hepatic/renal/renal

Dosage Adjustments*

"Usual dose" assumes normal renal/hepatic function. * For renal insufficiency, give usual dose × 1 followed by maintenance dose per CrCl. For dialysis patients, dose the same as for CrCl < 10 mL/min and give supplemental (post-HD/PD dose) immediately after dialysis. CrCl = creatinine clearance; CVVH = continuous veno-venous hemofiltration; HD/PD = hemodialysis/peritoneal dialysis. See pp. 509–513 for explanations, pp. xi–xii for abbreviations; Linezolid (↑ risk of serotonin syndrome, see p. 620).

CrCl 50–80 mL/min	No change
CrCl 10–50 mL/min	Avoid
CrCl < 10 mL/min	Avoid
Post–HD dose	Avoid
Post–PD dose	Avoid
CVVH dose	Avoid
Mild hepatic insufficiency	No information
Moderate or severe hepatic insufficiency	No information

Antiretroviral Dosage Adjustments:

Fosamprenavir/ ritonavir	An additional 100 mg/day (300 mg total) of ritonavir is recommended when ATRIPLA is administered with fosamprenavir/ ritonavir q24h. No change in ritonaviir dose when ATRIPLA is administered with fosamprenavir/ ritonavir q12h
Atazanavir	Atazanavir 300 mg q24h Ritonavir 100 mg q12h
Indinavir	Indinavir 1000 mg q8h
Lopinavir/ ritonavir	Increase lopinavir/ ritonavir to 600/150 mg (3 tablets) q12h
Ritonavir	No information
Saquinavir	Avoid
Didanosine	Avoid
Rifabutin	Rifabutin 450–600 mg q24h or 600 mg 2–3x/ week if not on protease inhibitor
Rifampin	No change

Drug Interactions: Antiretrovirals, rifabutin (see dose adjustment grid above); astemizole, cisapride, ergotamine, methylergonovine, midazolam, triazolam, St John's Wort (↓ efavirenz levels), voriconazole (↓ voriconazole levels; avoid); caspofungin (↓ caspofungin levels); carbamazepine, phenytoin, phenobarbital (monitor anticonvulsant levels; use with caution; potential for ↓ efavirenz levels); statins (may ↓ statin levels); methadone, (↓ methadone levels); clarithromycin (may ↓ clarithromycin effectiveness, consider using azithromycin). Should not be administered concurrently with astemizole, cisapride, midazolam, triazolam, or ergot derivatives. Significantly reduces voriconazole drug levels.

Adverse Effects: Dizziness, insomnia, impaired concentration, somnolence, abnormal dreaming, euphoria, confusion, agitation, amnesia, hallucinations, stupor, abnormal thinking, and depersonalization. Psychiatric symptoms of depression suicidal ideation, nonfatal suicide attempts, aggressive behavior, paranoid reactions, and manic reactions. Mild to moderate skin rash, Steven's Johnson syndrome. Pancreatitis can occur. Increase in lipids and cholesterol. Immune reconstitution syndrome and redistribution/ accumulation of body fat have been reported in patients treated with combination antiretroviral therapy.

"Usual dose" assumes normal renal/hepatic function. * For renal insufficiency, give usual dose × 1 followed by maintenance dose per CrCl. For dialysis patients, dose the same as for CrCl < 10 mL/min and give supplemental (post-HD/PD dose) immediately after dialysis. CrCl = creatinine clearance; CVVH = continuous veno-venous hemofiltration; HD/PD = hemodialysis/peritoneal dialysis. See pp. 509–513 for explanations, pp. xi–xii for abbreviations; Linezolid (↑ risk of serotonin syndrome, see p. 620).

Allergic Potential: High
Safety in Pregnancy: D
Comments: Rash/CNS effects usually resolve in a few weeks. Take at bedtime on empty stomach. High fat meals can ↑ efavirenz by 50%. Use with caution in patients with history of seizures (↑ risk of convulsions). May cause false positive tests for cannabanoids.
Cerebrospinal Fluid Penetration: 1%

REFERENCES:

Gallant JE, DeJesus E, Arribas JR, et al: Tenofovir DF, emtricitabine, and efavirenz vs. zidovudine, lamivudine, and efavirenz for HIV. N Engl J Med 354:251–260, 2006.

Izzedine H, Aymard G, Launay-Vacher V, et al. Pharmacokinetics of efavirenz in a patient on maintenance haemodialysis. AIDS 14:618–619, 2000.

Panel on Antiretroviral Guidelines for Adults and Adolescents. Guidelines for the use of antiretroviral agents in HIV-1 infected adults and adolescents. Department of Health and Human Services. November 3, 2008; 1–139. Available at http://www.aidsinfor.nih.gov/ContentFiles/AdultandAdolescentGL.pdf

ter Hofstede HJ, de Marie S, Foudraine NA. Clinical features and risk factors of lactic acidosis following long-term antiretroviral therapy: 4 fatal cases. Intl J STD AIDS 11:611–616, 2000.

Website: www.atripla.com

Emtricitabine (Emtriva) FTC

Drug Class: Antiretroviral NRTI (nucleoside reverse transcriptase inhibitor).
Usual Dose: 200 mg (PO) q24h.
Pharmacokinetic Parameters:
Peak serum level: 1.8 mcg/mL
Bioavailability: 93%
Excreted unchanged (urine): 86%
Serum half-life (normal/ESRD): 10 hrs/extended
Plasma protein binding: 4%
Primary Mode of Elimination: Renal
Dosage Adjustments*

CrCl ≥ 50 mL/min	200 mg (PO) q24h
CrCl 30–49 mL/min	200 mg (PO) q48h
CrCl 15–29 mL/min	200 mg (PO) q72h
CrCl < 15 mL/min	200 mg (PO) q96h
Post–HD dose	200 mg (PO) q96h
Post–PD dose	No information
CVVH dose	No information
Moderate or severe hepatic insufficiency	No change

Drug Interactions: No significant interactions with indinavir, stavudine, zidovudine, famciclovir, tenofovir.
Adverse Effects: Lactic acidosis hepatomegaly with steatosis, post treatment exacerbation of hepatitis B. Headache, diarrhea, nausea and rash as well as abdominal pain, fatigue, dizziness abnormal dreams. Rare cases of skin hyperpigmentation on palms and soles. Immune reconstitution syndrome may occur.
Allergic Potential: Low
Safety in Pregnancy: B
Comments: May be taken with or without food. Does not inhibit CYP450 enzymes. Mean intracellular half-live of 39 hours. Potential cross-resistance to lamivudine and zalcitabine. Low affinity for DNA polymerase-gamma. Should not be coadministered with drugs containing lamivudine.
Cerebrospinal Fluid Penetration: No data

"Usual dose" assumes normal renal/hepatic function. * For renal insufficiency, give usual dose × 1 followed by maintenance dose per CrCl. For dialysis patients, dose the same as for CrCl < 10 mL/min and give supplemental (post-HD/PD dose) immediately after dialysis. CrCl = creatinine clearance; CVVH = continuous veno-venous hemofiltration; HD/PD = hemodialysis/peritoneal dialysis. See pp. 509–513 for explanations, pp. xi–xii for abbreviations; Linezolid (↑ risk of serotonin syndrome, see p. 620).

REFERENCES:

Anderson PL. Pharmacologic perspectives for once-daily antiretroviral therapy. Ann Pharmacother 38:1924–34, 2004.

Benson CA, van der Horst C, Lamarca A, et al. A randomized study of emtricitabine and lamivudine in stable suppressed patients with HIV. AIDS 18:2269–2276, 2004.

Dando TM, Wagstaff AJ. Emtricitabine/tenofovir disoproxil fumarate. Drugs 64:2075–82, 2004.

Gallant JE, DeJesus D, Arribas JR, et al. Tenofovir DF, emtricitabine, and efavirenz vs. zidovudine, lamivudine, and efavirenz for HIV. N Engl J Med 354:251–60, 2006.

Lim SG, Ng TN, Kung N, et al. A double-blind placebo-controlled study of emtricitabine in chronic hepatitis B. Arch Intern Med 166:49–56, 2006.

Panel on Antiretroviral Guidelines for Adults and Adolescents. Guidelines for the use of antiretroviral agents in HIV-1 infected adults and adolescents. Department of Health and Human Services. November 3, 2008; 1–139. Available at http://www.aidsinfor.nih.gov/ContentFiles/AdultandAdolescentGL.pdf

Saag MS. Emtricitabine, a new antiretroviral agent with activity against HIV and hepatitis B virus. Clin Infect Dis 42:128–31, 2006.

Website: www.emtriva.com

Emtricitabine + Tenofovir disoproxil fumarate (Truvada) FTC/TDF

Drug Class: Antiretroviral NRTI (nucleoside reverse transcriptase inhibitor) + nucleotide analogue.

Usual Dose: One tablet (PO) q24h (each tablet contains 200 mg of emtricitabine + 300 mg of tenofovir).

Pharmacokinetic Parameters:

Peak serum level: 1.8/0.3 mcg/L

Bioavailability: 93%/27% if fasting (39% with high fat meal)

Excreted unchanged (urine): 86/32%

Serum half-life (normal/ESRD): (10 hrs/extended)/(17 hrs/no data)

Plasma protein binding: 4/0.7–7.2%

Volume of distribution (V_d): no data/1.3 L/kg

Primary Mode of Elimination: Renal/Renal

Dosage Adjustments*

CrCl ≥ 50 mL/min	No change
CrCl 30–49 mL/min	One capsule (PO) q48h
CrCl 15–29 mL/min	Avoid
CrCl < 15 mL/min	Avoid
Post–HD dose	Avoid
Post–PD dose	Avoid
CVVH dose	Avoid
Moderate or severe hepatic insufficiency	No change

Drug Interactions: No significant interactions with indinavir, stavudine, zidovudine, famciclovir, lamivudine, lopinavir/ritonavir, efavirenz, methadone, oral contraceptives. Tenofovir ↑ didanosine levels which may result in severe pancreatitis. Tenofovir reduces systemic exposure to atazanavir; whenever the two are co-administered, the recommended dose of atazanavir is 300 mg once daily with ritonavir 100 mg once daily. Atazanavir may increase tenofovir levels. Avoid coadministration with didanosine.

Adverse Effects: Headache, diarrhea, nausea, vomiting, GI upset, rash, lactic acidosis with hepatic steatosis (rare but potentially life-threatening with NRTI's). Decreases bone mineral density. May result in flare of hepatitis after stopping medication in patients with chronic hepatitis B infection. Cases of osteomalacia and renal tubular acidosis have occurred. Renal dysfunction is more common in diabetic patients. Immune reconstitution

---

"Usual dose" assumes normal renal/hepatic function. * For renal insufficiency, give usual dose × 1 followed by maintenance dose per CrCl. For dialysis patients, dose the same as for CrCl < 10 mL/min and give supplemental (post-HD/PD dose) immediately after dialysis. CrCl = creatinine clearance; CVVH = continuous veno-venous hemofiltration; HD/PD = hemodialysis/peritoneal dialysis. See pp. 509–513 for explanations, pp. xi–xii for abbreviations; Linezolid (↑ risk of serotonin syndrome, see p. 620).

syndrome and redistribution/accumulation of body fat have been reported in patients treated with combination antiretroviral therapy.

Allergic Potential: Low

Safety in Pregnancy: B

Comments: May be taken with or without food. Does not inhibit CYP450 enzymes. Mean intracellular half-life with emtricitabine is 39 hours. Potential cross-resistance to lamivudine, zalcitabine, abacavir, didanosine. Low affinity for DNA polymerase-gamma.

Cerebrospinal Fluid Penetration: No data

REFERENCES:

Dando TM, Wagstaff AJ. Emtricitabine/tenofovir disoproxil fumarate. Drugs 64:2075–82, 2004.

Gallant JE, DeJesus D, Arribas JR, et al. Tenofovir DF, emtricitabine, and efavirenz vs. zidovudine, lamivudine, and efavirenz for HIV. N Engl J Med 354:251–60, 2006.

Panel on Antiretroviral Guidelines for Adults and Adolescents. Guidelines for the use of antiretroviral agents in HIV-1 infected adults and adolescents. Department of Health and Human Services. November 3, 2008; 1–139. Available at http://www.aidsinfor.nih.gov/ContentFiles/AdultandAdolescentGL.pdf

Website: www.truvada.com

Enfuvirtide (Fuzeon) ENF

Drug Class: Antiretroviral fusion inhibitor.

Usual Dose: 90 mg (SC) q12h.

Pharmacokinetic Parameters:

Peak serum level: 4.9 mcg/mL

Bioavailability: 84.3%

Serum half-life (normal/ESRD): 3.8 hrs/no data

Plasma protein binding: 92%

Volume of distribution (V_d): 5.5 L

Primary Mode of Elimination: Metabolized

Dosage Adjustments*

CrCl > 35 mL/min	No change
CrCl < 35 mL/min	No data
Post–HD dose	No data
Post–PD dose	No data
CVVH dose	No data
Moderate or severe hepatic insufficiency	No data

Drug Interactions: No clinically significant interactions with other antiretrovirals. Does not inhibit CYP450 enzymes.

Adverse Effects: Local injection site reactions are common. Diarrhea, nausea, fatigue may occur. Laboratory abnormalities include mild/transient eosinophilia. Pneumonia may occur, but cause is unclear and may not be due to drug therapy. Pancreatitis, myalgia, conjunctivitis (rare).

Allergic Potential: Hypersensitivity reactions may occur, including fever, chills, hypotension, rash, ↑ serum transaminases. Do not rechallenge following a hypersensitivity reaction

Safety in Pregnancy: B

Comments: Enfuvirtide interferes with entry of HIV-1 into cells by blocking fusion of HIV-1 and CD_4 cellular membranes by binding to HR1 in the gp41 subunit of the HIV-1 envelope glycoprotein. Additive/synergistic with NRTI's, NNRTI's, and PI's, and no cross resistance to other antiretrovirals in cell culture. Reconstitute in 1.1 mL of sterile water. SC injection should be given into upper arm, anterior thigh, or abdomen. Rotate injection sites; do not inject into moles, scars, bruises. After reconstitution, use immediately or refrigerate and use within 24 hours (no preservatives added).

"Usual dose" assumes normal renal/hepatic function. * For renal insufficiency, give usual dose × 1 followed by maintenance dose per CrCl. For dialysis patients, dose the same as for CrCl < 10 mL/min and give supplemental (post-HD/PD dose) immediately after dialysis. CrCl = creatinine clearance; CVVH = continuous veno-venous hemofiltration; HD/PD = hemodialysis/peritoneal dialysis. See pp. 509–513 for explanations, pp. xi–xii for abbreviations; Linezolid (↑ risk of serotonin syndrome, see p. 620).

REFERENCES:

Coleman CI, Musial, BL, Ross, J. Enfuvirtide: the first fusion inhibitor for the treatment of patients with HIV-1 infection. Formulary 38:204–222, 2003.

Kilby JM, Lalezari JP, Eron JJ, et al. The safety, plasma pharmacokinetics, and antiviral activity of subcutaneous enfuvirtide (T-20), a peptide inhibitor of gp41-mediated virus fusion, in HIV-infected adults. AIDS Res Hum Retroviruses 18:685–93, 2002.

Lalezari JP, Eron JJ, Carlson M, et al. A phase II clinical study of the long-term safety and antiviral activity of enfuvirtide-based antiretroviral therapy. AIDS 17:691–8, 2003.

Lalezari JP, Henry K, O'Hearn M, et al. TORO 1 Study Group. Enfuvirtide, an HIV-1 fusion inhibitor, for drug-resistant HIV infection in North and South America. N Engl J Med 348:2175–85, 2003.

Lazzarin A, Clotet B, Cooper D, et al. TORO 2 Study Group. Efficacy of enfuvirtide in patients infected with drug-resistant HIV-1 in Europe and Australia. N Engl J Med 348:2186–95, 2003.

Leao J, Frezzini C, Porter S. Enfuvirtide: a new class of antiretroviral therapy for HIV infection. Oral Dis 10:327–9, 2004.

Leen C, Wat C, Nieforth K. Pharmacokinetics of enfuvirtide in a patient with impaired renal function. Clin Infect Dis 4:339–55, 2004.

Panel on Clinical Practices for Treatment of HIV Infection. Guidelines for the Use of Antiretroviral Agents in HIV-Infected Adults and Adolescents. Department of Health and Human Services. www.hivatis.org. January 29, 2008.

Website: www.fuzeon.com

Entecavir (Baraclude)

Drug Class: Antiviral (nucleoside analogue).

Usual Dose: 0.5 mg (PO) q24h; 1 mg (PO) q24h for lamivudine-refractory patients.

Pharmacokinetic Parameters:

Peak serum level: 4.2 ng/mL (for 0.5 mg dose)

Bioavailability: Similar for tablet and oral solution

Excreted unchanged (urine): 62–73%

Serum half-life (normal/ESRD): 128–139 hrs

Plasma protein binding: No information

Volume of distribution (V_d): No information

Primary Mode of Elimination: Renal

Dosage Adjustments* (based on 0.5 mg dose)

CrCl > 50 mL/min	No change
CrCl 30–50 mL/min	0.25 mg (PO) q24h
CrCl 10–30 mL/min	0.15 mg (PO) q24h
CrCl < 10 mL/min	0.05 mg (PO) q24h
Post-HD	None
Post–PD	No information
Moderate or severe hepatic insufficiency	No change

Drug Interactions: No information.

Adverse Effects: Fatigue, headache, upper respiratory tract infection, upper abdominal pain, ↑ ALT, cough, nausea.

Allergic Potential: No information

Safety in Pregnancy: C

Comments: Used to treat chronic hepatitis B infection. Effective in lamivudine-resistant patients. Administer on an empty stomach. Available as tablets and oral solution.

REFERENCES:

[No authors listed]. Entecavir (Baraclude) for chronic hepatitis B. Med Lett Drugs Ther 47:47–8, 2005.

[No authors listed]. Entecavir: A new nucleoside analogue for the treatment of chronic Hepatitis B. Drugs for Today. 43:201–220, 2007.

Chang TT, Gish RG, Hadziyannis SJ, et al. A dose-ranging study of the efficacy and tolerability of entecavir in lamivudine-refractory chronic hepatitis B patients. Gastroenterology 129:1198–209, 2005.

Honkoop P, De Man RA. Entecavir: a potent new antiviral drug for hepatitis B. Expert Opin Investig Drugs 12:683–8, 2003.

Marzella N. Entecavir (Baraclude) for the Treatment of Chronic Hepatitis B Virus (HBV) Infection. Pharmacy & Therapeutics. 31:313–20, 2006.

"Usual dose" assumes normal renal/hepatic function. * For renal insufficiency, give usual dose × 1 followed by maintenance dose per CrCl. For dialysis patients, dose the same as for CrCl < 10 mL/min and give supplemental (post-HD/PD dose) immediately after dialysis. CrCl = creatinine clearance; CVVH = continuous veno-venous hemofiltration; HD/PD = hemodialysis/peritoneal dialysis. See pp. 509–513 for explanations, pp. xi–xii for abbreviations; Linezolid (↑ risk of serotonin syndrome, see p. 620).

Rivkin A. A review of entecavir in the treatment of chronic hepatitis B infection. Curr Med Res Opin. 21:1845–56, 2005.
Rosmawati M, Lao J, et al. Entecavir is superior to lamivudine in reducing hepatitis B virus DNA in patients with chronic hepatitis B infection. Gastroenterology 123:1831–8, 2002.
Shaw T, Locarnini S. Entecavir for the treatment of chronic hepatitis B. Expert Rev Anti Infect Ther 2:853–71, 2004.
Sherman M, Yurdaydin C, et al. Entecavir therapy for lamivudine-refractory chronic hepatitis B: improved virologic, biochemical, and serology outcomes through 96 weeks. Hepatology 48:99–108, 2008.
Sims KA, Woodland AM. Entecavir: For the Treatment of Chronic Hepatitis B Infection. Pharmacotherapy 12:1745–57, 2006.
Website: www.baraclude.com

Ertapenem (Invanz)

Drug Class: Carbapenem.
Usual Dose: 1 gm (IV/IM) q24h.
Spectrum: (see ***Susceptibility Profiles*** pp. 194–199).
Pharmacokinetic Parameters:
Peak serum level: 150 mcg/mL
Bioavailability: 90% (IM)
Excreted unchanged (urine): 40%; 40% excreted as active metabolite
Serum half-life (normal/ESRD): 4/14 hrs
Plasma protein binding: 95%
Volume of distribution (V_d): 0.12 L/kg
Primary Mode of Elimination: Renal
Dosage Adjustments*

CrCl 30–80 mL/min	No change
CrCl < 30 mL/min	500 mg (IV) q24h
Post–HD dose	If dosed < 6 h prior to HD, give 150 mg (IV)
Post–PD dose	No information
CVVH dose	No information
SLEDD dose	500 mg (IV) q24h
Moderate hepatic insufficiency	No change
Severe hepatic insufficiency	No change

* If dosed > 6 h prior to HD, no Post–HD needed

Drug Interactions: Not a substrate/inhibitor of cytochrome P-450 enzymes; probenecid (↓ clearance of ertapenem). Valproic acid (↓ seizure threshold).
Adverse Effects: Mild headache, infrequent nausea or diarrhea. No seizures. Probenecid (↓ clearance of ertapenem).
Allergic Potential: Low
Safety in Pregnancy: B
Comments: Concentration-dependent protein binding. Compared to imipenem, **ertapenem has little activity vs. enterococci, Acinetobacter or P. aeruginosa. Probably safe to use in penicillin allergic patients**. For deep muscle (IM) injection, mix 1 gm with 3.2 mL of 1% lidocaine. Na^+ content = 6 mEq/g.
Cerebrospinal Fluid Penetration: ~5% (also see ***Antibiotic Pearls & Pitfalls*** pp. 495–508).

REFERENCES:

Curran M, Simpson D, Perry C. Ertapenem: a review of its use in the management of bacterial infections. Drugs 63:1855–78, 2003.
Decousser JW, Methlouthi I, Pina P, et al. In vitro activity of ertapenem against bacteremic pneumococci: report of a French multicentre study including 339 strains. Journal of Antimicrobial Chemotherapy 55:396–8, 2005.
Graham DR, Lucasti C, Malafaia O, et al. Ertapenem once daily versus piperacillin-tazobactam 4 times per day for treatment of complicated skin and

"Usual dose" assumes normal renal/hepatic function. * For renal insufficiency, give usual dose × 1 followed by maintenance dose per CrCl. For dialysis patients, dose the same as for CrCl < 10 mL/min and give supplemental (post-HD/PD dose) immediately after dialysis. CrCl = creatinine clearance; CVVH = continuous veno-venous hemofiltration; HD/PD = hemodialysis/peritoneal dialysis. See pp. 509–513 for explanations, pp. xi–xii for abbreviations; Linezolid (↑ risk of serotonin syndrome, see p. 620).

skin-structure infections in adults: results of a prospective, randomized, double-blind multicenter study. Clin Infect Dis 34:1460–8, 2002.

Itani KMF, Wilson SE, Awad SS, et al. Ertapenem versus Cefotetan Prophylaxis in Elective Colorectal Surgery. N Engl J Med 355:2640–51, 2006.

Itani KM, Wilson SE, Awad SS, et al. Polyethylene glycol versus sodium phosphate mechanical bowel preparation in elective colorectal surgery. Am J Surg 193:190–194, 2007.

Lipsky BA, Armstrong DG, Citron DM, et al. Ertapenem versus piperacillin/tazobactam for diabetic foot infections (SIDESTEP): prospective, randomized, controlled, double-blinded, multicentre trial. Lancet 366:1695–703, 2005.

Livermore DM, Sefton AM, Scott GM. Properties and potential of ertapenem. J Antimicrob Chemother 52:331–44, 2003.

Mody RM, Erwin DP, Summers AM, et al. Ertapenem susceptibility of extended spectrum beta-lactamase-producing organisms. Ann Clin Microbiol Antimicrob 6:6, 2007.

Murcia JM, Gonzalez-Comeche J, Marin A, et al. Clinical response to ertapenem in severe community-acquired pneumonia: a retrospective series in an elderly population. Clin Microbiol Infect. 15:1046–1050, 2009.

Musson DG, Majumdar A, Holland S, et al. Pharmacokinetics of total and unbound ertapenem in healthy elderly subjects. Antimicrob Agents Chemother 48:521–4, 2004.

Namias N, Solomkin JS, Jensen EH, et al. Randomized, multicenter, double-blind study of efficacy, safety, and tolerability of intravenous ertapenem versus piperacillin/tazobactam in treatment of complicated intra-abdominal infections in hospitalized adults. Surg Infect 8:15–28, 2007.

Pelak BA, Bartizal K, Woods GL, et al. Comparative in vitro activities of ertapenem against aerobic and facultative bacterial pathogens from patients with complicated skin and skin structure infections. Diagn Microbiol Infect Dis 43:129–33, 2002.

Pelak BA, Woods GI, Teppler H. Comparative in-vitro activities of ertapenem against aerobic bacterial pathogens isolated from patients with complicated intra-abdominal infections. J Chemother 14:227–33, 2002.

Shah PM, Isaacs RD. Ertapenem, the first of a new group of carbapenems. J Antimicrob Chemother 52:538–42, 2003.

Solomkin JS, Yellin AE, Rotstein OD, et al. Ertapenem versus piperacillin/tazobactam in the treatment of complicated intraabdominal infections: results of a double-blind, randomized comparative phase III trial. Ann Surg 237:235–45, 2003.

Teppler H, Gesser RM, Friedland Ir, et al. Safety and tolerability of ertapenem. J Antimicrob Chemother 53:75–81, 2004.

Tice AD, Turpin RS, Hoey CT, et al. Comparative costs of ertapenem and piperacillin-tazobactam in the treatment of diabetic foot infections. Am J Health Syst Pharm 64:1080–1086, 2007.

Vetter N, Cambronero-Hernandez E, Rohlf J, et al. A prospective, randomized, double-blind multicenter comparison of parenteral ertapenem and ceftriaxone for the treatment of hospitalized adults with community-acquired pneumonia. Clin Ther 24:1770–85, 2002.

Yakovlev SV, Stratchounskin LS, Woods GL, et al. Ertapenem versus cefepime for initial empirical treatment of pneumonia acquired in skilled-care facilities or in hospitals outside the intensive care unit. Eur J Clin Micro Inf Dis 25:633–641, 2006.

Yellin AE, Johnson J, Higareda I, et al. Ertapenem or ticarcillin/clavulanate for the treatment of intra-abdominal infections or acute pelvic infections in pediatric patients. Am J Surg 194:367–374, 2007.

Website: www.invanz.com

Erythromycin lactobionate, base (various)

Drug Class: Macrolide.

Usual Dose: 1 gm (IV) q6h; 500 mg (PO) q6h (Take without food).

Spectrum: (see ***Susceptibility Profiles*** pp. 183–187).

Pharmacokinetic Parameters:

Peak serum level: 12 (IV);1.2 (PO) mcg/mL

Bioavailability: 50%

"Usual dose" assumes normal renal/hepatic function. * For renal insufficiency, give usual dose × 1 followed by maintenance dose per CrCl. For dialysis patients, dose the same as for CrCl < 10 mL/min and give supplemental (post-HD/PD dose) immediately after dialysis. CrCl = creatinine clearance; CVVH = continuous veno-venous hemofiltration; HD/PD = hemodialysis/peritoneal dialysis. See pp. 509–513 for explanations, pp. xi–xii for abbreviations; Linezolid (↑ risk of serotonin syndrome, see p. 620).

Excreted unchanged (urine): 5%; 5% exerted as active metabolite
Serum half-life (normal/ESRD): 1.4/5.4 hrs
Plasma protein binding: 80%
Volume of distribution (V_d): 0.5 L/kg
Primary Mode of Elimination: Hepatic
Dosage Adjustments*

CrCl 50–80 mL/min	No change
CrCl 10–50 mL/min	No change
CrCl < 10 mL/min	No change
Post-HD/PD dose	None
CVVH dose	No change
Moderate or severe hepatic insufficiency	No change

Drug Interactions: Amiodarone, procainamide, sotalol, astemizole, terfenadine, cisapride, pimozide (may ↑ QT interval, torsade de pointes); carbamazepine (↑ carbamazepine levels, nystagmus, nausea, vomiting, diarrhea; avoid combination); cimetidine, digoxin, ergot alkaloids, felodipine, midazolam, triazolam, phenytoin, ritonavir, tacrolimus, valproic acid (↑ interacting drug levels); clozapine (↑ clozapine levels; CNS toxicity); corticosteroids (↑ corticosteroid effect); cyclosporine (↑ cyclosporine levels with toxicity); efavirenz (↓ erythromycin levels); rifabutin, rifampin (↓ erythromycin levels, ↑ interacting drug levels); statins (↑ risk of rhabdomyolysis); theophylline (↑ theophylline levels, nausea, vomiting, seizures, apnea); warfarin (↑ INR); zidovudine (↓ zidovudine levels).
Adverse Effects: Nausea, vomiting, GI upset, irritative diarrhea, abdominal pain, phlebitis. May ↑ QT_c; avoid with other medications that prolong the QT_c interval and in patients with cardiac arrhythmias/heart block.
Allergic Potential: Low
Safety in Pregnancy: B
Comments: Do not mix erythromycin with B/C vitamins, glucose solutions, cephalothin, tetracycline, chloramphenicol, heparin, or warfarin. Increases GI motility and QT_c interval. **Limited anti-Legionella activity. S. pneumoniae resistance problematic.**
Cerebrospinal Fluid Penetration: < 10% (also see ***Antibiotic Pearls & Pitfalls*** pp. 495–508).

REFERENCES:

Alvarez-Elcoro S, Enzler MJ. The macrolides: Erythromycin, clarithromycin and azithromycin. Mayo Clin Proc 74:613–34, 1999.

Amsden GW. Erythromycin, clarithromycin, and azithromycin: Are the differences real? Clinical Therapeutics 18:572, 1996.

Bergman M, Huikko S, Huovinen P, et al. Macrolide and azithromycin use are linked to increased macrolide resistance in *Streptococcus pneumoniae*. Antimicrob Agents Chemother 50:3646–3650, 2006.

Cunha BA. The virtues of doxycycline and the evils of erythromycin. Adv Ther 14:172–80, 1997.

Daneman N, McGeer A, Green K, et al. Macrolide resistance in bacteremic pneumococcal disease.: Implications for patient management. Clin Infect Dis 43:432–438, 2006.

Gagliotti C, Nobilio L, Milandri M, et al. Macrolide Prescriptions and Erythyromycin Resistance or Streptococcus pyogenes. Clin Infect Dis 42:1153–6, 2006.

Jain R, Danzinger LH. The macrolide antibiotics: a pharmacokinetic and pharmacodynamic overview. Curr Pharm Des 10:3045–53, 2004.

Jenkins SG, Farrell DJ. Increase in Pneumococcus Macrolide Resistance, United States. Emerging Infect Dis 15:1260–1264, 2009.

Mandell LA, Wunderdink RG, Anzuetto A, et al. Infectious Diseases Society of America/American Thoracic Society consensus guidelines on the management of community-acquired pneumonia in adults. Clin Infect Dis 44:S27–72, 2007.

"Usual dose" assumes normal renal/hepatic function. * For renal insufficiency, give usual dose × 1 followed by maintenance dose per CrCl. For dialysis patients, dose the same as for CrCl < 10 mL/min and give supplemental (post-HD/PD dose) immediately after dialysis. CrCl = creatinine clearance; CVVH = continuous veno-venous hemofiltration; HD/PD = hemodialysis/peritoneal dialysis. See pp. 509–513 for explanations, pp. xi–xii for abbreviations; Linezolid (↑ risk of serotonin syndrome, see p. 620).

Smilack JD, Wilson WE, Cocerill FR 3rd. Tetracycline, chloramphenicol, erythromycin, clindamycin, and metronidazole. Mayo Clin Proc 66:1270–80, 1991.
Suzuki S, Yamazaki T, Narita M. Clinical Evaluation of Macrolide-Resistant Mycoplasma pneumoniae. Antimocrobial Agents and Chemotherapy. 50:709–12, 2006.
Website: www.pdr.net

Ethambutol (Myambutol) EMB

Drug Class: Anti-TB drug.
Usual Dose: 15 mg/kg (PO) q24h (see comments).
Pharmacokinetic Parameters:
Peak serum level: 2–5 mcg/mL
Bioavailability: 80%
Excreted unchanged (urine): 50%
Serum half-life (normal/ESRD): 4/10 hrs
Plasma protein binding: 20%
Volume of distribution (V_d): 2 L/kg
Primary Mode of Elimination: Renal/hepatic
Dosage Adjustments*

CrCl > 40 mL/min	No change
CrCl < 40 mL/min	No change
Post-HD/PD dose	None
CVVH dose	No change
Moderate or severe hepatic insufficiency	No change

Drug Interactions: Aluminum salts, didanosine buffer (↓ ethambutol and interacting drug absorption).
Adverse Effects: Drug fever/rash, ↓ visual acuity, central scotomata, color blindness (red-green), metallic taste, mental confusion, peripheral neuropathy, ↑ uric acid.
Allergic Potential: Low
Safety in Pregnancy: B
Comments: Optic neuritis may occur with high doses (≥ 15 mg/kg/day). TB D.O.T. dose: 4 gm (PO) 2x/week or 3 gm (PO) 3x/week. MAI dose: 15 mg/kg (PO) q24h (with azithromycin 500 mg [PO] q24h)
Meningeal dose = 25 mg/kg (PO) q24h.
Cerebrospinal Fluid Penetration:
Non-Inflamed meninges = 1%
Inflamed meninges = 40%

REFERENCES:

Chaisson RE, Keiser P, Pierce M, et al. Clarithromycin and ethambutol with or without clofazimine for the treatment of bacteremic Mycobacterium avium complex disease in patients with HIV infection. AIDS 11:311–317, 1997.
Davidson PT, Le HQ. Drug treatment of tuberculosis 1992. Drugs 43:651–73, 1992.
Drugs for tuberculosis. Med Lett Drugs Ther 35:99–101, 1993.
McIlleron H, Wash P, Burger A, et al. Determinants of Rifampin, Isoniazid, Pyrazinamide and Ethambutol Pharmacokinetics in a Cohort of Tuberculosis Patients. Antimicrob Agents Chemother 50:1170–77, 2006.
Perlman DC, Segal Y, Rosenkranz S, et al. The clinical pharmacokinetics of rifampin and ethambutol in HIV-infected persons with tuberculosis. Clinical Infectious Disease 41:1638–47, 2005.
Schlossberg D. Treatment of multi-drug resistant tuberculosis. Antibiotics for Clinicians 9:317–21, 2005.
Van Scoy RE, Wilkowske CJ. Antituberculous agents. Mayo Clin Proc 67:179–87, 1992.

Ethionamide (Trecator)

Drug Class: Anti-TB drug.
Usual Dose: 500 mg (PO) q12h.
Pharmacokinetic Parameters:
Peak serum level: 5 mcg/mL
Bioavailability: 99%
Excreted unchanged (urine): 1%
Serum half-life (normal/ESRD): 2/9 hrs

"Usual dose" assumes normal renal/hepatic function. * For renal insufficiency, give usual dose × 1 followed by maintenance dose per CrCl. For dialysis patients, dose the same as for CrCl < 10 mL/min and give supplemental (post-HD/PD dose) immediately after dialysis. CrCl = creatinine clearance; CVVH = continuous veno-venous hemofiltration; HD/PD = hemodialysis/peritoneal dialysis. See pp. 509–513 for explanations, pp. xi–xii for abbreviations; Linezolid (↑ risk of serotonin syndrome, see p. 620).

Plasma protein binding: 30%
Volume of distribution (V_d): No data
Primary Mode of Elimination: Renal/hepatic
Dosage Adjustments*

CrCl 40–60 mL/min	No change
CrCl < 40 mL/min	No change
Post-HD/PD dose	No information
CVVH dose	No information
Moderate hepatic insufficiency	No change
Severe hepatic insufficiency	500 mg (PO) q24h

Drug Interactions: Cycloserine (↑ neurologic toxicity); ethambutol (↑ GI distress, neuritis, hepatotoxicity); INH (peripheral neuritis, hepatotoxicity); pyrazinamide, rifampin (hepatotoxicity).
Adverse Effects: ↑ SGOT/SGPT, headache, nausea/vomiting, abdominal pain, tremor, olfactory abnormalities, alopecia, gynecomastia, hypoglycemia, impotence, neurotoxicity (central/peripheral neuropathy).
Allergic Potential: Low
Safety in Pregnancy: C
Comments: Additive toxicity with thiacetazone.
Cerebrospinal Fluid Penetration: 100%

REFERENCES:
Davidson PT, Le HQ. Drug treatment of tuberculosis 1992. Drugs 43:651–73, 1992.
Drugs for tuberculosis. Med Lett Drugs Ther 35:99–101, 1993.
Furin J, Nardell EA. Multidrug-resistant tuberculosis: An update on the best regimens. J Respir Dis 27:172–82, 2006.
Iseman MD. Treatment of multidrug resistant tuberculosis. N Engl J Med 329:784–91, 1993.
Schlossberg D. Treatment of multi-drug resistant tuberculosis. Antibiotics for Clinicians 9:317–321, 2005.

Famciclovir (Famvir)

Drug Class: HSV Antiviral, (see comments).
Usual Dose:
HSV-1: Meningitis/Encephalitis: 500 mg (PO) q8h × 10 days.
VZV: Chickenpox: 500 mg (PO) q8h × 5 days.
VZV Pneumonia: 500 mg (PO) q8h × 7–10 days.
Pharmacokinetic Parameters:
Peak serum level: 3.3 mcg/mL
Bioavailability: 77%
Excreted unchanged (urine): 60%
Serum half-life (normal/ESRD): 2.5/13 hrs
Plasma protein binding: 20%
Volume of distribution (V_d): 1.1 L/kg
Primary Mode of Elimination: Renal
Dosage Adjustments for HSV/VZV* (based on 250 mg [PO] q8h/500 mg [PO] q8h)

CrCl 40–60 mL/min	No change 500 mg (PO) q12h
CrCl 20–40 mL/min	125 mg (PO) q24h 500 mg (PO) q24h
CrCl < 20 mL/min	125 mg (PO) q24h 250 mg (PO) q24h
Post–HD dose	125 mg (PO) 250 mg (PO)
Post–PD dose	No information
CVVH dose	No information
Moderate hepatic insufficiency	No change
Severe hepatic insufficiency	No information

Drug Interactions: Digoxin (↑ digoxin levels).

"Usual dose" assumes normal renal/hepatic function. * For renal insufficiency, give usual dose × 1 followed by maintenance dose per CrCl. For dialysis patients, dose the same as for CrCl < 10 mL/min and give supplemental (post-HD/PD dose) immediately after dialysis. CrCl = creatinine clearance; CVVH = continuous veno-venous hemofiltration; HD/PD = hemodialysis/peritoneal dialysis. See pp. 509–513 for explanations, pp. xi–xii for abbreviations; Linezolid (↑ risk of serotonin syndrome, see p. 620).

Adverse Effects: Headache, seizures/tremors (dose related), nausea, diarrhea.
Allergic Potential: Low
Safety in Pregnancy: B
Comments: 99% converted to penciclovir in liver/GI tract. ***Highly active against HSV, VZV, and HHV-6. Some activity against CMV. No activity against EBV, RSV or adenoviruses.*** Meningeal dose = VZV dose.
Cerebrospinal Fluid Penetration: 50%

REFERENCES:

Alrabiah FA, Sacks SL. New anti-herpesvirus agents. Their targets and therapeutic potential. Drugs 52:17–32, 1996.

Chakrabarty A, Tyring SK, Beutner K, et al. Recent clinical experience with famciclovir-a "third generation" nucleoside prodrug. Antivir Chem Chemother 15:251–3, 2004.

Luber AD, Flaherty JF Jr. Famciclovir for treatment of herpesvirus infections. Ann Pharmacother 30:978–85, 1996.

Smith DE, Gold J. Famciclovir or valacyclovir in the management of herpes simplex and varicella zoster infections: an attitudinal survey of clinician perceptions or differential activity. Sex Health 4:141–142, 2007.

Website: www.famvir.com

Fluconazole (Diflucan)

Drug Class: Antifungal.
Usual Dose: 400 mg (IV/PO) × 1 dose, then 200 mg (IV/PO) q24h (see comments).
Pharmacokinetic Parameters:
Peak serum level: 6.7 mcg/mL
Bioavailability: 90%
Excreted unchanged (urine): 80%; 11% excreted as active metabolite
Serum half-life (normal/ESRD): 27/100 hrs
Plasma protein binding: 12%
Volume of distribution (V_d): 0.7 L/kg

Primary Mode of Elimination: Renal
Dosage Adjustments*

CrCl 50–80 mL/min	No change
CrCl 10–50 mL/min	100 mg (IV/PO) q24h
CrCl < 10 mL/min	100 mg (IV/PO) q24h
Post–HD dose	200 mg (IV/PO)
Post–PD dose	200 mg (IV/PO)
CVVH dose	No change
Moderate hepatic insufficiency	No change
Severe hepatic insufficiency	No change

Drug Interactions: Astemizole, cisapride, terfenadine, amiodarone (may ↑ QT interval, torsades de pointes); cyclosporine, oral hypoglycemics, tacrolimus, theophylline, zidovudine (↑ interacting drug levels with possible toxicity); hydrochlorothiazide (↑ fluconazole levels); phenytoin, rifabutin, rifampin (↓ fluconazole levels, ↑ interacting drug levels); warfarin (↑ INR).
Adverse Effects: Not hepatotoxic. Hypokalemia.
Allergic Potential: Low
Safety in Pregnancy: C
Comments: Usual dose for candidemia (C. albicans) = 400 mg (IV/PO) q24h after loading dose of 800 mg (IV/PO). Not effective against most non-albicans candida. Meningeal dose = 400 mg (IV/PO) q24h. ***Highly active against C. albicans, C. tropicalis, C. parasilosis, and C. lusitaniae. Some activity (dose dependent) against C. glabrata. No activity against C. krusei or Aspergillus. Highly active against Candida, Cryptococcus, Histoplasmosis, Blastomycosis,***

"Usual dose" assumes normal renal/hepatic function. * For renal insufficiency, give usual dose × 1 followed by maintenance dose per CrCl. For dialysis patients, dose the same as for CrCl < 10 mL/min and give supplemental (post-HD/PD dose) immediately after dialysis. CrCl = creatinine clearance; CVVH = continuous veno-venous hemofiltration; HD/PD = hemodialysis/peritoneal dialysis. See pp. 509–513 for explanations, pp. xi–xii for abbreviations; Linezolid (↑ risk of serotonin syndrome, see p. 620).

Sporotrichosis, Penicillum marneffei, Paracoccidiomycosis, Coccidiomycosis.
Some activity against Fusarium, Naegleria, Leishmania, or Mucor.
No activity against C. lusitaniae, Pseudoallescheria, or Trichosporon.

Cerebrospinal Fluid Penetration:
Non-Inflamed meninges = 80%
Inflamed meninges = 80%

REFERENCES:

Bruggemann RJM, Alffenaar JWC, Blijlevens NMA, et al. Clinical Relevance of the Pharmoacokinetic Interactions of Azole Antifungal Drugs with Coadministered Agents. Clin Infect Dis 48:1441–1458, 2009.

Cha R, Sobel JD. Fluconazole for the treatment of candidiasis: 15 years experience. Expert Rev Anti Infect Ther 2:357–66, 2004.

Clancy CJ, Yu VL, Morris AJ, et al. Fluconazole MIC and fluconazole dose/MIC ratio correlate with therapeutic response among patients with candidemia. Antimicrobial Agents and Chemotherapy 49:3171–3177, 2005.

Hamza OJM, Matee MIN, Bruggemann RJM, et al. Single-Dose Fluconazole versus Standard 2-Week Therapy for Oropharyngeal Candidiasis in HIV-Infected Patients: A Randomized, Double-Blind, Double-Dummy Trial. Clin Infect Dis 47:1270–1276, 2008.

Goa KL, Barradell LB. Fluconazole: An update of its pharmacodynamics and pharmacokinetic properties and therapeutic use in major superficial and systemic mycoses in immunocompromised patients. Drugs 50:658–90, 1995.

Kauffman CA, Carver PL. Antifungal agents in the 1990s: Current status and future developments. Drugs 53:539–49, 1997.

Kobayashi CC, de Fernandes OF, Miranda KC, et al. Candiduria in hospital patients: a study prospective. Mycopathologia 158:49–52, 2004.

Koh LP, Kurup A, Goh YT, et al. Randomized trial of fluconazole versus low-dose amphotericin B in prophylaxis against fungal infections in patients undergoing hematopoietic stem cell transplantation. Am J Hematol 71:260–7, 2002.

Kowalsky SF, Dixon DM. Fluconazole: A new antifungal agent. Clin Pharmacol 10:179–94, 1991.

MacMillan ML, Goodman JL, DeFor Te, et al. Fluconazole to prevent yeast infections in bone marrow transplantation patients: a randomized trial of high versus reduced dose and determination of the value of maintenance therapy. Am J Med 112:369–79, 2002.

Nussbaum JC, Jackson A, Namarika D, et al. Combination Flucytosine and High-Dose Fluconazole Compared with Fluconazole Monotherapy for the Treatment of Cryptococcal Meningitis: A Randomized Trial in Malawi. Clin Infect Dis 50:338–344, 2010.

Owens RC, Ambrose PG. Fluconazole. Antibiotics for Clinicians 1:109–117, 1997.

Pappas PG, Chetchotisakd P, Larsen RA, et al. A Phase II Randomized Trial of Amphotericin B Alone or Combined with Fluconazole in the Treatment of HIV-Associated Cryptococcal Meningitis. Clin Infect Dis 48:1775–1784, 2009.

Perfect JR, Dismukes WE, Dromer F, et al. Clinical Practice Guidelines for the Management of Cryptococcal Disease: 2010 Update by the Infectious Disease Society of America. Clin Infect Dis 50:291–322, 2010.

Reboli AC, Rotstein C, Pappas PG, et al. Anidulafungin versus fluconazole for invasive candidiasis. N Engl J Med 356:2472–82, 2007.

Rex JH, Pappas PG, Karchmer AW, et al. National Institute of Allergy and Infectious Diseases Mycoses Study Group. A randomized and blinded multicenter trial of high-dose fluconazole plus placebo versus fluconazole plus amphotericin B as therapy for candidemia and its consequences in nonneutropenic subjects. Clin Infect Dis 36:1221–8, 2003.

Sabatelli F. Patel R, Mann PA, et al. In vitro activities of posaconazole, fluconazole, itraconazole, voriconazole, and amphotericin B against a large collection of clinically important molds and yeasts. Antimicrob Agents Chemother 50:2009–15, 2006.

Terrell CL. Antifungal agents: Part II. The azoles. Mayo Clin Proc 74:78–100, 1999.

"Usual dose" assumes normal renal/hepatic function. * For renal insufficiency, give usual dose × 1 followed by maintenance dose per CrCl. For dialysis patients, dose the same as for CrCl < 10 mL/min and give supplemental (post-HD/PD dose) immediately after dialysis. CrCl = creatinine clearance; CVVH = continuous veno-venous hemofiltration; HD/PD = hemodialysis/peritoneal dialysis. See pp. 509–513 for explanations, pp. xi–xii for abbreviations; Linezolid (↑ risk of serotonin syndrome, see p. 620).

Testore GP, Dori L, Buonomini AR, et al. In vitro fluconazole susceptibility of 1565 clinical isolates of candida species evaluated by the disk diffusion method performed using NCCLS M44-A guidelines. Diagn Microbiol Infect Dis 50:187–92, 2004.

Website: www.diflucan.com

Flucytosine (Ancobon) 5-FC

Drug Class: Antifungal.
Usual Dose: 25 mg/kg (PO) q6h.
Pharmacokinetic Parameters:
Peak serum level: 3.5 mcg/ml
Bioavailability: 80%
Excreted unchanged (urine): 90%
Serum half-life (normal/ESRD): 4/85 hrs
Plasma protein binding: 4%
Volume of distribution (V_d): 0.6 L/kg
Primary Mode of Elimination: Renal
Dosage Adjustments*

CrCl 50–80 mL/min	500 mg (PO) q12h
CrCl 10–50 mL/min	500 mg (PO) q18h
CrCl < 10 mL/min	500 mg (PO) q24h
Post–HD dose	500 mg (PO)
Post–PD dose	500 mg (PO)
CVVH dose	500 mg (PO) q18h
Moderate or severe insufficiency	No change

Drug Interactions: Cytarabine (↓ flucytosine effect); zidovudine (neutropenia).
Adverse Effects: Leukopenia, anemia, thrombocytopenia, nausea, vomiting, abdominal pain, ↑ SGOT/SGPT, drug fever/rashes.
Allergic Potential: High
Safety in Pregnancy: C
Comments: Always use in combination with amphotericin B for cryptococcal meningitis. ***Highly active against Cryptococcus neoformans. Some activity against C. albicans. No activity against other yeasts/fungi.*** Meningeal dose = usual dose.
Cerebrospinal Fluid Penetration:
Non-Inflamed meninges = 100%
Inflamed meninges = 100%

REFERENCES:

Lyman CA, Walsh TJ. Systemically administered antifungal agents. A review of their clinical pharmacology and therapeutic applications: Part I. Amphotericin B preparations and flucytosine. Mayo Clin Proc 73:1205–25, 1998.
Mosquera J, Shartt A, Moore CB, et al. In vitro interaction of terbinafine with itraconazole, fluconazole, amphotericin B and 5-flucytosine against Aspergillus spp. J Antimicrob Chemother 50:189–94, 2002.
Nussbaum JC, Jackson A, Namarika D, et al. Combination Flucytosine and High-Dose Fluconazole Compared with Fluconazole Monotherapy for the Treatment of Cryptococcal Meningitis: A Randomized Trial in Malawi. Clin Infect Dis 50:338–344, 2010.
Pfaller MA, Messer SA, Boyken L, et al. In vitro activities of 5-fluorocytosine against 8,803 clinical isolates of Candida spp.: Global assessment of primary resistance using National Committee for Clinical Laboratory Standards susceptibility testing methods. Antimicrob Agents Chemother 46:3518–3521, 2002.
Perfect JR, Dismukes WE, Dromer F, et al. Clinical Practice Guidelines for the Management of Cryptococcal Disease: 2010 Update by the Infectious Disease Society of America. Clin Infect Dis 50:291–322, 2010.
Te Dorsthorst DT, Verweij PE, Meletidis J, et al. In vitro interaction of flucytosine combined with amphotericin B or fluconazole against thirty-five yeast isolates determined by both the fractional inhibitory concentration index and the response surface approach. Antimicrob Agents Chemother 46:2982–9, 2002.

"Usual dose" assumes normal renal/hepatic function. * For renal insufficiency, give usual dose × 1 followed by maintenance dose per CrCl. For dialysis patients, dose the same as for CrCl < 10 mL/min and give supplemental (post-HD/PD dose) immediately after dialysis. CrCl = creatinine clearance; CVVH = continuous veno-venous hemofiltration; HD/PD = hemodialysis/peritoneal dialysis. See pp. 509–513 for explanations, pp. xi–xii for abbreviations; Linezolid (↑ risk of serotonin syndrome, see p. 620).

Wintermeyer SM, Mahata MC. Stability of flucytosine in an extemporaneously compounded oral liquid. Am J Health Syst Pharm 53:407–9, 1996.
Website: www.pdr.net

Fosamprenavir (Lexiva) FPV

Drug Class: Antiretroviral protease inhibitor.
Usual Dose: 1400 mg (PO) q12h (without ritonavir); in combination with ritonavir: either 1400 mg (PO) q24h plus ritonavir 200 mg (PO) q24h or 700 mg (PO) q12h plus ritonavir 100 mg (PO) q12h. For PI-experienced patients: 700 mg (PO) q12h plus ritonavir 100 mg (PO) q12h.
Pharmacokinetic Parameters:
Peak serum level: 4.8 mcg/mL
Bioavailability: No data
Excreted unchanged (urine) (urine): 1%
Serum half-life (normal/ESRD): 7 hrs/no data
Plasma protein binding: 90%
Volume of distribution (V_d): 6.1 L/kg
Primary Mode of Elimination: Hepatic
Dosage Adjustments*

CrCl 50–80 mL/min	No change
CrCl 10–50 mL/min	No change
CrCl < 10 mL/min	No change
Post–HD or PD dose	No change
CVVH dose	No change
Mild-moderate hepatic insufficiency (Child-Pugh score 5–8)	700 mg (PO) q12h if given without ritonavir; no data with ritonavir
Severe hepatic insufficiency (Child-Pugh score 9–12)	Avoid

Antiretroviral Dosage Adjustments:

Didanosine	Administer didanosine 1 hour apart
Delavirdine	Avoid combination
Efavirenz	Fosamprenavir 700 mg q12h + ritonavir 100 mg q12h + efavirenz; fosamprenavir 1400 mg q24h + ritonavir 200 mg q24h + efavirenz; no data for fosamprenavir 1400 mg q12h + efavirenz
Indinavir	No information
Lopinavir/ ritonavir	Avoid
Nelfinavir	No information
Nevirapine	Avoid
Saquinavir	No information
Rifampin	Avoid combination
Rifabutin	Reduce usual rifabutin dose by 50% (or 75% if given with fosamprenavir plus ritonavir; max. 150 mg q48h)

Drug Interactions: Antiretrovirals (see dose adjustment grid, above). Contraindicated with: ergot derivatives, cisapride, midazolam, triazolam, pimozide, (flecainide and propafenone if administered with ritonavir). Do not coadminister with: rifampin, lovastatin, simvastatin, St. John's wort, delavirdine. Dose reduction (of other drug): atorvastatin, rifabutin, sildenafil, vardenafil, ketoconazole, itraconazole. Concentration monitoring (of other drug): amiodarone, systemic lidocaine, quinidine, warfarin (INR), tricyclic antidepressants, cyclosporin, tacrolimus,

"Usual dose" assumes normal renal/hepatic function. * For renal insufficiency, give usual dose × 1 followed by maintenance dose per CrCl. For dialysis patients, dose the same as for CrCl < 10 mL/min and give supplemental (post-HD/PD dose) immediately after dialysis. CrCl = creatinine clearance; CVVH = continuous veno-venous hemofiltration; HD/PD = hemodialysis/peritoneal dialysis. See pp. 509–513 for explanations, pp. xi–xii for abbreviations; Linezolid (↑ risk of serotonin syndrome, see p. 620).

sirolimus. H_2 blockers and proton pump inhibitors interfere with absorption. Sildenafil (do not give > 25 mg/48 hrs); tadalafil (max. 10 mg/72 hrs); vardenafil (max. 2.5 mg/72 hrs). May increase methadone effect/decrease methadone dose.
Adverse Effects: Rash, Stevens-Johnson syndrome (rare), GI upset, headache, depression, diarrhea, hyperglycemia (including worsening diabetes, new-onset diabetes, DKA), ↑ cholesterol/triglycerides (evaluate risk for coronary disease/pancreatitis), fat redistribution, ↑ SGOT/SGPT, possible increased bleeding in hemophilia. Immune reconstitution syndrome.
Allergic Potential: High. Fosamprenavir is a sulfonamide; use with caution in patients with sulfonamide allergies
Safety in Pregnancy: C
Comments: Usually given in conjunction with ritonavir. May be taken with or without food. Fosamprenavir is a prodrug that is rapidly hydrolyzed to amprenavir by gut epithelium during absorption. Amprenavir inhibits CYP3A4. Fosamprenavir contains a sulfonamide moiety (as do darunavir and tipranavir).

REFERENCES:

Becker S, Thornton L. Fosamprenavir: advancing HIV protease inhibitor treatment options. Expert Opin Pharmacother 5:1995–2005, 2004.

Chapman TM, Plosker GL, Perry CM. Fosamprenavir: a review of its use in the management of antiretroviral therapy-naive patients with HIV infection. Drugs 64:2101–24, 2004.

Lexiva (fosamprenavir) approved. AIDS Treat News 31;2, 2003.

Panel on Antiretroviral Guidelines for Adults and Adolescents. Guidelines for the use of antiretroviral agents in HIV-1 infected adults and adolescents. Department of Health and Human Services. November 3, 2008; 1–139. Available at http://www.aidsinfor.nih.gov/ContentFiles/AdultandAdolescentGL.pdf

Rodriguez-French A, Boghossian J, Gray GE, et al. The NEAT study: a 48–week open-label study to compare the antiviral efficacy and safety of GW433908 versus nelfinavir in antiretroviral therapy-naive HIV-1-infected patients. J Acquir Immune Defic Syndr 35:22–32, 2004.

Website: www.TreatHIV.com

Foscarnet (Foscavir)

Drug Class: CMV Antiviral; (see comments).
Usual Dose: <u>HSV:</u> 40 mg/kg (IV) q12h × 2–3 weeks; <u>CMV:</u> 90 mg/kg (IV) q12h × 2 weeks (induction dose), then 90–120 mg/kg (IV) q24h (maintenance dose) for life-long suppression. Relapse/reinduction dose: 120 mg/kg (IV) q24h × 2 weeks.
Pharmacokinetic Parameters:
Peak serum level: 150 mcg/ml
Bioavailability: Not applicable
Excreted unchanged (urine): 85%
Serum half-life (normal/ESRD): 2–4/25 hrs
Plasma protein binding: 17%
Volume of distribution (V_d): 0.5 L/kg
Primary Mode of Elimination: Renal /hepatic
Dosage Adjustments*

Induction	
CrCl 50–80 mL/min	40–50 mg/kg (IV) q8h
CrCl 20–50 mL/min	20–30 mg/kg (IV) q8h
CrCl < 20 mL/min	Avoid
Maintenance	
CrCl 50–80 mL/min	60–70 mg/kg (IV) q24h
CrCl 20–50 mL/min	65–80 mg/kg (IV) q48h
CrCl < 20 mL/min	Avoid
Post–HD dose	60 mg/kg (IV)
Post–hi-flux HD dose	60 mg/kg (IV)
Post–PD dose	None

"Usual dose" assumes normal renal/hepatic function. * For renal insufficiency, give usual dose × 1 followed by maintenance dose per CrCl. For dialysis patients, dose the same as for CrCl < 10 mL/min and give supplemental (post-HD/PD dose) immediately after dialysis. CrCl = creatinine clearance; CVVH = continuous veno-venous hemofiltration; HD/PD = hemodialysis/peritoneal dialysis. See pp. 509–513 for explanations, pp. xi–xii for abbreviations; Linezolid (↑ risk of serotonin syndrome, see p. 620).

CVVH dose	Induction: 20–30 mg/kg (IV) q8h; maintenance: 65–80 mg/kg (IV) q48h
Mod. hepatic insufficiency	No change
Severe hepatic insufficiency	No change

Infusion pump must be used. Adequate hydration is recommended to prevent renal toxicity
† Higher doses may be considered for early reinduction due to progression of CMV retinitis, and for patients showing excellent tolerance

Drug Interactions: Ciprofloxacin (↑ risk of seizures); amphotericin B, aminoglycosides, cis-platinum, cyclosporine, other nephrotoxic drugs (↑ nephrotoxicity); pentamidine IV (severe hypocalcemia reported; do not combine); zidovudine (↑ incidence/severity of anemia).

Adverse Effects: Major side effects include nephrotoxicity and tetany (from ↓ Ca^{++}). Others include anemia, nausea, vomiting, GI upset, headache, seizures, peripheral neuropathy, hallucinations, tremors, nephrogenic DI, ↓ Ca^{++}, ↓ Mg^{++}, ↓ $PO_4^{=}$, oral/genital ulcers.

Allergic Potential: Low

Safety in Pregnancy: C

Comments: Renal failure prevented/minimized by adequate hydration. Dilute with 150 cc normal saline per 1 gm foscarnet. Do not mix with other types of solutions. Administer by IV slow infusion ≤ 1 mg/kg/min using an infusion pump. ***Highly active against CMV. Some activity against HSV and VZV. No activity against EBV, RSV or adenoviruses.*** Meningeal dose = usual dose.

Cerebrospinal Fluid Penetration:
Non-Inflamed meninges = 90%
Inflamed meninges = 100%

REFERENCES:

De Clercq E. Antiviral drugs in current clinical use. J Clin Virol 30:115–33, 2004.

Derary G, Martinez F, Katlama C, et al. Foscarnet nephrotoxicity: Mechanism, Incidence and prevention. Am J Nephrol 9:316–21, 1989.

Mattes FM, Hainsworth EG, Geretti AM, et al. A randomized, controlled trial comparing ganciclovir plus foscarnet (each at half dose) preemptive therapy of cytomegalovirus infection in transplant recipients. J Infect Dis 189:1355–61, 2004.

Website: www.pdr.net

Fosfomycin (Monurol)

Drug Class: Urinary antiseptic.

Usual Dose: 3 gm (PO) q24h.

Spectrum: (see ***Susceptibility Profiles*** pp. 194–199).

Pharmacokinetic Parameters:

Peak serum level: 26 mcg/ml
Bioavailability: 37%
Excreted unchanged (urine): 60%; 40% excreted as active metabolite
Serum half-life (normal/ESRD): 5.7/50 hrs
Plasma protein binding: 3%
Volume of distribution (V_d): 2 L/kg

Primary Mode of Elimination: Renal

Dosage Adjustments*

CrCl 50–80 mL/min	No change
CrCl 10–50 mL/min	No change
CrCl < 10 mL/min	Use with caution
Post–HD dose	3 gm (PO)
Post–PD dose	1 gm (PO)

"Usual dose" assumes normal renal/hepatic function. * For renal insufficiency, give usual dose × 1 followed by maintenance dose per CrCl. For dialysis patients, dose the same as for CrCl < 10 mL/min and give supplemental (post-HD/PD dose) immediately after dialysis. CrCl = creatinine clearance; CVVH = continuous veno-venous hemofiltration; HD/PD = hemodialysis/peritoneal dialysis. See pp. 509–513 for explanations, pp. xi–xii for abbreviations; Linezolid (↑ risk of serotonin syndrome, see p. 620).

CVVH dose	No change
Moderate or severe hepatic insufficiency	No change

Drug Interactions: Antacids, metoclopramide (↓ fosfomycin effect).

Adverse Effects: Nausea, vomiting, diarrhea, GI upset, ↑ SGOT/SGPT, thrombocytosis.

Allergic Potential: Low

Safety in Pregnancy: B

Comments: Take without food. **Useful for cystitis/CAB**, not pyelonephritis/urosepsis. Treat cystitis × 3 days in males, or single dose in females. **Only oral antibiotic active against MDR P. aeruginosa, MDR Klebsiella pneumoniae, and MDR Acinetobacter baumanii in urine** (*cystitis/CAB*). (also see ***Antibiotic Pearls & Pitfalls*** pp. 495–508).

REFERENCES:

Falagas ME, Kastoris AC, Kapaskelis AM, et al. Fosfamycin for the treatment of multidrug-resistant, including extended-spectrum B-lactamase producing, Enterobacteriaceae infections. The Lancet 10:43–50, 2010.

Gosden PE, Reeves DS. Fosfomycin. Antibiotics for Clinicians 2:121–28, 1998.

Monden K, Ando E, Iida M, et al. Role of fosfomycin in a synergistic combination with ofloxacin against Pseudomonas aeruginosa growing in a biofilm. J Infect Chemother 8:218–26, 2002.

Okazaki M, Suzuki K, Asano N, et al. Effectiveness of fosfomycin combined with other antimicrobial agents against multidrug-resistant Pseudomonas aeruginosa isolates using the efficacy time index assay. J Infect Chemother 8:37–42, 2002.

Patel SS, Balfour JA, Bryson HM. Fosfomycin tromethamine: Pharmacokinetic properties and therapeutic efficacy as a single-dose oral treatment for acute uncomplicated low urinary tract infections. Drugs 53:637–56, 1997.

Sauermann R, Karch R, Langenberger H, et al. Antibiotic abscess penetration: fosfomycin levels measured in pus and simulated concentration-time profiles. Antimicrobial Agents and Chemotherapy 49:4448–4454, 2005.

Shrestha NK, Chua JD, Tuohy MJ, et al. Antimicrobial susceptibility of vancomycin-resistant enterococcus faecium: potential utility of fosfomycin. Scand J Infect Dis 35:12–14, 2003.

Ungheri D, Albini E, Belluco G. In-vitro susceptibility of quinolone-resistant clinical isolates of Escherichia coli to fosfomycin trometamol. J Chemother 14:237–40, 2002.

Website: www.pdr.net

Ganciclovir (Cytovene)

Drug Class: CMV Antiviral; (see comments), nucleoside inhibitor/analogue.

Usual Dose: 5 mg/kg (IV) q12h × 2 weeks (induction), then 5 mg/kg (IV) q24h or 1 gm (PO) q8h (maintenance).

Pharmacokinetic Parameters:

Peak serum level: 8.3 (IV)/1.2 (PO) mcg/ml

Bioavailability: 5%

Excreted unchanged (urine): 90%

Serum half-life (normal/ESRD): 3.6/28 hrs

Plasma protein binding: 1%

Volume of distribution (V_d): 0.74 L/kg

Primary Mode of Elimination: Renal

Dosage Adjustments*

CrCl 50–80 mL/min	2.5 mg/kg (IV) q12h (induction); 2.5 mg/kg (IV) q24h (maintenance); 500 mg (PO) q8h
CrCl 25–50 mL/min	2.5 mg/kg (IV) q24h (induction); 1.25 mg/kg (IV) q24h (maintenance); 500 mg (PO) q12h

"Usual dose" assumes normal renal/hepatic function. * For renal insufficiency, give usual dose × 1 followed by maintenance dose per CrCl. For dialysis patients, dose the same as for CrCl < 10 mL/min and give supplemental (post-HD/PD dose) immediately after dialysis. CrCl = creatinine clearance; CVVH = continuous veno-venous hemofiltration; HD/PD = hemodialysis/peritoneal dialysis. See pp. 509–513 for explanations, pp. xi–xii for abbreviations; Linezolid (↑ risk of serotonin syndrome, see p. 620).

CrCl 10–25 mL/min	1.25 mg/kg (IV) q24h (induction); 0.625 mg/kg (IV) q24h (maintenance); 500 mg (PO) q24h
CrCl < 10 mL/min	1.25 mg/kg (IV) 3x/week (induction); 0.625 mg/kg (IV) 3x/week (maintenance); 500 mg (PO) 3x/week
Post–HD dose	1.25 mg/kg (IV) (induction); 0.625 mg/kg (IV) (maintenance); 500 mg (PO)
Post–PD dose	None
CVVH dose	see CrCl 50–80 mL/min
Moderate hepatic insufficiency	No change
Severe hepatic insufficiency	No change

Drug Interactions: Cytotoxic drugs (may produce additive toxicity: stomatitis, bone marrow depression, alopecia); imipenem (↑ risk of seizures); probenecid (↑ ganciclovir levels); zidovudine (↓ ganciclovir levels, ↑ zidovudine levels, possible neutropenia).

Adverse Effects: Headaches, hallucinations, seizures/tremor (dose related), drug fever/rash, diarrhea, nausea/vomiting, GI upset, leukopenia, thrombocytopenia, anemia, retinal detachment. Ventricular arrhythmias (VT/torsades de pointes).

Allergic Potential: High

Safety in Pregnancy: C

Comments: Induction doses usually given IV. Maintenance doses may be given IV or PO.

CMV CAP dose: 2.5 mg/kg (IV) q8h × 20 doses plus IVIG 500 mg/kg (IV) q48h × 10 doses; then follow with 5 mg/kg (IV) 3–5x/week × 20 doses plus IVIG 500 mg/kg (IV) 2x/week × 8 doses. Reduce dose with neutropenia/thrombocytopenia. Bioavailability increased with food: 5% fasting; 6–9% with food; 28–31% with fatty food. Na^+ content = 4.0 mEq/g. ***Highly active against CMV, HHV-6, and HSV. Some activity against VZV and adenoviruses. No activity against RSV.*** Meningeal dose = usual dose.

Cerebrospinal Fluid Penetration: 70%

REFERENCES:

Czock D, Scholle C, Rasche FM, et al. Pharmacokinetics of valganciclovir and ganciclovir in renal impairment. Clin Pharmacol Ther 72:142–50, 2002.

Matthews T, Boehme R. Antiviral activity and mechanism of action of ganciclovir. Rev Infect Dis 10:490–4, 1988.

Paya CV, Wilson JA, Espy MJ, et al. Preemptive use of oral ganciclovir to prevent cytomegalovirus infection in liver transplant patients: a randomized, placebo-controlled trial J Infect Dis 185:861–7, 2002.

Singh N. Preemptive therapy for cytomegalovirus with oral ganciclovir after liver transplantation. Transplantation 73:1977–78, 2002.

Tokimasa S, Hara J, Osugi Y, et al. Ganciclovir is effective for prophylaxis and treatment of human herpesvirus-6 in allogeneic stem cell transplantation. Bone Marrow Transplant 29:595–8, 2002.

Website: www.rocheusa.com/Products/

Gatifloxacin (Tequin)

Drug Class: Fluoroquinolone.

Usual Dose: 400 mg (IV/PO) q24h.

Pharmacokinetic Parameters:

Peak serum level: 4.6 (IV)/4.2 (PO) mcg/ml

Bioavailability: 96%

Excreted unchanged (urine): 70%

Serum half-life (normal/ESRD): 11/30 hrs

"Usual dose" assumes normal renal/hepatic function. * For renal insufficiency, give usual dose × 1 followed by maintenance dose per CrCl. For dialysis patients, dose the same as for CrCl < 10 mL/min and give supplemental (post-HD/PD dose) immediately after dialysis. CrCl = creatinine clearance; CVVH = continuous veno-venous hemofiltration; HD/PD = hemodialysis/peritoneal dialysis. See pp. 509–513 for explanations, pp. xi–xii for abbreviations; Linezolid (↑ risk of serotonin syndrome, see p. 620).

Plasma protein binding: 20%
Volume of distribution (V_d): 2 L/kg
Primary Mode of Elimination: Renal
Dosage Adjustments*

CrCl 50–80 mL/min	No change
CrCl 10–50 mL/min	200 mg (IV/PO) q24h
CrCl < 10 mL/min	200 mg (IV/PO) q24h
Post–HD/PD dose	200 mg (IV/PO)
CVVH dose	200 mg (IV/PO) q24h
Moderate hepatic insufficiency	No change
Severe hepatic insufficiency	No information

Drug Interactions: Al^{++}, Fe^{++}, Mg^{++}, Zn^{++} antacids, citrate/citric acid, dairy products (↓ absorption of gatifloxacin only if taken together); amiodarone, procainamide, sotalol (may ↑ QT_c interval, torsade de pointes); digoxin (↑ digoxin levels 18–56%, ↑ digoxin effects); insulin, oral hypoglycemics (hypoglycemia); probenecid (↑ gatifloxacin levels); NSAIDs (CNS stimulation).

Adverse Effects: Headache, dizziness, nausea, diarrhea, vomiting, vaginitis, hypoglycemia > hyperglycemia (*contraindicated in diabetics*). Does not lower seizure threshold or cause seizures.

Allergic Potential: Low
Safety in Pregnancy: C
Comments: Nausea common GI side effect. Take 4 hours before aluminum/magnesium-containing antacids; not affected by calcium-containing antacids. Does not ↑ QT_c interval > 3 msec. C8-methoxy group increases activity and decreases resistance potential. TB dose (alternate drug in multi-drug resistant TB drug regimen): 400 mg (PO) q24h. ***Contraindicated in diabetics***.
Cerebrospinal Fluid Penetration: 36%
Bile Concentration: 500%

REFERENCES:

Arguedas A, Sher L, Lopez E, et al. Open label, multicenter study of gatifloxacin treatment of recurrent otitis media and acute otitis media treatment failure. Pediatr Infect Dis J. 22:949–56, 2003.

Capparelli EV, Reed MD, Bradley JS, et al. Pharmacokinetics of gatifloxacin in infants and children. Antimicrobial Agents and Chemotherapy 49:1106–1112, 2005.

Correa JC, Badaro R, Bumroongkit C, et al. Randomized, open-label, parallel-group, multicenter study of the efficacy and tolerability of IV gatifloxacin with the option for oral stepdown gatifloxacin versus IV ceftriaxone (with or without erythromycin or clarithromycin) with the option for oral stepdown clarithromycin for treatment of patients with mild to moderate community-acquired pneumonia requiring hospitalization. Clin Ther. 25:1453–68, 2003.

Dawis MA, Isenberg HD, France KA, et al. In vitro activity of gatifloxacin alone and in combination with cefepime, meropenem, piperacillin and gentamicin against multidrug-resistant organisms. J Antimicrob Chemother 51:1203–11, 2003.

Fish DN, North DS. Gatifloxacin, an advanced 8-methoxy fluoroquinolone. Pharmacotherapy 21:35–59, 2001.

Mignot A, Guillaume M, Gohler K, et al. Oral bioavailability of gatifloxacin in healthy volunteers under fasting and fed conditions. Chemotherapy 48:111–5, 2002.

Nicolau DP, Ambrose PG. Pharmacodynamic profiling of levofloxacin and gatifloxacin using Monte Carlo simulation for community-acquired isolates of Streptococcus pneumoniae. Am J Med 111(Suppl 9A):13S–18S; discussion 36S–38S, 2001.

Nicholson SC, High KP, Gothelf S, Webb CD. Gatifloxacin in community-based treatment of acute respiratory tract infections in the elderly. Diagn Microbiol Infect Dis 44:109–16, 2002.

"Usual dose" assumes normal renal/hepatic function. * For renal insufficiency, give usual dose × 1 followed by maintenance dose per CrCl. For dialysis patients, dose the same as for CrCl < 10 mL/min and give supplemental (post-HD/PD dose) immediately after dialysis. CrCl = creatinine clearance; CVVH = continuous veno-venous hemofiltration; HD/PD = hemodialysis/peritoneal dialysis. See pp. 509–513 for explanations, pp. xi–xii for abbreviations; Linezolid (↑ risk of serotonin syndrome, see p. 620).

Nicholson SC, Webb CD, Andriole VT, et al. Haemophilus influenzae in respiratory tract infections in community-based clinical practice: therapy with gatifloxacin. Diagn Microbiol Infect Dis 44:101–7, 2002.
Pankey GA, Ashcraft DS. In vitro synergy of ciprofloxacin and gatifloxacin against ciprofloxacin-resistant pseudomonas aeruginosa. Antimicrobial Agents and Chemotherapy 49:2959–2964, 2005.
Perry CM, Ormrod D, Hurst M, et al. Gatifloxacin: a review of its use in the management of bacterial infections. Drugs 62:169–207, 2002.
Rolston KV, Vaziri I, Frisbee-Hume S, et al. In vitro antimicrobial activity of gatifloxacin compared with other quinolones against clinical isolates from cancer patients. Chemotherapy 50:214–20, 2004.
Saravolatz LD, Leggett J. Gatifloxacin, gemifloxacin, and moxifloxacin: the role of 3 newer fluoroquinolones. Clin Infect Dis 37:1210–5, 2003.
Sethi S. Gatifloxacin in community-acquired respiratory tract infection. Expert Opin Pharmacother. 4:1847–55, 2003.
Sher LD, McAdoo MA, Bettis RB, et al. A multicenter, randomized, investigator-blinded study of 5- and 10-day gatifloxacin versus 10-day amoxicillin/clavulanate in patients with acute bacterial sinusitis. Clin Ther 24:269–81, 2002.
Schlossberg D. Treatment of multi-drug resistant tuberculosis. Antibiotics for Clinicians 9:317–321, 2005.
Tarshis GA, Miskin BM, Jones TM, et al. Once-daily oral gatifloxacin versus oral levofloxacin in treatment of uncomplicated skin and soft tissue infections: double-blind, multicenter, randomized study. Antimicrob Agents Chemother 45:2358–62, 2001.
White RL, Enzweiler KA, Friedrich LV, et al. Comparative activity of gatifloxacin and other antibiotics against 4009 clinical isolates of Streptococcus pneumoniae in the United States during 1999–2000. Diagn Microbiol Infect Dis 43:207–17, 2002.
Website: www.tequin.com

Gemifloxacin (Factive)

Drug Class: Fluoroquinolone.
Usual Dose: 320 mg (PO) q24h.

Pharmacokinetic Parameters:
Peak serum level: 1.6 mcg/ml
Bioavailability: 71%
Excreted unchanged (urine): 36%; 36% excreted as active metabolites
Serum half-life (normal/ESRD): 7/10 hrs
Plasma protein binding: 55–73%
Volume of distribution (V_d): 4.2 L/kg
Primary Mode of Elimination: Renal
Dosage Adjustments*

CrCl > 40 mL/min	No change
CrCl < 40 mL/min	160 mg (PO) q24h
CrCl < 10 mL/min	160 mg (PO) q24h
Post–HD dose	160 mg (PO)
Post–PD dose	None
Post–CVVH dose	160 mg (PO) q24h
Moderate hepatic insufficiency	No change
Severe hepatic insufficiency	No change

Drug Interactions: Al^{++}, Fe^{++}, Mg^{++}, Zn^{++} antacids/multivitamins, didanosine, sucralfate (↓ gemifloxacin levels only if taken together); probenecid (↑ gemifloxacin levels); amiodarone, quinidine, procainamide, sotalol (may ↑ QTc interval, torsade de pointes; avoid).
Adverse Effects: Rash, ↑ LFTs (doses > 320 mg/d). Does not lower seizure threshold or cause seizures.
Allergic Potential: Low
Safety in Pregnancy: C
Comments: Take at least 3 hours before or 2 hours after calcium/magnesium containing antacids. Take at least 2 hours before sucralfate. May ↑ QT_c interval > 3 msec.; avoid taking with other medications that prolong the

"Usual dose" assumes normal renal/hepatic function. * For renal insufficiency, give usual dose × 1 followed by maintenance dose per CrCl. For dialysis patients, dose the same as for CrCl < 10 mL/min and give supplemental (post-HD/PD dose) immediately after dialysis. CrCl = creatinine clearance; CVVH = continuous veno-venous hemofiltration; HD/PD = hemodialysis/peritoneal dialysis. See pp. 509–513 for explanations, pp. xi–xii for abbreviations; Linezolid (↑ risk of serotonin syndrome, see p. 620).

QT_c interval, and in patients with prolonged QT interval/heart block. Do not exceed usual dose.
Cerebrospinal Fluid Penetration: < 10%.

REFERENCES:

Chagan L. Gemifloxacin for the treatment of acute bacterial exacerbation of chronic bronchitis and community-acquired pneumonia. P&T 28:769–79, 2003.

File Jr. TM, Clinical implications and treatment of multiresistant Streptococcus pneumoniae pneumonia. Clin Microbiol Infect. 12:31–41, 2006.

File TM Jr, Tillotson GS. Gemifloxacin: a new, potent fluoroquinolone for the therapy of lower respiratory tract infections. Expert Rev Anti Infect Ther 2:831–43, 2004.

Gemifloxacin (factive). Med Lett Drugs Ther 46:78–9, 2004.

Goldstein EJ. Review of the in vitro activity of gemifloxacin against gram-positive and gram-negative anaerobic pathogens. J Antimicrob Chemother 45:55–65, 2000.

Hammerschlag MR. Activity of gemifloxacin and other new quinolones against Chlamydia pneumoniae: A review. J Antimicrob Chemother 45:35–9, 2000.

Islinger F, Bouw R, Stahl M, et al. Concentrations of gemifloxacin at the target site in healthy volunteers after a single oral dose. Antimicrob Agents Chemother 48:4246–9, 2004.

Saravolatz LD, Leggett J. Gatifloxacin, gemifloxacin, and moxifloxacin: the role of 3 newer fluoroquinolones. Clin Infect Dis 37:1210–5, 2003.

Waites KB, Crabb DM, Duffy LB. Inhibitory and bactericidal activities of gemifloxacin and other antimicrobials against Mycoplasma pneumoniae. Int J Antimicrob Agents 21:574–7, 2003.

Wilson R, Langan C, Ball P, et al. Oral gemifloxacin once daily for 5 days compared with sequential therapy with i.v. ceftriaxone/oral cefuroxime (maximum of 10 days) in the treatment of hospitalized patients with acute exacerbations of chronic bronchitis. Respir Med 97:242–9, 2003.

Website: www.factive.com

Gentamicin (Garamycin)

Drug Class: Aminoglycoside.
Usual Dose: 5–7 mg/kg (IV) q24h or 240 mg (IV) q24h (preferred over q8h dosing) (see comments).
Spectrum: (see ***Susceptibility Profiles*** pp. 194–199).
Pharmacokinetic Parameters:
Peak serum levels: 4–8 mcg/ml (q8h dosing); 16–24 mcg/ml (q24h dosing)
Bioavailability: Not applicable
Excreted unchanged (urine): 95%
Serum half-life (normal/ESRD): 2.5/48 hrs
Plasma protein binding: < 5%
Volume of distribution (V_d): 0.3 L/kg
Primary Mode of Elimination: Renal
Dosage Adjustments (based on 5 mg/kg)*

CrCl 50–80 mL/min	2.5 mg/kg (IV) q24h or 120 mg (IV) q24h
CrCl 10–50 mL/min	2.5 mg/kg (IV) q48h or 120 mg (IV) q48h
CrCl < 10 mL/min	1.25 mg/kg (IV) q48h or 80 mg (IV) q48h
Post–HD dose	1 mg/kg (IV) or 80 mg (IV)
Post–PD dose	0.5 mg/kg (IV) or 40 mg (IV)
Post–HFHD dose	2.5 mg/kg or 120 mg (IV)
Post-SLEDD dose	2.5 mg/kg (IV) or 120 mg (IV)
CVVH dose	2.5 mg/kg (IV) or 120 mg (IV) q48h

"Usual dose" assumes normal renal/hepatic function. * For renal insufficiency, give usual dose × 1 followed by maintenance dose per CrCl. For dialysis patients, dose the same as for CrCl < 10 mL/min and give supplemental (post-HD/PD dose) immediately after dialysis. CrCl = creatinine clearance; CVVH = continuous veno-venous hemofiltration; HD/PD = hemodialysis/peritoneal dialysis. See pp. 509–513 for explanations, pp. xi–xii for abbreviations; Linezolid (↑ risk of serotonin syndrome, see p. 620).

Moderate hepatic insufficiency	No change
Severe hepatic insufficiency	No change

Drug Interactions: Amphotericin B, cephalothin, cyclosporine, enflurane, methoxyflurane, NSAIDs, polymyxin B, radiographic contrast, vancomycin (↑ nephrotoxicity); cis-platinum (↑ nephrotoxicity, ↑ ototoxicity); loop diuretics (↑ ototoxicity); neuromuscular blocking agents, magnesium sulfate (↑ apnea, prolonged paralysis); non-polarizing muscle relaxants (↑ apnea).

Adverse Effects: Neuromuscular blockade with rapid infusion/absorption. Nephrotoxicity only with prolonged/extremely high serum trough levels; may cause reversible non-oliguric renal failure (ATN). Ototoxicity associated with prolonged/extremely high peak serum levels (usually irreversible): Cochlear toxicity (1/3 of ototoxicity) manifests as decreased high frequency hearing, but deafness is unusual. Vestibular toxicity (2/3 of ototoxicity) develops before ototoxicity, and typically manifests as tinnitus.

Allergic Potential: Low

Safety in Pregnancy: C

Comments: Synergy dose: 2.5 mg/kg (IV) q24h or 120 mg (IV) q24h. **Single daily dosing virtually eliminates nephrotoxic/ototoxic potential**. Incompatible with solutions containing β-lactams, erythromycin, chloramphenicol, furosemide, sodium bicarbonate. IV infusion should be given slowly over 1 hour. **May be given IM. Avoid intraperitoneal infusion due to risk of neuromuscular blockade**. Avoid intratracheal/aerosolized intrapulmonary instillation, which predisposes to antibiotic resistance. V_d increases with edema/ascites, trauma, burns, cystic fibrosis; may require ↑ dose. V_d decreases with dehydration, obesity; may require ↓ dose. **Renal cast counts are the best indicator of aminoglycoside nephrotoxicity, not serum creatinine**. Dialysis removes ~ 1/3 of gentamicin from serum. **CAPD dose:** 2–4 mg/L dialysate (IP) with each exchange.

Therapeutic Serum Concentrations (for therapeutic efficacy, *not toxicity*):
Peak (q24h/q8h dosing) = 16–24/8–10 mcg/ml
Trough (q24h/q8h dosing) = 0/1–2 mcg/ml

Intrathecal (IT) dose: 5 mg (IT) q24h.

Cerebrospinal Fluid Penetration:
Non-Inflamed meninges = 0%
Inflamed meninges = 20%

Bile Penetration: 30%

(also see ***Antibiotic Pearls & Pitfalls*** pp. 495–508).

REFERENCES:

Bruss JB. Lack of evidence associating nephrotoxicity with low-dose gentamicin for *Staphylococcus aureus* bacteremia and endocarditis. Clin Infect Dis 49:806, 2009.

Cornely OA, Bethe U, Seifert H, et al. A randomized monocentric trial in febrile neutropenic patients: ceftriaxone and gentamicin vs cefepime and gentamicin. Ann Hematol 81:37–43, 2002.

Cosgrove SE,Vigliani GA, Campion M, et al. Initial Low-Dose Gentamicin for *Staphylococcus aureus* Bacteremia and Endocarditis is Nephrotoxic. Clin Infect Dis 48:713–721, 2009.

Cunha BA. Aminoglycosides: Current role in antimicrobial therapy. Pharmacotherapy 8:334–50, 1988.

Edson RS, Terrell CL. The aminoglycosides. Mayo Clin Proc 74:519–28, 1999.

Freeman CD, Nicolau DP, Belliveau PP, et al. Once-daily dosing of aminoglycosides: Review and recommendations for clinical practice. J Antimicrob Chemother 39:677–86, 1997.

Hassoun A, Spera R, Dunkel J. Tularemia and Once-Daily Gentamycin. Antimicrob Agents Chemother 50:824, 2006.

"Usual dose" assumes normal renal/hepatic function. * For renal insufficiency, give usual dose × 1 followed by maintenance dose per CrCl. For dialysis patients, dose the same as for CrCl < 10 mL/min and give supplemental (post-HD/PD dose) immediately after dialysis. CrCl = creatinine clearance; CVVH = continuous veno-venous hemofiltration; HD/PD = hemodialysis/peritoneal dialysis. See pp. 509–513 for explanations, pp. xi–xii for abbreviations; Linezolid (↑ risk of serotonin syndrome, see p. 620).

Krol V, Cunha BA, Schoch PE, Klein NC. Appropriateness of empiric gentamicin and vancomycin therapy for bacteremias in chronic dialysis outpatient units in the era of antibiotic resistance. J Chemother 18:490–3, 2006.
Roushan MRH, Mohraz M, Hajiahmadi M, et al. Efficacy of Gentamicin plus Doxycycline versus Streptomycin plus Doxycycline in the Treatment of Brucellosis in Humans. Clin Infect Dis 42:1075–1080, 2006.
Snydman, DR, McDermott LA, Jacobus NV. Evaluation of in vitro interaction of daptomycin with gentamicin or beta-lactam antibiotics against Staphylococcus aureus and Enterococci by FIC index and timed-kill curves. J Chemother 17:614–21, 2005.

Griseofulvin (Fulvicin, Grifulvin, Ultra, Gris-PEG, Grisactin)

Drug Class: Antifungal.
Usual Dose: 500 mg-1 gm (PO) q24h (microsize); 330–375 mg (PO) q24h (ultramicrosize).
Pharmacokinetic Parameters:
Peak serum level: 1–2 mcg/mL
Bioavailability: 50%
Excreted unchanged (urine): 1%
Serum half-life (normal/ESRD): 9/22 hrs
Plasma protein binding: 84%
Volume of distribution (V_d): No data
Primary Mode of Elimination: Hepatic
Dosage Adjustments*

CrCl 50–80 mL/min	No change
CrCl 10–50 mL/min	No change
CrCl < 10 mL/min	No change
Post–HD or PD dose	None
CVVH dose	No change
Moderate hepatic insufficiency	No change
Severe hepatic insufficiency	Use with caution

Drug Interactions: Alcohol (↑ griseofulvin toxicity); barbiturates (↓ griseofulvin levels); oral contraceptives, warfarin (↓ interacting drug levels).
Adverse Effects: Photosensitivity reactions, headache, nausea, vomiting, diarrhea, angular stomatitis, glossitis, leukopenia.
Allergic Potential: Moderate
Safety in Pregnancy: C
Comments: May exacerbate SLE/acute intermittent porphyria. Take microsize griseofulvin with fatty meal to ↑ absorption to ~ 70%. Ultramicrosize griseofulvin is absorbed 1.5 times better than microsize griseofulvin.

REFERENCES:

Trepanier EF, Amsden GW. Current issues in onychomycosis. Ann Pharmacotherapy 32:204–14, 1998.
Website: www.pdr.net

Imipenem/Cilastatin (Primaxin)

Drug Class: Carbapenem.
Usual Dose: 500 mg-1 gm (IV) q6h (see comments).
Spectrum: (see ***Susceptibility Profiles*** pp. 194–199).
Pharmacokinetic Parameters:
Peak serum level: 21–58 mcg/ml (500 mg dose)
Bioavailability: Not applicable
Excreted unchanged (urine): 70%

"Usual dose" assumes normal renal/hepatic function. * For renal insufficiency, give usual dose × 1 followed by maintenance dose per CrCl. For dialysis patients, dose the same as for CrCl < 10 mL/min and give supplemental (post-HD/PD dose) immediately after dialysis. CrCl = creatinine clearance; CVVH = continuous veno-venous hemofiltration; HD/PD = hemodialysis/peritoneal dialysis. See pp. 509–513 for explanations, pp. xi–xii for abbreviations; Linezolid (↑ risk of serotonin syndrome, see p. 620).

Serum half-life (normal/ESRD): 1/4 hrs
Plasma protein binding: 20% / 40% (cilastatin)
Volume of distribution (V_d): 0.2 L/kg
Primary Mode of Elimination: Renal
Dosage Adjustments* (based on 500 mg dose; for 1 gm dosing double dose shown in grid)

CrCl 50–80 mL/min	500 mg (IV) q6h
CrCl 10–50 mL/min	500 mg (IV) q8h
CrCl < 10 mL/min†	250 mg (IV) q12h
Post–HD dose	250 mg (IV)
Post–PD dose	250 mg (IV)
CVVH dose	500 mg (IV) q8h
Moderate hepatic insufficiency	No change
Severe hepatic insufficiency	No change

† Avoid if CrCl ≤ 5 mL/min unless dialysis is instituted within 48 hours.

Drug Interactions: Cyclosporine (↑ cyclosporine levels); ganciclovir (↑ risk of seizures); probenecid (↑ imipenem levels); valproic acid (↓ seizure threshold).
Adverse Effects: Seizures, phlebitis.
Allergic Potential: Low
Safety in Pregnancy: C
Comments: Imipenem:cilastatin (1:1). Infuse 500 mg (IV) over 20–30 minutes; 1 gm (IV) over 40–60 minutes. Imipenem is renally metabolized by dehydropeptidase I; cilastatin is an inhibitor of this enzyme, effectively preventing the metabolism of imipenem. Imipenem/cilastatin can be given IM (IM absorption: imipenem 75%; cilastatin 100%). ***Fully susceptible organisms dose: 500 mg (IV) q6h; Less susceptible organisms (e.g., P. aeruginosa) dose:*** *1 gm (IV) q6-8h.* Incompatible in solutions containing vancomycin or metronidazole. ***Seizures more likely in renal insufficiency/high doses (> 2 gm/d)***. Inhibits endotoxin release from gram-negative bacilli. Very low incidence of cross reactions with β-lactams. ***Use increases MRSA prevalence and P. aeruginosa resistance***. Na^+ content = 3.2 mEq/gm.
Cerebrospinal Fluid Penetration:
Non-Inflamed meninges = 10%
Inflamed meninges = 15%
Bile Penetration: 1%
(also see ***Antibiotic Pearls & Pitfalls*** pp. 495–508).

REFERENCES:

Balfour JA, Bryson HM, Brogden RN. Imipenem/cilastatin: An update of its antibacterial activity, pharmacokinetics, and therapeutic efficacy in the treatment of serious infections. Drugs 51:99–136, 1996.

Barza M. Imipenem: First of a new class of beta-lactam antibiotics. Ann Intern Med 103:552–60, 1985.

Bernabeu-Wittel M, Pichardo C, Garcia-Curial A, et al. Pharmacokinetic/pharmacodynamic assessment of the in-vivo efficacy of imipenem alone or in combination with amikacin for the treatment of experimental multiresistant Acinetobacter baumannii pneumonia. Clin Microbiol Infect 11:319–25, 2005.

Choi JY, Soo Park Y, Cho CH, et al. Synergic in-vitro activity of imipenem and sulbactam against Acinetobacter baumannii. Clin Microbiol Infect 10:1089–1104, 2004.

Fish DN, Teitelbaum, I, Abraham E. Pharmacokinetics and pharmacodynamics of imipenem during continuous renal replacement therapy in critically ill patients. Antimicrobial Agents and Chemotherapy 49:2421–2428, 2005.

Garbino J, Villiger P, Caviezel A, et al. A randomized prospective study of cefepime plus metronidazole with imipenem-cilastatin in the treatment of intra-abdominal infections. Infection 35:161–166, 2007.

"Usual dose" assumes normal renal/hepatic function. * For renal insufficiency, give usual dose × 1 followed by maintenance dose per CrCl. For dialysis patients, dose the same as for CrCl < 10 mL/min and give supplemental (post-HD/PD dose) immediately after dialysis. CrCl = creatinine clearance; CVVH = continuous veno-venous hemofiltration; HD/PD = hemodialysis/peritoneal dialysis. See pp. 509–513 for explanations, pp. xi–xii for abbreviations; Linezolid (↑ risk of serotonin syndrome, see p. 620).

Helinger WC, Brewer NS. Carbapenems and monobactams: Imipenem, meropenem, and aztreonam. Mayo Clin Proc 74:420–34, 1999.

Klastersky JA. Use of imipenem as empirical treatment of febrile neutropenia. Int J Antimicrob Agents 21:393–402, 2003.

Lamoth F, Erard V, Asner S, et al. High imipenem blood concentrations associated with toxic encephalopathy in a patient with mild renal dysfunction. Int J Antimicrob Agents. 34:386–388, 2009.

Lautenbach E, Weiner MG, Nachamkin I, Bilker WB, Sheridan A, Fishman NO. Imipenem Resistance Among Pseudomonas aeruginosa Isolates: Risk Factors for Infection and Impact of Resistance on Clinical and Economic Outcomes. Infection Control and Hosp Epidemiol. 27:893–900, 2006.

Maravi-Poma E, Gener J, Alvarez-Lerma F, et al. Spanish Group for the Study of Septic Complications in Severe Acute Pancreatitis. Early antibiotic treatment (prophylaxis) of septic complications in severe acute necrotizing pancreatitis: a prospective, randomized, multicenter study comparing two regimens with imipenem-cilastatin. Intensive Care Med 29:1974–80, 2003.

Wareham DW, Bean DC. In Vitro Activities of Polymyxin B, Imipenem and Rifampin against Multidrug-Resistant Acinetobacter baumannii. Antimicrob Agents Chemother 50:825–26, 2006.

Website: www.pdr.net

Indinavir (Crixivan) IDV

Drug Class: Antiretroviral protease inhibitor.
Usual Dose: 800 mg (PO) q8h.
Pharmacokinetic Parameters:
Peak serum level: 252 mcg/mL
Bioavailability: 65% (77% with food)
Excreted unchanged (urine): < 20%
Serum half-life (normal/ESRD): 2 hrs/no data
Plasma protein binding: 60 %
Volume of distribution (V_d): No data
Primary Mode of Elimination: Hepatic
Dosage Adjustments*

CrCl 50–80 mL/min	No change
CrCl 10–50 mL/min	No change
CrCl < 10 mL/min	No change
Post–HD dose	None
Post–PD dose	None
CVVH dose	No change
Moderate hepatic insufficiency	600 mg (PO) q8h
Severe hepatic insufficiency	400 mg (PO) q8h

Antiretroviral Dosage Adjustments:

Didanosine	Administer didanosine 1 hour apart
Delavirdine	Indinavir 600 mg q8h
Efavirenz	Indinavir 1000 mg q8h
Lopinavir/ritonavir	Indinavir 600 mg q12h
Nelfinavir	Limited data for indinavir 1200 mg q12h + nelfinavir 1250 mg q12h
Nevirapine	Indinavir 1000 mg q8h
Ritonavir	Indinavir 800 mg q12h + ritonavir 100–200 mg q12h, or 400 mg q12h of each drug
Saquinavir	No information
Rifampin	Avoid combination
Rifabutin	Indinavir 1000 mg q8h; rifabutin 150 mg q24h or 300 mg 2–3x/week

Drug Interactions: Antiretrovirals, rifabutin, rifampin (see dose adjustment grid, above); astemizole, terfenadine, benzodiazepines,

"Usual dose" assumes normal renal/hepatic function. * For renal insufficiency, give usual dose × 1 followed by maintenance dose per CrCl. For dialysis patients, dose the same as for CrCl < 10 mL/min and give supplemental (post-HD/PD dose) immediately after dialysis. CrCl = creatinine clearance; CVVH = continuous veno-venous hemofiltration; HD/PD = hemodialysis/peritoneal dialysis. See pp. 509–513 for explanations, pp. xi–xii for abbreviations; Linezolid (↑ risk of serotonin syndrome, see p. 620).

cisapride, ergot alkaloids, statins, St. John's wort (avoid if possible); calcium channel blockers (↑ calcium channel blocker levels); carbamazepine, phenobarbital, phenytoin (↓ indinavir levels, ↑ anticonvulsant levels; monitor); tenofovir (↓ indinavir levels, ↑ tenofovir levels); clarithromycin, erythromycin, telithromycin (↑ indinavir and macrolide levels); didanosine (administer indinavir on empty stomach 1 hour apart); ethinyl estradiol, norethindrone (↑ interacting drug levels; no dosage adjustment); grapefruit juice (↓ indinavir levels); itraconazole, ketoconazole (↑ indinavir levels); sildenafil (↑ or ↓ sildenafil levels; do not exceed 25 mg in 48 hrs), tadalafil (max. 10 mg/72 hrs), vardenafil (max 2.5 mg/72 hrs); theophylline (↓ theophylline levels); fluticasone nasal spray (avoid concomitant use).

Adverse Effects: Nephrolithiasis, nausea, vomiting, diarrhea, anemia, leukopenia, headache, insomnia, hyperglycemia (including worsening diabetes, new-onset diabetes, DKA), ↑ SGOT/SGPT, ↑ indirect bilirubin (2° to drug-induced Gilbert's syndrome; inconsequential), fat redistribution, lipid abnormalities (evaluate risk of coronary disease/pancreatitis), abdominal pain, possible ↑ bleeding in hemophilia, dry skin, chelitis, paronychiae. Immune reconstitution syndrome.

Allergic Potential: Low

Safety in Pregnancy: C

Comments: Renal stone formation may be prevented/minimized by adequate hydration (1–3 liters water daily); ↑ risk of nephrolithiasis with alcohol. Take 1 hour before or 2 hours after meals (may take with skim milk or low fat meal). Separate dosing with ddI by 1 hour.

Cerebrospinal Fluid Penetration: 16%

REFERENCES:

Acosta EP, Henry K, Baken L, et al. Indinavir concentrations and antiviral effect. Pharmacotherapy 19:708–712, 1999.

Antinori A, Giancola MI, Griserri S, et al. Factors influencing virological response to antiretroviral drugs in cerebrospinal fluid of advanced HIV-1-infected patients. AIDS 16:1867–76, 2002.

Deeks SG, Smith M, Holodniy M, et al. HIV-1 protease inhibitors: A review for clinicians. JAMA 277:145–53, 1997.

DiCenzo R, Forrest A, Fischl MA, et al. Pharmacokinetics of indinavir and nelfinavir in treatment-naive, human immunodeficiency virus-infected subjects. Antimicrob Agents Chemother 48:918–23, 2004.

Go J, Cunha BA. Indinavir: A review. Antibiotics for Clinicians 3:81–87, 1999.

Justesen US, Andersen AB, Klitgaard NA, et al. Pharmacokinetic interaction between rifampin and the combination of indinavir and low-dose ritonavir in HIV-infected patients. Clin Infect Dis 38:426–9, 2004.

Kopp JB, Falloon J, Filie A, et al. Indinavir-associated intestinal nephritis and urothelial inflammation: clinical and cytologic findings. Clin Infect Dis 34:1122–8, 2002.

Meraviglia P, Angeli E, Del Sorbo F, et al. Risk factors for indinavir-related renal colic in HIV patients: predicative value of indinavir dose-body mass index. AIDS 16:2089–2093, 2002.

McDonald CK, Kuritzkes DR. Human immunodeficiency virus type 1 protease inhibitors. Arch Intern Med 157:951–9, 1997.

Panel on Antiretroviral Guidelines for Adults and Adolescents. Guidelines for the use of antiretroviral agents in HIV-1 infected adults and adolescents. Department of Health and Human

---

"Usual dose" assumes normal renal/hepatic function. * For renal insufficiency, give usual dose × 1 followed by maintenance dose per CrCl. For dialysis patients, dose the same as for CrCl < 10 mL/min and give supplemental (post-HD/PD dose) immediately after dialysis. CrCl = creatinine clearance; CVVH = continuous veno-venous hemofiltration; HD/PD = hemodialysis/peritoneal dialysis. See pp. 509–513 for explanations, pp. xi–xii for abbreviations; Linezolid (↑ risk of serotonin syndrome, see p. 620).

Services. November 3, 2008; 1–139. Available at http://www.aidsinfor.nih.gov/ContentFiles/AdultandAdolescentGL.pdf
Website: www.crixivan.com

Isoniazid (INH)

Drug Class: Anti–TB drug.
Usual Dose: 5 mg/kg or 300 mg (PO) q24h (see comments).
Pharmacokinetic Parameters:
Peak serum level: 7 mcg/ml
Bioavailability: 90%
Excreted unchanged (urine): 50–70%
Serum half-life (normal/ESRD): 1/1 hr
Plasma protein binding: 15%
Volume of distribution (V_d): 0.75 L/kg
Primary Mode of Elimination: Hepatic
Dosage Adjustments*

CrCl 50–80 mL/min	No change
CrCl 10–50 mL/min	No change
CrCl < 10 mL/min	No change
Post–HD dose	300 mg
Post–PD dose	300 mg
CVVH dose	None
Moderate hepatic insufficiency	No change
Severe hepatic insufficiency	No change

Drug Interactions: Alcohol, rifampin (↑ risk of ↑ SGOT/SGPT); alfentanil (↑ duration of alfentanil effect); aluminum salts (↓ isoniazid absorption); carbamazepine, phenytoin (↑ interacting drug levels); itraconazole (↓ itraconazole levels); warfarin (↑ INR).
Adverse Effects: ↑ SGOT/SGPT, drug fever/rash, age-dependent hepatotoxicity (after age 60), drug-induced ANA/SLE, hemolytic anemia, neuropsychiatric changes in the elderly. Transient/reversible ↑ SGOT/SGPT frequently occur early (< 3 weeks) after INH use. If ↑ SGOT/SGPT, monitor twice weekly until levels peak, then monitor weekly until levels return to within normal range. Stop INH only if ↑ SGOT/SGPT ≥ 10 × upper limit of normal.
Allergic Potential: Low
Safety in Pregnancy: C
Comments: Administer with 50 mg of pyridoxine daily to prevent peripheral neuropathy. Increased blood pressure/rash with tyramine–containing products, e.g., cheese/wine. ↑ hepatotoxicity in slow acetylators. Slow acetylator dose: 150 mg (PO) q24h. TB D.O.T. dose: 15 mg/kg or 900 mg (PO) 3x/week. Meningeal dose = usual dose.
Cerebrospinal Fluid Penetration:
Non-Inflamed meninges = 90%
Inflamed meninges = 90%

REFERENCES:

Ahn C, Oh KH, Kim K, et al. Effect of peritoneal dialysis on plasma and peritoneal fluid concentrations of isoniazid, pyrazinamide, and rifampin. Perit Dial Int. 23:362–7, 2003.

Colebunders R, Apers L, Shamputa IC. Treatment of multidrug-resistant tuberculosis. Lancet 10:1240, 2004.

Ena J, Valls V. Short-course therapy with rifampin plus isoniazid, compared with standard therapy with isoniazid, for latent tuberculosis infection: A meta-analysis. Clin Infect Dis 40:670–6, 2005.

McIllerson H, Wash P, Burger A, et al. Determinants of Rifampin, Isoniazid, Pyrazinamide and Ethambutol Pharmacokinetics in a Cohort of Tuberculosis Patients. Antimicrob Agents Chemother 50:1170–77, 2006.

Schaller A, Sun Z, Yang Y, et al. Salicylate reduces susceptibility of Mycobacterium tuberculosis to multiple antituberculosis drugs. Antimicrob Agents Chemother 46:2533–9, 2002.

Schlossberg D. Treatment of multi-drug resistant tuberculosis. Antibiotics for Clinicians 9:317–321, 2005

Van Scoy RE, Wilkowske CJ. Antituberculous agents. Mayo Clin Proc 67:179–87, 1992.

"Usual dose" assumes normal renal/hepatic function. * For renal insufficiency, give usual dose × 1 followed by maintenance dose per CrCl. For dialysis patients, dose the same as for CrCl < 10 mL/min and give supplemental (post-HD/PD dose) immediately after dialysis. CrCl = creatinine clearance; CVVH = continuous veno-venous hemofiltration; HD/PD = hemodialysis/peritoneal dialysis. See pp. 509–513 for explanations, pp. xi–xii for abbreviations; Linezolid (↑ risk of serotonin syndrome, see p. 620).

Itraconazole (Sporanox)

Drug Class: Antifungal.

Usual Dose: 200 mg (PO, capsules or solution, solution produces better absorption) q12h or q24h **(take *without* food)** depending on disease; due to enhanced drug delivery, IV therapy begins with 200 mg IV q12h × 2 days (4 doses) and then continues with only 200 mg (IV) q24h; PO follow-up to IV therapy for serious infection is at 200 mg PO q12h. Each IV dose should be infused over 1 hour (see comments).

Pharmacokinetic Parameters:

Peak serum level: 2.8 mcg/ml
Bioavailability: 55% (capsules)/90% (solution- **take without food***)*
Excreted unchanged (urine): 1%
Serum half-life (normal/ESRD): 21–64/35 hrs
Plasma protein binding: 99.8%
Volume of distribution (V_d): 10 L/kg

Primary Mode of Elimination: Hepatic; metabolized predominantly by the cytochrome P450 3A4 isoenzyme system (CYP3A4)

Dosage Adjustments*

CrCl 50–80 mL/min	No change
CrCl 10–50 mL/min	No change
CrCl < 10 mL/min	No change
Post–HD dose	100 mg (IV/PO)
Post–PD dose	None
Post-CVVH dose	None
Moderate hepatic insufficiency	No change†
Severe hepatic insufficiency	No change†

† ↑ $t_{1/2}$ of itraconazole in patients with hepatic insufficiency should be considered when given with medications metabolized by P450 isoenzymes. Also see Adverse Effects for information regarding patients who develop liver dysfunction.

Drug Interactions: *Itraconazole may ↑ plasma levels of:* alfentanil, buspirone, busulfan, carbamazepine, cisapride, cyclosporine, digoxin, dihydropyridines, docetaxel, dofetilide, methylprednisolone, oral hypoglycemics (↑ risk of hypoglycemia), pimozide, quinidine, rifabutin, saquinavir, sirolimus, tacrolimus, trimetrexate, verapamil, vinca alkaloids, warfarin; alprazolam, diazepam, midazolam, triazolam (↑ sedative/hypnotic effects); atorvastatin, lovastatin, simvastatin (↑ risk of rhabdomyolysis); indinavir, ritonavir, saquinavir; coadministration of oral midazolam, triazolam, lovastatin, or simvastatin with itraconazole is contraindicated; coadministration of cisapride, pimozide, quinidine, amiodarone, or dofetilide with itraconazole is contraindicated due to the risk of ↑ QT_c/life-threatening ventricular arrhythmias. *Decreased itraconazole levels may occur with:* antacids, carbamazepine, H_2-receptor antagonists, isoniazid, nevirapine, phenobarbital, phenytoin, proton pump inhibitors, rifabutin, rifampin; coadministration of rifampin with itraconazole is not recommended. *Increased itraconazole levels may occur with:* clarithromycin, erythromycin, indinavir, ritonavir.

Adverse Effects: ≥ 2%: nausea, diarrhea, vomiting, headache, abdominal pain, bilirubinemia, rash, ↑ SGPT/SGOT, hypokalemia, ↑ serum creatinine. Rarely, itraconazole has been associated with serious hepatotoxicity (liver failure/death). If liver disease develops, discontinue treatment, perform liver function testing, and reevaluate risk/benefit of further treatment. Use itraconazole with caution in patients with ↑ liver enzymes, active liver disease, or previous drug-induced hepatotoxicity. Life-threatening ventricular arrhythmias/sudden death have occurred in patients using cisapride, pimozide, or

---

"Usual dose" assumes normal renal/hepatic function. * For renal insufficiency, give usual dose × 1 followed by maintenance dose per CrCl. For dialysis patients, dose the same as for CrCl < 10 mL/min and give supplemental (post-HD/PD dose) immediately after dialysis. CrCl = creatinine clearance; CVVH = continuous veno-venous hemofiltration; HD/PD = hemodialysis/peritoneal dialysis. See pp. 509–513 for explanations, pp. xi–xii for abbreviations; Linezolid (↑ risk of serotonin syndrome, see p. 620).

quinidine concomitantly with itraconazole; coadministration of these drugs with itraconazole is contraindicated. Use itraconazole with caution in patients with ventricular dysfunction. IV itraconazole may cause transient, asymptomatic ↓ in ejection fraction for ≤ 12 hours. If CHF develops, consider discontinuation of itraconazole.

Allergic Potential: Low

Safety in Pregnancy: C

Comments: ***Oral itraconazole***: Requires gastric acidity for absorption. When antacids are required, administer ≥ 1 hour before or 2 hours after itraconazole capsules. Oral solution is better absorbed without food; capsules are better absorbed with food. Capsule bioavailability is food dependent: 40% fasting/90% post-prandial. For oral therapy, bioavailability of 10 ml of solution without food = 100 mg capsule with food. Administer with a cola beverage in patients with achlorhydria or taking H_2-receptor antagonists/other gastric acid suppressors. While oral solution and capsules can be interchanged for treatment of systemic disease if adequate blood levels are achieved, oral solution produces more reliable blood levels and is definitely preferred for oral/esophageal candidiasis where the local effect of the solution on the infection seem helpful. ***IV itraconazole***: Hydroxypropyl-β-cyclodextrin stabilizer in IV formulation accumulates in renal failure. IV itraconazole should not be used in patients with CrCl < 30 mL/min; if possible, use the oral preparation. Infuse 60 ml of dilute solution (3.33 mg/ml = 200 mg itraconazole, pH ~ 4.8) IV over 60 minutes, using infusion set provided. After administration, flush the infusion set with 15–20 ml of normal saline injection. The compatibility of IV itraconazole with flush solutions other than normal saline is unknown. ***Highly active against C. albicans, non-albicans Candida, Cryptococcus, Histoplasmosis, Blastomycosis, Paracococcidiomycosis, Sporotrichosis. Active against dermatophytes. No activity against Pseudoallescheria/Scedosporium, Fusaria or Mucor.***

Cerebrospinal Fluid Penetration: < 10%

REFERENCES:

Boogaerts M, Winston DJ, Bow EJ, et al. Intravenous and oral itraconazole versus intravenous amphotericin B deoxycholate as empirical antifungal therapy for persistent fever in neutropenic patients with cancer who are receiving broad-spectrum antibacterial therapy. A randomized controlled trial. Ann Intern Med 135:412–22, 2001.

Bruggemann RJM, Alffenaar JWC, Blijlevens NMA, et al. Clinical Relevance of the Pharmoacokinetic Interactions of Azole Antifungal Drugs with Coadministered Agents. Clin Infect Dis 48:1441–1458, 2009.

Calvopina M, Guevara AG, Armijos RX, et al. Itraconazole in the treatment of New World mucocutaneous leishmaniasis. Int J Dermatol 43:659–63, 2004.

Caputo R. Itraconazole (Sporanox) in superficial and systemic fungal infections. Expert Rev Anti Infect Ther 1:531–42, 2004.

Conte JE Jr, Golden JA, Kipps J, et al. Intrapulmonary pharmacokinetics and pharmacodynamics of itraconazole and 14-hydroxyitraconazol steady state. Antimicrob Agents Chemother 48:3823–7, 2004.

Dominguez-Gil Hurle A, Sanchez Navarro A, Garcia Sanchez MJ. Therapeutic drug monitoring of itraconazole and the relevance of pharmacokinetic interactions. Clin Microbiol and Infection. 12:S97–106, 2006.

Glasmacher A, Prentice A. Current experience with itraconazole in neutropenic patients: a concise overview of pharmacological properties in use in prophylactic and empirical antifungal therapy. Clin Microbiol and Infection. 12:S84–90, 2006.

Go J, Cunha BA. Itraconazole. Antibiotics for Clinicians 3:61–70, 1999.

"Usual dose" assumes normal renal/hepatic function. * For renal insufficiency, give usual dose × 1 followed by maintenance dose per CrCl. For dialysis patients, dose the same as for CrCl < 10 mL/min and give supplemental (post-HD/PD dose) immediately after dialysis. CrCl = creatinine clearance; CVVH = continuous veno-venous hemofiltration; HD/PD = hemodialysis/peritoneal dialysis. See pp. 509–513 for explanations, pp. xi–xii for abbreviations; Linezolid (↑ risk of serotonin syndrome, see p. 620).

Horousseau JL, Dekker AW, et al. Itraconazole oral solution for primary prophylaxis of fungal infections in patients with hematological malignancy and profound neutropenia: a randomized, double-blind, double-placebo, multicenter trial comparing itraconazole and amphotericin B. Antimicrob Agents Chemother 44:1887–93, 2000.

Lewis, RE, Wiederhold NP, Klepser ME. In vitro pharmacodynamics of amphotericin B, itraconazole, and voriconazole against aspergillus, fusarium, and scedosporium spp. Antimicrobial Agents and Chemotherapy 49:945–951, 2005.

Mattiuzzi GN, Alvarado G, Giles FJ, et al. Open-label, randomized comparison of itraconazole versus caspofungin for prophylaxis in patients with hematologic malignancies. Antimicrob Agents Chemother 50:143–7, 2006.

Mosquera J, Shartt A, Moore CB, et al. In vitro interaction of terbinafine with itraconazole, fluconazole, amphotericin B and 5-flucytosine against Aspergillus spp. J Antimicrob Chemother 50:189–94, 2002.

Phillips EJ. Itraconazole was as effective as amphotericin B for fever and neutropenia in cancer and led to fewer adverse events. ACP J Club 136:58, 2002.

Rubin MA, Carroll KC, Cahill BC. Caspofungin in combination with itraconazole for the treatment of invasive aspergillosis in humans. Clin Infect Dis 34:1160–1, 2002.

Sabatelli F. Patel R, Mann PA, et al. In vitro activities of posaconazole, fluconazole, itraconazole, voriconazole, and amphotericin B against a large collection of clinically important molds and yeasts. Antimicrob Agents Chemother 50:2009–15, 2006.

Terrell CL. Antifungal agents Part II. The azoles. Mayo Clin Proc 74:78–100, 1999.

Urunsak M, Ilkit M, Evruke C, et al. Clinical and mycological efficacy of single-day oral treatment with itraconazole (400 mg) in acute vulvovaginal candidosis. Mycoses 47:422–7, 2004.

Winston DJ. Itraconazole vs. fluconazole for antifungal prophylaxis in allogeneic stem-cell transplant patients. 12:S91–96, 2006.

Winston DJ, Busuttil RW. Randomized controlled trial of oral itraconazole solution versus intravenous/oral fluconazole for prevention of fungal infections in liver transplant recipients. Transplantation 74:688–95, 2002.

Website: www.pdr.net

Ketoconazole (Nizoral)

Drug Class: Antifungal.
Usual Dose: 200 mg (PO) q24h.
Pharmacokinetic Parameters:
Peak serum level: 3.5 mcg/ml
Bioavailability: 82%
Excreted unchanged (urine): 70%
Serum half-life (normal/ESRD): 6/20 hrs
Plasma protein binding: 99%
Volume of distribution (V_d): 2 L/kg
Primary Mode of Elimination: Hepatic
Dosage Adjustments*

CrCl > 40 mL/min	No change
CrCl < 40 mL/min	No change
Post–HD dose	None
Post–PD dose	None
CVVH dose	No change
Moderate hepatic insufficiency	No information
Severe hepatic insufficiency	Avoid

Drug Interactions: Astemizole, cisapride, terfenadine, amiodarone (may ↑ QT interval, torsades de pointes); carbamazepine, INH (↓ ketoconazole levels); cimetidine, famotidine, nizatidine, ranitidine, omeprazole, INH (↓ ketoconazole absorption); cyclosporine, digoxin, loratadine, tacrolimus (↑ interacting drug levels with possible toxicity); didanosine (↓ ketoconazole levels); midazolam, triazolam (↑ interacting drug levels, ↑ sedative effects);

"Usual dose" assumes normal renal/hepatic function. * For renal insufficiency, give usual dose × 1 followed by maintenance dose per CrCl. For dialysis patients, dose the same as for CrCl < 10 mL/min and give supplemental (post-HD/PD dose) immediately after dialysis. CrCl = creatinine clearance; CVVH = continuous veno-venous hemofiltration; HD/PD = hemodialysis/peritoneal dialysis. See pp. 509–513 for explanations, pp. xi–xii for abbreviations; Linezolid (↑ risk of serotonin syndrome, see p. 620).

oral hypoglycemics (severe hypoglycemia); phenytoin, rifabutin, rifampin (↓ ketoconazole levels, ↑ interacting drug); statins (↑ statin levels; rhabdomyolysis reported); warfarin (↑ INR).

Adverse Effects: Nausea, vomiting, abdominal pain, pruritus.

Allergic Potential: Low

Safety in Pregnancy: C

Comments: Dose-dependent reduction in gonadal (androgenic) function. Decreased cortisol production with doses ≥ 800 mg/day, but **does not result in adrenal insufficiency**. Give oral doses with citric juices. ***Highly active against dermatophytes, Candida albicans. Some activity against Aspergillus Coccidiomycosis, Paracoccidiomycosis, Histoplasmosis. No activity against Pseudoallescheria/ Scedosporium, Fusaria or Mucor.***

Cerebrospinal Fluid Penetration: < 10%

REFERENCES:

Allen LV. Ketoconazole oral suspension. US Pharm 18:98–9, 1993.

Como JA, Dismukes WE. Oral azole drugs as systemic antifungal therapy. N Engl J Med 330:263–72, 1993.

Lyman CA, Walsh TJ. Systemically administered antifungal agents: A review of their clinical pharmacology and therapeutic applications. Drugs 44:9–35, 1992.

Terrell CL. Antifungal agents: Part II. The azoles. Mayo Clin Proc 74:78–100, 1999.

Website: www.pdr.net

Lamivudine (Epivir) 3TC

Drug Class: Antiretroviral NRTI (nucleoside reverse transcriptase inhibitor); antiviral (HBV).

Usual Dose: 150 mg (PO) q12h or 300 mg (PO) q24h (HIV); 100 mg (PO) q24h (HBV).

Pharmacokinetic Parameters:

Peak serum level: 1.5 mcg/mL

Bioavailability: 86%

Excreted unchanged (urine): 71%

Serum half-life (normal/ESRD): 5–7/20 hrs

Plasma protein binding: 36%

Volume of distribution (V_d): 1.3 L/kg

Primary Mode of Elimination: Renal

Dosage Adjustments*

CrCl 30–50 mL/min	150 mg (PO) q24h
CrCl 15–30 mL/min	100 mg (PO) q24h
CrCl 5–15 mL/min	50 mg (PO) q24h
CrCl < 5 mL/min	25 mg (PO) q24h
Post–HD dose	None
Post–PD dose	None
CVVH dose	100 mg (PO) q24h
Moderate hepatic insufficiency	No change
Severe hepatic insufficiency	No information

Drug Interactions: Didanosine, zalcitabine (↑ risk of pancreatitis); TMP–SMX (↑ lamivudine levels); zidovudine + lamivudine not recommended.

Adverse Effects: Lamivudine tablets and oral solution used to treat HIV infection contain a higher dose of lamivudine than Epivir-HBV® tablets and oral solution used to treat chronic hepatitis B. Severe acute exacerbations of hepatitis B have been reported in patients who are co-infected with hepatitis B virus (HBV) and HIV and have discontinued lamivudine. Hepatic function should be monitored closely for at least several months in patients who discontinue lamivudine. Most common

---

"Usual dose" assumes normal renal/hepatic function. * For renal insufficiency, give usual dose × 1 followed by maintenance dose per CrCl. For dialysis patients, dose the same as for CrCl < 10 mL/min and give supplemental (post-HD/PD dose) immediately after dialysis. CrCl = creatinine clearance; CVVH = continuous veno-venous hemofiltration; HD/PD = hemodialysis/peritoneal dialysis. See pp. 509–513 for explanations, pp. xi–xii for abbreviations; Linezolid (↑ risk of serotonin syndrome, see p. 620).

include headache, dizziness, malaise, nausea nasal congestion, cough, rash, neuropathy, leucopenia. Pancreatitis and or lactic acidosis with hepatic steatosis (rare but potentially life threatening toxicity with NRTI's). Immune reconstitution syndrome can occur.

Allergic Potential: Low

Safety in Pregnancy: C

Comments: Potential cross resistance with didanosine. Prevents development of AZT resistance and restores AZT susceptibility. May be taken with or without food. Although effective against HBV, lamivudine is no longer a first-line option because of the development of resistance in 70% of treated patients. A component of insew put Combivir, Trizivir, and Epzicom.

Cerebrospinal Fluid Penetration: 15%

REFERENCES:

Benson CA, van der Horst C, Lamarca A, et al. A randomized study of emtricitabine and lamivudine in stable suppressed patients with HIV. AIDS 18:2269–2276, 2004.

Eron JJ, Benoit SL, Jemsek J, et al. Treatment with lamivudine, zidovudine, or both in HIV-positive patients with 200 to 500 CD_4 cells per cubic millimeter. N Engl J Med 333:1662–9, 1995.

Keeffe EB, Dieterich DT, Pawlotsky JM, et al. Chronic hepatitis B: preventing, detecting, and managing viral resistance. Clin Gastroenterol Hepatol 6:268–274, 2008.

Lai Cl, Chien RN. Leung NW, et al. A one-year trial of lamivudine for chronic hepatitis B. N Engl J Med 339:61–8, 1998.

Lau GK, He ML, Fong DY, et al. Preemptive use of lamivudine reduces hepatitis B exacerbation after allogeneic hematopoietic cell transplantation. Hepatology 36:702–9, 2002.

Leung N. Lamivudine for chronic hepatitis B. Expert Rev Anti Infect Ther 2:173–80, 2004.

Liaw YF, Sung JY, Chow WC, et al. Lamivudine for patients with chronic hepatitis B and advanced liver disease. N Engl J Med 351:1521–31, 2004.

Lu Y, Wang B, Yu L, et al. Lamivudine in prevention and treatment of recurrent HBV after liver transplantation. Hepatobiliary Pancreat Dis Int 3:504–7, 2004.

Marrone A, Zampino R, D'Onofrio M, et al. Combined interferon plus lamivudine treatment in young patients with dual HBV (HbeAg positive) and HCV chronic infection. J Hepatol 41:1064–5, 2004.

Murphy RL, Brun S, Hicks C, et al. ABT-378/ritonavir plus stavudine and lamivudine for the treatment of antiretroviral-naive adults with HIV-1 infection: 48-week results. AIDS 15:F1–9, 2001.

Panel on Antiretorviral Guidelines for Adults and Adolescents. Guidelines for the use of antriretroviral agents in HIV-1 infected adults and adolescents. Department of Health and Human Services. November 3, 2008; 1–139. Available at http://www.aidsinfor.nih.gov/ContentFiles/AdultandAdolecentGL.pdf.

Perry CM, Faulds D. Lamivudine. A review of its antiviral activity, pharmacokinetic properties and therapeutic efficacy in the management of HIV infection. Drugs 53:657–80, 1997.

Rivkina A, Rybalov S. Chronic hepatitis B: current and future treatment options. Pharmacotherapy 22:721–37, 2002.

Schmilovitz-Weiss H, Ben-Ari Z, Sikuler E, et al. Lamivudine treatment for acute severe hepatitis B: a pilot study. Liver Int 24:547–51, 2004.

Staszewski S, Morales-Ramirez J, Trashima KT, et al. Efavirenz plus zidovudine and lamivudine, efavirenz plus indinavir, and indinavir plus zidovudine and lamivudine in the treatment of HIV-1 infection in adults. N Engl J Med 341:1865–1873, 1999.

Website: www.TreatHIV.com

Lamivudine + Zidovudine (Combivir) 3TC/ZDV

Drug Class: Antiretroviral NRTI's combination.

Usual Dose: Combivir tablet = 150 mg lamivudine + 300 mg zidovudine. Usual dose = 1 tablet (PO) q12h.

"Usual dose" assumes normal renal/hepatic function. * For renal insufficiency, give usual dose × 1 followed by maintenance dose per CrCl. For dialysis patients, dose the same as for CrCl < 10 mL/min and give supplemental (post-HD/PD dose) immediately after dialysis. CrCl = creatinine clearance; CVVH = continuous veno-venous hemofiltration; HD/PD = hemodialysis/peritoneal dialysis. See pp. 509–513 for explanations, pp. xi–xii for abbreviations; Linezolid (↑ risk of serotonin syndrome, see p. 620).

Pharmacokinetic Parameters:
Peak serum level: 2.6/1.2 mcg/mL
Bioavailability: 82/60%
Excreted unchanged (urine): 86/64%
Serum half-life (normal/ESRD): [6/1.1]/[20/2.2] hrs
Plasma protein binding: <36/<38%
Volume of distribution (V_d): 1.3/1.6 L/kg
Primary Mode of Elimination: Renal
Dosage Adjustments*

CrCl 50–80 mL/min	No change
CrCl 10–50 mL/min	Avoid
CrCl < 10 mL/min	Avoid
Post–HD dose	Avoid
Post–PD dose	Avoid
CVVH dose	Avoid
Moderate hepatic insufficiency	Avoid
Severe hepatic insufficiency	Avoid

Drug Interactions: Atovaquone (↑ zidovudine levels); stavudine (antagonist to stavudine; avoid combination); ganciclovir, doxorubicin (neutropenia); tipranavir (↓ zidovudine levels); TMP–SMX (↑ lamivudine and zidovudine levels); vinca alkaloids (neutropenia).

Adverse Effects: Zidovudine, one of the two active ingredients in combivir, has been associated with hematologic toxicity including neutropenia and severe anemia. Prolonged use of zidovudine has been associated with symptomatic myopathy. Lactic acidosis and severe hepatomegaly with steatosis, including fatal cases. Severe acute exacerbations of hepatitis B have been reported in patients who are co-infected with hepatitis B virus (HBV) and HIV and have discontinued lamivudine. Nausea, vomiting, diarrhea, anorexia, insomnia fever/chills, headache, malaise/fatigue, peripheral neuropathy and pancreatitis. Immune reconstitution syndrome and redistribution/accumulation of body fat have been reported in patients treated with combination antiretroviral therapy.

Allergic Potential: Low
Safety in Pregnancy: C.
Cerebrospinal Fluid Penetration:
Lamivudine = 12%; zidovudine = 60%

REFERENCES:

Drugs for AIDS and associated infections. Med Lett Drug Ther 35:79–86, 1993.

Hirsch MS, D'Aquila RT. Therapy for human immunodeficiency virus infection. N Engl J Med 328:1685–95, 1993.

McLeod GX, Hammer SM. Zidovudine: Five years later. Ann Intern Med 117:487–510, 1992.

Panel on Antiretroviral Guidelines for Adults and Adolescents. Guidelines for the use of antiretroviral agents in HIV-1 infected adults and adolescents. Department of Health and Human Services. November 3, 2008; 1–139. Available at http://www.aidsinfor.nih.gov/ContentFiles/AdultandAdolescentGL.pdf.

Staszewski S, Morales-Ramirez J, Trashima KT, et al. Efavirenz plus zidovudine and lamivudine, efavirenz plus indinavir, and indinavir plus zidovudine and lamivudine in the treatment of HIV-1 infection in adults. N Engl J Med 341:1865–1873, 1999.

Website: www.TreatHIV.com

Levofloxacin (Levaquin)

Drug Class: Fluoroquinolone.
Usual Dose: 500–750 mg (IV/PO) q24h (see comments).
Spectrum: (see ***Susceptibility Profiles*** pp. 194–199).

"Usual dose" assumes normal renal/hepatic function. * For renal insufficiency, give usual dose × 1 followed by maintenance dose per CrCl. For dialysis patients, dose the same as for CrCl < 10 mL/min and give supplemental (post-HD/PD dose) immediately after dialysis. CrCl = creatinine clearance; CVVH = continuous veno-venous hemofiltration; HD/PD = hemodialysis/peritoneal dialysis. See pp. 509–513 for explanations, pp. xi–xii for abbreviations; Linezolid (↑ risk of serotonin syndrome, see p. 620).

Pharmacokinetic Parameters:
Peak serum level: 5–8 mcg/ml
Bioavailability: 99%
Excreted unchanged (urine): 87%
Serum half-life (normal/ESRD): 7 hrs/prolonged
Plasma protein binding: 30%
Volume of distribution (V_d): 1.3 L/kg
Primary Mode of Elimination: Renal
Dosage Adjustments* (based on 500 mg q24h)

CrCl 50–80 mL/min	No change
CrCl 10–50 mL/min	250 mg (IV/PO) q24h
CrCl < 10 mL/min	250 mg (IV/PO) q48h
HD/CAPD	250 mg (IV/PO) q48h
Post–HD dose	250 mg (IV/PO)
Post–HFHD dose	250 mg (IV/PO)
Post–PD dose	250 mg (IV/PO)
CVVH dose	250 mg (IV/PO) q24h
SLEDD dose	250 mg (IV/PO) q24h
Moderate hepatic insufficiency	No change
Severe hepatic insufficiency	No change

Drug Interactions: Al^{++}, Fe^{++}, Mg^{++}, Zn^{++} antacids (↓ absorption of levofloxacin if taken together); NSAIDs (CNS stimulation); probenecid (↑ levofloxacin levels); warfarin (↑ INR).

Adverse Effects: Does not cause seizures. Headache, insomnia, nausea, constipation, C. difficile diarrhea/colitis. FQ use has an increased risk of tendinitis/tendon rupture. Risk in highest in the elderly, those on steroids, and those with heart, lung or renal transplants.

Allergic Potential: Low

Safety in Pregnancy: C

Comments: Take 2 hours before or after aluminum/magnesium-containing antacids. Does not increase digoxin concentrations. May QTc interval, particularly in patients with predisposing conditions or medications e.g., amiodarone. **Acute bacterial sinusitis dose:** 750 mg (PO) q24h × 5 days. **CAP dose:** 750 mg (IV/PO) q24h × 5 days. **Nosocomial pneumonia dose:** 750 mg (IV/PO) q24h × 7–14 days. **cSSSI dose:** 750 mg (IV/PO) q24h × 7–14 days. **TB dose** (alternate drug in MDR TB regimen): 500 mg (PO) q24h. **Complicated UTI/acute pylonephritis dose:** 750 mg (IV/PO) q24h × 5 days.

↑ incidence of C. difficile diarrhea/colitis with PPIs (for patients on PPIs during FQ therapy, switch to H_2 blocker for duration of FQ therapy).

Cerebrospinal Fluid Penetration: 16% (also see ***Antibiotic Pearls & Pitfalls*** pp. 495–508).

REFERENCES:

Alvarez-Lerma F, Grau S, Alvarez-Beltran. Levofloxacin in the treatment of ventilator-associated pneumonia. Clin Microbiol Infect. 12:81–92, 2006.

Antos D, Schneider-Brachert W, Bastlein E, et al. 7 day triple therapy of Helicobacter pylori infection with levofloxacin, amoxicillin, and high-dose omeprazole in patients with known antimicrobial sensitivity. Helicobacter. 11:39–45, 2006.

Benko R, Matuz M, Doro P, et al. Pharmacokinetics and pharmacodynamics of levofloxacin in critically ill patients with ventilator-associated pneumonia. Int J Antimicrob Agents 30:162–168, 2007.

Bucaneve G, Micozzi A, Menichetti F, et al. Levofloxacin to prevent bacterial infection in patients with cancer and neutropenia. N Engl J Med 353:977–87, 2005.

Drago L, DeVecchi E, Mombelli L, et al. Activity of levofloxacin and ciprofloxacin against urinary pathogens. J Antimicrob Chemother 48:37–45, 2001.

"Usual dose" assumes normal renal/hepatic function. * For renal insufficiency, give usual dose × 1 followed by maintenance dose per CrCl. For dialysis patients, dose the same as for CrCl < 10 mL/min and give supplemental (post-HD/PD dose) immediately after dialysis. CrCl = creatinine clearance; CVVH = continuous veno-venous hemofiltration; HD/PD = hemodialysis/peritoneal dialysis. See pp. 509–513 for explanations, pp. xi–xii for abbreviations; Linezolid (↑ risk of serotonin syndrome, see p. 620).

File TM Jr, Milkovich G, Tennenberg AM, et al. Clinical implications of 750 mg, 5-day levofloxacin for the treatment of community-acquired pneumonia. Curr Med Res Opin 20:1473–81, 2004.

Garcia-Vazquez E, Mensa J, Sarasa M, et al. Penetration of levofloxacin into the anterior chamger (aqueous humour) of the human eye after intravenous administration. Eur J Clin Microbiol Infect Dis 26:137–140, 2007.

Glasheen JJ, Prochazka AV. The safety of levofloxacin in patients on warfarin. Am J Med 120:e13, 2007.

Ho C-C, Chen Y-C, Hu F-C, et al. Safety of Fluoro quinolone Use in Patients with Hepatoxicity Induced by Anti-Tuberculosis Regimens. Clin Infect Dis 48:1526–1533, 2009.

Kiser TH, Hoody DW, Obritsch MD, et al. Levofloxacin pharmacokinetics and pharmacodynamics in patients with severe burn injury. Antimicrob Agents Chemother 50:1937–45, 2006.

Klausner HA, Brown P, Peterson J, et al. Double-blind, randomized comparison of levofloxacin 750 mg once daily for 5 days versus ciprofloxin for 10 days in the treatment of acute pyelonephritis. Curr Med Res Opin 23:2637–2645, 2007.

Kuriyama T, Williams DW, Yanagisawa M, et al. Antimicrobial susceptibility of 800 anaerobic isolates from patients with dentoalveolar infection to 13 oral antibiotics. Oral Microbiol Immunol 22:285–288, 2007.

Lee CK, Boyle MP, Diener-West M, et al. Levofloxacin pharmacokinetics in adult cystic fibrosis. Chest 131:796–802, 2007.

Marchetti F, Viale P. Current and Future Perspectives for Levofloxacin in Severe *Pseudomonas aeruginosa* Infections. J Chemotherapy. 15:315–322, 2003.

Maurin M, Raoult D. Bacteriostatic and bactericidal activity of levofloxacin against Rickettsia rickettsii, Rickettsia conorii, 'Israel spotted fever group rickettsii' and Coxiella burnetii. Journal of Antimicrobial Chemotherapy. 39:725–30, 1997.

Nightingale CH, Grant EM, Quintiliani R. Pharmacodynamics and pharmacokinetics of levofloxacin. Chemotherapy 46:6–14, 2000.

Nista EC, Candelli M, Zocco, MA, et al. Levofloxacin-based triple therapy in first-line treatment for Helicobacter pylori eradication. Am J Gastroenterol. 101:1985–90, 2006.

Ogrendik M. Levofloxacin treatment in patients with rheumatoid arthritis receiving methotrexate. South Med J 100:135–139, 2007.

Olapade-Olaopa EO, Adebayo SA. Re: Treatment of chronic bacterial prostatitis with levofloxacin and ciprofloxacin lowers serum prostate specific antigen. J. Urol. 175:2365–66, 2006.

Pea F, Marioni G, Pavan F, et al. Penetration of levofloxacin into paranasal sinuses mucosa of patients with chronic rhinosinusitis after a single 500 mg oral dose. Pharmacol Res 55:38–41, 2007.

Poole M, Anon J, Paglia M, et al. A trial of high dose, short-course levofloxacin for the treatment of acute bacterial sinusitis. Otolaryngol Head Neck Surg 134:10–17, 2006.

Sakamoto H, Sakamoto M, Hata Y, et al. Aqueous and vitreous penetration of levofloxacin after topical and/or oral administration. Eur J Ophthalmol 17:372–376, 2007.

Tennenberg AM, Davis NB, Wu SC, Kahn J. Pneumonia due to Pseudomonas aeruginosa: the levofloxacin clinical trials experience. Curr Med Res Opin. 22:843–50, 2006.

Website: www.levaquin.com

Linezolid (Zyvox)

Drug Class: Oxazolidinone.

Usual Dose: 600 mg (IV/PO) q12h.

Spectrum: (see ***Susceptibility Profiles*** pp. 194–199).

Pharmacokinetic Parameters:

Peak serum level: 15–21 mcg/ml

Bioavailability: 100% (IV and PO)

Excreted unchanged (urine): 30%

Serum half-life (normal/ESRD): 6.4/7.1 hrs

Plasma protein binding: 31%

Volume of distribution (V_d): 0.64 L/kg

Primary Mode of Elimination: Hepatic/metabolized

Dosage Adjustments*

"Usual dose" assumes normal renal/hepatic function. * For renal insufficiency, give usual dose × 1 followed by maintenance dose per CrCl. For dialysis patients, dose the same as for CrCl < 10 mL/min and give supplemental (post-HD/PD dose) immediately after dialysis. CrCl = creatinine clearance; CVVH = continuous veno-venous hemofiltration; HD/PD = hemodialysis/peritoneal dialysis. See pp. 509–513 for explanations, pp. xi–xii for abbreviations; Linezolid (↑ risk of serotonin syndrome, see p. 620).

CrCl 50–80 mL/min	No change
CrCl 10–50 mL/min	No change
CrCl < 10 mL/min	No change
Post–HD dose	600 mg (IV/PO)
Post–PD dose	None
CVVH dose	No change
Moderate hepatic insufficiency	No change
Severe hepatic insufficiency	No information

Drug Interactions: Pseudoephedrine, tyramine-containing foods (↑ risk of hypertensive crisis); serotonergic agents, e.g., SSRIs, MAOIs, St. John's wort, ritonavir (↑ risk of serotonin syndrome). Serotonin syndrome: fever, delerium, hypertension, tremor/clonus, hyperreflexia.

Adverse Effects: Mild, readily reversible thrombocytopenia, anemia, or leukopenia occurs usually after ≥ 2 weeks of therapy. Lactic acidosis (rare), optic/peripheral neuropathy (> 28 days of therapy, rare). Monitor visual function if symptomatic or therapy ≥ 2 weeks; monitor CBC weekly if therapy > 2 weeks.

Allergic Potential: Low

Safety in Pregnancy: C

Comments: ***Ideal for IV-to-PO switch programs***. Unlike vancomycin, ***linezolid does not increase VRE prevalence***. Unlike quinupristin/dalfopristin, linezolid is active against E. faecalis (VSE). **Effective oral therapy of MRSA, MRSE, and E. faecium (VRE) infections. *Alternate therapy for Nocardia and Listeria***. Meningeal dose = usual dose.

Cerebrospinal Fluid Penetration: 70% (also see ***Antibiotic Pearls & Pitfalls*** p. 505).

REFERENCES:

Aeziokoro CO, Cannon JP, Pachucki CT, et al. The effectiveness and safety of oral linezolid for the primary and secondary treatment of osteomyelitis. J Chemother 17:643–50, 2005.

Bassetti M, Vitale F, Melica G, et al. Linezolid in the treatment of gram-positive prosthetic joint infections. J Antimicrob Chemother 55:387–390, 2005.

Bouza E. New therapeutic choices for infections caused by methicillin-resistant *Staphylococcus aureus*. Clin Microbiol Infect Dis 15:44–52, 2009.

Cannon JP, Pachucki CT, Aneziokoro CO and Lentino JR. The Effectiveness and Safety of Oral Linezolid as Primary or Secondary Treatment of Bloodstream Infections. Infect Dis Clin Pract. 14:221–226, 2006.

Castro P, Soriano A, Escrich C, Villalba G, et al. Linezolid treatment of ventriculoperitoneal shunt infection without implant removal. Eur J Clin Microbiol Infect Dis 24:603–06, 2005.

Clark DB, Andrus MR, Byrd DC. Drug interactions between linezolid and selective serotonin reuptake inhibitors: case report involving sertraline and review of the literature. Pharmacotherapy. 26:269–76, 2006.

Colli A, Compodonico R, Gherli T. Early switch from vancomycin to oral linezolid for treatment of gram-positive heart valve endocarditis. Ann Thorac Surg. 84:87–91, 2007.

Conte JE Jr, Golden JA, Dipps J, et al. Intrapulmonary pharmacokinetics of linezolid. Antimicrob Agents Chemother 46:1475–80, 2000.

Cunha BA. Antimicrobial Therapy of Multidrug-Resistant Streptococccus pneumoniae, Vancomycin-Resistant Enterococci, and Methicillin-Resistant Staphlycoccus aureus. Med Clin N Am 90:1165–82, 2006.

Cunha BA. Oral Antibiotic Therapy of Serious Systemic Infections. Med Clin N Am 90:1197–1222, 2006.

Deville JG, Adler S, AZimi PH, et al. Linezolid versus vancomycin in the treatment of known or suspected resistant Gram-positive infections in neonates. The Pediatric Infect Disease J. 22:S158–63, 2003.

Falagas ME, Manta KG, Ntziora F, et al. Linezolid for the treatment of patients with endocarditis: a systematic review of published evidence. J Antimicrob Chemother 58:273–280, 2006.

"Usual dose" assumes normal renal/hepatic function. * For renal insufficiency, give usual dose × 1 followed by maintenance dose per CrCl. For dialysis patients, dose the same as for CrCl < 10 mL/min and give supplemental (post-HD/PD dose) immediately after dialysis. CrCl = creatinine clearance; CVVH = continuous veno-venous hemofiltration; HD/PD = hemodialysis/peritoneal dialysis. See pp. 509–513 for explanations, pp. xi–xii for abbreviations; Linezolid (↑ risk of serotonin syndrome, see p. 620).

Falagas ME, Siempos II, Vardakas KZ. Linezolid versus glycopeptide or B-lactam for treatment of Gram-positive bacterial infections: meta-analysis of randomized controlled trials. Lancet Infect Dis 8:53–66, 2008.

Hill EE, Herijgers P, Herregods MC, Peetermans WE. Infective endocarditis treated with linezolid: case report and literature review. Eur J Clin Microbiol Infect Dis 25:202–4, 2006.

Johnson JR. Linezolid versus vancomycin for methicillin-resistant Staphylococcus aureus infections. Clin Infect Dis 36:236–7, 2003.

Kaka AS, Rueda AM, Shelburne SA 3rd, Hamill RJ. Bactericidal activity of orally available agents against methicillin-resistant Staphylococcus aureus. J Antimicrob Chemother 58:680–3, 2006.

Kalil AC, Puumala S, Stoner J. Is Linezolid Superior to Vancomycin for Complicated Skin and Soft Tissue Infections Due to Methicillin-Resistant Staphylococcus aureus? Antimicrob Agents Chemother 50:1910–1911, 2006.

Kruse AJ, Peederman SM, Bet PM, Debets-Oseenkopp YJ. Successful treatment with Linezolid of meningitis due to methicillin-resistant Staphylococcus epidermidis refractory to vancomycin treatment. Eur J Clin Microb Infect 215:135–7, 2006.

Kutscha-Lissberg F, Hebler U, Muhr G, et al. Linezolid penetration into bone and joint tissues infected with methicillin-resistant staphylococci. Antimicrob Agents Chemother 47:3964–6, 2003.

Lawrence KR, Adra M, Gillman PK. Serotonin Toxicity Associated with the Use of Linezolid: A Review of Postmarketing Data. Clin Infect Dis 42:1578–83, 2006.

Lustberg ME, Schlesinger LS, Mangino JE. Concerns about "Complicated Skin and Skin-Structure Infections and Catheter-Related Bloodstream Infections: Noninferiority of Linezolid in a Phase 3 Study. Clin Infect Dis 49:313–314, 2009.

Manfredi R, Sabbatani S, Marinacci G, Salizzoni E, Chiodo F. Listeria monocytogenes Meningitis and Multiple Brain Abscesses in an Immunocompetent Host. Favorable Response to Combination Linezolid-Meropenem Treatment. J Chemother 18:331–33, 2006.

Moreillon P, Wilson WR, Leclercq R, et al. Single-dose oral amoxicillin or linezolid for prophylaxis of experimental endocarditis due to vancomycin-susceptible and vancomycin-resistant Enterococcus faecalis. Antimicrob Agents Chemother 51:1661–1665, 2007.

Moylett EH, Pacheco SE, Brown-Elliott BA, et al. Clinical experience with linezolid for the treatment of nocardia infection. Clin Infect Dis 36:313–8, 2003.

Myrianthefs P, Markantonis SL, Vlachos K, et al. Serum and Cerebrospinal Fluid Concentrations of Linezolid in Neurosurgical Patients. Antimicrob Agents Chemother 50:3971–76, 2006.

Nasraway SA, Shorr AF, Kuter DJ, et al. Linezolid does not increase the risk of thrombocytopenia in patients with nosocomial pneumonia: comparative analysis of linezolid and vancomycin use. Clin Infect Dis 11:1609–16, 2003.

Nathani N, Iles P, Elliott TS. Successful treatment of MRSA native valve endocarditis with oral linezolid therapy: a case report. J Infect 51:213–215, 2005.

Nguyen S, Pasquet A, Legout L, et al. Efficacy and tolerance of rifampin-linezolid compared with rifampin-cotrimoxazole combinations in prolonged oral therapy for bone and joint infections. Clin Microbiol Infect Dis 15:1163–1169, 2009.

Park IN, Hong SB, Oh YM, Kim MN, et al. Efficacy and tolerability of daily-half dose linezolid in patients with intractable multidrug-resistant tuberculosis. J Antimicrob Chemther. 58:701–4, 2006.

Ravindran V, John J, Kaye GC, et al. Successful use of oral linezolid as a single active agent in endocarditis unresponsive to conventional antibiotic therapy. J Infect. 47:164–6, 2003.

Rao N, Ziran BH, Hall RA, et al. Successful treatment of chronic bone and joint infections with oral linezolid. Clin Orthop 427:67–71, 2004.

Schecter GF, Scott C, True L, et al. Linezolid in the Treatment of Multidrug-Resistant Tuberculosis. Clin Infect Dis 50:49–55, 2010.

Siegel RE. Linezolid to decrease length of stay in the hospital for patients with methicillin-resistant Staphylococcus aureus infection. Clin Infect Dis 36:124–5, 2003.

"Usual dose" assumes normal renal/hepatic function. * For renal insufficiency, give usual dose × 1 followed by maintenance dose per CrCl. For dialysis patients, dose the same as for CrCl < 10 mL/min and give supplemental (post-HD/PD dose) immediately after dialysis. CrCl = creatinine clearance; CVVH = continuous veno-venous hemofiltration; HD/PD = hemodialysis/peritoneal dialysis. See pp. 509–513 for explanations, pp. xi–xii for abbreviations; Linezolid (↑ risk of serotonin syndrome, see p. 620).

Souli M, Pontikis K, Chryssouli Z, et al. Successful treatment of right-sided prosthetic valve endocarditis due to methicillin-resistant teicoplanin-heteroresistant Staphylococcus aureus with linezolid. Eur J Clin Microbiol Infect Dis 24:760–762, 2005.

Stalker DJ, Jungbluth GL. Clinical pharmacokinetics of linezolid, a novel oxazolidinone antibacterial. Clin Pharmacokinet. 42:1129–40, 2003.

Stein GE, Schooley SL, Havlichek DH, et al. Outpatient Intravenous Antibiotic Therapy Compared with Oral Linezolid in Patients with Skin and Soft Tissue Infections: A-Pharmacoeconomic Analysis. Infectious Dis in Clin Practice. 16:235–240, 2008.

Stevens DL, Herr D, Lampiris H, et al. Linezolid versus vancomycin for the treatment of methicillin-resistant Staphylococcus aureus infections. Clin Infect Dis 34:1481–90, 2002.

Taylor JJ, Wilson JW, Estes LL. Linezolid and serotonergic Drug Interactions: a retrospective survey. Clin Infect Dis 43:180–7, 2006.

Villani P, Pegazzi MB, Marubbi F, et al. Cerebrospinal fluid linezolid concentrations in postneurosurgical central nervous system infections. Antimicrob Agents Chemother 46:936–7, 2002.

Website: www.zyvox.com

Lopinavir + Ritonavir (Kaletra) LP/RTV

Drug Class: Antiretroviral protease inhibitor combination.

Usual Dose: Therapy-naive: 400/10 mg (2 tablets or 5 mL solution) q12h or 800/200 mg (4 tablets or 10 mL solution) q24h. Therapy-experienced: 400/100 mg q12h. New tablet formulation (lopinavir 200 mg + ritonavir 50 mg) replaces capsules (lopinavir 133.3 mg + ritonavir 33.3 mg), resulting in reduction in total number of pills from 6 capsules to 4 tablets per day. Also available as an oral solution (lopinavir 400 mg + ritonavir 100 mg per 5 mL).

Pharmacokinetic Parameters:

Peak serum level: 9.6/≤ 1 mcg/mL

Bioavailability: No data

Excreted unchanged (urine): 3%

Serum half-life (normal/ESRD): 5–6/5–6 hrs

Plasma protein binding: 99%

Volume of distribution (V_d): No data/ 0.44 L/kg

Primary Mode of Elimination: Hepatic

Dosage Adjustments*

CrCl 50–80 mL/min	No change
CrCl 10–50 mL/min	No change
CrCl < 10 mL/min	No change
Post–HD dose	None
Post–PD dose	None
CVVH dose	No change
Moderate hepatic insufficiency	No change
Severe hepatic insufficiency	Avoid

Antiretroviral Dosage Adjustments:

Fosamprenavir	Avoid
Delavirdine	No information
Efavirenz	Consider lopinavir/ ritonavir 600/150 mg (3 tablets) q12h
Indinavir	Indinavir 600 mg q12h
Nelfinavir	Same as for efavirenz
Nevirapine	Same as for efavirenz
Rifabutin	Max. dose of rifabutin 150 mg qod or 3 times per week
Saquinavir	Saquinavir 1000 mg q12h

"Usual dose" assumes normal renal/hepatic function. * For renal insufficiency, give usual dose × 1 followed by maintenance dose per CrCl. For dialysis patients, dose the same as for CrCl < 10 mL/min and give supplemental (post-HD/PD dose) immediately after dialysis. CrCl = creatinine clearance; CVVH = continuous veno-venous hemofiltration; HD/PD = hemodialysis/peritoneal dialysis. See pp. 509–513 for explanations, pp. xi–xii for abbreviations; Linezolid (↑ risk of serotonin syndrome, see p. 620).

Drug Interactions: Antiretrovirals, rifabutin, (see dose adjustment grid, above); Rifampin may significantly reduce lopinavir levels leading to drug failure and should be avoided. Sidenafil, tadalafil, and verdenafil levels will be greatly increased and their dosage must be decreased. Antiarhythmics such as amiodarone, bepredil, lidocaine and quinidine may increase. Tacrolimus, cyclosporine and rapamycin levels can be altered leading to increased toxicity. Methadone levels may be decreased leading to withdrawal reactions. Fluticasone levels may increase leading to Cushing like syndrome, astemizole, terfenadine, benzodiazepines, cisapride, ergotamine, flecainide, pimozide, propafenone, rifampin, statins, St. John's wort (contraindicated); tenofovir (↓ lopinavir levels, ↑ tenofovir levels). ↓ effectiveness of oral contraceptives. Insufficient data on other drug interactions listed for ritonavir alone. At end of drug interaction add lopinavir/resolution contains alcohol and can lead to a disulfram reaction when administered with metranidazole.
Adverse Effects: Diarrhea (very common), headache, nausea, vomiting, asthenia, ↑ SGOT/SGPT, hepatotoxicity, abdominal pain, pancreatitis, paresthesias, hyperglycemia (including worsening diabetes, new-onset diabetes, DKA), ↑ cholesterol/triglycerides (evaluate risk for coronary disease, pancreatitis), ↑ CPK, ↑ uric acid, fat redistribution, possible increased bleeding in hemophilia. Oral solution contains 42.4% alcohol. Immune reconstitution syndrome and redistribution/accumulation of body fat have been reported in patients treated with combination antiretroviral therapy.
Allergic Potential: Low
Safety in Pregnancy: C
Comments: New tablet formulation does not require refrigeration and may be taken with or without food. With oral solution, Lopinavir serum concentrations with moderately fatty meals are increased 54%.

REFERENCES:

Benson CA, Deeks SG, Brun SC, et al. Safety and antiviral activity at 48 weeks of lopinavir/ritonavir plus nevirapine and 2 nucleoside reverse-transcriptase inhibitors in human immunodeficiency virus type 1-infected protease inhibitor-experienced patients. J Infect Dis 185:599–607, 2002.

Fischl MA. Antiretroviral therapy in 1999 for antiretroviral-naive individuals with HIV infection. AIDS 13:49–59, 1999.

Manfredi R, Calza L, Chiodo F. First-line efavirenz versus lopinavir-ritonavir-based highly active antiretroviral therapy for naive patients. AIDS 18:2331–2333, 2004.

Panel on Antiretroviral Guidelines for Adults and Adolescents. Guidelines for the use of antiretroviral agents in HIV-1 infected adults and adolescents. Department of Health and Human Services. November 3, 2008; 1–139. Available at http://www.aidsinfor.nih.gov/ContentFiles/AdultandAdolescentGL.pdf.

Walmsley S, Bernstein B, King M, et al. Lopinavir-ritonavir versus nelfinavir for the initial treatment of HIV infection. N Engl J Med 346:2039–46, 2002.

Website: www.kaletra.com

Loracarbef (Lorabid)

Drug Class: 2nd generation oral cephalosporin.
Usual Dose: 400 mg (PO) q12h (see comments).
Spectrum: (see ***Susceptibility Profiles*** pp. 188–193).
Pharmacokinetic Parameters:
Peak serum level: 14 mcg/mL
Bioavailability: 90%
Excreted unchanged (urine): 90%
Serum half-life (normal/ESRD): 1.2/32 hrs
Plasma protein binding: 25%

"Usual dose" assumes normal renal/hepatic function. * For renal insufficiency, give usual dose × 1 followed by maintenance dose per CrCl. For dialysis patients, dose the same as for CrCl < 10 mL/min and give supplemental (post-HD/PD dose) immediately after dialysis. CrCl = creatinine clearance; CVVH = continuous veno-venous hemofiltration; HD/PD = hemodialysis/peritoneal dialysis. See pp. 509–513 for explanations, pp. xi–xii for abbreviations; Linezolid (↑ risk of serotonin syndrome, see p. 620).

Volume of distribution (V_d): 0.35 L/kg
Primary Mode of Elimination: Renal
Dosage Adjustments*

CrCl 50–80 mL/min	No change
CrCl 10–50 mL/min	200 mg (PO) q24h
CrCl < 10 mL/min	200 mg (PO) q72h
Post–HD dose	400 mg (PO)
Post–PD dose	200 mg (PO)
CVVH dose	200 mg (PO) q12h
Moderate hepatic insufficiency	No change
Severe hepatic insufficiency	No change

Drug Interactions: None.
Adverse Effects: Drug fever/rash, C. difficile diarrhea/colitis.
Allergic Potential: Low
Safety in Pregnancy: B
Comments: Take 1 hour before or 2 hours after meals. **CAP dose:** 400 mg (PO) q12h. **Sinusitis/tonsillitis dose:** 200 mg (PO) q12h.
Cerebrospinal Fluid Penetration: < 10%
(also see ***Antibiotic Pearls & Pitfalls*** pp. 495–508).

REFERENCES:
Bandak SI, Turnak MR, Allen BS, et al. Assessment of the susceptibility of Streptococcus pneumoniae to cefaclor and loracarbef in 13 cases. J Chemother 12:299–305, 2000.

Gooch WM 3rd, Adelglass J, Kelsey DK, et al. Loracarbef versus clarithromycin in children with acute otitis media with effusion. Clin her 21:711–22, 1999.

Paster RZ, McAdoo MA, Keyserling CH. A comparison of a five-day regimen of cefdinir with a seven-day regimen of loracarbef for the treatment of acute exacerbations of chronic bronchitis. Int J Clin Pract 64:293–9, 2000.

Vogel F, Ochs HR, Wettich K, et al. Effect of step-down therapy of ceftriazone plus loracarbef versus parenteral therapy of ceftriaxone on the intestinal microflora in patients with community-acquired pneumonia. Clin Microbiol Infect 7:376–9, 2001.

Website: www.pdr.net

Maraviroc (Selzentry)

Drug Class: HIV-1 chemokine receptor 5 (CCR5) antagonist.
Usual Dose: 150 mg, 300 mg, or 600 mg (PO) q12h, depending on concomitant medications (see below), in CCR5-tropic HIV-1 isolates. Available in 150 mg and 300 mg tablets.
Pharmacokinetic Parameters:
Peak serum level: 266–618 mcg/mL
Bioavailability: 23–33%
Excreted unchanged: 20% (urine); 76% (feces)
Serum half-life (normal/ESRD): 14–18 hrs/not studied
Plasma protein binding: 76%
Volume of distribution (V_d): 194 L
Primary Mode of Elimination: Fecal/renal
Dosage Adjustments*

CrCl 50–80 mL/min	No change
CrCl 10–25 mL/min	Use caution
CrCl < 10 mL/min	Use caution
Post–HD dose	No information
Post–PD dose	No information
CVVH dose	No information
Mild hepatic insufficiency	No information
Moderate or severe hepatic insufficiency	No information

"Usual dose" assumes normal renal/hepatic function. * For renal insufficiency, give usual dose × 1 followed by maintenance dose per CrCl. For dialysis patients, dose the same as for CrCl < 10 mL/min and give supplemental (post-HD/PD dose) immediately after dialysis. CrCl = creatinine clearance; CVVH = continuous veno-venous hemofiltration; HD/PD = hemodialysis/peritoneal dialysis. See pp. 509–513 for explanations, pp. xi–xii for abbreviations; Linezolid (↑ risk of serotonin syndrome, see p. 620).

Antiretroviral Dosage Adjustments:

protease inhibitors (except tipranavir/ritonavir), delavirdine, ketoconazole, itraconazole, clarithromycin, nefazodone, telithromycin	150 mg (PO) q12h
tipranavir/ritonavir, nevirapine, all NRTIs and enfuvirtide	300 mg (PO) q12h
efavirenz, rifampin, carbamazepine, phenobarbital, phenytoin	600 mg (PO) q12h

Drug Interactions: Maraviroc is a substrate of CYP3A and P-glycoprotein and is likely to be modulated by inhibitors and inducers of these enzymes/transporters.
Adverse Effects: Hepatotoxicity has been reported. A systemic allergic reaction (e.g., pruritic rash, eosinophilia, or elevated IgE) prior to the development of hepatotoxicity may occur. Other Adverse Effects: cough, infection, upper respiratory tract infection, rash, pyrexia, dizziness, abdominal pain, musculoskeletal symptoms (joint/muscle pain). Myocardial infarction/ ischemia reported in < 2% in clinical trials.
Allergic Potential: Low
Safety in Pregnancy: B
Comments: Indicated for treatment-experienced adult patients infected with only cellular chemokine receptor (CCR) 5-tropic HIV-1 virus detectable who have evidence of viral replication and HIV-1 strains resistant to multiple antiretroviral agents. Used in combination with other antiretroviral agents. Trofile phenotype test (performed at Monogram) is needed to confirm infection with CCR5-tropic HIV-1 (also known as "R5 virus"). May increase risk of infection (especially HSV) and risk of neoplasms.
Cerebrospinal Fluid Penetration: No data

REFERENCES:

Dorr P, Westby M, Dobbs S, et al. Maraviroc (UK-427,857), a potent, orally bioavailable, and selective small-molecule inhibitor of chemokine receptor CCR5 with broad-spectrum anti-human immunodeficiency virus type 1 activity. Antimicrob Agents Chemother 49:4721–4732, 2005.

Lalezari, J. Efficacy and Safety of Maraviroc plus Optimized Background Therapy in Viremic ART-experienced Patients Infected with CCR5-tropic HIV-1: 24-Week Results of a Phase 2b/3 Study in the US and Canada [Abstract 104bLB]. Conference on Retroviruses and Opportunistic Infections. Alexandria, VA. 2007. Available from URL: http://www.retroconference.org/2007/Abstracts/30635.htm.

Lederman MM, Penn-Nicholson A,Cho M, et al.Biology of CCR5 and its role in HIV infection and treatment. JAMA 296:815–826, 2006.

Nelson, M. Efficacy and Safety of Maraviroc plus Optimized Background Therapy in Viremic, ART-experienced Patients Infected with CCR5-tropic HIV-1 in Europe, Australia, and North America: 24-Week Results [Abstract 104aLB]. Conference on Retroviruses and Opportunistic Infections. Alexandria, VA. 2007. Available from URL: http://www.retroconference.org/2007/Abstracts/30636.htm.

Panel on Antiretroviral Guidelines for Adults and Adolescents. Guidelines for the use of antiretroviral agents in HIV-1 infected adults and adolescents. Department of Health and Human Services. November 3, 2008; 1–139. Available at http://www.aidsinfor.nih.gov/ContentFiles/AdultandAdolescentGL.pdf.

Product Information: SELZENTRY(R) oral tablets, maraviroc oral tablets. Pfizer Labs, New York, NY, 2007.

Website: www.selzentry.com

Meropenem (Merrem/Meronem)

Drug Class: Carbapenem.
Usual Dose: 500 mg–1 gm (IV) q8h (see comments).

"Usual dose" assumes normal renal/hepatic function. * For renal insufficiency, give usual dose × 1 followed by maintenance dose per CrCl. For dialysis patients, dose the same as for CrCl < 10 mL/min and give supplemental (post-HD/PD dose) immediately after dialysis. CrCl = creatinine clearance; CVVH = continuous veno-venous hemofiltration; HD/PD = hemodialysis/peritoneal dialysis. See pp. 509–513 for explanations, pp. xi–xii for abbreviations; Linezolid (↑ risk of serotonin syndrome, see p. 620).

Spectrum: (see ***Susceptibility Profiles*** pp. 194–199).
Pharmacokinetic Parameters:
Peak serum level: 49 mcg/ml
Bioavailability: Not applicable
Excreted unchanged (urine): 70%
Serum half-life (normal/ESRD): 1/7 hrs
Plasma protein binding: 2%
Volume of distribution (V_d): 0.35 L/kg
Primary Mode of Elimination: Renal
Dosage Adjustments* (based on 1 gm dose; for 500 mg dosing use half of dose shown in grid)

CrCl 25–50 mL/min	1 gm (IV) q12h
CrCl 10–25 mL/min	500 mg (IV) q12h
CrCl < 10 mL/min	500 mg (IV) q24h
Post–HD dose	500 mg (IV)
Post–HFHD dose	500 mg (IV)
Post–PD dose	500 mg (IV)
CVVH dose	1 gm (IV) q12h
SLEDD dose	1 gm (IV) q12h
Moderate hepatic insufficiency	No change
Severe hepatic insufficiency	No change

Drug Interactions: Probenecid (↑ meropenem half-life by 40%), Valproic acid (↓ seizure threshold).
Adverse Effects: Rarely, mild infusion site inflammation. No seizures. **No cross allergenicity with penicillins/β-lactams; safe to use in patients with a history of penicillin allergic reactions.**
Allergic Potential: Low
Safety in Pregnancy: B
Comments: ***MDR GNBs, cystic fibrosis/ meningitis dose:*** *2 gm (IV) q8h;* **cSSSIs, cIAIs or UTIs dose:** 500 mg (IV) q8h. Inhibits endotoxin release from gram-negative bacilli. **Meropenem is the *only carbapenem that may be given by IV bolus injection over 3–5 minutes*.** Na^+ content = 3.92 mEq/g. Meningeal dose = 2 gm (IV) q8h.
Cerebrospinal Fluid Penetration:
Non-Inflamed meninges = 10%
Inflamed meninges = 15%
Bile Penetration:
Without obstruction = 75%
With obstruction = 40%
(also see ***Antibiotic Pearls & Pitfalls*** pp. 495–508).

REFERENCES:

Berman SJ, Fogarty CM, Fabian T, et al. Meropenem monotherapy for the treatment of hospital-acquired pneumonia: results of a multicenter trial. J Chemother 16:362–71, 2004.
Cheng AC, Fisher DA, Anstey NM, et al. Outcomes of patients with melioidosis treated with meropenem. Antimicrob Agents Chemother 48:1763–5, 2004.
Conte JE Jr, Golden JA, Kelley MG, Zurlinden E. Intrapulmonary pharmacokinetics and pharmacodynamics of meropenem. Int J Antimicrob Agents. 26:449–56, 2005.
Cunha BA. Meropenem: Lack of Cross Reactivity in Penicillin Allergic Patients. Journal of Chemotherapy 20:233–237, 2008.
Cunha BA. Meropenem: Current Uses in Critical Care. Antibiotics for Clinicians 11:433–444, 2007.
Cunha BA. Pseudomonas aeruginosa: Resistance and therapy. Semin Respir Infect 17:231–9, 2002.
Cunha BA. The use of meropenem in critical care. Antibiotics for Clinicians 4:59–66, 2000.
Cunha BA. Cross allergenicity of penicillin with carbapenems and monobactams. J Crit Illness 13:344, 1998.
Cunha BA. The safety of meropenem in elderly and renally impaired patients. Intern J Antimicrob Ther 10:109–117, 1998.

"Usual dose" assumes normal renal/hepatic function. * For renal insufficiency, give usual dose × 1 followed by maintenance dose per CrCl. For dialysis patients, dose the same as for CrCl < 10 mL/min and give supplemental (post-HD/PD dose) immediately after dialysis. CrCl = creatinine clearance; CVVH = continuous veno-venous hemofiltration; HD/PD = hemodialysis/peritoneal dialysis. See pp. 509–513 for explanations, pp. xi–xii for abbreviations; Linezolid (↑ risk of serotonin syndrome, see p. 620).

Du X, Li C, Kuti JL, Nightingale CH, et al.Population pharmacokinetics and pharmacodynamics of meropenem in pediatric patients. J Clin Pharmacol. 46:69–75, 2006.

Edwards SJ, Campbell HE, Plumb JM. Cost-utility analysis comparing meropenem with imipenem plus cilastatin in the treatment of severe infections in intensive care. Eur J Health Econ 7:72–8, 2006.

Erdem I, Kucukercan M, Ceran N. In vitro activity of combination therapy with cefepime, piperacillin-tazobactam, or meropenem with ciprofloxacin against multidrug-resistant Pseudomonas aeruginosa strains. Chemotherapy 49:294–7, 2003.

Fabian TC, File TM, Embil HM, et al. Meropenem vs. imipenem-cilastatin for the treatment of hospitalized patients with complicated skin and skin structure infections: results of a multicenter, randomized, double-blind comparative study. Surgical Infections 6:269–282, 2005.

Fish DN, Singletary TJ. Meropenem: A new carbapenem antibiotic. Pharmacotherapy 17:644–69, 1997.

Garcia-Rodriguez JA, Jones RN. Antimicrobial resistance in gram-negative isolates from European intensive care units: data from the Meropenem Yearly Susceptibility Test Information Collection (MYSTIC) programme. J Chemother 14:25–32, 2002.

Hellinger WC, Brewer NS. Carbapenems and monobactams: Imipenem, meropenem, and aztreonam. Mayo Clin Proc 74:420–34, 1999.

Jaruratanasirikul S, Sriwiriyajan, Punyo J. Comparison of the pharmacodynamics of meropenem in patients with ventilator-associated pneumonia following administration by 3-hour infusion or bolus injection. Antimicrobial Agents and Chemotherapy 49:1337–39, 2005.

Kitzes-Cohen R, Farin D, Piva G, et al. Pharmacokinetics and pharmacodynamics of meropenem in critically ill patients. Int J Antimicrob Agents 19:105–10, 2002.

Li Cn Xiaoli D, Kuti JL, et al. Clinical pharmacodynamics of meropenem in patients with lower respiratory tract infections. Antimicrob Agents Chemother 51:1725–1730, 2007.

Lomaestro BM, Drusano GL. Pharmacodynamic evaluation of extending the administration time of meropenem using a Monte Carlo simulation. Antimicrobial Agents and Chemotherapy 49:461–463, 2005.

Manfredi R, Sabbatani S, Marinacci G, Salizzoni E, Chiodo F. Listeria monocytogenes Meningitis and Multiple Brain Abscesses in an Immunocompetent Host. Favorable Response to Combination Linezolid-Meropenem Treatment. Journal of Chemotherapy. 18:331–33, 2009.

Mattoes HM, Kuti JL, Drusano GL, et al. Optimizing antimicrobial pharmacodynamics: dosage strategies for meropenem. Clin Ther 26:1187–98, 2004.

Perez-Simon JA, Garcia-Escobar I, Martinez J, et al. Antibiotic prophylaxis with meropenem after allogeneic stem cell transplantation. Bone Marrow Transplant 33:183–7, 2004.

Rhomberg PR, Jones RN, Sades HS, et al. Antimicrobial resistance rates and clonality results from the meropenem yearly susceptibility test information collection (MYSTIC) programed: report of year five (2003). Diagn Microbiol Infect Dis 49:273–81, 2004.

Romano A, Viola M, Gueant-Rodriquez R, et al. Tolerability of meropenem in patients with IgE-mediated hypersensitivity of penicillins. Ann Intern Med 146:266–69, 2007.

Sodhi M, Axtell SS, Callahan J, et al. Is it safe to use carbapenems in patients with a history of allergy to penicillin? J Antimicrob Chemother 54:1155–7, 2004.

Unal S, Garcia-Rodriguez JA. Activity of meropenem and comparators against Pseudomonas aeruginosa and Acinetobacter spp. isolated in the MYSTIC Program, 2002–2004.Diagn Microbiol Infect Dis 53:265–71, 2006.

Website: www.MerremIV.com

Methenamine hippurate (Hiprex, Urex) Methenamine mandelate (Mandelamine)

Drug Class: Urinary antiseptic.

Usual Dose: 1 gm (PO) q6h (hippurate); 1 gm (PO) q6h (mandelate).

Pharmacokinetic Parameters:

Peak serum level: Not applicable

"Usual dose" assumes normal renal/hepatic function. * For renal insufficiency, give usual dose × 1 followed by maintenance dose per CrCl. For dialysis patients, dose the same as for CrCl < 10 mL/min and give supplemental (post-HD/PD dose) immediately after dialysis. CrCl = creatinine clearance; CVVH = continuous veno-venous hemofiltration; HD/PD = hemodialysis/peritoneal dialysis. See pp. 509–513 for explanations, pp. xi–xii for abbreviations; Linezolid (↑ risk of serotonin syndrome, see p. 620).

Bioavailability: 90%
Excreted unchanged (urine): 90%
Serum half-life (normal/ESRD): 4 hrs/no data
Plasma protein binding: Not applicable
Volume of distribution (V_d): Not applicable
Primary Mode of Elimination: Renal
Dosage Adjustments*

CrCl 50–80 mL/min	Avoid
CrCl 10–50 mL/min	Avoid
CrCl < 10 mL/min	Avoid
Post–HD dose	Avoid
Post–PD dose	Avoid
CVVH dose	Avoid
Moderate hepatic insufficiency	No change
Severe hepatic insufficiency	Avoid

Drug Interactions: Acetazolamide, sodium bicarbonate, thiazide diuretics (↓ antibacterial effect due to ↑ urinary pH ≥ 5.5).
Adverse Effects: GI upset.
Allergic Potential: Low
Safety in Pregnancy: C
Comments: Take with food to decrease GI upset. Effectiveness depends on maintaining an acid urine (pH ≤ 5.5) with acidifying agents (e.g., ascorbic acid). **Useful only for catheter-associated bacteriuria (CAB)**, not UTIs. **Forms formaldehyde in acid urine; resistance does not develop.**

REFERENCES:

Cunha BA, Comer JB, Pharmacokinetic considerations in the treatment of urinary tract infections. Conn Med 43:347–53, 1979.

Klinge D, Mannisto P, Mantyla R, et al. Pharmacokinetics of methenamine in healthy volunteers. J Antimicrob Chemother 9:209–16, 1982.

Musher DM, Griggith DP,Generation of formaldehyde from methenamine: Effect of pH and concentration, and antibacterial effect. Antimicrob Agents Chemother 6:708–11, 1974.

Musher DM, Griffith DP, Templeton GB, Further observations of the potentiation of the antibacterial effect of methenamine by acetohydroxamic acid. J Infect Dis 133:564–67, 1976.

Schiotz HA, Guttu K, Value of urinary prophylaxis with methenamine in gynecologic surgery. Acta Obstet Gynecol Scand 81:743–6, 2002.

Metronidazole (Flagyl)

Drug Class: Nitroimidazole antiparasitic/antibiotic.
Usual Dose: 1 gm (IV) q24h; 500 mg (IV/PO) q6-8h (see comments).
Spectrum: (see ***Susceptibility Profiles*** pp. 183–187).
Pharmacokinetic Parameters:
Peak serum level: 26 (IV)/12 (PO) mcg/ml
Bioavailability: 100%
Excreted unchanged (urine): 20%
Serum half-life (normal/ESRD): 8/14 hrs
Plasma protein binding: 20%
Volume of distribution (V_d): 0.25–0.85 L/kg
Primary Mode of Elimination: Hepatic
Dosage Adjustments*

CrCl 50–80 mL/min	No change
CrCl 10–50 mL/min	No change
CrCl < 10 mL/min	500 mg (IV) q24h 250 mg (PO) q12h
Post–HD dose	1 gm (IV) 500 mg (PO)
Post–PD dose	1 gm (IV) 500 mg (PO)

"Usual dose" assumes normal renal/hepatic function. * For renal insufficiency, give usual dose × 1 followed by maintenance dose per CrCl. For dialysis patients, dose the same as for CrCl < 10 mL/min and give supplemental (post-HD/PD dose) immediately after dialysis. CrCl = creatinine clearance; CVVH = continuous veno-venous hemofiltration; HD/PD = hemodialysis/peritoneal dialysis. See pp. 509–513 for explanations, pp. xi–xii for abbreviations; Linezolid (↑ risk of serotonin syndrome, see p. 620).

CVVH dose	No change
Moderate hepatic insufficiency	No change
Severe hepatic insufficiency	500 mg (IV/PO) q24h

Drug Interactions: Alcohol (disulfiram-like reaction); disulfiram (acute toxic psychosis); warfarin (↑ INR); phenobarbital, phenytoin (↑ metronidazole metabolism).

Adverse Effects: Encephalopathy, metallic taste, aseptic meningitis, seizures, peripheral neuropathy. With oral formulation, nausea, vomiting, GI upset. May discolor urine brown.

Allergic Potential: Low

Safety in Pregnancy: B (avoid in 1st trimester)

Comments: For intra-abdominal/pelvic sepsis (**plus anti-aerobic GNB drug**). **q24h dosing is preferred to q6h/q8h dosing because of long half-life** ($t_{1/2}$ = 8 h). For **C. difficile diarrhea**, use 250 mg (PO) q6h. For **C. difficile colitis**, use 500 mg (IV or PO) q6-8h or 1 gm (IV) q24h. **For severe C. difficile colitis, add anti-GNB coverage**, e.g., ertapenem or meropenem for microscopic/macroscopic perforation/peritonitis. **Use increases VRE prevalence**.

Meningeal dose = usual dose.

Cerebrospinal Fluid Penetration:

Non-Inflamed meninges = 30%

Inflamed meninges = 100%

(also see ***Antibiotic Pearls & Pitfalls*** p. 507).

REFERENCES:

Bouza E, Burillo A, Munoz P, Antimicrobial Therapy of Clostridium difficile-Associated Diarrhea. Med Clin N Am 90:1141–63, 2006.

Clay PG, Graham MR, Lindsey CC, et al. Clinical efficacy, tolerability, and cost savings associated with the use of open-label metronidazole plus ceftriaxone once daily compared with ticarcillin/clavulanate every 6 hours as empiric treatment for diabetic lower-extremity infections in older males. Am J Geriatr Pharmacother 2:181–9, 2004.

Cunha BA.Oral Antibiotic Therapy of Serious Systemic Infections. Med Clin N Am 90:1197–1222, 2006.

Falagas ME, Gorbach SL. Clindamycin and metronidazole. Med Clin North Am 79:845–67, 1995.

Freeman CD, Klutman NE. Metronidazole: A therapeutic review and update. Drugs 54:679–708, 1997.

Freeman CD, Nightingale CH, Nicolau DP, et al. Serum bactericidal activity of ceftriaxone plus metronidazole against common intra-abdominal pathogens. Am J Hosp Pharm 51:1782–7, 1994.

Garbino J, Villiger P, Caviezel A, et al. A randomized prospective study of cefepime plus metronidazole with imipenem-cilastatin in the treatment of intra-abdominal infections. Infection 35:161–166, 2007.

Hermsen ED, Hovde LB, Sprandel KA, et al. Levofloxacin plus metronidazole administered once daily versus moxifloxacin monotherapy against a mixed infection of Escherichia coli and Bacteroides fragilis in an in vitro pharmacodynamic model. Antimicrobial Agents and Chemotherapy 49:685–689, 2005.

Ishikawa T, Okamura S, Oshimoto H, et al. Metronidazole plus ciprofloxacin therapy for active Crohn's disease. Intern Med 42:318–21, 2003.

Kasten MJ. Clindamycin, metronidazole, and chloramphenicol. Mayo Clin Proc 74:825–33, 1999.

Musher DM, Aslam S, Logan N, et al. Relatively poor outcome after treatment of Clostridium difficile colitis with metronidazole. Clinical Infectious Disease 40:1586–90, 2005.

Sprandel KA, Drusano GL, Hecht DW, et al. Population pharmacokinetic modeling and Monte Carlo simulation of varying doses of intravenous metronidazole. Diag Microbiol And Infect Dis 55:303–9, 2006.

Sprandel KA, Schriever CA, Pendland SL, et al. Pharmacokinetics and pharmacodynamics of intravenous levofloxacin at 750 milligrams and

"Usual dose" assumes normal renal/hepatic function. * For renal insufficiency, give usual dose × 1 followed by maintenance dose per CrCl. For dialysis patients, dose the same as for CrCl < 10 mL/min and give supplemental (post-HD/PD dose) immediately after dialysis. CrCl = creatinine clearance; CVVH = continuous veno-venous hemofiltration; HD/PD = hemodialysis/peritoneal dialysis. See pp. 509–513 for explanations, pp. xi–xii for abbreviations; Linezolid (↑ risk of serotonin syndrome, see p. 620).

various doses of metronidazole in healthy adult subjects. Antimicrob Agents Chemother 48: 4597–605, 2004.
Vasa CV, Glatt AE. Effectiveness and appropriateness of empiric metronidazole for Clostridium difficile diarrhea. Am J Gastroenterol 98:354–8, 2003.
Wacha H, Warren B, Bassaris H, et al. Comparison of Sequential Intravenous/Oral Ciprofloxacin Plus Metronidazole with Intravenous Ceftriaxone Plus Metronidazole for Treatment of Complicated Intra-Abdominal Infections. Surgical Infections 7:341–54, 2006.
Wang S, Cunha BA, Hamid NS, Amato BM, Feuerman M, Malone B. Intravenous Metronidazole: Once Daily vs. Multiple Dosing in Intra-abdominal Infections. Journal of Chemotherapy 19:410–416, 2007.
Website: www.pdr.net

Mezlocillin (Mezlin)

Drug Class: Antipseudomonal penicillin.
Usual Dose: 3 gm (IV) q6h.
Pharmacokinetic Parameters:
Peak serum level: 300 mcg/ml
Bioavailability: Not applicable
Excreted unchanged (urine): 65%
Serum half-life (normal/ESRD): 1.1/4 hrs
Plasma protein binding: 30%
Volume of distribution (V_d): 0.18 L/kg
Primary Mode of Elimination: Renal
Dosage Adjustments*

CrCl > 30 mL/min	No change
CrCl 10–30 mL/min	3 gm (IV) q8h
CrCl < 10 mL/min	2 gm (IV) q8h
Post–HD dose	3 gm (IV)
Post–PD dose	None
CVVH dose	3 gm (IV) q8h
Moderate hepatic insufficiency	No change
Severe hepatic insufficiency	3 gm (IV) q12h

Drug Interactions: Aminoglycosides (inactivation of mezlocillin in renal failure); warfarin (↑ INR); oral contraceptives (↓ oral contraceptive effect); cefoxitin (↓ mezlocillin effect).
Adverse Effects: Drug fever/rash, E. multiforme/Stevens–Johnson syndrome, anaphylactic reactions (hypotension, laryngospasm, bronchospasm), hives; serum sickness. **Dose-dependent inhibition of platelet aggregation is minimal/absent** (usual dose is less than carbenicillin).
Allergic Potential: Low
Safety in Pregnancy: B
Comments: Dose-dependent half-life ($t_{1/2}$). Na^+ content = 1.8 mEq/g.
Cerebrospinal Fluid Penetration: < 10%

REFERENCES:
Donowitz GR, Mandell GL. Beta-lactam antibiotics. N Engl J Med 318:419–26, 490–500, 1993.
Wright AJ, Wirkowske CJ. The penicillins. Mayo Clin Proc 66:1047–63, 1991.
Wright AJ. The penicillins. Mayo Clin Proc 74:290–307, 1999.
Website: www.pdr.net

Micafungin (Mycamine)

Drug Class: Echinocandin antifungal.
Usual Dose: 100 mg (IV) q24h for candidemia; 150 mg q24h for treatment of esophageal candidiasis. 50 mg (IV) q24h for prevention of candidal infection in hematopoietic stem cell transplant recipients.

"Usual dose" assumes normal renal/hepatic function. * For renal insufficiency, give usual dose × 1 followed by maintenance dose per CrCl. For dialysis patients, dose the same as for CrCl < 10 mL/min and give supplemental (post-HD/PD dose) immediately after dialysis. CrCl = creatinine clearance; CVVH = continuous veno-venous hemofiltration; HD/PD = hemodialysis/peritoneal dialysis. See pp. 509–513 for explanations, pp. xi–xii for abbreviations; Linezolid (↑ risk of serotonin syndrome, see p. 620).

Pharmacokinetic Parameters:
Peak serum level: 5.1 mcg/ml (50 mg); 11.2 mcg/ml (100 mg); 16.4 mcg/ml (150 mg)
Bioavailability: Not applicable
Excreted unchanged (urine): 11%
Serum half-life (normal/ESRD): 10–15 hrs/no change
Plasma protein binding: > 99%
Volume of distribution (V_d): 0.39 L/kg
Primary Mode of Elimination: Liver
Dosage Adjustments

CrCl ≥ 50 mL/min	No change
CrCl 30–50 mL/min	No change
CrCl 15–30 mL/min	No change
CrCl < 15 mL/min	No change
Post–HD dose	None
Post–PD dose	None
CVVH dose	No change
Mild or Moderate hepatic insufficiency	No change
Severe hepatic insufficiency	No information

Drug Interactions: Sirolimus AUC ↑ by 21% with no change in Cmax (monitor for sirolimus toxicity), nifedipine AUC and Cmax ↑ by 18% and 42%, respectively (monitor for nifedipine toxicity).

Adverse Effects: Nausea, vomiting, ↑ SGOT/SGPT, rash.

Allergic Potential: Low

Safety in Pregnancy: C

Comments: Administer by IV infusion over one hour—do not give as a bolus as more rapid infusions may result in more frequent histamine mediated reactions. Do not mix or co-use with other medications; flush intravenous line with 0.9% saline prior to infusion.
Most cost effective parenteral antifungal for empiric therapy of systemic Candida/Aspergillus infections.

Cerebrospinal Fluid Penetration: < 1%

REFERENCES:

Andes D, Safdar N. Efficacy of micafungin for the treatment of candidemia. Eur J Clin Microbiol Infect Dis 24:662–664, 2005.

Bennett JE, Echinocandins for candidemia in adults without neutropenia. N Engl J Med 355:1154–9, 2006.

Chandraseka PH, Sobel JD. Micafungin: A New Echinocandin. Clin Infect Dis 42:1171–78, 2006.

Denning DW, Marr KA, Lau WM, et al. Micafungin (FK463), alone or in combination with other systemic antifungal agents, for the treatment of acute invasive aspergillosis. Journal of Infection 53:337–349, 2006.

de Wet N, Llanos-Cuentas A, Suleiman J, et al. A randomized, double-blind, parallel-group, dose-response study of micafungin compared with fluconazole for the treatment of esophageal candidiasis in HIV-positive patients. Clin Infect Dis 39:842–9, 2004.

de Wet N, Bester A, et al. A randomized, double blind, comparative trial of micafungin (FK463) vs. fluconazole for the treatment of oesophageal candidiasis. Aliment Pharmacol Ther 21:899–907, 2005.

Higashiyama Y, Kohno S. Micafungin: a therapeutic review. Expert Rev Anti Infect Ther 2:345–55, 2004.

Hirata K, Aoyama T, Matsumoto Y, et al. Pharmacokinetics of antifungal agent micafungin in critically ill patients receiving continuous hemodialysis filtration. Yakugaku Zasshi 127:897–901, 2007.

Ikeda F, Tanaka S, Ohki H, et al. Role of micafungin in the antifungal armamentarium. Curr Med Chem 14:1263–1275, 2007.

Isumikawa K, Ohtsu Y, Kawabata M, et al. Clinical efficacy of micafungin for chronic pulmonary aspergillosis. Med Mycol 45:273–278, 2007.

Joseph JM, Jain R, Danziger LH. Micafungin: a new echinocandin antifungal. Pharmacotherapy 27:53–67, 2007.

Keirns J, Sawamoto T. Holum M, et al. Steady-state pharmacokinetics of micafungin and voriconazole after

---

"Usual dose" assumes normal renal/hepatic function. * For renal insufficiency, give usual dose × 1 followed by maintenance dose per CrCl. For dialysis patients, dose the same as for CrCl < 10 mL/min and give supplemental (post-HD/PD dose) immediately after dialysis. CrCl = creatinine clearance; CVVH = continuous veno-venous hemofiltration; HD/PD = hemodialysis/peritoneal dialysis. See pp. 509–513 for explanations, pp. xi–xii for abbreviations; Linezolid (↑ risk of serotonin syndrome, see p. 620).

separate and concomitant dosing in healthy adults. Antimicrob Agents Chemother 51:787–790, 2007.
Kohno S, Masaoka T, et al. A multicenter, open-level clinical study of micafungin (FK463) in the treatment of deep-seated mycosis in Japan. Scand J Infect Dis 36:372–379, 2004.
Kuse ER, Chetchotisakd P, da Cunha CA, et al. Micafungin versus liposomal amphotericin B for candidaemia and invasive candidosis: a phase III radomised double-blind trial. Lancet 369:1519–1527, 2007.
Messer SA, Diekema DJ, Boyken L, Tendolkar S, et al. Activities of micafungin against 315 invasive clinical isolates of fluconazole-resistant Candida spp. J Clin Microbiol 44:324–6, 2006.
Morrison VA. Echinocandin antifungals: review and update. Expert Rev Anti Infect Ther 4:325–42, 2006.
Nakagawa Y, Ichii Y, Saeki Y, et al. Plasma concentration of micafungin in patients with hematologic malignancies. J Infect Chemother 13:39–45, 2007.
Okugawa S, Ota Y, Tatsuno K, et al. A case of invasive central nervous system aspergillosis treated with micafungin with monitoring of micafungin concentrations in the cerebrospinal fluid. Scand J Infect Dis 39:344–346, 2007.
Ostrosky-Zeichner L, Kontoyiannis D, Raffalli J, et al. International, open-label, noncomparative, clinical trial of micafungin alone and in combination for treatment of newly diagnosed and refractory candidemia. Eur J Clin Microbiol Infect Dis 24: 654–661, 2005.
Paderu P, Garcia-Effron G, Balashov S, et al. Serum differentially alters the antifungal properties of echinocandin drugs. Antimicrob Agents Chemother 51:2253–2256, 2007.
Pappas PG, Rotstein CM, Betts RF, et al. Micafungin versus caspofungin for treatment of candidemia and other forms of invasive candidiasis. Clin Infect Dis 45:883–893, 2007.
Pawlitz D, Young M, Klepser M. Micafungin. Formulary 38:354–67, 2003.
Pettengell K, Mynhardt J, et al. Successful treatment of oesophageal candidiasis by micafungin: a novel systemic antifungal agent. Aliment Pharmacol 20:475–481, 2004.
Seibel NL, Schwartz C, Arrieta A, et al. Safety, tolerability and pharmacokinetics of micafungin (FK463) in febrile neutropenic pediatric patients. Antimicrobial Agents and Chemotherapy 49:3317–3324, 2005.
Toubai T, Tanaka J, Ota S, et al. Efficacy and safety of micafungin in febrile neutropenic patients treated for hematological malignancies. Intern Med 46:3–9, 2007.
van Burik JA, Ratanatharathorn V, Stepan DE, et al. National Institute of Allergy and Infectious Diseases Mycoses Study Group. Micafungin versus fluconazole for prophylaxis against invasive fungal infections during neutropenia in patients undergoing hematopoietic stem cell trasnsplantation. Clin Infect Dis 39:1407–16, 2004.
Wiederhold NP, Lewis JS 2nd. The echinocandin micafungin: a review of the pharmacology, spectrum of activity, clinical efficacy and safety. Expert Opin Pharmacother 8:1155–1166, 2007.
Website: www.mycamine.com

Minocycline (Minocin)

Drug Class: 2nd generation tetracycline.
Usual Dose: 100 mg (IV/PO) q12h or 200 mg (IV/PO) q24h (see comments).
Spectrum: (see ***Susceptibility Profiles*** pp. 183–187).
Pharmacokinetic Parameters:
Peak serum level: 4 mcg/mL
Bioavailability: 95%
Excreted unchanged (urine): 10%
Serum half-life (normal/ESRD): 15/18–69 hrs
Plasma protein binding: 75%
Volume of distribution (V_d): 1.5 L/kg
Primary Mode of Elimination: Hepatic
Dosage Adjustments*

CrCl > 50 mL/min	No change
CrCl 10–50 mL/min	No change
CrCl < 10 mL/min	No change
Post–HD/PD dose	None

"Usual dose" assumes normal renal/hepatic function. * For renal insufficiency, give usual dose × 1 followed by maintenance dose per CrCl. For dialysis patients, dose the same as for CrCl < 10 mL/min and give supplemental (post-HD/PD dose) immediately after dialysis. CrCl = creatinine clearance; CVVH = continuous veno-venous hemofiltration; HD/PD = hemodialysis/peritoneal dialysis. See pp. 509–513 for explanations, pp. xi–xii for abbreviations; Linezolid (↑ risk of serotonin syndrome, see p. 620).

CVVH dose	No change
Moderate hepatic insufficiency	No change
Severe hepatic insufficiency	100 mg (IV/PO) q24h

Drug Interactions: Antacids, Al^{++}, Ca^{++}, Fe^{++}, Mg^{++}, Zn^{++}, multivitamins, sucralfate (↓ minocycline absorption); isotretinoin (pseudotumor cerebri); warfarin (↑ INR).

Adverse Effects: Nausea, GI upset if not taken with food, hyperpigmentation of skin with prolonged use, vestibular toxicity (dizziness), photosensitivity rare.

Allergic Potential: Low

Safety in Pregnancy: X

Comments: Infuse slowly over 1 hour. Dizziness due to high inner ear levels. Also ***effective against Nocardia.***

One of only two oral antibiotics effective against serious systemic MSSA/MRSA infections, e.g., MSSA/MRSA ABE, MSSA/MRSA meningitis. ***Preferable to doxycycline for MSSA, HA/CO MRSA, and CA-MRSA.***

May be preferable to doxycycline for neuroborreliosis.

Meningeal dose = usual dose.

Cerebrospinal Fluid Penetration:

Non-inflamed meninges = 50%

Inflamed meninges = 50%

Bile Penetration: 1000%

(also see ***Antibiotic Pearls & Pitfalls*** pp. 495–508).

REFERENCES:

Bernadino ALF, Kaushal D, Philipp MT. The Antibiotics Doxycycline and Minocycline Inhibit the Inflammatory Responses to the Lyme Disease Spirochete *Borrelia burgdorferi*. Journal of Infectious Disease 199:1379–1388, 2009.

Bouza E. New therapeutic choices for infections caused by methicillin-resistant *Staphylococcus aureus*. Clin Microbiol Infect Dis 15:44–52, 2009.

Cunha BA. New uses for older antibiotics: nitrofurantoin, amikacin, colistin, polymyxin B, doxycycline and minocycline revisited. Med Clin North Am 90:1089–107, 2006.

Cunha BA. Oral Antibiotic Therapy of Serious Systemic Infections. Med Clin N Am 90:1197–1222, 2006.

Cunha BA. Minocycline vs. doxycycline for the antimicrobial therapy of lyme neuroborreliosis. Clin Infect Dis 30:237–238, 2000.

Klein NC, Cunha BA. New uses for older antibiotics. Med Clin North Am 85:125–32, 2001.

Lewis KE, Ebden P, Wooster SL, et al. Multi-system Infection with Nocardia farcinica-therapy with linezolid and minocycline. J Infect 46:199–202, 2003.

Pavoni GL, Giannella M, Falcone M, et al. Conservative medical therapy of prosthetic joint infections: retrospective analysis of an 8-year experience. Clin Microbiol Infect 10:831–7 2004.

Schwartz BS, Graber CJ, Diep BA, et al. Doxycycline, not Minocycline, Induces Its Own Resistance in Multidrug-Resistant Community-Associated Methicillin-Resistant *Staphylococcus aureus* Clone USA300. Clin Infect Dis 48:1483–1484, 2009.

Website: www.pdr.net

Moxifloxacin (Avelox)

Drug Class: Fluoroquinolone.

Usual Dose: 400 mg (IV/PO) q24h (see comments).

Spectrum: (see ***Susceptibility Profiles*** pp. 194–199).

Pharmacokinetic Parameters:

Peak serum level: 4.4 (IV)/4.5 (PO) mcg/mL

Bioavailability: 90%

Excreted unchanged (urine): 20%

Serum half-life (normal/ESRD): 12/12 hrs

Plasma protein binding: 50%

Volume of distribution (V_d): 2.2 L/kg

Primary Mode of Elimination: Hepatic

"Usual dose" assumes normal renal/hepatic function. * For renal insufficiency, give usual dose × 1 followed by maintenance dose per CrCl. For dialysis patients, dose the same as for CrCl < 10 mL/min and give supplemental (post-HD/PD dose) immediately after dialysis. CrCl = creatinine clearance; CVVH = continuous veno-venous hemofiltration; HD/PD = hemodialysis/peritoneal dialysis. See pp. 509–513 for explanations, pp. xi–xii for abbreviations; Linezolid (↑ risk of serotonin syndrome, see p. 620).

Dosage Adjustments*

CrCl 50–80 mL/min	No change
CrCl 10–50 mL/min	No change
CrCl < 10 mL/min	No change
Post–HD dose	None
Post–PD dose	None
CVVH dose	No change
SLEDD dose	No change
Moderate hepatic insufficiency	No change
Severe hepatic insufficiency	No information

Drug Interactions: Al^{++}, Fe^{++}, Mg^{++}, Zn^{++} antacids, citrate/citric acid, dairy products (↓ absorption of fluoroquinolones only if taken together); amiodarone, procainamide, sotalol (may ↑ QT_c interval, torsade de pointes).
Adverse Effects: C. difficile diarrhea/colitis. May ↑ QT_c interval > 3 msec; avoid taking with medications e.g., amiodarone that prolong the QT_c interval, and in patients with cardiac arrhythmias/heart block. Does not cause seizures. FQ use has an increased risk of tendinitis/tendon rupture. Risk in highest in the elderly, those on steroids, and those with heart, lung or renal transplants.
Allergic Potential: Low
Safety in Pregnancy: C
Comments: *Only quinolone with anti–B. fragilis activity*. FQ with the highest activity against S. pneumoniae, VSE, and MSSA. Metabolized to microbiologically-inactive glucuronide (M1)/sulfate (M2) conjugates. Take 4 hours before or 8 hours after calcium or magnesium containing antacids or didanosine. No interactions with oral hypoglycemics. C8-methoxy group increases activity and decreases resistance potential. **TB dose** (*alternate drug in MDR TB drug regimens*): 400 mg (PO) q24h.
↑ incidence of C. difficile diarrhea/colitis with PPIs (for patients on PPIs during FQ therapy, switch to H_2 blocker for duration of FQ therapy).
Cerebrospinal Fluid Penetration: < 10% (also see ***Antibiotic Pearls & Pitfalls*** pp. 495–508).

REFERENCES:

Al-Nawas B, Walter C, Morbach T. Clinical and microbiological efficacy of moxifloxacin versus amoxicillin/clavulanic acid in severe odontogenic abscesses: a pilot study. Eur J Clin Microbiol Infect Dis 28:75–82, 2009.

Anzueto A, Niederman MS, Pearle J, et al. Community-Acquired Pneumonia Recovery in the Elderly Study Group. Community-Acquired Pneumonia Recovery in the Elderly (CAPRIE): efficacy and safety of moxifloxacin therapy versus that of levofloxacin therapy. Clin Infect Dis 42:73–81, 2006.

Arrieta JR, Galgano AS, Sakano E, et al. Moxifloxacin vs. amoxicillin/clavulanate in the treatment of acute sinusitis. Am J Otolaryngol 28:78–82, 2007.

Bassetti M, Rosso R, Tosi C, et al. Moxifloxacin in the treatment of hospitalized community acquired pneumonia in HIV-infected subjects. J Chemother 19:104–105, 2007.

Behra-Miellet J, Dubreuil L, Jumas-Bilak E. Antianaerobic activity of moxifloxacin compared with that of ofloxacin, ciprofloxacin, clindamycin, metronidazole and beta-lactams. Int J Antimicrob Agents 20:366–74, 2002.

Balfour JA, Wiseman LR. Moxifloxacin. Drugs 57:363–73, 1999.

Caeiro JP, Iannini PB. Moxifloxacin (Avelox): a novel fluoroquinolone with a broad spectrum of activity. Expert Rev Anti Infect Ther 1:363–70, 2004.

Cheon JH, Kim N, Lee DH, et al. Efficacy of moxifloxacin-based triple therapy as second-line treatment for Helicobacter pylori infection. Helicobacter 11:46–51, 2006.

"Usual dose" assumes normal renal/hepatic function. * For renal insufficiency, give usual dose × 1 followed by maintenance dose per CrCl. For dialysis patients, dose the same as for CrCl < 10 mL/min and give supplemental (post-HD/PD dose) immediately after dialysis. CrCl = creatinine clearance; CVVH = continuous veno-venous hemofiltration; HD/PD = hemodialysis/peritoneal dialysis. See pp. 509–513 for explanations, pp. xi–xii for abbreviations; Linezolid (↑ risk of serotonin syndrome, see p. 620).

Cunha BA. Oral Antibiotic Therapy of Serious Systemic Infections. Med Clin N Am 90:1197–1222, 2006.

Daneman N, McGeer, Green K, Low DE. Macrolide Resistance in Bacteremic Pneumococcal Disease: Implications for Patient Management. Clin Infect Dis 43:432–8, 2006.

Drummond MF, Becker DL, Hux M, et al. An economic evaluation of sequential i.v./po moxifloxacin therapy compared to i.v./po co-amoxiclav with or without clarithromycin in the treatment of community-acquired pneumonia Chest 124:526–35, 2003.

Giordano P, Song J, Pertel P, et al. Sequential intravenous/oral moxifloxacin versus intravenous piperacillin-tazobactam followed by oral amoxicillin-clavulanate for the treatment of complicated skin and skin structure infection. Int J Antimicrob Agents 26:357–65, 2005.

Gillespie SH, Gosling RD, Uison L, et al. Early bactericidal activity of a moxifloxacin and isoniazid combination in smear-positive pulmonary tuberculosis. J Antimicrob Chemother 56:1169–71, 2005.

Goldstein EJ, Citron DM, Warren YA, et al. In vitro activity of moxifloxacin against 923 anaerobes isolated from human intra-abdominal infections. Antimicrob Agents Chemother 50:148–55, 2006.

Haggerty CL, Ness RB. Newest approaches to treatment of pelvic inflammatory disease: a review of recent randomized clinical trials. Clin Infect Dis 44:953–960, 2007.

Hariprasad SM, Shah GK, Mieler WF, Feiner L, Blinder KJ, et al. Vitreous and aqueous penetration of orally administered moxifloxacin in humans. Arch Opthamol 124:178–82, 2006.

Hart D, Weinstein MP. Cross-over assessment of serum bactericidal activity of moxifloxacin and levofloxacin versus penicillin-susceptible and penicillin-resistant Streptococcus pneumoniae in healthy volunteers. Diagn Microbiol Infect Dis 58:375–378, 2007.

Ho C-C, Chen Y-C, Hu F-C, et al. Safety of Fluoro quinolone Use in Patients with Hepatoxicity Induced by Anti-Tuberculosis Regimens. Clin Infect Dis 48:1526–1533, 2009.

Hoeffken G, Talan D, Larsen LS, et al. Efficacy and safety of sequential moxifloxacin for treatment of community-acquired pneumonia associated with atypical pathogens. Eur J Clin Microbiol Infect Dis 23:772–5, 2004.

Katz E, Larsen LS, Fogarty CM, et al. Safety and efficacy of sequential I.V. to P.O. moxifloxacin versus conventional combination therapies the treatment of community-acquired pneumonia in patients requiring initial I.V. therapy. J Emerg Med 27:554–9, 2004.

Klutman NE, Culley CM, Lacy ME, et al. Moxifloxacin. Antibiotics for Clinicians 5:17–27, 2001.

Lode H, Grossman C, Choudhri S, et al. Sequential IV/PO moxifloxacin treatment of patients with severe community-acquired pneumonia. Respir Med 97:1134–42, 2003.

Malincarne L, Ghebtegzabher M, Moretti MV, et al. Penetration of moxifloxacin into bone in patients undergoing total knee arthroplasty. J Antimicrob Chemother 57:950–4, 2006.

Malingoni MA, Song J, Herrington J, et al. Randomized controlled trial of moxifloxacin compared with piperacillin-tazobactam and amoxicillin-clavulanate for the treatment of complicated intra-abdominal infections. Ann Surg 244:204–11, 2006.

Metlay JP, Fishman NO, Joffe MM, et al. Macrolide Resistance in Adults with Bacteremic Pneumococcal Pneumonia. Emerging Infect Dis 12:1223–30, 2006.

Miravitlles M, Llor C. Determining factors in the prescription of moxifloxacin in exacerbations of chronic bronchitis in the primary-care setting. Clin Drug Investig 27:95–104, 2007.

Nguyen HA, Grellet J, Dubois V, et al. Factors compromising the activity of moxifloxacin against intracellular Staphylococcus aureus. J Antimicrob Chemother 59:755–758, 2007.

Nijland HM, Ruslami R, Suroto AJ, et al. Rifampicin reduces plasma concentrations of moxifloxacin in patients with tuberculosis. Clin Infect Dis 45:1001–1007, 2007.

Rijnders BJ. Moxifloxacin for community-acquired pneumonia. Antimicrob Agents Chemother 47:444–445, 2003.

Saravolatz LD, Leggett J.Gatifloxacin, gemifloxacin, and moxifloxacin: the role of 3 newer fluoroquinolones. Clin Infect Dis 37:1210–5, 2003.

Schentag JJ. Pharmacokinetic and pharmacodynamic predictors of antimicrobial efficacy: moxifloxacin and Streptococcus pneumoniae. J Chemother 14(Suppl 2):13–21, 2002.

"Usual dose" assumes normal renal/hepatic function. * For renal insufficiency, give usual dose × 1 followed by maintenance dose per CrCl. For dialysis patients, dose the same as for CrCl < 10 mL/min and give supplemental (post-HD/PD dose) immediately after dialysis. CrCl = creatinine clearance; CVVH = continuous veno-venous hemofiltration; HD/PD = hemodialysis/peritoneal dialysis. See pp. 509–513 for explanations, pp. xi–xii for abbreviations; Linezolid (↑ risk of serotonin syndrome, see p. 620).

Schlossberg D. Treatment of multi-drug resistant tuberculosis. Antibiotics for Clinicians 9:317–321, 2005.

Solnick, JV. Treatment with moxifloxacin versus standard therapy for community-acquired pneumonia. 10 Clinics 41:1697–1705, 2005.

Speciale A, Musumeci R, Blandino G, et al. Minimal inhibitory concentrations and time-kill determination of moxifloxacin against aerobic and anaerobic isolates. Int J Antimicrob Agents 19:111–8, 2002.

Stass, H, Rink AD, Delesen H, et al. Pharmacokinetics and peritoneal penetration of moxifloxacin in peritonitis. J Antimicrob Chemother 58:693–6, 2006.

Stein GE, Goldstein EJC. Fluoroquinolones and Anaerobes. Clin Infect Dis 42:1598–607, 2006.

Torres A, Muir JF, Corris P, et al. Effectiveness of oral moxifloxacin in standard first-line therapy in community-acquired pneumonia. Eur Respir J 21:135–43, 2003.

Walter S, Kuchenbecker J, Banditt P, et al. Concentration of moxifloxacin in serum and human aqueous humor following a single 400 mg oral dose. J Cataract Refract Surg 33:553–555, 2007.

Welte T, Petermann W, Schurmann D, et al. Treatment with sequential intravenous or oral moxifloxacin was associated with faster clinical improvement that the standard therapy for hospitalized patients with community-acquired pneumonia who received initial parenteral therapy. Clin Infect Dis 41:1697–705, 2005.

Zervos M, Martinez FJ, Amsden GW, et al. Efficacy and safety of 3-day azithromycin versus 5-day moxifloxacin for the treatment of acute bacterial exacerbations of chronic bronchitis. Int J Antimicrob Agents 29:56–61, 2007.

Website: www.avelox.com

Nafcillin (Unipen)

Drug Class: Antistaphylococcal penicillin.
Usual Dose: 2 gm (IV) q4h.
Spectrum: (see ***Susceptibility Profiles*** pp. 183–187).

Pharmacokinetic Parameters:
Peak serum level: 80 mcg/ml
Bioavailability: Not applicable
Excreted unchanged (urine): 10–30%
Serum half-life (normal/ESRD): 0.5/4 hrs
Plasma protein binding: 90%
Volume of distribution (V_d): 0.24 L/kg
Primary Mode of Elimination: Hepatic
Dosage Adjustments*

CrCl 10–80 mL/min	No change
CrCl < 10 mL/min	No change
Post-HD/PD dose	None
CVVH dose	No change
Moderate or severe hepatic insufficiency	No change

Drug Interactions: Cyclosporine (↓ cyclosporine levels); nifedipine, warfarin (↓ interacting drug effect).
Adverse Effects: Not hepatotoxic. Drug fever/ rash, leukopenia.
Allergic Potential: High
Safety in Pregnancy: B
Comments: Avoid oral formulation (not well absorbed/erratic serum levels).
Meningeal dose = usual dose.
Cerebrospinal Fluid Penetration:
Non-Inflamed meninges = 1%
Inflamed meninges = 20%
Bile Penetration: 100%
(also see ***Antibiotic Pearls & Pitfalls*** pp. 495–508).

REFERENCES:

Donowitz GR, Mandell GL. Beta-lactam antibiotics. N Engl J Med 318:419–26 490–500, 1993.

Wright AJ. The penicillins. Mayo Clin Proc 74:290–307, 1999.

Website: www.pdr.net

"Usual dose" assumes normal renal/hepatic function. * For renal insufficiency, give usual dose × 1 followed by maintenance dose per CrCl. For dialysis patients, dose the same as for CrCl < 10 mL/min and give supplemental (post-HD/PD dose) immediately after dialysis. CrCl = creatinine clearance; CVVH = continuous veno-venous hemofiltration; HD/PD = hemodialysis/peritoneal dialysis. See pp. 509–513 for explanations, pp. xi–xii for abbreviations; Linezolid (↑ risk of serotonin syndrome, see p. 620).

Nelfinavir (Viracept) NFV

Drug Class: Antiretroviral protease inhibitor.
Usual Dose: 1250 mg (PO) q12h (two 625-mg tablets per dose) with meals, or five 250-mg tabs or 750 mg (three 250-mg tabs) (PO) q8h.
Pharmacokinetic Parameters:
Peak serum level: 35 mcg/mL
Bioavailability: 20–80%
Excreted unchanged (urine): 1–2%
Serum half-life (normal/ESRD): 4 hrs/no data
Plasma protein binding: 98%
Volume of distribution (V_d): 5 L/kg
Primary Mode of Elimination: Hepatic
Dosage Adjustments*

CrCl 50–80 mL/min	No change
CrCl 10–50 mL/min	No change
CrCl < 10 mL/min	No change
Post–HD dose	None
Post–PD dose	None
CVVH dose	No change
Moderate hepatic insufficiency	No information
Severe hepatic insufficiency	No information – use caution

Antiretroviral Dosage Adjustments:

Delavirdine	No information (monitor for neutropenia)
Efavirenz	No changes
Indinavir	Limited data for nelfinavir 1250 mg q12h + indinavir 1200 mg q12h
Lopinavir/ritonavir	Nelfinavir 1000 mg q12h or lopinavir/r 600/150 mg q12h
Nevirapine	No information
Ritonavir	No information
Saquinavir	Saquinavir 1200 mg q12h
Rifampin	Avoid combination
Rifabutin	Nelfinavir 1250 mg q12h; rifabutin 150 mg q24h or 300 mg 2–3x/week

Drug Interactions: Antiretrovirals, rifabutin, rifampin (see dose adjustment grid, above); amiodarone, quinidine, astemizole, terfenadine, benzodiazepines, cisapride, ergot alkaloids, statins, St. John's wort (avoid if possible); carbamazepine, phenytoin, phenobarbital (↓ nelfinavir levels, ↑ anticonvulsant levels; monitor); caspofungin (↓ caspofungin levels, may ↓ caspofungin effect); clarithromycin, erythromycin, telithromycin (↑ nelfinavir and macrolide levels); didanosine (dosing conflict with food; give nelfinavir with food 2 hours before or 1 hour after didanosine); itraconazole, voriconazole, ketoconazole (↑ nelfinavir levels); lamivudine (↑ lamivudine levels); methadone (may require ↑ methadone dose); oral contraceptives, zidovudine (↓ zidovudine levels); sildenafil (↑ or ↓ sildenafil levels; do not exceed 25 mg in 48 hrs, tadalafil (max. 10 mg/72 hrs, vardenafil (max. 2.5 mg/72 hrs)
Adverse Effects: Impaired concentration, nausea, abdominal pain, secretory diarrhea, ↑ SGOT/SGPT, rash, ↑ cholesterol/triglycerides (evaluate risk for coronary disease/pancreatitis), fat redistribution, hyperglycemia (including

---

"Usual dose" assumes normal renal/hepatic function. * For renal insufficiency, give usual dose × 1 followed by maintenance dose per CrCl. For dialysis patients, dose the same as for CrCl < 10 mL/min and give supplemental (post-HD/PD dose) immediately after dialysis. CrCl = creatinine clearance; CVVH = continuous veno-venous hemofiltration; HD/PD = hemodialysis/peritoneal dialysis. See pp. 509–513 for explanations, pp. xi–xii for abbreviations; Linezolid (↑ risk of serotonin syndrome, see p. 620).

worsening diabetes, new-onset diabetes, DKA), possible increased bleeding in hemophilia
Allergic Potential: Low
Safety in Pregnancy: B
Comments: Take with food (absorption increased 300%). 625-mg tablet available.
Cerebrospinal Fluid Penetration: Undetectable

REFERENCES:

Albrecht MA, Bosch RJ, Hammer SM, et al. Nelfinavir, efavirenz, or both after the failure of nucleoside treatment of HIV infection. N Engl J Med 345:398–407, 2001.

Clotet B, Ruiz L, Martinez-Picado J, et al. Prevalence of HIV protease mutations on failure of nelfinavir-containing HAART: a retrospective analysis of four clinical studies and two observational cohorts. HIV Clin Trials 3:316–23, 2002.

Deeks SG, Smith M, Holodniy M, et al. HIV-1 protease inhibitors: A review for clinicians. JAMA 277:145–53, 1997.

DiCenzo R, Forrest A, Fischl MA, et al. Pharmacokinetics of indinavir and nelfinavir in treatment-naive, human immunodeficiency virus-infected subjects. Antimicrob Agents Chemother 48:918–23, 2004.

Go J, Cunha BA. Nelfinavir: A review. Antibiotics for Clinicians 4:17–23, 2000.

Kaul DR, Cinti SK, Carver PL, et al. HIV protease inhibitors: Advances in therapy and adverse reactions, including metabolic complications. Pharmacotherapy 19:281–98, 1999.

Panel on Antiretroviral Guidelines for Adults and Adolescents. Guidelines for the use of antiretroviral agents in HIV-1 infected adults and adolescents. Department of Health and Human Services. November 3, 2008; 1–139. Available at http://www.aidsinfor.nih.gov/ContentFiles/AdultandAdolescentGL.pdf.

Perry CM, Benfield P. Nelfinavir. Drugs 54:81–7, 1997.

Simpson KN, Luo MP, Chumney E, et al. Cost-effective of lopinavir/ritonavir versus nelfinavir as the first-line highly active antiretroviral therapy regimen for HIV infection. HIV Clin Trials 5:294–304, 2004.

Walmsley S, Bernstein B, King M, et al. Lopinavir-ritonavir versus nelfinavir for the initial treatment of HIV infection. N Engl J Med 346:2039–46, 2002.

Website: www.viracept.com

Nevirapine (Viramune) NVP

Drug Class: Antiretroviral NNRTI (non-nucleoside reverse transcriptase inhibitor).
Usual Dose: 200 mg (PO) q24h × 2 weeks, then 200 mg (PO) q12h.
Pharmacokinetic Parameters:
Peak serum level: 0.9–3.6 mcg/mL
Bioavailability: 90%
Excreted unchanged (urine): 5%
Serum half-life (normal/ESRD): 40 hrs/no data
Plasma protein binding: 60%
Volume of distribution (V_d): 1.4 L/kg
Primary Mode of Elimination: Hepatic
Dosage Adjustments*

CrCl 50–80 mL/min	No change
CrCl 10–50 mL/min	No change
CrCl < 20 mL/min	No change; use caution
Post–HD dose	200 mg (PO)
Post–PD dose	None
CVVH dose	No change
Moderate hepatic insufficiency	Use caution
Severe hepatic insufficiency	Avoid

Antiretroviral Dosage Adjustments:

Delavirdine	No information
Efavirenz	No information
Indinavir	Indinavir 1000 mg q8h

"Usual dose" assumes normal renal/hepatic function. * For renal insufficiency, give usual dose × 1 followed by maintenance dose per CrCl. For dialysis patients, dose the same as for CrCl < 10 mL/min and give supplemental (post-HD/PD dose) immediately after dialysis. CrCl = creatinine clearance; CVVH = continuous veno-venous hemofiltration; HD/PD = hemodialysis/peritoneal dialysis. See pp. 509–513 for explanations, pp. xi–xii for abbreviations; Linezolid (↑ risk of serotonin syndrome, see p. 620).

Lopinavir/ritonavir (l/r)	Consider l/r 600/150 mg q12h in PI-experienced patients
Nelfinavir	No information
Ritonavir	No changes
Saquinavir	No information
Rifampin	Not recommended
Rifabutin	Use caution

Drug Interactions: Antiretrovirals, rifabutin, rifampin (see dose adjustment grid, above); carbamazepine, phenobarbital, phenytoin (monitor anticonvulsant levels); caspofungin (↓ caspofungin levels, may ↓ caspofungin effect); ethinyl estradiol (↓ ethinyl estradiol levels; use additional/alternative method); ketoconazole (avoid); voriconazole (↑ nevirapine levels); methadone (↓ methadone levels; titrate methadone dose to effect); tacrolimus (↓ tacrolimus levels).

Adverse Effects: Severe, life-threatening, and in some cases fatal hepatotoxicity, particularly in the first 18 weeks, has been reported in patients treated with nevirapine. In some cases, patients presented with non-specific prodromal signs or symptoms of hepatitis and progressed to hepatic failure. These events are often associated with rash. Female gender and higher CD_4 counts at initiation of therapy place patients at increased risk; women with CD_4 counts > 250 cells/mm^3, including pregnant women receiving nevirapine in combination with other antiretrovirals for the treatment of HIV infection, are at the greatest risk. However, hepatotoxicity associated with mevirapine use can occur in both genders, all CD_4 counts and at any time during treatment. Severe, life-threatening skin reactions, including fatal cases, have occurred in patients treated with nevirapine. These have included cases of Stevens-Johnson syndrome, toxic epidermal necrolysis, and hypersensitivity reactions characterized by rash, constitutional findings, and organ dysfunction. Extra vigilance is warranted during the first 6 weeks of therapy, which is the period of greatest risk of these events. Do not restart nevirapine following severe hepatic, skin or hypersensitivity reactions. Take out all the rest under adverse reactions.

Allergic Potential: High

Safety in Pregnancy: C

Comments: Absorption not affected by food. Not to be used for post-exposure prophylaxis because of potential for fatal hepatitis.

Cerebrospinal Fluid Penetration: 45%

REFERENCES:

D'Aquila RT, Hughes MD, Johnson VA, et al. Nevirapine, zidovudine, and didanosine compared with zidovudine and didanosine in patients with HIV-1 infection. Ann Intern Med 124:1019–30, 1996.

Hammer SM, Kessler HA, Saag MS. Issues in combination antiretroviral therapy: A review. J Acquired Immune Defic Syndr 7:24–37, 1994.

Havlir DV.Lange JM. New antiretrovirals and new combinations. AIDS 12:165–74, 1998.

Herzmann C, Karcher H. Nevirapine plus zidovudine to prevent mother-to-child transmission of HIV. N Engl J Med 351:2013–5, 2004.

Johnson S, Chan J, Bennett CL. Hepatotoxicity after prophylaxis with a nevirapine-containing antiretroviral regimen. Ann Intern Med 137:146–7, 2002.

Milinkovic A, Martinez E. Nevirapine in the treatment of HIV. Expert Rev Anti Infect Ther 2:367–73, 2004.

Montaner JS, Reiss P, Cooper D, et al. A randomized, double-blind trial comparing combinations of nevirapine, didanosine, and zidovudine for HIV-infected patients: The INCAS trial. Italy, the Netherlands, Canada and Australia Study. J Am Med Assoc 279:930–937, 1998.

"Usual dose" assumes normal renal/hepatic function. * For renal insufficiency, give usual dose × 1 followed by maintenance dose per CrCl. For dialysis patients, dose the same as for CrCl < 10 mL/min and give supplemental (post-HD/PD dose) immediately after dialysis. CrCl = creatinine clearance; CVVH = continuous veno-venous hemofiltration; HD/PD = hemodialysis/peritoneal dialysis. See pp. 509–513 for explanations, pp. xi–xii for abbreviations; Linezolid (↑ risk of serotonin syndrome, see p. 620).

Negredo E, Ribalta J, Paredes R, et al. Reversal of atherogenic lipoprotein profile in HIV-1 infected patients with lipodystrophy after replacing protease inhibitors by nevirapine. AIDS 16:1383–9, 2002.

Panel on Antiretroviral Guidelines for Adults and Adolescents. Guidelines for the use of antiretroviral agents in HIV-1 infected adults and adolescents. Department of Health and Human Services. November 3, 2008; 1–139. Available at http://www.aidsinfor.nih.gov/ContentFiles/AdultandAdolescentGL.pdf.

Weverling GJ, Lange JM, Jurriaans S, et al. Alternative multidrug regimen provides improved suppression of HIV-1 replication over triple therapy. AIDS 12:117–22, 1998.

Website: www.viramune.com

Nitazoxanide (Alinia)

Drug Class: Antiprotozoal.

Usual Dose: 500 mg (PO) q12h.

Pharmacokinetic Parameters:

Peak serum level: 9.1–10.6 mcg/mL; tizoxanile/tizoxanile glucuronide (metabolites)

Bioavailability: No data

Excreted unchanged (urine): < 10%

Serum half-life (normal/ESRD): No data

Plasma protein binding: 99%

Volume of distribution (V_d): No data

Primary Mode of Elimination: Hepatic (66%); renal (34%)

Dosage Adjustments*

CrCl 50–80 mL/min	No change
CrCl 10–50 mL/min	No change
CrCl < 10 mL/min	Use with caution
Post–HD dose	None
Post–PD dose	None
CVVH dose	No change
Mild/moderate	No change
Mild hepatic insufficiency	No change
Moderate or severe hepatic insufficiency	Use with caution

Drug Interactions: Avoid in patients with hypersensitivity to salicylates.

Adverse Effects: Dizziness, headache, nausea/vomiting, abdominal pain, flu-like syndrome, yellow discoloration of sclera/urine.

Allergic Potential: Low

Safety in Pregnancy: B

Comments: Nitazoxanide concentrates in GI tract but is not present in serum. **Give with food**; absorption greatly increased with food (↑ plasma levels of metabolites ~ 50%). Contains 1.4 gm sucrose/5 mL of reconstituted suspension. **Preferred therapy for *Cryptosporidia* and giardiasis. Also Effective against *Cyclospora*. *Effective for severe C. difficile diarrhea/colitis unresponsive to metronidazole or vancomycin*.** *Also useful for H. pylori or B. hominis.*

REFERENCES:

Abboud P, Lemee V, Gargala G, et al. Successful Treatment of Metronidazole and Albendazole-Resistant Giardiasis with Nitazoxanide in a Patient with Acquired Immunodeficiency Syndrome. Clin Infect Dis 32:1792–4, 2001.

Aslam S, Hamill RJ, Musher DM. Treatment of Clostridium difficile-associated disease: old therapies and new strategies. Lancet Infect Dis 5:549–57, 2005.

Bailey JM, Erramouspe J. Nitazoxanide treatment for giardiasis and cryptosporidiosis in children. Ann Pharmacother 38:634–40, 2004.

Bouza E, Burillo A, Munoz P. Antimicrobial Therapy of Clostridium difficile-Associated Diarrhea. Med Clin N Am 90:1141–63, 2006.

Cohen SA. Use of nitazoxanide as a new therapeutic option for persistent diarrhea: a pediatric perspective. Curr Med Res Opin 21:999–1004, 2005.

"Usual dose" assumes normal renal/hepatic function. * For renal insufficiency, give usual dose × 1 followed by maintenance dose per CrCl. For dialysis patients, dose the same as for CrCl < 10 mL/min and give supplemental (post-HD/PD dose) immediately after dialysis. CrCl = creatinine clearance; CVVH = continuous veno-venous hemofiltration; HD/PD = hemodialysis/peritoneal dialysis. See pp. 509–513 for explanations, pp. xi–xii for abbreviations; Linezolid (↑ risk of serotonin syndrome, see p. 620).

Gilles HM, et al. Treatment of intestinal parasitic infections: a review of nitazoxanide. Trends in Parasitology 18:95–7, 2002.

Hoffman PS, Sisson G, Croxen MA, et al. Antiparasitic drug nitazoxanide inhibits the pyruvate oxidoreductases of Helicobacter pylori, selected anaerobic bacteria and parasites, and Campylobacter jejuni. Antimicrob Agents Chemother 51:868–876, 2007.

Musher DM, Logan N, Hamill RJ, et al. Nitazoxanide for the Treatment of Clostridium difficile Colitis. Clin Infect. Dis 43:421–30, 2006.

Rossignol JF, et al. Treatment of diarrhea caused by Cryptosporidium parvum: a prospective randomized, double-blind, placebo-controlled study of nitazoxanide. J Infect Dis 184:103, 2001.

White CA Jr. Nitazoxanide: a new broad spectrum antiparasitic agent. Expert Rev Anti Infect Ther 2:43–9, 2004.

Web site: www.romark.com

Nitrofurantoin (Macrodantin, Macrobid)

Drug Class: Urinary antiseptic.
Usual Dose: 100 mg (PO) q12h.
Spectrum: (see ***Susceptibility Profiles*** pp. 194–199).
Pharmacokinetic Parameters:
Peak serum level: 1 mcg/mL
Bioavailability: 80%
Excreted unchanged (urine): 25%
Serum half-life (normal/ESRD): 0.5/1 hrs
Plasma protein binding: 40%
Volume of distribution (V_d): 0.8 L/kg
Primary Mode of Elimination: Renal
Dosage Adjustments*

CrCl 50–80 mL/min	100 mg (PO) q12h
CrCl 30–50 mL/min	100 mg (PO) q24h
CrCl < 30 mL/min	Avoid
Post–HD dose	Not applicable
Post–PD dose	Not applicable
CVVH dose	Not applicable
Moderate hepatic insufficiency	No change
Severe hepatic insufficiency	No change

Drug Interactions: Antacids, magnesium (↓ nitrofurantoin absorption); probenecid (↑ nitrofurantoin levels).
Adverse Effects:
Acute hypersensitivity reactions (reversible): pneumonitis
Chronic reactions (irreversible): chronic hepatitis, peripheral neuropathy, interstitial fibrosis.
Allergic Potential: Moderate
Safety in Pregnancy: B
Comments: For CAB/lower UTIs only, not systemic infection. GI upset minimal with microcrystalline preparations. Useful in asymptomatic bacteriuria of pregnancy; **No transplacental transfer**. Chronic toxicities associated with prolonged use/renal insufficiency; avoid in severe renal insufficiency. **Active against most aerobic GNB uropathogens, except P. aeruginosa and Proteus sp. Effective for VSE/VRE catheter-associated bacteriuria (CAB)/lower UTIs**. (also see ***Antibiotic Pearls & Pitfalls*** pp. 495–508).

REFERENCES:

Cunha BA. New uses for older antibiotics: nitrofurantoin, amikacin, colistin, polymyxin B, doxycycline, and minocycline revisited. Med Clin North Am. 90:1089–107, 2006.

"Usual dose" assumes normal renal/hepatic function. * For renal insufficiency, give usual dose × 1 followed by maintenance dose per CrCl. For dialysis patients, dose the same as for CrCl < 10 mL/min and give supplemental (post-HD/PD dose) immediately after dialysis. CrCl = creatinine clearance; CVVH = continuous veno-venous hemofiltration; HD/PD = hemodialysis/peritoneal dialysis. See pp. 509–513 for explanations, pp. xi–xii for abbreviations; Linezolid (↑ risk of serotonin syndrome, see p. 620).

Cunha BA. Nitrofurantoin: A review. Adv Ther 6:213–36, 1989.
Cunha BA. Nitrofurantoin: An update. OB/GYN 44:399–406, 1989.
Cunha BA. Nitrofurantoin: Bioavailability and therapeutic equivalence. Adv Ther 5:54–63, 1988.
Klein NC, Cunha BA. New uses for older antibiotics. Med Clin North Am 85:125–32, 2001.
Linden PK. Treatment options for vancomycin-resistant enterococcal infections. Drugs 62:425–41, 2002.
Mendez JL, Nadrous HF, Hartman TE, et al. Chronic nitrofurantoin–induced lung disease. Mayo Clin Proc 80:1298–1302, 2005.
Nicolle LE. Urinary tract infection: traditional pharmacologic therapies. Am J Med 113(Suppl 1A):35S-44S, 2002.

Ofloxacin (Oflox)

Drug Class: Fluoroquinolone.
Usual Dose: 400 mg (IV/PO) q12h (see comments).
Pharmacokinetic Parameters:
Peak serum level: 5.5–7.2 mcg/ml
Bioavailability: 95%
Excreted unchanged (urine): 90%
Serum half-life (normal/ESRD): 6/40 hrs
Plasma protein binding: 32%
Volume of distribution (V_d): 2 L/kg
Primary Mode of Elimination: Renal
Dosage Adjustments*

CrCl 50–80 mL/min	400 mg (IV/PO) q12h
CrCl 10–50 mL/min	400 mg (IV/PO) q24h
CrCl < 10 mL/min	200 mg (IV/PO) q24
Post–HD dose	200 mg (IV/PO)
Post–PD dose	200 mg (IV/PO)
CVVH dose	400 mg (IV/PO) q24h
Moderate hepatic insufficiency	No change
Severe hepatic insufficiency	400 mg (IV/PO) q24h

Drug Interactions: Al^{++}, Ca^{++}, Fe^{++}, Mg^{++}, Zn^{++} antacids, citrate/citric acid, dairy products (↓ absorption of ofloxacin only if taken together); cimetidine (↑ ofloxacin levels); cyclosporine (↑ cyclosporine levels); NSAIDs (CNS stimulation); probenecid (↑ ofloxacin levels); warfarin (↑ INR).
Adverse Effects: Drug fever/rash, mild neuroexcitatory symptoms. C. difficile diarrhea/colitis. FQ use has an increased risk of tendinitis/tendon rupture. Risk in highest in the elderly, those on steroids, and those with heart, lung or renal transplants.
Allergic Potential: Low
Safety in Pregnancy: C
Comments: H_2 antagonist increases half-life by ~ 30%. Levofloxacin has improved pharmacokinetics/pharmacodynamics and greater antimicrobial activity. Take ofloxacin 2 hours before or after calcium/magnesium containing antacids. **PPNG dose:** 400 mg (PO) × 1 dose. NGU/cervicitis dose: 300 mg (PO) q12h × 1 week.
Cerebrospinal Fluid Penetration: < 10%
Bile Penetration: 1500%

REFERENCES:
Absalon J, Domenico PD, Ortega AM, Cunha, BA. The antibacterial activity of ofloxacin versus ciprofloxacin against Pseudomonas aeruginosa in human urine. Adv Ther 13:191–4, 1996.

"Usual dose" assumes normal renal/hepatic function. * For renal insufficiency, give usual dose × 1 followed by maintenance dose per CrCl. For dialysis patients, dose the same as for CrCl < 10 mL/min and give supplemental (post-HD/PD dose) immediately after dialysis. CrCl = creatinine clearance; CVVH = continuous veno-venous hemofiltration; HD/PD = hemodialysis/peritoneal dialysis. See pp. 509–513 for explanations, pp. xi–xii for abbreviations; Linezolid (↑ risk of serotonin syndrome, see p. 620).

Fuhrmann V, Schenk P, Thalhammer F. Ofloxacin clearance during continuous hemofiltration. Am J Kidney Dis 42:1327–8, 2003.

Hooper DC, Wolfson JS. Fluoroquinolone antimicrobial agents. N Engl J Med 324:384–94, 1991.

Monk JP, Campoli-Richards DM. Ofloxacin: A review of its antibacterial activity, pharmacokinetics properties, and therapeutic use. Drugs 33:346–91, 1987.

Pendland SL, Messick CR, Jung R. In vitro synergy testing of levofloxacin, ofloxacin, and ciprofloxacin in combination with aztreonam, ceftazidime, or piperacillin against Pseudomonas aeruginosa. Diagn Microbiol Infect Dis 42:75–8, 2002.

Schwartz M, Isenmann R, Weikert E, et al. Pharmacokinetic basis for oral perioperative prophylaxis with ofloxacin in general surgery. Infection 29:222–7, 2001.

Walker RC, Wright AJ, The fluoroquinolones. Mayo Clin Proc 66:1249–59, 1991.

Website: www.pdr.net

Oseltemavir (Tamiflu)

Drug class: Neuraminidase inhibitor.

Usual dose: Treatment: 75 mg (PO) q12L × 5 days; Prophylaxis: 75 mg (PO) q24h × 10 days.

Pharmacokinetic Parameters:

Peak serum level: 65.2 mcg/L

Bioavailability: 75%

Excreted unchanged: 1%

Serum half-life (normal/ESRD): 1–3 hours/no data

plasma protein binding: 42%

Volume of distribution (V_d): 23–26 L

Primary Mode of Elimination: Renal (oseltamivir carboxylate)

Dosage Adjustments*

CrCl ≥ 50 mL/min	No adjustment
CrCl ~ 30–49 mL/min	No adjustment
CrCl ~ 10–29 mL/min	75 mg (PO) q24h (treatment) 75 mg (PO) q48h or 30 mg (PO) q24h (prophylaxis)
CrCl < 10 mL/min	No data
Post-HD dose	No data
Post-PD dose	No data
CVVH dose	No data
Moderate or severe hepatic insufficiency	None

Drug Interactions: Live attenuated influenza vaccine 2 weeks before or 2 days after oseltemavir.

Adverse Effects: nausea, vomiting, serious skin reactions, diplopia, visual disturbances, palpitations, atrial fibrillation, supraventricular/ventricular tachycardias neuropsychiatric events.

Allergic Potential: Low

Safety in Pregnancy: C

Comments: Begin prophylaxis within 3 days of exposure. **Pediatric treatment doses:** ≤ 15 kg = 30 mg (PO) q12h, 16–23 kg = 45 mg (PO) q12h, 24–40 kg = 60 mg (PO) q12h, > 40 kg = 75 mg (PO) q12h. **Pediatric prophylaxis dose** ≤ 15 kg = 30 mg (PO) q24h, 16–23 kg = 45 mg (PO) q24h, 24–40 kg = 60 mg (PO) q24h, > 40 kg = 75 mg (PO) q24h. Available as 30, 45 and 75 mg capsules and 300 mg oral suspension.

REFERENCES:

Chen H, Cheung CL, Tai H, et al. Oseltamivir-Resistant Influenza A Pandemic (H1N1) 2009 Virus, Hong Kong, China. Emerg Infect Dis 15:1970–1972, 2009.

Sotos JG. Emergence of Oseltamivir-Resistant Pandemic H1N1 Virus during Prophylaxis. N Engl J Med 361:2296–2298, 2009.

"Usual dose" assumes normal renal/hepatic function. * For renal insufficiency, give usual dose × 1 followed by maintenance dose per CrCl. For dialysis patients, dose the same as for CrCl < 10 mL/min and give supplemental (post-HD/PD dose) immediately after dialysis. CrCl = creatinine clearance; CVVH = continuous veno-venous hemofiltration; HD/PD = hemodialysis/peritoneal dialysis. See pp. 509–513 for explanations, pp. xi–xii for abbreviations; Linezolid (↑ risk of serotonin syndrome, see p. 620).

Oxacillin (Prostaphlin)

Drug Class: Antistaphylococcal penicillin.
Usual Dose: 1–2 gm (IV) q4h.
Pharmacokinetic Parameters:
Peak serum level: 43 mcg/ml
Bioavailability: Not applicable
Excreted unchanged (urine): 39–66%
Serum half-life (normal/ESRD): 0.5/1 hrs
Plasma protein binding: 94%
Volume of distribution (V_d): 0.2 L/kg
Primary Mode of Elimination: Renal
Dosage Adjustments* (based on 2 gm q4h):

CrCl 10–80 mL/min	No change
CrCl < 10 mL/min	No change
Post–HD dose	None
Post–PD dose	None
CVVH dose	No change
Moderate hepatic insufficiency	No change
Severe hepatic insufficiency	No change

Drug Interactions: Cyclosporine (↓ cyclosporine levels); nifedipine, warfarin (↓ interacting drug effect).
Adverse Effects: Drug fever/rash, leukopenia, ↑ SGOT/SGPT, interstitial nephritis.
Allergic Potential: High
Safety in Pregnancy: B
Comments: Avoid oral formulation (not well absorbed/erratic serum levels). Na^+ content = 3.1 mEq/g. Meningeal dose = 2 gm (IV) q4h.
Cerebrospinal Fluid Penetration:
Non-inflamed meninges = 1%
Inflamed meninges = 10%
Bile Penetration: 25%

REFERENCES:

Al-Homaidhi H, Abdel-Haq NM, El-Baba M, et al. Severe hepatitis associated with oxacillin therapy. South Med J 95:650–2, 2002.
Donowitz GR, Mandell GL. Beta-lactam antibiotics. N Engl J Med 318:419–26 and 318:490–500, 1993.
Jensen AG, Wachmann CH, Espersen F, et al. Treatment and outcome of Staphylococcus aureus bacteremia: a prospective study of 278 cases. Arch Intern Med 162:25–32, 2002.
Jones ME, Mayfield DC, Thronsberry C, et al. Prevalence of oxacillin resistance in Staphylococcus aureus among inpatients and outpatients in the United States during 2000. Antimicrob Agents Chemother 46:3104–5, 2002.
Wright AJ. The penicillins. Mayo Clin Proc 74:290–307, 1999.
Website: www.pdr.net

Pegylated Interferon alfa-2a (Pegasys) + Ribavirin

Drug Class: Interferon/antiviral.
Usual Dose: Pegasys: 180 mcg once weekly (SQ) × 48 weeks; ribavirin: 500 mg (< 75 kg) or 800 mg (> 75 mg) (PO) q12h × 48 weeks (see comments).
Pharmacokinetic Parameters:
Trough level: 16 ng/ml
Bioavailability: No data
Excreted unchanged (urine): No data
Serum half-life (normal/ESRD): 80/100–120 hrs
Plasma protein binding: No data
Volume of distribution (V_d): 8–12 L/kg
Primary Mode of Elimination: Renal
Dosage Adjustments*

"Usual dose" assumes normal renal/hepatic function. * For renal insufficiency, give usual dose × 1 followed by maintenance dose per CrCl. For dialysis patients, dose the same as for CrCl < 10 mL/min and give supplemental (post-HD/PD dose) immediately after dialysis. CrCl = creatinine clearance; CVVH = continuous veno-venous hemofiltration; HD/PD = hemodialysis/peritoneal dialysis. See pp. 509–513 for explanations, pp. xi–xii for abbreviations; Linezolid (↑ risk of serotonin syndrome, see p. 620).

CrCl 40–60 mL/min	Pegasys: no change. Avoid ribavirin if CrCl < 50 mL/min
CrCl 10–40 mL/min	Avoid ribavirin
CrCl < 10 mL/min	Pegasys: 135 mcg q week; avoid ribavirin
Post–HD dose	Pegasys: 135 mcg q week; avoid ribavirin
Post–PD dose	No information
CVVH dose	No information
Moderate hepatic insufficiency	135 mcg if ALT ↑
Severe hepatic insufficiency	Avoid
Moderate depression	↓ Pegasys to 135 mcg (90 mcg in some); evaluate once weekly
Severe depression	Discontinue Pegasys; immediate psychiatric consult

Pegasys Adjustment for Hematologic Toxicity:

Absolute neutrophil count < 750/mm^3	↓ Pegasys to 135 mcg
Absolute neutrophil count < 500/mm^3	Discontinue Pegasys until neutrophils > 1000/mm^3. Reinstitute at 90 mcg and monitor neutrophil count
Platelets < 50,000/mm^3	↓ Pegasys to 90 mcg
Platelets < 25,000/mm^3	Discontinue Pegasys

Ribavirin Adjustment for Hematologic Toxicity

Hgb < 10 gm/dL and no cardiac disease	↓ Ribavirin to 600 mg/day†
Hgb < 8.5 gm/dL and no cardiac disease	Discontinue ribavirin
Hgb ≥ 2 gm/dL ↓ during 4-week treatment period and stable cardiac disease	↓ Ribavirin to 600 mg/day*
Hgb < 12 gm/dL despite 4 weeks at reduced dose and stable cardiac disease	Discontinue ribavirin

* One 200-mg tablet in a.m. and two 200-mg tablets in p.m.

Drug Interactions: Inhibits CYP IA2. May ↑ theophylline levels.

Adverse Effects: Flu-like symptoms, neuropsychiatric disturbances, bone marrow toxicity, nausea/vomiting/diarrhea, alopecia, hypothyroidism, ARDS.

Allergic Potential: Low

Safety in Pregnancy: Pegasys: C (ribavirin: X; also avoid in partners of pregnant women)

Comments: Ribavirin dose with Pegasys for HCV (genotypes 2, 3) is 800 mg/d. The optimal ribavirin dose for HCV (genotype 1) has not been determined but 800–1400 mg/d has been used. Combination therapy is more effective than monotherapy. Avoid in autoimmune hepatitis and decompensated cirrhosis. Check CBC weekly. For genotypes 2 and 3, duration of therapy is 24 weeks and ribavirin dose is 400 mg (PO) bid (rather than q12h). Ribavirin should be taken with breakfast and dinner to ↑ bioavailability/↓ nausea. Ribavirin taken after dinner may cause insomnia. Ribavirin's long serum half-life allows q24h dosing, but ↑ nausea.

"Usual dose" assumes normal renal/hepatic function. * For renal insufficiency, give usual dose × 1 followed by maintenance dose per CrCl. For dialysis patients, dose the same as for CrCl < 10 mL/min and give supplemental (post-HD/PD dose) immediately after dialysis. CrCl = creatinine clearance; CVVH = continuous veno-venous hemofiltration; HD/PD = hemodialysis/peritoneal dialysis. See pp. 509–513 for explanations, pp. xi–xii for abbreviations; Linezolid (↑ risk of serotonin syndrome, see p. 620).

Cerebrospinal Fluid Penetration: No data
Bile Penetration: No data

REFERENCES:

[No authors listed]. Peginterferon alfa-2a (Pegasys) for chronic hepatitis C. Med Lett Drugs Ther 45:19–20, 2003.

Davis GL. Combination treatment with interferon and ribavirin for chronic hepatitis C. Clin Liver Dis 1:811–26, 1999.

Ferenci P. Peginterferon alfa-2a (40KD) (Pegasys) for the treatment of patients with chronic hepatitis C. Int J Clin Pract 57:610–5, 2003.

Fried MN, et al. Peg-interferon alfa-2a plus ribavirin for chronic hepatitis C virus infection. N Engl J Med 347:975–82, 2002.

Kamal SM, et al. Peg-interferon alone or with ribavirin enhances HCV-specific CD_4 T-helper responses in patients with chronic hepatitis C. Gastroenterology 123:1070–83, 2002.

Plosker GL, Keating GM. Peginterferon-alpha-2a (40kD) plus ribavirin: a review of its use in hepatitis C virus and HIV co-infection. Drugs 64:2823–43, 2004.

Rajender Reddy K, Modi MW, Pedder S. Use of peginterferon alfa-2a (40 KD) (Pegasys) for the treatment of hepatitis C. Adv Drug Deliv Rev 54:571–86, 2002.

Rasenack J, Zeuzem S, Feinman SV, et al. Peginterferon alpha-2a (40kD) [Pegasys] improves HR-QOL outcomes compared with unmodified interferon alpha-2a [Roferon-A]: in patients with chronic hepatitis C. Pharmacoeconomics 21:341–9, 2003.

Torriani FJ, Rodriguez-Torres M, Rockstroh JK, et al. Peginterferon alfa-2a plus ribavirin for chronic hepatitis C virus infection in HIV-infected patients. N Engl J Med 351:438–50, 2004.

Website: www.pegasys.com

Pegylated Interferon alfa-2b (Peg-Intron) + Ribavirin

Drug Class: Interferon/antiviral.
Usual Dose: See pp. 95–96.
Pharmacokinetic Parameters:

Peak serum level: 30 IU/ml / 3680 ng/ml
Bioavailability: No data/64%
Excreted unchanged (urine): No data/17%
Serum half-life (normal/ESRD): [40 hrs/no data] / [298 hrs/no data]
Plasma protein binding: No data
Volume of distribution (V_d): 0.99 L/kg

Primary Mode of Elimination: Renal/renal
Dosage Adjustments*

CrCl 50–80 mL/min	No change
CrCl 10–50 mL/min	Avoid ribavirin
CrCl < 10 mL/min	Avoid ribavirin
Post–HD dose	No information
Post–PD dose	No information
CVVH dose	No information
Moderate hepatic insufficiency	None
Severe hepatic insufficiency	None
Moderate depression	↓ Peg-Intron by 50%; evaluate once weekly
Severe depression	Discontinue both drugs; immediate psychiatric consult

Dosage Adjustments for Hematologic Toxicity

Hgb < 10 gm/dL	↓ ribavirin by 200 mg/day
Hgb < 8.5 gm/dL	Permanently discontinue both drugs
WBC < 1.5×10^9/L	↓ Peg-Intron by 50%
WBC < 1.0×10^9/L	Permanently discontinue both drugs

"Usual dose" assumes normal renal/hepatic function. * For renal insufficiency, give usual dose × 1 followed by maintenance dose per CrCl. For dialysis patients, dose the same as for CrCl < 10 mL/min and give supplemental (post-HD/PD dose) immediately after dialysis. CrCl = creatinine clearance; CVVH = continuous veno-venous hemofiltration; HD/PD = hemodialysis/peritoneal dialysis. See pp. 509–513 for explanations, pp. xi–xii for abbreviations; Linezolid (↑ risk of serotonin syndrome, see p. 620).

Neutrophils < 0.75 × 10^9/L	↓ Peg-Intron by 50%
Neutrophils < 0.5 × 10^9/L	Permanently discontinue both drugs
Platelets < 80 × 10^9/L	↓ Peg-Intron by 50%
Platelets < 50 × 10^9/L	Permanently discontinue both drugs
Hgb ≥ 2 gm/dL ↓ during 4-week treatment period and stable cardiac disease	↓ Peg-Intron by 50% and ribavirin by 200 mg/day
Hgb < 12 gm/dL despite ribavirin dose reduction	Permanently discontinue both drugs

Drug Interactions: Nucleoside analogs: fatal/non-fatal lactic acidosis. May ↑ levels of theophylline. Overlapping toxicity with other bone marrow suppressants.

Adverse Effects: Hemolytic anemia, psychological effects, cytopenias, pulmonary symptoms, pancreatitis, hypersensitivity reactions, ↑ triglycerides, flu-like symptoms, nausea/vomiting, alopecia, rash, hypothyroidism.

Allergic Potential: Low

Safety in Pregnancy: Peg-Intron: C (ribavirin: X; also avoid in partners of pregnant women)

Comments: Avoid in autoimmune hepatitis. Check CBC pretreatment and at 2 and 4 weeks (must adjust doses for ↓ WBC, ↓ neutrophils, ↓ platelets, ↓ hemoglobin). Poorly tolerated in decompensated cirrhosis or recurrent hepatitis C after transplant. Be alert for severe depression/psychiatric changes.

Cerebrospinal Fluid Penetration: No data

Bile Penetration: No data

REFERENCES:

Alfaleh FZ, Hadad Q, Khuroo MS, et al. Peginterferon alpha-2b plus ribavirin compared with interferon alpha-2b plus ribavirin for initial treatment of chronic hepatitis C in Saudi patients commonly infected with genotype 4. Liver Int 24:568–74, 2004.

Fried MN. Side effects of therapy of hepatitis C and their management. Hepatology 36:S237–44, 2002.

Jaeckel E, Cornberg M, Wedemeyer H, et al. Treatment of acute hepatitis C with interferon alfa-2b. N Engl J Med 345:1452–7, 2001.

Wright TL. Treatment of patients with hepatitis C and cirrhosis. Hepatology 36:S185–91, 2002.

Website: www.pegintron.com

Penicillin G (various)

Drug Class: Natural penicillin.

Usual Dose: 2–4 mu (IV) q4h (see comments).

Spectrum: (see ***Susceptibility Profiles*** pp. 183–187).

Pharmacokinetic Parameters:

Peak serum level: 20–40 mcg/ml

Bioavailability: Not applicable

Excreted unchanged (urine): 80%

Serum half-life (normal/ESRD): 0.5/5.1 hrs

Plasma protein binding: 60%

Volume of distribution (V_d): 0.3 L/kg

Primary Mode of Elimination: Renal

Dosage Adjustments*

CrCl 50–80 mL/min	2–4 mu (IV) q4h
CrCl 10–50 mL/min	1–2 mu (IV) q4h
CrCl < 10 mL/min	1 mu (IV) q6h
Post–HD dose	2 mu (IV)
Post–PD dose	0.5 mu (IV)
CVVH dose	2 mu (IV) q6h

"Usual dose" assumes normal renal/hepatic function. * For renal insufficiency, give usual dose × 1 followed by maintenance dose per CrCl. For dialysis patients, dose the same as for CrCl < 10 mL/min and give supplemental (post-HD/PD dose) immediately after dialysis. CrCl = creatinine clearance; CVVH = continuous veno-venous hemofiltration; HD/PD = hemodialysis/peritoneal dialysis. See pp. 509–513 for explanations, pp. xi–xii for abbreviations; Linezolid (↑ risk of serotonin syndrome, see p. 620).

Moderate hepatic insufficiency	No change
Severe hepatic insufficiency	No change

Drug Interactions: Probenecid (↑ penicillin G levels).

Adverse Effects: Drug fever/rash, E. multiforme/ Stevens–Johnson syndrome; anaphylactic reactions (hypotension, laryngospasm, bronchospasm), hives, serum sickness.

Allergic Potential: High

Safety in Pregnancy: B

Comments: Incompatible in solutions containing erythromycin, aminoglycosides, calcium bicarbonate, or heparin. Penicillin G (potassium): K^+ content = 1.7 mEq/g; Na^+ content = 0.3 mEq/g. Penicillin G (sodium): Na^+ content = 2 mEq/g. **1°, 2°, early latent syphilis dose:** PCN benzathine 2.4 mu (IM) × 1 dose. **Late latent syphilis dose:** PCN benzathine 2.4 mu (IM) q8h once weekly × 3. **Neurosyphilis dose:** PCN G 4 mu (IV) q4h × 2 weeks. Meningeal dose = 4 mu (IV) q4h.

Cerebrospinal Fluid Penetration:
Non-inflamed meninges ≤ 1%
Inflamed meninges = 5%

Bile Penetration: 500%
(also see ***Antibiotic Pearls & Pitfalls*** p. 496).

REFERENCES:

Falco V, Almirante B, Jordano Q, et al. Influence of penicillin resistance of outcome in adult patients with invasive pneumococcal pneumonia. Is penicillin useful against intermediately resistant strains? J Antimicrob Chemother 54:481–8, 2004.

Giachetto G, Pirez MC, Nanni L, et al. Ampicillin and penicillin concentration in serum and pleural fluid of hospitalized children with community-acquired pneumonia. Pediatr Infect Dis J 7:625–9, 2004.

Steininger C, Allerberger F, Gnaiger E. Clinical significance of inhibition kinetics for Streptococcus pyogenes in response to penicillin. J Antimicrob Chemother 50:517–23, 2002.

Wendel Jr GD, Sheffield JS, Hollier LM, et al. Treatment of syphilis in pregnancy and prevention of congenital syphilis. Clin Infect Dis 35(Suppl2):S200–9, 2002.

Wright AJ. The penicillins. Mayo Clin Proc 74:290–307, 1999.

Penicillin V (various)

Drug Class: Natural penicillin.

Usual Dose: 500 mg (PO) q6h. (Take without food)

Spectrum: (see ***Susceptibility Profiles*** pp. 183–187).

Pharmacokinetic Parameters:
Peak serum level: 5 mcg/ml
Bioavailability: 60%
Excreted unchanged (urine): 80%
Serum half-life (normal/ESRD): 0.5/8 hrs
Plasma protein binding: 70%
Volume of distribution (V_d): 0.5 L/kg

Primary Mode of Elimination: Renal

Dosage Adjustments*

CrCl 50–80 mL/min	No change
CrCl 10–50 mL/min	No change
CrCl < 10 mL/min	250–500 mg (PO) q8h
Post–HD dose	250 mg (PO)
Post–PD dose	250 mg (PO)
CVVH dose	500 mg (PO) q6h
Moderate hepatic insufficiency	No change
Severe hepatic insufficiency	No change

Drug Interactions: Probenecid (↑ penicillin V levels).

"Usual dose" assumes normal renal/hepatic function. * For renal insufficiency, give usual dose × 1 followed by maintenance dose per CrCl. For dialysis patients, dose the same as for CrCl < 10 mL/min and give supplemental (post-HD/PD dose) immediately after dialysis. CrCl = creatinine clearance; CVVH = continuous veno-venous hemofiltration; HD/PD = hemodialysis/peritoneal dialysis. See pp. 509–513 for explanations, pp. xi–xii for abbreviations; Linezolid (↑ risk of serotonin syndrome, see p. 620).

Adverse Effects: Drug fever/rash, E. multiforme/Stevens-Johnson syndrome, anaphylactic reactions (hypotension, laryngospasm, bronchospasm), hives, serum sickness C. difficile diarrhea/colitis.

Allergic Potential: High

Safety in Pregnancy: B

Comments: Jarisch–Herxheimer reactions when treating spirochetal infections, e.g., Lyme disease, syphilis, yaws.

Cerebrospinal Fluid Penetration: < 10% (also see ***Antibiotic Pearls & Pitfalls*** p. 496).

REFERENCES:

Bisno AL, Gerber MA, Swaltney JM, et al. Practice guidelines for the diagnosis and management of group A streptococcal pharyngitis. Infectious Diseases Society of America. Clin Infect Dis 35:113–25, 2002.

Chiou CC, Does Penicillin Remain the Drug of Choice for Pneumococcal Pneumonia in View of Emerging in Vitro Resistance? Clin Infect Dis 42:234–7, 2006.

Donowitz GR, Mandell GL. Beta-lactam antibiotics. N Engl J Med 318:419–26 and 490–500, 1993.

Klugman KP, Yu VL. No Impact of Penicillin Resistance on Mortality. Clin Infect Dis 43:261, 2006.

Peterson LR. Penicillin for Treatment of Pneumococcal Pneumonia: Does In Vitro Resistance Really Matter? Clin Infect Dis 42:224–33, 2006.

Portier H, Filipecki J, Weber P, et al. Five day clarithromycin modified release versus 10 day penicillin V for group A streptococcal pharyngitis: a multi-centre, open-label, randomized study. J Antimicrob Chemother 49:337–44, 2002.

Wright AJ. The penicillins. Mayo Clin Proc 74:290, 1999.

Pentamidine (Pentam 300, NebuPent)

Drug Class: Antiparasitic.

Usual Dose: 4 mg/kg (IV) q24h (see comments).

Pharmacokinetic Parameters:

Peak serum level: 0.6–1.5 mcg/mL

Bioavailability: Not applicable

Excreted unchanged (urine): 50%

Serum half-life (normal/ESRD): 6.4/90 hrs

Plasma protein binding: 69%

Volume of distribution (V_d): 5 L/kg

Primary Mode of Elimination: Metabolized

Dosage Adjustments*

CrCl 50–80 mL/min	No change
CrCl 10–50 mL/min	No change
CrCl < 10 mL/min	No change
Post–HD dose	None
Post–PD dose	None
CVVH dose	No change
Moderate or severe hepatic insufficiency	No change

Drug Interactions: Alcohol, valproic acid, didanosine, (↑ risk of pancreatitis); foscarnet (severe hypocalcemia reported; do not combine); amphotericin B, aminoglycosides, capreomycin, cis-platinum, colistin, methoxyflurane, polymyxin B, vancomycin, other nephrotoxic drugs (↑ nephrotoxicity).

Adverse Effects: Severe hypotension, hypocalcermia, hypoglycemia, increase in creatinine, pancreatitis, severe leukopenia, anemia and thrombocytopenia. May increase the QT interval with IV administration and cause ventricular tachycardia. Severe hypoglycemic episodes may result in later diabetes mellitus. IV extravasation may cause severe skin necrosis and IM injections can be severely painful and should be avoided if possible. The following tests should be carried out at regular intervals; Daily blood urea nitrogen and serum creatinine, blood glucose, complete blood count and platelet count as well as every other day

"Usual dose" assumes normal renal/hepatic function. * For renal insufficiency, give usual dose × 1 followed by maintenance dose per CrCl. For dialysis patients, dose the same as for CrCl < 10 mL/min and give supplemental (post-HD/PD dose) immediately after dialysis. CrCl = creatinine clearance; CVVH = continuous veno-venous hemofiltration; HD/PD = hemodialysis/peritoneal dialysis. See pp. 509–513 for explanations, pp. xi–xii for abbreviations; Linezolid (↑ risk of serotonin syndrome, see p. 620).

bilirubin, alkaline phosphatase, AST (SGOT, and ALT (SGPT). An electrocardiogram should be done at regular intervals to calculate the QT_c interval. If creatinine starts to rise the dose should be cut back to 3 or 2 mg/kg. The medication should be held if hypoglycemia occurs and or if the QT_c interval increases.

Allergic Potential: High

Safety in Pregnancy: C

Comments: Well absorbed IM, but painful. Administer IV slowly in D_5W over 1 hour, not saline/may be used at a dose of 300 mg aerosol q month to prevent aerosol pentamidine. Caution should be used with inhalent pentamidine especially around pregnant employees as it can induce spontaneous abortion. Special attention should be made to the proper aerosolization of medication so that it is distributed evenly through the lung. Adverse effects with aerosolized pentamidine include chest pain, arrhythmias, dizziness, wheezing, coughing, dyspnea, headache, anorexia, nausea, diarrhea, rash, pharyngitis. **If PCP patient also has pulmonary TB, aerosolized pentamidine treatments may expose medical personnel to TB via droplet inhalation**. Nebulizer dose: Inhaled pentamidine isethionate (NebuPent) 300 mg monthly via Respirgard II nebulizer can be used for PCP prophylaxis. **Nebulized pentamidine less effective than IV/IM pentamidine and is not effective against extrapulmonary PCP**. Use with caution in renal disease. Subtle creatinine changes may be associated with severe toxicity.

Cerebrospinal Fluid Penetration: < 10%

REFERENCES:

Chan C, Montaner J, LeFebvre BA, et al. Atovaquone suspension compared with aerosolized pentamidine for prevention of Pneumocystis carinii pneumonia in human immunodeficiency virus infected subsets intolerant of trimethoprim or sulfamethoxazole. J Infect Dis 180:369–376, 1999.

Goa KL, Campoli-Richards DM. Pentamidine isethionate: A review of its antiprotozoal activity, pharmacokinetic properties and therapeutic use in Pneumocystis carinii pneumonia. Drugs 33:242–58, 1987.

Guerin PJ, Alar P, Sundar S, et al. Visceral leishmaniasis: current status of control, diagnosis, and treatment, and a proposed research and development agenda. Lancet Infect Dis 2:494–501, 2002.

Lionakis MS, Lewis RE, Samonis G, et al. Pentamidine is active in vitro against Fusarium species. Antimicrob Agents Chemother 47:3252–9, 2003.

Monk JP, Benfield P. Inhaled pentamidine: An overview of its pharmacological properties and a review of its therapeutic use in Pneumocystis carinii pneumonia. Drugs 39:741–56, 1990.

Rodriquez M, Fishman JA. Prevention of infection due to Pneumocystis spp. in human immunodeficiency virus-negative immunocompromised patients. Clin Microbiol Rev 17:770–82, 2004.

Sattler FR, Cowam R. Nielsen DM, et al. Trimethoprim-sulfamethoxazole compared with pentamidine for treatment of Pneumocystis carinii pneumonia in the acquired immunodeficiency syndrome. Ann Intern Med 109:280–7, 1988.

Website: www.pdr.net

Peramivir

Drug class: Neuroaminidase inhibitor.

Usual dose: 400 mg (IV) q24h or 10 mg/kg (IV) q24h, maximum dose 600 mg/day (IV) over 30 minutes.

Pharmacokinetic Parameters:

Peak serum level: 17–44 mcg/mL/13 mcg/mL

Bioavailability: not applicable

Excreted unchanged: no data

Serum half-life (normal/ESRD): 7–20 hrs/no data

Plasma protein binding: no data

Volume of distribution (V_d): no data

Primary Mode of Elimination: Renal

"Usual dose" assumes normal renal/hepatic function. * For renal insufficiency, give usual dose × 1 followed by maintenance dose per CrCl. For dialysis patients, dose the same as for CrCl < 10 mL/min and give supplemental (post-HD/PD dose) immediately after dialysis. CrCl = creatinine clearance; CVVH = continuous veno-venous hemofiltration; HD/PD = hemodialysis/peritoneal dialysis. See pp. 509–513 for explanations, pp. xi–xii for abbreviations; Linezolid (↑ risk of serotonin syndrome, see p. 620).

Dosage Adjustments*

CrCl > 49 mL/min	600 mg (IV) q24h
CrCl 31–49 mL/min	150 mg (IV) q24h
CrCl 10–30 mL/min	100 mg (IV) q24h
CrCl < 10 mL/min	15 mg (IV) q24h
Post-HD dose	15 mg (IV) q24h
Post-PD dose	No data
CVVH dose	No data
Moderate or severe hepatic insufficiency	No adjustment needed

Drug Interactions: No data

Adverse Effects: Diarrhea, nausea, vomiting, neutropenic fever, rare cause of anaphylaxis

Allergic Potential: Low—do not use if severely allergic to other neuroaminidase inhibitors

Safety in Pregnancy: No data

Comments: Emergency use authorization (EUA) for the investigational antiviral drug peramivir intravenous (IV) in certain adult and pediatric patients with confirmed or suspected 2009 H1N1 influenza infection who are admitted to a hospital. **IV peramivir is authorized only for hospitalized adult and pediatric patients for whom therapy with an IV drug is clinically appropriate, based on one or more of the following reasons: 1. the patient is not responding to either oral or inhaled antiviral therapy, or 2. when drug delivery by a route other than an intravenous route—eg., enteral (absorbed by the intestines) or 3. for adults only, when the clinician judges IV therapy is appropriate due to other circumstances**. To obtain peramivir go to www.cdc.gov/h1niflu/eua. Should be used within 72 of symptom onset. Do not use if oseltamivir resistance. Do not exceed 40 mg/minute infusion rate. ***Highly active against swine influenza (H1N1)***.

Cerebrospinal Fluid Penetration: no data

REFERENCES:

Birnkrant D, Cox E. The Emergency Use Authorization of Peramivir for Treatment of 2009 H1N1 Influenza. N Engl J Med 361:2204–2207, 2009.

Website: www.cdc.gov

Website: www.fda.gov

Piperacillin (Pipracil)

Drug Class: Antipseudomonal penicillin.

Usual Dose: 3 gm (IV) q4-6h (see comments).

Spectrum: (see ***Susceptibility Profiles*** pp. 183–187).

Pharmacokinetic Parameters:

Peak serum level: 412 mcg/ml

Bioavailability: Not applicable

Excreted unchanged (urine): 50–70%

Serum half-life (normal/ESRD): 1/3 hrs

Plasma protein binding: 16%

Volume of distribution (V_d): 0.24 L/kg

Primary Mode of Elimination: Renal

Dosage Adjustments* (based on 4 gm q8h):

CrCl 50–80 mL/min	No change
CrCl 10–50 mL/min	3 gm (IV) q8h
CrCl < 10 mL/min	3 gm (IV) q12h
Post–HD dose	1 gm (IV)
Post–PD dose	2 gm (IV)
CVVH dose	3 gm (IV) q8h
Moderate or severe hepatic insufficiency	No change

Drug Interactions: Aminoglycosides (inactivation of piperacillin in renal failure); warfarin (↑ INR); oral contraceptives (↓ oral contraceptive effect); cefoxitin (↓ piperacillin effect).

Adverse Effects: Drug fever/rash, anaphylactic reactions (hypotension, laryngospasm, bronchospasm), hives, serum sickness, leukopenia, C. difficile diarrhea/colitis.

"Usual dose" assumes normal renal/hepatic function. * For renal insufficiency, give usual dose × 1 followed by maintenance dose per CrCl. For dialysis patients, dose the same as for CrCl < 10 mL/min and give supplemental (post-HD/PD dose) immediately after dialysis. CrCl = creatinine clearance; CVVH = continuous veno-venous hemofiltration; HD/PD = hemodialysis/peritoneal dialysis. See pp. 509–513 for explanations, pp. xi–xii for abbreviations; Linezolid (↑ risk of serotonin syndrome, see p. 620).

Allergic Potential: High
Safety in Pregnancy: B
Comments: 75% absorbed when given IM. Do not mix/administer with aminoglycosides. **Most active antipseudomonal penicillin against P. aeruginosa. Nosocomial pneumonia/P. aeruginosa dose:** 3 gm (IV) q4h. Meningeal dose = usual dose.
Cerebrospinal Fluid Penetration:
Non-Inflamed meninges = 1%
Inflamed meninges = 30%
Bile Penetration: 1000%
(also see ***Antibiotic Pearls & Pitfalls*** pp. 495–508).

REFERENCES:

Donowitz GR, Mandell GL. Beta-lactam antibiotics. N Engl J Med 318:419–26 and 318:490–500, 1993.

Kim MK, Capitano B, Mattoes HM, et al. Pharmacokinetic and pharmacodynamic evaluation of two dosing regimens for piperacillin-susceptible organisms. Pharmacotherapy 22:569–77, 2002.

Peacock JE, Herrington DA, Wade JC, et al. Ciprofloxacin plus piperacillin compared with tobramycin plus piperacillin as empirical therapy in febrile neutropenic patients. A randomized, double-blind trial. Ann Intern Med 137:120, 2002.

Tan JS, File TM, Jr. Antipseudomonal penicillins. Med Clin North Am 79:679–93, 1995.

Website: www.pdr.net

Piperacillin/tazobactam (Zosyn, Tazocin)

Drug Class: Antipseudomonal penicillin.
Usual Dose: 3.375 gm (IV) q6h (see comments).
Spectrum: (see ***Susceptibility Profiles*** pp. 183–187).
Pharmacokinetic Parameters:
Peak serum level: 298/34 mcg/ml
Bioavailability: Not applicable
Excreted unchanged (urine): 60/80%
Serum half-life (normal/ESRD): [1.5/8] / [1/7] hrs
Plasma protein binding: 30/30%
Volume of distribution (V_d): 0.3/0.21 L/kg
Primary Mode of Elimination: Renal
Dosage Adjustments* (also see comments):

CrCl > 40 mL/min	No change
CrCl 20–40 mL/min	2.25 gm (IV) q6h
CrCl < 20 mL/min	2.25 gm (IV) q8h
Hemodialysis	2.25 gm (IV) q8h
Post–HD dose	0.75 gm (IV)
Post–PD dose	None
CVVH dose	2.25 gm (IV) q6h
Moderate or severe hepatic insufficiency	No change

Drug Interactions: Aminoglycosides (↓ aminoglycoside levels); vecuronium (↑ vecuronium effect); probenecid (↑ piperacillin/tazobactam levels); methotrexate (↑ methotrexate levels).
Adverse Effects: Drug fever/rash, eosinophilia, ↓/↑ platelets, leukopenia (with prolonged use > 21 days), ↑ PT/PTT, mild transient ↑ SGOT/SGPT, insomnia, nausea, headache, constipation, hypertension, C. difficile diarrhea/colitis.
Allergic Potential: High
Safety in Pregnancy: B
Comments: P. aeruginosa/nosocomial pneumonia doses: For CrCl > 40 mL/min use 4.5 gm (IV) q6h. For CrCl 20–40 mL/min use 3.375 gm (IV) q6h. For CrCl < 20 mL/min use 2.25 gm (IV) q6h. **Hemodialysis (HD) doses:** 2.25 gm (IV) q8h; give 0.75 gm (IV) Post–HD on HD days. Do not mix with Ringers lactate.
Cerebrospinal Fluid Penetration:
Non-Inflamed meninges = 1%

"Usual dose" assumes normal renal/hepatic function. * For renal insufficiency, give usual dose × 1 followed by maintenance dose per CrCl. For dialysis patients, dose the same as for CrCl < 10 mL/min and give supplemental (post-HD/PD dose) immediately after dialysis. CrCl = creatinine clearance; CVVH = continuous veno-venous hemofiltration; HD/PD = hemodialysis/peritoneal dialysis. See pp. 509–513 for explanations, pp. xi–xii for abbreviations; Linezolid (↑ risk of serotonin syndrome, see p. 620).

Inflamed meninges = 30%
Bile Penetration: 6000%
(also see ***Antibiotic Pearls & Pitfalls*** pp. 495–508).

REFERENCES:

Bow EJ, Rotstein C, Noskin GA, et al. A Randomized, Open-Label, Multicenter Comparative Study of the Efficacy and Safety of Piperacillin-Tazobactam and Cefepime for the Empirical Treatment of Febrile Neutropenic Episodes in Patients with Hematologic Malignancies. Clin Infect Dis 43:447–59, 2006.

Del Real GA, Rose ME, Ramirez-Atamoros MT, et al. Penicillin skin testing in patients with a history of beta-lactam allergy. Ann Allergy Asthma Immunol 98:355–359, 2007.

Frei CR, Hampton SL, Burgess DS. Influence of culture site-specific MIC distributions on the pharmacokinetic and pharmacodynamic properties of piperacillin/tazobactam and piperacillin: a data analysis. Clin Ther. 28:1035–40, 2006.

Gin A, Dilay L, Karlowsky JA, et al. Piperacillin-tazobactam: a beta-lactam/beta-lactamase inhibitor combination. Expert Rev Anti Infect Ther 5:365–383, 2007.

Harter C, Schulze B, Goldschmidt H, et al. Piperacillin/tazobactam vs ceftazidime in the treatment of neutropenic fever in patients with acute leukemia or following autologous peripheral blood stem cell transplantation: a prospective randomized trial. Bone Marrow Transplant. 37:373–379, 2006.

Lau WK, Mercer D, Itani KM, et al. Randomized, Open-Label, Comparative Study of Piperacillin-Tazobactam Administered by Continuous Infusion versus Intermittent Infusion for Treatment of Hospitalized Patients with Complicated Intra-Abdominal Infection. Antimicrob Agents and Chemother 50:3556–61, 2006.

Lodise TP Jr, Lomaestro B, Drusano GL. Piperacillin-tazobactam for Pseudomonas aeruginosa infection: clinical implications of an extended-infusion dosing strategy. Clin Infect Dis 44:357–363, 2007.

Mattoes HM, Capitano B, Kim MK, et al. Comparative pharmacokinetic and pharmacodynamic profile of piperacillin/tazobactam 3.375 G Q4H and 4.5 G Q6H. Chemotherapy 458:59–63, 2002.

Minnaganti VR, Cunha BA. Piperacillin/tazobactam. Antibiotics for Clinicians 3:101–8, 1999.

Sader HS, Hsiung A, Fritsche TR, et al. Comparative activities of cefepime and piperacillin/tazobactam tested against a global collection of Escherichia coli and Klebsiella spp. With an ESBL phenotype. Diagn Microbiol Infect Dis 57:341–344, 2007.

Sanders WE Jr, Sanders CC. Piperacillin/tazobactam: A critical review of the evolving clinical literature. Clin Infect Dis 22:107–23, 1996.

Schoonover LL, Occhipinti DJ, Rodvold KA, et al. Piperacillin/tazobactam: A new beta-lactam/beta-lactamase inhibitor combination. Ann Pharmacother 29:501–14, 1995.

Scheetz MH, McKoy JM, Parada JP, et al. Systematic review of piperacillin-induced neutropenia. Drug Saf 30:295–306, 2007.

Simon A, Lehrnbecher T, Bode U, et al. Piperacillin-tazobactam in pediatric cancer patients younger than 25 months: a retrospective multicenter survey. Eur J Clin Microbiol Infect Dis 26:801–806, 2007.

Wiesmayr S, Stelzmueller I, Muehlmann MW. Experience with the use of piperacillin-tazobactam in pediatric non-renal solid organ transplantation. Pediatr Transplant 11:38–48, 2007.

Winston LG, Charlebois ED, Pang S, et al. Impact of a formulary switch from ticarcillin-clavulanate to piperacillin-tazobactam on colonization with vancomycin-resistant enterococci. Am J Infect Control 32:462–9, 2004.

Website: www.zosyn.com

Polymyxin B

Drug Class: Cell membrane-altering antibiotic.
Usual Dose: 1–1.25 mg/kg (IV) q12h (1 mg = 10,000 units) (see comments).
Spectrum: (see ***Susceptibility Profiles*** pp. 194–199).
Pharmacokinetic Parameters:
Peak serum level: 8 mcg/ml
Bioavailability: Not applicable
Excreted unchanged (urine): 60%
Serum half-life (normal/ESRD): 6/48 hrs

"Usual dose" assumes normal renal/hepatic function. * For renal insufficiency, give usual dose × 1 followed by maintenance dose per CrCl. For dialysis patients, dose the same as for CrCl < 10 mL/min and give supplemental (post-HD/PD dose) immediately after dialysis. CrCl = creatinine clearance; CVVH = continuous veno-venous hemofiltration; HD/PD = hemodialysis/peritoneal dialysis. See pp. 509–513 for explanations, pp. xi–xii for abbreviations; Linezolid (↑ risk of serotonin syndrome, see p. 620).

Plasma protein binding: < 10%
Volume of distribution (V_d): *No data*
Primary Mode of Elimination: Renal
Dosage Adjustments*

CrCl 50–80 mL/min	0.5–1 mg/kg (IV) q12h
CrCl 10–50 mL/min	0.5 mg/kg (IV) q12h
CrCl < 10 mL/min	0.2 mg/kg (IV) q12h
Post–HD/PD dose	No information
CVVH dose	0.5 mg/kg (IV) q12h
Moderate or severe hepatic insufficiency	No change

Drug Interactions: Amphotericin B, amikacin, gentamicin, tobramycin, vancomycin (↑ nephrotoxicity).
Adverse Effects: Renal failure. Neurotoxicity associated with very prolonged/high serum levels; neuromuscular blockade potential with renal failure/neuromuscular disorders.
Allergic Potential: Low
Safety in Pregnancy: B
Comments: Inhibits endotoxin release from gram-negative bacilli. Avoid intraperitoneal infusion due to risk of neuromuscular blockade. Increased risk of reversible non–oliguric renal failure (ATN) when used with other nephrotoxic drugs. No ototoxic potential. May be given IM with procaine, but painful. Nebulizer dose for multidrug resistant P. aeruginosa in cystic fibrosis/bronchiectasis: 80 mg in saline via aerosol/nebulizer q8h (for recurrent infection use 160 mg). Intrathecal (IT) polymyxin B dose = 5 mg (50,000 u) q24h × 3 days, then q48h × 2 weeks. Dissolve 50 mg (500,000 u) into 10 ml for IT administration.
Cerebrospinal Fluid Penetration: < 10% (also see ***Antibiotic Pearls & Pitfalls*** pp. 495–508).

REFERENCES:

Bratu S, Quale J, Cebular S, et al. Multidrug-resistant Pseudomonas aeruginosa in Brooklyn, New York: molecular epidemiology and in vitro activity of polymyxin B. Eur J Clin Microbiol Infect Dis 24:196–201, 2005.

Cruz DN, Antonelli M, Fumagalli R, et al. Early use of Polymyxin B Hemoperfusion in Abdominal Septic Shock. The EUPHAD Randomized Controlled Trial. JAMA. 301:2445–2452, 2009.

Cunha BA. New uses for older antibiotics: nitrofurantoin, amikacin, colistin, polymyxin B, doxycycline, and minocycline revisited. Med Clin North Am. 90:1089–107, 2006.

Evans ME, Feola DJ, Rapp RP. Polymyxin B sulfate and colistin: Old antibiotics for emerging multiresistant gram-negative bacteria. Ann Pharmacother 33:960–7, 1999.

Falagas ME, Kasiakou SK. Colistin: the revival of polymyxins for the management of multidrug-resistant gram-negative bacterial infections. Clin Infect Dis 40:1333–41, 2005.

Kunin CM. The Pharmacokinetics of Polymyxin B are Dependent on Binding and Release from Deep-Tissue Compartments. Clin Infect Dis 48:842–844, 2009.

Li J, Nation RL. Old Polymyxins are Back: Is Resistance Close? Clin Infect Disease. 43:663–64, 2006.

Menzies D, Minnaganti VR, Cunha BA. Polymyxin B. Antibiotics for Clinicians 4:33–40, 2000.

Parchuri S, Mohan S, Young S, Cunha BA. Chronic ambulatory peritoneal dialysis associated peritonitis ESBL producing Klebsiella pneumoniae successfully treated with polymyxin B. Heart & Lung 34:360, 2005.

Segal-Maurer S, Mariano N, Qavi A, et al. Successful treatment of ceftazidime-resistant Klebsiella pneumoniae ventriculitis with intravenous meropenem and intraventricular polymyxin B: Case report and review. Clin Infect Dis 28:1134–8, 1999.

Wareham DW, Bean DC. In Vitro Activities of Polymyxin B, Imipenem and Rifampin against Multidrug-Resistant Acinetobacter baumannii. Antimicrob Agents Chemother 50:825–26, 2006.

Posaconazole (Noxafil)

Drug Class: Antifungal (triazole).
Usual Dose: Prophylaxis of invasive Aspergillus and Candida infections in high-risk patients (graft-vs-host disease, prolonged neutropenia from chemotherapy) ≥ 13 years of age: 200 mg (PO) q8h. **Treatment of oropharyngeal candidiasis:** 100 mg (PO) q12h × 1 day, then 100 mg (PO) q24h × 13 days; for fluconazole- and/or itraconazole-resistant strains, use 400 mg (PO) q12h with duration of therapy based on underlying condition and clinical response. Available as a 40 mg/mL oral suspension. Take with a meal or 240 mL of a nutritional supplement.
Pharmacokinetic Parameters:
Peak serum level: 3 mcg/mL
Bioavailability: Absorption is ↑ 2–6-fold by food
Excreted unchanged (feces): 66%
Serum half-life (normal/ESRD): 35/35 hrs
Plasma protein binding: 98.2%
Volume of distribution (V_d): 1774 L
Primary Mode of Elimination: Hepatic
Dosage Adjustments*

CrCl 50–80 mL/min	No change
CrCl 10–50 mL/min	No change
CrCl < 10 mL/min	No change
Post–HD dose	None
Post–PD dose	None
CVVH dose	None
Moderate or severe hepatic insufficiency	Insufficient data; use with caution

Drug Interactions: Posaconazole is metabolized by hepatic glucuronidation. Inducers (e.g., rifampin, phenytoin) may alter disposition. Amiodarone, rifabutin, phenytoin, cimetidine (↓ posaconazole levels 50%). Posaconazole inhibits hepatic CYP3A4 and can increase levels of drugs metabolized by this enzyme. QT prolonging drugs terfenadine, astemizole, cisapride, pimozide, halofantrine, quinidine (↑ interacting drug levels, ↑ risk of cardiac arrhythmias); ergot (↑ ergot levels); statins (↑ statin levels and risk of rhabdomyolysis); vinca alkaloids (↑ vinca alkaloid levels and risk of neurotoxicity); cyclosporine, tacrolimus, sirolimus, midazolam and other benzodiazapines metabolized by CYP3A4, calcium channel blockers metabolized by CYP3A4 (diltiazem, verapamil, nifedipine, nisoldipine); digoxin, sulfonylureas, ritonavir, indinavir (↑ interacting drug levels).
Adverse Effects: Nausea, vomiting, diarrhea, headache, ↑ SGOT/SGPT; ↑ QTc.
Allergic Potential: Low
Safety in Pregnancy: C
Comments: Posaconazole (200 mg 3x/d) reduced aspergillosis/mortality in hematopoietic stem cell transplant recipients with severe graft vs. host disease. ***Highly active against Candida albicans, most non-albicans Candida, Aspergillus, Crypotococcus, Histoplasmosis, Blastomycocis, Sporotrichosis, Paracoccidiomycosis. Some activity against Coccidiomycosis, Fusarium, Pseudoallescheria, or C. glabrata. No activity against Mucor***. Blood levels not increased with higher dosages.
Cerebrospinal Fluid Penetration: No data

REFERENCES:

Alffenaar JWC, van Assen S, van der Werf TS. Omeprazole Significantly Reduces Poconazole Serum Through Level. Clin Infect Dis 48:839–840, 2009.

Bruggemann RJM, Alffenaar JWC, Blijlevens NMA, et al. Clinical Relevance of the Pharmoacokinetic Interactions of Azole Antifungal Drugs with Coadministered Agents. Clin Infect Dis 48: 1441–1458, 2009.

Chen A, Sobel JD. Emerging azole antifungals. Expert Opin Emerg Drugs 10:21–33, 2005.

"Usual dose" assumes normal renal/hepatic function. * For renal insufficiency, give usual dose × 1 followed by maintenance dose per CrCl. For dialysis patients, dose the same as for CrCl < 10 mL/min and give supplemental (post-HD/PD dose) immediately after dialysis. CrCl = creatinine clearance; CVVH = continuous veno-venous hemofiltration; HD/PD = hemodialysis/peritoneal dialysis. See pp. 509–513 for explanations, pp. xi–xii for abbreviations; Linezolid (↑ risk of serotonin syndrome, see p. 620).

Cornely OA, Maertens J, Winston DJ, et al. Posaconazole vs. fluconazole or itraconazole prophylaxis in patients with neutropenia. N Engl J Med 356:348–59, 2007.

Courtney R, Pai S, Laughlin M, et al. Pharmacokinetics, safety, and tolerability of oral posaconazole in single and multiple doses in healthy adults. Antimicrob Agents Chemother 47:2788–2795, 2003.

Courtney R, Sansone A, Smith W, et al. Posaconazole pharmacokinetics, safety, and tolerability in subjects with varying degrees of chronic renal disease. J Clin Pharmacol 45:185–192, 2005.

Dodds Ashley ES, Alexander BD. Posaconazole. Drugs Today 41:393–400, 2005.

Ezzet F, Wexler D, Courtney R, et al. Oral bioavailability of posaconazole in fasted healthy subjects-comparison between three regimens and basis for clinical dosage recommendations. Clin Pharmacokinet 44:211–220, 2005.

Golan Y, Overview of transplant mycology. Am J Health Syst Pharm 62:S17–21, 2005.

Greenberg RN, Mullane K, van Burik JA, et al. Posaconazole as salvage therapy for zygomycosis. Antimicrob Agents Chemother 50:126–33, 2006.

Gubbins PO, Krishna G, Sansone-Parsons A, et al. Pharmacokinetics and safety of oral posaconazole in neutropenic stem cell transplant recipients. Antimicrob Agents Chemother 50:1993–9, 2006.

Herbrecht R, Nivoix Y, Fohrer C, et al. Management of systemic fungal infections: alternatives to itraconazole. J Antimicrob Chemother 56:139–148, 2005.

Keating GM, Posaconazole. Drugs 65:1553–69, 2005.

Kontoyiannis DP, Lewis RE. Posaconazole prophylaxis in hematologic cancer. N Engl J Med 24:2214–2215, 2007.

Krieter P, Flannery B, Musick T, et al. Disposition of posaconazole following single-dose oral administration in healthy subjects. Antimicrob Agents Chemother 48:3543–51, 2004.

Mullane K, Toor AA, Kalnicky C, et al. Posaconazole salvage therapy allows successful allogeneic hematopoietic stem cell transplantation in patients with refractory invasive mold infections. Transpl Infect Dis 9:89–96, 2007.

Raad II, Graybill JR, Bustamante AB, et al. Safety of long-term oral posaconazole use in the treatment of refractory invasive fungal infections. Clin Infect Dis 42:1726–34, 2006.

Radd II, Hachem RY, Herbrecht R, et al. Posaconazole as salvage treatment for invasive fusariosis in patients with underlying hematologic malignancy and other conditions. Clin Infect Dis 42:1398–403, 2006.

Restrepo A, Tobon A, Clark B, et al. Salvage treatment of histoplasmosis with posaconazole. Salvage treatment of histoplasmosis with posaconazole. J Infect 54:319–327, 2007.

Sabatelli F. Patel R, Mann PA, et al. In vitro activities of posaconazole, fluconazole, itraconazole, voriconazole, and amphotericin B against a large collection of clinically important molds and yeasts. Antimicrob Agents Chemother 50:2009–15, 2006.

Ullmann AJ, Cornely OA, Burchardt A, et al. Pharmacokinetics, safety, and efficacy of posaconazole in patients with persistent febrile neutropenia or refractory invasive fungal infection. Antimicrob Agents Chemother 50:658–66, 2006.

Ullmann AJ, Lipton JH, Vesole DH, et al. Posaconazole or fluconazole for prophylaxis in severe graft-versus-host disease. N Engl J Med 356:335–47, 2007.

van Burik JA, Role of new antifungal agents in prophylaxis of mycoses in high risk patients. Curr Opin Infect Dis 18:479–83, 2005.

Vazquez JA, Skiest DJ, Nieto L, et al. A multicenter randomized trial evaluating posaconazole versus fluconazole for the treatment of oropharyngeal candidiasis in subjects with HIV/AIDS. Clin Infect Dis 42:1179–86, 2006.

Walsh TJ, Raad I, Patterson TF, et al. Treatment of invasive Aspergillosis with posaconazole in patients who are refractory to or intolerant of conventional therapy: an externally controlled trial. Clin Infect Dis 44:2–12, 2007.

Wexler D, Courtney R, Richards W, et al. Effect of posaconazole on cytochrome P450 enzymes: a randomized, open-label, two-way crossover study. Eur J Pharm Sci 21:645–653, 2004.

Website: www.noxafil.com

"Usual dose" assumes normal renal/hepatic function. * For renal insufficiency, give usual dose × 1 followed by maintenance dose per CrCl. For dialysis patients, dose the same as for CrCl < 10 mL/min and give supplemental (post-HD/PD dose) immediately after dialysis. CrCl = creatinine clearance; CVVH = continuous veno-venous hemofiltration; HD/PD = hemodialysis/peritoneal dialysis. See pp. 509–513 for explanations, pp. xi–xii for abbreviations; Linezolid (↑ risk of serotonin syndrome, see p. 620).

Primaquine

Drug Class: Antimalarial/Anti-PCP.
Usual Dose: **Antimalarial dose:** 15 mg (base 26.3 mg) (PO) q24h. **PCP dose:** 15–30 mg (PO) q24h plus clindamycin 600 mg (IV) or 300 mg (PO) q6h.
Pharmacokinetic Parameters:
Peak serum level: 30–100 mcg/ml
Bioavailability: 90%
Excreted unchanged (urine): 3.6%
Serum half-life (normal/ESRD): 3.7–9.6/3.7–9.6 hrs
Plasma protein binding: 75%
Volume of distribution (V_d): No data
Primary Mode of Elimination: Hepatic
Dosage Adjustments*

CrCl < 80 mL/min	No change
Post–HD/Post–PD dose	None
CVVH dose	No change
Hepatic insufficiency	No change

Drug Interactions: Avoid in patients receiving bone marrow suppressive drugs (↑ risk of agran-ulocytosis), alcohol (↑ GI side effects), quinacrine (↑ primaquine levels/ toxicity).
Adverse Effects: Nausea/vomiting, headache, abdominal pain, leukopenia (dose dependent), agranulocytosis, pruritus. Hemolytic anemia in G6PD deficiency; methemoglobinemia in NADH reductase deficiency.
Allergic Potential: Low
Safety in Pregnancy: C
Comments: Take with food to ↓ GI side effects. Use with caution in (and screen for) G6PD deficiency. Use with caution in NADH reductase deficiency.
Cerebrospinal Fluid Penetration: No data

REFERENCES:

Baird JK. Effectiveness of antimalarial drugs. N Engl J Med 352:1565–77, 2005.
Chen LH, Keystone JS. New strategies for the prevention of malaria in travelers. Infect Dis Clin North Am 19:185–210, 2005.
Korraa H, Saadeh C. Options in the management of pneumonia caused by Pneumocystis carinii in patients with acquired immune deficiency syndrome and intolerance to trimethoprim/sulfamethoxazole. South Med J 89:272–7, 1996.
Safrin S, Finkelstein DM, Feinberg J, et al. Comparison of three regimens for treatment of mild to moderate Pneumocystis carinii pneumonia in patients with AIDS. A double-blind randomized trial of oral TMP–SMX, dapsone-TMP & clinda-primaquine. Ann Intern Med 124:792–802, 1996.
Warren E, George S, You J, Kazanjian P. Advances in the treatment and prophylaxis of Pneumocystis carinii pneumonia. Pharmacotherapy 17:900–16, 1997.

Pyrazinamide (PZA)

Drug Class: Anti–TB drug.
Usual Dose: 25 mg/kg (PO) q24h (max. 2 gm) (see comments).
Pharmacokinetic Parameters:
Peak serum level: 30–50 mcg/ml
Bioavailability: 90%
Excreted unchanged (urine): 10%
Serum half-life (normal/ESRD): 9/26 hrs
Plasma protein binding: 10%
Volume of distribution (V_d): 0.9 L/kg
Primary Mode of Elimination: Hepatic
Dosage Adjustments*

CrCl 50–80 mL/min	No change
CrCl 10–50 mL/min	No change
CrCl < 10 mL/min	No change
Post–HD dose	25 mg/kg (PO) or 1 gm (PO)

"Usual dose" assumes normal renal/hepatic function. * For renal insufficiency, give usual dose × 1 followed by maintenance dose per CrCl. For dialysis patients, dose the same as for CrCl < 10 mL/min and give supplemental (post-HD/PD dose) immediately after dialysis. CrCl = creatinine clearance; CVVH = continuous veno-venous hemofiltration; HD/PD = hemodialysis/peritoneal dialysis. See pp. 509–513 for explanations, pp. xi–xii for abbreviations; Linezolid (↑ risk of serotonin syndrome, see p. 620).

Post–PD dose	No change
CVVH dose	No information
Moderate hepatic insufficiency	No information
Severe hepatic insufficiency	Avoid

Drug Interactions: INH, rifabutin, rifampin (may ↑ risk of hepatoxicity).

Adverse Effects: Drug fever/rash, malaise, nausea, vomiting, anorexia, ↑ SGOT/SGPT, ↑ uric acid, sideroblastic anemia.

Allergic Potential: Low

Safety in Pregnancy: C

Comments: Avoid in patients with gout (may precipitate acute attacks). **TB D.O.T. dose:** 4 gm (PO) 2x/week or 3 gm (PO) 3x/week. Meningeal dose = usual dose.

Cerebrospinal Fluid Penetration: 100%

REFERENCES:

Ahn C, Oh KH, Kim K, et al. Effect of peritoneal dialysis on plasma and peritoneal fluid concentrations of isoniazid, pyrazinamide, and rifampin. Perit Dial Int. 23:362–7, 2003.

Davidson PT, Le HQ. Drug treatment of tuberculosis 1992. Drugs 43:651–73, 1992.

Drugs for tuberculosis. Med Lett Drugs Ther 35:99–101, 1993.

Furin J, Nardell EA. Multidrug-resistant tuberculosis: An update on the best regimens. J Respir Dis 27:172–82, 2006.

Havlir DV, Barnes PF. Tuberculosis in patients with human immunodeficiency virus infection. N Engl J Med 340:367–73, 1999.

Iseman MD. Treatment of multidrug-resistant tuberculosis. N Engl J Med 329:784–91, 1993.

Ijaz K, McElroy PD, Navin TR. Short course rifampin and pyrazinamide compared with isoniazid for latent tuberculosis infection: a cost-effectiveness analysis based on a multicenter clinical trial. Clin Infect Dis 39:289, 2004.

McIlleron H, Wash P, Burger A, et al. Determinants of Rifampin, Isoniazid, Pyrazinamide and Ethambutol Pharmacokinetics in a Cohort of Tuberculosis Patients. Antimicrob Agents Chemother 50:1170–77, 2006.

Van Scoy RE, Wilkowske CJ. Antituberculous agents. Mayo Clin Proc 67:179–87, 1992.

Pyrimethamine (Daraprim)

Drug Class: Antiparasitic.

Usual Dose: 75 mg (PO) q24h (see comments).

Pharmacokinetic Parameters:

Peak serum level: 0.4 mcg/ml

Bioavailability: 90%

Excreted unchanged (urine): 25%

Serum half-life (normal/ESRD): 96/96 hrs

Plasma protein binding: 87%

Volume of distribution (V_d): 2.5 L/kg

Primary Mode of Elimination: Hepatic

Dosage Adjustments*

CrCl 50–80 mL/min	No change
CrCl 10–50 mL/min	No change
CrCl < 10 mL/min	No change; use caution
Post–HD dose	None
Post–PD dose	25 mg (PO)
CVVH dose	No change
Moderate hepatic insufficiency	No change
Severe hepatic insufficiency	No change; use caution

Drug Interactions: Folic acid (↓ pyrimethamine effect); lorazepam (↑ risk of hepatotoxicity); sulfamethoxazole, trimethoprim, TMP–SMX (↑ risk of thrombocytopenia, anemia, leukopenia).

"Usual dose" assumes normal renal/hepatic function. * For renal insufficiency, give usual dose × 1 followed by maintenance dose per CrCl. For dialysis patients, dose the same as for CrCl < 10 mL/min and give supplemental (post-HD/PD dose) immediately after dialysis. CrCl = creatinine clearance; CVVH = continuous veno-venous hemofiltration; HD/PD = hemodialysis/peritoneal dialysis. See pp. 509–513 for explanations, pp. xi–xii for abbreviations; Linezolid (↑ risk of serotonin syndrome, see p. 620).

Adverse Effects: Megaloblastic anemia, leukopenia, thrombocytopenia, ataxia, tremors, seizures.
Allergic Potential: Low
Safety in Pregnancy: C
Comments: Antacids decrease absorption. **Toxoplasmosis dose:** 200 mg (PO) × 1 dose, then 50–75 mg/kg (PO) q24h (with folinic acid 20 mg PO q24h plus either sulfadiazine or clindamycin).
Cerebrospinal Fluid Penetration: 10–25%

REFERENCES:

Drugs for Parasitic Infections. Med Lett Drugs Ther 40: 1–12, 2000.

Lemnge MM, Ali AS, Malecela EK, et al. Therapeutic Efficacy of Sulfadoxine Pyrimethamine and Amodiaquine Among Children with Uncomplicated Plasmodium Falciparum Malaria in Zanzibar, Tanzania. Am. J. Trop. Med Hyg. 73:681–5, 2005.

Podzamczer D, Salazar A, Jiminez J, et al. Intermittent trimethoprim-sulfamethoxazole compared with dapsone-pyrimethamine for the simultaneous primary prophylaxis of Pneumocystis pneumonia and toxoplasmosis in patients infected with HIV. Ann Intern Med 122:755–61, 1995.

Porter SB, Sande MA. Toxoplasmosis of the central nervous system in the acquired-immunodeficiency syndrome. N Engl J Med 327:1643–8, 1992.

Website: www.pdr.net

Quinine sulfate

Drug Class: Antimalarial.
Usual Dose: 650 mg (PO) q8h (see comments).
Pharmacokinetic Parameters:
Peak serum level: 3.8 mcg/ml
Bioavailability: 80%
Excreted unchanged (urine): 5%
Serum half-life (normal/ESRD): 7/14 hrs
Plasma protein binding: 95%
Volume of distribution (V_d): 3 L/kg

Primary Mode of Elimination: Renal/hepatic
Dosage Adjustments*

CrCl 50–80 mL/min	No change
CrCl 10–50 mL/min	650 mg (PO) q12h
CrCl < 10 mL/min	650 mg (PO) q12h
Post–HD dose	None
Post–PD dose	650 mg (PO)
CVVH dose	650 mg (PO) q12h
Moderate hepatic insufficiency	325 mg (PO) q8h; use caution
Severe hepatic insufficiency	325 mg (PO) q12h; use caution

Drug Interactions: Amiodarone, Aluminum-based antacids (↓ quinidine absorption); astemizole, cisapride, terfenadine (↑ interacting drug levels, torsade de pointes; avoid); cimetidine, ritonavir (↑ quinidine toxicity: headache, deafness, blindness, tachycardia); cyclosporine (↓ cyclosporine levels); digoxin (↑ digoxin levels); dofetilide, flecainide (arrhythmias); mefloquine (seizures, may ↑ QT interval, torsade de pointes, cardiac arrest, ↓ mefloquine efficacy); metformin (↑ risk of lactic acidosis); pancuronium, succinylcholine, tubocurarine (neuromuscular blockade); warfarin (↑ INR).
Adverse Effects: Drug fever/rash, ↑ QT_c interval, arrhythmias, drug-induced SLE, lightheadedness, diarrhea, abdominal discomfort, nausea, vomiting, cinchonism with chronic use. Avoid in patients with G6PD deficiency.
Allergic Potential: High
Safety in Pregnancy: D
Comments: **PO malaria dose:** 650 mg (PO) q8h (*plus doxycycline* 100 mg PO q12h) × 3–7 days).

"Usual dose" assumes normal renal/hepatic function. * For renal insufficiency, give usual dose × 1 followed by maintenance dose per CrCl. For dialysis patients, dose the same as for CrCl < 10 mL/min and give supplemental (post-HD/PD dose) immediately after dialysis. CrCl = creatinine clearance; CVVH = continuous veno-venous hemofiltration; HD/PD = hemodialysis/peritoneal dialysis. See pp. 509–513 for explanations, pp. xi–xii for abbreviations; Linezolid (↑ risk of serotonin syndrome, see p. 620).

IV malaria dose: quinine hydrochloride 600 mg (IV) q8h × 3–7 days, or quinidine gluconate 10 mg/kg (IV) × 1 dose (infuse over 1–2 hours) then 0.02 mg/kg/min (IV) × 72 hours or until parasitemia < 1%.
Cerebrospinal Fluid Penetration: 2–5%

REFERENCES:

Corpelet C, Vacher P, Coudor F, et al. Role of quinine in life-threatening Babesia divergens infection successfully treated with clindamycin. Eur J Clin Microbiol Infect Dis 24:74–75, 2005.

Croft AM, Herxheimer A. Tolerability of antimalaria drugs. Clin Infect Dis 34:1278; discussion 1278–9, 2002. Drugs for Parasitic Infections. Med Letter. March, 2000.

Panisko DM, Keystone JS. Treatment of malaria. Drugs 39:160–89, 1990.

Wyler DJ, Malaria: Overview and update. Clin Infect Dis 16:449–56, 1993.

Quinupristin/dalfopristin (Synercid)

Drug Class: Streptogramin.
Usual Dose: 7.5 mg/kg (IV) q8h.
Spectrum: (see ***Susceptibility Profiles*** pp. 194–199).
Pharmacokinetic Parameters:
Peak serum level: 3.2/8 mcg/ml
Bioavailability: Not applicable
Excreted unchanged: 20% (urine); 80% (feces)
Serum half-life (normal/ESRD): [3.1/1]/[3.1/1] hrs
Plasma protein binding: 55/15%
Volume of distribution (V_d): 0.45/0.24 L/kg
Primary Mode of Elimination: Hepatic
Dosage Adjustments*

CrCl 50–80 mL/min	No change
CrCl 10–50 mL/min	No change
CrCl < 10 mL/min	No change
Post–HD dose	None
Post–PD dose	None
CVVH dose	No change
Moderate hepatic insufficiency	No change
Severe hepatic insufficiency	No information

Drug Interactions: Amiodarone, Amlodipine (↑ amlodipine toxicity); astemizole, cisapride (may ↑ QT interval, torsades de pointes); carbamazepine (↑ carbamazepine toxicity: ataxia, nystagmus, diplopia, headache, seizures); cyclosporine, delavirdine, indinavir, nevirapine (↑ interacting drug levels); diazepam, midazolam (↑ interacting drug effect); diltiazem, felodipine, isradipine (↑ interacting drug toxicity: dizziness, hypotension, headache, flushing); disopyramide (↑ disopyramide toxicity: arrhythmias, hypotension, syncope); docetaxel (↑ interacting drug toxicity: neutropenia, anemia, neuropathy); lidocaine (↑ lidocaine toxicity: neurotoxicity, arrhythmias, seizures); methylprednisolone (↑ methylprednisolone toxicity: myopathy, diabetes mellitus, cushing's syndrome); nicardipine, nifedipine, nimodipine (↑ interacting drug toxicity: dizziness, hypotension, flushing, headache); statins (↑ risk of rhabdomyolysis).
Adverse Effects: Pain, inflammation, and swelling at infusion site (dose related), severe/prolonged myalgias, hyperbilirubinemia. Hepatic insufficiency increases concentration (AUC) of metabolites by 180%/50%.
Allergic Potential: Low
Safety in Pregnancy: B

"Usual dose" assumes normal renal/hepatic function. * For renal insufficiency, give usual dose × 1 followed by maintenance dose per CrCl. For dialysis patients, dose the same as for CrCl < 10 mL/min and give supplemental (post-HD/PD dose) immediately after dialysis. CrCl = creatinine clearance; CVVH = continuous veno-venous hemofiltration; HD/PD = hemodialysis/peritoneal dialysis. See pp. 509–513 for explanations, pp. xi–xii for abbreviations; Linezolid (↑ risk of serotonin syndrome, see p. 620).

Comments: Administer in D_5W or sterile water, not in saline. Requires central IV line for administration. ***Not effective against E. faecalis (VSE). May be useful for daptomycin resistant MSSA/MRSA infections.***

Cerebrospinal Fluid Penetration: < 10% (also see ***Antibiotic Pearls & Pitfalls*** p. 506).

REFERENCES:

Abb J, Comparative activity of linezolid, quinupristin-dalfopristin and newer quinolones against Streptococcus pneumoniae. Int J Antimicrob Agents. 21:289–91, 2003.

Blondeau JM, Sanche Se. Quinupristin/dalfopristin. Expert Opin Pharmacother 3:1341–64, 2002.

Bouza E. New therapeutic choices for infections caused by methicillin-resistant *Staphylococcus aureus*. Clin Microbiol Infect Dis 15:44–52, 2009.

Bryson HM, Spencer CM. Quinupristin/dalfopristin. Drugs 52:406–15, 1996.

Chant C, Ryback MH. Quinupristin/dalfopristin (RP 59500): A new streptogramin antibiotic. Ann Pharmacother 29:1022–7, 1995.

Goff DA, Sierawski SJ. Clinical experience of quinupristin-dalfopristin for the treatment of antimicrobial-resistant gram-positive infections. Pharmacotherapy 22:748–58, 2002.

Griswold MW, Lomaestro BM, Briceland LL. Quinupristin-dalfopristin (RP 59500): An injectable streptogramin combination. Am J Health Syst Pharm. 53:2045–53, 1996.

Kim MK, Nicolau DP, Nightingale CH, et al. Quinupristin/dalfopristin: A treatment option for vancomycin-resistant enterococci. Conn Med 64:209–12, 2000.

Klastersky J. Role of quinupristin/dalfopristin in the treatment of Gram-positive nosocomial infections in haematological or oncological patients. Cancer Treat Rev. 29:431–40, 2003.

Nadler H, Dowzicky MJ, Feger C, et al. Quinupristin/dalfopristin: A novel selective-spectrum antibiotic for the treatment of multi-resistant and other gram-positive pathogens. Clin Microbiol Newslett 21:103–12, 1999.

Scotton PG, Rigoli R, Vaglia A. Combination of quinupristin/dalfopristin and glycopeptide in severe methicillin-resistant staphylococcal infections failing previous glycopeptide regimen. Infection 30:161–3, 2002.

Website: www.synercid.com

Raltegravir (Isentress)

Drug Class: HIV-1 integrase inhibitor.

Usual Dose: 400 mg (PO) q12h.

Pharmacokinetic Parameters:

Peak serum level: 6.5 μM

Bioavailability: ~ 32% (20–43%)

Excreted unchanged: 51% (feces); 9% (urine)

Serum half-life (normal/ESRD): 9–12 hrs/ no data

Plasma protein binding: 83%

Volume of distribution (V_d): not studied

Primary Mode of Elimination: Fecal/renal

Dosage Adjustments*

CrCl 50–80 mL/min	No change
CrCl 10–50 mL/min	No change
CrCl < 10 mL/min	No information
Post–HD dose	No information
Post–PD dose	No information
CVVH dose	No information
Mild/moderate hepatic insufficiency	No change
Severe hepatic insufficiency	No information

"Usual dose" assumes normal renal/hepatic function. * For renal insufficiency, give usual dose × 1 followed by maintenance dose per CrCl. For dialysis patients, dose the same as for CrCl < 10 mL/min and give supplemental (post-HD/PD dose) immediately after dialysis. CrCl = creatinine clearance; CVVH = continuous veno-venous hemofiltration; HD/PD = hemodialysis/peritoneal dialysis. See pp. 509–513 for explanations, pp. xi–xii for abbreviations; Linezolid (↑ risk of serotonin syndrome, see p. 620).

Antiretroviral Dosage Adjustments:

Atazanavir	No change
Atazanavir/ritonavir	No change
Efavirenz	No change
Rifampin	Avoid
Ritonavir	No change
Tenofovir	No change
Tipranavir/ritonavir	No change

Drug Interactions: Rifampin (↓ raltegravir levels, use with caution). In-vitro, raltegravir does not inhibit CYP1A2, CYP2B6, CYP2C8, CYP2C9, CYP2C19, CYP2D6 or CYP3A and does not induce CYP3A4. In addition, raltegravir does not inhibit P-glycoprotein-mediated transport. Raltegravir is therefore not expected to affect the pharmacokinetics of drugs that are substrates of these enzymes or P-glycoprotein (e.g., protease inhibitors, NNRTIs, methadone, opioid analgesics, statins, azole antifungals, proton pump inhibitors, oral contraceptives, anti-erectile dysfunction agents).
Adverse Effects: Nausea, headache, diarrhea, pyrexia.
Allergic Potential: Low
Safety in Pregnancy: C
Comments: May be taken with or without food. CPK elevations, myopathy and rhabdomyolysis have been reported—use with caution in patients at increased risk for myopathy or rhabdomyolysis, such as those receiving concomitant medications known to cause these conditions (e.g., statins). Raltegravir is indicated for treatment-experienced adult patients who have evidence of viral replication and HIV-1 strains resistant to multiple antiretroviral agents. Slight increase in cancer is severly immunocompromised hosts.
Cerebrospinal Fluid Penetration: No data

REFERENCES:

Cooper, D. Results of BENCHMRK-1, a Phase III Study Evaluating the Efficacy and Safety of MK-0518, a Novel HIV-1 Integrase Inhibitor, in Patients with Triple-class Resistant Virus [Abstract 105aLB]. Conference on Retroviruses and Opportunistic Infections. Alexandria, VA. 2007. Available from URL: http://www.retroconference.org/2007/Abstracts/30687.htm.

Grinsztejn B, Nguyen BY, Katlama C, et al. Safety and efficacy of the HIV-1 integrase inhibitor raltegravir (MK-0518) in treatment-experienced patients with multidrug-resistant virus: a phase II randomised controlled trial. Lancet 369:1261–1269, 2007.

Hicks C, Gulick RM. Raltegravir: The First HIV Type 1 Integrase Inhibitor. Clin Infect Dis 48:931–940, 2009.

Iwamoto M, Wenning LA, Petry AS, et al. Safety, tolerability, and pharmacokinetics of raltegravir after single and multiple doses in healthy subjects. Clin Pharmacol Ther 2007.

Kassahun K, McIntosh I, Cui D, et al. Metabolism and Disposition in Humans of Raltegravir (MK-0518), an Anti-AIDS Drug Targeting the HIV-1 Integrase Enzyme. Drug Metab Dispos Epub: 1–28, 2007.

Markowitz M, Morales-Ramirez JO, Nguyen BY, et al. Antiretroviral activity, pharmacokinetics, and tolerability of MK-0518, a novel inhibitor of HIV-1 integrase, dosed as monotherapy for 10 days in treatment-naive HIV-1–infected individuals. J Acquir Immune Defic Syndr 43:509–515, 2006.

Palmisano L, Role of integrase inhibitors in the treatment of HIV disease. Expert Rev Anti Infect Ther 5:67–75, 2007.

Panel on Antiretroviral Guidelines for Adults and Adolescents. Guidelines for the use of antiretroviral agents in HIV-1 infected adults and adolescents. Department of Health and Human Services. November 3, 2008; 1–139. Available at http://www.aidsinfor.nih.gov/ContentFiles/AdultandAdolescentGL.pdf.

Steigbigel, R. Results of BENCHMRK-2, a Phase III Study Evaluating the Efficacy and Safety of MK-0518, a Novel HIV-1 Integrase Inhibitor, in Patients with Triple-class Resistant Virus [Abstract 105bLB]. Conference on Retroviruses and Opportunistic Infections. Alexandria, VA. 2007. Available from URL: http://www.retroconference.org/2007/Abstracts/30688.htm.

Website: www.isentress.com

Ribavirin (Rebetol) (Copegus)

Drug Class: RSV, HCV Antiviral; (see comments).

Usual Dose: 600 mg (PO) q12h (see comments).

Pharmacokinetic Parameters:

Peak serum level: 0.07–0.28 mcg/ml

Bioavailability: 64%

Excreted unchanged (urine): 40%

Serum half-life (normal/ESRD): 120 hrs/no data

Plasma protein binding: 0%

Volume of distribution (V_d): 10 L/kg

Primary Mode of Elimination: Hepatic

Dosage Adjustments*

CrCl 50–80 mL/min	No change
CrCl 10–50 mL/min	Avoid
CrCl < 10 mL/min	Avoid
Post–HD dose	Avoid
Post–PD dose	Avoid
CVVH dose	Avoid
Moderate hepatic insufficiency	No change
Severe hepatic insufficiency	No change

Drug Interactions: Ribavirin may antagonize the *in vitro antiviral* activity of stavudine and zidovudine against *HIV*. Pegylated interferon (Pegasys) in HIV patients (↓ CD_4 counts).

Adverse Effects: Primary toxicity of ribavirin is hemolytic anemia. The *anemia* associated with ribavirin therapy may result in worsening of cardiac disease that has led to fatal and nonfatal myocardial infarctions. Patients with a history of significant or unstable cardiac disease should not be treated with ribavirin. Patient whose hemoglobin level falls below 10 g/dL have his/her ribavirin dose reduced to 600 mg daily. Patients whose hemoglobin falls below 8.5 should have ribavirin discontinued. When combined with interferon there are significant adverse events caused by ribavirin/intron A and or PegIntron therapy, including severe depression and suicidal ideation, hemolytic anemia, suppression of bone marrow function, autoimmune and infectious disorders, pulmonary dysfunction, pancreatitis, and diabetes. Drug fever/rash, nausea, vomiting, GI upset, leukopenia, hyperbilirubinemia, hemolytic anemia, ↑ uric acid.

Allergic Potential: Low

Safety in Pregnancy: X (Extreme care must be taken to avoid pregnancy during therapy and for 6 months after completion of therapy in both female patients and in female partners of male patients who are taking ribavirin therapy)

Comments: Nebulizer dose for RSV: 20 mg/ml aerosolized over 12 hours administered once daily × 3–7 days. Also as activity against Lassa fever and HPS. ***Highly active against HCV and RSV. Some activity against HBV. No activity against CMV, adenoviruses, HSV, VZV, or influenza.***

Cerebrospinal Fluid Penetration: No data

"Usual dose" assumes normal renal/hepatic function. * For renal insufficiency, give usual dose × 1 followed by maintenance dose per CrCl. For dialysis patients, dose the same as for CrCl < 10 mL/min and give supplemental (post-HD/PD dose) immediately after dialysis. CrCl = creatinine clearance; CVVH = continuous veno-venous hemofiltration; HD/PD = hemodialysis/peritoneal dialysis. See pp. 509–513 for explanations, pp. xi–xii for abbreviations; Linezolid (↑ risk of serotonin syndrome, see p. 620).

REFERENCES:

Keating MR, Antiviral agents. Mayo Clin Proc 67:160–78, 1992.

Ottolini MG, Hemming VG. Prevention and treatment recommendations for respiratory syncytial virus infection: Background and clinical experience 40 years after discovery. Drugs 54:867–84, 1997.

Ventre K, Randolph A. Ribavirin for respiratory syncytial virus infection of the lower respiratory tract in infants and young children. Cochrane Database Syst Rev 18:CD000181, 2004.

Website: www.rocheusa.com/products/

Rifabutin (Mycobutin)

Drug Class: Anti-MAI drug.

Usual Dose: 5 mg/kg or 300 mg (PO) q24h (see comments).

Pharmacokinetic Parameters:

Peak serum level: 0.38 mcg/ml
Bioavailability: 20–50%
Excreted unchanged (urine): 10%
Serum half-life (normal/ESRD): 45/45 hrs
Plasma protein binding: 85%
Volume of distribution (V_d): 9.3 L/kg

Primary Mode of Elimination: Hepatic

Dosage Adjustments*

CrCl 50–80 mL/min	No change
CrCl 10–50 mL/min	No change
CrCl < 10 mL/min	No change
Post–HD dose	None
Post–PD dose	None
CVVH dose	None
Moderate hepatic insufficiency	No change
Severe hepatic insufficiency	No change

Drug Interactions: Atovaquone, amprenavir, indinavir, nelfinavir, ritonavir, clarithromycin, erythromycin, telithromycin, fluconazole, itraconazole, ketoconazole (↓ interacting drug levels, ↑ rifabutin levels); beta-blockers, clofibrate, cyclosporine, enalapril, oral contraceptives, quinidine, sulfonylureas, tocainide, warfarin (↓ interacting drug effect); corticosteroids (↑ corticosteroid requirement); delavirdine (↓ delavirdine levels, ↑ rifabutin levels; avoid); digoxin, phenytoin, propafenone, theophylline, zidovudine (↓ interacting drug levels); methadone (↓ methadone levels, withdrawal); mexiletine (↑ mexiletine clearance); protease inhibitors (↓ protease inhibitor levels, ↑ rifabutin levels; caution).

Adverse Effects: Headache, nausea, vomiting. ↑ SGOT/SGPT, leukopenia, anemia, thrombocytopenia, drug fever/rash. Brown/orange discoloration of body fluids.

Allergic Potential: High

Safety in Pregnancy: C

Comments: Avoid in leukopenic patients with WBC ≤ 1000 cells/mm^3. Always use as part of a multi-drug regimen, never as monotherapy. **Rifabutin doses when co-administered with antiretrovirals:** 450 mg (PO) q24h with EFV; 150 mg (PO) q24h with AVP, IDV, NFV, FPN; 150 mg (PO) q48h with RTV/LPV combination. Meningeal dose = usual dose.

Cerebrospinal Fluid Penetration: 50–70%

REFERENCES:

Benson CA, Williams PL, Cohn DL, and the ACTG 196/CPCRA 009 Study Team. Clarithromycin or rifabutin alone or in combination for primary prophylaxis of Mycobacterium avium complex disease in patients with AIDS: A randomized, double-blinded, placebo-controlled trial. J Infect Dis 181:1289–97, 2000.

"Usual dose" assumes normal renal/hepatic function. * For renal insufficiency, give usual dose × 1 followed by maintenance dose per CrCl. For dialysis patients, dose the same as for CrCl < 10 mL/min and give supplemental (post-HD/PD dose) immediately after dialysis. CrCl = creatinine clearance; CVVH = continuous veno-venous hemofiltration; HD/PD = hemodialysis/peritoneal dialysis. See pp. 509–513 for explanations, pp. xi–xii for abbreviations; Linezolid (↑ risk of serotonin syndrome, see p. 620).

Centers for Disease Control and Prevention. Notice to readers: Updated guidelines for the use of rifabutin or rifampin for the treatment and prevention of tuberculosis among HIV-infected patients taking protease inhibitors or nonnucleoside reverse transcriptase inhibitors. MMWR 49:183–189, 2000.

Drugs for AIDS and associated infections. Med Lett Drug Ther 35:79–86, 1993.

Finch CK, Chrisman CR, Baciewicz AM, et al. Rifampin and rifabutin Drug Interactions: an update. Arch Intern Med 162:985–92, 2002.

Hoy J, Mijch A, Sandland M, et al. Quadruple-drug therapy for Mycobacterium avium-intracellulare bacteremia in AIDS patients. J Infect Dis 161:801–5, 1990.

Nightingale SD, Cameron DW, Gordin FM, et al. Two controlled trials of rifabutin prophylaxis against Mycobacterium avium complex infection in AIDS. N Engl J Med 329:828–33, 1993.

Panel on Clinical Practices for Treatment of HIV Infection. Guidelines for the use of antiretroviral agents in HIV-infected adults and adolescents. Department of Health and Human Services. www.hivatis.org. January 29, 2008.

Website: www.pdr.net

Rifampin (Rifadin, Rimactane)

Drug Class: Antibiotic/anti-TB drug.

Usual Dose: 600 mg (PO) q24h (see comments).

Spectrum: (see ***Susceptibility Profiles*** pp. 183–187).

Pharmacokinetic Parameters:

Peak serum level: 7 mcg/ml

Bioavailability: 95%

Excreted unchanged (urine): 15%

Serum half-life (normal/ESRD): 3.5/11 hrs

Plasma protein binding: 80%

Volume of distribution (V_d): 0.93 L/kg

Primary Mode of Elimination: Hepatic

Dosage Adjustments*

CrCl 50–80 mL/min	No change
CrCl 10–50 mL/min	No change
CrCl < 10 mL/min	No change
Post–HD dose	None
Post–PD dose	None
CVVH dose	No change
Moderate hepatic insufficiency	No change; use caution
Severe hepatic insufficiency	Avoid

Drug Interactions: Amprenavir, indinavir, nelfinavir (↑ rifampin levels); beta-blockers, clofibrate, cyclosporine, oral contraceptives, quinidine, sulfonylureas, tocainamide, warfarin (↓ interacting drug effect); caspofungin (↓ caspofungin levels, may ↓ caspofungin effect); clarithromycin, ketoconazole (↑ rifampin levels, ↓ interacting drug levels); corticosteroids (↑ corticosteroid requirement); delavirdine (↑ rifampin levels, ↓ delavirdine levels; avoid); disopyramide, itraconazole, phenytoin, propafenone, theophylline, methadone, nelfinavir, ritonavir, tacrolimus, drugs whose metabolism is induced by rifampin, e.g., ACE inhibitors, dapsone, diazepam, digoxin, diltiazem, doxycycline, fluconazole, fluvastatin, haloperidol, nifedipine, progestins, triazolam, tricyclics, zidovudine (↓ interacting drug levels); fluconazole, TMP–SMX (↑ rifampin levels); INH (INH converted into toxic hydrazine); mexiletine (↑ mexiletine clearance); nevirapine (↓ nevirapine levels; avoid).

Adverse Effects: Flu–like symptoms, ↑ SGOT/SGPT, drug fever/rash, thrombocytopenia. Red/orange discoloration of body secretions.

Allergic Potential: Moderate

Safety in Pregnancy: Probably safe

"Usual dose" assumes normal renal/hepatic function. * For renal insufficiency, give usual dose × 1 followed by maintenance dose per CrCl. For dialysis patients, dose the same as for CrCl < 10 mL/min and give supplemental (post-HD/PD dose) immediately after dialysis. CrCl = creatinine clearance; CVVH = continuous veno-venous hemofiltration; HD/PD = hemodialysis/peritoneal dialysis. See pp. 509–513 for explanations, pp. xi–xii for abbreviations; Linezolid (↑ risk of serotonin syndrome, see p. 620).

Comments: Potent CYP 3A4 inducer. Contraindicated in HIV. For anti–TB prophylaxis/therapy, monitor potential hepatotoxicity with serial SGOT/SGPTs weekly × 3, then monthly × 3. Take 1 hour before or 2 hours after meals. **TB D.O.T. dose:** 10 mg/kg or 600 mg (PO) 2–3x/week. **Do not use as monotherapy for S. aureus. Of no proven clinical advantage when combined with another anti–MSSA/MRSA antibiotic. With another anti-staphylococcal drug, dose:** 300 mg (PO) q12h. **Nasal carriage dose:** 600 mg (PO) q12h × 72 hours.
Meningeal dose = usual dose.

Cerebrospinal Fluid Penetration:
Non-Inflamed meninges = 50%
Inflamed meninges = 50%

Bile Penetration: 7000%

(also see ***Antibiotic Pearls & Pitfalls*** pp. 495–508).

REFERENCES:

Cascio A, Scarlata F, Giordano S, et al. Treatment of human brucellosis with rifampin plus minocycline. J Chemother 15:248–52, 2003.

Castahneira D, Rifampin. Antibiotics for Clinicians 6:89–100, 2001.

Centers for Disease Control and Prevention. Notice to readers: Updated guidelines for the use of rifabutin or rifampin for the treatment and prevention of tuberculosis among HIV-infected patients taking protease inhibitors or nonnucleoside reverse transcriptase inhibitors. MMWR 49:183–189, 2000.

Curry SR, Marsh JW, Shutt KA, et al. High Frequency of Rifampin Resistance Identified in an Epidemic *Clostridium difficile* Clone from a Large Teaching Hospital. Clin Infect Dis 48:425–430, 2009.

Davidson PT, Le HQ. Drug treatment of tuberculosis 1992. Drugs 43:651–73, 1992.

Ena J, Valls V. Short-course therapy with rifampin plus isoniazid compared with standard therapy with isoniazid, for latent tuberculosis infection: a meta-analysis. Clin Infect Dis 40:670–6, 2005.

Euga G, Murillo O, Fernandez-Sabe N, et al. Treatment of Chronic Staphylococcal Osteomyelitis: Intravenous or Oral? How Long? Antimicrob Agents Chemother 53:2672–2676, 2009.

Giamarellos-Bourboulis EJ, Sambatakou H, Galani I, et al. In vitro interaction of colistin and rifampin on multidrug-resistant Pseudomonas aeruginosa. J Chemother 15:235–8, 2003.

Havlir DV, Barnes PF. Tuberculosis in patients with human immunodeficiency virus infection. N Engl J Med 340:367–73, 1999.

Ijaz K, Jereb JA, Lambert LA, et al. Severe or Fatal Injury in 50 Patients in the United States Taking Rifampin and Pyrazinamide for Latent Tuberculosis Infection. Clin Infect Dis 42:346–56, 2006.

Ijaz K, McElroy PD, Navin TR. Short course rifampin and pyrazinamide compared with isoniazid for latent tuberculosis infection: a cost-effectiveness analysis based on a multicenter clinical trial Clin Infect Dis 39:289, 2004.

Krause PJ, Corrow CL, Bakken JS. Successful treatment of human granulocytic ehrlichiosis in children using rifampin. Pediatrics. 112:e252–3, 2003.

Lundstrom TS, Sobel JD. Vancomycin, trimethoprim - sulfamethoxazole, and rifampin. Infect Dis Clin North Am 91:747–67, 1995.

McIlleron H, Wash P, Burger A, et al. Determinants of Rifampin, Isoniazid, Pyrazinamide and Ethambutol Pharmacokinetics in a Cohort of Tuberculosis Patients. Antimicrob Agents Chemother 50:1170–77, 2006.

Nguyen S, Pasquet A, Legout L, et al. Efficacy and tolerance of rifampin-linezolid compared with rifampin-cotrimoxazole combinations in prolonged oral therapy for bone and joint infections. Clin Microbiol Infect Dis 15:1163–1169, 2009.

Panel on Clinical Practices for Treatment of HIV Infection. Guidelines for the use of antiretroviral agents in HIV-infected adults and adolescents. Department of Health and Human Services. www.hivatis.org. January 29, 2008.

Perlman DC, Segal Yoniah, Rosenkranz S, et al. The clinical pharmacokinetics of rifampin and ethambutol in HIV-infected persons with tuberculosis. Clin Infect Dis 41:1638–47, 2005.

Schlossberg D, Treatment of multi-drug resistant tuberculosis. Antibiotics for Clinicians 9:317–321, 2005.
Van Scoy RE, Wilkowske CJ. Antituberculous agents. Mayo Clin Proc 67:179–87, 1992.
Vesely JJ, Pien FD, Pien BC. Rifampin, a useful drug for nonmyocobacterial infections. Pharmacotherapy 18:345–57, 1998.
Wareham DW, Bean DC. In Vitro Activities of Polymyxin B, Imipenem and Rifampin against Multidrug-Resistant Acinetobacter baumannii. Antimicrob Agents Chemother 50:825–26, 2006.
Website: www.pdr.net

Rimantadine (Flumadine)

Drug Class: Antiviral.
Usual Dose: 100 mg (PO) q12h (see comments).
Pharmacokinetic Parameters:
Peak serum level: 0.7 mcg/ml
Bioavailability: 90%
Excreted unchanged (urine): 25%
Serum half-life (normal/ESRD): 25/38 hrs
Plasma protein binding: 40%
Volume of distribution (V_d): 4.5 L/kg
Primary Mode of Elimination: Hepatic
Dosage Adjustments*

CrCl 50–80 mL/min	No change
CrCl 10–50 mL/min	No change
CrCl < 10 mL/min	100 mg (PO) q24h
Post–HD dose	None
Post–PD dose	None
CVVH dose	None
Moderate hepatic insufficiency	No change
Severe hepatic insufficiency	100 mg (PO) q24h

Drug Interactions: Alcohol (↑ CNS effects); benztropine, trihexyphenidyl, scopolamine (↑ interacting drug effect: dry mouth, ataxia, blurred vision, slurred speech, toxic psychosis); cimetidine (↓ rimantadine clearance); CNS stimulants (additive stimulation); digoxin (↑ digoxin levels); trimethoprim (↑ rimantadine and trimethoprim levels).
Adverse Effects: Dizziness, headache, insomnia, anticholinergic effects (blurry vision, dry mouth, orthostatic hypotension, urinary retention, constipation).
Allergic Potential: Low
Safety in Pregnancy: C
Comments: Less anticholinergic side effects than amantadine. Patients ≥ 60 years old or with a history of seizures should receive 100 mg (PO) q24h. **Influenza dose (prophylaxis):** 100 mg (PO) q12h for duration of exposure/outbreak. **Influenza dose (therapy):** 100 mg (PO) q12h × 7 days. **May improve peripheral airway function/oxygenation in severe influenza pneumonia. *Highly active against influenza A. No activity against other viruses.***
Cerebrospinal Fluid Penetration: No data

REFERENCES:

Antiviral drugs for prophylaxis and treatment of influenza. Med Lett Drugs Ther 46:85–7, 2004.
Dolin R, Reichman RC, Madore HP, et al. A controlled trial of amantadine and rimantadine in the prophylaxis of Influenza A infection. N Engl J Med 307:580–4, 1982.
Gravenstein S, Davidson HE. Current strategies for management of influenza in the elderly population. Clin Infect Dis 35:729–37, 2002.
Jefferson T, Deeks JJ, Demicheli V, et al. Amantadine and rimantadine for preventing and treating influenza A in adults. Cochrane Database Syst Rev 3:CD001169, 2004.
Keating MR, Antiviral agents. Mayo Clin Proc 67:160–78, 1992.

"Usual dose" assumes normal renal/hepatic function. * For renal insufficiency, give usual dose × 1 followed by maintenance dose per CrCl. For dialysis patients, dose the same as for CrCl < 10 mL/min and give supplemental (post-HD/PD dose) immediately after dialysis. CrCl = creatinine clearance; CVVH = continuous veno-venous hemofiltration; HD/PD = hemodialysis/peritoneal dialysis. See pp. 509–513 for explanations, pp. xi–xii for abbreviations; Linezolid (↑ risk of serotonin syndrome, see p. 620).

Schmidt AC, Antiviral therapy for influenza: a clinical and economic comparative review. Drugs 64:2031–46, 2004.

Wintermeyer SM, Nahata MC. Rimantadine: A clinical perspective. Ann Pharmacotherapy 29:299–310, 1995.

Website: www.pdr.net

Ritonavir (Norvir) RTV

Drug Class: Antiretroviral protease inhibitor.
Usual Dose: 600 mg (PO) q12h (see comments).
Pharmacokinetic Parameters:
Peak serum level: 11 mcg/ml
Bioavailability: No data
Excreted unchanged (urine): 3.5%
Serum half-life (normal/ESRD): 4 hrs/no data
Plasma protein binding: 99%
Volume of distribution (V_d): 0.41 L/kg
Primary Mode of Elimination: Hepatic
Dosage Adjustments*

CrCl 50–80 mL/min	No change
CrCl 10–50 mL/min	No change
CrCl < 10 mL/min	No change
Post–HD dose	None
Post–PD dose	None
CVVH dose	None
Moderate hepatic insufficiency	No change
Severe hepatic insufficiency	No change; use caution

Antiretroviral Dosage Adjustments:

Atazanavir	Ritonavir 100 mg q24h + atazanavir 300 mg q24h with food
Delavirdine	Delavirdine: no change; ritonavir: No information
Efavirenz	Ritonavir 600 mg q12h (500 mg q12h for intolerance)
Fosamprenavir	Fosamprenavir 1400 mg + ritonavir 200 mg q24h
Indinavir	Ritonavir 100–200 mg q12h + indinavir 800 mg q12h, or 400 mg q12h of each drug
Nelfinavir	Ritonavir 400 mg q12h + nelfinavir 500–750 mg q12h
Nevirapine	No changes
Saquinavir	Ritonavir 400 mg q12h + saquinavir 400 mg q12h
Ketoconazole	Caution; do not exceed ketoconazole 200 mg q24h
Rifampin	Avoid
Rifabutin	Rifabutin 150 mg q48h or 3x/week

Drug Interactions: Antiretrovirals, rifabutin, rifampin (see dose adjustment grid, above); alprazolam, diazepam, estazolam, flurazepam, midazolam, triazolam, zolpidem, meperidine, propoxyphene, piroxicam,

"Usual dose" assumes normal renal/hepatic function. * For renal insufficiency, give usual dose × 1 followed by maintenance dose per CrCl. For dialysis patients, dose the same as for CrCl < 10 mL/min and give supplemental (post-HD/PD dose) immediately after dialysis. CrCl = creatinine clearance; CVVH = continuous veno-venous hemofiltration; HD/PD = hemodialysis/peritoneal dialysis. See pp. 509–513 for explanations, pp. xi–xii for abbreviations; Linezolid (↑ risk of serotonin syndrome, see p. 620).

quinidine, amiodarone, encainide, flecainide, propafenone, astemizole, bepridil, bupropion, cisapride, clorazepate, clozapine, pimozide, St. John's wort, terfenadine (avoid); alfentanil, fentanyl, hydrocodone, tramadol, disopyramide, lidocaine, mexiletine, erythromycin, clarithromycin, warfarin, dronabinol, ondansetron, metoprolol, pindolol, propranolol, timolol, amlodipine, diltiazem, felodipine, isradipine, nicardipine, nifedipine, nimodipine, nisoldipine, nitrendipine, verapamil, etoposide, paclitaxel, tamoxifen, vinblastine, vincristine, loratadine, tricyclic antidepressants, paroxetine, nefazodone, sertraline, trazodone, fluoxetine, venlafaxine, fluvoxamine, cyclosporine, tacrolimus, chlorpromazine, haloperidol, perphenazine, risperidone, thioridazine, clozapine, pimozide, methamphetamine (↑ interacting drug levels); voriconazole (↓ voriconazole levels); telithromycin (↑ ritonavir levels); codeine, hydromorphone, methadone, morphine, ketoprofen, ketorolac, naproxen, diphenoxylate, oral contraceptives, theophylline (↓ interacting drug levels); carbamazepine, phenytoin, phenobarbital, clonazepam, dexamethasone, prednisone (↓ ritonavir levels, ↑ interacting drug levels; monitor anticonvulsant levels); metronidazole (disulfiram-like reaction); tenofovir, tobacco (↓ ritonavir levels); sildenafil (do not exceed 25 mg in 48 hrs); tadalafil (max. 10 mg/72 hrs); vardenafil (max. 2.5 mg/72 hrs).

Adverse Effects: Anorexia, anemia, leukopenia, hyperglycemia (including worsening diabetes, new-onset diabetes, DKA), ↑ cholesterol/triglycerides (evaluate risk for coronary disease/pancreatitis), fat redistribution, ↑ CPK, nausea, vomiting, diarrhea, abdominal pain, circumoral/extremity paresthesias, ↑ SGOT/SGPT, pancreatitis, taste perversion, possible increased bleeding in hemophilia.

Allergic Potential: Low

Safety in Pregnancy: B

Comments: Usually used at low dose (100–200 mg/day) as pharmacokinetic "booster" of other PI's. GI intolerance decreases over time. Take with food if possible (serum levels increase 15%, fewer GI side effects). Dose escalation regimen: day 1–2 (300 mg q12h), day 3–5 (400 mg q12h), day 6–13 (500 mg q12h), day 14 (600 mg q12h). Separate dosing from ddI by 2 hours. Refrigerate capsules (not oral solution) if temperature to exceed 78°F.

Cerebrospinal Fluid Penetration: < 10%

REFERENCES:

Cameron DW, Japour AJ, Xu Y, et al. Ritonavir and saquinavir combination therapy for the treatment of HIV infection. AIDS 13:213–224, 1999.

Deeks SG, Smith M, Holodniy M, et al. HIV-1 protease inhibitors: A review for clinicians. JAMA 277:145–53, 1997.

Kaul DR, Cinti SK, Carver PL, et al. HIV protease inhibitors: Advances in therapy and adverse reactions, including metabolic complications. Pharmacotherapy 19:281–98, 1999.

Lea AP, Faulds D. Ritonavir. Drugs 52:541–6, 1996.

McDonald CK, Kuritzkes DR. Human immunodeficiency virus type 1 protease inhibitors. Arch Intern Med 157:951–9, 1997.

Panel on Antiretroviral Guidelines for Adults and Adolescents. Guidelines for the use of antiretroviral agents in HIV-1 infected adults and adolescents. Department of Health and Human Services. November 3, 2008; 1–139. Available at http://www.aidsinfor.nih.gov/ContentFiles/AdultandAdolescentGL.pdf

Piliero PJ. Interaction between ritonavir and stains. Am J Med 112:510–1, 2002.

Rathbun RC, Rossi DR. Low-dose ritonavir for protease inhibitor pharmacokinetic enhancement. Ann Pharmacother 36:702–6, 2002.

Shepp DH, Stevens RC. Ritonavir boosting of HIV protease inhibitors. Antibiotics for Clinicians 9:301–311, 2005.

Website: www.TreatHIV.com

"Usual dose" assumes normal renal/hepatic function. * For renal insufficiency, give usual dose × 1 followed by maintenance dose per CrCl. For dialysis patients, dose the same as for CrCl < 10 mL/min and give supplemental (post-HD/PD dose) immediately after dialysis. CrCl = creatinine clearance; CVVH = continuous veno-venous hemofiltration; HD/PD = hemodialysis/peritoneal dialysis. See pp. 509–513 for explanations, pp. xi–xii for abbreviations; Linezolid (↑ risk of serotonin syndrome, see p. 620).

Saquinavir (Invirase) SQV

Drug Class: Antiretroviral protease inhibitor.
Usual Dose: 1000 mg (PO) q12h (see comments) with ritonavir 100 mg (PO) q12h, or 400 mg (PO) q12h with ritonavir 400 mg (PO) q12h.
Pharmacokinetic Parameters:
Peak serum level: 0.07 mcg/mL
Bioavailability: hard-gel (4%)
Excreted unchanged (urine): 13%
Serum half-life (normal/ESRD): 13 hrs/no data
Plasma protein binding: 98%
Volume of distribution (V_d): 10 L/kg
Primary Mode of Elimination: Hepatic
Dosage Adjustments*

CrCl 50–80 mL/min	No change
CrCl 10–50 mL/min	No change
CrCl < 10 mL/min	No change
Post–HD dose	None
Post–PD dose	None
CVVH dose	No change
Moderate hepatic insufficiency	No change
Severe hepatic insufficiency	Use caution

Antiretroviral Dosage Adjustments:

Darunavir	Avoid
Delavirdine	No Information
Efavirenz	Avoid use as sole PI
Indinavir	No information
Lopinavir/ritonavir 3 capsules q12h	Saquinavir 500 mg q12h
Nelfinavir	Saquinavir 1 gm q12h or 1200 mg q12h
Nevirapine	No information
Ritonavir	Ritonavir 100 mg q12h + saquinavir 1 gm q12h
Rifampin	Contraindicated
Rifabutin	Avoid

Drug Interactions: Antiretrovirals, rifabutin, rifampin (see dose adjustment grid, above); astemizole, terfenadine, benzodiazepines, cisapride, ergotamine, statins, St. John's wort (avoid if possible); carbamazepine, phenytoin, phenobarbital, dexamethasone, prednisone (↓ saquinavir levels, ↑ interacting drug levels; monitor anticonvulsant levels); clarithromycin, erythromycin, telithromycin (↑ saquinavir and macrolide levels); grapefruit juice, itraconazole, voriconazole, ketoconazole (↑ saquinavir levels); sildenafil (do not give > 25 mg/48 hrs); tadalafil (max. 10 mg/72 hrs), vardenafil (max. 2.5 mg/72 hrs).
Adverse Effects: Anorexia, headache, anemia, leukopenia, hyperglycemia (including worsening diabetes, new-onset diabetes, DKA), ↑ cholesterol/triglycerides (evaluate risk for coronary disease/pancreatitis), ↑ SGOT/SGPT, hyperuricemia, fat redistribution, possible increased bleeding in hemophilia.
Allergic Potential: Low
Safety in Pregnancy: B
Comments: Take with food. Avoid garlic supplements, which ↓ saquinavir levels ~ 50%. Boosted dose: 1 gm saquinavir/100 mg ritonavir (PO) q12h. Preferred formulation

"Usual dose" assumes normal renal/hepatic function. * For renal insufficiency, give usual dose × 1 followed by maintenance dose per CrCl. For dialysis patients, dose the same as for CrCl < 10 mL/min and give supplemental (post-HD/PD dose) immediately after dialysis. CrCl = creatinine clearance; CVVH = continuous veno-venous hemofiltration; HD/PD = hemodialysis/peritoneal dialysis. See pp. 509–513 for explanations, pp. xi–xii for abbreviations; Linezolid (↑ risk of serotonin syndrome, see p. 620).

is 500 mg hard-gel capsule (Invirase 500). Soft-gel capsules (Fortovase) no longer available.

Cerebrospinal Fluid Penetration: < 1%

REFERENCES:

Borck C. Garlic supplements and saquinavir. Clin Infect Dis 35:343, 2002.

Cameron DW, Japour AJ, Xu Y, et al. Ritonavir and saquinavir combination therapy for the treatment of HIV infection. AIDS 13:213–224, 1999.

Cardiello PF, van Heeswijk RP, Hassink EA, et al. Simplifying protease inhibitor therapy with once-daily dosing of saquinavir soft-gelatin capsules/ritonavir (1600/100 mg): HIVNAT 001.3 study. J Acquir Immune Defic Syndr 29:464–70, 2002.

Hsu A, Granneman GR, Cao G, et al. Pharmacokinetic interactions between two human immunodeficiency virus protease inhibitors, ritonavir and saquinavir. Clin Pharmacol Ther 63:453–64, 1998.

Murphy RL, Brun S, Hicks C, et al. ABT-378/ritonavir plus stavudine and lamivudine for the treatment of antiretroviral-naive adults with HIV-1 infection: 48-week results. AIDS 15:F1-9, 2001.

Noble S, Faulds D. Saquinavir: A review of its pharmacology and clinical potential in the management of HIV infection. Drugs 52:93–112, 1996.

Perry CM, Noble S. Saquinavir soft-gel capsule formation: A review of its use in patients with HIV infection. Drugs 55:461–86, 1998.

Panel on Clinical Practices for Treatment of HIV Infection. Guidelines for the use of antiretroviral agents in HIV-infected adults and adolescents. Department of Health and Human Services. www.hivatis.org. January 29, 2008.

Vella S, Floridia M. Saquinavir: Clinical pharmacology and efficacy. Clin Pharmacokinet 34:189–201, 1998.

Website: www.fortovase.com

Spectinomycin (Spectam, Trobicin)

Drug Class: Aminocyclitol.

Usual Dose: 2 gm (IM) × 1 dose.

Pharmacokinetic Parameters:

Peak serum level: 100 mcg/ml

Bioavailability: Not applicable

Excreted unchanged (urine): 80%

Serum half-life (normal/ESRD): 1.6/16 hrs

Plasma protein binding: 20%

Volume of distribution (V_d): 0.25 L/kg

Primary Mode of Elimination: Renal

Dosage Adjustments*

CrCl 50–80 mL/min	No change
CrCl 10–50 mL/min	No change
CrCl < 10 mL/min	No change
Post–HD dose	None
Post–PD dose	None
CVVH dose	None
Moderate hepatic insufficiency	No change
Severe hepatic insufficiency	No change

Drug Interactions: None.

Adverse Effects: Local pain at injection site.

Allergic Potential: Low

Safety in Pregnancy: B

Comments: Ineffective in pharyngeal GC (poor penetration into secretions).

Cerebrospinal Fluid Penetration: < 10%

"Usual dose" assumes normal renal/hepatic function. * For renal insufficiency, give usual dose × 1 followed by maintenance dose per CrCl. For dialysis patients, dose the same as for CrCl < 10 mL/min and give supplemental (post-HD/PD dose) immediately after dialysis. CrCl = creatinine clearance; CVVH = continuous veno-venous hemofiltration; HD/PD = hemodialysis/peritoneal dialysis. See pp. 509–513 for explanations, pp. xi–xii for abbreviations; Linezolid (↑ risk of serotonin syndrome, see p. 620).

REFERENCES:

Fiumara NJ. The treatment of gonococcal proctitis: An evaluation of 173 patients treated with 4 gm of spectinomycin. JAMA 239:735–7, 1978.

Holloway WJ. Spectinomycin. Med Clin North Am 66:169–173, 1995.

McCormack WM, Finland M. Spectinomycin. Ann Intern Med 84:712–16, 1976.

Tapsall J. Current concepts in the management of gonorrhoea. Expert Opin Pharmacother 3:147–57, 2002.

Website: www.pdr.net

Stavudine (Zerit) d4t

Drug Class: Antiretroviral NRTI (nucleoside reverse transcriptase inhibitor).

Usual Dose: ≥ 60 kg: 40 mg (PO) q12h; < 60 kg: 30 mg (PO) q12h.

Pharmacokinetic Parameters:

Peak serum level: 4.2 mcg/mL

Bioavailability: 86%

Excreted unchanged (urine): 40%

Serum half-life (normal/ESRD): 1.0/5.1 hrs

Plasma protein binding: 0%

Volume of distribution (V_d): 0.5 L/kg

Primary Mode of Elimination: Renal

Dosage Adjustments* ≥ 60 kg/[≤ 60 kg]

CrCl 50–80 mL/min	40 mg (PO) q12h [30 mg (PO) q12h]
CrCl 25–50 mL/min	20 mg (PO) q12h [15 mg (PO) q12h]
CrCl ~ 10–25 mL/min	20 mg (PO) q24h [15 mg (PO) q24h]
Post–HD dose	20 mg (PO) [15 mg (PO)]
Post–PD dose	No information
CVVH dose	20 mg (PO) q24h [15 mg (PO) q24h]
Moderate hepatic insufficiency	No change
Severe hepatic insufficiency	No change

Drug Interactions: Ribavirin (↓ stavudine efficacy, ↑ risk of lactic acidosis); dapsone, INH, other neurotoxic agents (↑ risk of neuropathy), didanosine (↑ risk of neuropathy, lactic acidosis). Avoid combining zidovudine with stavudine.

Adverse Effects: Lactic acidosis and severe hepatomegaly with steatosis, including fatal cases, have been reported with the use of nucleoside analogues alone or in combination, including stavudine and other antiretrovirals. Fatal lactic acidosis has been reported in pregnant women who reveived the combination of stavudine and didanosine with other antiretroviral agents. The combination of stavudine and didanosine sould be used with great caution during pregnancy and only when necessary. Drug fever/rash, nausea, vomiting, GI upset, diarrhea, headache, insomnia, dose dependent peripheral neuropathy, myalgias, pancreatitis, ↑ SGOT/SGPT, ↑ cholesterol, facial fat pad wasting, lipodystrophy, thrombocytopenia, leukopenia, lactic acidosis with hepatic steatosis. There is an increased risk of hepatotoxicity may occur in patients treated with stavudine in combination with didanosine and hydroxyurea. Immune reconstitution syndrome can occur.

Allergic Potential: Low

Safety in Pregnancy: C

Comments: Pancreatitis may be severe/ fatal. Avoid coadministration with AZT or ddC.

"Usual dose" assumes normal renal/hepatic function. * For renal insufficiency, give usual dose × 1 followed by maintenance dose per CrCl. For dialysis patients, dose the same as for CrCl < 10 mL/min and give supplemental (post-HD/PD dose) immediately after dialysis. CrCl = creatinine clearance; CVVH = continuous veno-venous hemofiltration; HD/PD = hemodialysis/peritoneal dialysis. See pp. 509–513 for explanations, pp. xi–xii for abbreviations; Linezolid (↑ risk of serotonin syndrome, see p. 620).

Decrease dose in patients with peripheral neuropathy to 20 mg (PO) q12h. Pregnant women may be at increased risk for lactic acidosis/liver damage when stavudine is used with didanosine (ddI).

Cerebrospinal Fluid Penetration: 30%

REFERENCES:

Berasconi E, Boubaker K, Junghans C, et al. Abnormalities of body fat distribution in HIV-infected persons treated with antiretroviral drugs: The Swiss HIV Cohort Study. J Acquir Immune Defic Syndr 31:50–5, 2002.

Dudley MN, Graham KK, Kaul S, et al. Pharmacokinetics of stavudine in patients with AIDS and AIDS-related complex. J Infect Dis 166:480–5, 1992.

FDA notifications. FDA changes information for stavudine label. Aids Alert 17:67, 2002.

Joly V, Flandre P, Meiffredy V, et al. Efficacy of zidovudine compared to stavudine, both in combination with lamivudine and indinavir, in human immunodeficiency virus-infected nucleoside-experienced patients with no prior exposure to lamivudine, stavudine, or protease inhibitors (Novavir trial). Antimicrob Agents Chemother 46:1906–13, 2002.

Lea AP, Faulds D. Stavudine: A review of its pharmacodynamic and pharmacokinetic properties and clinical potential in HIV infection. Drugs 51:846–64, 1996.

Miller KD, Cameron M, Wood LV, et al. Lactic acidosis and hepatic steatosis associated with use of stavudine: Report of four cases. Ann Intern Med 133:192–196, 2000.

Murphy RL, Brun S, Hicks C, et al. ABT-378/ritonavir plus stavudine and lamivudine for the treatment of antiretroviral-naive adults with HIV-1 infection: 48-week results. AIDS 15:F1-9, 2001.

Panel on Clinical Practices for Treatment of HIV Infection. Guidelines for the use of antiretroviral agents in HIV-infected adults and adolescents. Department of Health and Human Services. www.hivatis.org. January 29, 2008.

Website: www.ze\rit.com

Streptomycin

Drug Class: Anti-TB aminoglycoside.

Usual Dose: 15 mg/kg (IM) q24h or 1 gm (IM) q24h (see comments).

Pharmacokinetic Parameters:

Peak serum level: 25–50 mcg/ml

Bioavailability: Not applicable

Excreted unchanged (urine): 90%

Serum half-life (normal/ESRD): 2.5/100 hrs

Plasma protein binding: 35%

Volume of distribution (V_d): 0.26 L/kg

Primary Mode of Elimination: Renal

Dosage Adjustments*

CrCl 50–80 mL/min	No change
CrCl 10–50 mL/min	15 mg/kg (IM) q72h or 1 gm (IM) q72h
CrCl < 10 mL/min	15 mg/kg (IM) q72h or 1 gm (IM) q72h
Post–HD dose	7.5 mg/kg (IM) or 500 mg (IM) 2–3 x/week
Post–PD dose	7.5 mg/kg (IM) or 500 mg (IM) or 20–40 mg/ml in dialysate q24h
CVVH dose	15 mg/kg (IM) or 1 gm (IM) q72h
Moderate hepatic insufficiency	No change
Severe hepatic insufficiency	No change

Drug Interactions: Amphotericin B, cephalothin, cyclosporine, enflurane,

"Usual dose" assumes normal renal/hepatic function. * For renal insufficiency, give usual dose × 1 followed by maintenance dose per CrCl. For dialysis patients, dose the same as for CrCl < 10 mL/min and give supplemental (post-HD/PD dose) immediately after dialysis. CrCl = creatinine clearance; CVVH = continuous veno-venous hemofiltration; HD/PD = hemodialysis/peritoneal dialysis. See pp. 509–513 for explanations, pp. xi–xii for abbreviations; Linezolid (↑ risk of serotonin syndrome, see p. 620).

methoxyflurane, NSAIDs, polymyxin B, radiographic contrast, vancomycin (↑ nephrotoxicity); cis-platinum (↑ nephrotoxicity, ↑ ototoxicity); loop diuretics (↑ ototoxicity); neuromuscular blocking agents (↑ apnea, prolonged paralysis); non-polarizing muscle relaxants (↑ apnea).

Adverse Effects: Most ototoxic aminoglycoside (usually vestibular ototoxicity); least nephrotoxic aminoglycoside.

Allergic Potential: Low

Safety in Pregnancy: D

Comments: May be given IV slowly over 1 hour. **TB D.O.T. dose:** 20–30 mg/kg (IM) 2–3x/week. **Tularemia dose:** 1 gm (IV/IM) q12h. **Plague dose:** 2 gm (IV/IM) q12h.

Cerebrospinal Fluid Penetration: 20%

REFERENCES:

Akaho E, Maekawa T, Uchinashi M. A study of streptomycin blood level information of patients undergoing hemodialysis. Biopharm Drug Dispos 23:47–52, 2002.

Davidson PT, Le HQ. Drug treatment of tuberculosis 1992. Drugs 43:651–73, 1992.

Kim-Sing A, Kays MB, Vivien EJ, et al. Intravenous streptomycin use in a patient infection with high-level gentamicin-resistant Streptococcus faecalis. Ann Pharmacother 27:712–4, 1993.

Morris JT, Cooper RH. Intravenous streptomycin: A useful route of administration. Clin Infect Dis 19:1150–1, 1994.

Roushan MRH, Mohraz M, Hajiahmadi M, et al. Efficacy of Gentamicin plus Doxycicline versus Streptomycin plus Doxycicline in the Treatment of Brucellosis in Humans. Clin Infect Dis 42:1075–80, 2006.

Van Scoy RE, Wilkowske CJ. Antituberculous agents. Mayo Clin Proc 67:179–87, 1992.

Ormerod P. The clinical management of the drug-resistant patient. Ann NY Acad Sci 953:185–91, 2001.

Telavancin (Vibativ)

Drug class: Lipolycopeptide

Usual dose: 10 mg/kg (IV) q24h

Spectrum: (see ***Susceptibility Profiles*** pp. 194–199).

Pharmacokinetic Parameters:

Peak serum level: 93–108 mcg/mL

Bioavailability: not applicable

Excreted unchanged: 76%

Serum half-life (normal/ESRD): 6–9 hrs/no data

Plasma protein binding: 93%

Volume of distribution (V_d): 0.133-0.145 mL/kg

Primary Mode of Elimination: Renal

Dosage Adjustments*

CrCl > 50 mL/min	No change
CrCl 30–50 mL/min	7.5 mg/kg (IV) q24h
CrCl 10–29 mL/min	10 mg/kg (IV) q48h
CrCl < 10 mL/min	No data
Post–HD dose	No data
Post–PD dose	No data
CVVH dose	7.5 mg/kg (IV) q24h
Moderate or severe hepatic insufficiency	No change

Drug Interactions: Drugs that prolong QT_c (additive effect); PT, INR, PTT (↑ levels); other interactions unlikely because is not metabolized through CYP450 system

Adverse Effects: Headache, taste disturbance, nausea, vomiting, diarrhea, nephrotoxicity, "red-man syndrome".

Allergic Potential: Low

Safety in Pregnancy: C

"Usual dose" assumes normal renal/hepatic function. * For renal insufficiency, give usual dose × 1 followed by maintenance dose per CrCl. For dialysis patients, dose the same as for CrCl < 10 mL/min and give supplemental (post-HD/PD dose) immediately after dialysis. CrCl = creatinine clearance; CVVH = continuous veno-venous hemofiltration; HD/PD = hemodialysis/peritoneal dialysis. See pp. 509–513 for explanations, pp. xi–xii for abbreviations; Linezolid (↑ risk of serotonin syndrome, see p. 620).

Comments: Infuse over at least 60 minutes to minimize infusion-related reactions. **Effective for MSSA/MRSA cSSSIs. Efficacy decreased in renal insufficiency with CrCl < 50 ml/min.**

Cerebrospinal Fluid Penetration:

Inflamed meninges: 2%

Non-inflamed meninges: 1%

(also see ***Antibiotic Pearls & Pitfalls*** p. 508).

REFERENCES:

Bouza E. New therapeutic choices for infections caused by methicillin-resistant *Staphylococcus aureus*. Clin Microbiol Infect Dis 15:44–52, 2009.

Charneski L, Patel PN, Sym D. Telavancin: a novel lipoglycopeptide antibiotic. Annals Pharmacother 43:928–38, 2009.

Gotfried M., Shaw J, Spencer E, et al. Intrapulmonary distribution of intravenous telavancin in healthy subjects and effect of pulmonary surfactant on in vitro activities of telavancin and other antibiotics. Antimicrob Agents Chemother 52:92–7, 2008.

Saravolatz LD, Stein GE, Johnson LB. Telavancin: A Novel Lipoglycopeptide. Clin Infect Dis 49:1908–1914, 2009.

Stryjewski ME, Chu VH, O-Rierdan WD, et al. Fast-2 Investigator Group. Telavancin versus standard therapy for treatment of complicated skin and skin structure infection caused by gram-positive bacteria: FAST 2 study. Antimicrob Agents Chemother 50:862–7, 2006.

Stryjewski ME, Graham DR, Wilson SE, et al. Telavancin versus vancomycin for the treatment of complicated skin and skin-structure infections caused by gram-positive organisms. Clin Infect Dis 46:1683–1693, 2008.

Stryjewski ME, O'Rierdan WD, Lau WK, et al. Telavancin versus standard therapy for treatment of complicated skin and soft-tissue infections caused by gram-positive bacteria. Clin Infect Dis 40:1601–1607, 2005.

Stucki A, Gerber P, Acosta F, et al. Efficacy of telavancin against penicillin-resistant pneumococci and *Staphylococcus aureus* in a rabbit meningitis model and determination of kinetic parameters. Antimicrob Agents Chemother 50:770–3, 2006.

Wilson SE, O'Rierdan W, Hopkins A, et al. Telavancin versus vancomycin for the treatment of complicated skin and skin-structure infections associated with surgical procedures. Am J Surg 197:791–796, 2009.

Website: www.vibativ.com

Telithromycin (Ketek)

Drug Class: Ketolide.

Usual Dose: Acute sinusitis/AECB: 800 mg (PO) q24h × 5 days. Community-acquired pneumonia: 800 mg (PO) q24h × 7–10 days. 800 mg (PO) dose taken as two 400-mg tablets (PO) at once.

Spectrum: (see ***Susceptibility Profiles*** pp. 183–187).

Pharmacokinetic Parameters:

Peak serum level: 2.27 mcg/ml

Bioavailability: 57%

Excreted unchanged (urine): 13%

Serum half-life (normal/ESRD): 9.8/11 hrs

Plasma protein binding: 65%

Volume of distribution (V_d): 2.9 L/kg

Primary Mode of Elimination: Hepatic

Dosage Adjustments*

CrCl 30–80 mL/min	No change
CrCl 10–30 mL/min	600 mg (PO) q24h
CrCl < 10 mL/min	600 mg (PO) q24h
CrCl < 30 mL/min + hepatic impairment	400 mg (PO) q24h
Post–HD/Post–PD dose	No information
CVVH dose	No information

"Usual dose" assumes normal renal/hepatic function. * For renal insufficiency, give usual dose × 1 followed by maintenance dose per CrCl. For dialysis patients, dose the same as for CrCl < 10 mL/min and give supplemental (post-HD/PD dose) immediately after dialysis. CrCl = creatinine clearance; CVVH = continuous veno-venous hemofiltration; HD/PD = hemodialysis/peritoneal dialysis. See pp. 509–513 for explanations, pp. xi–xii for abbreviations; Linezolid (↑ risk of serotonin syndrome, see p. 620).

Moderate hepatic insufficiency	No change
Severe hepatic insufficiency	No change

Drug Interactions: Digoxin (↑ interacting drug levels); ergot derivatives (acute ergot toxicity); itraconazole, ketoconazole (↑ telithromycin level); midazolam, triazolam (↑ interacting drug levels, sedation); oral anticoagulants (may ↑ anticoagulant effects; monitor PT/INR); simvastatin (↑ risk of rhabdomyolysis; giving simvastatin 12h after telithromycin decreases the ↑ in simvastatin levels ~ 50%); theophylline (additive nausea). CYP 3A4 inhibitor/substate. Telithromycin is contraindicated with cisapride and pimozide.

Adverse Effects: Nausea, diarrhea, dizziness, syncope, eye accomodation difficulties. ***Contraindicated in patients with history of hepatitis/jaundice*** (rarely fatal acute/fulminant hepatitis or acute liver failure in those with pre-existing liver disease). Avoid with myasthenia gravis (↑ risk of respiratory failure).

Resistance Potential: Low.

Allergic Potential: Low

Safety in Pregnancy: C

Comments: May take with or without food. New smaller tablets minimize potential GI upset.

(also see ***Antibiotic Pearls & Pitfalls*** pp. 495–508).

REFERENCES:

Aubier M, Aldons PM, Leak A, et al. Telithromycin is as effective as amoxicillin/clavulanate in acute exacerbations of chronic bronchitis. Respir Med 96:862–71, 2002.

Brown SD, Farrell DJ. Antibacterial susceptibility among streptococcus pneumoniae isolated from paediatric and adult patients as part of the PROTECT US study in 2001–2002. Journal of Antimicrobial Chemotherapy 54 (Suppl. S1):23–29, 2004.

Brown SD, Rybak MJ. Antimicrobial susceptibility of streptococcus pneumoniae, streptococcus pyogenes and haemophilus influenzae collected from patients across the USA, in 2001–2002, as part of the PROTECT US study. Journal of Antimicrobial Chemotherapy 54 (Suppl. S1):7–15, 2004.

Carbon C, Moola S, Velancsics I, et al. Telithromycin 800 mg once daily for seven to ten days is an effective and well-tolerated treatment for community-acquired pneumonia. Clin Microbiol Infect 9:691–703, 2003.

Dunbar LM, Carbon C, van Rensburg D, et al. Efficacy of telithromycin in community-acquired pneumonia caused by atypical and intracellular pathogens. Infect Dis Clin Pract 13:10–16, 2005.

Ferguson BJ, Guzzetta RV, Spector SL, et al. Efficacy and safety of oral telithromycin once daily for 5 days versus moxifloxacin one daily for 10 days in the treatment of acute bacterial rhinosinusitis. Otolaryngol Head Neck Surg 131:207–14, 2004.

Hagberg L, Torres A, van Rensburg D, et al. Efficacy and tolerability of once-daily telithromycin compared with high-dose amoxicillin for treatment of community-acquired pneumonia. Infection 30:378–386, 2002.

Jacobs MR. In vivo veritas: in vitro macrolide resistance in systemic S. pneumoniae infections does result in clinical failure. Clin Infect Dis 35:565–9, 2002.

Kim, DM, Yu KD, Lee JH, et al. Controlled trial of 5-day course of telithromycin versus doxycycline for treatment of mild to moderate scrub typhus. Antimicrob Agents Chemother 51:2011–2015, 2007.

Klugman KP, Lonks JR. Hidden epidemic of macrolide-resistant pneumococci. Emerg Infect Dis 11:802–807, 2005.

Low DE, Brown S, Felmingham D. Clinical and bacteriology efficacy of the ketolide telithromycin against isolates of key respiratory pathogens: a pooled analysis of phase III studies. Clin Microbiol Infect 10:27–36, 2004.

Ortega M, Marco F, Almela M, et al. Activity of telithromycin against erythromycin-susceptible resistant Streptococcus pneumoniae is from adults with invasive infections. Int J Antimicrob Agents 24:616–8, 2004.

Roos K, Tellier G, Baz M, et al. Clinical and bacteriological efficacy of 5-day telithromycin in acute maxillary sinusitis: a pooled analysis. www.elsevierhealth.com/journals/jinf.

Tellier G, Niederman MS, Nusrat R, et al. Clinical and bacteriological efficacy and safety of 5 and 7 day regimens of telithromycin once daily compared with a 10 day regimen of clarithromycin twice daily in patients with mild to moderate community-acquired pneumonia. Journal of Antimicrobial Chemotherapy 54:515–523, 2004.

van Rensburg D, Fogarty C, De Salvo MC, et al. Efficacy of oral telithromycin in community-acquired pneumonia caused by resistant Streptococcus pneumoniae. Journal of Infection 51:201–5, 2005.

Zervos MJ, Heyder AM, Leroy B. Oral telithromycin 800 mg once daily for 5 days versus cefuroxime axetil 500 mg twice daily for 10 days in adults with acute exacerbations of chronic bronchitis. J Int Med Res 31:157–69, 2003.

Website: www.ketek.com

Tenofovir disoproxil fumarate (Viread) TDF

Drug Class: Antiretroviral (nucleotide analogue). Anti-HBV drug.

Usual Dose: 300 mg (PO) q24h.

Pharmacokinetic Parameters:

Peak serum level: 0.29 mcg/mL

Bioavailability: 25%/39% (fasting/high fat meal)

Excreted unchanged (urine): 32%

Serum half-life (normal/ESRD): 17 hrs/no data

Plasma protein binding: 0.7–7.2%

Volume of distribution (V_d): 1.3 L/kg

Primary Mode of Elimination: Renal

Dosage Adjustments*

CrCl ≥ 50 mL/min	No change
CrCl 30–49 mL/min	300 mg (PO) q48h
CrCl 10–29 mL/min	300 mg (PO) 2x/week
CrCl < 10 mL/min	No information
Post–HD dose	300 mg q7d or after 12 hours on HD
Post–PD dose	No information
CVVH dose	No information
Moderate hepatic insufficiency	No change
Severe hepatic insufficiency	No change

Drug Interactions: Didanosine (if possible, avoid concomitant didanosine due to impaired CD_4 response and increased risk of virologic failure); valganciclovir (↑ tenofovir levels); atazanavir, lopinavir/ritonavir (↑ tenofovir levels) (↓ atazanavir levels; use atazanavir 300 mg/ritonavir 100 mg with tenofovir); no clinically significant interactions with lamivudine, efavirenz, methadone, oral contraceptives. Not a substrate/inhibitor of cytochrome P-450 enzymes.

Adverse Effects: Lactic acidosis and severe hepatomegaly with steatosis, including fatal cases, have been reported with the nucleoside analogs. Severe acute exacerbations of hepatitis have been reported in HBV-infected patients who have discontinued antihepatitis B therapy, including teonfovir. Mild nausea, vomiting, GI upset, asthenia, headache, diarrhea renal tubular acidosis, decrease bone density occur. It is recommended that creatinine clearance be calculated in all patients prior to initiating therapy and as clinically appropriate during therapy with tenofovir. Routine

---

"Usual dose" assumes normal renal/hepatic function. * For renal insufficiency, give usual dose × 1 followed by maintenance dose per CrCl. For dialysis patients, dose the same as for CrCl < 10 mL/min and give supplemental (post-HD/PD dose) immediately after dialysis. CrCl = creatinine clearance; CVVH = continuous veno-venous hemofiltration; HD/PD = hemodialysis/peritoneal dialysis. See pp. 509–513 for explanations, pp. xi–xii for abbreviations; Linezolid (↑ risk of serotonin syndrome, see p. 620).

monitoring of calculated creatinine clearance and serum phosphorus should be performed in patients at risk for renal impairment. Immune constitution syndrome can occur.

Allergic Potential: Low

Safety in Pregnancy: B

Comments: Eliminated by glomerular filtration/tubular secretion. May be taken with or without food. If possible, avoid concomitant didanosine (see drug interactions). **Effective therapy of chronic HBV.**

Cerebrospinal Fluid Penetration: No data

REFERENCES:

Gallant JE, DeJesus D, Arribas JR, et al. Tenofovir DF, emtricitabine, and efavirenz vs. zidovudine, lamivudine, and efavirenz for HIV. N Engl J Med 354:251–60, 2006.

Gallant JE. Efficacy and safety of tenofovir DF vs stavudine in combination therapy in antiretroviral-naive patients: a 3-year randomized trial. JAMA 292:191–201, 2004.

Gallant JE, Deresinski S. Tenofovir disoproxil fumarate. Clin Infect Dis 37:944–50, 2003.

Jullien V, Treluye JM, Rey E, et al. Population pharmacokinetics of tenofovir in human immunodeficiency virus-infected patients taking highly active antiretroviral therapy. Antimicrobial Agents and Chemotherapy 49:3361–3366, 2005.

Panel on Antiretroviral Guidelines for Adults and Adolescents. Guidelines for the use of antiretroviral agents in HIV-1 infected adults and adolescents. Department of Health and Human Services. November 3, 2008; 1–139. Available at http://www.aidsinfor.nih.gov/ContentFiles/AdultandAdolescentGL.pdf.

Terrault NA. Treatment of recurrent hepatitis B infection in liver transplant recipients. Liver Transpl 8(Suppl 1):S74–81, 2002.

Thromson CA. Prodrug of tenofovir diphosphate approved for combination HIV therapy. Am J Health Syst Pharm 59:18, 2002.

Website: www.viread.com

Terbinafine (Lamisil, Daskil)

Drug Class: Antifungal.

Usual Dose: 250 mg (PO) q24h.

Pharmacokinetic Parameters:

Peak serum level: 1 mcg/ml

Bioavailability: 70%

Excreted unchanged (urine): 75%

Serum half-life (normal/ESRD): 24 hrs/no data

Plasma protein binding: 99%

Volume of distribution (V_d): 13.5 L/kg

Primary Mode of Elimination: Renal/hepatic

Dosage Adjustments*

CrCl ~ 50–60 mL/min	No change
CrCl < 50 mL/min	Avoid
Post–HD dose	Avoid
Post–PD dose	Avoid
CVVH dose	Avoid
Moderate or severe hepatic insufficiency	Avoid

Drug Interactions: Cimetidine (↓ terbinafine clearance, ↑ terbinafine levels); phenobarbital, rifampin (↑ terbinafine clearance, ↓ terbinafine levels).

Adverse Effects: Drug fever/rash, lymphopenia, leukopenia, ↑ SGOT/SGPT, visual disturbances, nausea, vomiting, GI upset.

Allergic Potential: Low

Safety in Pregnancy: B

Comments: May cause green vision and changes in the lens/retina.

Cerebrospinal Fluid Penetration: < 10%

REFERENCES:

Abdel-Rahman SM, Nahata MC. Oral terbinafine: A new antifungal agent. Ann Pharmacother 31:445–56, 1997.

Amichai B, Grunwald MH. Adverse drug reactions of the new oral antifungal agents – terbinafine,

"Usual dose" assumes normal renal/hepatic function. * For renal insufficiency, give usual dose × 1 followed by maintenance dose per CrCl. For dialysis patients, dose the same as for CrCl < 10 mL/min and give supplemental (post-HD/PD dose) immediately after dialysis. CrCl = creatinine clearance; CVVH = continuous veno-venous hemofiltration; HD/PD = hemodialysis/peritoneal dialysis. See pp. 509–513 for explanations, pp. xi–xii for abbreviations; Linezolid (↑ risk of serotonin syndrome, see p. 620).

fluconazole, and itraconazole. Int J Dermatol 37:410–5, 1998.
Darkes MJ, Scott LJ, Goa KL. Terbinafine: a review of its use in onychomycosis in adults. Am J Clin Dermatol. 4:39–65, 2003.
Jain S, Sehgal VN. Itraconazole versus terbinafine in the management of onychomycosis: an overview. J Dermatolog Treat. 14:30–42, 2003.
Mosquera J, Shartt A, Moore CB, et al. In vitro interaction of terbinafine with itraconazole, fluconazole, amphotericin B and 5-flucytosine against Aspergillus spp. J Antimicrob Chemother 50:189–94, 2002.
Salo H, Pekurinen M. Cost effectiveness or oral terbinafine (Lamisil) compared with oral fluconazole (Diflucan) in the treatment of patients with toenail onychomycosis. Pharmacoeconomics 20:319–24, 2002.
Trepanier EF, Amsden GW. Current issues in onychomycosis. Ann Pharmacother 32:204–14, 1998.
Website: www.pdr.net

Tetracycline (various)

Drug Class: Tetracycline.
Usual Dose: 500 mg (PO) q6h (Take without food).
Spectrum: (see ***Susceptibility Profiles*** pp. 183–187).
Pharmacokinetic Parameters:
Peak serum level: 1.5 mcg/ml
Bioavailability: 60%
Excreted unchanged (urine): 60%
Serum half-life (normal/ESRD): 8/108 hrs
Plasma protein binding: 5%
Volume of distribution (V_d): 0.7 L/kg
Primary Mode of Elimination: Renal
Dosage Adjustments*

CrCl 50–80 mL/min	No change
CrCl < 50 mL/min	Avoid
Post–HD/Post–PD dose	Avoid
CVVH dose	Avoid
Moderate hepatic insufficiency	No change
Severe hepatic insufficiency	≤ 1 gm (PO) q24h

Drug Interactions: Antacids, Al^{++}, Ca^{++}, Fe^{++}, Mg^{++}, Zn^{++}, multivitamins, sucralfate (↓ absorption of tetracycline); barbiturates, carbamazepine, phenytoin (↓ half-life of tetracycline); bicarbonate (↓ absorption and ↑ clearance of tetracycline); digoxin (↑ digoxin levels); insulin (↑ insulin effect); methoxyflurane (↑ nephrotoxicity).
Adverse Effects: Nausea, vomiting, GI upset, diarrhea, hepatotoxicity, vaginal candidiasis, photosensitizing reactions, benign intracranial hypertension (pseudotumor cerebri).
Allergic Potential: Low
Safety in Pregnancy: D
Comments: Take without food. *Hepatotoxicity dose dependent (≥ 2 gm/day), especially in pregnancy/renal failure. Avoid prolonged sun exposure. Doxycycline or minocycline preferred for all tetracycline indications.*
Cerebrospinal Fluid Penetration:
Non-Inflamed meninges = 5%
Inflamed meninges = 5%
Bile Penetration: 1000%
(also see ***Antibiotic Pearls & Pitfalls*** pp. 495–508).

REFERENCES:

Agwuh KN, MacGowan A. Pharmacokinetics and pharmacodynamics of the tetracyclines including glycylcyclines. J of Antimicrob Chemotherapy. 58:256–265, 2006.
Cunha BA, Comer J, Jonas M. The tetracyclines. Med Clin North Am 66:293–302, 1982.
Dahl EL, Shock JL, Shenai BR, Gut J, DeRisi JL, Rosenthal PJ. Tetracyclines Specifically Target the Apicoplast of the Malaria Parasite Plasmodium falciparum. Antimicrob Agents Chemother 50:3124–31, 2006.

"Usual dose" assumes normal renal/hepatic function. * For renal insufficiency, give usual dose × 1 followed by maintenance dose per CrCl. For dialysis patients, dose the same as for CrCl < 10 mL/min and give supplemental (post-HD/PD dose) immediately after dialysis. CrCl = creatinine clearance; CVVH = continuous veno-venous hemofiltration; HD/PD = hemodialysis/peritoneal dialysis. See pp. 509–513 for explanations, pp. xi–xii for abbreviations; Linezolid (↑ risk of serotonin syndrome, see p. 620).

Donovan BJ, Weber DJ, Rublein JC, et al. Treatment of tick-borne diseases. Ann Pharmacother 36:1590–1597, 2002.

Pugliese A, Cunha BA. Tetracyclines. Int J Urogyn 5:221–7, 1994.

Smilack JD, Wilson WE, Cocerill Fr 3rd. Tetracycline, chloramphenicol, erythromycin, clindamycin, and metronidazole. Mayo Clin Proc 66:1270–80, 1991.

Ticarcillin (Ticar)

Drug Class: Antipseudomonal penicillin.
Usual Dose: 3 gm (IV) q6h.
Spectrum: (see ***Susceptibility Profiles*** pp. 183–187).
Pharmacokinetic Parameters:
Peak serum level: 118–300 mcg/ml
Bioavailability: Not applicable
Excreted unchanged (urine): 95%
Serum half-life (normal/ESRD): 1/5 hrs
Plasma protein binding: 45%
Volume of distribution (V_d): 0.2 L/kg
Primary Mode of Elimination: Renal
Dosage Adjustments*

CrCl 50–80 mL/min	No change
CrCl 10–50 mL/min	2 gm (IV) q8h
CrCl < 10 mL/min	2 gm (IV) q12h
Post–HD dose	2 gm (IV)
Post–PD dose	3 gm (IV)
CVVH dose	2 gm (IV) q8h
Moderate hepatic insufficiency	No change
Severe hepatic insufficiency	No change

Drug Interactions: Aminoglycosides (inactivation of ticarcillin in renal failure); warfarin (↑ INR); oral contraceptives (↓ oral contraceptive effect); cefoxitin (↓ ticarcillin effect).

Adverse Effects: Drug fever/rash; E. multiforme/Stevens-Johnson syndrome, anaphylactic reactions (hypotension, laryngospasm, bronchospasm), hives, serum sickness. Dose-dependent inhibition of platelet aggregation is minimal/absent (usual dose is less than carbenicillin). C. difficile diarrhea/colitis.
Allergic Potential: High
Safety in Pregnancy: B
Comments: Administer 1 hour before or after aminoglycoside. Na^+ content = 5.2 mEq/g. Meningeal dose = usual dose.
Cerebrospinal Fluid Penetration:
Non-Inflamed meninges = 1%
Inflamed meninges = 30%
(also see ***Antibiotic Pearls & Pitfalls*** pp. 495–508).

REFERENCES:

Donowitz GR, Mandell GL. Beta-lactam antibiotics. N Engl J Med 318:419–26 and 318:490–500, 1993.

Tan JS, File TM, Jr. Antipseudomonal penicillins. Med Clin North Am 79:679–93, 1995.

Wright AJ. The penicillins. Mayo Clin Proc 74:290–307, 1999.

Ticarcillin/clavulanate (Timentin)

Drug Class: Antipseudomonal penicillin.
Usual Dose: 3.1 gm (IV) q6h.
Spectrum: (see ***Susceptibility Profiles*** pp. 183–187).
Pharmacokinetic Parameters:
Peak serum level: 330 mcg/ml
Bioavailability: Not applicable
Excreted unchanged (urine): 95/45%
Serum half-life (normal/ESRD): [1/13]/[1/2] hrs
Plasma protein binding: 45/25%
Volume of distribution (V_d): 0.2/0.3 L/kg

"Usual dose" assumes normal renal/hepatic function. * For renal insufficiency, give usual dose × 1 followed by maintenance dose per CrCl. For dialysis patients, dose the same as for CrCl < 10 mL/min and give supplemental (post-HD/PD dose) immediately after dialysis. CrCl = creatinine clearance; CVVH = continuous veno-venous hemofiltration; HD/PD = hemodialysis/peritoneal dialysis. See pp. 509–513 for explanations, pp. xi–xii for abbreviations; Linezolid (↑ risk of serotonin syndrome, see p. 620).

Primary Mode of Elimination: Renal

Dosage Adjustments*

CrCl 50–80 mL/min	2 gm (IV) q4h
CrCl 10–50 mL/min	2 gm (IV) q8h
CrCl < 10 mL/min	2 gm (IV) q12h
Post–HD dose	2 gm (IV)
Post–PD dose	3.1 gm (IV)
CVVH dose	3.1 gm (IV) q8h
Moderate hepatic insufficiency	If CrCl < 10 mL/min: 2 gm (IV) q24h
Severe hepatic insufficiency	If CrCl < 10 mL/min: 2 gm (IV) q24h

Drug Interactions: Aminoglycosides (↓ aminoglycoside levels); methotrexate (↑ methotrexate levels); vecuronium (↑ vecuronium effect).

Adverse Effects: Drug fever/rash, E. multiforme/Stevens-Johnson syndrome, anaphylactic reactions (hypotension, laryngospasm, bronchospasm), hives, serum sickness. C. difficile diarrhea/colitis.

Allergic Potential: High

Safety in Pregnancy: B

Comments: 20% of clavulanate removed by dialysis. Na^+ content = 4.75 mEq/g. K^+ content = 0.15 mEq/g.

Cerebrospinal Fluid Penetration: < 10%

Bile Penetration:

Without obstruction = 100%

With obstruction = 10%

(also see ***Antibiotic Pearls & Pitfalls*** pp. 495–508).

REFERENCES:

Donowitz GR, Mandell GL. Beta-lactam antibiotics. N Engl J Med 318:419–26 and 318:490–500, 1993.

Graham DR, Talan DA, Nichols RL, et al. Once-daily, high-dose levofloxacin versus ticarcillin-clavulanate alone or followed by amoxicillin-clavulanate for complicated skin and skin-structure infections: a randomized, open-label trial. Clin Infect Dis 35:381–9, 2002.

Itokazu GS, Danziger LH. Ampicillin-sulbactam and ticarcillin-clavulanic acid: A comparison of their in vitro activity and review of their clinical efficacy. Pharmacotherapy 11:382–414, 1991.

Winston LG, Charlebois ED, Pang S, et al. Impact of a formulary switch from ticarcillin-clavulanate to piperacillin-tazobactam on colonization with vancomycin-resistant enterococci. Am J Infect Control. 32:462–9, 2004.

Website: www.timentin.com

Tigecycline (Tygacil)

Drug Class: Glycylcycline.

Usual Dose: 100 mg (IV) × 1 dose, then 50 mg (IV) q12h.

Spectrum: (see ***Susceptibility Profiles*** pp. 194–199).

Pharmacokinetic Parameters:

Peak serum level: 1.45 mcg/ml (100 mg dose); 0.87 mcg/ml (50 mg dose)

Bioavailability: Not applicable

Excreted unchanged (urine): 22%

Serum half-life (normal/ESRD): 42/42 hrs

Plasma protein binding: 89%

Volume of distribution (V_d): 8 L/kg

Primary Mode of Elimination: Biliary

Dosage Adjustments*

CrCl 50–80 mL/min	No change
CrCl 10–50 mL/min	No change
CrCl < 10 mL/min	No change
Post–HD dose	None
Post–PD dose	None
CVVH dose	No change

"Usual dose" assumes normal renal/hepatic function. * For renal insufficiency, give usual dose × 1 followed by maintenance dose per CrCl. For dialysis patients, dose the same as for CrCl < 10 mL/min and give supplemental (post-HD/PD dose) immediately after dialysis. CrCl = creatinine clearance; CVVH = continuous veno-venous hemofiltration; HD/PD = hemodialysis/peritoneal dialysis. See pp. 509–513 for explanations, pp. xi–xii for abbreviations; Linezolid (↑ risk of serotonin syndrome, see p. 620).

Moderate hepatic insufficiency	No change
Severe hepatic insufficiency (Child Pugh C)	100 mg (IV) × 1 dose, then 25 mg (IV) q12h

Drug Interactions: Warfarin (↑ INR). Does not inhibit and is not metabolized by CYP450.
Adverse Effects: N/V, dyspepsia, diarrhea, dizziness, asthenia, thrombocytosis, ↑ SGOT, ↑ alkaline phosphatase, pancreatitis, (↑ amylase/ lipase), ↑ LDH, ↑ BUN, ↓ total protein.
Allergic Potential: Low
Safety in Pregnancy: D
Comments: Effective for cSSSIs/cIAIs. **Often the only antibiotic effective against MDR Klebsiella pneumoniae or MDR Acinetobacter baumanii.** Higher doses may be needed to treat MDR GNB pathogens. After the loading dose the maintenance dose i.e., 50 mg (IV) of q12h, may also be given as 100 mg (IV) of q24h. **Tigecycline effective monotherapy for severe C. difficile colitis** (anti-C. difficile ***and*** anti-GNB/B. fragilis activity for microscopic/ gross peritonitis). Infuse over 30–60 minutes; mix with D5W or 0.9% pathogens. Safe to use in penicillin/sulfa-allergic patients.
Cerebrospinal Fluid Penetration: No data
Bile Penetration: 3800%
(also see ***Antibiotic Pearls & Pitfalls*** p. 506).

REFERENCES:

Akcam FZ, Kaya O, Basoglu N, et al. E-test minimum inhibitory concentrations for tigecycline against nosocomial Acinetobacter baumannii strains. J Chemother 19:2310–231, 2007.

Alriksson NT, Akerlund I, Burman LG, et al. In vitro susceptibility to 17 antimicrobials among clinical Clostridium difficile isolates collected 1993–2007 in Sweden. Clin MIcrobiolog Infect. (Epub ahead of print). 2009.

Aslam S, Trautner BW, Ramanathan V, et al. Combination of tigecycline and N-acetylcysteine reduces biofilm-embedded bacteria on vascular catheters. Antimicrob Agents Chemother 51:1556–1558, 2007.

Babinchak T, Ellis-Grosse E, Dartois N, et al. The efficacy and safety of tigecycline for the treatment of complicated intra-abdominal infections: analysis of pooled clinical trial data. Clin Infect Dis 41(Suppl 5:S3):54–67, 2005.

Baines SD, Saxton K, Freeman K, et al. Tigecycline does not induce proliferation or cytotoxin production by epidemic Clostridium difficile strains in a human gut model. J Antimicrob Chemother 58:1062–1065, 2006.

Bendu C, Culebras E, Gomez M, et al. In vitro activity of tigecycline against Bacteroides species. J Antimicrob Chemother 56:349–52, 2005.

Bergallo C, Jasovich A, Teglia O, et al. Safety and efficacy of intravenous tigecycline in Treatment of community-acquired pneumonia: results from a double-blind randomized Phase 3 comparison study with levofloxacin. Diagn Microbiol Infect Dis 63:52–61, 2009.

Biedenbach DJ, Beach ML, Jones RN. In vitro antimicrobial activity of GAR-936 tested against antibiotic-resistant gram-positive blood stream infection isolates and strains producing extended-spectrum beta-lactamases. Diagn Microbiol Infect Dis 40:173–7, 2001.

Bolmstrom A, Karlsson A, Engelhardt A, et al. Validation and reproducibility assessment of tigecycline MIC determinations by Etest. J Clin Microbiol 45:2474–2479, 2007.

Bouchillon SK, Hoban DJ, Johnson BM, et al. In vitro evaluation of tigecycline and comparative agents in 3049 clinical isolates: 2001 to 2002. Diagn Microbial Infect Dis 51:291–5, 2005.

Bouza E. New therapeutic choices for infections caused by methicillin-resistant *Staphylococcus aureus*. Clin Microbiol Infect Dis 15:44–52, 2009.

Bradford PA, Peterson PJ, Tuckman M, et al. In vitro activity of tigecycline and occurrence of tetracycline resistance determinants in isolates from patients enrolled in phase 3 clinical trials for community-acquired pneumonia. Clin Microbiol Infect 14:882–886, 2008.

Bradford PA, Weaver-Sands DT, Petersen PJ. In vitro activity of tigecycline against isolates from patients enrolled in phase 3 clinical trials of treatment for complicated skin and skin-structure infections and complicated intra-abdominal infections. Clin Infect Dis 41(Suppl 5):S315–32, 2005.

Bradford PA. Tigecycline: A first in class glycylcycline. Clinical Microbiology Newsletter 26:163–168, 2004.

Bratu S, Tolaney P, Karumudi U, et al. Carbapenemase-producing Klebsiella pneumoniae in Brooklyn, NY: molecular epidemiology and in vitro activity of polymyxin B and other agents. J Antimicrob Chemother 56:128–32, 2005.

Breedt J, Teras J, Gardovskis J, et al. Safety and efficacy of tigecycline in treatment of skin and skin structure infections: results of a double-blind phase 3 comparison study with vancomycin-aztreonam. Antimicrobial Agents Chemother 49:4658–4666, 2005.

Cercenado E, Cercenado S, Gomez JA, et al. In vitro activity of tigecycline (GAR-936), a novel glycylcycline, against vancomycin-resistant enterococci and staphylococci with diminished susceptibility to glycopeptides. J Antimicrob Chemother 52:138–9, 2003.

Chemaly RF, Hanmod S, Jiang Y, et al. Tigecycline Use in Cancer Patients with Serious Infections: A Report of 110 Cases from a Single Institution. Medicine. 88:211–220, 2009.

Cunha BA, McDermott B, Nausheen S. Single once daily high dose therapy of tigecycline in a urinary tract infection due to multi-drug resistant (MDR) Klebsiella pneumoniae and MDR Enterobacter agglomerans. Journal of Chemotherapy 19:753–754, 2008.

Cunha BA. Once daily tigecycline therapy of multidrug-resistant and non-multidrug resistant gram-negative bacteremias. J of Chemother 19:232–33, 2007.

Cunha BA. Antimicrobial Therapy of Multidrug-Resistant Streptococcus pneumoniae, Vancomycin-Resistant Enterococci, and Methicillin-Resistant Staphlycoccus aureus. Med Clin N Am 90:1165–82, 2006.

Curcio D, Fernandez F, Jones RN, et al. Tigecycline disk diffusion breakpoints of Acinetobacter spp.: a clinical point of view. J Clin Microbiol 45:2095–2096, 2007.

Daly MW, Riddle DJ, Ledeboer NA, et al. Tigecycline for treatment of pneumonia and empyema caused by carbapenems-producing Klebsiella pneumoniae. Pharmacotherapy 27:1052–1057, 2007.

Dandache P, Nicolau DP, Sakoulas G. Tigecycline for the Treatment of Multidrug-Resistant *Klebsiella pneumoniae* Meningitis. Infect Dis in Clin Practice. 17:66–68, 2009.

Dartois N, Castiang N, Gandjini H, et al. Tigecycline versus levofloxacin for the treatment of community-acquired pneumonia: European experience. J Chemother 20:28–35, 2008.

Dizbay M, Kilic S, Hizel K, et al. Tigecycline: its potential for treatment of brucellosis. Scand J Infect Dis 39:432–434, 2007.

Dominguez EA. Single Agent Therapy With Tigecycline in the Treatment of Complicated Skin and Skin Structure and Complicated Intraabdominal Infections. Infectious Diseases in Clinical Practice. 17:144–149, 2009.

Ellis-Grosse EJ, Babinchak T, Dartois N, et al. The efficacy and safety of tigecycline in the treatment of skin and skin-structure infections: results of 2 double-blind phase 3 comparison studies with vancomycin-aztreonam. Clin Infect Dis 41(Suppl 5):S341–53, 2005.

Fraise AP. Tigecycline: The answer to beta-lactam and fluoroquinolone resistance? Journal of Infection. 53:293–300, 2006.

Fritache TR, Kirby JT, Jones RN. In vitro activity of tigecycline (GAR-936) tested against 11,859 recent clinical isolates associated with community-acquired respiratory tract and gram-positive cutaneous infections. Diagn Microbiol Infect Dis 49:201–9, 2004.

Gardiner D, Dukart G, Cooper A, et al. Safety and Efficacy of Intravenous Tigecycline in Subjects with Secondary Bacteremia: Pooled Results from 8 Phase III Clinical Trials. Clin Infect. Dis. 50:229–238, 2010.

Garrison MW, Neumiller JJ, Setter SM. Tigecycline: an investigational glycylcycline antimicrobial with activity against resistant gram-positive organisms. Clin Ther 27:12–22, 2005.

Hawkey P, Finch R. Tigecycline: in-vitro performance as a predictor of clinical efficacy. Clin Microbiol Infect 13:354–362, 2007.

Hawser SP. Activity of tigecycline against recent European clinical isolates of Clostridium difficile. Int J Antimicrob Agents. 3: (Epub ahead of print), 2009.

Herpers BL, Vlaminckx B, Burkhardt O, et al. Intravenous Tigecycline as Adjunctive or Alternative Therapy for Severe Refractory *Clostridium difficile* Infection. Clin Infect Dis 48:1732–1735, 2009.

Hoban DJ, Bouchillon SK, Dowzicky MJ. Antimicrobial susceptibility of extended-spectrum beta-lactamase producers and multidrug-resistant Acinetobacter baumannii throughout the United States and comparative in vitro activity of tigecycline, a new glycylcyline antimicrobial. Diagn Microbiol Infect Dis 57:423–428, 2007.

Hope R, Warner M, Potz NA, et al. Activity of tigecycline against ESBL-producing and AmpC-hyperproducing Enterobacteriaceae from south-east England. J Antimicrob Chemother 58:1312–1314, 2006.

Insa R, Cercenado E, Goyanes MJ, et al. In vitro activity of tigecycline against clinical isolates of Acinetobacter baumannii and Stenotrophomonas maltophilia. J Antimicrob Chemother 59:583–585, 2007.

Jacobus NV, McDermott LA, Ruthazer R, et al. In vitro activities of tigecycline against the Bacteroides fragilis group. Antimicrob Agents Chemother 48:1034–6, 2004.

Jenkins I. Linezolid- and vancomycin-resistant Enterococcus faecium endocarditis: successful treatment with tigecycline and daptomycin. J Hosp Med 2:343–344, 2007.

Jones RN, Ferraro MJ, Reller LB, et al. Multicenter studies of tigecycline disk diffusion susceptibility results for Acinetobacter spp. J Clin Microbiol 45:227–230, 2007.

Koomanachai P, Crandon JL, Banevicius. Pharmacodynamic Profile of Tigecycline against Methicillin-Resistant Staphylococcus aureus in an Experimental Pneumonia Model. Antimicrob Agents Chemother 53:5060–5063, 2009.

Kresken M, Leitner E, Brauers J, et al. Susceptibility of common aerobic pathogens to tigecycline: results of a surveillance study in Germany. Eur J Clin Microbiolg Infec Dis 28:83–90, 2009.

McKeage K, Keating GM. Tigecycline: in community-acquired pneumonia. Drugs. 68:2633–2644, 2008.

Meagher AK, Ambrose PG, Grasela TH, et al. The pharmacokinetic and pharmacodynamic profile of tigecycline. Clin Infect Dis 41(Suppl 5):S333–40, 2005.

Meagher AK, Passarell JA, Cirincione BB, et al. Exposure-response analyses of tigecycline efficacy in patients with complicated skin and skin-structure infections. Antimicrob Agents Chemother 51:1939–1945, 2007.

Muralidharan G, Fruncillo RJ, Micalizzi M, et al. Effects of age and sex on single-dose pharmacokinetics of tigecycline in healthy subjects. Antimicrob Agents Chemother 49:1656–1659, 2005.

Muralidharan G, Micalizzi M, Speth J, et al. Pharmacokinetics of tigecycline after single and multiple doses in healthy subjects. Antimicrob Agents Chemother 49:220–9, 2005.

Nord CE, Sillerstrom E, Wahlund E. Effect of Tigecycline on Normal Oropharyngeal and Intestinal Microflora. Antimicrob Agents Chemother 50:3375–80, 2006.

Noskin GA. Tigecycline: a new glycylcycline for treatment of serious infections. Clin Infect Dis 41(Suppl 5):S303–14, 2005.

Noviello S, Ianniello F, Leone S, et al. *In Vitro* Activity of Tigecycline: MICs, MBCs, Time-Kill Curves and Post-Antibiotic Effect. J Chemotherapy. 20:577–580, 2008.

Pankey GA. Tigecycline. J Antimicrob Chemother 53:470–80, 2005.

Pankey GA, Steele RW. Tigecycline: a single antibiotic for polymicrobial infections. Pediatr Infect Dis J 26:77–78, 2007.

Peleg AY, Potoski BA, Rea R, et al. Acinetobacter baumannii bloodstream infection while receiving tigecycline: a cautionary report. J Antimicrob Chemother 59:128–31, 2007.

Petersen PJ, Jones CH, Bradford PA. In vitro antibacterial activities of tigecycline and comparative agents by time-kill kinetic studies in fresh Mueller-Hinton broth. Diagn Microbiol Infect Dis 59:347–349, 2007.

Raad I, Hanna H, Jiang Y, et al. Comparative activities of daptomycin, linezolid, and tigecycline against catheter-related methicillin-resistant Staphylococcus bacteremic isolates embedded in biofilm. Antimicrob Agents Chemother 51:1656–1660, 2007.

Rodvold KA, Gotfried MH, Cwik M, et al. Serum, tissue and body fluid concentrations of tigecycline after a single 100 mg dose. J Antimicrob Chemother 58:1221–1229, 2006.

Rubinstein E, Vaughan D. Tigecycline: a novel glycylcycline. Drugs 65:1317–36, 2005.

Sands M, McCarter Y, Sanchez W. Synergy testing of multidrug resistant Acinetobacter baumannii against tigecycline and polymyxin using an E-test methodology. Eur J Clin Microbiol Infect Dis 26: 521–522, 2007.

Schafer JJ, Goff DA, Stevenson KB, et al. Early experience with tigecycline for ventilator-associated pneumonia and bacteremia caused by multidrug-resistant acinetobacter baumannii. Pharmacotherapy 27:980–987, 2007.

Scheetz MH, Q Chao, Warren JR, et al. In vitro activities of various antimicrobials alone and in combination with tigecycline against carbapenem-intermediate or -resistant Acinetobacter baumannii. Antimicrob Agents Chemother 51:1621–1626, 2007.

Slover CM, Rodvold KA, Danziger LH. Tigecycline: a novel broad-spectrum antimicrobial. Ann Pharmacother 41:965–972, 2007.

Sotto A, Bouziges N, Jourdan N, et al. In vitro activity of tigecycline against strains isolated from diabetic foot ulcers. Pathol Biol 55:398–406, 2007.

Souli M, Kontopidou FV, Koratzanis E, Antoniadou A, et al. In Vitro Activity of Tigecycline against Multi-Drug-Resistant, Including Pan-Resistant, Gram-Negative and Gram-Positive Clinical Isolates from Greek Hospitals. Antimicrob Agents Chemother 50:3166–69, 2006.

Stein GE, Craig WA. Tigecycline: A Critical Analysis. Clin Infect Dis 43:518–24, 2006.

Swoboda S, Ober M, Hainer C, et al. Tigecycline for the treatment of patients with severe sepsis of septic shock: a drug use evaluation in a surgical intensive care unit. J Antimicrob Chemother 61:729–733, 2008.

Sym D. Tigecycline (Tygacil). Antibiotics for Clinicians. 11:349–52, 2006.

Taccone FS, Rodriguez-Villalobos H, DeBacker D, et al. Successful treatment of septic shock due to pan-resistant Acinetobacter baumannii using combined antimicrobial therapy including tigecycline. Eur J Clin Microbiol Infect Dis 25:257–60, 2006.

Tanaseanu C, Bergallo C, Teglia O, et al. Integrated results of 2 phase studies comparing tigecycline and levofloxacin in community-acquired pneumonia. Diagn Microbiol Infect Dis 61:329–338, 2008.

Van Wart SA, Owen JS, Ludwig EA, et al. Population Pharmacokinetics of Tigecycline in Patients with Complicated Intra-Abdominal or Skin and Skin Structure Infections. Antimicrob Agents and Chemother 50:3701–07, 2006.

Waites KB, Duffy LB, Dowzicky MJ. Antimicrobial Susceptibility among Pathogens Collected from Hospitalized Patients in the United States and In Vitro Activity of Tigecycline, a New Glycylcylcine Antimicrobial. Antimicrob Agents Chemother 50:3479–84, 2006.

Wilcox MH. Evidence for low risk of Clostridium difficile infection associated with tigecycline. Clin Microbiol Infect 13:949–952, 2007.

Woodford N, Hill RL, Livermore DM. In vitro activity of tigecycline against carbapenem-susceptible and resistant isolates of Klebsiella spp. And Enterobacter spp. J Antimicrob Chemother 59:582–583, 2007.

Zinner SH. Overview of antibiotic use and resistance: setting the stage for tigecycline. Clin Infect Dis 41(Suppl 5):S289–92, 2005.

Website: www.tygacil.com

Tipranavir (Aptivus) TIP

Drug Class: Protease inhibitor.

Usual Dose: 500 mg (PO) with ritonavir 200 mg (PO) q12h.

Pharmacokinetic Parameters:

Peak serum level: 77–94 mcg/mL

Bioavailability: No data

Excreted unchanged (urine): 44%

Serum half-life (normal/ESRD): 5.5–6/5.5–6 hrs

Plasma protein binding: 99.9%

Volume of distribution (V_d): 7–10 L/kg

Primary Mode of Elimination: Hepatic

Dosage Adjustments*

"Usual dose" assumes normal renal/hepatic function. * For renal insufficiency, give usual dose × 1 followed by maintenance dose per CrCl. For dialysis patients, dose the same as for CrCl < 10 mL/min and give supplemental (post-HD/PD dose) immediately after dialysis. CrCl = creatinine clearance; CVVH = continuous veno-venous hemofiltration; HD/PD = hemodialysis/peritoneal dialysis. See pp. 509–513 for explanations, pp. xi–xii for abbreviations; Linezolid (↑ risk of serotonin syndrome, see p. 620).

CrCl 50–80 mL/min	No change
CrCl 10–50 mL/min	No change
CrCl < 10 mL/min	No change
Post–HD dose	No change
Post–PD dose	No change
CVVH dose	No change
Mild hepatic insufficiency	No change
Moderate or severe hepatic insufficiency	Avoid

Drug Interactions: Rifabutin (↑ levels), clarithromycin (↑ levels), loperamide (↓ levels), statins (↑ risk of myopathy); abacavir, saquinavir, tenofovir, zidovudine, amprenavir/RTV, lopinavir/RTV (↓ levels). Aluminum/magnesium antacids (↓ absorption 25–30%). Ritonavir (↑ risk of hepatitis). St. John's Wort (↓ tipranavir levels). Keep refrigerated 2–8°C. Metabolized via CYP 3A4.

Adverse Effects: Contraindicated in moderate/severe hepatic insufficiency. ↑ risk of hepatotoxicity in HIV patients co-infected with HBV/HCV. Case reports of intracerebral hemorrhage–use with caution in patients with coagulopathies.

Allergic Potential: High. Tipranavir is a sulfonamide; use with caution in patients with sulfonamide allergies

Safety in Pregnancy: C

Comments: Should be taken with food. Increased bioavailability when taken with meals. Must be co-administered with 200 mg ritonavir. Tipranavir contains a sulfonamide moiety (as do darunavir and fosamprenavir).

Cerebrospinal Fluid Penetration: No data

REFERENCES:

Barbaro G, Scozzafava A, Mastrolorenzo A, et al. Highly active antiretroviral therapy: current state of the art, new agents and their pharmacological interactions useful for improving therapeutic outcome. Curr Pharm Des 11:1805–43, 2005.

Clotet B. Strategies for overcoming resistance in HIV-1 infected patients receiving HAART. AIDS Rev 6:123–30, 2004.

Croom KF, Keam SJ. Tipranavir: a ritonavir-boosted protease inhibitor. Drugs 65:1669–79, 2005.

de Mendoza C, Soriano V. Resistance to HIV protease inhibitors: mechanisms and clinical consequences. Curr Drug Metab 5:321–8, 2004.

Gulick RM. New antiretroviral drugs. Clin Microbiol Infect 9:186–93, 2003.

Kandula VR, Khanlou H, Farthing C. Tipranavir: a novel second-generation nonpeptidic protease inhibitor. Expert Rev Anti Infect Ther 3:9–21, 2005.

Kashuba AD. Drug-drug interactions and the pharmacotherapy of HIV infection. Top HIV Med 13:64–9, 2005.

Panel on Antiretroviral Guidelines for Adults and Adolescents. Guidelines for the use of antiretroviral agents in HIV-1 infected adults and adolescents. Department of Health and Human Services. November 3, 2008; 1–139. Available at http://www.aidsinfor.nih.gov/ContentFiles/AdultandAdolescentGL.pdf

Plosker GL, Figgitt DP. Tripanavir. Drugs 63:1611–8, 2003.

Turner D, Schapiro JM,Brenner BG, Wainberg MA. The influence of protease inhibitor profiles on selection of HIV therapy in treatment-naïve patients. Antivir Ther 9:301–14, 2004.

Yeni P. Tipranovir: a protease inhibitor from a new class with distinct antiviral activity. J Acquir Immune Defic Syndr 34 (Suppl 1):S91–4, 2003.

Website: www.aptivus.com

TMP–SMX (Bactrim, Septra)

Drug Class: Folate antagonist/sulfonamide.

Usual Dose: 2.5–5 mg/kg (IV/PO) q6h.

"Usual dose" assumes normal renal/hepatic function. * For renal insufficiency, give usual dose × 1 followed by maintenance dose per CrCl. For dialysis patients, dose the same as for CrCl < 10 mL/min and give supplemental (post-HD/PD dose) immediately after dialysis. CrCl = creatinine clearance; CVVH = continuous veno-venous hemofiltration; HD/PD = hemodialysis/peritoneal dialysis. See pp. 509–513 for explanations, pp. xi–xii for abbreviations; Linezolid (↑ risk of serotonin syndrome, see p. 620).

Spectrum: (see ***Susceptibility Profiles*** pp. 183–187).

Pharmacokinetic Parameters:

Peak serum level: 2–8/40–80 mcg/ml

Bioavailability: 98%

Excreted unchanged (urine): 67/85%

Serum half-life (normal/ESRD): (10/8)/40–80 hrs

Plasma protein binding: 44–70%

Volume of distribution (V_d): 1.8/0.3 L/kg

Primary Mode of Elimination: Renal

Dosage Adjustments*

CrCl 50–80 mL/min	No change
CrCl 10–50 mL/min	1.25–2.5 mg/kg (IV/PO) q6h
CrCl < 10 mL/min	Avoid (except for PCP use 1.25–2.5 mg/kg [IV/PO] q8h)
Post–HD dose	5 mg/kg (IV/PO)
Post–PD dose	0.16 mg/kg (IV/PO)
CVVH dose	2.5 mg/kg (IV/PO) q6h
Moderate or severe hepatic insufficiency	No change

Drug Interactions: *TMP component:* Azathioprine (leukopenia); amantadine, dapsone, digoxin, methotrexate, phenytoin, rifampin, zidovudine (↑ interacting drug levels, nystagmus with phenytoin); diuretics (↑ serum K^+ with K^+-sparing diuretics, ↓ serum Na^+ with thiazide diuretics); warfarin (↑ INR, bleeding). *SMX component*: Cyclosporine (↓ cyclosporine levels); phenytoin (↑ phenytoin levels, nystagmus, ataxia); methotrexate (↑ antifolate activity); sulfonylureas, thiopental (↑ interacting drug effect); warfarin (↑ INR, bleeding).

Adverse Effects: Common cause of drug induced aseptic meningitis.

TMP: Folate deficiency, hyperkalemia

SMX: Leukopenia, thrombocytopenia, hemolytic anemia ± G6PD deficiency, aplastic anemia, ↑ SGOT/SGPT, severe hypersensitivity reactions (E. multiforme/Stevens–Johnson syndrome), ↑ risk of hypoglycemia in chronic renal failure.

Allergic Potential: Very high (SMX); none (TMP)

Safety in Pregnancy: X

Comments: Drug fever/rash increased in HIV/AIDS. **Excellent bioavailability (IV = PO).** 1 SS tablet = 80 mg TMP + 400 mg SMX. 1 DS tablet = 160 mg TMP + 800 mg SMX. 1 SS tablet (PO) q6h = 10 mg/kg (IV) q24h. 1 DS tablet (PO) q6h = 20 mg/kg (IV) q24h. **Oral TMP–SMX has the same spectrum as ceftriaxone IV. In sulfa allergic patients, use TMP which is equally effective of TMP–SMX.** Meningeal dose = 5 mg/kg (IV/PO) q6h.

Cerebrospinal Fluid Penetration:

Non-Inflamed meninges = 40%

Inflamed meninges = 40%

Bile Penetration: 100%

(also see ***Antibiotic Pearls & Pitfalls*** p. 503).

REFERENCES:

Bouza E. New therapeutic choices for infections caused by methicillin-resistant *Staphylococcus aureus*. Clin Microbiol Infect Dis 15:44–52, 2009.

Cockerill FR, Edson RS. Trimethoprim-sulfamethoxazole. Mayo Clin Proc 66:1260–9, 1991.

Cunha BA. Oral Antibiotic Therapy of Serious Systemic Infections. Med Clin N Am 90:1197–1222, 2006.

Euga G, Murillo O, Fernandez-Sabe N, et al. Treatment of Chronic Staphylococcal Osteomyelitis: Intravenous or Oral? How Long? Antimicrob Agents Chemother 53:2672–2676, 2009.

"Usual dose" assumes normal renal/hepatic function. * For renal insufficiency, give usual dose × 1 followed by maintenance dose per CrCl. For dialysis patients, dose the same as for CrCl < 10 mL/min and give supplemental (post-HD/PD dose) immediately after dialysis. CrCl = creatinine clearance; CVVH = continuous veno-venous hemofiltration; HD/PD = hemodialysis/peritoneal dialysis. See pp. 509–513 for explanations, pp. xi–xii for abbreviations; Linezolid (↑ risk of serotonin syndrome, see p. 620).

Francis P, Patel VB, Bill PL, et al. Oral trimethoprim-sulfamethoxazole in the treatment of cerebral toxoplasmosis in AIDS patients-a prospective study. S Afr Med J 94:51–3, 2004.

Giannakopoulos G Johnson ES. TMP–SMX. Antibiotics for Clinicians 1:63–9, 1997.

Hooton TM, Besser R, Foxman B, et al. Acute uncomplicated cystitis in an era of increasing antibiotic resistance: a proposed approach to empirical therapy. Clin Infect Dis 39:75–80, 2004.

Lundstrom TS, Sobel JD. Vancomycin, trimethoprim-sulfamethoxazole, and rifampin. Infect Dis Clin North Am 9:747–67, 1995.

Masters PA, O'Bryan TA, Zurlo JM, et al. Trimethoprim-sulfamethoxazole revisited. Arch Intern Med 163:402–10, 2003.

McLaughlin SP, Carson CC. Urinary tract infections in women. Med Clin North Am 88:417–29, 2004.

Miller LG, Tang AW. Treatment of uncomplicated urinary tract infections in an era of increasing antimicrobial resistance. Mayo Clin Proc 79:1048–53, 2004.

Nguyen S, Pasquet A, Legout L, et al. Efficacy and tolerance of rifampin-linezolid compared with rifampin-cotrimoxazole combinations in prolonged oral therapy for bone and joint infections. Clin Microbiol Infect Dis 15:1163–1169, 2009.

Nicolle LE. Urinary tract infection: traditional pharmacologic therapies. Am J Med 113(Suppl 1A):35S–44S, 2002.

Para MF, Dohn M, Frame P, et al., for the ACTG 268 dapsone study Team. Reduced toxicity with gradual initiation of trimethoprim-sulfamethoxazole as primary prophylaxis for Pneumocystis carinii pneumonia: AIDS Clinical Trials Group 268. J Acquire Immune Defic Syndr 24:337–43, 2000.

Schaffer AJ. Empiric use of trimethoprim-sulfamethoxazole (TMP–SMX) in the treatment of women with uncomplicated urinary tract infections, in a geographic area with a high prevalence of TMP–SMX-resistance uropathogens. J Urol 168 (4 Pt 1):1652–3, 2002.

Thomas CF Jr, Limper AH. Pneumocystis pneumonia. N Engl J Med 350:2487–98, 2004.

Website: www.pdr.net

Tobramycin (Nebcin)

Drug Class: Aminoglycoside.

Usual Dose: 5 mg/kg (IV) q24h or 240 mg (IV) q24h (preferred over q8h dosing) (see comments).

Spectrum: (see ***Susceptibility Profiles*** pp. 194–199).

Pharmacokinetic Parameters:

Peak serum levels: 4–8 mcg/ml (q8h dosing); 16–24 mcg/ml (q24h dosing)

Bioavailability: Not applicable

Excreted unchanged (urine): 95%

Serum half-life (normal/ESRD): 2.5/56 hrs

Plasma protein binding: 10%

Volume of distribution (V_d): 0.24 L/kg

Primary Mode of Elimination: Renal

Dosage Adjustments*

CrCl 50–80 mL/min	2.5 mg/kg (IV) q24h or 120 mg (IV) q24h
CrCl 10–50 mL/min	2.5 mg/kg (IV) q48h or 120 mg (IV) q48h
CrCl < 10 mL/min	1.25 mg/kg (IV) q48h or 60 mg (IV) q48h
Post–HD dose	1 mg/kg (IV) or 80 mg (IV)
Post–HFHD dose	2.5 mg/kg (IV) or 120 mg (IV)
Post–PD dose	0.5 mg/kg (IV) or 40 mg (IV) or 2–4 mg/L in dialysate q24h
CVVH dose	2.5 mg/kg (IV) or 120 mg (IV) q48h
Moderate hepatic insufficiency	No change
Severe hepatic insufficiency	No change

"Usual dose" assumes normal renal/hepatic function. * For renal insufficiency, give usual dose × 1 followed by maintenance dose per CrCl. For dialysis patients, dose the same as for CrCl < 10 mL/min and give supplemental (post-HD/PD dose) immediately after dialysis. CrCl = creatinine clearance; CVVH = continuous veno-venous hemofiltration; HD/PD = hemodialysis/peritoneal dialysis. See pp. 509–513 for explanations, pp. xi–xii for abbreviations; Linezolid (↑ risk of serotonin syndrome, see p. 620).

Drug Interactions: Amphotericin B, cyclosporine, enflurane, methoxyflurane, NSAIDs, polymyxin B, radiographic contrast, vancomycin (↑ nephrotoxicity); cis-platinum (↑ nephrotoxicity, ↑ ototoxicity); loop diuretics (↑ ototoxicity); neuromuscular blocking agents (↑ apnea, prolonged paralysis); non-polarizing muscle relaxants (↑ apnea).

Adverse Effects: Neuromuscular blockade with rapid infusion/absorption. Nephrotoxicity only with prolonged/extremely high serum trough levels; may cause reversible non–oliguric renal failure (ATN). Ototoxicity associated with prolonged/extremely high peak serum levels (usually irreversible): Cochlear toxicity (1/3 of ototoxicity) manifests as decreased high frequency hearing, but deafness is unusual. Vestibular toxicity (2/3 of ototoxicity) develops before ototoxicity, and typically manifests as tinnitus.

Allergic Potential: Low

Safety in Pregnancy: C

Comments: Single daily dosing greatly reduces nephrotoxic/ototoxic potential. Incompatible with solutions containing β–lactams, erythromycin, chloramphenicol, furosemide, sodium bicarbonate. IV infusion should be given slowly over 1 hour. May be given IM. ***Avoid intraperitoneal infusion due to risk of neuromuscular blockade. Avoid intratracheal/ aerosolized intrapulmonary instillation, which predisposes to antibiotic resistance***. V_d increases with edema/ascites, trauma, burns, cystic fibrosis; may require ↑ dose. V_d decreases with dehydration, obesity; may require ↓ dose. **Renal cast counts are the best indicator of aminoglycoside nephrotoxicity, not serum creatinine**. Dialysis removes ~ 1/3 of tobramycin from serum. Tobramycin nebulizer dose: 300 mg via nebulizer q12h ***(not recommended due to ↑ risk of resistance)***.

CAPD dose: 2–4 mg/L in dialysate (I.P.) with each exchange.

Therapeutic Serum Concentrations (for therapeutic efficacy, *not toxicity*):

Peak (q24h/q8h dosing) = 16–24/8–10 mcg/ml
Trough (q24h/q8h dosing) = 0/1–2 mcg/ml

Synergy dose: 2.5 mg/kg (IV) q24h or 120 mg (IV) q24h

Intrathecal (IT) dose: 5 mg (IT) q24h

Cerebrospinal Fluid Penetration:
Non-inflamed meninges = 0%
Inflamed meninges = 20%

Bile Penetration: 30%

(also see ***Antibiotic Pearls & Pitfalls*** pp. 495–508).

REFERENCES:

Begg EJ, Barclay ML. Aminoglycosides - 50 years on. Br J Clin Pharmacol 39:597–603, 1995.

Buijk SE Mouton JW, Gyssens IC, et al. Experience with a once-daily dosing program of aminoglycosides in critically ill patients. Intensive Care Med 28:936–42, 2002.

Cheer SM, Waugh J, Noble S. Inhaled tobramycin (TOBI): a review of its use in the management of Pseudomonas aeruginosa infections in patients with cystic fibrosis. Drugs. 63:2501–20, 2003.

Cunha BA. Aminoglycosides: Current role in antimicrobial therapy. Pharmacotherapy 8:334–50, 1988.

Dupuis LL, Sung L, Taylor T, et al. Tobramycin pharmacokinetics in children with febrile neutropenia undergoing stem cell transplantation once-daily versus thrice-daily administration. Pharmacotherapy 24:564–73, 2004.

Edson RS, Terrel CL. The aminoglycosides. Mayo Clin Proc 74:519–28, 1999.

Geller DE, Pistlick WH, Nardella PA, et al. Pharmacokinetics and bioavailability of aerosolized tobramycin in cystic fibrosis. Chest 122:219–26, 2002.

Gilbert DN. Once-daily aminoglycoside therapy. Antimicrob Agents Chemother 35:399–405, 1991.

Hustinx WN, Hoepelman IM. Aminoglycoside dosage regimens: Is once a day enough? Clin Pharmacokinet 25:427–32, 1993.

Kahler DA, Schowengerdt KO, Fricker FJ, et al. Toxic serum trough concentrations after administration of nebulized tobramycin. Pharmacotherapy. 23:543–5, 2003.

Lortholary O, Tod M, Cohen Y, et al. Aminoglycosides. Med Clin North Am 79:761–87, 1995.

McCormack JP, Jewesson PJ. A critical reevaluation of the "therapeutic range" of aminoglycosides. Clin Infect Dis 14:320–39, 1992.

Moss RB. Long-term benefits of inhaled tobramycin in adolescent patients with cystic fibrosis. Chest 121:55–63, 2002.

Whitehead A, Conway SP, Etherington C, et al. Once-daily tobramycin in the treatment of adult patients with cystic fibrosis. Eur Respir J 19:303–9, 2002.

Wood GC, Chapman JL, Boucher BA, et al. Tobramycin bladder irrigation for treating a urinary tract infection in a critically ill patient. Ann Pharmacother 38:1318–9, 2004.

Website: www.pdr.net

Trimethoprim (Proloprim, Trimpex)

Drug Class: Folate antagonist.
Usual Dose: 100 mg (PO) q12h (see comments).
Pharmacokinetic Parameters:
Peak serum level: 2–8 mcg/ml
Bioavailability: 98%
Excreted unchanged (urine): 67%
Serum half-life (normal/ESRD): 8/24 hrs
Plasma protein binding: 44%
Volume of distribution (V_d): 1.8 L/kg
Primary Mode of Elimination: Renal
Dosage Adjustments*

CrCl 50–80 mL/min	No change
CrCl 10–50 mL/min	50 mg (PO) q12h
CrCl < 10 mL/min	Avoid (except for PCP, see TMP–SMX)
Post–HD dose	Avoid (except for PCP, see TMP–SMX)
Post–PD dose	100 mg (PO)
CVVH dose	50 mg (PO) q12h
Moderate or severe hepatic insufficiency	No change

Drug Interactions: Azathioprine (leukopenia); amantadine, dapsone, digoxin, methotrexate, phenytoin, rifampin, zidovudine (↑ interacting drug levels, nystagmus with phenytoin); diuretics (↑ serum K^+ with K^+-sparing diuretics, ↓ serum Na^+ with thiazide diuretics); warfarin (↑ INR, bleeding).
Adverse Effects: Folate deficiency, hyperkalemia
Allergic Potential: Low
Safety in Pregnancy: X
Comments: Useful in sulfa-allergic patients unable to take TMP–SMX. PCP dose: 5 mg/kg (PO) q8h plus dapsone 100 mg (PO) q24h.
Meningeal dose: 5 mg/kg or 300 mg (PO) q6h.
Cerebrospinal Fluid Penetration: 40%
Bile Penetration: 100%

REFERENCES:

Brogden RN, Carmine AA, Heel RC, et al. Trimethoprim: A review of its antibacterial activity, pharmacokinetics and therapeutic use in urinary tract infections. Drugs 23:405–30, 1982.

Friesen WT, Hekster YA, Vree TB. Trimethoprim: Clinical use and pharmacokinetics. Drug Intelligence & Clinical Pharmacy 15:325–30, 1981.

Neu HC. Trimethoprim alone for treatment of urinary tract infection. Rev Infect Dis 4:366–71, 1982.

Website: www.pdr.net

"Usual dose" assumes normal renal/hepatic function. * For renal insufficiency, give usual dose × 1 followed by maintenance dose per CrCl. For dialysis patients, dose the same as for CrCl < 10 mL/min and give supplemental (post-HD/PD dose) immediately after dialysis. CrCl = creatinine clearance; CVVH = continuous veno-venous hemofiltration; HD/PD = hemodialysis/peritoneal dialysis. See pp. 509–513 for explanations, pp. xi–xii for abbreviations; Linezolid (↑ risk of serotonin syndrome, see p. 620).

Trimethoprim-Sulfamethoxazole, see TMP–SMX (Bactrim, Septra)

Valacyclovir (Valtrex)

Drug Class: HSV, VZV Antiviral (see comments).

Usual Dose:

HSV–1: HSV–1 late onset VAP**:** 1 gm (PO) q8h × 10 days.

VZV: *VZV Pneumonia*: 1–2 gm (PO) q8h × 10 days.

Pharmacokinetic Parameters:

Peak serum level: 3.7–5 mcg/ml

Bioavailability: 55%

Excreted unchanged (urine): 1%

Serum half-life (normal/ESRD): 3/14 hrs

Plasma protein binding: 15%

Volume of distribution (V_d): 0.7 L/kg

Primary Mode of Elimination: Renal

Dosage Adjustments* (based on 1 gm q8h):

CrCl 10–50 mL/min	1 gm (PO) q12h
CrCl < 10 mL/min	500 mg (PO) q24h
Post–HD dose	1 gm (PO)
Post–PD dose	500 mg
CVVH dose	500 mg (PO) q24h
Moderate hepatic insufficiency	No change
Severe hepatic insufficiency	No change

Drug Interactions: Cimetidine, probenecid (↑ acyclovir levels).

Adverse Effects: Headache, nausea, diarrhea, abdominal pain, weakness. Rarely, HUS/TTP (only in HIV).

Allergic Potential: Low

Safety in Pregnancy: B

Comments: Converted to acyclovir in liver. ***Highly active against HSV and VZV. Some activity against CMV. No activity against EBV, RSV or adenoviruses.***

Meningeal dose = 1 gm (PO) q6h.

Cerebrospinal Fluid Penetration: 50%

REFERENCES:

Acost EP, Fletcher CV. Valacyclovir. Ann Pharmacotherapy 31:185–91, 1997.

Alrabiah FA, Sacks SL. New antiherpesvirus agents: Their targets and therapeutic potential. Drugs 52:17–32, 1996.

Dworkin RH, Johnson RW, Breuer J, et al. Recommendations for the management of herpes zoster. Clin Infect Dis 44(S1):S1–S26, 2007.

Fiddian P, Sabin CA, Griffiths PD. Valacyclovir provides optimum acyclovir exposure for prevention of cytomegalovirus and related outcomes after argan transplantation. J Infect Dis 186(Suppl 1):S110–5, 2002.

Ljungman P, de La Camara R, Milpied N, et al. Randomized study of valacyclovir as prophylaxis against cytomegalovirus reactivation in recipients of allogeneic bone marrow transplants. Blood 99:3050–6, 2002.

MacDougall C, Guglielmo BJ. Pharmacokinetics of valaciclovir. J Antimicrob Chemother 53:899–901, 2004.

Perry CM, Faulds D. Valacyclovir: A review of its antiviral activity, pharmacokinetic properties, and therapeutic efficacy in herpesvirus infections. Drugs 52:754–72, 1996.

Website: www.valtrex.com

Valganciclovir (Valcyte)

Drug Class: CMV, HSV, HHV-6 antiviral (see comments).

Usual Dose: 900 mg (PO) q12h × 21 days (induction), then 900 mg (PO) q24h for life (maintenance). 900 mg dose taken as two 450-mg tablets once daily with food.

Pharmacokinetic Parameters:

Peak serum level: 5.6 mcg/ml

Bioavailability: 59.4%

"Usual dose" assumes normal renal/hepatic function. * For renal insufficiency, give usual dose × 1 followed by maintenance dose per CrCl. For dialysis patients, dose the same as for CrCl < 10 mL/min and give supplemental (post-HD/PD dose) immediately after dialysis. CrCl = creatinine clearance; CVVH = continuous veno-venous hemofiltration; HD/PD = hemodialysis/peritoneal dialysis. See pp. 509–513 for explanations, pp. xi–xii for abbreviations; Linezolid (↑ risk of serotonin syndrome, see p. 620).

Excreted unchanged (urine): 90%
Serum half-life (normal/ESRD): 4.1/67.5 hrs
Plasma protein binding: 1%
Volume of distribution (V_d): 15.3 L/kg
Primary Mode of Elimination: Renal
Dosage Adjustments*

CrCl 40–60 mL/min	450 mg (PO) q12h (induction), then 450 mg (PO) q24h (maintenance)
CrCl 25–40 mL/min	450 mg (PO) q24h (induction), then 450 mg (PO) q48h (maintenance)
CrCl 10–25 mL/min	450 mg (PO) q48h (induction), then 450 mg (PO) 2x/ week (maintenance)
CrCl < 10 mL/min	Avoid
Post–HD dose	Avoid
Post–PD dose	Use CrCl 25–40 mL/ min dose
CVVH dose	No information
Moderate hepatic insufficiency	No change
Severe hepatic insufficiency	No change

Drug Interactions: Cytotoxic drugs (may produce additive toxicity: stomatitis, bone marrow depression, alopecia); imipenem (↑ risk of seizures); probenecid (↑ valganciclovir levels); zidovudine (↓ valganciclovir levels, ↑ zidovudine levels, possible neutropenia).
Adverse Effects: Drug fever/rash, diarrhea, nausea, vomiting, GI upset, leukopenia, anemia, thrombocytopenia, paresthesias/peripheral neuropathy, retinal detachment, aplastic anemia.
Allergic Potential: Low
Safety in Pregnancy: C
Comments: Valganciclovir exposures (AUC) larger than for IV ganciclovir. Tablets should be taken with food. Valganciclovir is rapidly hydrolyzed to ganciclovir. Not interchangeable on a tablet-to-tablet basis with oral ganciclovir. Much higher bioavailability than ganciclovir capsules; serum concentration equivalent to IV ganciclovir. Indicated for induction/maintenance therapy of CMV infection. Preferred to ganciclovir for all indications except for CMV prophylaxis in liver transplants. ***Highly active for CMV, HHV-6, and HSV. Some activity against VZV and adenoviruses. No activity against EBV or RSV.*** Meningeal dose = usual dose.
Cerebrospinal Fluid Penetration: 70%

REFERENCES:

Cocohoba JM, McNicholl IR. Valganciclovir: an advance in cytomegalovirus therapeutics. Ann Pharmacother 36:1075–9, 2002.

Czock D, Scholle C, Rasche FM, et al. Pharmacokinetics of valganciclovir and ganciclovir in renal impairment. Clin Pharmacol Ther 72:142–50, 2002.

Jung D, Dorr A. Single-dose pharmacokinetics of valganciclovir in HIV and CMV seropositive subjects. J Clin Pharmacol 39:800–804, 1999.

Khoury JA, Storch GA, Bohl DL, et al. Prophylactic verus preemptive oral valganciclovir for the management of cytomegalovirus infection in adult renal transplant recipients. Am J Transplant. 6:2134–43, 2006.

Len O, Gavalda J, Agnado, JM, et al. Valganciclovir as treatment for cytomegalovirus disease in solid organ transplant recipients. Clin Infect Dis 46:20–27, 2008.

Lopau K, Greser A, Wanner C. Efficacy and safety of preemptive anti-CMV therapy with valganciclovir after kidney transplantation. Clin Transplant 21:80–85, 2007.

"Usual dose" assumes normal renal/hepatic function. * For renal insufficiency, give usual dose × 1 followed by maintenance dose per CrCl. For dialysis patients, dose the same as for CrCl < 10 mL/min and give supplemental (post-HD/PD dose) immediately after dialysis. CrCl = creatinine clearance; CVVH = continuous veno-venous hemofiltration; HD/PD = hemodialysis/peritoneal dialysis. See pp. 509–513 for explanations, pp. xi–xii for abbreviations; Linezolid (↑ risk of serotonin syndrome, see p. 620).

Razonable RR, Paya CV. Valganciclovir for the prevention and treatment of cytomegalovirus disease in immunocompromised hosts. Expert Rev Anti Infect Ther 2:27–41, 2004.

Rubin RH. Cytomegalovirus infection in the liver transplant recipient. Epidemiology, pathogenesis, and clinical management. Clin Liver Dis 1:439–52, 2004.

Slifkin M, Doron S, Snydman DR. Viral prophylaxis in organ transplant patients. Drugs 64:2763–92, 2004.

Taber DJ, Ashcraft E, Baillie GM, et al. Valganciclovir prophylaxis in patients at high risk for the development of cytomegalovirus disease. Transpl Infect Dis 6:101–9, 2004.

Website: www.rocheusa.com/products/

Vancomycin (Vancocin)

Drug Class: Glycopeptide.
Usual Dose: 1 gm (IV) q12h (see comments).
Spectrum: (see ***Susceptibility Profiles*** pp. 194–199).
Pharmacokinetic Parameters:
Peak serum level: 63 mcg/ml
Bioavailability: IV (not applicable)/PO (0%)
Excreted unchanged (urine): 90%
Serum half-life (normal/ESRD): 6/180 hrs
Plasma protein binding: 55%
Volume of distribution (V_d): 0.7 L/kg
Primary Mode of Elimination: Renal
Dosage Adjustments*

CrCl 50–80 mL/min	500 mg (IV) q12h
CrCl 10–50 mL/min	500 mg (IV) q24h
CrCl < 10 mL/min	1 gm (IV) qweek
Post–HD dose	None
Post–HFHD dose	500 mg (IV)
Post–PD dose	None
Post–SLEDD dose	500 mg (IV)
CVVH dose	1 gm (IV) q24h
Moderate hepatic insufficiency	No change
Severe hepatic insufficiency	No change

Drug Interactions: Aminoglycosides, amphotericin B, polymyxin B (↑ nephrotoxicity).
Adverse Effects: "Red man/neck syndrome" with rapid IV infusion (histamine mediated), leukopenia, thrombocytopenia, cardiac arrest, hypotension.
Allergic Potential: Low
Safety in Pregnancy: C
Comments: Not nephrotoxic. "Red man/neck syndrome" can be prevented/minimized by infusing IV vancomycin slowly over 1–2 hours. Intraperitoneal absorption = 40%. **IV vancomycin use increases VRE prevalence. C. difficile diarrhea dose:** oral vancomycin 250 mg (PO) q6h. *If no response in 72 hours, ≠ dose to 500 mg (PO) q6h to complete therapy.* **C. difficile relapse dose:** 500 mg (PO) q6h × 1 month and reevaluate. Should C. difficle later recur, treat × 2 or 3 months with 500 mg (PO) q6h. **Do *not* taper dose.** Vancomycin (IV/PO) is ineffective for C. difficile colitis. Vancomycin doesn't penetrate well into the CSF with non-inflamed meninges. For therapeutic CSF concentrations, use IT administration. **Intrathecal (IT) dose:** 20 mg (IT) in preservative free NaCl.
Therapeutic Serum Concentrations (for therapeutic efficacy, *not toxicity*):
Peak = 25–40 mcg/ml
Trough = 5–12 mcg/ml
There are **no convincing data that vancomycin is ototoxic or nephrotoxic. CrCl, not serum levels, should be used to adjust vancomycin dosing**. Prolonged/high dose vancomycin (60 mg/kg/day or 2 gm [IV] q12h) has been

---

"Usual dose" assumes normal renal/hepatic function. * For renal insufficiency, give usual dose × 1 followed by maintenance dose per CrCl. For dialysis patients, dose the same as for CrCl < 10 mL/min and give supplemental (post-HD/PD dose) immediately after dialysis. CrCl = creatinine clearance; CVVH = continuous veno-venous hemofiltration; HD/PD = hemodialysis/peritoneal dialysis. See pp. 509–513 for explanations, pp. xi–xii for abbreviations; Linezolid (↑ risk of serotonin syndrome, see p. 620).

useful in treating S. aureus osteomyelitis, S. aureus infections with high MICs (VISA), and infections in difficult-to-penetrate tissues without toxicity. In bone or CSF, vancomycin tissue concentrations are ~ 15% of serum levels.

Cerebrospinal Fluid Penetration:
Non-Inflamed meninges = 0%
Inflamed meninges = 15%

Bile Penetration: 50%

(also see ***Antibiotic Pearls & Pitfalls*** p. 505).

REFERENCES:

Anderson BJ, Allegaert K, Van den Anker JN, Cossey V, et al. Vancomycin pharmacokinetics in preterm neonates and the prediction of adult clearance. Br J Clin Pharmacol 63:75–84, 2007.

Bouza E. New therapeutic choices for infections caused by methicillin-resistant *Staphylococcus aureus*. Clin Microbiol Infect Dis 15:44–52, 2009.

Cantu TG, Yamanaka-Yuen NA, Lietman PS. Serum vancomycin concentrations: Reappraisal of their clinical value. Clin Infect Dis 18:533–43, 1994.

Cosgrove SE, Carroll KC, Perl TM. Staphylococcus aureus with reduced susceptibility to vancomycin. Clin Infect Dis 39:539–45, 2004.

Cruciani M, Gatti G, Lazzarini L, et al. Penetration of vancomycin into human lung tissue. Journal of Antimicrobial Chemotherapy. 38:865–69, 1996.

Cunha BA. Vancomycin Revisisted: A Reappraisal of Clinical Use. Critical Care Clinics of North America 24:394–420, 2008.

Cunha BA, Mohan SS, Hamid N, McDermott GP, Daniels P. Cost Ineffectiveness of Serum Vancomycin Levels. Eur J Clin Microbiol Infect Dis 13:509–511, 2007.

Cunha BA. Vancomycin serum levels: unnecessary, unhelpful, and costly. Antibiotics for Clinicians 8:273–77, 2004.

Cunha BA. Vancomycin. Med Clin North Am 79:817–31, 1995.

Cunha BA, Deglin J, Chow M, et al. Pharmacokinetics of vancomycin in patients undergoing chronic hemodialysis. Rev Infect Dis 3:269–72, 1981.

Decker BS, Mueller BA, Sowinski KM. Drug dosing considerations in alternative hemodialysis. Adv Chronic Kidney Dis 14:e17–e26, 2007.

DelDot ME, Lipman J, Tett SE. Vancomycin pharmacokinetics in critically ill patients receiving continuous venovenous haemodiafiltration. Br J Clin Pharmacol 58:259–68, 2004.

del Mar Fernandez de Gatta Garcia, Revilla N, Calvo MV, et al. Pharmacokinetic/pharmacodynamic analysis of vancomycin in ICU patient. Intensive Care Med 33:279–285, 2007.

Deresinski S. Vancomycin: does it still have a role as an antistaphylococcal agent? Expert Rev Anti Infect Ther 5:393–401, 2007.

El Amari EB, Vuagnat A, Stern R, et al. High versus standard dose vancomycin for osteomyelitis. Scand J Infect Dis 36:712–7, 2004.

Hidayat LK, Hsu DI, Quist R, Shriner KA, Wong-Beringer A. High-Dose Vancomycin Therapy for Methicillin-Resistant Staphylococcus aureus Infections. Arch Inter Med 166:2138–44, 2006.

Johnson JR. Vancomycin levels, efficacy, and toxicity. Arch Intern Med 167:1207–1209, 2007.

Krol V, Cunha BA, Schoch PE, Klein NC. Appropriateness of empiric gentamicin and vancomycin therapy for bacteremias in chronic dialysis outpatient units in the era of antibiotic resistance. J Chemother 18:490–3, 2006.

Menzies D. Goel K, Cunha BA. Vancomycin. Antibiotics for Clinicians 2:97–9, 1998.

Moellering RC Jr. Monitoring serum vancomycin levels: climbing the mountain because it is there? Clin Infect Dis 18:544–6, 1994.

Moreillon P, Wilson WR, Leclercq R, et al. Single-dose oral amoxicillin or linezolid for prophylaxis of experimental endocarditis due to vancomycin-susceptible and vancomycin-resistant Enterococcus faecalis. Antimicrob Agents Chemother 51:1661–1665, 2007.

Okamoto H. Vancomycin-induced immune thrombocytopenia. N Engl J Med 356:2537–2538, 2007.

"Usual dose" assumes normal renal/hepatic function. * For renal insufficiency, give usual dose × 1 followed by maintenance dose per CrCl. For dialysis patients, dose the same as for CrCl < 10 mL/min and give supplemental (post-HD/PD dose) immediately after dialysis. CrCl = creatinine clearance; CVVH = continuous veno-venous hemofiltration; HD/PD = hemodialysis/peritoneal dialysis. See pp. 509–513 for explanations, pp. xi–xii for abbreviations; Linezolid (↑ risk of serotonin syndrome, see p. 620).

Patanwala AE, Erstad BL, Nix DE. Cost-effectiveness of linezolid and vancomycin in the treatment of surgical site infections. Curr Med Res Opin 23:185–193, 2007.

Patel N, Lubanski P, Ferro S, et al. Correlation between Vancomycin MIC Values and Those of Other Agents against Gram-Positive Bacteria among Patients with Bloodstream Infections Caused by Methicillin-Resistant *Staphylococcus aureus*. Antimicrob Agents Chemother 53:5141–5144, 2009.

Pope SD, Roecker A. Vancomycin for treatment of invasive, multi-drug resistant Staphylococcus aureus infections. Exp Opin Pharmacother 8:1245–1261, 2007.

Ricard JD, Wolff M, Lacerade JC, et al. Levels of vancomycin in cerebrospinal fluid of adult patients receiving adjunctive corticosteroids to treat pneumococcal meningitis: a prospective multicenter observational study. Clin Infect Dis 44:250–255, 2007.

Rybak MJ. The pharmacokinetic and pharmacodynamic properties of vancomycin. Clin Infect Dis 42:S35–9, 2006.

Rybak MJ, Lomaestro B, Rotschafer J, et al. Continuous Infusion of Vancomycin Less Effective and Safe than Intermittent Infusion, Based on Pharmacodynamic and Pharmacokinetic Principles. Clin Infect Dis 49:1964, 2009.

Rybak MJ. Lomaestro B, Rotschafer JC, et al. Therapeutic Monitoring *of vancomycin* in adult patients: A concensus review of the American Society of Health-System Pharmacists, the Infectious Diseases Society of America, and the Society of Infectious Diseases Pharmacists. Am J Health-Syst Pharm 66:82–98, 2009.

Saribas S, Bagdatli Y. Vancomycin tolerance in enterococci. Chemotherapy 50:250–4, 2004.

Skhirtladze K, Hutschala, Fleck T, Thalhammer F, Ehrlich M, et al. Impaired Target Site Penetration of Vancomycin in Diabetic Patients following Cardiac Surgery. Antimicrob Agents Chemother 50:1372–75, 2006.

Stevens DL. The role of vancomycin in the treatment paradigm. Clin Infect Dis 42:S51–7, 2006.

Stryjewski ME, Szczech LA, Benjamin DK Jr, et al. Use of vancomycin or first-generation cephalosporins for the treatment of hemodialysis-dependent patients with methicillin-susceptible Staphylococcus aureus bacteremia. Clin Infect Dis 44:190–196, 2007.

Tenover FC, Moellering RC. The rationale for revising the clinical and laboratory standards institute vancomycin minimal inhibitory concentration interpretive criteria for staphylococcus aureus. Clin Infect Dis 44:1208–1215, 2007.

Valle MJ, Gonzalez-Lopez F, Dominquez-Gill Hurle A, et al. Pulmonary versus systemic delivery of antibiotics: comparison of vancomycin dispositions in the isolated rat lung. Antimicrob Agents and Chemother 51:3771–3774, 2007.

Von Drygalski A, Curtis BR, Bougie DW, et al. Vancomycin-Induced Immune Thrombocytopenia. N Engl J Med 356:904–10, 2007.

Wang G, Hindler JF, Ward KW, Bruckner DA. Increased Vancomycin MICs for Staphylococcus aureus Clinical Isolates from a University Hospital during a 5-Year Period. Journal of Clinical Microbiology. 44:3883–86, 2006.

Website: www.pdr.net

Voriconazole (Vfend)

Drug Class: Triazole antifungal.

Usual Dose: IV dosing: Loading dose of 6 mg/kg (IV) q12h × 1 day, then maintenance dose of 4 mg/kg (IV) q12h. Can switch to weight-based PO maintenance dosing anytime while on maintenance IV dose (see comments)
PO dosing: *Weight ≥ 40 kg*: Loading dose of 400 mg (PO) q12h × 1 day, then maintenance dose of 200 mg (PO) q12h. If response is inadequate, the dose may be increased to 300 mg (PO) q12h. *Weight* < 40 kg: Loading dose of 200 mg (PO) × 1 day, then maintenance dose of 100 mg (PO) q12h. If response is inadequate, the dose may be increased to 150 mg (PO) q12h. For chronic/non-life-threatening infections, loading dose may be given PO (see comments).

"Usual dose" assumes normal renal/hepatic function. * For renal insufficiency, give usual dose × 1 followed by maintenance dose per CrCl. For dialysis patients, dose the same as for CrCl < 10 mL/min and give supplemental (post-HD/PD dose) immediately after dialysis. CrCl = creatinine clearance; CVVH = continuous veno-venous hemofiltration; HD/PD = hemodialysis/peritoneal dialysis. See pp. 509–513 for explanations, pp. xi–xii for abbreviations; Linezolid (↑ risk of serotonin syndrome, see p. 620).

Pharmacokinetic Parameters:
Peak serum level: 2.3–4.7 mcg/ml
Bioavailability: 96%
Excreted unchanged (urine): 2%
Serum half-life (normal/ESRD): 6/6 hrs
Plasma protein binding: 58%
Volume of distribution (V_d): 4.6 L/kg
Primary Mode of Elimination: Hepatic
Dosage Adjustments*

CrCl 50–80 mL/min	No change
CrCl 10–50 mL/min	No change PO; do not use IV
CrCl < 10 mL/min	No change PO; do not use IV
Post–HD dose	Usual dose (IV/PO)
Post–PD dose	No information
CVVH dose	Use 10–50 mL/min dosing
Moderate hepatic insufficiency	6 mg/kg (IV) q12h × 1 day or 200 mg (PO) q12h × 1 day, then 2 mg/kg (IV) q12h or 100 mg (PO) q12h (> 40 kg)
Severe hepatic insufficiency	No information

Drug Interactions: Benzodiazepines, vinca alkaloids (↑ interacting drug levels); carbamazepine, ergot alkaloids, rifampin, rifabutin, sirolimus, long-acting barbiturates (contraindicated with voriconazole); cyclosporine, omeprazole (↑ interacting drug levels, ↓ interacting drug dose by 50%); tacrolimus (↑ tacrolimus levels, ↓ tacrolimus dose by 66%); phenytoin (↓ voriconazole levels); ↑ voriconazole dose from 4 mg/kg [IV] to 5 mg/kg [IV] and from 200 mg [PO] to 400 mg [PO]; warfarin (↑ INR); statins (↑ risk of rhabdomyolysis); dihydropyridine calcium channel blockers (hypotension); sulfonylureas (hypoglycemia). Voriconazole has not been studied with protease inhibitors or NNRTIs, but ↑ voriconazole levels are predicted (↑ hepatotoxicity/adverse effects).

Adverse Effects: ↑ SGOT/SGPT; visual events (blurring vision, ↑ brightness, pain; occurs soon after ingestion and usually resolves quickly (~ ½ hour), hallucinations, hypoglycemia, dose-dependent arrhythmias, ↑ QT_c interval; rash, including Stevens-Johnson Syndrome; photosensitivity reactions (avoid direct sunlight).
Allergic Potential: High
Safety in Pregnancy: D
Comments: If intolerance to therapy develops, the IV maintenance dose may be reduced to 3 mg/kg and the PO maintenance dose may be reduced in steps of 50 mg/d to a minimum of 200 mg/d q12h (weight ≥ 40 kg) or 100 mg q12h (weight < 40 kg). Non-linear kinetics (doubling of oral dose = 2.8-fold increase in serum levels). 10–15% of patients have serum levels > 6 mcg/ml. Food decreases bioavailability; take 1 hour before or after meals. Do not use IV voriconazole if CrCl < 50 mL/min to prevent accumulation of voriconazole IV vehicle, sulphobutyl ether cyclodextrin (SBECD); instead use oral formulation, which has no SBECD. Loading dose may be given PO for chronic/non-life-threatening infections. Because of visual effects, do not drive or operate machinery. Monitor LFTs before and during therapy. ***Highly active against C. albicans, non-albicans Candida, Aspergillus, Fusaria, and Pseudoallescheria/Scedosporium. Some***

"Usual dose" assumes normal renal/hepatic function. * For renal insufficiency, give usual dose × 1 followed by maintenance dose per CrCl. For dialysis patients, dose the same as for CrCl < 10 mL/min and give supplemental (post-HD/PD dose) immediately after dialysis. CrCl = creatinine clearance; CVVH = continuous veno-venous hemofiltration; HD/PD = hemodialysis/peritoneal dialysis. See pp. 509–513 for explanations, pp. xi–xii for abbreviations; Linezolid (↑ risk of serotonin syndrome, see p. 620).

activity against Penicillium marneffei. No activity against Mucor. **Most effective Aspergillus antifungal (IV/PO) available.**
Meningeal dose = usual dose.
Cerebrospinal Fluid Penetration: 90%

REFERENCES:

Alffenaar JWC, van Assen S, van der Werf TS. Omeprazole Significantly Reduces Poconazole Serum Through Level. Clin Infect Dis 48:839–840, 2009.

Bruggemann RJM, Alffenaar JWC, Blijlevens NMA, et al. Clinical Relevance of the Pharmoacokinetic Interactions of Azole Antifungal Drugs with Coadministered Agents. Clin Infect Dis 48:1441–1458, 2009.

Camuset J, Nunes H, Dombret MC, et al. Treatment of chronic pulmonary aspergillosis by voriconazole in nonimmunocompromised patients. Chest 131:1435–1441, 2007.

Capitano B, Potoski BA, Husain S, et al. Intrapulmonary penetration of voriconazole in patients receiving an oral prophylactic regimen. Antimicrob Agents Chemother 50:1878–80, 2006.

den Hollander JG, van Arkel C, Rijnders BJ, et al. Incidence of voriconazole hepatotoxicity during intravenous and oral treatment for invasive fungal infections. J Antimicrob Chemother 57:1248–50, 2006.

Denes E, Boumediene A, Durox H, et al. Voriconazole concentrations in synovial fluid and bone tissues. J Antimicrob Chemother 59:818–819, 2007.

Denning DW, Ribaud P, Milpied N, et al. Efficacy and safety of voriconazole in the treatment of acute invasive aspergillosis. Clin Infect Dis 34:563–71, 2002.

Dodds Ashley ES, Zaas AK, Fang AF, et al. Comparative pharmacokinetics of voriconazole administered orally as either crushed or whole tablets. Antimicrob Agents Chemother 51:877–880, 2007.

Dominguez-Gil A, Martin I, Garcia Vargas M, et al. Economic evaluation of voriconazole versus caspofungin for the treatment of aspergillosis in Spain. Clin Drug Investig 27:197–205, 2007.

Elter T, Sieniawski M, Gossmann A, et al. Voriconazole brain tissue levels in rhinocerebral aspergillosis in a successfully treated young woman. Int J Antimicrob Agents. 28:262–5, 2006.

Herbrecht R, Denning DW, Patterson TF, et al. Voriconazole versus amphotericin B for primary therapy of invasive aspergillosis. N Engl J Med 347:408–15, 2002.

Ho DY, Lee JD, Rosso F, et al. Treating disseminated fusariosis: amphotericin B, voriconazole or both? Mycoses. 50:227–231, 2007.

Hoffman HL, Rathbun RC. Review of the safety and efficacy of voriconazole. Expert Opin Investig Drugs 11:409–29, 2002.

Jain LR, Denning DW. The efficacy and tolerability of voriconazole in the treatment of chronic cavitary pulmonary aspergillosis. J Infect 52: e133–7, 2006.

Jurkunas UV, Langston DP, Colby K. Use of voriconazole in the treatment of fungal keratitis. Int Ophthalmol Clin 47:47–59, 2007.

Keirns J, Sawamoto T, Holum M, et al. Steady-state pharmacokinetics of micafungin and voriconazole after separate and concomitant dosing in healthy adults. Antimicrob Agents Chemother 51:787–790, 2007.

Leveque D, Nivoix Y, Jehl F, Herbrecht R. Clinical pharmacokinetics of voriconazole. Int J Antimicrob Agents. 27:274–84, 2006.

Liu P, Foster G, Labadie R, et al. Pharmacokinetic interaction between voriconazole and methadone at steady state in patients on methadone therapy. Antimcrob Agents Chemother 51:110–118, 2007.

Poza G, Montoya J, Redondo C, et al. Meningitis caused by Pseudallescheria boydii treated with voriconazole. Clin Infect Dis 30:981–2, 2000.

Sambatakou H, Dupont B, Lode H, Denning DW. Voriconazole treatment for subacute invasive and chronic pulmonary aspergillosis. Am J Med 119:527, 2006.

Schwartz S, Ruhnke M, Ribaud P, et al. Improved outcome in central nervous system aspergillosis, using voriconazole treatment. Amer Soc of Hematology. 106:2641–5, 2006.

"Usual dose" assumes normal renal/hepatic function. * For renal insufficiency, give usual dose × 1 followed by maintenance dose per CrCl. For dialysis patients, dose the same as for CrCl < 10 mL/min and give supplemental (post-HD/PD dose) immediately after dialysis. CrCl = creatinine clearance; CVVH = continuous veno-venous hemofiltration; HD/PD = hemodialysis/peritoneal dialysis. See pp. 509–513 for explanations, pp. xi–xii for abbreviations; Linezolid (↑ risk of serotonin syndrome, see p. 620).

Scott LJ, Simpson D. Voriconazole: a review of its use in the management of invasive fungal infections. Drugs 67:269–98, 2007.

Schwartz S, Ruhnke M, Ribaud P, et al. Poor efficacy of amphotericin B-based therapy in CNS aspergillosis. Mycoses 50:196–200, 2007.

Shehab N, DePestel DD, Mackler ER, et al. Institutional experience with voriconazole compared with liposomal amphotericin B as empiric therapy for febrile neutropenia. Pharmacotherapy 27:970–979, 2007.

Smith J, Safdar N, Knasinski V, et al. Voriconazole Therapeutic Drug Monitoring. Antimicrob Agents Chemother 50:1570–72, 2006.

Supparatpinyo K, Schlamm HT. Voriconazole as therapy for systemic Penicillium marneffei infections in AIDS patients. Am J Trop Med Hyg 77:350–353, 2007.

Tan K, Brayshaw N, Tomaszewski K, et al. Investigation of the potential relationships between plasma voriconazole-concentrations and visual adverse events or liver function test abnormalities. J Clin Pharmacol. 46:235–43, 2006.

Tattevin P, Bruneel F, Lellouche F, et al. Successful treatment of brain aspergillosis with voriconazole. Clin Microbiol Infect 10:928–31, 2004.

Trifilio S, Pennick G, Pi J, et al. Monitoring plasma voriconazole levels may be necessary to avoid subtherapeutic levels in hematopoietic stem cell transplant recipients. Cancer 109:1532–1535, 2007.

Walsh TJ, Anaissie EJ, Denning DW, et al. Treatment of Aspergillosis: Clinical Practice Diseases Society of America. Clin Infect Dis 46:327–360, 2008.

Walsh TJ, Pappas P, Winston DJ, et al. Voriconazole compared with liposomal amphotericin B for empirical antifungal therapy in patients with neutropenia and persistent fever. N Engl J Med 346:225–34, 2002.

Wandroo F, Stableforth P, Hasan Y. Aspergillus brain abscess in a patient with acute myeloid leukemia successfully treated with voriconazole. Clin Lab Haematol 28:130–3, 2006.

Website: www.vfend.com

Zalcitabine (HIVID) ddC

Drug Class: Antiretroviral NRTI (nucleoside reverse transcriptase inhibitor).

Usual Dose: 0.75 mg (PO) q8h.

Pharmacokinetic Parameters:

Peak serum level: 0.08 mcg/ml

Bioavailability: 80%

Excreted unchanged (urine): 75%

Serum half-life (normal/ESRD): 2/8.5 hrs

Plasma protein binding: 0%

Volume of distribution (V_d): 0.54 L/kg

Primary Mode of Elimination: Renal

Dosage Adjustments*

CrCl 50–80 mL/min	No change
CrCl 10–50 mL/min	0.75 mg (PO) q12h
CrCl < 10 mL/min	0.75 mg (PO) q24h
Post–HD dose	No information
Post–PD dose	No information
CVVH dose	0.75 mg (PO) q12h
Moderate hepatic insufficiency	No change
Severe hepatic insufficiency	No change

Drug Interactions: Cimetidine, probenecid, TMP–SMX (↑ zalcitabine levels); dapsone, didanosine, stavudine, INH, phenytoin, metronidazole, other neurotoxic agents or history of neuropathy (↑ risk of peripheral neuropathy); magnesium/aluminum containing antacids, metoclopramide (↓ bioavailability of zalcitabine); pentamidine IV, valproic

"Usual dose" assumes normal renal/hepatic function. * For renal insufficiency, give usual dose × 1 followed by maintenance dose per CrCl. For dialysis patients, dose the same as for CrCl < 10 mL/min and give supplemental (post-HD/PD dose) immediately after dialysis. CrCl = creatinine clearance; CVVH = continuous veno-venous hemofiltration; HD/PD = hemodialysis/peritoneal dialysis. See pp. 509–513 for explanations, pp. xi–xii for abbreviations; Linezolid (↑ risk of serotonin syndrome, see p. 620).

acid, alcohol, other agents known to cause pancreatitis (↑ risk of pancreatitis).

Adverse Effects: Drug fever/rash, leukopenia, anemia, thrombocytopenia, hepatomegaly, hepatotoxicity/hepatic necrosis, peripheral neuropathy, pancreatitis, stomatitis, oral/genital ulcers, dysphagia, arthritis, hyperglycemia, lipotrodystrophy, wasting, lactic acidosis with hepatic steatosis (rare, but potentially life-threatening toxicity with use of NRTIs).

Allergic Potential: High

Safety in Pregnancy: C

Comments: Foscarnet may increase toxicity. Do not use with stavudine, didanosine, or lamivudine to avoid additive toxicities. Food decreases absorption by 39%. Effective antiretroviral therapy consists of at least 3 antiretrovirals (same/different classes).

Cerebrospinal Fluid Penetration: 25%

REFERENCES:

Drugs for AIDS and associated infections. Med Lett Drug Ther 35:79–86, 1993.

HIV Trialists' Collaborative Group. Zidovudine, didanosine, and zalcitabine in the treatment of HIV infection: Meta-analyses of the randomised evidence. Lancet 353:2014–2025, 1999.

Panel on Antiretroviral Guidelines for Adults and Adolescents. Guidelines for the use of antiretroviral agents in HIV-1 infected adults and adolescents. Department of Health and Human Services. November 3, 2008; 1–139. Available at http://www.aidsinfor.nih.gov/ContentFiles/AdultandAdolescentGL.pdf

Shelton MJ, O'Donnell AM, Morse GD. Zalcitabine. Ann Pharmacotherapy 27:480–9, 1993.

Skowron G, Bozzette SA, Lim L, et al. Alternating and intermittent regimens of zidovudine and dideoxycytidine in patients with AIDS or AIDS-related complex. Ann Intern Med 118:321–30, 1993.

Website: www.rocheusa.com/products/

Zidovudine (Retrovir) ZDV Azidothymidine AZT

Drug Class: Antiretroviral NRTI (nucleoside reverse transcriptase inhibitor).

Usual Dose: 300 mg (PO) q12h (see comments). IV solution 10 mg/mL (dose 1 mg/kg 5–6 x/day).

Pharmacokinetic Parameters:

Peak serum level: 1.2 mcg/mL
Bioavailability: 64%
Excreted unchanged (urine): 16%
Serum half-life (normal/ESRD): 1.1/1.4 hrs
Plasma protein binding: < 38%
Volume of distribution (V_d): 1.6 L/kg

Primary Mode of Elimination: Hepatic

Dosage Adjustments*

CrCl 50–80 mL/min	No change
CrCl 10–50 mL/min	No change
CrCl < 10 mL/min	300 mg (PO) q24h
HD/PD	100 mg (PO) q6-8h
Post–HD/PD dose	None
CVVH dose	300 mg (PO) q24h
Moderate or severe hepatic insufficiency	No information

Drug Interactions: Acetaminophen, atovaquone, fluconazole, methadone, probenecid, valproic acid (↑ zidovudine levels); clarithromycin, nelfinavir, rifampin, rifabutin (↓ zidovudine levels); dapsone, flucytosine, ganciclovir, interferon alpha, bone marrow suppressive/cytotoxic agents (↑ risk of hematologic toxicity); indomethacin (↑ levels of zidovudine toxic metabolite); phenytoin

"Usual dose" assumes normal renal/hepatic function. * For renal insufficiency, give usual dose × 1 followed by maintenance dose per CrCl. For dialysis patients, dose the same as for CrCl < 10 mL/min and give supplemental (post-HD/PD dose) immediately after dialysis. CrCl = creatinine clearance; CVVH = continuous veno-venous hemofiltration; HD/PD = hemodialysis/peritoneal dialysis. See pp. 509–513 for explanations, pp. xi–xii for abbreviations; Linezolid (↑ risk of serotonin syndrome, see p. 620).

(↑ zidovudine levels, ↑ or ↓ phenytoin levels); ribavirin (↓ zidovudine effect; avoid).

Adverse Effects: Zidovudine, has been associated with hematologic toxicity including neutropenia and severe anemia. Prolonged use of zidovudine has been associated with symptomatic myopathy as well as lactic acidosis and severe hepatomegaly with steatosis, including fatal cases. May cause nausea, vomiting, GI upset, diarrhea, malaise, anorexia, macrocytosis, headachese, insomnia, blue/black nail discoloration and asthenia. Nausea, vomiting, GI upset, diarrhea, malaise, anorexia, leukopenia, severe anemia, macrocytosis, thrombocytopenia, headaches, ↑ SGOT/SGPT, hepatotoxicity, myalgias, myositis, symptomatic myopathy, insomnia, blue/black nail discoloration, asthenia, lactic acidosis with hepatic steatosis (rare, but potentially life-threatening toxicity with use of NRTI's).

Allergic Potential: Low

Safety in Pregnancy: C

Comments: Antagonized by ganciclovir or ribavirin. Also a component of Combivir and Trizivir. Patients on IV therapy should be switched to PO as soon as able to take oral medication. For IV administration, dilute in D5W to a concentration no greater than 4 mg/mL and infuse over 1 hour.

Cerebrospinal Fluid Penetration: 60%

REFERENCES:

Barry M, Mulcahy F, Merry C, et al. Pharmacokinetics and potential interactions amongst antiretroviral agents used to treat patients with HIV infection. Clin Pharmacol 36:289–304, 1999.

Been-Tiktak AM, Boucher CA, Brun-Vezinet F, et al. Efficacy and safety of combination therapy with delavirdine and zidovudine: A European/Australian phase II trial. Intern J Antimcrob Agents 11:13–21, 1999.

McDowell JA, Lou Y, Symonds WS, et al. Multiple-dose pharmacokinetics and pharmacodynamics of abacavir alone and in combination with zidovudine in human immunodeficiency virus-infected adults. Antimicrob Agents Chemother 44:2061–7, 2000.

Montaner JS, Reiss P, Cooper D, et al. A randomized, double-blind trial comparing combinations of nevirapine, didanosine, and zidovudine for HIV-infected patients: The INCAS trial. Italy, the Netherlands, Canada and Australia Study. J Am Med Assoc 279:930–937, 1998.

Mushatt DM, Mihm LB, Dreisbach AW, et al. Antibiotic dosing in slow extended daily dialysis. Clin Infect Dis 49:433–437, 2009.

Panel on Antiretroviral Guidelines for Adults and Adolescents. Guidelines for the use of antiretroviral agents in HIV-1 infected adults and adolescents. Department of Health and Human Services. November 3, 2008; 1–139. Available at http://www.aidsinfor.nih.gov/ContentFiles/AdultandAdolescentGL.pdf.

Piscitelli SC, Gallicano KD. Interactions among drugs for HIV and opportunistic infections. N Engl J Med 344:984–996, 2001.

Roberts JA, Lipman J. Pharmokinetic Issues for antibiotics in the critically ill patient. Crit Care Med 37:840–847, 2009.

Roberts JA, Webb S, Paterson D, et al. A systematic review of clinical benefits of continuous administration of B-lactam antibiotics. Crit Care Med 37:2071–2078, 2009.

Simpson DM. Human immunodeficiency virus-associated dementia: A review of pathogenesis, prophylaxis, and treatment studies of zidovudine therapy. Clin Infect Dis 29:19–34, 1999.

Website: www.TreatHIV.com

"Usual dose" assumes normal renal/hepatic function. * For renal insufficiency, give usual dose × 1 followed by maintenance dose per CrCl. For dialysis patients, dose the same as for CrCl < 10 mL/min and give supplemental (post-HD/PD dose) immediately after dialysis. CrCl = creatinine clearance; CVVH = continuous veno-venous hemofiltration; HD/PD = hemodialysis/peritoneal dialysis. See pp. 509–513 for explanations, pp. xi–xii for abbreviations; Linezolid (↑ risk of serotonin syndrome, see p. 620).

REFERENCES AND SUGGESTED READINGS

TEXTBOOKS

Ambrose P, Nightingale AT (eds). Principles of Pharmacodynamics. Marcel Dekker, Inc., New York, 2001.

Baddour L, Gorbach SL (eds). Therapy of Infectious Diseases. Saunders, Philadelphia, 2003.

Bartlett JG (ed). The Johns Hopkins Hospital Guide to Medical Care of Patients with HIV Infection, Lippincott Williams & Wilkins, Philadelphia, 2005.

Bartlett JG, Auwaerter PG, Pham PA (eds). The ABX Guide, 1st Edition. Thomson PDR, Montvale, NJ, 2005.

Bennet WM, Aronoff GR, Golper TA, Morrison G, Brater DC, Singer I (eds). Drug Prescribing in Renal Failure, 2nd Edition. American College of Physicians, Philadelphia, 2000.

Bryskier A (ed). Antimicrobial Agents. ASM Press, Washington, D.C., 2005.

Finch RG, Greenwood D, Norrby SR, Whitley RJ (eds). Antibiotic and Chemotherapy. Churchill Livingstone, United Kingdom, 2003.

Gorbach SL, Bartlett JG, Blacklow NR (eds). Infectious Diseases, 4th Edition. Lippincott Williams Wilkins, Philadelphia, 2004.

Kucers A, Crowe S, Grayson ML, Hoy J (eds). The Use of Antibiotics: A Clinical Review of Antibacterial, Antifungal, and Antiviral Drugs, 5th Edition. Butterworth-Heinemann, Oxford, 1997.

Mandell GL, Bennett JE, Dolin R (eds). Mandell, Douglas and Bennett's Principles and Practice of Infectious Disease, 7th Edition. Elsevier, Philadelphia, 2010.

Pai MP, Momary KM, Rodvold KA. Antibiotic Drug Interactions. Med Clin N Am 90:1223–55, 2006.

Perfect JR, Dismukes WE, Dromer F, et al. Clinical Practice Guidelines for the Management of Cryptococcal Disease: 2010 Update by the Infectious Disease Society of America. Clin Infect Dis 50:291–322, 2010.

Physicians' Desk Reference, 64th Edition. Thompson PDR, Montvale, NJ, 2010.

Piscitelli SC, Rodvold KE (eds). Drug Interactions in Infectious Diseases. Humana Press, Totowa, 2001.

Ristuccia AM, Cunha BA (eds). Antimicrobial Therapy. Raven Press, New York, 1984.

Root RK (ed). Clin Infect Dis: A Practical Approach. Oxford University Press, New York, 1999.

Sax PE, Cohen CJ, Kuritzkes DR (eds). HIV Essentials. 3rd edition. Jones & Bartlett, Sudbury, MA, 2010.

Schlossberg D (ed). Current Therapy of Infectious Disease, 3rd Edition. Mosby-Yearbook, St. Louis, 2008.

Schlossberg D (ed). Tuberculosis and Non-Tuberculous Mycobacterial Infections, 6th Edition. McGraw-Hill, New York, 2006.

Scholar EM, Pratt WB (eds). The Antimicrobial Drugs, 2nd Edition. Oxford University Press, New York, 2000.

Wormser GP (ed). AIDS, 4th Edition. Elsevier, Philadelphia, 2004.

Yoshikawa TT, Rajagopalan S (eds). Antibiotic Therapy for Geriatric Patients. Taylor & Francis, New York, 2006.

Yoshikawa TT, Norman DC (eds). Antimicrobial Therapy in the Elderly. Marcel Dekker, New York, 1994.

Yu VL, Merigan, Jr. TC, Barrier SL (eds). Antimicrobial Therapy and Vaccines, 2nd edition. Williams & Wilkins, Baltimore, 2005.

Zinner SH, Young LS, Acar JF, Ortiz-Neu C (eds). New Considerations for Macrolides, Azalides, Streptogramins, and Ketolides. Marcel Dekker, Inc., New York, 2000.

INDEX

NOTES

NOTES

NOTES

NOTES

NOTES

NOTES

NOTES